PRIMARY CARE OF THE
CHILD *with a*
CHRONIC CONDITION

PRIMARY CARE OF THE
CHILD *with a*
CHRONIC CONDITION

FOURTH EDITION

Patricia Jackson Allen, RN, MS, PNP, FAAN
Clinical Professor
Yale University, School of Nursing
New Haven, Connecticut

Clinical Professor, Emeritus
University of California, San Francisco
San Francisco, California

Judith A. Vessey, RN, PhD, MBA, DPNP, FAAN
Leila Holden Carroll Professor of Nursing
Boston College, William F. Connell School of Nursing
Chestnut Hill, Massachusetts

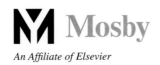 Mosby

An Affiliate of Elsevier

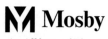

An Affiliate of Elsevier

11830 Westline Industrial Drive
St. Louis, Missouri 63146

Photo Credits
The editors wish to thank the numerous contributors who submitted photos for chapter openers, as well as the following:

Photo Disc: Chapter opener photos for Chapters 5, 14, 25, 28, 36, and 38.
Photos.com: Chapter opener photo for Chapter 4.
Wong DL et al: Whaley and Wong's Nursing Care of Infants and Children, ed. 6, St. Louis, 1999, Mosby, Chapter opener for Chapter 6.
Ken Hatfield: Chapter opener for Ch. 14 and figure 14-3.

NOTICE

Pharmacology is an ever-changing field. Standard safety precautions must be followed, but as new research and clinical experience broaden our knowledge, changes in treatment and drug therapy may become necessary or appropriate. Readers are advised to check the most current product information provided by the manufacturer of each drug to be administered to verify the recommended dose, the method and duration of administration, and contraindications. It is the responsibility of the licensed health care provider, relying on experience and knowledge of the patient, to determine dosages and the best treatment for each individual patient. Neither the publisher nor the author assumes any liability for any injury and/or damage to persons or property arising from this publication.

Previous editions copyrighted 1992, 1996, 2000

ISBN-13: 978–0–323–02364–1   ISBN-10: 0–323–02364–9

Executive Vice President, Nursing & Health Professions: Sally Schrefer
Executive Publisher: Barbara Nelson Cullen
Editor: Sandra Clark Brown
Developmental Editor: Sophia Oh Gray
Publishing Services Manager: Catherine Albright Jackson
Project Manager: Celeste Clingan
Design Manager: Amy Buxton
Cover Designer: Studio Montage

ISBN-13: 978–0–323–02364–1
ISBN-10: 0–323–02364–9

Printed in China

Last digit is the print number: 9   8   7   6   5   4

To my children, Heather, Robert, and Scott,
who have grown up to be wonderful caring adults,

To my husband, Rick, who has become my soul mate and new partner in life's
journey, and

To all the children with chronic health conditions and their families, especially
Aidan and his parents, who have been the inspiration for this text.

PJA

In loving memory of my parents, Leora and Eric Vessey.

JAV

CONTRIBUTORS

Patricia Jackson Allen, RN, MS, PNP, FAAN
Lecturer,
Yale University, School of Nursing,
New Haven, Connecticut
*Chapter 1   The Primary Care Provider and Children with
    Chronic Conditions*
Chapter 5   School and the Child with a Chronic Condition
Chapter 36   Prematurity

Erin Powell Alving, MSN, CDE, PNP
Clinical Faculty,
University of Washington School of Nursing;
Pediatric Nurse Practitioner,
Children's Hospital and Regional Medical Center,
Seattle, Washington
Chapter 20   Congenital Adrenal Hyperplasia

Christina R. Baggott, MN, RN-CNS, PNP, CPON
Pediatric Nurse Practitioner, Pediatric Oncology,
Packard Children's Hospital at Stanford,
Palo Alto, California
Chapter 17   Cancer

Betsy Haas-Beckert, RN, MSN, PNP
Pediatric Nurse Practitioner, Pediatric Gastroenterology,
University of California at San Francisco,
San Francisco, California
Chapter 30   Inflammatory Bowel Disease

Joan L. Blair, MSN, RN, APRN-BC
Pediatric Nurse Practitioner,
Division of Neurology,
AI du Pont Hospital for Children,
Wilmington, Delaware
Chapter 25   Epilepsy

Anne Boekelheide, RN, MHSL, MSN, PNP
Nurse Coordinator for the Center for Craniofacial Anomalies,
Children's Hospital,
University of California at San Francisco,
San Francisco, California
Chapter 19   Cleft Lip and Palate

Elizabeth A. Boland, MSN, APRN, CDE
Pediatric Nurse Practitioner,
Yale University, School of Medicine,
New Haven, Connecticut
Chapter 23   Diabetes Mellitus (Types 1 and 2)

Elizabeth A. Bryson, RN, MSN, CNP, CS
Adjunct Clinical Faculty,
Kent State University,
Kent, Ohio;
Pediatric Subspecialty Manager,
Advanced Cystic Fibrosis Clinical Nurse Specialist, Nurse
    Practitioner,
Children's Hospital Medical Center of Akron
Akron, Ohio
Chapter 22   Cystic Fibrosis

Rhonda Burton, RN, MS, PNP
Pediatric Nurse Practitioner,
Children's Hospital Oakland, Neurology,
Oakland, California
Chapter 27   Head Injury

Barbara A. Carroll, MN, RN, CPNP
Pediatric Nurse Practitioner, Sickle Cell Program,
Children's Healthcare of Atlanta, AFLAC Cancer and Blood
    Disorders Service,
Atlanta, Georgia
Chapter 39   Sickle Cell Disease

Renee M. Charbonneau, MS, CPNP
Metabolism Nurse Practitioner,
Children's Hospital,
Boston, Massachusetts
Chapter 35   Phenylketonuria

Elizabeth H. Cook, MS, RNC, PNP
Adjunct Assistant Professor,
Samuel Merritt College School of Nursing,
Oakland, California
Chapter 21   Congenital Heart Disease

Ann W. Cox, PhD, RN, FAAN
Director of Preservice Training,
Virginia Institute for Developmental Disabilities;
Assistant Professor of Education and Nursing,
Virginia Commonwealth University,
Richmond, Virginia
Chapter 9   Transition to Adulthood

Randy Q. Cron, MD, PhD
Assistant Professor,
Children's Hospital of Philadelphia,
Division of Rheumatology,
Philadelphia, Pennsylvania
*Chapter 31   Juvenile Rheumatoid Arthritis and Juvenile
    Spondyloarthropathy*

Ginny Curtin, MS, RNC, PNP
Pediatric Nurse Practitioner,
Pediatric Otolaryngology,
Packard Children's Hospital at Stanford,
Palo Alto, California
Chapter 19   Cleft Lip and Palate

Susan Ditmyer, MSN, RN, PNP
Pediatric Nurse Practitioner, Neurosurgery,
Children's Hospital Oakland,
Oakland, California
Chapter 29   Hydrocephalus

Mary Alice Dragone, MS, RN, CS, PNP
Pediatric Clinical Consultant,
Degge Group, Inc.,
Arlington, Virginia
Chapter 17   Cancer

Rita Fahrner, RN, MS, PNP
Clinical Nurse Specialist,
San Francisco General Hospital, Occupational Health Service
San Francisco, California
Chapter 28   HIV Infection and AIDS

Margaret Grey, DrPH, FAAN, CPNP
Independence Foundation Professor of Nursing, Associate
   Dean for Research Affairs,
Yale University, School of Nursing,
New Haven, Connecticut
Chapter 23   Diabetes Mellitus (Types 1 and 2)

Daniel F. Gunther, MD, MA
Assistant Professor of Pediatrics,
University of Washington;
Pediatric Endocrinologist,
Children's Hospital & Regional Medical Center,
Seattle, Washington
Chapter 20   Congenital Adrenal Hyperplasia

Randi J. Hagerman, MD
Medical Director, M.I.N.D. Institute,
University of California at Davis, Medical Center,
Sacramento, California
Chapter 26   Fragile X Syndrome

Melvin B. Heyman, MD, MPh
Professor of Clinical Pediatrics,
Chief, Division of Pediatric Gastroenterology, Hepatology,
   and Nutrition,
Director, Training Program in Pediatric Gastroenterology and
   Nutrition,
University of California at San Francisco, School of Medicine,
San Francisco, California
Chapter 30   Inflammatory Bowel Disease

Sarah S. Higgins, PhD, RN, FAAN
Associate Professor,
University of San Francisco,
San Francisco, California
Chapter 21   Congenital Heart Disease

June Andrews Horowitz, PhD, FAAN, CS
Associate Professor,
Boston College, William F. Connell School of Nursing
Chestnut Hill, Massachusetts
Chapter 32   Mood Disorders

Susan Karp, RN, MS
Hemophilia Clinical Nurse Specialist,
University of California at San Francisco,
San Francisco, California
Chapter 14   Bleeding Disorders

Gail Kieckhefer, PhD, ARNP
Associate Professor,
University of Washington, School of Nursing
Seattle, Washington
Chapter 11   Asthma

Melanie Klein, RN, MSN, CNP
Nurse Practitioner,
Rainbow Babies and Children's Hospital,
Cleveland, Ohio
Chapter 34   Organ Transplantation
Chapter 38   Renal Failure, Chronic

Kathy Knafl, PhD, FAAN
Professor,
Yale University, School of Nursing,
New Haven, Connecticut
Chapter 3   Chronic Conditions and the Family

Karen Marie Kristovich, RN, PNP
Pediatric Nurse Practitioner, Hematology/Oncology,
Packard Children's Hospital,
Palo Alto, California
Chapter 15   Bone Marrow Transplantation

Barbara J. Kruger, RN, MPH, PhD (c.)
Assistant Professor,
University of North Florida, College of Health,
Jacksonville, Florida
Chapter 7   Care Coordination

Elizabeth A. Kuehne, PNP, MSN
Pediatric Nurse Practitioner, Nurse Consultant,
Children's Aid and Family Services, Inc.,
Paramus, New Jersey
Chapter 37   Prenatal Cocaine Exposure

Kathy S. Lawrence MN, RN
Clinical Nurse Specialist,
Children's Hospital of Pittsburgh, Cardiology Division
Pittsburgh, Pennsylvania
Chpater 34   Organ Transplantation

Cynthia Colen Lazzaretti
Spina Bifida Clinic Coordinator,
Spina Bifida Clinic,
University of California at San Francisco,
San Francisco, California
Chapter 33   Myelodysplasia

Mary E. Lynch, RN, PNP, MS, MPH
Clinical Professor,
University of California at San Francisco, School of Nursing,
San Francisco, California
Chapter 36   Prematurity

Carol Anne Marchetti, RN, BS, MS
Registered Nurse,
New England Medical Center,
Boston, Massachusetts
Chapter 32   Mood Disorders

Ann H. McMullen, RN, MS, CPNP
Associate Professor of Clinical Nursing,
University of Rochester School of Nursing;
Senior Advanced Practice Nurse, Pediatric Nurse Practitioner,
Gallisano Children's Hospital at Strong,
Rochester, New York
Chapter 22   Cystic Fibrosis

Stephanie L. Merhar, BA
Medical Student,
University of Pennsylvania,
Philadelphia, Pennsylvania
*Chapter 31   Juvenile Rheumatoid Arthritis and Juvenile
    Spondyloarthropathy*

Stephanie G. Metzger, MS, RN, CS, PNP
Advanced Practice Nurse,
Children's Hospital,
Richmond, VA;
Clinical Assistant Professor,
School of Nursing, Virginia Commonwealth University,
Richmond, Virginia
Chapter 9   Transition to Adulthood

Beverly Capper-Michel, RN, MSN
Care Manager, Outreach Educator NICU,
Rainbow Babies & Children's Hospital,
Cleveland, Ohio
Chapter 16   Bronchopulmonary Dysplasia

Kimberely Moffatt, RN, MS, CPNP
Pediatric Nurse Practitioner, Neurology,
Children's Hospital Oakland,
Oakland, California
Chapter 27   Head Injury

Carol Kerrigan Moore, MS, RN, FNP-BC
Faculty,
University of Delaware Graduate Program,
Department of Nursing,
Newark, Delaware
Chapter 12   Attention Deficit Hyperactivity Disorder

Alicia S. Namrow, RN, MSN, CCRN, CNP
Nurse Practitioner,
University Hospital of Cleveland,
Rainbow Babies and Children's Hospital,
Cleveland, Ohio
Chapter 38   Renal Failure, Chronic

Wendy M. Nehring, RN, PHD
Associate Dean for Academic Affairs and Associate
    Professor,
Rutgers, The State University of New Jersey,
College of Nursing,
Newark, New Jersey
Chapter 18   Cerebral Palsy
Chapter 24   Down Syndrome

Beverly Kosmach-Park, MSN, CRNP
Clinical Nurse Specialist,
Department of Transplant Surgery,
Children's Hospital of Pittsburgh,
Pittsburgh, Pennsylvania
Chapter 34   Organ Transplantation

Caroline Pearson, RN, PNP
Pediatric Nurse Practitioner,
Department of Pediatric Neurosurgery,
University of California at San Francisco,
San Francisco, California
Chapter 33   Myelodysplasia

Marijo Ratcliffe, RN, MN, PNP
Pediatric Nurse Practitioner, Pulmonary Department,
Children's Hospital and Medical Center;
Lecturer, Family and Child Nursing,
University of Washington in Seattle
Seattle, Washington
Chapter 11   Asthma

Catherine Yetter Read, RN, PhD
Assistant Professor,
Boston College, William F. Connell School of Nursing,
Chestnut Hill, Massachusetts;
Adjunct Staff,
Children's Hospital,
Boston, Massachusetts
Chapter 35   Phenylketoruria

Elizabeth O. Record, CPNP
Certified Pediatric Nurse Practitioner, Sickle Cell,
Children's Healthcare of Atlanta,
Atlanta, Georgia
Chapter 39   Sickle Cell Disease

Roberta S. Rehm, RN, PhD
Assistant Professor,
Department of Family Health Care Nursing,
School of Nursing,
University of California at San Francisco,
San Francisco, California
Chapter 4   Family Culture and Chronic Conditions

Marianne W. Reilly, BSN, MSN, CPNP
Clinical Instructor, PNP Program,
Columbia University,
New York, New York;
Pediatric Nurse Practitioner,
Holy Name Hospital,
Teaneck, New Jersey
Chapter 37   Prenatal Cocaine Exposure

Patricia Rettig, RN, MSN, CRNP
Nurse Practitioner and Nurse Manager,
Division of Pediatric Rheumatology,
Children's Hospital of Philadelphia,
Philadelphia, Pennsylvania
*Chapter 31   Juvenile Rheumatoid Arthritis and Juvenile
  Spondyloarthropathy*

Sostena Romano MSN, APRN
Clinical Coordinator, Pediatric AIDS Care Project,
Yale New Haven Hospital,
New Haven, Conneticut
Chapter 28   HIV Infection and AIDS

Melissa Rumsey, BSN
Research Assistant
Boston College, William F. Connell School of Nursing,
Chestnut Hill, Massachusetts
Chapter 2   Chronic Conditions and Child Development

Cindy Hylton Rushton, DNSc, RN, FAAN
Assistant Professor of Nursing,
Johns Hopkins University, School of Nursing,
Baltimore, Maryland
Chapter 6   Ethics and the Child with a Chronic Condition

Sheila Judge Santacroce, PhD, APRN, CPNP
Assistant Professor, Pediatric Nurse Practitioner Specialty,
Yale University, School of Nursing,
New Haven, Connecticut
Chapter 3   Chronic Conditions and the Family

Kathleen J. Sawin, DNS, RN, CPNP, FAAN
Associate Professor,
School of Nursing, Virginia Commonwealth University;
Pediatric Nurse Practitioner, Spina Bifida Program,
Children's Hospital,
Richmond, Virginia
Chapter 9   Transition to Adulthood

Teresa A. Savage, PhD, RN
Associate Director,
Center for the Study of Disability Ethics,
Rehabilitation Institute of Chicago;
Assistant Professor, Research, Maternal-Child Nursing,
University of Illinois at Chicago, College of Nursing,
Chicago, Illinois
Chapter 6   Ethics and the Child with a Chronic Condition

Naomi A. Schapiro, RN, MS, CPNP
Assistant Clinical Professor,
University of California at San Francisco,
School of Nursing,
San Francisco, California
*Chapter 40   Tourette's Syndrome & Obsessive-Compulsive
  Disorder*

Janice Selekman, DNSc, RN
Professor and Chair,
Department of Nursing, University of Delaware,
Newark, Delaware
Chapter 12   Attention Deficit Hyperactivity Disorder
Chapte 25   Epilepsy

Maureen Sheehan, BA, RN, MS, CPNP
Pediatric Nurse Practitioner,
Pediatric Neurology and Epilepsy,
Stanford University Medical Center,
Packard Children's Hospital at Stanford,
Stanford, California
Chapter 13   Autism

Elizabeth Sloand, MS, CRNP
Assistant Professor,
John's Hopkins University, School of Nursing,
Baltimore, Maryland
Chapter 10   Allergies

Jenna A. Thate, RN, BSN, MSN
Clinical Instructor
University of Maryland School of Nursing
Baltimore, Maryland
Chaper 10   Allergies

Judith A. Vessey, RN, PhD, MBA, DPNP, FAAN
Leila Holden Carroll Professor of Nursing,
Boston College, William F. Connell School of Nursing,
Chestnut Hill, Massachusetts
Chapter 2   Chronic Conditions and Child Development
Chapter 5   School and the Child with a Chronic Condition
*Chapter 8   Financing Health Care for Children with
  Chronic Conditions*

REVIEWERS

Elizabeth Downey, BSN, MSN, CS, PNP
Pediatric Nurse Practitioner
Ranken Jordan Pediatric Rehabilitation Center
St. Louis, Missouri

Katherine Rossiter, MSN, CDE, APRN, CPNP
Pediatric Nurse Practitioner
Children's Hospital of Omaha
Omaha, Nebraska

Lisa South, RN, DSN
The University of Alabama in Huntsville,
Huntsville, Alabama

PREFACE

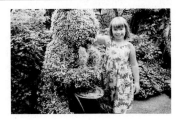

Growing up is not easy. Seemingly limitless potential is juxtaposed with devastating possibilities. Medical advances over the past 60 years have dramatically decreased the mortality and morbidity rates in children, especially from infectious diseases that annually killed thousands in previous decades. With many devastating illnesses controlled, pediatric health care providers shifted their focus of care from illness management to prevention, with the goal of maximizing each child's potential through health promotion, disease and injury prevention, and growth and development counseling.

During this same period, however, a new childhood morbidity profile emerged. Children with chronic conditions and special health care needs who would have died decades ago as a result of their condition are now surviving. Their medical care is often complex and costly, frequently requiring multiple treatment modalities. In addition, treatments that were previously only provided by professionals in acute care hospitals are now being provided by family members at home, shifting medical responsibilities from hospital professionals to community providers. The need to improve the quality of care for children with special health care needs through care coordination and preventive health services has resulted in the Institute of Medicine identifying the care of children with special health care needs as one of the top 20 priority areas for health system change (Institute of Medicine, *Priority Areas for National Action: Transforming Health Care Quality*, 2003).

In an attempt to keep pace with the rapid developments in medical and surgical treatment for children with chronic conditions, care has often become specialized, focused on the disease process instead of on holistic care for the child. Frequently multiple specialists are involved in the child's plan of care to address the associated problems of the underlying condition. The importance of preventative care can be overlooked by both health care providers and families. Developing, implementing, and monitoring a care plan that ensures comprehensive, culturally sensitive, and family centered care of the child, not the disease, is critical in improving the quality of care.

Growing up with a chronic condition or disability is inherently more difficult. A child's growth and development may be compromised by the stress of the illness and treatments; a child's susceptibility to common childhood illnesses, behavioral dysfunctions, and injuries may be increased as a result of the chronic condition. Many children with chronic conditions also come from families with little or no access to preventive health care, increasing the potential morbidity from the chronic condition, as well as the general health risks.

This book provides pediatric health care professionals with the knowledge necessary to provide comprehensive primary preventative care to children with special health care needs.

Part I addresses the major issues common to care of all children with chronic conditions: the role of the primary care provider, effect of a chronic condition on a child's development and on a family, school issues, transition to adulthood, ethical and cultural concerns, care coordination, and the financial resources—or lack thereof—available and necessary to support the care of a child with a chronic condition. This knowledge is not condition-specific but forms the framework for delivery of care to all children with chronic conditions.

Part II identifies 31 chronic conditions found in children that necessitate alterations in standard primary care practices. Each condition-specific chapter was written by health care professionals with extensive experience in caring for the complex needs of children with the condition. The information provided briefly covers causes and clinical manifestations of the chronic condition but mainly focuses on how these affect the primary care needs of the child, i.e., health maintenance, common illness management, and developmental issues common in childhood. The primary care needs are summarized at the end of each chapter for quick reference and each chapter has consistent headings, development of content, and formatting to facilitate the use of the book as a reference.

Decisions about which chronic conditions were included in this text were based on two criteria. First, the prevalence of the condition needed to be at least 1 in 10,000 or would likely reach this level if underreporting were not a problem. For a few other conditions, the decision of inclusion was based on how rapidly the incidence was increasing. The second criterion for inclusion was that the condition requires significant adaptations in primary care. In the fourth edition of this text we have included two new chapters addressing mental health conditions, i.e., Mood Disorders and Tourette's Syndrome and Obsessive-Compulsive Disorder, recognizing the growing incidence and awareness of psychosocial and mental health conditions in children, and chapters on Allergies and Bone Marrow Transplantation. Each condition-specific chapter also has new headings for content on known genetic etiology of the condition and complementary and alternative therapies currently being used by professionals or families, both areas of significant growth in knowledge in the past few years and expected growth in the near future.

Whenever possible, inclusive language regarding health care providers has been used throughout the text. We have extended this terminology to include nurse practitioners, physicians, and other health care providers because individuals with a variety of professional preparations provide primary care to children with chronic conditions. Readers will also note that the terms *patient* and *chronic illness* are rarely used and, whenever possible, we have used the wording "the child with (condition name)" rather than the "(condition name) child." Although we recognize that this sometimes makes for awkward grammar, it reflects our philosophy that children are children first instead of being defined by their condition and that wellness and illness are relative.

It would be presumptuous to edit such a text without acknowledging its scope and limitations. First, we assume that readers have a basic knowledge of growth and development and of common pediatric conditions and their management. Second, we believe there are many excellent texts available that review the diagnostic process required to determine a chronic condition in a child so have not included this content. Our intent is to provide the health care provider with a review of the condition's etiology, known genetic causes, incidence, clinical manifestations and associated problems, treatment, including complementary and alternative therapies, and prognosis as a foundation for establishing a plan for primary health care. And thirdly, it is impossible to provide detailed information on treatment options for all secondary problems that may occur in conjunction with those highlighted. Wherever possible, readers are referred to another chapter of the text. If referral was not feasible, readers should consult the general pediatric literature for management protocols and review the extensive reference list accompanying each chapter.

The preparation of this text has been a professionally challenging and personally rewarding endeavor for us. As with any text, its successful completion depended on the help of numerous others. We wish to extend our gratitude to the contributors for their excellent careful and timely work and to all past contributors who's work and early development of each chapter has been so important in the evolution of this text. The contributions of the Yale University School of Nursing, University of California, San Francisco, Department of Family Health Care Nursing, and the Boston College, William F. Connell School of Nursing are recognized and sincerely appreciated. The assistance and support of the Elsevier staff editors, Barbara Nelson Cullen, Sandra Brown, and Sophia Gray, are also acknowledged.

In summary, we hope the information provided in this book will help ensure that children with chronic conditions receive more holistic family centered primary care that will help them stay healthy, live successfully with their condition, promote their growth and development and maximize their potential in all areas. This care can only be accomplished if health care professionals are willing to assume the challenge of providing comprehensive care to these children so they can reach their biological, intellectual and social potential – and beyond.

Patricia Jackson Allen
Judith A. Vessey

TABLE OF CONTENTS

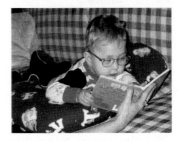

PART ONE

Concepts in Pediatric Primary Care

1 The Primary Care Provider and Children with Chronic Conditions

Patricia Jackson Allen

The Health of America's Children

Health Statistics for Children

Nationwide the number of children grew 14% between 1990 and 2000 (from 63.6 million to 72.3 million) with minority children accounting for 98% of the growth (O'Hare, 2001). In 2000, 64% of children were non-Hispanic white; 16% were Hispanic; 15% were black; 4% were Asian/Pacific Islander; and 1% were American Indian/Alaska Native (ChildStats.gov, 2002). It is estimated that by 2025, half of the children in America will be from a "racial minority."

During the past decade many indicators of child health and well-being in the United States have improved, moving closer to the goals and objectives of *Healthy People 2000*. The Centers for Disease Control and Prevention (2002) reports infant mortality rates declined to a record low in 2000 of 6.9 per 1000 live births (Figure 1-1) but infant mortality for black infants (13.9 per 1000 live births) continues to be over twice the rate for non-Hispanic white infants (5.7 per 1000 live births) and four times the rate for infants of Chinese mothers (3.5 per 1000 live births). There continues to be disparity along racial lines of characteristics of mothers known to be associated with poorer outcomes of newborns, that is, young age, limited education, unmarried,

and delayed or limited health care utilization (Table 1-1) (MacDorman et al, 2002; O'Hare, 2001). About one fifth of the children in the United States are immigrants or children of immigrants with 19% of children living with at least one foreign-born parent (Childstats.gov, 2002). Families with foreign-born parents are more likely to live below the poverty level (28%) and have parents with less than a high school degree (42%), both factors contributing to increased health risks in children. Multiple factors (biologic, environmental, societal) affect health, and there is growing recognition that situations affecting fetal and early childhood health have continued health implications into adulthood (Joseph & Kramer, 1996).

During the past 2 decades mortality among children and young adults (ages 1 to 24 years) has declined, in part because of improved medical and surgical care for children with cancer, heart disease, congenital birth defects, and infectious disease and improved trauma services for children with unintentional and intentional injuries (Table 1-2) (Pastor et al, 2002). Although the incidence of congenital birth defects does not vary significantly across racial groups, chronic health conditions and the incidence of injuries with their subsequent health problems or disabilities are more prevalent in children of racial minority groups. Gender discrepancies are now also being

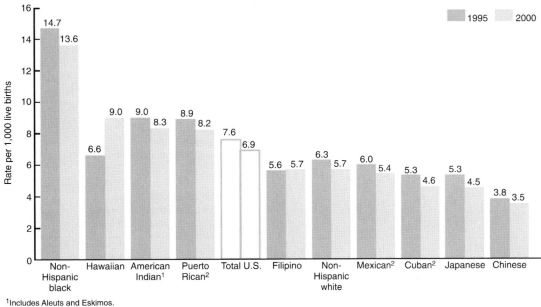

[1] Includes Aleuts and Eskimos.
[2] Persons of Hispanic origin may be of any race.
NOTE: Differences are significant for total U.S., non-Hispanic white, non-Hispanic black, and Mexican mothers.

FIGURE 1-1 Infant mortality rates by race and ethnicity, United States, 1995 and 2000. (From Centers for Disease Control and Prevention (CDC): Infant mortality statistics from the 2000 period linked birth/infant death data set, National Vital Statistics Reports [NVSS] 50[12]:1, 2002; Web site: http://www.cdc.gov/nchs/data/nvsr/nvsr50/nvsr50_12.pdf.)

tracked for mortality and indicate a higher mortality rate for males in all ages and racial groups (Table 1-3).

Health Care Coverage for Children

Recently released data from the 2001 National Health Interview Survey (NHIS) show a continued increase in the number of children less than 18 years of age with some form of health

care coverage (Ni & Cohen, 2003) (see Chapter 8). The rise in health care coverage was the result of increased public health plan coverage; 35% of Hispanic children, 42.5% of non-Hispanic black children, and 15.9% of non-Hispanic white children were covered by some form of public health insurance in 2001. This increase was accompanied by a decrease in children covered by private insurance from 69.1% in 1999 to 67.1% in 2001, possibly reflecting the downturn in the national economy and the continued increase in health care costs resulting in reduction of health care coverage for employed parents. A sluggish economy and continued rise in health care costs increase the likelihood of even working families being without health care coverage for periods of time. Analysis of census data for 2001 to 2002 found over 75 million people under age 65 years were without insurance at some point during that 2-year period and that included over 27% of children from birth to age 18 years (Meckler, 2003).

The Welfare Reform Act of 1996 curtails eligibility of children of immigrant parents—even those residing in the United States legally—from income assistance, including Supplemental Security Income (SSI), food stamps, Women, Infants, and Children (WIC) programs, and general health

TABLE 1-1

Percentage of Births with Selected Characteristics by Race of Mothers and Infants, United States, 2000

	All Races	Non-Hispanic White	Black	Hispanic
Mother <20 yr of age	11.8	8.7	19.7	16.2
Mother unmarried	33.8	22.1	68.5	42.7
Mother: <12 completed yr of school	16.4	8.1	16.9	44.4
First trimester prenatal care	83.2	88.5	74.3	74.4
Infants with low birth weight	7.6	6.6	13.0	6.4
Infants with very low birth weight	1.4	1.1	3.1	1.1

TABLE 1-2

Leading Causes of Death and Numbers of Death in Children from Birth to 24 Years, United States, 1980 and 2000

Age and Rank Order	1980 Cause of Death	Deaths	2000 Cause of Death	Deaths
UNDER 1 YR				
1	Congenital anomalies	9,220	Congenital malformations, deformations, and chromosomal abnormalities	5,743
2	Sudden infant death syndrome	5,510	Disorders related to short gestation and low birth weight, not elsewhere classified	4,397
3	Respiratory distress syndrome	4,989	Sudden infant death syndrome	2,523
4	Disorders relating to short gestation and unspecified low birth weight	3,648	Newborn affected by maternal complications of pregnancy	1,404
5	Newborn affected by maternal complications of pregnancy	1,572	Newborn affected by complications of placenta, cord, and membranes	1,062
1-4 YR				
1	Unintentional injuries	3,313	Unintentional injuries	1,826
2	Congenital anomalies	1,026	Congenital malformations, deformations, and chromosomal abnormalities	495
3	Malignant neoplasms	573	Malignant neoplasms	420
4	Diseases of heart	338	Homicide	356
5	Homicide	319	Diseases of heart	181
5-14 YR				
1	Unintentional injuries	5,224	Unintentional injuries	2,979
2	Malignant neoplasms	1,497	Malignant neoplasms	1,014
3	Congenital anomalies	561	Congenital malformations, deformations, and chromosomal abnormalities	399
4	Homicide	415	Homicide	371
5	Diseases of heart	330	Suicide	307
15-24 YR				
1	Unintentional injuries	26,206	Unintentional injuries	14,113
2	Homicide	6,537	Homicide	4,939
3	Suicide	5,239	Suicide	3,994
4	Malignant neoplasms	2,683	Malignant neoplasms	1,713
5	Diseases of heart	1,223	Diseases of heart	1,031

From Pastor PN: Chartbook on trends in the health of Americans. Health, United States, 2002, Hyattsville, Md, 2002, National Center for Health Statistics.

care through Medicaid, dramatically increasing the number of children without health insurance and at risk for complications of health conditions associated with inconsistent health care and poverty (Children's Defense Fund, 1997; Geltman et al, 1996; Mihaly, 1997; National Research Council, Institute of Medicine, 1998; The Henry J. Kaiser Family Foundation, 2002). In 1999, Medicaid use by low-income legal immigrant families with children and low-income immigrant citizen families with children did not vary appreciably testifying to the success of programs such as Title XXI, State Children's Health Insurance Program (SCHIP) (see Chapter 8) to broaden health insurance eligibility for children (Fix & Passel, 2002). However, there was a 28% decrease in Medicaid coverage for noncitizen children of undocumented parents and a 43% drop in Medicaid coverage for children of refugee parents between 1994 and 1999 (Fix & Passel, 2002). More than 27% of

citizen children of legal permanent residents (LPRs) were uninsured in 1999, and 39.3% of citizen children of undocumented parents were uninsured in 1999 (Figure 1-2). Their numbers continue to increase as immigration, legal and illegal, continues and may increase dramatically as states that currently elect to provide social benefits and health insurance to immigrant families eliminate these support programs because of state budget deficits.

Availability of insurance is important to child health. Children covered by public health insurance are in families with limited financial resources and are therefore susceptible to the multiple effects associated with poverty. The National Survey of Early Childhood Health (Halfon et al, 2002) found 90% of children 4 to 35 months who were privately insured were reported by parents to be in excellent or very good health as compared with publicly insured children whose parents

TABLE 1-3
Death Rates for all Causes by Sex, Age 0-24 Years, and Race, United States, 1980 and 2000

Sex, Race, and Age	Deaths per 100,000 Resident Population		Sex, Race, and Age	Deaths per 100,000 Resident Population	
	1980	2000		1980	2000
ALL PERSONS			5-14 yr	—	20.2
<1 yr	1288.3	728.7	15-24 yr	—	100.5
1-4 yr	63.9	32.9			
5-14 yr	30.6	18.7	**WHITE FEMALE**		
15-24 yr	115.4	81.6	<1 yr	962.5	537.9
			1-4 yr	49.3	25.4
WHITE MALE			5-14 yr	22.9	14.4
<1 yr	1230.3	656.2	15-24 yr	55.5	41.6
1-4 yr	66.1	32.5			
5-14 yr	35.0	20.4	**BLACK FEMALE**		
15-24 yr	167.0	107.6	<1 yr	2123.7	1352.7
			1-4 yr	84.4	50.8
BLACK MALE			5-14 yr	30.5	21.7
<1 yr	2586.7	1653.2	15-24 yr	70.5	59.6
1-4 yr	100.5	61.2			
5-14 yr	47.4	30.6	**AMERICAN INDIAN OR**		
15-24 yr	209.1	181.4	**ALASKA NATIVE FEMALE**		
			<1 yr	1352.6	592.4
AMERICAN INDIAN OR			1-4 yr	87.5	52.1
ALASKA NATIVE MALE			5-14 yr	33.5	22.7
<1 yr	1598.1	867.2	15-24 yr	90.3	68.4
1-4 yr	82.7	59.4			
5-14 yr	43.7	25.8	**ASIAN OR PACIFIC ISLANDER FEMALE**		
15-24 yr	311.1	167.0	<1 yr	755.8	375.3
			1-4 yr	35.4	18.4
ASIAN OR PACIFIC ISLANDER MALE			5-14 yr	21.5	11.3
<1 yr	816.5	468.8	15-24 yr	32.3	25.1
1-4 yr	50.9	21.2			
5-14 yr	23.4	12.3	**HISPANIC FEMALE**		
15-24 yr	80.8	63.6	<1 yr	746.6	575.0
			1-4 yr	42.1	28.8
HISPANIC MALE			5-14 yr	17.3	14.5
<1 yr	—	666.6	15-24 yr	40.6	35.2
1-4 yr	—	33.1			
5-14 yr	—	19.6	**WHITE, NON-HISPANIC FEMALE**		
15-24 yr	—	131.2	<1 yr	655.3	509.3
			1-4 yr	34.0	23.9
WHITE, NON-HISPANIC MALE			5-14 yr	17.6	14.0
<1 yr	—	635.4	15-24 yr	46.0	42.2
1-4 yr	—	31.8			

From Pastor PN: Chartbook on trends in the health of Americans. Health, United States, 2002, Hyattsville, Md, 2002, National Center for Health Statistics.

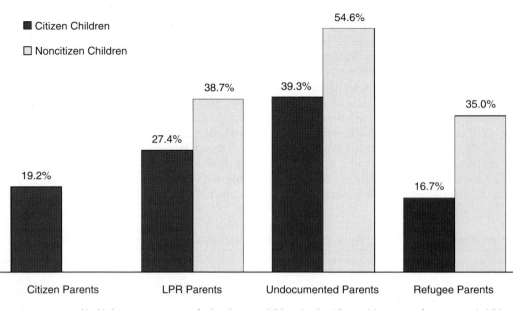

Percent Without Health Insurance Among Children (Under 18) in Families with Incomes Under 200% of Poverty (2000 CPS)

Note: All categories are significantly different from citizen parents, except citizen children of refugees.

FIGURE 1-2 Health insurance coverage for low-income children (under 18 years) by status of parents and children: 1999. *LPR,* Legal permanent resident. (From Fix M and Passel JS: The scope and impact of welfare reform's immigrant provisions, Washington, DC, 2002, The Urban Institute; Web site: www.urban.org/url.cfm?ID=410412. Reprinted with permission.)

reported only 77% of the children this age were in excellent to very good health. Uninsured children were nearly three times as likely to have not seen a health care provider in the past year as children with insurance (30% compared with 11%), and 39% of parents of uninsured children reported having trouble paying for health and medical benefits and delayed getting needed care (Halfon et al, 2002). Even when insurance is available, studies have found overall 18.7% of children have no usual source of care (care is sought and received at a variety of clinics), but black children were more than twice as likely (12.5%) as white children (6.0%) and Hispanic children were three times as likely (17.2%) as white children to have no source of usual care (Weinick & Krauss, 2000). The National Survey of Early Childhood Health (Halfon et al, 2002) found that fewer than one half of the children saw a particular provider when they sought health care. Lack of a regular source and provider of care prevents continuity in health care delivery and is associated with decreased screening and diagnosis of chronic conditions and appropriate and timely referrals (Committee on Children with Disabilities, 1998).

Although health status is an important predictor of children's use of services (e.g., the sicker the child, the more frequent the use of health services), poor, minority, and uninsured children, as well as those with their primary language being other than English (Weinick & Krauss, 2000), were most likely to experience barriers to access or were less apt to seek care than other children with comparable needs.

If a child is covered by insurance, access to care is usually improved, but out-of-pocket medical expenses for the family (i.e., deductibles, co-payments, pharmaceutical costs, noncovered services or equipment) can be significant. The average

American consumer paid 17% of medical expenses out-of-pocket in 2000, and families with members with chronic conditions can be expected to have higher out-of-pocket expenses (Pastor et al, 2002). Even families on federal assistance with Medicaid health insurance, living at or below the poverty level, incur direct out-of-pocket health care expenses to care for their children with chronic conditions, expenses that represent a substantial burden for these families (Lukemeyer et al, 2000; Meyers et al, 2000).

Effect of Poverty on Children's Health

In 2001 the percent of Americans living in poverty rose to 11.7% (32.9 million people) (Proctor & Dalaker, 2002). Income thresholds for poverty by family size and composition are found in Table 1-4. This was the first year-to-year rise in poverty since 1991 to 1992 and coincides with the recession beginning in March 2001 (Proctor & Dalaker, 2002). In 2001, 11.7 million children under 18 years of age (16.3%) were poor, a higher rate than any other age-group including people 65 years and older (Proctor & Dalaker, 2002). Younger children are even more vulnerable to poverty, with 18.2% of related children under age 6 years living in poverty and 48.9% of children under age 6 years in households headed by single women living in poverty, over five times the number of children living in married-couple families. More than one quarter of black and Hispanic children were poor (family income less than 100% of poverty level), and more than one half were poor or near poor (near poor being defined as 100% to 199% of poverty level) (ChildStats.gov, 2002). Many low-income working parents and their children remain poor. In 2001, 40% of children lived in families classified as "working poor" (Child Trends, 2002) with

TABLE 1-4

Poverty Thresholds (in Dollars) in 2001 by Size of Family and Number of Related Children Under 18 Yr

Size of Family Unit	Related Children Under 18 yr								
	None	**One**	**Two**	**Three**	**Four**	**Five**	**Six**	**Seven**	**Eight or More**
One person (unrelated individual)									
Under 65 yr	9214								
65 yr and over	8494								
Two people									
Householder under 65 yr	11,859	12,207							
Householder 65 yr and over	10,705	12,161							
Three people	13,853	14,255	14,269						
Four people	18,267	18,566	17,960	18,022					
Five people	22,029	22,349	21,665	21,135	20,812				
Six people	25,337	25,438	24,914	24,411	23,664	23,221			
Seven people	29,154	29,386	28,708	28,271	27,456	26,505	25,462		
Eight people	32,606	32,894	32,302	31,783	31,047	30,112	29,140	28,893	
Nine people or more	39,223	39,413	38,889	38,449	37,726	36,732	35,833	35,610	34,238

From US Census Bureau.

12% of Hispanic families and 9% of black families meeting this definition. Poverty is associated with no or limited health insurance and lack of regular health care. Children from low-income families and minorities are more likely to be uninsured, to receive fewer health care services, and to be hospitalized more often than children who are not poor (Center for The Future of Children, 1997; McConnochie et al, 1997; Newacheck et al, 1996, 1997).

Inequities in Health Care and Health Status for Children

The Institute of Medicine released an extensive report titled *Unequal Treatment: Confronting Racial and Ethnic Disparities in Health Care* (2003). This report compiles evidence of broad-based health care disparities and individual racial discrimination in health care and health care systems, legal and regulatory, that result in discrimination and poor quality of care provided to minority people. Although the majority of this report focused on disparities in health care for adults, the report does include discussion and analysis of research showing discrepancy in parents' reports of pediatric care under managed care by race/ethnicity (Moralis et al, 2001), variable access to kidney transplant by race/ethnicity (Furth et al, 2000), use of psychotropic medications (Zito et al, 1998), and use of prescription medications (Hahn, 1995). Additional recent reports support the disparity in health outcomes for children based on race/ethnicity and language (Flores et al, 2002a, 2002b; Keppel et al, 2002; Newacheck et al, 2002; Wood, 2002). Race, family structure (single parent vs. two parent), parent education, poverty, and culture/language are closely linked in the United States; and many professionals question whether disparities in health care are more related to poverty, family structure, or parent education than minority status (Committee on Pediatric Research, 2000; Fujiura, 1999; Fujiura & Yamaki, 2000; Williams, 2002).

Poverty has a profound effect on family well-being in the domains of health, productivity, physical environment, emotional well-being, and family interaction (Park et al, 2002)

BOX 1-1

Impact of Poverty on Family Life Domains

FAMILY HEALTH
Undernutrition during pregnancy and childhood
Food insecurity
Limited access to health care/supplies
Lack of continuity in health care

FAMILY PRODUCTIVITY
Delayed cognitive development
Inferior schooling, daycare
Decreased cognitive stimulation in the home
Increased incidence of parent with limited education
Limited opportunities for leisure and recreation

FAMILY PHYSICAL ENVIRONMENT
Housing insecurity
Poor and unsafe housing units
Lack of adequate heat, water, electricity, sanitation
Increased exposure to community health hazards (i.e., environmental toxins, community violence)

FAMILY EMOTIONAL WELL-BEING
Stress related to financial insecurity
Increased unhappiness, anxiety, dependence
Decrease in self-esteem, self-worth

FAMILY INTERACTION
Decreased marital and family satisfaction
Increased aversive and coercive discipline
Decreased support systems

Data from Park J et al: Impacts of poverty on quality of life in families of children with disabilities, *Exceptional Children* 68(2):151-170, 2002.

(Box 1-1). This impact is compounded when the family has a child with a chronic or disabling condition. The goals of *Healthy People 2010* reflect the need to address health disparities not just based on race, as was done in *Healthy People 2000*, but also based on the multiple factors now thought to impact health status in the United States (Box 1-2).

BOX 1-2
Goals for Healthy People 2010

1. Increase quality and years of healthy life.
   a. Life expectancy
   b. Quality of life
      (1) Personal sense of physical and mental health
      (2) Global assessment of health (i.e., poor, good)
      (3) Healthy days (i.e., days perceived as healthy)
      (4) Years of healthy life (i.e., years perceived as healthy)
2. Eliminate health disparities related to:
   a. Gender
   b. Race and ethnicity (focus of *Healthy People 2000*)
   c. Income and education
   d. Disability
   e. Geographic location
   f. Sexual orientation

Chronic and Disabling Conditions in Children

There are basic differences in the type and profile of chronic conditions in children and adults. Children are affected by a large number of rare diseases and genetic or prenatal conditions, and adults are affected by a relatively small number of common diseases (e.g., heart disease, emphysema, hypertension, diabetes) that increase in morbidity with age (Halfon & Hochstein, 1997; Perrin, 2002). Children with chronic conditions have unique health and social needs. Chronic illness in children is often not stable but subject to acute exacerbations and remissions that are superimposed on the child's growth and development. Children also depend on adults for care. Parent/family health, ethnicity, culture, socioeconomic status, education, and source of health care insurance all affect the child's access to services, use of services, and adherence to management plans.

Chronic Conditions in Children

The number of children who have a chronic condition and the relative severity of the conditions are unknown. Estimates of children with chronic conditions depend on the definition and method used to identify them (Stein & Silver, 2002). Stein defined chronic conditions in children as conditions that at the time of diagnosis or during their expected course will produce one or more of the following current or future long-term sequelae: limitation of functions appropriate for age and development, disfigurement, dependency on medication or special diet for normal functioning or control of condition, dependency on medical technology for functioning, need for more medical care or related services than usual for the child's age, or special ongoing treatments at home or in school (Stein, 1992). Perrin (2002, p. 303) defined chronic conditions in children as simply "health conditions that at the time of diagnosis are predicted to last longer than 3 months."

The National Health Interview Survey on Child Health (NHIS-CH), which was conducted by the National Center for Health Statistics in 1988, estimated that 31% of children under 18 years of age, or almost 20 million children nationwide, had one or more chronic conditions—not including mental health conditions—based on parent reports (Aday, 1992; Newacheck

et al, 1991; Newacheck & Taylor, 1992). The majority of the children (66%) in the NHIS-CH study reportedly had only mild conditions that resulted in little or no "bother" or limitation of activity. The high incidence of reported respiratory, skin, and digestive allergies probably accounts for the significant number of mild chronic conditions.

Children with Special Health Care Needs

Although 31% of children studied had chronic physical conditions, only a portion of these children required additional health, education, or social services. In 1995, the federal Maternal and Child Health Bureau's Division of Services for Children with Special Health Care Needs (DSCSHCN) established a group of professionals to develop a definition of children with special health care needs (McPherson et al, 1998). Health, education, and social policy changes, as well as changes in child health and disability patterns, warranted a definition that was easily understood and used by federal and state programs for planning and developing comprehensive community-based, family-centered services for children with special health care needs. While this new definition was being created, eligibility criteria for existing state and federal Title V programs, special education, and Supplemental Security Income (SSI) programs were reviewed. The following definition was developed:

Children with special health care needs are those who have or are at risk for a chronic physical, developmental, behavioral, or emotional condition and who also require health and related services of a type or amount beyond that required by children generally (McPherson et al, 1998, p. 138).

This definition of children with special health care needs focuses on the criterion of need for additional services instead of an identified medical condition or functional impairment, recognizing the variability in disease severity, degree of impairment, and service needs among children with the same or differing diagnosis. This definition also recognizes that children at risk for developing chronic physical, developmental, behavioral, or emotional conditions because of biologic or environmental characteristics also require health and related services beyond those generally required by children (McPherson et al, 1998).

In 1998 the Child and Adolescent Health Measurement Initiative (CAHMI), a national collaborative coordinated by the Foundation for Accountability, brought together a task force of federal and state policymakers, pediatric health care providers, researchers, and consumer groups to develop a method to identify children with special health care needs based on the new definition. The Children with Special Health Care needs (CSHCN) Screener was developed by this task force (Box 1-3) (Bethell et al, 2002a, 2002b; van Dyck et al, 2002). This short five-question parent report screening tool identifies children based not on diagnosis but on functional limitation or service use needs that are the direct result of an ongoing physical, emotional, behavioral, developmental, or other health condition and should determine more accurately the prevalence of children with special health care needs in studied populations, be they national surveys or clinic populations. To date the CSHCN Screener has been successful in identifying all, or nearly all, children with more severe or complex conditions and only those children whose milder condition (i.e., asthma, allergies,

BOX 1-3

Children with Special Health Care Needs (CSHCN) Screening Tool (Mail or Telephone)

1. Does your child currently need or use *medicine prescribed by a doctor* (other than vitamins)?
   Yes → Go to Question 1a
   No → Go to Question 2
   1a. Is this because of ANY medical, behavioral, or other health condition?
   Yes → Go to Question 1b
   No → Go to Question 2
   1b. Is this a condition that has lasted or is expected to last for *at least* 12 months?
   Yes
   No

2. Does your child need or use more *medical care, mental health, or educational services* than are usual for most children of the same age?
   Yes → Go to Question 2a
   No → Go to Question 3
   2a. Is this because of ANY medical, behavioral, or other health condition?
   Yes → Go to Question 2b
   No → Go to Question 3
   2b. Is this a condition that has lasted or is expected to last for *at least* 12 months?
   Yes
   No

3. Is your child *limited or prevented* in any way in his or her ability to do the things most children of the same age can do?
   Yes → Go to Question 3a
   No → Go to Question 4
   3a. Is this because of ANY medical, behavioral, or other health condition?
   Yes → Go to Question 3b
   No → Go to Question 4
   3b. Is this a condition that has lasted or is expected to last for *at least* 12 months?
   Yes
   No

4. Does your child need or get *special therapy*, such as physical, occupational, or speech therapy?
   Yes → Go to Question 4a
   No → Go to Question 5
   4a. Is this because of ANY medical, behavioral, or other health condition?
   Yes → Go to Question 4b
   No → Go to Question 5
   4b. Is this a condition that has lasted or is expected to last for *at least* 12 months?
   Yes
   No

5. Does your child have any kind of emotional, developmental, or behavioral problem for which he or she needs or gets *treatment or counseling*?
   Yes → Go to Question 5a
   No
   5a. Has this problem lasted or is it expected to last for *at least* 12 months?
   Yes
   No

SCORING THE CHILDREN WITH SPECIAL HEALTH CARE NEEDS (CSHCN) SCREENING TOOL

Conceptual Background

The CSHCN screener uses consequences-based criteria to screen for children with chronic or special health needs. To qualify as having chronic or special health needs, the following set of conditions must be met:

1. The child currently experiences a specific consequence.
2. The consequence is due to a medical or other health condition.
3. The duration or expected duration of the condition is 12 months or longer.

The first part of each screener question asks whether a child experiences one of five different health consequences:

1. Use or need of prescription medication
2. Above-average use or need of medical, mental health, or educational services
3. Functional limitations compared with others of same age
4. Use or need of specialized therapies (occupational therapy, physical therapy, speech, etc.)
5. Treatment or counseling for emotional or developmental problems

The second and third parts* of each screener question ask those responding "yes" to the first part of the question whether the consequence is due to any kind of health condition and if so, whether that condition has lasted or is expected to last for at least 12 months.

All three parts of at least one screener question (or in the case of question 5, the two parts) must be answered "yes" in order for a child to meet CSHCN screener criteria for having a chronic condition or special health care need.

The CSHCN screener has three "definitional domains":

1. Dependency on prescription medications
2. Service use above that considered usual or routine
3. Functional limitations

The definitional domains are not mutually exclusive categories. A child meeting the CSHCN screener criteria for having a chronic condition may qualify for one or more definitional domains (see diagram below).

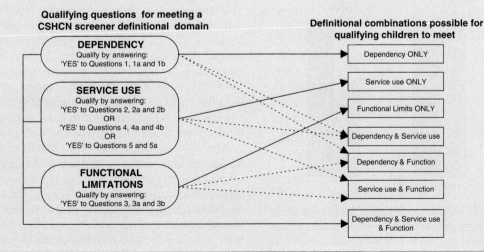

Qualifying questions for meeting a CSHCN screener definitional domain

DEPENDENCY
Qualify by answering:
'YES' to Questions 1, 1a and 1b

SERVICE USE
Qualify by answering:
'YES' to Questions 2, 2a and 2b
OR
'YES' to Questions 4, 4a and 4b
OR
'YES' to Questions 5 and 5a

FUNCTIONAL LIMITATIONS
Qualify by answering:
'YES' to Questions 3, 3a and 3b

Definitional combinations possible for qualifying children to meet

Dependency ONLY
Service use ONLY
Functional Limits ONLY
Dependency & Service use
Dependency & Function
Service use & Function
Dependency & Service use & Function

From FACCT—Foundation For Accountability: CAMHI project/chronic condition screener, January 2000. Reprinted with permission.
*NOTE: CSHCN screener question 5 is a two-part question. Both parts must be answered "yes" to qualify.

learning disabilities) results in elevated service needs. Unfortunately, the questionnaire does not identify children at risk.

In 2000 the Maternal and Child Health Bureau (MCHB) partnered with the National Center for Health Statistics (NCHS) to develop a new national and state survey, using the new definition of children with special health care needs, to determine the prevalence and impact of special health care needs among children (van Dyck et al, 2002). The State and Local Integrated Telephone Survey (SLAITS) of Children with Special Health Care Needs (CSHCN) provides baseline data for *Healthy People 2010* and will be repeated during the coming decade to show change in service needs and family needs. The initial parent telephone survey, conducted in 12% languages, was collected between October 2000 and March 2002. Preliminary findings from this national telephone survey indicate 30% of children have a chronic condition but of those children only a national prevalence of 13% of children from 0-17 years of age are "children with special health care needs" as defined by the Maternal and Child Health Bureau (Centers for Disease Control and Prevention [CDC], National Center for Health Statistics [NCHS], 2003). The previous NHIS-CH study indicated the majority of children were reported to have respiratory conditions, learning disabilities, behavior or conduct disorders, vision or hearing problems, or musculoskeletal conditions, but over one half of the children were only mildly affected and did not require "health and related services of a type or amount beyond that required by children generally." The 12.8% with special health care needs are estimated to be responsible for 45% of the pediatric health care expenditures, reflecting their increased utilization of services. Prevalence of children with special health care needs by gender, race, and age is found in Figure 1-3 and generally mirrors other studies on child health. The dramatic increase in children with special health care needs during the school years reflects the increased identification of children with chronic conditions limiting school participation or requiring related special services (see Chapter 5). Significant variations by minority grouping were found with parents of Hispanic children reporting fewer special health care needs than parents of either white or black children. The reasons for this finding are unknown, and further analysis is necessary.

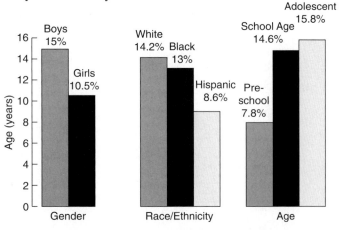

FIGURE 1-3 Prevalence by gender, race, and age of children with special health care needs. (From Centers for Disease Control and Prevention, National Center for Health Statistics: National survey of children with special health care needs, 2003, Maternal and Child Health Bureau; Web site: http://www.cdc.gov/nchs/about/major/slaits/cshcn.htm.)

Disabilities in Children

Definitions of disability have also been changing in an attempt to standardize data collection to determine prevalence estimates and characteristics of children with disabilities. Common components of most definitions of disabilities are as follows: having a particular need for services (i.e., daily medication, respiratory therapy, routine catheterization); having a diagnosis of a physical or mental condition commonly associated with being disabled (i.e., mental retardation, hearing loss, cystic fibrosis); and/or exhibiting specific functional deficits (i.e., needing a wheelchair for mobility, needing gavage feedings, being blind) (Westbrook et al, 1998). The World Health Organization has also been trying to standardize the definition and screening method for determining disabilities in people all over the world (Mbogoni & Me, 2002). Cultural variations in expected functions and recognition of the stigma often associated with disability have resulted in an International Classification of Functioning, Health and Disability (ICF) (Clancy & Andersen, 2002). The current definition of disability used by the World Health Organization is "a person who is limited in the kind or amount of activities that he or she can do because of ongoing difficulties due to a long-term physical condition, mental conditions or health problems" (United Nations, 1998). The classic functions used to determine disability in adults (the ability to work, to perform household chores, and to care for oneself independently) are not appropriate in determining ability in children. Limitations in activities associated with play, the ability to attend and succeed in school, and the ability to develop self-care activities are more appropriate indicators of ability or limitations in ability for children.

The National Health Interview Survey (NHIS) for the years 1992 to 1994 indicated that 6.5% of children under 18 years of age (i.e., 4.4 million children) had some disability, with 0.7% of this group having a severe disability that made them unable to participate in a major, age-appropriate activity (e.g., playing for younger children; attending school for older children) (Newacheck & Halfon, 1998). The survey results were further delineated: 4% of the children were limited in their ability to perform expected activities, and 1.8% were able to perform major activities but were restricted in other activities. The three major condition categories resulting in disability were respiratory conditions (i.e., principally asthma), impairment of speech or intelligence (i.e., principally mental retardation), and mental and nervous system disorders (i.e., principally learning disabilities). Children with identified disabilities had physician contact three times as often as other children and spent eight times as many days in the hospital (Newacheck & Halfon, 1998). Although some chronic conditions and disabilities have minimal effect on a child's daily activities, 1.5 million children and adolescents under the age of 22 years were deemed severely disabled and required daily assistive care (McNeil, 1997).

The 2000 census, for the first time in more than a century, tracked children ages 5 to 20 years to determine the prevalence of disability. Figures indicate 1 in 12 children (5.2 million children) has some physical or mental disability (Cohn, 2002). The disabilities ranged from mild asthma to serious mental illness or retardation requiring extensive services. The National Health Interview Survey has tracked reporting by parents of limitation of activity because of chronic physical, mental, or emotional disorders and need for special education or early intervention

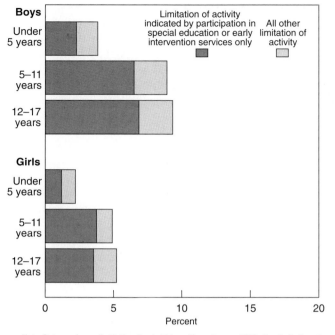

FIGURE 1-4 Limitation of activity caused by one or more chronic health conditions among children by gender and age: United States, 1998 to 2000. (From Pastor PN: Chartbook on trends in the health of Americans. Health, United States, 2002, Hyattsville, Md, 2002, National Center for Health Statistics.)

services between 1997 and 2000 (Pastor et al, 2002). The surveys found a fairly stable frequency of reported limitations in activity (overall for children under 18 years of 6.0%) but significant variation by gender and age (Figure 1-4).

A large retrospective longitudinal cohort study of children with developmental disability found that over 65% had one or more chronic health conditions (9-fold increase in central nervous system and ear, nose, and throat problems; 5-fold increase in gastrointestinal problems; 1.5- to 2-fold increase in respiratory and malignant conditions) than a matched cohort of children without developmental delays (Gallaher et al, 2002). Children in this study with developmental disabilities and additional chronic health conditions were more than seven times as likely to be hospitalized and had approximately three times the physician visits. There is clearly a hierarchy of health and social risk among children with chronic and disabling conditions, as well as a hierarchy of those with increased service needs.

Changing Patterns of Chronic and Disabling Conditions in Children

The patterns of childhood morbidity and mortality have changed because of advances in technology, pharmacotherapeutics, pediatric emergency trauma services, improved prevention and treatment of infectious diseases that were previously fatal, improved diagnoses and case findings of children with previously unrecognized illnesses, and implementation of public and preventive health measures that have saved the lives of infants and children who would have previously

died (Kleiman & Perloff, 1997; Perrin, 2002). The overall incidence of most childhood chronic conditions has not changed significantly over the past 20 years, but this improved life expectancy results in an increased prevalence of children living with chronic and disabling conditions. Infants, children, and adolescents are surviving, requiring additional health care and social services. Many women born with birth defects now survive to have children of their own with an increased incidence of the same birth defect (Skjaerven et al, 1999). Each year an estimated 50,000 children acquire a permanent disability as a result of serious injury or acute illness (Guyer & Ellers, 1990; MacKenzie, 2000; Valadka et al, 2000).

The prevalence of children and adolescents requiring care for chronic conditions has increased dramatically. For example, children with cystic fibrosis now frequently survive into adulthood (see Chapter 22). Improved surgical intervention and control of urinary tract infections have prolonged the life expectancy of children with spina bifida (see Chapter 33). Newborn screening programs and early dietary intervention have dramatically improved the quality of life and reproductive capability of children with phenylketonuria (see Chapter 35). Advanced trauma care has enabled children to survive severe brain injury, which often results in a chronic disability (see Chapter 27). Recognition of the increasing incidence or diagnosis of mental and behavioral problems in children and new treatment modalities have increased the service demand for these children and demand for community/primary care (see Chapters 12, 13, 32, 40).

New categories of childhood chronic conditions are also emerging. Infants surviving extreme prematurity or very low birth weight are posing new medical and management problems (see Chapter 36). The dramatic rise in childhood obesity has resulted in an increased prevalence of type 2 diabetes, virtually unheard of 1 decade ago (see Chapter 23). Children with acquired immunodeficiency syndrome (AIDS) are living longer because of advances in treatment (see Chapter 28). The health care system with its advanced technology has created a spectrum of children with chronic iatrogenic conditions (e.g., infants with bronchopulmonary dysplasia [see Chapter 16], children with immune suppression as a result of drug therapy following organ or bone marrow transplantation [see Chapters 34 and 15], survivors of childhood cancer who later experience the residual effects of treatment [see Chapter 17]). And many congenital birth defects and acquired health conditions with previously unknown etiology are now being linked to prenatal and childhood exposure to environmental toxins (Woodruff et al, 2003).

Inequities in Distribution of Chronic and Disabling Conditions in Children

Not all children in the United States are equally affected by chronic and disabling conditions. Socioeconomic status and ethnicity play important roles in the incidence and severity of chronic conditions (Committee on Pediatric Research, 2000; Flores et al, 2002a; Institute of Medicine, 2002; Keppel et al, 2002). Poor children have a significantly higher incidence rate and severity level of disability (Newacheck et al, 2002; Perrin, 2002), and a child's disability has a major impact on a family's finances because of increased health care expenditures and decreased ability of parents to work as a result of child care needs.

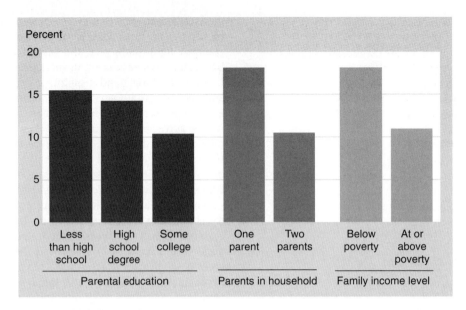

FIGURE 1-5 Percentage of children ages 5 to 17 years who have difficulty performing everyday activities by socio-economic status, 1994. (From Centers for Disease Control and Prevention [CDC], National Center for Health Statistics: National health interview survey on disability. Retrieved January 19, 2003 from http://childstats.gov/ac1999/spectxt.asp.)

Males, children from families with incomes below the poverty level, and children in single-parent families have an increased prevalence of disability and these factors exert an independent effect on the probability of disability (Fujiura & Yamaki, 2000; Newacheck & Halfon, 1998). Figure 1-5 shows that 15.5% of children in households where neither parent was a high school graduate had difficulty performing everyday activities as compared with 10.3% of children in households where at least one parent had some college education; 18.1% of children in single-parent households as compared with 10.4% of children in households with two parents had difficulties; and in families with incomes below the poverty level 18.1% of children had difficulty performing activities of daily living as compared with 10.9% in families at or above the poverty level (Centers for Disease Control and Prevention, National Center for Health Statistics, 1999). Looking at just the population of children with disabilities, 28% are living in poor families (Park et al, 2002).

Barriers to Quality Comprehensive Care for Children with Chronic and Disabling Conditions

Unmet Health Care Needs. Health care needs can go unmet for a variety of reasons; that is, the need is unrecognized, access is restricted because of lack of insurance or financial means to pay for the service, the appropriate provider is not available, or the client/family needing service is unable to access service (language barriers, transportation, other competing needs). Unmet health needs are an indicator of available health services and need for health policy intervention (Newacheck et al, 2000). Overall, more than 7% of American children are estimated to have an unmet health care need annually (Newacheck et al, 2000). Poor and near-poor children and children without insurance were three times more likely to have an unmet health care need than nonpoor and insured children. Children with chronic

conditions often have needs for services above and beyond children in general (i.e., the definition of children with special health care needs), and therefore it can be anticipated they will have a greater frequency of unmet needs.

The SLAITS Survey of Children with Special Health Care Needs (Centers for Disease Control and Prevention, National Center for Health Statistics, Health Resources and Services Administration, Maternal and Child Health Bureau, 2003) revealed 17.7% of the children had an unmet health care need in the past year with 14.5% of the parents reporting their insurance did not cover needed services. Family Voices, a national parent support and advocacy organization for families with children with special health care needs, surveyed members in 1999 and 2000 to determine health care utilization and needs (Wells et al, 2000). Families reported 48% had difficulty receiving home health care; 43% of children receiving mental health services had problems finding a skilled provider, obtaining referrals, or having insurance coverage for needed visits; 27% had trouble obtaining speech therapy or physical therapy; 26% had difficulty obtaining occupational therapy; and 23% had problems obtaining specialty services. Families also were dissatisfied or did not get respite services (46%), nutritional supplements (38%), durable medical equipment (31%), disposable medical supplies (26%), and dental care (18%).

Dental health care needs and mental health services are two areas of unmet needs commonly identified (Committee on Children with Disabilities and Committee on Psychosocial Aspects of Child and Family Health, 1993; Committee on Psychosocial Aspects of Child and Family Health, 2001; Newacheck et al, 2000). Children with chronic conditions often have special diets or eating patterns that can affect oral health. Medications may affect tooth or gum development, and dental hygiene may be very difficult in children with severe disabilities or oral aversion. Dentists skilled in the care of children with complex conditions are often difficult to find but important in helping to maintain oral health and long-term adequate nutrition.

As providers become more aware of mental and behavioral health problems in children the identified need for comprehensive mental health services has become more apparent (Committee on Psychosocial Aspects of Child and Family Health, 2001). It is estimated that 7% to 18% of children in primary care settings have identifiable psychosocial problems (Kelleher et al, 2000). The American Psychiatric Association (1999) estimates more than 13 million children are in need of mental health or substance abuse services. A recent review of three national household health surveys found only 2% to 3% of 3- to 5-year-old children and 6% to 9% of children 6 to 17 years old used mental health services; 80% of the children identified as in need of mental health services did not receive services, and the rate of unmet need was greater for Hispanic children than white children and for uninsured children (Kataoka et al, 2002).

Children with chronic conditions are twice as likely as other children to have behavioral or emotional problems (Committee on Children with Disabilities and Committee on Psychosocial Aspects of Child and Family Health, 1993). Co-morbidity of chronic conditions and mental health problems is more common in children with neurologic and/or developmental conditions but can occur in any child (Vessey, 1999). The child's general health status or severity of illness is not highly correlated with development of mental health problems (Committee on Children with Disabilities, 1993). Males, children with visible disabilities, children with a poor or uncertain prognosis, and families with mental health conditions, minimal support systems, and minimal financial resources have all been associated with a higher prevalence of mental health problems (Northam, 1999). Unfortunately, as the identification of need for mental health services has increased, the services have not (American Academy of Pediatrics, 2000). Attempts to restrain health care costs have often resulted in decreased availability of mental health and substance abuse services for children and adolescents even when research has indicated intervention can help children and families cope with the psychologic and social consequences of chronic health conditions (Bauman et al, 1997).

Concern over the large number of children without adequate health care caused the American Academy of Pediatrics, Committee on Child Health Financing, to release a policy statement on access to health care for infants, children, adolescents, and pregnant women (Committee on Child Health Financing, 1998). The American Academy of Pediatrics advocates universal access to quality health care, which includes preventive care services, acute and chronic care services, emergency care services, and all necessary services that (1) are appropriate for the child's age and health status; (2) will prevent or ameliorate the effects of a condition, illness, injury, or disorder; (3) will aid in the overall physical and mental development of the individual; and/or (4) will assist in achieving or maintaining functional capacity (Committee on Child Health Financing, 1998).

Inadequate Continuity of Care. The SLAITS Survey of Children with Special Health Care Needs (Centers for Disease Control and Prevention, National Center for Health Statistics, Health Resources and Services Administration, Maternal and Child Health Bureau, 2003) found that of the children identified as having special health care needs, 9.2% had no source of regular care and an additional 11% did not have a regular provider (physician or nurse) at the health facility they attended. Over 8.8% of the parents reported having great difficulty obtaining referrals to specialists, 12.3% reported their insurance did not permit them to see providers they felt they needed for their child, and 14.5% had health care service needs not covered by insurance. Lack of continuity care or reliance on community clinics may result in poor identification of chronic health conditions, inconsistency in management, and lack of appropriate referrals. When hospital records were reviewed for unscheduled intensive care unit admission, children with chronic conditions were three times more likely to be admitted for treatment than previously healthy children and health care system deficiencies were estimated to account for 64% of these potentially preventable severe acute illnesses (Dosa et al, 2001). Access to health care—even for those children with chronic or disabling conditions—is more likely to be sporadic and delayed if a family does not have a continuity provider or adequate insurance. Many services required to prevent or ameliorate the effects of the child's condition, to aid in the child's overall physical and mental development, or to assist the child in achieving or maintaining functional capacity may not be provided or covered by the family's insurance.

Fragmentation of Care. Many children with chronic conditions receive the majority of their medical care in specialty clinics that do not provide routine health care management (Stein, 1997). Shuffled from specialist to specialist, children often miss the screenings, developmental assessments, anticipatory guidance, and immunizations that healthy children of the same age receive. This lack of routine health care appears to cross disease categories. Jessop & Stein (1994) interviewed mothers of children with a variety of chronic conditions and found that although 56% could identify a usual source of care, few could identify a provider who would listen to their concerns (27%), provide them with general advice about the child's condition (24%), or facilitate case-management services with other agencies (22%) (Table 1-5).

The development of medical specialization, which has improved the disease control and life expectancy of children with special health care needs, has also resulted in fragmentation of health care delivery and increased medical costs (Ireys et al, 1997; Stein, 1997). The families of these children—far more than other families—have to interact with multiple institutions providing some aspect of care for their child (e.g., early intervention programs; equipment vendors; social services; special education programs; federal, state, or private financial providers of care). In addition, there are often medical subspecialists whose expectations may or may not be realistic for the family or child. Demands are sometimes conflicting, uncoordinated, and incomprehensible to the family. Subspecialists rarely address primary health care needs, developmental concerns, or common illness management, resulting in parents needing to seek additional health care services (Miller et al, 2000). Primary care providers, on the other hand, frequently cite lack of adequate time with children and families, lack of adequate reimbursement for care of children with complex medical or behavioral conditions, and unavailability of subspecialists in their community as barriers to their

TABLE 1-5

Health Services Provided to Families with Children with Chronic Conditions and the Questions Used to Elicit Them

Area	Question	% Indicating Services Currently Provided
Usual source of care	Is there a place you usually go for care and a particular person you usually see there?	56
Coordination with specialists	Does this provider make arrangements if the child needs to see a specialist?	50
Coordination with other agencies	Does this provider talk to other agencies (e.g., school, daycare center, Medicaid)?	22
General advice	Does anyone give general advice about your child and things such as special schooling, handicaps, behavior problems, and what to expect later in childhood or adulthood?	24
Family risk	Does anyone discuss with you whether the child's illness runs in the family or could occur in other family members?	38
Listen to concerns	Does anyone listen to your concerns about your child and understand the problems of raising a child with an illness?	27
Explanation of illness	Has the child's illness been explained to you?	62
Intercurrent illness	Is there someone you go to when the child has a fever, an ear infection, or something similar?	72
Health care maintenance	Does anyone measure the child's height and weight, talk about development and eating, etc.?	80

From Jessop DJ and Stein RE: Providing comprehensive health care to children with chronic illness, Pediatrics 93(4):602-607, 1994. Modified with permission.

provision of comprehensive care to children with chronic conditions (Barclay, 2003).

Knowledge Barriers. Knowledge barriers to optimal health care can be present for both the family and the practitioner. A study of caretakers' knowledge about their children's medical problems found that only one half of the caretakers interviewed in specialty clinics could provide a lay diagnosis of the condition, 29% could not provide an accurate list of current medications, and 25% could not identify the subspecialist providing care to the child (Carraccio et al, 1998). This lack of knowledge jeopardizes the child's health care if continuity providers are not available for care. A recent study of racial and ethnic differences in accessing health care identified a marked disadvantage among Hispanic families and postulated this was related to "language ability and characteristics associated with being a non-English speaker, including differing knowledge of and beliefs about the health care system and primary care" (Weinick & Krauss, 2000, p. 1773). Not knowing the need for, or value of, early intervention may delay the initiation of care. Not knowing how to access services with proper referrals and eligibility identification may prevent families from obtaining the care they are entitled to receive. Parents may not appreciate the need for health maintenance care in addition to subspecialty care.

Because of the explosive growth of medical knowledge and technology, it is difficult for practitioners to stay abreast of the current management techniques for children with chronic conditions. The specific condition and its severity, the availability of subspecialists in the community, and parental requests all affect a primary care provider's perceived ability and role in caring for children with chronic conditions. This recognition of knowledge limitations, possibly coupled with concern over potential legal consequences if subtle but important changes in a chronic condition are not recognized early, may be the reason some primary care practitioners do not want to assume medical or health care responsibilities for children with chronic conditions.

A survey of pediatric primary care physicians in a new model program for children with special health care needs found that although more than 80% were satisfied with their relationship with subspecialists and the care their clients received in the emergency room, less than 50% were satisfied with the amount and quality of information services they could provide families, their access to quality home care and community services, case management, and the ability to provide or access psychologic and mental health services (Davidson et al, 2002). Fifty percent or more of the physicians responding to the survey identified the need for additional training or support on (1) public programs, (2) parent-to-parent support groups, (3) community resource material, (4) accessing mental health services, (5) transitional health care services, and (6) development of individualized health care plans. Although the survey participants reflected a cohort of physicians committed to caring for children with special health care needs they did not feel they had the knowledge, resources, infrastructure, or reimbursement to provide comprehensive services, especially for the children with complex health conditions (Davidson et al, 2002).

Managed Care and Children with Chronic Conditions

Managed care health plans have become the dominant form of health care coverage. From their inception, managed care plans were designed to provide services for adults, whose care consumed 86% of health care dollars, so the needs of children received little attention (Deal et al, 1998) (see Chapter 8). With the rapid expansion of managed care, especially for Medicaid-eligible clients, the roles and responsibilities of state Title V programs for children with special health care needs are also changing (McManus et al, 1996). Across the United States, the direct services provided by specialty clinics funded through Title V have decreased while managed care systems attempt to provide services to children within the managed care organization (Newacheck et al, 1995). The consequences of these changes are unknown. Managed care plans have the potential to establish a "medical home for care," decrease out-of-pocket expenses for health care, and offer increased and coordinated services (e.g., preventive health care and specialty care at a fixed price for enrolled families) to children with special health care needs (Committee on Children with Disabilities, 1998; Newacheck et al, 2001). The provision of coordinated services within one system of care can increase access to services and reduce the number of bureaucracies with which families must negotiate.

Managed care plans are constructed to be cost-efficient, however, and focus on providing services to relatively healthy populations. Private health care plans can discourage the enrollment of high-risk individuals by excluding enrollment of individuals with certain preexisting conditions, having higher rates of cost sharing for out-of-plan referrals, restricting the use of specialists or choice of hospitals, and having a narrow interpretation of what is medically necessary (Berman, 1997; Fowler & Anderson, 1996; Walker, 1998). Many conditions of children with special health care needs are fairly rare, so providers assigned to care for them who were not trained in pediatric specialty centers will not be as knowledgeable in caring for the child, prioritizing services that could prevent or ameliorate the effects of the condition, aiding the overall physical and mental growth and development of the child, or using the available community resources to support the child and family. Therefore the quality of care may be decreased (Committee on Child Health Financing, 1998; Ireys et al, 1996; Newacheck et al, 1996) although a recent comparison of self-reported outcomes of access, satisfaction, use, or quality of care for a general child population showed no difference between children enrolled in managed care and traditional health plans (Newacheck et al, 2001). A similar study for children with chronic conditions needs to be performed.

Providing care to children with chronic or disabling conditions is expensive, but clear standards of care or clinical guidelines have not been established to mandate a higher expenditure for services (Committee on Children with Disabilities, 1998; Fowler & Anderson, 1996; Ireys et al, 1997; Neff & Anderson, 1995). Changing technology and limited outcomes data, especially regarding mental health and rehabilitation services to promote normal growth and development, often result in arbitrary caps on services provided by managed care organizations (Committee on Children with Disabilities, 1998). Increased capitation fees for providers willing to care for children with special health care needs and continued fee-for-service "carve outs" for these children are two of the risk adjustment methods that have been tried. Any risk adjustment method must recognize the increased time and frequency of health care visits, service referrals and coordination, and family counseling necessary for quality care (Committee on Children with Disabilities, 1998).

Primary care providers have a central role in managed care systems. Clients are often assigned a primary care provider who is a gatekeeper to health services. This central role increases the responsibility of primary care providers to care for children with chronic or disabling conditions and requires that providers be more knowledgeable about the direct care of these children and the availability and effectiveness of potential referrals. The primary care provider must be able to articulate and advocate for "medically necessary" care and services that enhance the child's health, growth, and development (Ireys et al, 1999). In conjunction with the family, primary care providers are now more responsible for accessing services through a system of care predicated on cost savings and demonstrated outcomes.

Role of the Primary Care Provider in Caring for Children with Chronic Conditions

Few professionals would argue that the pediatric subspecialists with advanced training and skills gained from caring for many children with similar conditions are not the best professionals to deal with the medical complexities of many chronic conditions. On the other hand, if the broader needs of the child and family (i.e., education, support, advocacy, health promotion)— needs that families have regardless of the specific chronic condition—are seen as the major focus of care, there is an obvious role for a primary care provider.

The primary care provider should be an integral part—if not the leading force—in the care of children with chronic conditions for the following reasons. (1) Holistic health care of children requires that they be viewed first and primarily as children with the health care and developmental needs of any child. (2) The family must be seen as an integral part of the child's growth and development and recognized for its individual strengths and weaknesses. The development of partnership with families in the care of their children is a fundamental tenet of pediatric primary care. (3) Health promotion, disease prevention, and anticipatory guidance have even greater significance when children already have a condition putting them at increased risk. Subspecialists are experts in their area of disease management but often have limited knowledge of normal growth and development and standard health care practices for health maintenance. (4) Primary care providers most likely know a family's community resources better than subspecialists, who may have practices many miles from the family's home. This knowledge of community resources is extremely important in helping families receive optimal care and support for their children.

To address the complexity of care provision needed by children with special health care needs the American Academy of Pediatrics, the Maternal Child Health Bureau, and Family Voices have developed the goals of a community-based system of care in the document "All Aboard the 2010 Express: A 10-Year Action Plan to Achieve Community-based Service Systems for Children and Youth with Special Health Care Needs and their Families" (Maternal Child Health Bureau, Health Resources and Services Administration, 2001) (Box 1-4). The SLAITS Survey of Children with Special Health Care Needs (CDC, NCHS, and Health Resources and Services Administration, Maternal and Child Health Bureau, 2003) attempted to measure current levels of attainment for key attributes of these goals. Over 57% of parents reported the child's physician made them feel like a partner in the child's care by spending enough time with them, being culturally sensitive, providing needed information, and listening to their concerns. Goal 2 refers to families having access to a "medical home." A "medical home" (the term "health care home" is preferable because it connotes the importance of health maintenance and health promotion) is the term used to connote an ideal health care practice in the child's community that offers a source of ongoing, comprehensive, family-centered care for children with special health care needs. A health care home offers the child and family preventive primary care services as well as management of chronic and acute conditions, 24 hours

BOX 1-4

Goals Identified To Achieve Community-Based Service Systems for Children with Special Health Care Needs to Meet Healthy People 2010 Goals

Goal 1: Families of children with special health care needs will partner in decision making at all levels and will be satisfied with the services they receive.

Goal 2: All children with special health care needs will receive coordinated, ongoing, comprehensive care within a medical home.

Goal 3: All families of children with special health care needs will have adequate private and/or public insurance to pay for the services they need.

Goal 4: All children will be screened early and continuously for special health care needs.

Goal 5: Community-based services systems will be organized so families can use them easily.

Goal 6: All youth with special health care needs will receive the services necessary to make transitions to all aspects of adult life, including adult health care, work, and independence.

From US Department of Health and Human Services, Maternal and Child Health Bureau: All aboard the 2010 express: a 10-year action plan to achieve community-based service systems for children and youth with special health care needs and their families, 2001.

per day, 7 days per week. Care coordination and collaboration among primary care providers, specialists, and community resources, in partnership with the child and family, are fundamental components of a health care home. Fifty-two percent of parents in this recent survey indicated their child had a regular care provider (physician or nurse), experienced no problems obtaining referrals, and received care coordination, all components of a "medical home." Goal 3, availability of adequate insurance to meet health care needs, was reported by 60% of parents. Early, regular, and comprehensive screening for children with special health care needs is goal 4; fifty-two percent of families in the SLAITS survey reported their children had annual preventive health visits and dental visits, the two selected indicators for determining attainment of this goal. Seventy-four percent of parents reported services were organized for easy use, goal 5, but less than 6% of parents reported they received services needed to support their child's transition to adulthood. Clearly, the pediatric health care systems have a long way to go to reach the *Healthy People 2010* targets for children with special health care needs and their families.

Levels of Primary Care Intervention for Children with Chronic or Disabling Conditions

Caring for children with chronic conditions is a challenging, rewarding, and time-consuming proposition. It requires a commitment to service beyond that required for routine ambulatory pediatric care, increased knowledge about children with chronic conditions, and additional interpersonal communication and organizational skills necessary to provide optimal child and family care.

Levels of intervention in the primary care of children, as well as the knowledge base and skills primary care providers need at each level of intervention, are outlined in Box 1-5. These levels of intervention are cumulative (i.e., level 3 intervention cannot be attained until the knowledge base and skills

of levels 1 and 2 are mastered). As the levels increase, so do the commitment of the provider and the comprehensiveness of care for the child and family. This model of care was inspired by work done in the area of family-centered care by Doherty & Baird (1987).

Level 1 care is the provision of routine health care maintenance and common illness management to healthy children and their families. Some health care providers may elect not to care for children with chronic conditions because of practice restrictions, a knowledge base limited to the care of normal children, or a lack of skills necessary to adequately manage more complex medical and psychosocial problems. Optimal care can be provided at level 1 but only to children and families without complex health care needs.

Level 2 care is task-oriented care requiring minimal interaction with the child or family and no commitment to continuity care. Level 2 care is not primary care but may be used to supplement primary care when a certain task must be accomplished. The knowledge base and skill level needed for task-oriented care are limited to those necessary to complete the task efficiently, effectively, and safely. Examples of this level of care include the primary care provider administering immunizations, ordering laboratory tests, or performing a prehospitalization physical examination at the request of the managing subspecialist.

Level 3 care is provided when health care professionals offer routine primary care to children with chronic conditions, recognizing the unique health care needs of the child and family. Providers are able to assess the child's chronic condition but refer this care to other individuals or agencies. Because of the complexity of some conditions, the provider's personal interest and/or knowledge base, or practice restriction, primary care providers may elect to manage some children with chronic conditions at this level while managing children with other conditions at a higher level.

Level 4 care is comprehensive primary health care that incorporates the unique complexities of the chronic condition, the child, and the family. At this level the practitioner assumes the primary health care responsibilities of the child and family and uses consultations or referrals for complex situations. This is the level of care often expected of primary care providers serving as gatekeepers in managed care systems. Practitioners do not abdicate care to subspecialists but work with them and the family to provide optimal care. As the health professional with the greatest knowledge of the family, the child, the health care system, and the community, the primary care provider assumes a leadership role in providing comprehensive continuity care.

Level 5 care takes the role of the primary provider one step further to that of care coordinator. A care coordinator assesses, plans, facilitates, implements, coordinates, monitors, and evaluates the education and service needs of a child and family (Committee on Children with Disabilities, 1999; Lindeke et al, 2002). The care coordinator must know the available resources and how to access them, provide linkage between services, integrate services so they are not duplicative, and be able to set measurable goals to determine effectiveness of individual interventions. As systems of care for children with special health care needs become more complex, multiple interdisciplinary

BOX 1-5

Hierarchic Intervention Framework for Practitioners Caring for Children with Chronic Conditions

LEVEL 1
Ongoing health care and illness management for children without chronic conditions

Knowledge Base Needed
Routine health care maintenance and common illness management for children without chronic conditions and their families

Skills Needed
1. The ability to collect subjective and objective data related to child health maintenance and common pediatric illnesses
2. The ability to elicit relevant family data related to family structure, medical history, and current health problems and concerns
3. The ability to listen effectively
4. The ability to assess the information obtained
5. The ability to identify a treatment plan for an individual child without a chronic condition and family
6. The ability to effectively communicate the treatment plan to the child and family
7. The ability to identify children with more complex needs requiring additional services
8. The ability to provide culturally sensitive care to the child and family

LEVEL 2
Task-oriented care for children with chronic conditions; primary care needs and specialty care needs managed by other professionals

Additional Knowledge Base Needed
Task-related knowledge

Additional Skill Needed
Performance of task in efficient, correct manner

LEVEL 3
Management of routine health care needs for children with chronic conditions; collaboration or referral for care related to the chronic condition

Additional Knowledge Base Needed
1. Basic pathophysiology of chronic conditions
2. Child and family reactions to the stress of chronic conditions
3. Noncategorical effect of chronic conditions on child development
4. Collaborative role function
5. Specialists, community agencies, tertiary care centers, and other professionals to assume responsibility for care of child's chronic condition

Additional Skills Needed
1. The ability to educate the child and family about health care maintenance needs, management plans, and accessing services
2. The ability to work with family members in their efforts to manage the child's normal growth and development
3. The ability to assess the child with a chronic condition, identifying change requiring consultation or referral to a specialist
4. The ability to identify family dysfunction requiring referral
5. The ability to communicate physical or psychosocial changes in the child or family to the appropriate professional
6. The ability to provide culturally sensitive care to the child and family experiencing a chronic health condition

LEVEL 4
Comprehensive primary care of children with chronic conditions and their families

Additional Knowledge Base Needed
1. In-depth pathophysiology of chronic conditions
2. Unique primary care needs of children with chronic conditions
3. Common associated problems found in chronic conditions and effective management
4. Differential diagnosis for common pediatric illnesses occurring in children with chronic conditions
5. Specific stressors for child and family with chronic condition
6. Effect of chronic condition on child's growth, development, and activities of daily living
7. Health care system resources and consultants available to assist child and family
8. Resource needs associated with chronic condition and means of accessing services
9. Basic cost of services provided to family and health system
10. Community resources, including educational resources, available to assist child and family and means of accessing these services

Additional Skills Needed
1. The ability to systematically assess the medical condition and health care needs of the child with a chronic condition
2. The ability to plan and implement primary health care, including common illness management, that is individualized for the child, the family, and the chronic condition
3. The ability to identify complications of the chronic condition requiring more complex care and to make appropriate referrals
4. The ability to educate the family on the special health care needs of the child with a chronic condition, management plans, and accessing of services
5. The ability to access services within the health care system and community, including educational system, to meet child's health care needs
6. The ability to work with families to plan short- and long-term care consistent with medical needs and family function
7. The ability to assist parents and child in problem solving both medical and family concerns
8. The ability to help families recognize the needs of individual members and balance these needs
9. The ability to assist families in planning services and activities to reduce stress
10. The ability to make interdisciplinary referrals communicating child and family needs and expectations
11. The ability to provide consistent, available, long-term care

LEVEL 5
Care coordination of families and children with chronic conditions

Additional Knowledge Base Needed
1. Service network available to child and family
2. Information systems available to collect and evaluate outcome data
3. Cost of resources
4. Quality outcome measures
5. Service planning and systems coordination
6. Team building and coordination
7. Eligibility requirements, referral process, and utilization measures for agencies or services that might benefit the family and child

Additional Skills Needed
1. The ability to identify outcome measures of quality care for children with chronic conditions
2. The ability to develop an alliance with family and child to work together to plan and provide optimum care

Continued

BOX 1-5

Hierarchic Intervention Framework for Practitioners Caring for Children with Chronic Conditions—cont'd

Additional Skills Needed—cont'd

3. The ability to make a comprehensive needs assessment for child and family
4. The ability to plan and initiate appropriate and successful referrals for services within the health care system and community
5. The ability to analyze cost/benefit ratio for services provided
6. The ability to coordinate services and personnel working with the family and child
7. The ability to utilize information systems to collect and evaluate outcome data
8. The ability to measure and monitor child and family progress
9. The ability to make changes in management and service plan as necessary
10. The ability to communicate findings from multiple interdisciplinary sources to family, child, and other involved personnel or agencies
11. The willingness to function as child and family advocate

LEVEL 6
Advocate for children with chronic conditions and their families

Additional Knowledge Base Needed

1. Institutional structure governing practice priorities
2. Community leadership network
3. Legislative process
4. Legislative policymakers
5. Research on evidence-based practice

Additional Skills Needed

1. Ability to identify and articulate important child health issues that are measurable and achievable
2. Ability to influence decision making with available data
3. Ability to build coalitions of individuals around particular child health issues
4. Ability to compromise
5. Ability to work within the political system and with politicians

---

professionals may act as care coordinators, each assuming responsibility for their component of the child's care; that is, the primary care provider may assume the coordination of the health care system, the school nurse the coordination of the services delivered in the school setting, and the social worker the coordination of social services (Committee on Children with Disabilities, 1999). Care coordination of children with complex health care needs has become more critical as managed care and capitation require coordinated, efficient, cost-effective, team-based approaches to care.

Primary care providers may assume the role of care coordinator for the child's health services. This role is not defined with specific tasks but is dynamic and determined by the needs of the child and family (see Chapter 7). Barriers to the provision of care coordination by primary care providers include lack of knowledge about the specific condition and available community resources, lack of communication between health care professionals and organizations, and the time required to perform care coordination, which is usually not reimbursable by private and public insurance plans (Committee on Children with Disabilities, 1999). Subspecialty providers or treatment teams may also assume this role in children with complex conditions, such as organ transplantation. The need for care coordination has been recognized as critical to ensure quality continuity care. The Institute of Medicine identified care coordination for people with chronic conditions as one of the 20 priority areas to improve health care quality and delivery (Adams & Corrigan, 2002).

In many instances, parents become the central care coordinator, becoming the "coordinator of the coordinators." Parents who are knowledgeable about their child's condition and the health care systems involved can become empowered to perform this role but should always feel they are partnered with concerned professionals. They should be assured that during

times of high intensity care coordination needs, such as during hospital discharge, a new diagnosis or complication, entrance into school, or transition to adulthood, additional care coordination will be available from the appropriate health professional (Committee on Children with Disabilities, 1999). Respectful partnerships between professional care coordinators and families are necessary. "At all times, care coordinators must remember that the families are the continuous influence in children's lives and respect the parents' roles, needs, and culture" (Lindeke et al, 2002, p. 294).

As the complexity of medical management increases with knowledge and technology and the health care financial system becomes overtaxed with health care costs, service efficiency and cost effectiveness will be central concerns. In the past, practitioners have been more likely to emphasize the quality of services and intensive care needs of clients, while administrators and funding sources often viewed service efficiency and cost effectiveness as more important (Weil & Karls, 1985). The term "case management" has assumed the connotation of "cost containment" whereas care coordination assumes a broader role for systems organization. Primary care providers functioning as care coordinators must learn to assess and document the effectiveness of the treatment programs used by their clients to support the continuation of these programs in this era of shrinking health care dollars and rising incidences of chronic conditions in children.

Level 6 care goes beyond direct health care services and management of services to the policies and political activism of child advocacy. Provision of quality health care services to individual children with special health care needs is critical and requires knowledgeable and skilled providers willing to take on the additional care requirements of these children. The barriers to optimal health for children with chronic conditions will not be altered, however, without significant changes in health care delivery systems, community awareness and acceptance of the special needs of such children, and legislative mandates for improved health care for all children.

Pediatric primary care providers must become leaders in child advocacy at the institutional, community, state, and federal level—especially during periods of financial competition for service priorities (Berman, 1998). The barriers to optimal health care identified earlier (i.e., poverty, lack of insurance, minority/immigrant status, fragmentation of care) will not be reduced without fundamental changes in society's awareness and recognition of the health care needs of children. Pediatric health care providers can become effective child advocates by getting involved in the governing structure of health care organizations to ensure that the needs of children are addressed, by conducting or participating in research to determine outcome measures of quality care, by performing community service as professional and community leaders, by getting involved in the legislative process to change laws or regulations affecting children's health care, and by becoming pediatric health care experts in development of policies governing pediatric health care (Berman, 1998).

Summary

Primary care providers working with children with complex needs must identify their role and the roles of other health care professionals working with the child and family and communicate this role to all concerned, including the family. If primary care providers plan to only intervene at levels 1 to 3, the family must be informed of this decision and an appropriate professional identified to provide level 4 and 5 care. Leaders in the care of children with special health care needs should aspire to level 6 care in order to have the greatest effect on these children.

If the chronic condition is medically complicated, uses complex technology, or requires prolonged use of resources housed in a tertiary care center, the primary subspecialist (i.e., often more than one subspecialist is working with a child) may be the appropriate professional to assume the leadership role in total health care management of the child. In this situation the subspecialist is required to consult with or refer to a pediatric primary practitioner for normal health care maintenance appropriate for the child. Many specialty clinics are now using advanced nurse practitioners knowledgeable in both the specialty area and primary care to help facilitate communication and care among the specialty clinic, the primary provider, and the family.

Most chronic conditions of childhood are not so complex that the primary care practitioner with additional knowledge about the chronic condition and its implications for primary care, as well as a commitment to effective communication, cannot assume a leadership role in health care management. In many managed care plans, this is a requirement of the primary care provider as a gatekeeper to additional services. Providers of pediatric health care have long embraced the philosophy that it encompasses much more than disease management (Green, 1994). Regionalized systems of care that link high-quality specialized health services with community-based primary care

services are needed to coordinate the special needs of children with chronic conditions (Perrin et al, 1994). The primary care provider must play a key role in establishing, organizing, and participating in these systems if they are to exist and provide the holistic, family-centered, health care maintenance needed to ensure the maximum health and potential of each child. Care—rather than cure—assumes greater meaning when working with children with chronic conditions, but there is much care in common with that needed by all children and their families.

The goal of health care maintenance for these children is to promote normal growth and development; to maximize the child's potential in all areas; to prevent or diminish the behavioral, social, and family dysfunction frequently accompanying a chronic condition; and to confine or minimize the biologic disorder and its sequelae (Committee on Children with Disabilities, 1993, 1998; Stein, 1997). The primary care provider who knows the child and family well, knows the resources of the community, and specializes in health care maintenance is most often the appropriate health care professional to assume leadership in the often complex care and care coordination of these children.

REFERENCES

Adams, K. & Corrigan, J.M. (Eds.). (2002). *Priority areas for national action. Transforming health care quality*. Washington, DC: The National Academies Press.

Aday, L.A. (1992). Health insurance and utilization of medical care for chronically ill children with special needs: health of our nation's children, United States, 1988. *Advanced Data from the Centers for Disease Control/National Center for Health Statistics, 215*, 1-8.

American Academy of Pediatrics. (2000). Insurance coverage of mental health and substance abuse services for children and adolescents: A consensus statement. *Pediatrics, 106*(4), 860-862.

American Psychiatric Association. (1999). *Issues affecting mental health coverage for children*. Washington, DC: American Psychiatric Association.

Barclay, L. (2003, February 4). Limited time for pediatric visits compromises care: A newsmaker interview with Peter Holbrook, MD. *Medscape: Medical News* [online] Available: http://www.medscape.com/viewarticle/448898.

Bauman, L.J., Drotar, D., Leventhal, J.M., Perrin, E.C., & Pless, I.B. (1997). A review of psychosocial interventions for children with chronic health conditions. *Pediatrics, 100*(2), 244-251.

Berman, S. (1997). A pediatric perspective on medical necessity. *Arch Pediatr Adolesc Medicine, 51*, 858-859.

Berman, S. (1998). Training pediatricians to become child advocates. *Pediatrics, 102*(3), 632-636.

Bethell, C.D., Read, D., Neff, J., Blumberg, S.J., Stein, R.E., et al. (2002a). Comparison of the children with special health care needs screener to the questionnaire for identifying children with chronic conditions-revised. *Ambul Pediatr, 2*(1), 49-57.

Bethell, C., Read, D., Stein, R.E.K., Blumberg, S.J., Wells, N., et al. (2002b). Identifying children with special health care needs: Development and evaluation of a short screening instrument. *Ambul Pediatr, 2*(1), 38-48.

Carraccio, C.L., Dettmer, K.S., duPont, M.L., & Sacchetti, A.D. (1998). Family member knowledge of children's medical problems: the need for universal application of an emergency data set. *Pediatrics, 102*(2), 367-370.

Centers for Disease Control and Prevention (CDC). (2002). Infant mortality statistics from the 2000 period linked birth/infant death data set. *National Vital Statistics Reports (NVSS), 50*(12), 1. [online]. Available: http://www.cdc.gov/nchs/data/nvsr/nvsr50_12.pdf.

Centers for Disease Control and Prevention (CDC), National Center for Health Statistics (NCHS). (2002, July 15). *HHS report shows more American children with health coverage. Progress reflects success of bi-partisan state children's health insurance program* [online]. Available: http://www.cdc.gov/nchs/releases/02news/release200207.htm.

Centers for Disease Control and Prevention (CDC), National Center for Health Statistics (NCHS). (2002, September 12). *HHS issues report showing dramatic improvements in America's health over past 50 years* [online]. Available: http://www.cdc.gov/nchs/releases/02news/hus02.htm.

Centers for Disease Control and Prevention (CDC), National Center for Health Statistics (NCHS), & Health Resources and Services Administration, Maternal and Child Health Bureau. (n.d.). *State and Local Area Integrated Telephone Survey (SLAITS) Survey of Children with Special Health Care Needs (CSHCN)*, [online]. Available: http://ftp.cdc.gov/pub/Health_Statistics/NCHS/slaits/other%20info/factsheet_cshcn.pdf.

Centers for Disease Control and Prevention (CDC), National Center for Health Statistics. (2003). *National health interview survey on disability* [online]. Available: http://childstats.gov/ac1999/spectxt.asp.

Center for the Future of Children. (1997). The David and Lucile Packard Foundation: Children and poverty. *Future Child, 7*(2).

The Child and Adolescent Health Measurement Initiative (CAHMI), & Foundation for Accountability (FACCT). (2000). *The children with special health care needs (CSHCN) Screener*. Portland, OR: Author.

ChildStats.gov. (n.d.). Children of at least one foreign-born parent. *America's Children 2002* [online]. Available: http://childstats.gov/ac2002/indicators.asp?IID=40&id=7.

ChildStats.gov. (n.d.). Child poverty and family income. *America's Children 2002* [online]. Available: http://childstats.gov/ac2002/indicators.asp?IID=14&id=3.

ChildStats.gov. (n.d.). Racial and ethnic composition. *America's Children 2002* [online]. Available: http://childstats.gov/ac2002/indicators.asp?IID=10&id=1.

ChildStats.gov. (n.d.). Table ECON1.A: Child poverty: Percentage of related children under age 18 living below selected poverty levels by age, family structure, race, and Hispanic origin, selected years 1980-2000 [online]. Available: http://childstats.gov/ac2002/tbl.asp?iid=14&id=3&indcode=ECON1A.

Child Trends DataBank. (n.d.) [online]. Available: http://www.childtrendsdatabank.org.

Clancy, C.M., & Andersen, E.M. (2002). Meeting the health care needs of persons with disabilities. *Milbank Q, 80*(2), 381-391.

Cohn, D. (2002, July 5). U.S. counts one in 12 children as disabled. Census reflects increase of handicapped youth. *The Washington Post*, B1(2).

Committee on Child Health Financing, American Academy of Pediatrics. (1998). Principles of child health care financing. *Pediatrics, 102*(4), 994-995.

Committee on Children with Disabilities, American Academy of Pediatrics. (1993). Pediatric services for infants and children with special health care needs, *Pediatrics, 92*(1), 163-165.

Committee on Children with Disabilities, American Academy of Pediatrics. (1998). Managed care and children with special health care needs: A subject review, *Pediatrics, 102*(3), 657-659.

Committee on Children with Disabilities, American Academy of Pediatrics. (1999). Care coordination: Integrating health and related systems of care for children with special health care needs. *Pediatrics, 104*(4), 978-981.

Committee on Children with Disabilities, & Committee on Psychosocial Aspects of Child and Family Health, American Academy of Pediatrics. (1993). Psychosocial risks of chronic health conditions in childhood and adolescence (RE9338). *Pediatrics, 92*(6), 876-878.

Committee on Pediatric Research, American Academy of Pediatrics. (2000). Race/ethnicity, gender, socioeconomic status—Research exploring their effects on child health: A subject review (RE9848). *Pediatrics, 105*(6), 1349-1351.

Committee on Psychosocial Aspects of Child and Family Health, American Academy of Pediatrics. (2001). The new morbidity revisited: A renewed commitment to the psychosocial aspects of pediatric care. *Pediatrics, 108*(5), 1227-1230.

Davidson, E.J., Silva, T.J., Sofis, L.A., Ganz, M.L., & Palfrey, J.S. (2002). The doctor's dilemma: Challenges for the primary care physician caring for the child with special health care needs. *Ambul Pediatr, 2*(3), 218-223.

Deal, L.W., Shiono, P.H., & Behrman, R.E. (1998). Children and managed health care: analysis and recommendations. *Future Child, 8*(2).

Doherty, W. & Baird, M.A. (1987). *Family centered medical care: a clinical casework*. New York: Guilford Press.

Dosa, N.P., Boeing, N.M., & Kanter, R.K. (2001). Excess risk of severe acute illness in children with chronic health conditions. *Pediatrics, 107*(3), 499-504.

Fix, M., & Passel, J.S. (2002). *The scope and impact of welfare reform's immigrant provisions*. Washington, DC: The Urban Institute [online]. Available: http://newfederalism.urban.org/pdf/discussion02-03.pdf.

Flores, G., Fuentes-Afflick, E., Barbot, O., Carter-Pokras, O., Claudio, L., et al. (2002a). The health of Latino children: Urgent priorities, unanswered questions, and a research agenda. *J Am Med Assoc, 288*(1), 82-90.

Flores, G., Rabke-Verani, J., Pine, W., & Sabharwal, A. (2002b). The importance of cultural and linguistic issues in the emergency care of children. *Pediatr Emerg Care, 18*(4), 271-284.

Fowler, E.J. & Anderson, G.F. (1996). Capitation adjustment for pediatric populations. *Pediatrics, 98*(1), 10-17.

Fujiura, G.T. (1999). The implications of emerging demographics: A commentary on the meaning of race and income inequity to disability policy. Paper presented at the Switzer Memorial Seminar, East Lansing, MI [online]. Available: http://www.mswitzer.org/sem99/papers/fujiura.html.

Fujiura, G.T., & Yamaki, K. (2000). Trends in demography of childhood poverty and disability. *Exceptional Children, 66*(2), 187-199.

Furth, S.L., Garg, P.P., Neu, A.M., Hwang, W., Fivush, B.A., et al. (2000). Racial differences in access to the kidney transplant waiting list for children and adolescents with end-stage renal disease. *Pediatrics, 106*(4), 756-761.

Gallaher, M.M., Christakis, D.A., & Connell, F.A. (2002). Health care use by children diagnosed as having developmental delay. *Arch Pediatr Adolesc Med, 156*, 246-251.

Green, M. (Ed.) (1994). *1994 Bright futures: national guidelines for health supervision of infants, children, and adolescent*. Arlington, VA: National Center for Education in Maternal and Child Health.

Guyer, B. & Ellers, B. (1990). Childhood injuries in the United States: mortality, morbidity, and cost. *J Dis Child, 144*(6), 649-652.

Guyer, B., MacDorman, M.F., Martin, J.A., Peters, K.D., & Strobino, D.M. (1998). Annual summary of vital statistics 1997. *Pediatrics, 102*(6), 1333-1349.

Hahn, B.A. (1995). Children's health: Racial and ethnic differences in the use of prescription medications. *Pediatrics, 95*(5), 727-732.

Halfon, N. & Hochstein, M. (1997). Developing a system of care for all: what the needs of vulnerable children tell us. In R. Stein (Ed.) *Health care for children: what's right, what's wrong, what's next*. New York: United Hospital Fund.

Halfon, N., Olson, L., Inkelas, M., Mistry, R., Sareen, H., et al. (2002, January-Final Draft). *Summary statistics from the National Survey of Early Childhood Health, 2000. National Survey of Early Childhood Health (NSECH)*. Washington, DC: U.S. Department of Health and Human Services, Centers for Disease Control and Prevention, National Center for Health Statistics [online]. Available: http://www.cdc.gov/nchs/data/slaits/summary_sech00.pdf.

The Henry J. Kaiser Family Foundation (2002, August 27). Capital Hill Watch: The uninsured will be the 'next great health debate,' congressional, business leaders say. *Kaiser Daily Health Policy Report* [online]. Available: http://www.kaisernetwork.org/daily_reports/rep_hpolicy_recent_rep.cfm?dr_cat=3&show=yes&dr_DateTime=08-27-02.

Institute of Medicine. (2002). *Unequal treatments confronting racial and ethnic disparities in health care*. Washington, DC: The National Academies Press.

Ireys, H.T., Anderson, G.F., Shaffer, T.J., & Neff, J.M. (1997). Expenditures for care of children with chronic illnesses enrolled in the Washington state Medicaid program fiscal year 1993. *Pediatrics, 100*(2), 197-204.

Ireys, H.T., Grason, H., & Gwyer, B. (1996). Assuring quality of care for children with special needs in managed care organization: roles for pediatricians. *Pediatrics, 98*, 178-185.

Ireys, H.T., Wehr, E., & Cooke, R.E. (1999). *Defining medical necessity. Strategies for promoting access to quality care for persons with developmental disabilities, mental retardation, and other special health care needs*. Arlington, VA: National Center for Education in Maternal and Child Health.

Jessop, D.J. & Stein, R.E. (1994). Providing comprehensive health care to children with chronic illness. *Pediatrics, 93*(4), 602-607.

Joseph, K.S., & Kramer, M.S. (1996). Review of the evidence on fetal and early childhood antecedents of adult chronic disease. *Epidemiol Rev, 18*(2), 158-174.

Kataoka, S.H., Zhang, L., & Wells, K.B. (2002). Unmet need for mental health care among U.S. children: Variation by ethnicity and insurance status. *Am J Psychiatry, 159*(9), 1548-1555.

Kelleher, K.J., McInerny, T.K., Gardner, W.B., Childs, G.E., & Wasserman, R.C. (2000). Increasing identification of psychosocial problems: 1979-1996. *Pediatrics, 105*, 1313-1321.

Keppel, K.G., Pearcy, J.N., & Wagener, D.K. (2002). Trends in racial and ethnic-specific rates for the health status indicators: United States, 1990-98. *Statistical Notes, 23*, 1-16 [online]. Available: http://www.cdc.gov/nchs/data/statnt/statnt23.pdf.

Kleiman, L. & Perloff, J.D. (1997). Recent trends in the health of U.S. children. In R. Stein (Ed.) *Health care for children: what's right, what's wrong, what's next.* New York: United Hospital Fund.

Lindeke, L.L., Leonard, B.J., Presler, B., & Garwick, A. (2002). Family-centered care coordination for children with special needs across multiple settings. *J Pediatr Health Care, 16*(6), 290-297.

Lukemeyer, A., Meyers, M.K., & Smeeding, T. (2000). Expensive children in poor families: Out-of-pocket expenditures for the care of disabled and chronically ill children in welfare families. *J Marriage Fam, 62*, 399-415.

MacDorman, M.F., Minino, A.M., Strobino, D.M., & Guyer, B. (2002). Annual summary of vital statistics — 2001. *Pediatrics, 110*(6), 1037-1052.

MacKenzie, E.J. (2000). Epidemiology of injuries: Current trends and future challenges. *Epidemiol Rev, 22*(1), 112-119.

Maternal and Child Health Bureau, Health Resources and Services Administration. (2001). *All aboard the 2010 express: A 10-year action plan to achieve community-based service systems for children and youth with special health care needs and their families.* Rockville, MD: MCHB, HRSA. [online]. Available: http://www.mchb.hrsa.gov/html/cshcn10plan.htm.

Mbogoni, M., & Me, A. (2002, February 18-20). *Revising the United Nations census recommendations on disability.* Paper prepared for the First meeting of the Washington Group on Disability Statistics, Washington, DC [online]. Available: http://www.cdc.gov/nchs/about/otheract/citygroup/products/me_mbogoni1.thm.

McConnochie, K.M., Roghmann, K.J., & Liptak, G.S. (1997). Socioeconomic variation in discretionary and mandatory hospitalization of infants: an ecological analysis. *Pediatrics, 99*(6), 774-784.

McManus, P. et al. (1996). *Strengthening partnerships between state programs for children with special health needs and managed care organizations.* Washington, DC: US Department of Health and Human Services, Public Health Service, Health Resources & Services Administration, Maternal and Child Health Bureau.

McNeil, J.M. (1997). *Current population reports: Americans with disabilities: 1994-1995.* Maryland: US Census Bureau.

McPherson, M., Arango, P., Fox, H., Lauver, C., McManus, M., et al. (1998). A new definition of children with special health care needs. *Pediatrics, 102*(1), 137-140.

Meckler, L. (2003, March 5). Uninsured population continues to expand. Slow economy, rising health costs blamed. *San Francisco Chronicle,* A4.

Meyers, M.K., Brady, H.E., & Seto, E.Y. (2000). *Expensive children in poor families: The intersection of childhood disabilities and welfare.* San Francisco, CA: Public Policy Institute of California [online]. Available: http://www.ppic.org/publications/PPIC140/index.html.

Miller, M.R., Forrest, C.B., & Kan, J.S. (2000). Parental preferences for primary and specialty care collaboration in the management of teenagers with congenital heart disease. *Pediatrics, 106*(2), 264-269.

Morales, L.S., Spritzer, K., Elliott, M., Hays, R.D., & Weech-Maldonado, R. (2001). Racial and ethnic differences in parents' assessments of pediatric care in Medicaid managed care. *Health Serv Res, 36*(3), 575-594.

Neff, J.M. & Anderson, G. (1995). Protecting children with chronic illness in a competitive market place. *JAMA, 274*(23), 1866-1869.

Newacheck, P.W., et.al. (1997). Children's access to health care: the role of social and economic factors. In R. Stein (Ed.) *Health care for children: what's right, what's wrong, what's next.* New York: United Hospital Fund.

Newacheck, P.W., Hughes, D.C., English, A., Fox, H.B., Perrin, J., & Halfon, N. (1995). The effect on children of curtailing Medicaid spending. *JAMA, 274*, 1468-1471.

Newacheck, P.W., Stein, R.E., Walker, D.K., Gortmaker, S.L., Kuhlthau, K., et al. (1996). Monitoring and evaluating managed care for children with chronic illness and disabilities. *Pediatrics, 98*(5), 952-958.

Newacheck, P.W. & Halfon, N. (1998). Prevalence and impact of disabling chronic conditions in childhood. *Am J Pub Health, 88*(4), 610-617.

Newacheck, P.W., Hughes, D.C., & Stoddard, J.J. (1996). Children's access to primary care: differences by race, income, and insurance status. *Pediatrics, 97*(1), 26-32.

Newacheck, P.W., Hughes, D.C., Hung, Y., Wong, S., & Stoddard, J.J. (2000). The unmet health needs of America's children. *Pediatrics, 105*(4), 989-997.

Newacheck, P.W., Hung, Y., Marchi, K.S., Hughes, D.C., Pitter, C., et al. (2001). The impact of managed care on children's access, satisfaction, use and quality of care. *Health Serv Res, 36*(2), 315-334.

Newacheck, P.W., Hung, Y., & Wright, K.K. (2002). Racial and ethnic disparities in access to care for children with special health care needs. *Ambul Pediatr, 2*(4), 247-254.

Newacheck, P.W., McManus, M.A., & Fox, H.B. (1991). Prevalence and impact of chronic illness among adolescents. *Am J Dis Child, 145*, 1367-1373.

Newacheck, P.W. & Taylor, W.R. (1992). Childhood chronic illness: prevalence, severity, and impact. *Am Public Health, 82*(3), 364-371.

Ni, H., & Cohen, R. (n.d.). *Trends in health insurance coverage by race/ethnicity among persons under 65 years of age: United States, 1997-2001* [online]. Available: http://www.cdc.gov/nchs/products/pubs/pubd/hestats/healthinsur.htm.

Northam, E.A. (1997). Psychosocial impact of chronic illness in children. *J Paediatr Child Health, 33*, 369-372.

O'Hare, W.P. (2001, June). *The child population: First data from the 2000 census* [online]. Available: http://www.aecf.org/kidscount/trends_children.pdf or http://www.ameristat.org.

Park, J., Turnbull, A.P., & Turnbull, H.R. (2002). Impacts of poverty on quality of life in families of children with disabilities. *Except Child, 68*(2), 151-170.

Pastor, P.N., Makuc, D.M., Reuben, C., & Xia, H. (2002). *Chartbook on trends in the health of Americans. Health, United States,* 2002. Hyattsville, MD: National Center for Health Statistics.

Perrin, J.M. (2002). Health services research for children with disabilities. *Milbank Q, 80*(2), 303-324.

Perrin, J.M., Kahn, R.S., Bloom, S.R., Davidson, S., Guyer, B., et al. (1994). Health care reform and the special needs of children, *Pediatrics, 93*(3), 504-506.

Procter, B.D. & Dalaker, J. (2002). *U.S. Census Bureau, Current Population Reports, P60-219, Poverty in the United States: 2001.* Washington, DC: Government Printing Office.

Skjaerven, R., Wilcox, A.J., & Lie, R.T. (1999). A population-based study of survival and childbearing among female subjects with birth defects and the risk of recurrence in their children. *N Engl J Med, 340*(14), 1057-1062.

Stein, R. (1997). *Health care for children: what's right, what's wrong, what's next.* New York: United Hospital Fund.

Stein, R.E. (1992). Chronic physical disorders. *Pediatr Review, 13*(6), 224-229.

Stein, R.E. & Silver, E.J. (2002). Comparing different definitions of chronic conditions in a national data set. *Ambul Pediatr, 2*(1), 63-70.

United Nations. (1998). Principles and recommendations for population and housing censuses, Revision 1. United Nations Publication, Sales No. E.98.XVII.8.

U.S. Census Bureau. (1997, December). Disabilities affect one-fifth of all Americans. Proportion could increase in coming decades. *Census Brief* (CENBR/97-5) [online]. Available: http://www.census.gov/prod/3/97pubs/cenbr975.pdf.

Valadka, S., Poenaru, D., & Dueck, A. (2000). Long-term disability after trauma in children. *J Pediatr Surg, 35*, 684-687.

van Dyck, P.C., McPherson, M., Strickland, B.B., Nesseler, K., Blumberg, S.J., et al. (2002). The national survey of children with special health care needs. *Ambul Pediatr, 2*(1), 29-37.

Vessey, J.A. (1999). Psychological comorbidity in children with chronic conditions. *Pediatr Nurs, 25*(2), 211-214.

Walker, W.A. (1998). A subspecialist's view of training and pediatric practice in the next millennium, Part I. *Pediatrics, 102*(3), 636-644.

Weil, M. & Karls, J. (1985). *Case management in human service practice.* San Francisco: Jossey-Bass.

Weinick, R.M., & Krauss, N.A. (2000). Racial/ethnic difference in children's access to care. *Am J Public Health, 90*(11), 1771-1774.

Wells, N., Krauss, M.W., Anderson, B., Gulley, S., Leiter, V., et al. (2000). *What do families say about health care for children with special health care needs? Your voice counts!! The Family Partners Project Report to Families.* Unpublished manuscript. Boston, MA: Family Voices at the Federation for Children with Special Health Care Needs.

Westbrook, L.E., Silver, E.J., & Stein, R.E. (1998). Implications for estimates of disability in children: A comparison of definitional components. *Pediatrics, 101*(6), 1025-1030.

Williams, D.R. (2002, November 1). *Closing the gap in health disparities.* Keynote address presented at the American Academy of Nursing, 2002

Annual Conference and Meeting, Naples, Florida, on Closing the Gap in Health Disparities: Creating an Action Agenda for Nursing.

Wood, B.P. (2002). Latinos: A neglected group of children (Commentary). *AAP Grand Rounds, 8*(4), 37-38.

Woodruff, T.J., Axelrad, D.A., Kyle, A.D., Nweke, O., & Miller, G.G. (2003). *America's children and the environment: Measures of contaminants, body burdens, and illness* (2nd Ed.) (EPA 240-R-03-001). Washington, DC: U.S. Environmental Protection Agency.

Zito, J.M., Safer, D.J., Riddle, M.A., Johnson, R.E., Speedie, S.M., et al. (1998). Prevalence variations in psychotropic treatment of children. *J Child Adolesc Psychopharmacol, 8*(2), 99-105.

2 Chronic Conditions and Child Development

Judith A. Vessey and Melissa Rumsey

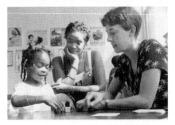

DEVELOPMENT does not exist in a vacuum; children's developmental domains are significantly influenced by their physiologic state, psychologic competence, and external environment (Hertzman, 1998). The presence of a chronic condition adds a dimension of developmental and behavioral risk (Patterson & Blum, 1996). Because children with chronic conditions are more similar than different (Gartstein et al, 1999; Stein & Silver, 1999), a noncategorical approach focusing on the commonalties of these children rather than just on the disease process will serve as the foundation for this chapter.

Children with chronic conditions may experience developmental lags in acquiring cognitive, communicative, motor, adaptive, and social skills compared with their unaffected peers. These maturational alterations may range from minor to all-encompassing and from transient to permanent. The presence of a chronic condition, while complicating the attainment of developmental tasks, does not necessarily connote the presence of a developmental disturbance or permanent disability. The development of many children with chronic conditions progresses without interruption.

The maturational alterations that accompany chronic conditions may be manifested within a single area of development (e.g., motor difficulty in a child with juvenile rheumatoid arthritis) or globally, affecting all developmental domains (e.g., those seen in a child with Down syndrome). Children whose developmental trajectory is delayed may advance through the normal sequence of milestones but at a rate slower than that of their peers of the same chronologic age. Such is the case of a child with an uncorrected congenital heart defect. Discrepancies in development across domains result from unevenly developed or damaged neurologic processes and result in disruptions in selected developmental sequences (e.g., a child with autism) (Reeve, 2001). The greater the severity of a condition, the more likely that the child will face global delays, with some domains being more affected than others.

Development is ongoing and the maturation of structures and functions interdependent. For example, an integrated nervous system is modeled through repeated use, such as is seen with the development of normal 20/20 vision or, in the absence of repeated use, amblyopia (Reeve, 2001). Numerous physiologic and psychologic variables can contribute to the occurrence and severity of maturational alterations associated with chronic conditions. For example, infants and mothers may have difficulty forming long-term emotional bonds with each other if they are physically, cognitively (e.g., brain damage), or emotionally (e.g., postpartum depression) separated from each other.

Characteristics of the Condition

The severity, pathophysiology, visibility, and prognosis of the condition, as well as any iatrogenic insults that may have occurred, influence a child's developmental outcome (Patterson & Blum, 1996).

Severity and Pathophysiology

The severity of the condition and numerous specific pathophysiologic mechanisms (e.g., chronic hypoxemia, aberrant serum glucose levels, or malabsorption) can alter development. The correlation between physiologic severity and developmental attainment is neither causal nor highly robust, with psychologic qualities and social supports serving as moderating variables (Wallander & Thompson, 1995). It appears that children in the least and most disabled groups are at greater risk than those at intermediate levels of severity (Northam, 1997).

The pathophysiologic changes that children with mild conditions experience lack sufficient severity or are ameliorated by treatment so they readily adapt to them, and thus the potential for developmental insult is minimized. When conditions are marked by only occasional exacerbations, have limited visibility, or appear to cause only marginal problems, they may be ignored or denied by children and their families (Joachim & Acorn, 2000; Patterson & Blum, 1996). This denial is often motivated by an effort to normalize the child's condition; yet when mild conditions are not recognized by others but do affect a child's performance, the child may be held to unrealistic expectations, such as frequently seen in children with attention deficit hyperactivity disorder (ADHD). Unfortunately, children may have poorer developmental outcomes when denial interferes with symptom recognition, ongoing management regimens, and appropriate expectations of behavior.

Children experiencing significant disability related to neurologic impairment or multisystem involvement are at significantly greater developmental risk because their condition physically, mentally, or psychologically limits or prohibits them from completing developmental tasks. The interaction of pathophysiologic changes, availability for learning, and contact with the environment further compromises developmental attainment.

Developmental sequelae secondary to prolonged disease states are also emerging. As research continues to advance health care technology, the mortality previously associated with many chronic conditions has been reduced. Usually, reductions in mortality initially result in escalating morbidity. The morbidity associated with survival of very low birth weight infants is an example (Malloy & Freeman, 2000; Petrini et al, 2002) (see Chapter 36).

Other developmental limitations are secondarily imposed by the condition's pathophysiology and management. Conditions that are painful, embarrassing, or energy depleting place a child at greater developmental risk (Patterson & Blum, 1996). Tremendous exertion may be necessary to cope with intensive treatment protocols or the time-consuming activities of daily life. For example, children with cystic fibrosis may spend more than 3 hours each day receiving pulmonary care. Additional energy is also required in adjusting to new or exacerbated symptoms (e.g., persistent pain, malaise, and/or fatigue). The activities of children who depend on technology are limited by physical constraints and the time needed to care for equipment such as ventilators and infusion pumps. Such expenditures of time and energy may limit children's opportunities to engage in recreational activities or predispose them to significant fatigue because participation requires too much effort. Moreover, in families where caregiving needs become the primary focus of daily living, parent-child interactions and other social activities are restricted.

Visibility

The visibility of a chronic condition may place the child at risk for stigmatization. Stigmatization is "a process in which a social meaning is attached to behaviours and individuals" (Joachim & Acorn, 2000, p. 244). Jones (as cited in Joachim & Acorn, 2000) lists six dimensions of stigma that can affect children's psychosocial development (Box 2-1). Visible conditions (e.g., Down syndrome, myelodysplasia [see Chapters 24 and 33]) place a child at risk for immediate stigmatization, and adults may discredit the child's other capabilities. For conditions that are invisible, such as inflammatory bowel disease (see Chapter 30), children may try to hide their condition but by trying to "pass" as normal create stress for fear of discovery. "Passing" may also require ignoring aspects of condition management, such as adolescents with diabetes or phenylketonuria (PKU) (see Chapters 23 and 35) who ignore dietary recommendations, thus impairing their health status. Choosing to disclose one's condition may promote stigmatization, as frequently occurs in children with human immunodeficiency virus/acquired immunodeficiency syndrome (HIV/AIDS)

(see Chapter 28). For children with deteriorating conditions, accidental disclosure is always a fear.

Prognosis

Maturational progression is superimposed on the natural course of the condition. In conditions associated with ongoing pathophysiologic deterioration, children may initially achieve milestones but lose them as the condition worsens. This is always noted when there is progressive degeneration of the neurologic system (e.g., as with muscular dystrophy), but this is also a problem with any seriously compromised physiologic state. Even in nonprogressive conditions, developmental lags become noticeable as children mature and developmental expectations are higher. In part, the ability to sustain development depends on effectively managing the effects of the disease and promoting the child's functional status and psychosocial adjustment.

The uncertainty associated with a condition's trajectory that parents and children face is a major stressor and may influence a child's developmental outcomes (Burke et al, 2000; Garwick et al, 2002; Stewart & Mishel, 2000). Children who have limited or uncertain futures or whose significant others (i.e., family, teachers) consider them to have a poor prognosis for reaching adulthood may be deprived of a past-present-future perspective of learning about one's cultural heritage or forming goals and personal aspirations. This longitudinal perspective plays an integral role in shaping cognitive processes. If individuals are misguided into thinking that such information is not worth transmitting or would be unduly upsetting, especially for children who recognize their potentially diminished longevity, this lack of information limits children's ability to learn. Children may also be held to differing behavioral expectations than their peers by sympathetic but misguided adults. Differing expectations can create anxiety in the child and resentment in siblings and peers.

Predicting prognoses is a risky business in light of rapid advances in medical science; nearly 90% of children with chronic conditions live into adulthood (Newacheck & Halfon, 1998). The life expectancies for children with cystic fibrosis, organ transplantation, cancer, HIV, and numerous other conditions continue to increase at dramatic rates. If a poor medical prognosis is communicated to the family without a broader perspective of the child's future, it may become a self-fulfilling prophecy, resulting in poorer psychologic outcomes as well.

Iatrogenic Insults

Selected treatment protocols impose their own risks (Northam, 1997). Developmental iatrogeny refers to health care interventions that hinder children from progressing through their normal developmental milestones. Therapeutic interventions commonly associated with developmental iatrogeny are the associations between aminoglycosides and hearing loss (Narla et al, 1998); cancer therapies, transplantation, and late effects (Ganz, 2001); and oxygen administration and retinopathy of prematurity (Clarkson, 2001). Numerous other interventions, however, directly or indirectly influence development. Many classes of drugs (e.g., anticonvulsants, steroids) have been shown to alter cognition, perceptual abilities, and/or

---

BOX 2-1	
Dimensions of Stigma	
Concealability	The degree to which the condition is hidden or visible
Course of the condition	The extent to which a condition changes over time
Strain	The effect of the condition's visibility and qualities on interpersonal relationships
Aesthetic qualities	The extent to which a condition affects a child's appearance
Cause of stigma	Whether the condition is congenital or acquired
Peril	Dangers associated with being affiliated with a stigmatized child

From Joachim, G. & Acorn, S. (2000). Stigma of visible and invisible chronic conditions, *J Adv Nurs* 32:243-248, 2000. Reprinted with permission.

behavior and make children less available for learning (Kutcher, 2002).

Characteristics of the Child

Each age-group gives rise to different sets of challenges for children with chronic conditions. The child's age at onset of a condition, however, affects progression from one stage of development to the next. Achieving a developmental task that has never been acquired is very different from regaining a skill mastered and then lost. Overall, children with congenital conditions have greater developmental plasticity and more readily adjust to condition-imposed limitations because greater adaptive mechanisms come into play (Weiss & Wagner, 1998); yet evidence suggests that the risk of behavioral difficulty associated with chronic conditions is inversely correlated with age (Frank et al, 1998), with younger children being at higher risk.

Infancy

The major developmental tasks of infancy include establishing trust and learning about the environment through sensorimotor exploration. For infants with congenital chronic conditions, these tasks may be difficult to accomplish. Parents who are mourning the loss of their perfect child have little energy to care for their infants whose needs may be complex and demanding. If parents find little gratification in trying to meet their child's basic needs despite their best efforts, they may begin to view their child as vulnerable because of the extensive care required, and this attitude can affect future development. A poor prognosis may lead some parents to emotionally divorce themselves from their infants in an effort to insulate themselves from further emotional hurt. Infants subjected to prolonged or frequent hospitalizations may encounter repeated separations, the unpredictability associated with numerous caregivers, potentially unreliable or inadequate care, and painful experiences. All these factors can inhibit attachment and the subsequent development of a trusting relationship. For infants whose conditions are physically limiting or painful, exploration and interaction with their environment are limited, further curtailing development.

Toddlerhood

The major developmental tasks of toddlerhood include acquiring a sense of autonomy, developing self-control, and forming symbolic representation through the acquisition of language. If a child's chronic condition requires careful limit setting and control of activities of daily living, independence in tasks such as toileting, feeding, or acquiring larger social networks may not be encouraged. For example, toddlers who are immunosuppressed need to be restricted in their social contacts and play arenas. Mandatory prolonged dependency can make separation difficult and contribute to a fragile self-image. Developmental tasks that have just been mastered are often easily lost in toddlers experiencing acute exacerbations of disease—with or without hospitalization. This behavioral regression is a means of social and emotional adaptation whereby children revert to earlier, previously abandoned stages when they do not have the necessary psychic energy to maintain functioning at developmental levels already achieved (Freud, 1966). Behavioral

regression is exacerbated by psychic and physiologic stress associated with fear, separation, pain, and other symptomatology. Although regression can happen at any point along the developmental continuum, it is most commonly noted in this age-group.

Preschool Children

The primary developmental task for preschoolers is acquiring a sense of initiative to successfully meet the challenges of their ever-expanding world. Preschoolers with chronic conditions may not have the physical energy or motivation to design and perform such activities; therefore opportunities for learning about the environment, developing social relationships, and cultivating self-confidence and a sense of purpose are diminished. They may have difficulty forming a healthy self-concept, body image, and sexual identity, particularly if most of their body awareness is associated with disability and discomfort. The egocentricity and naive reasoning processes of preschoolers directly influence their understanding and interpretation of their condition. Although their understanding of illness and its relationship to morality is less enmeshed than previously thought (Kato et al, 1998), preschoolers still may think that their thoughts or behaviors cause their symptoms. Regardless, developing self-esteem and motivation to undertake new tasks may be compromised by their condition.

School-Aged Children

For school-aged children, increasing independence and mastery over their environment are important developmental landmarks. Such activities contribute to gaining social skills, developing a sense of accomplishment, learning to effectively cope with stress, and acquiring the skills that result in self-sufficiency. Functional limitations in self-care, communication, mobility, stamina, and learning hinder children with chronic conditions from successfully participating in school and extracurricular activities that help develop independence and mastery (Msall et al, 2003).

Parental and child perceptions of the impact of their condition affect a child's developing sense of self-worth and psychologic adjustment (Immelt, 2000). Enforced dependency—whether required by the treatment regimen or instituted by overprotective parents—creates additional social and emotional barriers between these children and their unaffected peers.

Children with a condition that is not highly visible may try to hide its existence until forced by circumstances to admit otherwise when they recognize that it distinguishes them from their peers, placing them at risk for stigmatization, ostracism, and/or bullying (Joachim & Acorn, 2000; Vessey et al, 2003). When provided with the necessary skills to be socially competent, including communicating condition-specific information to their peers, these youth will be able to build and sustain friendships and thwart bullying attempts. Failure to do so frequently results in withdrawal, anxiety and depression, and other risks to their psychosocial well-being.

Adolescence

Adolescence is the transitional period from childhood to adulthood where a primary developmental task of youth is to become increasingly independent of their parents. Adolescents need to begin to make decisions about future career and personal goals. For adolescents with chronic conditions, this requires expanding their networks for social support and assistance beyond their immediate family and friends to include help from an array of interdisciplinary services and professionals (Betz & Redcay, 2002). Adolescents are prone to two dangers in planning for the future: they may (1) overemphasize the potential barriers that accompany their condition and succumb to a sense of futility or despair or (2) deny realistic limitations and set themselves up for failure by holding unrealistic expectations. Chapter 9 more fully discusses these issues.

Adolescence is the time for assuming responsibility for care, but adolescents' relative inexperience and the complexity of care needs may preclude this from happening (Vessey & Miola, 1997). Parental support and peer support have a profound impact on the success of youth in making this transition (Kef, 2002). Christian et al (1999) identify three themes in the process of gaining self-responsibility. *Making it fit* refers to youth learning how to integrate condition management into their daily lives. *Ready and willing* reflects adolescents' acceptance of self-responsibility. *Having a safety net of friends* underscores the importance of supportive peers in condition management and assistance in case difficulties (e.g., insulin reaction) are encountered. When realistic expectations and meaningful social support are available, adolescents can learn from their choices and the natural consequences they experience (Reeve, 2001). For an adolescent who requires complex care or has a limited life expectancy, the developmental task of transitioning from parental care to self-care is more difficult to achieve and may go unmet.

Puberty, a time of rapid change and uncertainty for adolescents, may be more difficult for teens with chronic conditions. Delayed puberty accompanies many conditions, emphasizing the differences between affected and unaffected adolescents. Integrating limitations into a changing body image and self-concept amplifies these differences. This is a particularly difficult time to be viewed as different by one's peers, and some adolescents may withdraw from social activities and relationships that promote healthy psychosexual development (Bolyard, 2001; Cheng & Udry, 2002). Others may choose to engage in risky behaviors (e.g., smoking, unprotected sex) despite the potentially damaging effects to be accepted by peers (Britto et al, 1998). The exposure to sex education is generally consistent, but often insufficient, across youths with chronic conditions. Although pubertal development may be slower and social isolation more common, youths with disabilities are as interested in pursuing intimate sexual relationships and as sexually experienced as their counterparts (Berman et al, 1999; Cheng & Udry, 2002). Youths with disabilities also may be at higher risk for sexual exploitation.

Individualism

Despite great odds, many children have intrapsychic and interpersonal resources that allow them to conquer virtually any disability and excel in life. A child's individualism, or the rubric of those relatively stable behavioral attributes that underlie a child's behavior (i.e., temperament, motivation, resilience, locus of control, intellect, attitudinal qualities, interpersonal

skills), influences developmental attainment and adaptation to the child's condition (Frank et al, 1998; Meijer et al, 2002; Zeanah et al, 1997).

Children with chronic conditions display the same scope of individual differences and developmental assets as children without chronic conditions. Some behavioral traits, such as temperament, are inborn, and others, such as self-concept, develop over time. A child's individualism is influenced by social and other environmental factors, although there is little correlation between familial attitudes and practices and a child's psychosocial development.

A child's self-esteem is linked to fully mastering a variety of physical, intellectual, social, and emotional tasks during the appropriate developmental period. Failing such tasks does not bode well for physical or psychosocial health. Although children with chronic conditions are at a somewhat higher risk for developing a vulnerable personality, many are remarkably resilient and approach life's challenges with aplomb. Many learn to rapidly identify threats to their integrity, respond with justifiable anger to those who are prejudiced against them, and reject biased individuals as inferior. These children often work to simultaneously educate those around them, dispelling myths and inaccuracies that might interfere with their own developmental competence.

Co-morbidity is common in children with chronic conditions. Co-morbidity refers to the co-occurrence of two of more conditions, either within the same domain—chronic illnesses, developmental disabilities, or mental health problems—or across domains (Figure 2-1) (Vessey, 1999). Children with multiple chronic conditions are especially at increased risk for psychosocial problems, although condition severity alone does not affect a child's psychologic outcome. Factors known to place children at greater risk for psychologic co-morbidity are as follows: (1) poor self-esteem, (2) inappropriate or under-developed coping mechanisms, (3) a dysfunctional family, (4) familial or geographic isolation, and (5) poverty (Costello et al, 2001; Melnyk et al, 2001; Newacheck et al, 1998; Silver et al, 1999).

Although the information on the influence of gender and co-morbidity is meager, boys experiencing behavioral problems

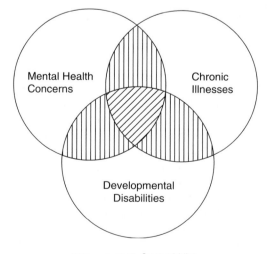

Figure 2-1 Co-morbidity.

tend toward externalizing disorders (e.g., conduct or oppositional disorders), and girls tend toward internalizing disorders (e.g., depression). Externalized disorders are more readily detected and diagnosed. Girls, however, tend to report more symptoms of distress (Wallander & Thompson, 1995).

The interrelationships of a child's positive self-esteem, perceived autonomy, easy temperament, internal locus of control, at least normal intelligence, adequate perceptual and communication skills, accurate cognitive appraisal of the condition, and coping skills in conjunction with environmental and family support all purport better adaptation (Meijer et al, 2002; Northam, 1997). When children are provided with the protective factors needed to balance out risk exposure, improved resilience and developmental attainment will result (Patterson & Blum, 1996; Rink & Tricker, 2003).

Role of Family and Social Networks

Healthy development depends on repeated, varied positive interactions between the growing child and the environment. Such reciprocity results in a spiral of mutually effective interactions. A child's family is the most important influence on development during early childhood (Wallander & Thompson, 1995). Most parents are tremendously resilient despite the demands of the child's condition and effectively balance their role in normative parenting with meeting specific demands of the condition. For a minority of parents, the converse is also true. Parental guilt, despair, or unfinished grief over the loss of the fantasied child may negatively affect a child's development. Other factors include maternal depression, "nerves," poor self-esteem, and a chronically stressful environment (Dadds et al, 1995; Thompson & Gustafson, 1996). Well-functioning families enhance their child's development, whereas those with discordant functioning curtail it (Patterson & Blum, 1996). Differences between children and families who successfully adapt are related to their coping abilities and access to needed resources (see Chapter 3).

Differing cultural orientation, social class, and economic status of the family influence development in children with chronic conditions (Sterling et al, 1997). As these orientations vary, so do the symbolic significance and semantic significance of the events, perceived origins, and potential consequences. Practitioners working with children from varied circumstances need to recognize the variations in intrafamily communication patterns, temporal orientation, religiousness, and the value placed on childhood because these are known to influence development (see Chapters 3 and 4).

As children mature, their environments and social networks naturally expand, and extended family members, teachers, friends, and acquaintances influence their developmental attainment. Informal and voluntary support appears to be the most critical. Individuals who offer practical, tangible support, provide intellectual stimulation, plan activities that help the child excel, and take pride in the child's accomplishments truly serve as the child's advocates. Unfortunately, some individuals have had few experiences with children with special needs and may overcompensate for or reject a child's limitations. For children whose conditions are associated with disfigurement, their development may be unwittingly at risk because of the reactions of others. Many uninformed individuals automatically assume that a physical handicap is associated with cognitive impairment. Children may be spoken of as if they are not present, or questions may be addressed to nearby family members or peers. The damage that can be done to a child's sense of self-worth is inestimable. The family can be helped to educate significant others about the child's strengths and limitations, mainstream their child into community activities, and use effective methods for working with insensitive individuals.

Developmental Perspectives of the Body, Illness, Medical Procedures, and Death

Children's perspectives about their bodies, illness, medical procedures, and death differ depending on age and experience. Early research investigating how children conceptualized topics used a developmental approach (Bibace & Walsh, 1981) and was influenced by cognitive stage theory. However, knowledge in these studies depends not only on cognitive level but also on a child's previous experiences (Crisp et al, 1996). Children with chronic conditions may develop expertise about selected topics within the range of their experiences and beyond that expected at their cognitive levels, but they may hold less sophisticated views about general concepts of anatomy, physiology, illness, procedures, and treatments. Children may use advanced terminology that could confuse others into thinking that their comprehension exceeds what is normally expected. For example, a 4-year-old stated that he was receiving "methotrexate intravenously" but thought his blood filled an empty body cavity because blood vessels were an unknown entity.

Children's self-concepts, interpersonal abilities, and therapeutic adherence to treatment regimens are related to the beliefs they hold. For those who perceive their chronic condition as totally negative and restricting, functional status, school performance, and psychosocial competence are more likely to be compromised. These perspectives need to be taken into account when children are taught about their condition and their help is enlisted in therapeutic adherence.

Understanding of the Body

Toddlers can point to various body parts, but by the preschool period, children have well-defined concepts of their external bodies and the relationships of its parts. Their understanding of anatomy and physiology, however, is primitive in keeping with experience, cognitive level, and perceptual abilities. By the early school years, children can name several internal body parts, with the heart, brain, bones, and blood being the most common. Children's descriptions of the parts and how they function tend to be global, undifferentiated, and laced with fantasy, although there is a great deal of variation among children about their specific ideas. Knowledge of the interrelationships of the parts and their functions is equally hazy. Physiologic processes are seen as a series of static states, with each organ having a singular, autonomous function. By middle to late grade school age, when children's causal reasoning and ability to differentiate mature, they begin to understand the complexities of anatomy and physiology. Levels of the body's organization are differentiated and hierarchically integrated with each other. Progressively more complex information about body functions, much of it from required academic classes, is incorporated throughout adolescence. Children with chronic conditions hold a slightly different—although not necessarily more sophisticated—view of their internal bodies than that of their unaffected peers. They may focus on the affected part of the body but do not identify fewer organs or organ systems (Schmidt, 2001; Vessey & O'Sullivan, 2000).

Understanding of Illness

If children are considered by their parents to be sick, their developing views and personalization of illness will significantly influence how they interpret their condition. As children mature and their view of illness evolves, primary care practitioners and significant others can assist them in developing positive images of their condition.

Infants are concerned about illness only as it directly interferes with their comfort and attachment to their parents. By toddlerhood, children begin to understand the concept of illness. For children with chronic conditions, this is usually interpreted by how the condition interferes with desired activities. Many condition-specific tasks (e.g., injections of insulin, wearing a seizure helmet) are particularly onerous for this age-group. As children mature, they form ideas and articulate their feelings about illness. Preschoolers' understanding of illness—although naive—is more sophisticated than once thought. A child's understanding of illness, however, is related to the difficulty of comprehending why things are happening to them (Kato et al, 1998). Relying on phenomenism (i.e., attributing illness to any external concrete phenomenon) or ascribing the causes of illness to another temporally occurring event is common. As children reach school age, their view of illness begins to reflect their evolving causal reasoning. Illness is initially perceived as occurring from contamination of or physical contact with the causal agent. Over time their understanding matures, and the cause of illness is believed to be external (e.g., germs that enter the body). With the development of formal operations in adolescents, illness causation is seen as a complex, multifaceted process. Biologic and physiologic explanations initially emerge as the basis for illness and later evolve into psychophysiologic explanations. The relationship of behavior and emotion to illness is usually acknowledged during adolescence.

Understanding of Medical Procedures and Treatments

Children's understanding of medical procedures and treatments is intrinsically linked to their knowledge about their body and illness. Infants and young children have no specific initial understanding of procedures, which are only interpreted in light of how they intrude on personal comfort. By preschool age, children's comprehension of medical procedures is marked by magical thinking, transductive reasoning, and overgeneralization. The purpose of a procedure is independent of a child's health status, and little discrimination about its diagnostic or therapeutic purpose is made except by children who have undergone repetitive procedures. All procedures are designed to make them "better" or "sicker." Many associate treatment with punishment (Kato et al, 1998); and because preschoolers' understanding of body boundaries is not well developed,

virtually all invasive procedures are perceived as threats to their body integrity.

As children mature, their view of medical procedures evolves from overgeneralization to overdiscrimination and then to correct identification of their functions. Multistep procedures and their purposes can be understood by school-age children, who can classify and order variables. Information may be interpreted quite literally, however, and misunderstandings can occur if the content taught is not validated. Children of grade school age respect health care personnel and their hierarchic position, but expressions of affection are often ambivalent. Often intrigued with understanding medical procedures, children are usually pleased when asked to participate in their own care.

Adolescents can understand the efficacy of specific medical procedures and the relationships between procedures and their health status, although their sense of invincibility and desire for experimentation affect their decision making. Informed decisions about alternative treatments are possible. Adolescents view the health care provider's authority as extending only as far as their willingness to adhere to the therapeutic regimen. Although the need for therapeutic adherence is understood, treatments are not automatically affectively and behaviorally assimilated into an adolescent's daily activities.

Understanding of Death

Death is the ultimate experience of separation and loss for children and their families. Children's understanding of death is formed along a developmental progression and reflects their cognitive maturation (Karns, 2002). Infants do not comprehend death per se but react to phenomena (e.g., pain, separation) associated with death. By late toddlerhood and preschool age, children may talk freely about death but may describe its occurrence and attributes with magical thinking and an egocentric viewpoint. They may perceive their impending death as punishment yet do not view death as permanent but rather as "sleep" or departure from the family. The permanence of death is not realized until the grade school–age period, when the concepts of reversibility and irreversibility are learned. Children in this age-group tend to personify death as the bogeyman or some kind of monster. For children who are dying, this newly found knowledge can enhance their fears of the unknown. Adolescents, with their new metacognitive abilities, conceptualize death as a process of the life cycle, readily comprehending the emotional, social, and financial implications of the loss occurring from death for themselves and their families. Of all age-groups, adolescents have the most difficulty in dealing with death.

Children with chronic conditions are often subjected to many intrusive and painful experiences and may have experienced the death of friends in the hospital. These experiences often exacerbate their anxieties about death. Depending on individual experience, a child's understanding of death may not follow the projected trajectory. Although information about how affected children's views of death differ from their nonaffected peers is limited, it appears that the fears associated with death are remarkably similar to the fears of hospitalization and intrusive procedures. Even preschool-aged children may express fear of separation, despite the fact that death may not yet be conceptualized as irreversible.

For the dying child, how issues such as separation, mutilation, and loss of control are handled plays an important role in their personal conceptualization of death. Care must be taken to prevent unnecessary separation and help these children maintain their autonomy, sense of mastery, and other developmental skills whenever possible.

Primary Care Provider's Role in Promoting Development

Because a cure is not possible for many chronic conditions, practitioners must focus on care. The goal of care is to minimize the manifestations of the disease and maximize the child's physical, cognitive, and psychosocial potential. Realization of this goal is facilitated by appreciating the family's ecology and adopting a family-centered approach to care. Family-centered care recognizes that the family is the constant in the child's life and as such is vital to children successfully meeting their potential. Practicing family-centered care requires professionals to do the following: (1) recognize and respect a family's strengths and individuality, (2) promote a family's confidence and competence in caring for the child, and (3) empower a family to advocate for their child when working with the health care system. A noncategorical approach, incorporated with specific strategies for disease management and mitigating functional limitations (Msall et al, 2003), provides a nexus on which to base assessments and develop holistic management plans. A good maxim to follow is to generalize developmental information across diagnostic groups and then individualize it for each child and family (Stein & Jessop, 1989).

Assessment and Management

In today's climate of cost constraint, children are being discharged earlier—and often medically more fragile—than before. This places increased care demands on family members who may feel unprepared to handle these increased responsibilities. The primary care provider can assist during this transition.

Maturational alterations are rarely immutable and should not be thought of as such. Children with chronic conditions require comprehensive care to achieve their optimal level of functioning. Therefore a developmental surveillance program must be established. Developmental surveillance is a broader approach than detection; it is comprehensive and continuous and contains the following components: (1) general and condition-specific screening, (2) child and parental observation, (3) identification of concerns, and (4) general primary care guidance (Gilbride, 1995). Although developmental surveillance falls under the primary care provider's purview, it can involve input from an interdisciplinary group of professionals. The composition of the group is dynamic and varies depending on the child's age, disability, level of impairment, familial involvement, and environmental resources. Coordination is critical to preventing omissions and duplications of services. Involvement of the primary care provider helps ensure consistency across the disciplines.

Ideally, children at risk for developmental lags and/or behavioral problems should be identified as soon as possible and observed closely (Committee on Children with Disabilities, 2001a). Primary care providers should anticipate and, whenever possible, vigorously intervene before significant aberrations occur. This is best accomplished by identifying and initiating treatment in the preclinical period when slight indications of developmental impairment may be detected but gross manifestations are not yet evident. A "wait and see" attitude is never warranted because these children are at developmental risk. Early intervention may prevent or ameliorate many secondary problems or those resulting from neglect or mistreatment of the original condition. Although a child may experience hearing loss from aminoglycosides, for example, subsequent language and cognitive delays may be prevented with aggressive intervention. Because a chronic condition generally persists throughout a child's life, ongoing surveillance of physical development and psychosocial adjustment is helpful.

Assessment of the child's physical development normally consists of evaluating basic indicators of health, including growth measures and vital signs, performing a comprehensive physical examination, and noting any changes in the status of the chronic condition. Additional dimensions of assessment should include screening specific developmental domains (e.g., language, perceptual motor skills), rating the child's functional status, and directed questioning designed to elicit specific parental concerns (Bosch, 2002; Glascoe, 1997, 1999). An evaluation of functional status provides information about the child's ability to engage in the activities of daily living that heavily influence developmental outcomes. Expressed parental concerns are highly correlated to developmental differences of their children and identify areas that need further evaluation (Glascoe, 1999).

Although the tendency may be to focus attention on the child's physical status, assessing the child's psychosocial adjustment is of critical importance. Not all the psychosocial stresses experienced by children with chronic conditions are caused by their condition, nor do only affected children experience stress. These children, however, are at increased risk of psychologic difficulties, many of which can be attributed to the child's condition (Wallander & Thompson, 1995). It is estimated that two to three times as many children with chronic conditions have behavioral problems as their nonaffected peers. Moreover, over one third of these children also have school-related problems, only one half of which are directly related to their condition.

Assessment has traditionally focused on identifying how children with chronic conditions differ from their nonaffected peers. This information is useful in developing an explanatory theory about the effects of chronic conditions but does little to help an individual child. Evaluating if a child is effectively coping with the condition and adjusting to school, peer groups, and the like provides guidelines on which interventions can be based.

Standardized assessment instruments are useful, necessary adjuncts to a complete history and physical examination for a comprehensive developmental evaluation. When used at regular intervals, these instruments provide objective data so that small developmental changes can be detected. Considering the ever-growing number of children with special needs being cared for in the community, primary care practitioners need to have a compendium of readily administered standardized instruments from which to draw (Table 2-1). They also should not rely only

Text continued on p. 36

TABLE 2-1

Instruments Used in Developmental Assessment

Types of Screening Tools	Test/Score	Age Level	Method	Comments
General development	Alberta Infant Motor Scale *Authors:* M Piper, J Darrah, L Pinnell, T Maguire, P Byrne *Source:* Piper MC, Darrah J: Motor assessment of the developing infant, Philadelphia, 1993, WB Saunders.	Birth-18 mo	Observation	*General Information* Measures gross motor developmental milestones Assesses postural control in supine, prone, and sitting positions *Time Required:* varies*
	Battelle Developmental Inventory (BDI) (1984) *Authors:* J Newborg, J Stock, L Wnek, J Guidubaldi, J Svinicki *Source:* Riverside Publishing Co, 8420 Bryn Mawr Ave, Chicago, IL 60631	Birth-8 yr	Structured test format Parent and teacher interview Observation	*General Information* Includes a screening test that can be used to identify areas of development in need of a complete comprehensive BDI Full BDI consists of 341 test items in five domains: personal-social, adaptive, motor, communication, and cognitive Screening test consists of 96 items taking 20-35 min to administer *Time Required:* 1-1½ hr to administer*
	Bayley Scales of Infant Development, ed 2 (1993) *Author:* N Bayley *Source:* The Psychological Corporation, Harcourt, Brace, Jovanovich, Inc, 6277 Sea Harbor Dr, Orlando, FL 32887 *Phone:* 1-800-211-8378 *Web site:* www.psychcorp.com	1-42 mo	Observation/ demonstration	*General Information* Evaluates motor, mental, and social behavior of infants and toddlers Diagnoses normal vs. delayed development New scoring procedures allow examiners to determine a child's developmental age equivalent for each ability domain Requires a qualified practitioner to examine and evaluate an infant *Time Required:* <15 mo, 25-35 min; >15 mo, 60 min
	Bender Visual Motor Gestalt Test *Author:* L Bender *Source:* American Orthopsychiatric Association, Inc, Seventh Ave, 18th Floor, New York, NY 10001 *Phone:* 212-564-5930 *Web site:* www.amerortho.org	≥3 yr	Demonstration	*General Information* A drawing test for evaluating developmental problems, learning disabilities, retardation, psychosis, organic brain disorders in children Requires a qualified practitioner *Time Required:* 10-20 min to administer
	Brigance Diagnostic Inventory of Early Development (Revised) (1991) *Author:* A Brigance *Source:* Curriculum Associates, Inc, 5 Esquire Rd, North Billerica, MA 01862-2589 *Phone:* 978-667-8000 *Web site:* www. curriculumassociates.com	Birth-7 yr	Performance task by child	Assesses skills in all areas required for PL 101-476 eligibility Criterion and normative referenced, curriculum based May be administered by a paraprofessional with supervision *Time Required:* varies
	Developmental Profile II *Authos:* G Alpern, T Boll, M Shearer *Source:* Western Psychological Services, 12031 Wilshire Blvd, Los Angeles, CA 90025-1251	Birth-9½ yr	Parent or teacher report	*General Information* Screens children for delays in five domains: physical (motor and muscle development), self-help, social, academic, and communication Can be computer scored *Time Required:* 186 items take 20-40 min to administer
	The Early Screening Inventory (Revised) (1997) *Authors:* S Meisels, D Marsden, M Wiske, L Henderson *Source:* Rebus, Inc, PO Box 479, Ann Arbor, MI 48106 *Phone:* 1-800-435-3085 *Web site:* mail@rebusinc.com	3-6 yr	Observation	*General Information* Two separate tests: one for age 3-4½ yr, and one for 4½-6 yr Assesses visual-motor/adaptive skills, language cognition, and gross motor Also includes a parental checklist Must be administered by a trained professional *Time Required:* 15-20 min

*Can be administered by a professional or paraprofessional. Some special training required. Must understand testing procedures and develop rapport with children.

TABLE 2-1

Instruments Used in Developmental Assessment—cont'd

Types of Screening Tools	Test/Score	Age Level	Method	Comments
General development—cont'd	Hawaii Early Learning Profile (HELP) (1979) *Authors:* SF Furuno, KA O'Reilly, CM Hosaka, TT Inatsuka, TL Allman, B Zeisloft, S Parks *Source:* Vort Corporation, PO Box 60880, Palo Alto, CA 94306	Birth-36 mo	Observation and parent interview	*General Information* 685 developmental tasks used to assess six domains: cognition, language, gross motor, fine motor, social-emotional, and self-help Criterion referenced, curriculum based *Time Required:* Each domain takes 15-30 min to administer; domains may be selected for individual use
	Minnesota Infant Development Inventory (1988) Minnesota Early Child Development Inventory (1988) Minnesota Preschool Development Inventory (1984) *Authors:* H Ireton, E Thwing *Source:* Behavior Science Systems, PO Box 1108, Minneapolis, MN 55458	Birth-15 mo 1-3 yr 3-6 yr	Observation/interview Parent report True/false	*General Information* A first-level screening tool Measures the infant's development in five domains: gross motor, fine motor, language, comprehension, and personal-social Provides a profile of the child's strengths and weaknesses 60-80 items on each inventory *Time Required:* varies
	Movement Assessment of Infants *Authors:* LS Chandler, MW Swanson, MS Andrews *Source:* Infant Movement Research, PO Box 4631, Rolling Bay, WI 18060	Birth-12 mo	Observation	*General Information* Provides uniform approach to the evaluation of high-risk infants Assesses muscle tone, reflexes, automatic reactions, volitional movement Must be administered by a trained professional *Time Required:* varies
	Peabody Developmental Motor Scales, ed 2 *Authors:* M Folio, R Fewell *Source:* DLM Teaching Resources, One DLM Park, Allen, TX 75002	Birth-6 yr	Observation	*General Information* Assesses reflexes, stationary, locomotion, object manipulation, grasping, and visual-motor integration skills Must be administered by a trained professional *Time Required:* 20 min
	Rapid Developmental Screening Checklist *Authors:* Committee on Children with Handicaps, American Academy of Pediatrics *Source:* MJ Giannini, MD Director, Mental Retardation Institute, New York Medical College, Valhalla, NY 10595 Phone: 914-493-8215	1 mo-5 yr	Checklist	*General Information* Tests general developmental milestones and tasks *Time Required:* minimal time allotment
	Riley Motor Problems Inventory (RMPI) *Author:* GD Riley *Source:* Western Psychological, 12031 Wilshire Blvd, Los Angeles, CA 90025	≥4 yr	Performance tasks by the child	*General Information* Provides a quantified system for observation and measurement of neurologic signs that lead to problems in speech, language, learning, and behavior Needs to be administered by a qualified practitioner *Time Required:* varies
	Wheel Guide to Normal Milestones of Development *Author:* U Hayes *Source:* A Developmental Approach to Case Findings, ed 2, U.S. Dept of Health and Human Services, Superintendent of Documents, Washington, DC 20402 Phone: 202-690-6782 *Web site:* www.acf.dhhs.gov	1-3 yr	Observation	*General Information* Assesses basic reflexes and developmental milestones Reinforces the normal growth and development patterns of children *Time Required:* varies

Continued

TABLE 2-1

Instruments Used in Developmental Assessment—cont'd

Types of Screening Tools	Test/Score	Age Level	Method	Comments
Adaptive behavior	AAMR Adaptive Behavior Scale-School, ed 2; ABS-S:2 (1981-1993) *Authors:* N Lambert, K Nihira, H Leland *Source:* PRO-ED, Inc, 8700 Shoal Creek Blvd, Austin, TX 76758-6897 *Phone:* 512-451-3246 *Web site:* www.Proedinc.com	3-18 years	Performance tasks, observation, and parent report	*General Information* Used as a screening tool and for instructional planning Can be an indicator in assessing children whose adaptive behavior indicates possible mental retardation, learning difficulties, or emotional disturbances; provides 16 domain scores Previously called AAMD Adaptive Behavior Scale Software for scoring available *Time Required:* 15-30 min
	Vineland Adaptive Behavior Scales *Authors:* SS Sparrow, DA Balla, DV Cicchetti *Source:* American Guidance Services Inc, 4201 Woodland Road, Circle Pines, MN 55014-1796 *Phone:* 612-786-4343 *Web site:* www.agsnet.com	Birth-19 yr	Semistructured interview with caregiver observation	*General Information* Assesses adaptive behavior in four sectors: communication, daily living skills, socialization, and motor skills Can be used with mentally retarded and disabled individuals *Time Required:* 20-40 min to administer; 20-40 min for interview edition; 60-90 min for expanded edition
Temperament	Temperament Assessment Battery for Children (TABC) (1988) *Author:* RP Martin *Source:* Clinical Psychology Publishing Co, Inc, #4 Conant Square, Brandon, VT 05733	3-7 yr	Structured test format	*General Information* Measures basic personality-behavioral dimensions in the areas of activity, adaptability, approach/withdrawal, intensity, distractibility, persistence *Time Required:* 10-25 min to administer
	Carey and McDevitt Revised Temperament Questionnaire: Toddler Temperament Scale *Authors:* W Fullard, SC McDevitt, WB Carey *Source:* W Fullard, PhD, Dept of Educational Psychology, Temple University, Philadelphia, PA 19122 *Phone:* 215-204-8087	1-3 yr	Interview	*General Information* Provides an objective measure of the child's temperament profile Fosters more effective interaction between parent and child 95 items, 6-point frequency scale *Time Required:* varies
	Carey and McDevitt Revised Temperament Questionnaire: Behavior Style Questionnaire *Authors:* SC McDevitt, WB Carey *Source:* SC McDevitt, PhD, Dev Profile II, Devereaux Center, 6436 E Sweetwater, Scottsdale, AZ 85254 *Phone:* 602-922-5440	3-7 yr	Interview	*General Information* Provides and objective measure of the child's temperament profile Fosters more effective interactions between parent and child *Time Required:* varies
	Early Infancy Temperament Questionnaire (EITQ) Revised Infant Temperament Questionnaire (RITQ) Toddler's Temperament Scale (TTS) Behavioural Style Questionnaire (BSQ) Middle Childhood Questionnaire (MCYQ) *Authors:* WB Carey, SC McDevitt *Source:* WB Carey, MD, 319 West Front St. Media, PA 19063 *Phone:* 610-543-0818	1-4 mo 4-11 mo 1-3 yr 3-7 yr 8-12 yr	Interview and parent report	*General Information* Provides an objective measure of the infant/child's temperament profile Fosters more effective interaction between parent and child *Time Required:* 20 min
Vision	Allen Picture Card Test of Visual Acuity *Author:* HF Allen *Source:* LADOCA Project and Publishing Foundation, E 51st Ave and Lincoln St, Denver, CO 80216 *Phone:* 303-295-6379	2½-6 yr	Observation	*General Information* Preschooler screening test for visual acuity Must teach child names of pictures before testing *Time Required:* varies
	Denver Eye Screening Test (DEST) (1973)	6 mo-6 yr	Observation	*General Information* Includes 3 different tests according to age

TABLE 2-1

Instruments Used in Developmental Assessment—cont'd

Types of Screening Tools	Test/Score	Age Level	Method	Comments
Vision—cont'd	*Authors:* WK Frankenberg, AD Goldstein, J Barker *Source:* LADOCA Project and Publishing Foundation, E 51st Ave and Lincoln St, Denver, CO 80216 *Phone:* 303-295-6379			Identifies children with acuity problems 6 mo-2½ yr—fixation test 2½-3 yr (preschool-age children unable to respond to the Snellen Illiterate E Test): do a picture card test—takes 5 min 3-6 yr—Snellen Illiterate E Test *Time Required:* 6 mo-3 yr—5 min; 3-6 yr—10 min
	HOTV (matching symbol test) *Author:* O Lippmann *Source:* Wilson Ophthalmic Corp, PO Box 49, Mustang, OK 73064 *Phone:* 405-376-9114	≥2½ yr or when the child can identify shapes	Flashcards	*General Information* Good for young children or those who do not like to verbalize Children name the four letters *H, O, T,* and *V* on a chart for testing at 10-20 ft and match them to a demonstration card Avoids the problem with image reversal and eye-hand coordination that can occur with the letter E *Time Required:* varies
	Picture Card Test (adaptation of the Preschool Vision Test) *Author:* HF Allen *Source:* LADOCA Project and Publishing Foundation, E 51st Ave and Lincoln St, Denver, CO 80216 *Phone:* 303-295-6379	≥2½ yr	Interview—"name the picture"	*General Information* Identifies children with acuity problems *Time Required:* 10 min
	Snellen Illiterate E Test *Author:* H Snellen *Source:* National Society for Blindness; American Association of Ophthalmology, 1100 17th St NW, Washington, DC 20036	≥3 yr	Observation using two persons as a team in screening	*General Information* Intended as a screening measure for central acuity of preschool-aged children and other children who have not learned to read *Time Required:* varies
Speech and language	The Bzoch-League Receptive Expressive Emergent Language Scale (REEL) *Authors:* KR Bzoch, R League *Source:* University Park Press, 360 N Charles St, Baltimore, MD 21201	Birth-3 yr	Paper-pencil inventory; parent interview	*General Information* Identifies children needing further follow-up in language *Time Required:* 15-20 min to administer
	Denver Articulation Screening Exam (DASE) (1971-1973) *Authors:* AF Drumwright, WK Frankenberg *Source:* Denver Developmental Materials, Inc, PO Box 6919, Denver, CO 80206-0919 *Phone:* 303-355-4777	2½-7 yr	Observation	*General Information* Designed to identify significant developmental delay in the acquisition of speech sounds Good for screening children who may be economically disadvantaged and have a potential speech problem with articulation or pronunciation Administered by a qualified professional or a non-professional with special training *Time Required:* 5-15 min to administer
	Early Language Milestone Scale, ed 2 (ELM Scale-2) *Source:* Education Corporation, PO Box 721, Tulsa, OK 74101	Birth-36 mo	Interview/observation	*General Information* Screening instrument for auditory expressive, auditory receptive, and visual components of language 43 items arranged in 3 divisions: expressive, receptive, and visual components of language *Time Required:* 1-10 min
	McCarthur Communicative Development Inventory *Authors:* L Fenson, PS Dale, D Thal, E Bates, JP Harding, S Pethick, JS Reily	8-30 mo and older developmentally delayed children	Parent report measuring vocabulary development	*General Information* Measures vocabulary development (words and sentences) in children with and without developmental delays Includes an extensive vocabulary checklist

Continued

TABLE 2-1

Instruments Used in Developmental Assessment—cont'd

Types of Screening Tools	Test/Score	Age Level	Method	Comments
Speech and language—cont'd	*Source:* Singular Publishing Group Inc, San Diego, CA			containing words that children typically produce in the second and third years of life; parents are asked to review and check all words that their child can spontaneously produce Must be administered by a speech therapist or pathologist, physician, or nurse *Time Required:* varies
	Peabody Picture Vocabulary Test, Revised (PPVT-R) (1981) *Authors:* LM Dunn, LM Dunn *Source:* American Guidance Service, 4201 Woodland Rd, Circle Pine, MN 55014-1796 *Phone:* 612-786-4343 *Web site:* www.agsnet.com	2½-40 yr	Individual "point to" response test	*General Information* IQ used to assess receptive vocabulary; not a measure of speech and language skills Measures hearing vocabulary for standard American English Used with non-English-speaking students to screen for mental retardation or giftedness Requires a qualified practitioner to administer *Time Required:* 10-20 min to administer
	Riley Articulation and Language Test, Revised (RALT-R) *Author:* GD Riley *Source:* Western Psychological, 12031 Wilshire Blvd, Los Angeles, CA 90025	≥4 yr (kindergarten-grade 2)	Performance tasks by the child	*General Information* 2- to 3-min screening test that identifies children in need of speech therapy Uses 3 subjects: language proficiency and intelligibility, articulation function, and language function Provides a quantified system for observing and measuring neurologic signs leading to problems in speech, language, learning, and behavior Must be administered by a qualified clinician *Time Required:* 3 min
Hearing	Noise Stik *Author:* LH Eckstein *Source:* Eckstein Bros, Inc, 4807 W 118th Pl, Hawthorne, CA 90250 *Phone:* 310-772-6113	Birth-3 yr	Behavioral response to auditory stimulation	*General Information* Hand-held free-field screener for early detection of infant hearing loss *Time Required:* varies
Child behavior and cognition	Kaufman Brief Intelligence Test (K-BIT) (1990) *Authors:* AS Kaufman, NL Kaufman *Source:* American Guidance Service, 4201 Woodlawn Rd, Circle Pines, MN 55014-1796 *Phone:* 612-786-4343 *Web site:* www.agsnet.com	4-90 yr	Structured test format	*General Information* Quick measure of verbal and nonverbal intelligence may not be substituted for comprehensive measure of intelligence Assesses expressive vocabulary, definitions, matrices *Time Required:* 15-30 min to administer
	Brazelton Neonatal Behavioral Assessment Scale *Author:* TB Brazelton *Source:* JB Lippincott, 227 Washington Square, Philadelphia, PA 19106-3780 *Phone:* 215-238-4200	3 days-4 wks		*General Information* Used as a predictive tool in clinical practice and research for behavioral and neurologic assessment Tests 28 behavioral, 18 reflexive items in the areas of habituation, orientation, motor maturity, variation, self-quieting, and social Requires a trained examiner *Time Required:* 20-30 min
	Child Behavior Checklist *Author:* TM Achenbach *Source:* Center for Children, Youth, and Families, University of Vermont, 1 S Prospect St. Burlington, VT 05401	4-18 yr	Observation/interview	*General Information* Provides an overview of the child's behavior Parent and teacher forms available *Time Required:* administrative form—15 min; scoring—3 min via computer, 20 min by hand

TABLE 2-1

Instruments Used in Developmental Assessment—cont'd

Types of Screening Tools	Test/Score	Age Level	Method	Comments
Child behavior and cognition—cont'd	Pediatric Symptom Checklist *Authors:* M Murphy, M Jellinek *Source:* Dr. Mike Jellinek, Child Psychology Service, Massachusetts General Hospital in Boston ACC725, Boston, MA 02114 *Phone:* 617-726-2724	6-18 yr	Completed by parent	*General Information* Used to screen for areas of weakness requiring more detailed diagnostic testing in scholastic achievement Parent-completed form A child self-report version Version for children 2- to 5 yr also available *Time Required:* 5 min to administer
	Peabody Individual Achievement Test: Revised (PIAT-R) (1970-1989) *Authors:* LM Dunn, FC Markwardt, Jr *Source:* American Guidance Service, 4201 Woodland Rd, Circle Pines, MN 55014-1796 *Phone:* 612-786-4343 *Web site:* www.agsnet.com	Kindergarten-grade 12	Interview and written test	*General Information* Content areas: general information, reading recognition, reading comprehension, math, spelling, and written expression Used to screen for areas of weakness requiring more detailed diagnostic testing in scholastic achievement Assesses reading recognition comprehension, total reading, mathematics, spelling, written expression Must be administered by a psychologist *Time Required:* 50-70 min to administer
	Riley Preschool Development Screening Inventory (RPDSI) *Author:* CMD Riley *Source:* Western Psychological, 12031 Wilshire Blvd, Los Angeles, CA 90025	3-5 yr	Observation	*General Information* For children who tend to have academic problems Used to screen for emotional, learning, and behavioral problems Requires a qualified clinician to administer *Time Required:* varies
	Wide Range Achievement Test (WRAT) 3 (1940-1993) *Author:* GS Wilkinson *Source:* Jastak Associates, Wide Range Inc, PO Box 3410, Wilmington, DE 19804-0250 *Phone:* 302-652-4990	5-75 yr	Paper-pencil subtests	*General Information* Used for education placement, vocational assessment, and job placement training Large print edition is available Measures the skills needed to learn reading, spelling, and arithmetic *Time Required:* 15-30 min to administer
Stress anxiety	State-Trait Anxiety Inventory for Children (STAIC) (1970-1973) *Authors:* CD Spielberg, CD Edwards, RE Lushene, J Montuori, D Platzek *Source:* Mind Garden, 1690 Woodside Rd, Redwood, CA 94061 *Phone:* 650-261-3500 *Web site:* www.mindgarden.com	Grades 4-6	Self-administered in groups or individually	*General Information* Measures anxiety in elementary school children Title on test is "How I Feel Questionnaire" *Time Required:* 20 min to administer
	State-Trait Anxiety Inventory (STAI) (1968-1984) *Authors:* CD Spielberg, RL Gorsuch, RE Lushene, PR Vagg, D Platzek *Source:* Mind Garden, 1690 Woodside Rd, Redwood, CA 94061 *Phone:* 650-261-3500 *Web site:* www.mindgarden.com	9-16 yr and adults	Group administration; test booklet available in Spanish and English	*General Information* Designed to assess anxiety as an emotional state (S-Anxiety) and individual differences in anxiety proneness as a personality trait (T-Anxiety) *Time Required:* 10-20 min to administer
Self-concept	Piers-Harris Children's Self-Concept Scale (The Way I Feel About Myself) (PHCSCS) (1969-1984), ed 2 *Authors:* EV Piers, DB Harris *Source:* Western Psychological Services, 12031 Wilshire Blvd, Los Angeles, CA 90025	7-18 yr	Descriptive statements used by groups or individual	*General Information* 80 questions requiring yes-no response Assesses a raw self-concept score plus cluster scores for 60 items 6 scales: behavioral adjustment, freedom from anxiety, intellectual and school status, happiness and satisfaction, physical appearance and attributes, popularity *Time Required:* 10-15 min

Continued

TABLE 2-1

Instruments Used in Developmental Assessment—cont'd

Types of Screening Tools	Test/Score	Age Level	Method	Comments
Family function	Feetham Family Functioning Survey (FFFS) (1982) *Authors:* S Feetham, S Humenick *Source:* Nursing Systems and Research Children's National Medical Center 111 Michigan Avenue NW Washington, DC 20010 *Phone:* 312-996-8008	Family	Self-reporting instrument	*General Information* 25 questions evaluating 6 areas of functioning: household tasks, child care, sexual and moral relations, interaction with family and friends, community involvement, sources of support Used for identifying specific areas of dysfunction in a stressed family *Time Required:* 10 min to administer
	Home Observation for Measurement of the Environment (HOME) (1984) *Authors:* R Bradley, B Caldwell *Source:* Center for Research on Teaching & Learning, University of Arkansas at Little Rock, 2801 S University Ave, Little Rock, AR 72204-1099 *Phone:* 501-569-8542	Birth-3 yr; 3-6 yr; Middle childhood (6-10 yr) Early adolescence (10-15 yr)	Interview and direct observation of the interaction between the caretaker and the child	*General Information* Two separate instruments designed to assess the quantity and quality of social, emotional, and cognitive support available to a child within the home The inventory for children at birth-3 yr contains 45 items; the inventory for 3- to 6-yr contains 55 items, the inventory for 6-10 yr contains 59 items; the inventory for 10-15 yr contains 40 items *Time Required:* each inventory takes about 1 hr

on basic developmental screening instruments that are designed to identify global delay rather than provide in-depth information on the type and severity of developmental problems. Focused instruments provide specific information that is useful as part of an in-depth evaluation.

Instruments should be carefully chosen and results thoroughly interpreted because most of these are norm referenced instead of criterion referenced. Other instruments and/or results are invalid if they measure one developmental construct based on performance in a different arena of development (e.g., the cognitive development of a child with a tracheostomy should not be assessed by an instrument requiring verbal responses). Timed tests may also bias results, particularly if a child has a motor or learning deficit. If a child tires easily, it is best to perform developmental assessments in short intervals so as not to obscure the child's true capabilities.

In general, children with chronic conditions who are at risk for developmental deviations but have no indications of problems should participate in developmental surveillance programs similar to those of their unaffected peers. For those children exhibiting warning signs of developmental problems, more frequent assessments are appropriate. If at-risk but non-symptomatic children are assessed too frequently, parents' perceptions may be altered so that they believe their child is unduly vulnerable, creating a self-fulfilling prophecy. Practitioners need to walk the fine line between errors of commission and those of omission when determining the frequency and intensity of assessment. The best defense is to place efforts on prevention rather than detection.

When untoward developmental manifestations are detected, the pediatric primary care provider can either provide treatment or, more likely, refer the child to subspecialists with expertise in the area of concern. Referrals should ideally be made to individuals who are parts of the specialty team or within the child's school setting, but additional local referrals may be necessary

if the specialty team is far away or school services are inadequate. Adding another layer of care providers requires exquisite coordination of services if the child is to receive appropriate care without overlaps, gaps, or too many demands to cause fatigue (see Chapter 7).

Obtaining services may require that the child's condition and associated problems be diagnostically labeled, although recent legislation has made this less common. Providing a label may help validate the concerns of children and families and direct future interventions and activities but must be done judiciously. Labeling often sets children apart from their peers and may result in different treatment by family members, teachers, and significant others. Diagnostic labels assigned in childhood follow children into adulthood and might prevent them from pursuing selected careers, joining the military, or being eligible for insurance. Although it is usually feasible to label specific disease entities, labeling associated with developmental manifestations should be done carefully. The ultimate long-term goal of care is for a child to reach and sustain optimal levels of functioning. Developing precise, measurable, short-term goals helps ensure that optimal functioning is obtained.

Fostering Psychosocial Health

Therapeutic intervention can improve the child's psychosocial well-being and prevent or mitigate the effects of psychologic co-morbidity. When a child's coping style is one to seek social support and have good social skills, he or she will likely have improved psychosocial functioning and be less likely to encounter developmental problems (Meijer et al, 2002). Health promotion includes fostering resilience in both children and their families. Fostering a good parent-child relationship is the gateway to promoting childhood resilience (Letourneau et al, 2001). Other strategies are listed in Box 2-2.

The role of schools should not be undervalued since they provide a measure of independence and opportunities for self-mastery and self-esteem building that are not readily achieved at home (see Chapter 5). Specialty camps help youth cope with their condition, improve self-care skills, and foster healthy self-esteem (Briery & Rabian, 1999; Thomas & Gaslin, 2001). Other extracurricular activities that showcase children's skills and encourage peer interaction are equally useful. Companion animals also help children adapt to their chronic condition (Spence & Kaiser, 2002). Suggestions for school reentry (see Chapter 5) can be adapted for returning to extracurricular activities as well.

Education

Primary care providers need to help prepare children in self-care behaviors and development of self-advocacy skills for dealing with the health care community. This is important for children and adolescents with chronic conditions because they are likely to use the health care system often throughout their lives. The transition between pediatric and adult care is a complex endeavor that is exacerbated by provider and system obstacles (Betz & Redcay, 2002) (see Chapter 9). Educating children and adolescents helps empower them to negotiate with the health care system effectively.

To accomplish the objectives of primary care, children must develop age-appropriate knowledge of anatomy, physiology, associated pathophysiology, and intricacies of the health care system. It is often incorrectly assumed that children are well versed about these topics because they know the jargon, appear comfortable with the health care environment, and have been diagnosed "for years." Accurate, developmentally appropriate information needs to be incorporated into the primary care of all children with chronic conditions since learning is more likely to occur in a nonthreatening environment where children are in a comparatively good state of health rather than when they are sick and/or hospitalized. A comprehensive plan managed by the primary care provider in conjunction with parents, subspecialty providers, and the school support services (see Chapter 8) will help ensure that this learning occurs. Teaching methods must be altered to fit the child's developmental age. Children will learn best when the material presented to them remains within one level above their current cognitive functioning.

A multisensory approach (i.e., one that brings all of the child's senses to bear on the learning task at hand) is more likely to be effective with preschool and school-aged children than more traditional lecture methods. Materials need to be selected according to their age appropriateness and accuracy of information. For example, anatomically correct rag dolls or models, doll hospitals, and play equipment are highly effective teaching aids to use with younger children. For older youths, an ever-expanding array of professionally developed audiovisual media (e.g., books, videos, interactive computer programs, Web sites) are available and are useful adjuncts to individualized teaching plans. The Starbright Foundation (see Resources), for example, is dedicated to developing and disseminating projects that empower children to deal with the medical and emotional challenges they face. Practitioners should examine all materials in advance to determine if the information presented will correspond to the child's experiences and treatment plan. There is little sense in providing cute but inaccurate information to a child, because these myths will just need to be dispelled when the child matures. This is of particular significance for younger children who have not developed causal reasoning, engage in fantasy, and tend to interpret their environment from a singular perspective.

Therapeutic Adherence

Promoting therapeutic adherence is a critical role of the primary care provider, especially in light of current health care trends shifting the onus of treatment responsibilities to the client. Therapeutic adherence is enhanced when youths actively participate in health care decisions; feel supported by parents, peers, and practitioners; and have the energy, motivation, and willpower to manage their treatment regimen (Kyngas & Rissanen, 2001). Practitioners who gradually involve children and adolescents in decisions about their care improve their therapeutic adherence and self-care abilities. Considering a child's individualism when determining treatment regimens can improve adherence. For example, a child who has a low activity level, is given appropriate autonomy, and adapts easily to new situations is more likely to comply with a regimen of bedrest and nutritional restrictions than a very active child who has difficulty adapting to new situations.

Assistive aids may help promote independence and therapeutic adherence. For example, beepers and watches with alarms help youths remember to take medications, and personal digital assistants (PDAs) can be used in dietary decision making. For youth with physical or emotional disabilities, companion animals help with long-term adaptation to their condition (Spence & Kaiser, 2002). Therapeutic adherence can be encouraged through open discussion and adoption of activities such as those listed in Box 2-3.

In evaluating therapeutic adherence, the clinician should seek information from both the child and parents and, when appropriate, other sources as well. Besides inquiring about the prescribed treatment plan, information regarding the use of complementary and alternative therapies needs to be sought (Committee on Children with Disabilities, 2001b), since families and/or youths frequently use these as adjunct or replacement measures. Evidence indicates that neither parents nor children are necessarily accurate in their reports, particularly as the child begins to move in social spheres exclusive of their parents

---

BOX 2-3

Promoting Therapeutic Adherence

Teach Children in a Developmentally Appropriate Manner About:
Anatomy and physiology
The pathophysiology of their condition
Medication and treatment effectiveness

Explore the Thoughts and Feelings of Children and Parents about the Treatment Plan.

Adjust the Treatment Plan to Fit within the Child's and Family's Lifestyle.

Suggest the Use of "Props" to Serve as Reminders:
Use wristwatch alarms for medication reminders.
Coordinate medications with mealtimes.
Use sticker charts or tokens with younger children.

(Burkhart et al, 2001). When nonadherence is an issue, determining the reason is critical before instituting any action. Nonadherence is usually not deliberate or consistent but due to misunderstanding the instructions, poor time management, forgetfulness, or other related behaviors. Some families with consistent but not deliberate nonadherence may be too disorganized to maintain a management plan. Smaller groups of children (and their parents) deliberately do not adhere to a treatment regimen because they believe it is inefficacious, fear side effects, find it too costly, or have similar reasons. Other families choose certain treatments as priorities and adhere to them while not adhering to others that they feel are of little value. Still others remain in denial as to the severity or ramifications of the condition. Interventions must specifically address the reason for nonadherence.

Advocacy

Many professionals are called on to care for the complex needs of children with chronic conditions. Although all have the same goal—to help the child reach maximum potential—conflicts may arise over the best approach for realizing it. Primary care providers are in the unique position to advocate for a child by identifying the range of treatment options and their implications, informing the child and family of available resources, and helping coordinate these interdisciplinary services (see Chapters 1 and 7). Advocacy extends to helping families acquire and maintain health insurance needed for receiving necessary services. This is especially critical in light of the changing service delivery and reimbursement patterns for chronic conditions (see Chapter 8).

Children with chronic conditions are at higher risk for severe acute illnesses, often potentially preventable and tangential to the condition (Dosa et al, 2001). They are also at higher risk for neglect or abuse from family members and others (Committee on Child Abuse and Neglect and Committee on Children with Disabilities, 2001). Clinicians can advocate for children's physiologic and psychologic safety by helping ensure ongoing assessments and instituting appropriate interventions. Providers should also help families prepare for emergency care of their child should it be necessary. Because children with chronic conditions may require different and complex services not usually needed by the typical child, the American Academy of Pediatrics (Committee on Pediatric Emergency Medicine, 1999) has published guidelines and an Emergency Information

Form (see Box 2-4 or www.aap.org/advocacy/blankform/pdf) to serve as the foundation for a child's plan of care in the event of an emergency. Condition-specific forms also are available at www.aap.org/advocacy/emergencyprep.htm.

Counseling. Because children with chronic conditions have a higher percentage of psychosocial problems, careful attention must be paid to the child's mental and emotional health (Pless et al, 1993). Growing up is difficult, and the incidence of violence, substance abuse, depression, suicide, and other risks continues to climb among all children. Children with chronic conditions—especially those with diminished self-esteem—may be particularly vulnerable, although research findings on this point remain controversial and unclear (Vessey, 1999). Proactive efforts to prevent mental health problems from occurring include the following: (1) encouraging normal life experiences, (2) improving coping and adaptive abilities, (3) helping children empower themselves, (4) expanding social support networks, (5) addressing parental identified needs, and (6) coordinating care (Committee on Children with Disabilities and Committee on Psychosocial Aspects of Child and Family Health, 1993; Perrin et al, 2000).

Despite the prevalence of mental health concerns among children, only 2% receive services from a mental health professional in a given year. The burden of identifying psychosocial problems falls on primary care providers. The longitudinal relationship that such individuals have with children and families is critical in helping to recognize that mental health problems might develop or may already exist. Unfortunately, the mental health problems of many children are overshadowed by the symptoms associated with their chronic condition and may go unrecognized and undiagnosed.

The first step for all pediatric providers is to recognize and appreciate the scope of psychologic co-morbidity in children with chronic conditions. Mental health problems may present as global behavioral or achievement problems or aberrant behaviors (e.g., psychosomatic complaints, extreme apprehension, deliberate therapeutic nonadherence, or dysfunctional communication) to family members and others. Adopting a healthy suspicion, conducting a careful health history, and providing an atmosphere for discussion will help identify children at risk. Research has shown that mental health concerns are missed if only the parents or the child is interviewed (Canning et al, 1992). Moreover, less than one half of parents will initiate discussions about psychosocial concerns, so it is important to explore this possibility in discussions with all family members. Standardized behavioral screening instruments also have low sensitivity with populations of children with chronic conditions (Canning & Kelleher, 1994).

If no problems are apparent, the focus is on primary prevention with a community-centered approach (Committee on Children with Disabilities and Committee on Psychosocial Aspects of Child and Family Health, 1993). Primary prevention programs are directed toward high-risk children without psychiatric diagnoses for whom measures can be undertaken to avoid onset of emotional disturbance or enhance mental health. Programs may be based on counseling, skills training, health education, discussion groups, or combinations of these and are designed to develop resilience and coping skills. Most of these approaches have been shown to be effective (Bauman et al,

BOX 2-4

Emergency Information Form for Children with Special Needs

American College of Emergency Physicians*	American Academy of Pediatrics		Date form completed By Whom	Revised Revised	Initials Initials

Name:		Birth date:		Nickname:
Home Address:		Home/Work Phone:		
Parent/Guardian:		Emergency Contact Names & Relationship:		
Signature/Consent*:				
Primary Language:		Phone Number(s):		

Physicians:

Primary care physician:	Emergency Phone:
	Fax:
Current specialty physician: Specialty:	Emergency Phone:
	Fax:
Current specialty physician: Specialty:	Emergency Phone:
	Fax:
Anticipated Primary ED:	Pharmacy:
Anticipated Tertiary Care Center:	

Diagnoses/Past Procedures/Physical Exam:

1.	Baseline physical findings:
2.	
3.	Baseline vital signs:
4.	
Synopsis:	
	Baseline neurological status:
Medications:	Significant baseline ancillary findings (lab, x-ray, ECG):
1.	
2.	
3.	
4.	Prostheses/Appliances/Advanced Technology Devices:
5.	
6.	

© American College of Emergency Physicians and American Academy of Pediatrics.
*Consent for release of this form to health care providers.

Continued

BOX 2-4

Emergency Information Form for Children with Special Needs—cont'd

Management Data:

Allergies: Medications/Foods to be avoided   **and why:**

1.

2.

3.

Procedures to be avoided   **and why:**

1.

2.

3.

Immunizations

Dates						Dates					
DPT						Hep B					
OPV						Varicella					
MMR						TB status					
HIB						Other					

Antibiotic prophylaxis: Indication: Medication and dose:

Common Presenting Problems/Findings With Specific Suggested Managements

Problem	Suggested Diagnostic Studies	Treatment Considerations

Comments on child, family, or other specific medical issues:

Physician/Provider Signature: **Print Name:**

LAST NAME:

1997). Referral may also be appropriate to help a child adapt to a new diagnosis or deteriorating prognosis; deal with school, family, and peer group issues; or clarify interpersonal and career goals, which are usually very private concerns for older children and adolescents.

Secondary prevention seeks to treat symptoms of emotional distress early to prevent long-term sequelae of mental illness. When problems exist, an accurate diagnosis in accordance with the *Diagnostic and Statistical Manual of Mental Disorders IV-TR* (American Psychiatric Association, 2000) is important. After the diagnosis is made, appropriate interventions must begin without delay. Individual or group counseling, judicious use of psychotropic medications, and/or referral to a mental health provider are appropriate measures. Unfortunately, the current insurance and health care delivery infrastructure, accompanied by family resistance to mental health intervention, is a significant barrier to the referral process. Moreover, seeking help while maintaining privacy may be difficult for

children and families if their mobility around the community is limited. Primary care providers can facilitate such help.

Hospitalization. Hospitalization is not uncommon with this population of children, and so care is usually transferred to the subspecialty team during this time. Pediatric primary care providers can assist in a smooth transition. In addition to giving information about the child's physical condition, parents must be encouraged to inform the subspecialty team of developmental stimulation programs or schooling that the child is receiving. If the hospitalization is planned, every effort should be made for hospital-based educators or tutors to confer with school officials before the child's admission so that schooling is not interrupted. Properly preparing the child and family—especially for new situations—also smooths the adjustment to hospitalization. Preparation must include procedural information about situations the child and family will encounter, definitions of medical jargon specific to the condition, and opportunities to process (i.e., through play, role playing, or discussion) new situations they may experience. For families who are nonassertive or overly aggressive, primary care providers can help to appropriately empower the child and family members for self-advocacy by working through these tasks.

Monitoring the child's adjustment to hospitalization and how it affects the child's future development is also an important part of advocacy. The individualism of the child and the severity of the condition affect adaptation to hospitalization. Hospitalization is an intrusion into the lives of many children with chronic conditions, but other children have positive memories of previous hospitalizations and may see the hospital as a safe environment. These children may perceive the staff as friends and are often relieved to have a temporary respite from the stress of school, the harassment of other children, or the demands of daily activities. Primary care providers need to recognize that children will occasionally try to become hospitalized to remove themselves from home or school situations that are particularly onerous, although this is uncommon.

Dying. Despite everyone's best efforts, some children will die. For children with a downward clinical course, early discussions of palliative care before all curative options are exhausted are appropriate (Committee on Bioethics and Committee on Hospital Care, 2000). Hospitalization and home care both have advantages and disadvantages, and the decision of which to pursue must be made in concert with the child's wishes and the family's capabilities. Although some parents and children may feel more secure being in the hospital and surrounded by professionals they trust, increasingly families are choosing for children to die at home, where they are in familiar surroundings, separation is minimized, care is individualized, and they are in greater control of their situation (Feudtner et al, 2002). Primary care providers can be instrumental in facilitating either option.

For families who choose for their child to die at home, primary care providers, as members of the larger interdisciplinary team, help in planning for a seamless transition from hospital to home and providing supportive/palliative care during this difficult time. Key responsibilities are to initiate intensive symptom management that alleviates the child's pain and suffering, facilitating the family's ability to provide this care, and arranging for necessary support services. Throughout, the primary care provider needs to be sensitive to the family's culture and spiritual belief system and rituals. Available hospice services may not have pediatric expertise, underscoring the importance of the pediatric primary care provider's contributions.

Children should participate in decision making to the fullest extent possible (Committee on Bioethics and Committee on Hospital Care, 2000). Primary care providers need to acknowledge that children frequently are aware of their impending death and help them communicate their wishes to their families and others. The psychosocial and emotional needs and fears of children need to be addressed from their cognitive level of development (Kane et al, 2000). Children must be reassured that they are not responsible for their illness and encouraged to talk about their feelings or express them through art or music therapy. Primary care providers can help family members with this by modeling ways to communicate these sensitive issues and offering insights on how children's developmental levels

affect their ability to conceptualize death. Children's questions are often upsetting to parents, such as when a 6-year-old requests detailed information about death rituals or a preschooler asks, "Who will read me stories after I die?" Many children are deeply spiritual, and their faith should not be left unexplored or unattended (Kane et al, 2000). Helping family members and other significant individuals communicate effectively with the child and each other makes death easier to bear. The child's death does not conclude the primary care provider's responsibility since parents and siblings benefit from additional empathetic support in the following months.

Summary

Children with chronic conditions are at a higher risk for negative developmental sequelae than their nonaffected peers. The severity of the condition, the child's individual traits, family functioning, and the available network of social supports all influence the child's developmental outcomes. Comprehensive prospective care often can eliminate or significantly ameliorate negative outcomes. Careful assessment using an interdisciplinary, integrated approach helps identify potential or emerging problems associated with the child's disease progression, functional status, social interactions, or global development. Individualized intervention strategies—including therapeutic management, education, counseling, and advocacy—can then be designed and implemented to help children with chronic conditions reach their developmental potential.

RESOURCES

Family Voices
3411 Candelaria NE, Suite M
Albuquerque, NM 87107
888-835-5669
505-872-4780 (fax)
www.familyvoices.org

Starbright Foundation
1850 Sawtelle Blvd, Suite 450
Los Angeles, CA 90025
800-315-2580
310-479-1235 (fax)
www.starbright.org

REFERENCES

American Psychiatric Association. (2000). *Diagnostic and statistical manual of mental disorder. DSM-IV-TR.* Washington DC: The Association.

Bauman, L.J., Drotar, D., Leventhal, J.M., Perrin, E.C., & Pless, I.B. (1997). A review of psychosocial interventions for children with chronic health conditions. *Pediatrics, 100,* 244-251.

Berman, H., Harris, D., Enright, R., Gilpin, M., Cathers, T., et al. (1999). Sexuality and the adolescent with a physical disability: Understandings and misunderstandings. *Issues Compr Pediatr Nurs, 22,* 183-196.

Betz, C.L. & Redcay, G. (2002). Lessons learned from providing transition services to adolescents with special health care needs. *Issues Compr Pediatr Nurs, 25,* 129-149.

Bibace, R. & Walsh M. (Eds). (1981). *New directions for child development: children's conceptions of health, illness, and bodily functions.* San Francisco: Jossey-Bass.

Bolyard, D.R. (2001). Sexuality and cystic fibrosis. *MCN, 26,* 39-41.

Bosch, J.J. (2002). Use of directed history and behavioral indicators in the assessment of the child with a developmental disability. *Pediatr Health Care, 16,* 170-179.

Briery, B.G. & Rabian, B. (1999). Psychosocial changes associated with participation in a pediatric summer camp. *J Pediatr Psychol, 24*, 183-190.

Britto, M.T., Garrett, J.M., Dugliss, M.A., Daeschner, C.W. Jr., Johnson, C.A., et al. (1998). Risky behavior in teens with cystic fibrosis or sickle cell disease: a multicenter study. *Pediatrics, 101*, 250-256.

Burke, S.O., Kauffmann, E., LaSalle, J., Harrison, M.B., & Wong, C. (2000). Parents' perceptions of chronic illness trajectories. *Can J Nurs Res, 32*, 19-36.

Burkhart, P.V., Dunbar-Jacob, J.M., & Rohay, J.M. (2001). Accuracy of children's self-reported adherence to treatment. *J Nurs Scholarsh, 33*, 27-32.

Canning, E.H. & Kelleher, K. (1994). Performance of screening tools for mental health problems in chronically ill children. *Arch Pediatr Adolesc Med, 148*, 272-278.

Canning, E.H., Hanser, S.B., Shade, K.A., & Boyce, W.T. (1992). Mental disorders in chronically ill children: parent-child discrepancy and physician identification. *Pediatrics, 90*, 692-696

Cheng, M.M. & Udry, J.R. (2002). Sexual behaviors of physically disabled adolescents in the United States. *J Adolesc Health, 31*, 48-58.

Christian, B.J., D'Auria, J.P., & Fox, L.C. (1999). Gaining freedom: Self-responsibility in adolescents with diabetes. *Pediatrics, 25*, 255-260, 266.

Clarkson, L.J. (2001). Retinopathy of prematurity: part I. A fresh look at its cause. *Journal of Neonatal Nursing, 7*, 186-189.

Committee on Bioethics and Committee on Hospital Care. (2000). Palliative care for children. *Pediatrics, 106*, 351-172.

Committee on Child Abuse and Neglect and Committee on Children with Disabilities. (2001). Assessment of maltreatment of children with disabilities. *Pediatrics, 108*, 508-512.

Committee on Children with Disabilities. (2001a). Developmental surveillance and screening of infants and young children. *Pediatrics, 108*, 192-196.

Committee on Children with Disabilities. (2001b). Counseling families who choose complementary and alternative medicine for their child with chronic illness or disability. *Pediatrics, 107*, 598-601.

Committee on Children with Disabilities and Committee on Psychosocial Aspects of Child and Family Health. (1993). Psychosocial risks of chronic health conditions in childhood and adolescence. *Pediatrics, 92*, 876-877.

Committee on Emergency Medicine. (1999). Emergency preparedness of children with special health care needs. *Pediatrics, 104*, e53.

Costello, E.J., Keeler, G.P., & Angold, A. (2001). Poverty, race/ethnicity, and psychiatric disorder: A study of rural children. *Am J Public Health, 91*, 1494-1498.

Crisp, J., Ungerer, J.A., & Goodnow J.J. (1996). The impact of experience on children's understanding of illness. *J Pediatr Psychol, 21*, 57-72.

Dadds, M.R., Stein, R.E., & Silver, E.J. (1995). The role of maternal psychological adjustment in the measurement of children's functional status. *J Pediatr Psychol, 20*, 527-544.

Dosa, N.P., Boeing, N.M., & Kanter, R.K. (2001). Excess risk of severe acute illness in children with chronic health conditions. *Pediatrics, 107*, 499-504.

Feudtner, C., Silveira, M.J., & Christakis, D.A. (2002). Where do children with complex chronic conditions die? Patterns in Washington State, 1980-1998. *Pediatrics, 109*, 656-660.

Frank, R.G., Thayer, J.F., Hagglund, K.J., Vieth, A.Z., Schopp, L.H., et al. (1998). Trajectories of adaptation in pediatric chronic illness: the importance of the individual. *J Consult Clin Psychol, 66*, 521-532.

Freud, A. (1966). *The ego mechanism of defense*. New York: International Universities Press.

Ganz, P.A. (2001). Late effects of cancer and its treatment. *Semin Oncol Nurs, 17*, 241-248.

Gartstein, M.A., Short, A.D., Vannatta, K., & Noll, R.B. (1999). Psychosocial adjustment of children with chronic illness: An evaluation of three models. *J Dev Behav Pediatr, 20*, 157-163.

Garwick, A.W., Patterson, J.M., Meschke, L.L., Bennett, F.C., & Blum, R.W. (2002). The uncertainty of preadolescents' chronic health conditions and family distress. *J Child Fam Nurs, 8*, 11-31.

Gilbride, K.E. (1995). Developmental testing. *Pediatr Rev, 16*, 338-345.

Glascoe, F.P. (1999). Using parents' concerns to detect and address developmental and behavioral problems. *J Soc Pediatr Nurs, 4*, 24-35.

Glascoe, F.P. (1997). Parents' concerns about children's development: Prescreening technique or screening test? *Pediatrics, 99*, 522-528.

Hertzman, C. (1998). The case for child development as a determinant of health. *Can J Public Health, 89*, S14-S19.

Immelt, S.C. (2000). *Correlates of global self-worth in young children with chronic medical conditions* [online]. Available: http://80-newfirstsearch.oclc.org.metaliab.bc.edu.

Joachim, G. & Acorn, S. (2000). Stigma of visible and invisible chronic conditions. *J Adv Nurs, 32*, 243-248.

Kane, J.R., Barber, R.G., Jordan, M., Tichenor, K.T., & Camp, K. (2000). Supportive/palliative care of children suffering from life-threatening and terminal illness. *Am J Hosp Palliat Care, 17*, 165-172.

Karns, J.T. (2002). Children's understanding of death. *Journal of Clinical Activities Assignments and Handouts in Psychotherapy Practice, 2*, 43-50.

Kato, P.M., Lyon, T.D., & Rasco, C. (1998). Reasoning about moral aspects of illness and treatment by preschoolers who are healthy or who have a chronic illness. *J Dev Behav Pediatr, 19*, 68-76.

Kef, S. (2002). Psychosocial adjustment and the meaning of social support for visually impaired adolescents. *Journal of Visual Impairment and Blindness, 96*, 22-37.

Kutcher, S. (2002). *Practical child and adolescent pyschopharmacology*. Cambridge, United Kingdom: Cambridge University Press.

Kyngas, H. & Rissanen, M. (2001). Support as a crucial predictor of good compliance of adolescents with a chronic illness. *J Clin Nurs, 10*, 767-773.

Letourneau, N., Drummond, J.U., Flemming, D., Kysela, G., McDonald, L., et al. (2001). Supporting parents: Can intervention improve parent-child relationships? Two pilot studies. *J Child Fam Nurs, 7*, 159-187.

Malloy, M.H. & Freeman, D.H. (2000). Respiratory distress syndrome mortality in the United States, 1987-1995. *J Perinatol, 20*, 414-420.

Meijer, S.A., Sinnema, G., Bijstra, J.O., Mellenbergh, G.J., & Wolters, W.M. (2002). Coping styles and locus of control as predictors for psychological adjustment of adolescents with a chronic illness. *Soc Sci Med, 54*, 1453-1461.

Melnyk, B.M., Moldenhauer, Z., Veenema, T., Gullo, S., McMurtrie, M., et al. (2001). The KySS (Keep your children/yourself Safe and Secure) Campaign: A national effort to reduce psycho-social morbidities in children and adolescents. *J Pediatr Health Care, 15*, 31A-34A.

Msall, M.E., Avery, R.C., Tremont, M.R., Lima, J.C., Rogers, M.L., et al. (2003). Functional disablity and school activity limitations in 41,300 school-age children: relationship to medical impairments. *Pediatrics, 111*, 548-553.

Narla, L.D., Spottswood, S.S., Hingsbergen, E.A. (1998). Iatrogenic complications of drugs in children. *Appl Radiol, 27*, 11-13, 16-18.

Newacheck, P.W., & Halfon, N. (1998). Prevalence and impact of disabling chronic conditions in childhood. *Am J Public Health, 88*, 610-617.

Newacheck, P.W., Strickland, B., Shonkoff, J.P., Perrin, J.M., McPherson, M., et al. (1998). An epidemiologic profile of children with special health care needs. *Pediatrics, 102*, 117-121.

Northam, E. (1997). Psychosocial impact of chronic illness in children. *J Paediatr Child Health, 33*, 369-372.

Patterson, J. & Blum, R.W. (1996). Risk and resilience among children and youth with disabilities. *Arch Pediatr Adolesc Med, 150*, 692-698.

Perrin, E.C., Lewkowicz, C. & Young, M.H. (2000). Shared vision: Concordance among fathers, mothers, and pediatricians about unmet needs. *Pediatrics, 105*, 277-285.

Petrini, J., Damus, K., Russell, R., Poschman, K., Davidoff, M.J., et al. (2002). Contribution of birth defects to infant mortality in the United States. *Teratology, 66*(Suppl 1), S3-6.

Pless, I.B., Power, C., & Peckham, C.S. (1993). Long-term psychosocial sequelae of chronic physical disorders in childhood. *Pediatrics, 91*, 1131-1136.

Reeve, A. (2001). Understanding the adolescent with developmental disabilities. *Pediatr Ann, 30*, 104-108.

Rink, E. & Tricker, R. (2003). Reliency-base research and adolescnet health behaviors. *The Prevention Researcher, 10*(1), 1-4.

Schmidt, C.K. (2001). Development of children's body knowledge, using knowledge of the lungs as an exemplar. *Issues Compr Pediatr Nurs, 24*, 177-191.

Silver, E.J., Stein, R.E., & Bauman, L.J. (1999). Sociodemographic and condition-related characteristics associated with conduct problems in school-aged children with chronic health conditions. *Arch Pediatr Adolesc Med, 153*, 815-820.

Spence, L.J. & Kaiser, L. (2002). Companion animals and adaptation in chronically ill children. *West J Nurs Res, 24*, 639-656.

Stein, R.E. & Jessop, D.J. (1989). What diagnosis does not tell: the case for a noncategorical approach to chronic illness in children. *Soc Sci Med, 29*, 769-778.

Stein, R.E. & Silver, E.G. (1999). Operationalizing a conceptually based noncategorical definition: A first look at US children with chronic conditions. *Arch Pediatr Adolesc Med, 153*, 68-74.

Sterling, Y.V., Peterson, J., & Weekes, D.P. (1997). African-American families with chronically ill children: oversights and insights. *J Pediatr Nurs, 12,* 292-300.

Stewart, J.L. & Mishel, M.H. (2000). Uncertainty in childhood illness: A synthesis of the parent and child literature. *Sch Inq Nurs Pract, 14,* 299-319.

Thomas, D. & Gaslin, T.C. (2001). "Camping up" self-esteem in children with hemophilia. *Issues Compr Pediatr Nurs, 24,* 253-263.

Thompson, R.J. & Gustafson, K.E. (1996). *Models of adaptation, adaptation to chronic childhood illness.* Washington DC: American Psychological Association.

Vessey, J.A. (1999). Psychologic comorbidity and chronic conditions. *Pediatr Nurs, 25,* 211-214.

Vessey, J.A., Carlson, K., & David, J. (2003). Helping children who are being teased or bullied. *Nurs Spectr, 7,* 14-16.

Vessey, J.A. & Miola, E.S. (1997). Teaching adolescents self-advocacy skills. *Pediatr Nurs, 23,* 53-56.

Vessey, J.A. & O'Sullivan, P. (2000). A study of children's concepts of their internal bodies: a comparison of children with and without congenital heart disease. *J Pediatr Nurs, 15,* 292-298.

Wallander, J.L. & Thompson, R.J. (1995). Psychosocial adjustment of children with chronic physical conditions. In M.C. Roberts (Ed.), *Handbook of pediatric psychology (2nd edition).* New York: Guilford Press.

Weiss, M.J. & Wagner, S.H. (1998). What explains the negative consequences of adverse childhood experiences on adult health? *Am J Prev Med, 14,* 356-360.

Zeanah, C.H., Boris, N.W., & Larrieu, J.A. (1997). Infant development and developmental risk: a review of the past 10 years. *J Am Acad Child Adolesc Psychiatry, 36,* 165-178.

3 Chronic Conditions and the Family

Kathleen Knafl and Sheila Santacroce

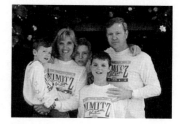

MORE than 4 million children in the United States are estimated to have a chronic condition, and for most it is experienced in the context of the family (Newacheck, 1998). There is considerable evidence in the literature for the existence of a strong reciprocal relationship between illness and child and family functioning (Austin, 1991; Faux, 1998; Feetham, 1997; Gilliss & Knafl, 1999; Knafl & Gilliss, 2002; Wallander & Varni, 1998). Attention to this reciprocal relationship is predicated on a view of the family as a system interacting with other systems.

Children with a chronic condition, along with their families, face multiple challenges that are of concern to both the families and the health care providers with whom they interact. Typically, parents are expected to master new, often sophisticated, medical information and complex regimens, and children are expected to cooperate with and adhere to treatments and the lifestyle changes that may ensue. The literature indicates that families respond in varying ways to a child's chronic condition. Although many families report they are able to lead normal, satisfying lives despite the challenges of their child's condition, others describe their lives as an ongoing struggle that takes its toll on both individual and family well-being (Austin & Sims, 1998; Faux & Seideman, 1996; Gilliss & Knafl, 1999; Knafl & Gilliss, 2002).

A unique array of strengths and limitations shapes each family's condition management efforts, and the difficulties they experience are varied as well. For example, some families struggle to master a child's treatment regimen, whereas others who have mastered the regimen remain stymied in their efforts to make condition management a less intrusive or conflict-laden aspect of their family life. This diversity of family responses necessitates individualized interventions if optimal child and family functioning is to be supported.

In order to understand the varying ways in which families and children respond to the challenges of a child's chronic condition, it is useful to understand the broader social context of the contemporary American family, current research on family responses to childhood chronic conditions, and key family concepts and conceptual frameworks that can guide the primary care of children with chronic conditions. Knowledge in these three areas provides the evidence base for practice and contributes to the practitioner's ability to develop individualized interventions. Ideally interventions address the unique needs of individual children and families and contribute to the family's ability to manage childhood chronic conditions in ways that result in both disease control and healthy child and family functioning.

The Contemporary American Family

Families of children with health conditions and practitioners interact in the social context of contemporary American society. Changes over the past 40 years in marital roles, prevailing family structures, and the cohesiveness of the family unit touch all families, including those experiencing a child's chronic condition. These changes in concert with the sociocultural diversity of the American family mean that practitioners are more likely than ever to encounter a varied array of family types and circumstances. Both the popular literature and the professional literature are replete with statistics meant to convey important information about the current state of children and family life in America, such as those listed in Box 3-1, which summarizes data from the National Survey of America's Families (Institute, 2000). Typically, statistics such as these are linked to concerns about the current well-being of children and the ability of the family to provide a safe environment that supports healthy child development. As such, the statistics provide useful information for shaping policies and programs. Knowing that growing numbers of children are in need of child care and that single parents are more likely to express considerable difficulty with their parental role suggests a need for certain kinds of services and supports. The statistics inform us about current trends, high-risk groups, and broad social needs. However, they are less useful in guiding direct practice and the kinds of interactions that take place among practitioners, children, and family members. Knowing that single parents statistically are more likely to live in poverty and express frustration with their parenting role tells the practitioner that the single parents they encounter fall into a high-risk group but nothing more. The statistics can alert the practitioner to key areas for assessment, but they reveal nothing about the unique needs of individual children and families, and population level data never replace the need for careful assessment of individual children and their families.

Moreover, although the statistics raise concerns about the ability of the American family to provide a safe and healthy environment for children, another considerable body of literature indicates that family members are highly involved in the care of ill members and health care providers increasingly encourage them to be so. As Campbell (2000, p. 166) noted "families, not health care providers, are the primary caretakers of patients with chronic illness." Such involvement is seen as both cost effective and in the affected child's best interest, and families typically prefer high levels of involvement in managing their members' health care needs. As a nation, we are not

Demographic Characteristics of the Contemporary American Family

In 2000, 69% of American children lived with two parents, down from 77% in 1980.

In 2000, 77% of white, non-Hispanic children lived with two parents compared with 38% of black children and 65% of children of Hispanic origin.

In 1999, 33% of all births were to unmarried women, including 4 in 10 first births. Single mothers are disproportionately more likely to be poor, and poverty has been associated with multiple negative outcomes for children (McLoyd, 1998).

In 1999, 54% of all children from birth through third grade received some form of child care on a regular basis from persons other than their parents.

In 1999, 12.5% of all children lacked health insurance.

In 1999, 10% of all children lived with a parent who reported that their child was particularly hard to care for.

waiting to resolve the current concerns about the ability of the American family to take an active role in caring for ill members. Providers and health insurance carriers typically encourage, and increasingly require, that families take considerable responsibility for managing the health care requirements of children with chronic conditions.

Statistics also are used to highlight the ethnic and cultural diversity of the American family. An early national census conducted in 1860 included only three ethnic categories: black, white, and "quadroon," or persons of mixed racial heritage. In contrast, the most recent 2000 census listed 30 ethnic categories, including 11 subcategories under "Hispanic." This striking change in census reporting reflects the growing recognition of ethnicity as a key aspect of identity, one that often is linked to beliefs about family, child rearing, illness behavior, and health care.

The 2000 census reported that as a nation, we are approximately 71% white, 12% black, 12% Hispanic, 4% Asian and Pacific Islander, and less than 1% American Indian, Eskimo, and Aleut Islander. However, these national figures mask considerable regional variation. For example, Maine, New Hampshire, and Vermont all are more than 95% white, whereas Hawaii and the District of Columbia are less than 30% white. California, New York, Illinois, and Florida are among the most diverse states with multiple ethnic groups comprising a large percent of the population. However, as with the statistics on characteristics of families, these figures provide an overview of national and regional trends but are of little direct use in guiding practice. The statistics point to the likelihood that practitioners will need to take into account ethnically based beliefs about health and illness when caring for families in which a child has a chronic condition, but they provide minimal, if any, guidance on how to address ethnically based health care beliefs.

The array of ethnic groups in the United States today, including recently arrived immigrants, presents a considerable challenge to practitioners who are committed to providing culturally sensitive care. How do practitioners meet the needs of diverse families confronting diverse illness situations? How do practitioners integrate our clinical and academic expertise of families and chronic conditions in order to help families meet illness-specific demands while sustaining a satisfying family life? The diversity of families speaks against the likelihood of

coming up with definitive guidelines for helping certain kinds of families facing certain kinds of health care challenges. The individuality of each family precludes the development of specific guidelines for assessment and intervention. On the other hand, a number of useful concepts and conceptual models are available that contribute to understanding how families experience chronic conditions and that suggest important topics and issues to take into account when interacting, assessing, and developing interventions that support family management of chronic conditions.

The remainder of this chapter addresses the current evidence base for working with families in which a child has a chronic condition by providing an overview of current research and discussing conceptual models that have proven useful in guiding practice with families of children with chronic conditions. The concepts and framework we discuss are useful in that they tell us where to look without telling us what to see in our assessment of individual families. In other words, they provide insights into what is important with regard to the nature of the challenges families face when a child member has a chronic condition. At the same time, the concepts and frameworks we discuss accommodate family diversity because they do not prescribe what we should expect to see or what judgments we should make about our observations. As such, they are meant to guide efforts to encourage families to share their experiences and work collaboratively with practitioners to develop effective interventions.

Families and Chronic Conditions: the Evidence Base for Practice

Transition to Living with the Diagnosis of a Pediatric Chronic Health Condition

Almost all of what is known about the transition to living with the diagnosis of a pediatric chronic health condition and initial responses to such diagnoses has to do with parents. The related literature about children addresses their responses to specific illness-related events and circumstances, such as painful procedures and hospitalization, rather than to the diagnosis. The focus on parental responses is justified because parents play a critical role in delivering medical treatments to the child with a chronic health condition, mediating condition-related distress for the affected child and healthy siblings, promoting child psychologic and social adaptation to a chronic condition, and managing day-to-day family life. Optimal care for children with chronic health conditions and their families requires an understanding of usual parental responses to the diagnosis of a pediatric chronic condition and the development of supports for parents.

Prediagnostic Stage. The transition to living with the diagnosis of a pediatric chronic health condition does not occur at the point in time when a clinician meets with the parents to formally pronounce the child's medical diagnosis, give population-based estimates for the child's prognosis and long-term survival, and make recommendations for the child's medical treatment. More accurately, this transition is a process that begins when parents become aware of changes in their child and is completed when family members absorb the implications of the condition for the child and the family. Davis (1963) first

---

BOX 3-2

The Transition to Living with the Diagnosis of Chronic Conditions

1. Prediagnostic stage
   a. Parents aware of changes in the child
   b. Parents and primary care provider (PCP) define symptoms as normal and attempt to manage
   c. Parents and PCP redefine symptoms as serious and seek subspecialty evaluation
2. Diagnostic stage
   a. Subspecialty evaluation is initiated.
   b. Formal pronouncement of the diagnosis and treatment recommendations
   c. Initiation of treatment
3. Living with the diagnosis
   a. Parents responsible for administering treatment
   b. Parental awareness of the implications of the diagnosis for child and family

---

described the process that families experience as it applied to families of children with poliomyelitis. Cohen (1993a, 1995a) found support for Davis's depiction and extended his work through family interviews and review of the autobiographic literature about families of children with a broad array of chronic health conditions. Clarke-Steffen (1993a) has developed a picture of the process as it occurred for families of children with cancer. Research about children with type 1 diabetes (Grey et al, 1995; Hatton et al, 1995) and children diagnosed at birth with a chronic health condition (Sharkey, 1995) shows that the transition process is realized when the family undertakes implementation of the child's medical regimen and develops an acute sense of the implications of the health condition for the affected child and family life.

According to Cohen (1995a), the onset of the transition to living with the diagnosis of a pediatric chronic health condition, which she referred to as the prediagnostic period, comprises three stages (Box 3-2). The onset of the transition begins with a parent's awareness that something is going on with the child and continues until the formal diagnostic announcement. Before the first, or lay-explanatory, stage, the child's symptoms (i.e., bone aches, irritability) are so ordinary as not to be noticed. The lay-explanatory stage begins when the child's symptoms enter the parent's awareness and become a focus of attention. Parents, especially those with little experience with serious pediatric health conditions, commonly apply a normal developmental explanation, such as growing pains or a desire for attention, or a benign medical explanation, such as the flu, to account for the symptoms; primary care providers may do the same thing. When the child's symptoms are defined as evidence of a nonmedical problem, parents use interactional strategies, such as ignoring, nagging, punishing, or paying extra attention to the child, to manage the child's symptoms. When the symptoms are defined as evidence of a medical problem, parents use medical strategies such as rest and over-the-counter medications for symptom management (Cohen, 1995a).

After symptom management strategies are initiated, parents wait to see improvement in the child's symptoms. If the problem

gets worse or does not resolve within a reasonable amount of time, parents question the plausibility of the lay explanation and start to legitimate the need for medical intervention. The second, or legitimizing, stage of the acute phase of the transition to living with the diagnosis of a pediatric chronic health condition commences when the parent redefines the child's symptoms as worrisome and originates a strategic plan in anticipation of a parent-provider interaction. Parents devote considerable effort to developing a strategic plan to guide their interactions with professionals. Parents do this for reasons such as fear of being made to feel alarmist, fear of the child's symptoms being dismissed by health care providers just as the parents had previously dismissed the symptoms, and, particularly in the current health care climate, to quickly gain the referral that many insurers require from a primary care provider before setting an appointment for evaluation by a specialist. Parents use a broad range of strategies to enact the strategic plan for interactions with providers, including raising their concerns during a routine health care visit, acquiring knowledge to counter a provider's appraisal of the child's symptoms as normal, using cash to obtain the care they believe is indicated, and embellishing the nature or severity of the child's symptoms (Cohen, 1995a). An adverse consequence of the prolonged lay-explanatory or legitimizing phases is loss of parents' confidence in their ability (1) to perform the parental role as it applies to monitoring the child's physical health, (2) distinguish normal variations from symptoms of illness, and (3) apply consistent expectations for child behavior. This loss of confidence applies to parenting not only affected children but also their healthy siblings (Cohen & Martinson, 1988).

The third, or medical diagnostic stage of the transition to diagnosis, begins when the parent makes an appointment for the child to be seen by a physician or other specialist and ends when the diagnosis is certain and formally announced to the family. The duration of this stage is determined by the extent to which there are unambiguous physical findings in the child, the degree to which the provider acknowledges parental concerns, and the degree to which a provider allows the relative frequency of a condition to influence diagnostic testing. For example, the relatively low incidence of childhood leukemia vs. viral illness may cause a health care provider to attribute the general symptoms of fever, bone pain, and pallor to viral illness and delay blood tests for leukemia.

When the medical diagnosis phase is protracted, the long wait for diagnostic certainty becomes unbearable, causing existential agony and extreme psychosocial stress for parents (Clarke-Steffen, 1993a). Adverse consequences of a prolonged medical diagnosis phase consist of parental anger with providers, institutions, and systems of care; lack of parental confidence in the provider's ability to assess and treat the child; and hypersensitivity to provider statements and behaviors (Clarke-Steffen, 1993a; Davis, 1963) that can be so extreme as to resemble paranoia. When the medical diagnostic phase has been prolonged, parents have reported extreme relief in response to the diagnoses of even potentially fatal pediatric health conditions (Cohen, 1995b; Santacroce, 2000). Parental relief is supported by provider statements reflecting the expectation that the condition can be managed by available treatment, specific treatment recommendations, the health care team's expertise with delivering treatment and supportive care, and a plan for initiating treatment (Santacroce, 2000) (Box 3-2).

Diagnostic Stage. Parents have likened the diagnosis of a chronic health condition in their child to a "physical assault by a powerful force" (Cohen, 1995a, p. 47). In 1994, the American Psychological Association (American Psychiatric Association [APA], 1994) recognized the diagnosis of a life-threatening disease in a child as a traumatic event for parents. The diagnosis may be particularly traumatic in the contemporary sociomedical context because of cognitive dissonance between what is expected and what is experienced. In the past, families expected to experience childhood death from disease. There were few available means to prevent or treat infectious diseases. Available technologies did not allow for early diagnosis of life-threatening disease, and there were few available means to manage late-stage disease or the side effects of crude treatments. Preparation for the child's certain and usually imminent death often followed the diagnostic announcement. Given medical and technologic developments over the past 4 decades, today's parents expect healthy children who will outlive them. Modern Western beliefs include personal responsibility for health, healthy living as a way to ensure personal and family health, and the availability of definitive cures for disease and other health conditions through widespread access to state-of-the-science medicine (Comaroff & Maguire, 1981). With the diagnosis of a pediatric chronic health condition that has no definitive cure, or when the application of available "curative" treatments generates a distinct set of problems, the previously taken for granted world comes apart and parents' beliefs about themselves, science, the world, and sometimes God are shattered. Uncertainty about the nature of the problem that existed during the prediagnostic phase changes to uncertainty that permeates every aspect of daily family life. Parents experience intense helplessness with being unable to prevent the child's health condition and protect the child from harm, guilt at their real or imagined role in causing or failing to recognize the disease, horror at witnessing the child's suffering and thoughts that the child may die, and fear about what the child and the family will have to endure in the future (Clarke-Steffen, 1997; Cohen, 1993a). These parental reactions may be heightened when there is a genetic component to the chronic condition. Grandparents may also respond to the child's diagnosis with helplessness, guilt, horror, and fear and be overcome by their intense distressing emotions. They may not be as emotionally or physically available to mediate parental or child distress as parents or children may need or desire.

Posttraumatic Stress Disorder Response to Diagnosis. Four to six weeks after the diagnosis of cancer in their child, parents have reported symptoms similar to those seen in persons with an extreme response to traumatic stressors, such as combat, natural disaster, or sexual assault: posttraumatic stress disorder (PTSD) (Santacroce, 2002). Symptoms of PSTD include insomnia, irritability, difficulty concentrating and remembering; recurrent intrusive daytime thoughts or night-mares about the traumatic event, detachment and inability to experience loving or pleasurable feelings, amnesia for important aspects of the trauma, careful avoidance of cues that recall the trauma, intense

reactivity with exposure to these cues, a sense of a foreshortened future, and separation of cognition and emotion (APA, 2000). Such symptoms imply full-blown PTSD when symptoms in each of three clusters (i.e., reexperiencing, avoidance/numbing, and heightened arousal) are present for 1 month or more with significant psychologic or social impairment as a result of the symptoms (APA, 2000). Some parents may be more vulnerable than others to developing full-blown PTSD or long-term PTSD-associated symptoms following the diagnosis of a childhood chronic condition. Risk factors for developing full-blown PTSD include female gender, acute emotional distress, depression and lack of social support after the trauma, and a history of exposure to interpersonal trauma (Bisson, 2002; Kessler, 2000). Mothers may be at greater risk for the development of PTSD than fathers by virtue of their gender and because, generally, mothers assume greater responsibility for the day-to-day care of their children and are thus more likely to experience cyclic retraumatization during treatments, procedures, and health care visits. Across a range of traumatic events, children are more likely to develop full-blown PTSD or its symptoms when their parents have the full-blown disorder or its symptoms (Santacroce, 2003). For parents of long-term survivors of childhood cancer, higher trait anxiety, smaller social network, and greater perceived intensity of treatment and threat to the child's life predicted PTSD-associated symptoms (Kazak et al, 1998).

In the immediate period following diagnosis, especially when there is an acute threat to the child's life, PTSD-associated symptoms are normative and protective in that they restrict parental awareness of upsetting events, dampen potentially overwhelming distressing emotions, and allow parents to make treatment decisions and take other steps to preserve child and family life. Conversely, PTSD-associated symptoms can impede parental ability to comprehend and remember detailed information about their child's condition and its treatment, learn critical disease-management skills, mediate their child's emotional distress, utilize social support, and plan for the future (Santacroce, 2002). Over time, as immediate threats to the child's life are eliminated, protective "symptoms" generally abate, allowing more comprehensive cognitive awareness of condition-related events.

Living with the Diagnosis

It is also when the child's condition is stabilized that parents usually assume responsibility for managing the child's medical regimen. Hatton & colleagues (1995) found that when parents of children with type 1 diabetes assumed responsibility for managing the child's medical regimen at home, they more completely absorbed the diagnosis, including an understanding of the widespread implications and pervasive influence of the condition on each member of the family. In children with type 1 diabetes, Grey & colleagues (1995) found increased levels of depressive symptoms and reduced levels of self-efficacy over the second year following the diagnosis. The researchers attributed the increased levels of depression and reduced self-efficacy to experience with managing the medical regimen and the development of an understanding of the meaning of the diagnosis and its implications, that is, that diabetes and diabetes self-management are forever.

In a study about families of children with conditions requiring home care, Sharkey (1995) found that the child's discharge home was associated with heightened awareness of the physical work and family environmental and lifestyle changes required to accommodate the child's health condition while maintaining some sense of normal family life.

Taken together, these findings indicate that the transition to living with the diagnosis of a pediatric chronic health condition is not complete when the diagnosis is announced. Instead, the transition is complete when responsibility for managing the child's disease-related and usual daily care is assumed by family members and the child and family develop genuine awareness of the implications of the diagnosis and the medical treatment regimen for individual and family life over the longer term. Clinical experience suggests that this idea is applicable beyond families of children with diabetes or children requiring home care.

The transition to living with the diagnosis of a pediatric health condition is a process that begins when the child's symptoms enter the parent's awareness and is complete when parental understanding of the meaning of the diagnosis for child and family life develops with experience managing the child's care. There may be parallel critical points in the child's transition to living with the diagnosis of a chronic health condition. That is, the child's transition may be advanced during late school age with the experience of beginning responsibility for self-management and completed during late adolescence or young adulthood with cognitive awareness of both the immediate and future implications of the disease and its treatment.

Impact of a Chronic Condition on Child and Family Functioning. Research on the interplay between childhood chronic conditions and child and family functioning has focused on the family's contribution to the child's functioning, the quality of family functioning in the context of childhood illness, and the patterns of family response to chronic illness. Studies in these areas have generated considerable knowledge with regard to child and family functioning and provide the practitioner with an understanding of the range of child and family responses likely to be encountered in practice. These studies also highlight family and child characteristics that may lead to adjustment difficulties as well as concepts that are likely to help the primary care providers understand the family context of childhood chronic conditions and support families' efforts to care for their child's condition in a way that contributes to healthy child development and family functioning.

Impact of a chronic condition on child functioning. The relationship between family and child functioning when a child has a chronic condition typically is discussed in terms of the family's impact on the child's psychosocial adjustment, disease control, and treatment adherence. A large body of research has focused on children's psychosocial adjustment to a chronic condition. Studies carried out over the past 20 years have shown that children with chronic physical problems are at increased risk for emotional and behavioral problems, suggesting that primary care providers need to be alert to the special needs of this particular group of children. A meta-analysis of 87 studies that compared the psychologic adjustment of children with chronic conditions with that of either study controls or normative data found a mean difference in overall psychologic adjustment of approximately one half of a standard deviation (Lavigne & Faier-Routman, 1992), indicating that a chronic condition puts children at significant risk for psychosocial problems. In a more recent review, Wallander & Varni (1998) concluded that prior research, including major epidemiologic surveys, has established the risk status of children with chronic conditions. At the same time, they, along with other investigators, are quick to point out that "although the prevalence of maladjustment is higher, only a minority of children with chronic disorders appeared maladjusted" (Wallander & Varni, 1998, p. 31).

Research consistently has shown that family functioning is an important predictor of adjustment in children with chronic conditions (Hamlett et al, 1992; Morris et al, 1997; Patterson et al, 1994; Perrin et al, 1993; Thompson et al, 1999; Wallander & Varni, 1998). Although different studies have linked varying characteristics of the family to child adjustment, the variables of family cohesion and absence of conflict consistently have been associated with better adjustment in children. As a group, these studies indicate that providers should expect the majority of children with chronic conditions in their practice to be well adjusted. On the other hand, they also point to the importance of including family variables in any assessment of adjustment difficulties a child may be experiencing. Moreover, a growing body of literature demonstrates the benefits of normalization as a coping strategy that helps both the child and the family adjust to the chronic condition (Amer, 1999; Clawson, 1996; Deatrick et al, 1999). As discussed later in this chapter, health care professionals can play a key role in helping parents create normal lives for children with a chronic condition and the families in which they live.

Impact of condition on family functioning. Numerous studies have addressed family functioning when a child has a chronic condition. Investigators have addressed how childhood chronic conditions impact family life as well as the quality of family functioning in the context of chronic conditions (Knafl & Gilliss, 2002). Studies address various aspects of family functioning, including problem solving, communication, and coping. The coping function of families or their ability to maintain stability in the face of change has been a particular concern of researchers interested in family. The results of these studies, which typically used standardized measures to assess family functioning, present a mixed picture of the impact of a chronic condition on family life. Some authors found evidence that families continue to function well when a member has a chronic condition (Bohachick & Anton, 1990; Donnelly, 1994; Rehm & Catanzaro, 1998; Sawyer, 1992; Youngblut et al, 1994). These authors found that families expressed satisfaction with family life and did not perceive the chronic condition to be the dominant focus of their life. In contrast, other studies documented negative outcomes for family functioning (Cornman, 1993; Ferrell et al, 1994; Kopp et al, 1995; Park & Martinson, 1998) as a result of a child's chronic illness. These studies suggest that families who are facing multiple stressors or whose child has a condition characterized by an uncertain disease course are more likely to experience impaired family functioning. Other studies have reported differential illness effects across different subsystems in the family, with the marital subsystem appearing to be especially at risk for negative outcomes (Dashiff, 1993; Gallo, 1990). Dashiff (1993), for example, found that parents reported an increase in family closeness but a decrease in couple closeness as a result of their daughter's diabetes.

Descriptive studies have provided insights into the cognitive and behavioral strategies that support optimal family functioning over the course of a child's chronic condition. As such, they serve to guide the assessment of key aspects of family life. These studies provide evidence that adaptation is a process that often occurs in a series of stages (Gilliss & Knafl, 1999; Knafl & Gilliss, 2002). For example, Horner (1998) in a qualitative study of 12 families in which a school-aged child had asthma identified three phases of adaptation: learning the ropes, dealing with asthma, and coming to terms with the asthma. She described how, over time, families mastered the treatment regimen and were able to balance asthma care with other aspects of family life. Other investigators have noted the importance of developing a routine for carrying out the treatment regimen that minimizes its intrusiveness on family life. These authors also noted that families typically were able to develop such a routine but often struggled to do so during the first few months following the diagnosis and during subsequent developmental transitions as the child's responsibility for self-care increased.

Helping families to master the treatment regimen and develop a management routine that accommodates other family activities and responsibilities is an important goal for health care providers. Burke & colleagues (1999) have developed a useful tool for helping families manage a child's condition. The Burke Assessment Guide to Stressors and Tasks in Families with a Child with a Chronic Condition was based on a series of interviews with more than 300 parents of children with a chronic condition and is meant to support the comprehensive assessment by health care providers of critical issues for families as a way to focus ongoing interventions. Box 3-3 lists the 11 major areas of stressors and tasks included in the Burke assessment guide.

Underlying Dimensions of Chronic Conditions. Researchers and clinicians also have identified general characteristics of chronic conditions that often play an important role in shaping the family's response to illness. Much of the research on family response to chronic conditions addresses the challenges that specific diseases present to children (Wallander & Varni, 1998) and families. However, some researchers have noted the limitations of focusing exclusively on disease categories when one's primary interest is the psychosocial as opposed to the physiologic consequences of chronic conditions (Rolland, 1994; Stein & Jessop, 1982; Wallander & Varni, 1998).

As early as 1975, Pless & Pinkerton discussed the benefits of taking a noncategorical approach to the care and study of children with chronic conditions and their families. They argued that it is neither possible nor particularly useful to try to chronicle the distinct challenges posed by each chronic condition. Since their seminal work, clinicians and researchers have identified underlying dimensions of chronic conditions that cut across disease entities and play an important role in shaping individual and family response. In their review of the effects of chronic physical illness on children and their families, Wallander & Varni (1998, p. 29) noted that an approach that "focuses on commonalities in the class of chronic physical disorders could enhance the understanding of the impact on the psychosocial adjustment of children and their families and could improve care." Several frameworks have been devised that highlight generic dimensions of the chronic illness experience (Jessop & Stein, 1985; LoBato et al, 1988; Rolland, 1994; Stein & Jessop, 1982). Although varied, these frameworks reveal some common themes and identify the nature of the condition's onset, course, functional limitations, and visibility as important psychosocial dimensions of a chronic illness that increase family stress (Box 3-4).

The illness onset dimension has to do with the abruptness with which the condition presents. Conditions such as diabetes and spinal cord injury have a sudden onset, allowing little time for family adaptation and requiring immediate changes in family life. On the other hand, conditions such as arthritis, muscular dystrophy, and attention deficit hyperactivity disorder permit more gradual adjustments in family life, although the uncertainty surrounding the diagnostic period may be the source of considerable stress. Disease course directs our attention to the relative stability and predictability of the condition. In general, conditions such as lupus and epilepsy that are unstable or unpredictable impose greater psychosocial demands on the family. The degree and nature of functional limitation associated with the condition also have implications for the quality of child and family adaptation. Rolland (1984) goes so far as

---

BOX 3-3

Major Stressors and Tasks Included in the Burke Assessment Guide

1. Gaining and interpreting knowledge, skills, and experience to manage the child's problem
2. Acquiring and managing physical resources and services to manage the child's health problem
3. Acquiring and managing financial resources to care for the child's health problem
4. Establishing and maintaining effective social supports
5. Rearing a child with a chronic condition
6. Developing beliefs, values, and philosophy of life
7. Managing the care of the child
8. Identifying and managing sibling issues
9. Managing spousal, parental, and nuclear family relationships
10. Maintaining health of other family members
11. Maintaining effective relationships with the health care system and other sources of care

---

BOX 3-4

Characteristics of Chronic Conditions Resulting in Increased Family Stress

1. Sudden onset
2. Instability in course of condition
3. Functional limitations
4. Visibility of condition

to say that it is the presence or absence of any major incapacitation rather than the exact nature of the incapacitation that is the salient functional dimension of a chronic condition. Visibility also has been identified as an important dimension of the chronic condition experience, although the nature of its influence is somewhat unclear, with some authors linking visibility with better and some with poorer adaptation (Wallander & Varni, 1998).

An advantage of taking a noncategorical perspective is that it provides direction for assessing the kinds of challenges the family and the ill child may be confronting. For example, using a noncategorical approach, the practitioner would question the family regarding the onset and course of the condition in an effort to uncover what family members identified as particularly difficult aspects of living with the condition. Noncategorical frameworks are particularly useful because they direct the clinician's attention away from an exclusive focus on the presenting disease to the experience of living with the condition.

Key Concepts for Understanding Family Response to Illness. Health care providers have a number of concepts to draw on to help them understand how families experience and respond to childhood chronic conditions. Uncertainty, stigma, normalization, and survivorship are concepts that capture important aspects of many families' experiences (Box 3-5).

Uncertainty. Uncertainty has been identified as the single greatest source of psychosocial stress for people affected by chronic health conditions (Koocher, 1985). For parents, uncertainty pervades the experience of pediatric chronic health conditions, from the time around diagnosis (Clarke-Steffen, 1993b; Cohen, 1993a, 1995a; Santacroce, 2000), through treatment (Clarke-Steffen, 1993a, 1997; Cohen, 1993b), with disease progression (Hinds et al, 1996), and during survivorship (Koocher, 1985; Sparacino et al, 1997) or bereavement (Cohen & Martinson, 1988). Over the course of pediatric chronic conditions, parents experience uncertainty as an unbearable urge to know what is not knowable about their child's future: what the child will be asked to suffer, whether or not the child will ultimately survive, and, if the child survives, the child's quality of life and ability to function in the future (Clarke-Steffen, 1993a; Cohen & Martinson, 1988).

Parental uncertainty has been defined as a parent's or other family caregiver's inability to determine meaning relative to illness events in a family member, specifically a child (Mishel, 1983; Santacroce, 2001). Uncertainty in adult illness has been shown to have four dimensions: (1) ambiguity about the illness state; (2) lack of information about the illness, its treatment and side effects, and their management; (3) complexity in what information is known, the health care system, and relationships with health care providers; and (4) unpredictability of the future (Mishel, 1981, 1997). Parental uncertainty in child chronic health conditions has been shown to share these features (Mishel, 1983; Santacroce, 2001). Different situations and events can trigger uncertainty (Box 3-6).

Uncertainty is inherently neutral but can be appraised as dangerous or beneficial. The appraisal of uncertainty is influenced by characteristics of the person, the environment, and the condition (Mishel, 1988). Adults initially tend to appraise uncertainty as being dangerous. When they appraise uncertainty as dangerous, people next evaluate whether they have the skills and resources to reduce uncertainty. When their skills and resources seem sufficient, adults take steps to resolve uncertainty. In the perceived absence of skills and resources, or when distressing emotions and negative beliefs impede action, people manage uncertainty by restricting their awareness of what produces uncertainty (Mishel, 1988). Uncertainty has been consistently associated with higher levels of emotional distress, reduced quality of life, and poorer psychosocial adjustment (Mishel, 1997). Higher levels of distressing emotions have predicted less functional coping with illness (Mishel, 1997).

Review of the literature shows that parents attempt to manage uncertainty primarily through information management (Stewart & Mishel, 2000). Information management typically takes two distinct forms. The first form of information management is intensive pursuit of information concerning the child's condition with hypervigilance to cues regarding the state of the child's health and potential threats in the environment. The second form of information management is careful avoidance of social encounters or cues that call to mind the child's condition and draw attention to negative aspects of uncertainty (Clarke-Steffen, 1993b; Cohen, 1993b, 1995b; Cohen & Martinson, 1988; Davis, 1963; Hinds et al, 1996; Santacroce et al, 2002). Overly intense pursuit of information can exhaust parents emotionally and physically and impede child development through overrestriction of child and family activities beyond what is medically indicated. Overreliance on avoidance of social encounters and reminders of the child's

---

BOX 3-5

Key Concepts in Family Responses to Childhood Chronic Conditions

1. _Uncertainty_ about nature of child's problem spreads to every aspect of family life at diagnosis.
2. _Stigma_ interferes with accessing available social supports and health care utilization.
3. _Normalization_ includes integrating condition with usual life to maximize medical outcomes and promote family function.
4. _Survivorship_ applies to affected child as well as family members.

BOX 3-6

Triggers of Uncertainty

Anniversaries, birthdays, holidays
Changes in the treatment regimen
Communications with health care providers
Nighttime
Onset of symptoms of minor illness
Questions from family and friends
Routine medical appointments
Stories in the media
Usual life transitions
Variations in mood or behavior
Waiting for the results of tests and procedures

condition can lead to lack of adherence to the medical treatment regimen, social isolation, and diminished communications about the condition within the family.

It has been shown that over the course of adult illness, people evolve in the appraisal of uncertainty as dangerous to beneficial and filled with opportunities. This development is supported through interactions with health care providers and members of a social network who acknowledge uncertainty in chronic conditions and focus on its positive features. For example, families of children with chronic health conditions may say that the child's condition has helped them grow stronger as a family unit and, with potentially fatal conditions, uncertainty about the ultimate prognosis for a particular child sustains family hope that their child will survive over the long term.

Change in appraisal of uncertainty from danger to opportunity is encumbered by social isolation and sizeable family caregiving responsibilities (Mishel, 1990, 1999). Parents of children with chronic health conditions are often socially isolated and carry considerable responsibility for the care of their children and maintenance of usual family life. As such, they are in particular need of assistance with the development of a broader range of functional strategies for managing uncertainty that is appraised as dangerous and support for acknowledging the positive features of uncertainty in childhood chronic conditions.

Stigma. In ancient Greece, stigma referred to body signs designed and inflicted to warn the larger community about the inferior moral state of an individual. Early Christians used the words "stigma" or "stigmata" to refer to both corporal signs of God's grace and signs of internal physical ailments. Present-day negative views of differences in personal or group characteristics have their roots in late nineteenth century American beliefs that immigrants' obvious physical and cultural distinctions from the Anglo-Saxon majority would lead to the destruction of society. Stigma has come to refer to social and personal intolerance of characteristics that are viewed as either undesirable or not stereotypical and thus deeply discredits a person's social identity (Goffman, 1963).

Children with chronic health conditions often have characteristics that differ from norms and set the children and their families apart in undesirable ways from age and role peers, as well as from life before the onset of the condition. These characteristics can potentially stigmatize, or disgrace, people with chronic conditions or disability, their families, and their caregivers. This stigmatization can interfere with the communication of important information, utilization of available social supports, formation of trusting relationships with health care providers, and maximal management of the underlying condition.

Childhood chronic health conditions are stigmatizing in that their occurrence can be viewed as parents' failure of their personal responsibility to protect their own health and the health of their children. Mothers of chronically ill children may be more stigmatized than fathers are since mothers bear and deliver the children, but there is no evidence to support this idea. The assumption that those who possess potentially stigmatizing characteristics have internalized the larger society's negative views about these traits and are aware of the shame is inherent in the idea of stigma.

Goffman (1963) has proposed a typology of stigma that can be applied to understanding family responses to childhood chronic illness: discredited and discreditable. Discrediting stigma are those that are readily evident. Among pediatric chronic conditions, discrediting conditions are those with obvious physical deformities, developmental disabilities, medication and equipment requirements, and diet or activity restrictions. A discreditable stigma is one that is unperceivable or not easily perceived. Discreditable pediatric chronic conditions are those that are not readily apparent.

People with discreditable stigma and their families tend to expend great effort to obscure traces of the potentially stigmatizing characteristic from others for as long as possible through use of strategies that include information management, impression management, and "passing" (Goffman, 1963). Gallo & colleagues (1991) found that healthy boys and girls tried to avoid stigma for themselves and help their siblings with chronic conditions "pass" as normal, especially in the absence of visible illness signs, by making careful decisions concerning who they told about the condition. Nehring et al (2000) have reported that both biologic and foster mothers of children with human immunodeficiency virus (HIV) delayed discussing the specific nature of the child's diagnosis with other people until the physical and relational costs outweighed the social benefits of not telling given the potentially stigmatizing nature of HIV. The stigma associated with a childhood chronic condition can make parents of children who are newly diagnosed reluctant to "join the club" of such parents and seek information, advice, and support even from parent peers (Moore, 1998). Moreover, Santacroce et al (2002) found that mothers of children with perinatally acquired HIV infection were reluctant to initiate state of the art medical treatment for their children when they believed that multidrug regimens would make a nonapparent condition readily obvious, that is, shift the stigma from discreditable to discredited. Thus stigma has the potential to compromise not only psychosocial outcomes for those affected by childhood chronic health conditions, but also medical outcomes when best available treatments are not implemented because of negative expectations about stigma.

Health care providers are also susceptible to stigma and engagement in stigmatizing behaviors. Stigma can be imparted to providers who work with children and families affected by health conditions that, given their nature, usually make people anxious or uncomfortable (i.e., children who are dying or children with contagious diseases). The public may attribute extraordinary personality characteristics or professional motives to such providers in order to explain the choices and in effect stigmatize the provider. Providers can also feel extremely anxious and aware of their own vulnerability when working with populations that include children who are terminally ill, are severely disabled, or harbor disease that can be transmitted through health care contacts.

Providers may create "stigma theories" to account for why such afflictions have been visited on certain families and why providers and their families are not vulnerable to the affliction. These stigma theories usually involve attribution of undesirable traits and behaviors to affected families. The theories serve to decrease the provider's anxiety and permit continued professional activities in the area, but they stigmatize children with

BOX 3-7
Attributes of Normalization

1. Acknowledge the condition and its potential to threaten lifestyle.
2. Adopt a "normalcy lens" for defining the child and the family.
3. Engage in parenting behaviors and a family routine that are consistent with a "normalcy lens."
4. Develop a treatment regimen that is consistent with a "normalcy lens."
5. Interact with others based on a view of their child and family as normal.

the condition and their families. Finally, providers may feel so emotionally distressed by childhood chronic health conditions that they go out of their way to pay special attention to and make exceptions for affected families. As a consequence, the families may perceive that they are pitied or viewed as unable to meet usual behavioral standards and thus feel stigmatized by the provider.

Normalization. As noted in the prior discussion of the family's transition to having a child with a chronic condition, the events surrounding the diagnostic process and the family's initial period of adjustment can be a difficult, stressful time. However, over time many families are able to incorporate the treatment regimen into their ongoing family routine and life resumes a taken-for-granted quality. Robinson (1993, p. 7) noted that "the preferred or dominant story for many individuals and families managing a chronic condition is one of normalization, that is, essentially normal persons leading normal lives." The concept of normalization has received considerable attention in the literature and can help guide practitioners' efforts to help families balance condition-related demands with the responsibilities of ongoing family life.

Based on a comprehensive review of research related to normalization of family life in the context of a childhood chronic condition, Deatrick et al (1999) identified five defining attributes of the concept (Box 3-7). They indicate that for many families of children with a chronic condition normalization is a valued goal and the five defining attributes can guide the practitioner's assessment of the family's normalization status. The attributes also can help to pinpoint areas where the family is experiencing normalization difficulties. For example, are difficulties the result of the failure of other systems, such as the school or health care system, to support the family's normalization efforts, or are difficulties based on problems with carrying out the treatment regimen? Assessing which attributes are reflective of normalization and which reflect barriers can direct intervention efforts. For example, if parents no longer view their child with diabetes as a "normal" 10-year-old, the practitioner can help them to recognize the many usual activities the child can still participate in and work with the family to develop a treatment routine that accommodates these usual activities. On the other hand, if the barrier to normalization is the school's reluctance to let the child continue participation on a sports team, the practitioner could strategize with the parents about how best to allay the school system's misgivings. In intervening to support the family's ability to normalize their situation, it is important to remember that the five attributes are based on the assumption that views of normalcy are highly subjective

and are likely to vary considerably across families and family members.

The five defining attributes indicate that families who normalize their life recognize the seriousness of their child's condition and the importance of the treatment regimen. However, families who normalize also believe that the chronic condition is only one aspect of their family and child. They see themselves as essentially normal with a particular problem that has to be managed. Moreover, they often are quick to point out that although not all families have a child with a chronic condition, all families do, in fact, have problems that must be managed. The adoption of a "normalcy lens" for viewing themselves and the world contributes to the family's illness management efforts as well as their interactions with others. Families who normalize the illness are likely to develop a flexible approach to adhering to the treatment regimen. In their article on the "tricks of the trade" parents develop for managing the treatment regimen, Gallo and Knafl (1998) noted that parents not only modified the treatment plan to make life more livable, but also relied on the advice and support of health care providers to do so.

As indicated by the fifth attribute listed in Box 3-7, families who normalize life in the context of a childhood chronic condition also expect others, both individuals and systems, to treat them and their child as normal. For example, health care providers are expected to help in the modification of treatment regimens so the child can participate in usual childhood activities, and school systems are expected to be flexible in restrictions placed on the child as a result of the condition.

Although a considerable body of literature indicates that many families achieve normalization, there also is evidence of families who view normalization as an impossible or inappropriate goal (Knafl & Deatrick, 2002). In these families, the child may be viewed as different from peers in multiple, important ways, or the treatment regimen may be experienced as a significant burden. Normalizing families experience illness as one of many concerns of family life. Families who are unable to normalize family life experience the illness as the pervasive focus of family life.

Families' varying experiences of normalization suggest that the health care provider is likely to work with families whose primary need is support for the normalized routine they have developed as well as with families who are struggling to achieve or sustain a normalized family life. Parents who indicate that they have been successful in incorporating the condition into everyday family life appreciate being commended for their efforts. Moreover, they need to know that health care providers understand their desire for flexibility in the treatment regimen and are willing to work with them to develop a routine that supports optimal disease control without making the condition the sole focus of family life. On the other hand, families who see normalization as an unattainable goal may need help in recognizing the many normal aspects of their child and the various family strengths they have to draw on to make life in the context of chronic illness more livable. The Calgary Family Assessment and Intervention Models (Box 3-8) (Wright & Leahey, 2000) described later in this chapter provide guidelines for identifying and building on family strengths. Knafl & Deatrick (2002) also have discussed how the model can be used

Calgary Family Assessment and Intervention Models

Assessment of family life
  Major aspects of family life
    Structural: internal, external, social context
    Developmental: stages of family and individual development
    Functional: routines of daily living and chronic condition management
  Use of genograms and ecograms
  Intervention model for solution-focused care
    Domains of family life
      Cognitive: family and individual beliefs
      Affective: family and individual emotions
      Behavioral: family and individual activities

to develop interventions directed to helping families achieve and sustain a normalized life.

Both parents and practitioners should recognize that normalization is a process that is likely to be achieved by different strategies at different points in the child's and family's development. It also is important to bear in mind that normalization may not always be an appropriate goal and that there are times when it is necessary to focus on the condition because of an exacerbation or change in the usual treatment routine. However, a temporary focusing on the condition need not signal the end of a normal family life (Knafl & Deatrick, 2002).

Survivorship. The National Coalition on Cancer Survivorship (NCCS) has defined cancer survivorship as the experience of living with, through, and beyond a cancer diagnosis. Because family members, friends, and caregivers are greatly affected by a cancer diagnosis, people who have been diagnosed with cancer, as well as their families, friends, and caregivers, are considered survivors from the point of diagnosis and for the balance of life (NCCS). This definition of survivorship and its application are germane not only to childhood cancer, a chronic condition, but also to the entire set of chronic health conditions that can affect families.

In clinical pediatric oncology, the term "long-term survivorship" has been used to denote the phase in the illness trajectory when the child with cancer has successfully completed all recommended cancer treatment, as well as a period of intensive monitoring for recurrent disease, and is considered "cured." This does not mean that the risk for disease recurrence is nothing during long-term survivorship nor that residual effects of the disease or its treatment resolve when treatment and intensive monitoring for recurrence end. There is mounting evidence that childhood health conditions and their treatment have lifelong physical, psychologic, social, and economic effects that may be subclinical during childhood and obvious in young adulthood (Hobbie et al, 2000). Long-term complications have been observed in young people who have been successfully treated for childhood cancer as well as in their family members (Barakat et al, 1997). Beneficial long-term effects of childhood chronic health conditions have been noted, including a new appreciation for life, accelerated maturity, and enhanced relationships within the family. However, there is also evidence of adverse effects, including long-term physical complications (Chiarelli et al, 1999), cognitive impairment and learning difficulties (Challinor et al, 2000), and symptoms of posttraumatic stress, impaired general physical and mental health, and reduced quality of life (Meeske et al, 2001).

Survivorship in the clinical sense of the word has become increasingly relevant with the development of surgical cures, such as cardiac repair or solid organ transplantation, and improved medical regimens for the management of conditions such as childhood cancer, type 1 diabetes, cystic fibrosis, HIV/acquired immunodeficiency syndrome (AIDS), infectious diseases, Down syndrome, and preterm birth. As a result, more and more children with chronic health conditions are becoming long-term survivors and experiencing the implications of their disease and its treatment for themselves, their families, and their future offspring. In response to survivors' needs for lifelong medical surveillance and assistance with managing the physical, psychologic, and socioeconomic complications of their underlying condition and its treatment, programs have been developed that provide comprehensive long-term follow-up care for children who have been successfully treated (Keene, 2002), transitional care for young adult survivors (Hobbie & Ogle, 2001), and care for adult survivors of childhood cancer (Oeffinger et al, 1998). The development of these programs rests on the view that childhood cancer survivors and their families have unique needs that deserve attention from experts who have an interest in survivorship and knowledge of the usual treatments for childhood cancer and their potential long-term adverse effects. The programs have also originated from an awareness that, when seen in the clinical setting alongside children who are newly diagnosed, in active treatment, or making decisions about end-of-life care, long-term survivors' concerns are viewed as nonurgent and therefore assigned lesser priority in terms of time and attention.

Ideally, comprehensive long-term follow-up programs are located within broader academic pediatric subspecialty programs, meet at least twice monthly at a time that is distinct from the rest of the subspecialty program, are multidisciplinary in nature, and serve families, not individuals, who have survived childhood cancer. Long-term follow-up programs should also offer information about health risks that are inherent in an individual survivor's situation, anticipatory monitoring and guidance, and education about healthy lifestyle to reduce the risks and empower survivors to take charge of their health. Finally, long-term follow-up programs must include active planning for transitioning young adult survivors of childhood health conditions to care by a knowledgeable community or adult specialty health care provider who has a particular interest in issues of relevance to survivors (Harvey et al, 1999) (see Chapter 9).

Conceptual Models for Understanding Families and Guiding Practice

A number of well-established models exist to help the health care provider to understand important dimensions of the family experience of a childhood chronic condition and develop interventions that support healthy child and family functioning. These models incorporate multiple concepts in an effort to provide a comprehensive framework for guiding nursing practice and research. Stress and coping models address family functioning in the context of childhood chronic illness. In contrast, the family management model focuses more narrowly on the treatment regimen and how the family incorporates the illness into daily family life. The Calgary Assessment and Intervention Models provide a framework for intervening to help families cope with the challenges of childhood chronic illness.

Stress and Coping Models. As generally applied to the study of human responses to illness, stress and coping models utilize an information-processing perspective to explain how individuals cognitively process illness events to create meaning and adapt. Stress and coping models assume that stress is not inherent in an illness event but depends on the individual's cognitive appraisal of stress, that is, that the demands of the event exceed available personal and environmental resources. Variation in what individuals appraise as stress has been largely attributed to personal differences in internal and external characteristics and resources for coping.

The Family Resilience Framework (FRF) represents a research and clinical practice–informed derivative of stress and coping models for use with families experiencing events that are generally recognized as extreme stressors: natural disasters, interpersonal violence including war, and serious illness or chronic condition. When employed in the study of family responses to chronic conditions, FRF addresses how the family as a unit responds and adapts. The FRF assumes that no single model will fit all families or one family across time and situations. The feature that distinguishes FRF is its emphasis on strengths and protective factors and functional coping strategies, such as resilience and problem-solving communication patterns, rather than on pathology. The overarching goal for assessments and interventions derived from the FRF is the identification and development of existing and potential internal and environmental strengths and competencies to enhance family function and well-being. Some challenges to using FRF as the basis for interventions with families include the need to consider within the family unit variations in individual family members' responses to stress, effectiveness of coping strategies, and adaptation to adversity (Coleman & Ganong, 2002).

Resilience, the central construct in FRF, had previously been viewed as an impervious characteristic possessed by extraordinary individuals. Within this perspective, studies of resilient individuals highlighted the role of extrafamilial caring adults and mentors in helping resilient individuals rise above their hopelessly dysfunctional families (Walsh, 2002). Gradually, informed by research about multiple adverse conditions, resilience came to be seen as ordinary rather than exceptional, arising from the operation of normative human adaptive functions by individuals, families, and communities (Masten, 2001).

Resilience is most currently conceptualized as the dynamic process of beneficial adaptation in the context of significant stress. Resilience is the beneficial behavioral patterns and functional competencies that individuals and families demonstrate under difficult circumstances. These patterns and competencies support a family's ability to ensure the well-being of individual family members and maintain the integrity of the family as a whole (McCubbin et al, 1996). Implicit in the current conceptualizations is exposure to extreme stress and the achievement of favorable adaptation despite the stress and its inherent challenges to key developmental processes (Coleman & Ganong, 2002). The current view incorporates both ecologic and developmental perspectives, seeing the family as an open system that is influenced by the broader sociocultural context with the potential for change and growth over time. Stress emerges from interactions among individual and family vulnerabilities, life experiences, and the sociocultural context. Family distress arises from unsuccessful attempts to cope with stress. The pileup of internal and external stressors can overwhelm the family and heighten risk for future problems (McCubbin & Patterson, 1983).

According to the FRF, assessment is multisystemic and should attend to concurrent and multiple family stressors over time, multigenerational influences, family processes for coping with adversity, and family functioning in the context of both normative and unpredictable stressful events. Interventions can be focused at the level of the individual, couple, family, multiple family groups, or the larger system, for example, school and health care systems, depending on the relevance of the system level to resolution of the problem. In the present view, parents, rather than extrafamilial adults, are the key mediators of individual and family stress and a focus of interventions to enhance family resilience. The current perspective recognizes growth as a potential outcome of stress or adversity and emphasizes preventive and intervention efforts that enhance families' abilities to not only overcome specific current challenges but also broadly apply their skills and resources to handle future situations more effectively (Walsh, 2002).

The stressors associated with serious pediatric chronic conditions pose a significant challenge to families and require considerable amounts of resilience and other resources for functional coping, adaptation, and growth. The FRF is then a suitable framework for studying family responses to chronic childhood conditions and designing strength-based interventions to promote functional family coping in the context of serious childhood chronic conditions. There is evidence of the utility of the FRF in studying the predictors of functional family coping with the stressors and demands associated with the diagnosis and active treatment phases of childhood cancer (McCubbin et al, 2002). Six resilience factors for families of children with cancer have been identified: (1) rapid mobilization and reorganization; (2) support from the health care team in the form of availability, information, and respect; (3) support from extended family in the form of respite care, transportation, and emotional support; (4) support from the community in the form of financial assistance, home maintenance, and emotional assistance; (5) support from the workplace in the form of flexible scheduling, time off, and job assurance; and (6) personal and family beliefs that allowed a focus on the positive. These factors indicate areas for assessment of resilience in families of children with serious health conditions, as well as targets for interventions to promote resilience and functional coping with serious childhood chronic illness (McCubbin et al, 2002).

Family Management Models. Much of the research in an earlier section of the chapter on the evidence base for practice addressed the identification of specific variables associated with child and family response to chronic conditions. However, Fisher & colleagues (2000, p. 54) have argued that it often is difficult to translate knowledge of specific variables into practice, since "for the clinician to apply customized interventions with relevance to individual patients, it may be more important to identify patterns and profiles of disease management than to review each disease management indicator separately." Following Fisher's lead, in recent years there has been a growing interest in uncovering patterns of family response to childhood chronic conditions and developing typologies of response that can be used to guide individualized interventions. Because they are based on multiple aspects of family life, typologies have the advantage of preserving and conveying how the family as a unit responds to a chronic condition.

Over the past 40 years, a number of investigators have identified patterns or typologies of response to childhood chronic conditions. For example, Davis (1963) reported two overarching patterns of response (normalization, disassociation), and Darling (1979) identified four patterns of response (normalization, altruism, crusadership, resignation). Both these typologies support the observation made in the previous section on normalization that some but not all families report being able to lead a normal family life despite their child's illness. More recently, Chesla (1991) developed a typology of caring practices in families in which a young adult had schizophrenia that included engaged, conflicted, managed, and distanced caring. Her work indicates that families develop varying strategies for accomplishing the work of managing a member's chronic condition.

Building on early efforts to identify typologies of family response to chronic conditions, Knafl & Deatrick (1990) formulated the Family Management Style Framework (FMSF) to guide research efforts directed toward further typology development as well as clinical assessment of families in which there is a child with a chronic condition. Since the initial publication of the FMSF, subsequent studies by the developers and others have provided evidence of the usefulness of the framework for identifying important elements and specifying different patterns of family illness management.

As noted above, the FMSF is composed of three conceptual dimensions: definition of the situation, management behaviors, and perceived consequences. *Definition of the situation* is the subjective meaning family members attribute to important elements of their situation. *Management behaviors* are the discrete behavioral accommodations that family members use to manage the condition on a daily basis. These include efforts directed to caring for the condition as well as those aimed at adapting family life to condition-related demands. Definitions of the situation and management behaviors are highly interrelated with the definition of the situation influencing which management behaviors are adopted. At the same time, the *perceived consequences* of the condition influence definitions of the situation and management behaviors. The framework conceptualizes sociocultural context as family members' subjective perceptions of factors influencing their approach to illness management. At any point, family members may identify sociocultural influences, such as past experiences with health care providers, culturally based beliefs about illness, or family rules and boundaries as exerting an influence on how they define and

manage their child's chronic condition and how they perceive its consequences.

The most current version of the framework (Knafl & Deatrick, in press) conceptualizes family management style (FMS) as the pattern formed by individual family members' definitions of the situation, management behaviors, and perceived illness consequences. The FMSF directs the researcher or clinician to focus on how family members are actively engaged in the management of the illness and how their subjective views of their situation and the impact of the chronic condition on family life shape their management efforts. The framework takes into account the definitions of the situation, management behaviors, and perceived consequences of all or a subset of family members. The actual management style is the pattern formed across family members. Family members' perceptions of sociocultural factors shape the FMS, which, in turn, interacts with individual and family functioning.

Research across a broad range of chronic conditions has contributed to the further specification of themes that comprise the three major components of the framework. These themes are summarized in Table 3-1. The themes defined in Table 3-1 are based on research with families experiencing varied chronic conditions and can guide assessment (Knafl & Deatrick, in press). By questioning families about the four themes in the definition component, the clinician develops a comprehensive understanding of the family's beliefs about the child, the condition, and their ability to work as a family unit to manage the condition. The management behavior themes provide insights into the extent to which condition management is

TABLE 3-1

Major Components and Conceptual Themes of the Family Management Style Framework

Conceptual Component	Conceptual Themes
Definition of the Situation	**Child identity:** Parents' views of the child and the extent to which those views focus on illness or normalcy and capabilities or vulnerabilities **Illness view:** Parents' beliefs about the cause, seriousness, predictability, and course of the illness **Management mindset:** Parents' views of the ease or difficulty of carrying out the treatment regimen and their ability to manage effectively **Parental mutuality:** Parents' beliefs about the extent to which they have shared or discrepant views of the child, the illness, their parenting philosophy, and their approach to illness management
Management Behaviors	**Parenting philosophy:** Parents' goals, priorities, and values that guide the overall approach and specific strategies for illness management **Management approach:** Parents' assessment of the extent to which they have developed a routine and related strategies for managing the illness and incorporating it into family life
Perceived Consequences	**Family focus:** Parents' assessment of the balance between illness management and other aspects of family life **Future expectation:** Parents' assessment of the implications of the illness for their child's and family's future

guided by a particular set of goals and has been integrated into everyday family routines. Questions addressing the perceived consequences themes provide information on whether the condition is viewed as foreground or background in family life and if family members see the condition as shaping their child's and their family's future. An understanding of how these themes are manifested in individual families contributes to the practitioner's understanding of both family strengths and areas of difficulty with regard to condition management. For example, assessment may reveal that parents' lack of mutuality with regard to their view of the child is the source of considerable conflict in the family and it is this conflict that leads to the condition being the focus of family life. In this case, work with the family may focus on resolving parental conflicts or referral to counseling. On the other hand, assessment may reveal that parents have shared views of the child, the illness, and their management goals but are struggling to develop a routine that accommodates the treatment regimen and other family life responsibilities. Based on this assessment, the practitioner might decide to direct interventions to developing a flexible condition management routine that lessens the family's focus on illness management. The FMSF provides a structure for identifying areas of strength and difficulty related to important aspects of families' illness management efforts.

Assessment and Intervention Models. For over 25 years, faculty associated with the Family Nursing Unit of the University of Calgary nursing program have provided direct care to families experiencing a member's chronic condition and training for practitioners interested in applying the Calgary assessment and intervention models. The models have been described in major publications (Wright & Leahey, 2000; Wright et al, 1996), and additional training is available through videotapes and an annual externship program. Detailed information about programs and resources can be found on the Web site for the Family Nursing Unit (www.ucalgary.ca/nu/fnu/html).

Directed toward practitioners in a variety of primary care settings (community, pediatric, maternity, mental health), the Calgary models were intended to be practical guidelines for practitioners committed to providing family-centered nursing care (Box 3-8). The Calgary Family Assessment Model (CFAM) and Family Intervention Model (CFIM) are grounded in core assumptions about the nature of family-practitioner relationships (Leahey & Harper-Jaques, 1996) as well as a number of theoretic constructs, including systems, communication, and change theories. The underlying assumptions emphasize the reciprocal, nonhierarchic nature of the family-practitioner relationship. Following these models, it is assumed that both practitioners and families have important areas of expertise related to the family's illness experiences, that there is no single, correct solution to any problem, and that practitioners and family members work together to construct solutions to condition-related problems. The theoretic underpinnings of the models support a view of reality as socially constructed and changing through the course of human interaction. Although the family unit is the focus of these models, the developers acknowledge that family assessment and intervention often are occurring in concert.

The intent of the CFAM is to provide a "map of the family . . . so that family strengths and problems can be identified"

(Wright & Leahey, 2000). Assessment occurs across three major aspects of family life: structural, developmental, and functional. Wright & Leahey (2000) specify categories of data that might be relevant in each area and provide examples of questions that could be used to elicit data. For example, structural family data include information on the internal family (e.g., composition, subsystems), the external family (e.g., extended family, other systems), and the family's social context (e.g., ethnicity, spirituality). Developmental assessment directs the practitioner's attention to the tasks associated with different stages of the family's life cycle. Functional assessment focuses on routine aspects of daily living such as meal preparation and treatment regimen management as well as the roles and interactions associated with carrying out usual family activities.

CFAM offers a comprehensive "menu of possibilities" for assessment, and the practitioner is advised to be selective in determining what are relevant and appropriate areas for assessment. For example, the assessment of developmental issues may be especially relevant in a family of a child with diabetes who is making the transition to adolescence. On the other hand, functional assessment targeting the family's usual routine may be more appropriate in families who are having difficulty carrying out a prescribed treatment regimen. Wright & Leahey (2000) advocate the use of family genograms and ecomaps as useful strategies for engaging families in the assessment process and eliciting considerable information about key aspects of family life. The genogram is a diagram of the family tree, usually including three generations of family members. The ecomap is a diagram of each family member's ties to persons and systems outside the family. Taken together, the genogram and ecomap efficiently summarize considerable information about the family's internal and external structure.

The CFIM is a problem- and solution-focused approach for promoting or sustaining family functioning in the context of a condition-related challenge. CFIM is not a long-term therapy approach, and its focus on solving current problems makes it a useful tool for the primary care practitioner. CFIM assumes that families have the ability to solve their own problems related to living with a chronic condition and that the role of the provider is to offer, rather than prescribe, possibly helpful solutions. The model conceptualizes interventions as taking place across three domains of family life: cognitive, affective, and behavioral. Cognitive interventions target family beliefs that make living with the condition more difficult. For example, the practitioner might note parents' firmly held beliefs about the fatal nature of cancer and provide information on survivorship programs in order to change beliefs about the condition and lessen fears about the future. Wright & Leahey (2000) note that commendations that identify family strengths are especially powerful cognitive interventions, which help family members form a more positive view of themselves and their ability to address health-related problems.

In contrast to cognitive interventions, which focus on family beliefs, affective interventions focus on decreasing emotional response to the condition as a way that sets the stage for effective problem solving. For example, acknowledging the normalcy of an intense emotional response can help family members consider when such responses are appropriate and when they impede problem solving. The third category of interventions, behavioral, invites family members to do certain things, such as become more directly involved in condition care or take a respite from caregiving, both of which can contribute to a parent's sense of competence as a caregiver.

Wright & Leahey (2000, p. 159) point out that questions that encourage families to think about their situation in new ways can be "one of the most powerful interventions for families experiencing health problems." For example, family members can be asked to speculate regarding how different members of the family view this situation or to consider the hypothetic outcomes of managing the condition in a different way. Questions such as these can set the stage for discussing differences that are a source of conflict among family members as well as possibilities for changing current problematic behaviors.

As the Calgary models have developed and been used by practitioners in various settings, researchers have begun to test their effectiveness and explore the ways in which they support family functioning. Robinson (1996) interviewed family members who had been clients on the Calgary family nursing unit in order to understand their perceptions of how their interactions with the practitioner addressed problems with managing the condition. Family members noted that the practitioner's ability to ask relevant questions, to balance closeness and distance, to remain nonjudgmental, and to mirror family strengths all contributed to positive changes in the family's ability to adapt to the illness. For primary care practitioners interacting with families in which a child has a chronic illness, the Calgary assessment and intervention models can provide a practical, comprehensive guide that promotes both problem solving and a positive working relationship between the practitioner and the family.

The Family and Primary Care

The challenges presented by chronic conditions for primary care practitioners are clearly different from those facing the family. For the practitioner, the challenge is identifying interventions that contribute to optimal child and family adaptation. The research, concepts, and frameworks presented in this chapter provide useful knowledge and tools for understanding families and developing interventions to promote optimal child and family functioning. However, knowledge alone does not guarantee a positive working relationship between the primary care provider and the family. The quality of the interactions between the practitioner and the family, as well as the nature of the interventions, is critical to establishing a positive working relationship. Robinson (1996) found that the effectiveness of interventions to help families identify and build on their strengths was linked to interactions that family members viewed as nonjudgmental and appropriate in terms of balancing closeness and distance. Other authors have noted the interplay between the interactional and more technical dimensions of health care. For example, Hobbs et al (1985, p. 238) identified five basic skills needed by professionals who work with families. These are the "ability to provide technically competent care, to communicate with families, to participate as an effective team member, to be sensitive to ethical issues, and to conceptualize problems in ecological terms." Their emphasis on

taking an ecologic perspective mirrors the focus of this chapter. Chronic conditions in childhood are best understood and cared for in the context of the child's family, while taking into account the family's particular sociocultural situation. Hobbs et al (1985) point out that the ability to communicate with families in a sensitive, concerned manner and to include families as members of the health care team is an especially important aspect of care. The five basic skills identified for professionals mirror the kinds of behavioral and interactional competencies valued by parents (Knafl et al, 1992; Robinson, 1996) and are consistent with the core principles of family-centered health care. Primary care practitioners are well positioned to make an important contribution to the family's ability to adapt to the challenges of a child's condition in a way that sustains the child's and family's quality of life.

REFERENCES

Amer, K. (1999). Children's adaptation to insulin dependent diabetes mellitus: A critical review of the literature. *Pediatr Nurs, 25*, 627-641.
American Psychiatric Association. (1994). *Diagnostic and statistical manual of mental disorders: DSM IV* (4th ed.). Washington, DC: Author.
American Psychiatric Association. (2000). *Diagnostic statistical manual of mental disorders: DSM IV-TR* (5th ed.). Washington, DC: Author.
Austin, J. (1991). Family adaptation to a child's chronic illness. *Annu Rev Nurs Res*, 103-120.
Austin, J., & Sims, S. (1998). Integrative review of assessment models for examining children's and families' responses to chronic illness. In M. Broome, K. Knafl, K. Pridham, & S. Feetham (Eds.), *Children and Families in Health and Illness*. Thousand Oaks, CA: Sage.
Barakat, L., Kazak, A., Meadows, A., Casey, R., Meeske, K., et al. (1997). Families surviving childhood cancer: Comparison of posttraumatic stress symptoms with families of healthy children. *J Pediatr Psychol, 22*, 843-859.
Bisson, J. (2002). Post-traumatic stress disorder. In S. Barton (Ed.), *Clinical evidence* (7th ed., pp. 177-178). London: BMJ Publishing Group.
Bohachick, P., & Anton, B.B. (1990). Psychosocial adjustment of patients and spouses to severe cardiomyopathy. *Res Nurs Health, 13*(6), 385-392.
Burke, S., Kauffman, E., Harrison, M., & Wiskin, N. (1999). Assessment of stressors in families with a child who has a chronic condition. *MCN, The Journal of Maternal/Child Nursing, 24*(2), 98-106.
Campbell, T. (2000). Physical illness: Challenges to families. In P. McKenry & S. Price (Eds.), *Families and change: Coping with stressful events and transitions*. Thousand Oaks, CA: Sage.
Challinor, J., Miaskowski, C., Moore, I., Slaughter, R., & Franck, L. (2000). Review of research studies that evaluated the impact of childhood cancer survivors on neurocognitions and behavioral social competence: Nursing implications. *J Soc Pediatr Nurs, 5*, 57-74.
Chesla, C. (1991). Parents caring practices for the schizophrenic offspring. *Qual Health Res, 1*(4), 446-468.
Chiarelli, A., Marrett, L., & Darlington, G. (1999). Early menopause and infertility in females after treatment for childhood cancer diagnosed in 1964-1988 in Ontario Canada. *Am J Epidemiol, 150*, 245-254.
Clarke-Steffen, L. (1993a). A model of the family transition to living with childhood cancer. *Cancer Pract, 1*(4), 285-292.
Clarke-Steffen, L. (1993b). Waiting and not knowing: The diagnosis of cancer in a child. *J Pediatr Oncol Nurs, 10*(4), 146-153.
Clarke-Steffen, L. (1997). Reconstructing reality: Family strategies for managing childhood cancer. *J Pediatr Nurs, 12*(5), 278-287.
Clawson, J. (1996). A child with chronic illness and the process of family adaptation. *J Pediatr Nurs, 11*, 52-60.
Cohen, M. (1993a). Diagnostic closure and the spread of uncertainty. *Issues Compr Pediatr Nurs, 16*, 135-146.
Cohen, M. (1993b). The unknown and the unknowable—managing sustained uncertainty. *West J Nurs Res, 15*(1), 77-96.
Cohen, M. (1995a). The stages of the prediagnostic period in chronic, life threatening childhood illness: A process analysis. *Res Nurs Health, 18*, 39-48.
Cohen, M. (1995b). The triggers of heightened parental uncertainty in chronic, life-threatening childhood illness. *Qual Health Res, 5*(1), 63-77.

Cohen, M. & Martinson, I. (1988). Chronic uncertainty: Its effects on parental appraisal of a child's health. *J Pediatr Nurs, 3*(2), 89-96.

Coleman, M. & Ganong, L. (2002). Resilience and families. *Fam Relat, 51*, 101-102.

Comaroff, J., & Maguire, P. (1981). Ambiguity and the search for meaning: Childhood leukemia in the modern clinical context. *Soc Sci Med, 15B*, 115-123.

Committee on Children with Disabilities and Committee on Adolescence. (1996). Transition of care provided for adolescents with special health care needs. *Pediatrics, 98*, 1203-1206.

Cornman, B. (1993). Childhood cancer: Differential effects on the family members. *Oncol Nurs Forum, 20*(10), 1559-1566.

Darling, R. (1979). *Families against society: A study of reactions to children with birth defects.* Beverly Hills, CA: Sage.

Dashiff, C.J. (1993). Parents' perceptions of diabetes in adolescent daughters and its impact on the family. *J Pediatr Nurs, 8*(6), 361-369.

Davis, F. (1963). *Passage through crisis: Polio victims and their families.* Minneapolis: Bobbs-Merrill.

Deatrick, J., Knafl, K., & Murphy-Moore, C. (1999). Clarifying the concept of normalization. *Image. The Journal of Nursing Scholarship, 31*(3), 209-214.

Donnelly, E. (1994). Parents of children with asthma: An examination of family hardiness, family stressors, and family functioning. *J Pediatr Nurs, 9*(6), 398-408.

Faux, S. (1998). Historical overview of responses of children and their families to chronic illness. In M. Broome, K. Knafl, K. Pridham, & S. Feetham (Ed.), *Children and Families in Health and Illness* (pp. 179-195). Thousand Oaks, CA: Sage.

Faux, S. & Seideman, R. (1996). Health care professionals and their relationships with families who have members with developmental disabilities. *J Child Fam Nurs, 2*(2), 217-238.

Feetham, S.L. (1997). Families and health in the urban environment: Implications for programs, research and policy. In O. Reyes, H. Wallberg, & R. Weissberg (Eds.), *Children and youth: Interdisciplinary perspectives* (pp. 321-362). Thousand Oaks, CA: Sage.

Ferrell, B., Rhiner, M., Shapiro, B., & Dierkes, M. (1994). The experience of pediatric cancer pain, Part I: Impact of pain on the family. *J Pediatr Nurs, 9*(6), 368-379.

Fisher, L., Chesla, C., Skaff, M., Gilliss, C., Kanter, R., Lutz, C., & Bartz, R. (2000). Disease management status: A typology of Latino and Euro-American Patients with type 2 diabetes. *Behav Med, 26*, 53-65.

Gallo, A.M. Breitmayer, B., Knafl, K., & Zoeller, L. (1991). Well siblings of children with chronic illness: Parents' reports of their psychological adjustment. *Pediatr Nurs, 18*(23-27).

Gallo, A.M. (1990). Family management style in juvenile diabetes: A case illustration. *J Pediatr Nurs, 5*(1), 23-32.

Gallo, A.M. & Knafl, K. (1998). Parents' reports of "tricks of the trade" for managing childhood chronic illness. *J Soc Pediatr Nurs, 3*(3), 93-100.

Gilliss, C. & Knafl, K. (1999). Nursing care of families in non-normative transitions: The state of the science and practice. In A. Hinshaw, S. Feetham, & J. Shaver (Eds.), *Handbook for clinical nursing research.* Newbury Park, CA: Sage.

Goffman, E. (1963). *Stigma: Notes on the management of spoiled identity.* Englewood Cliffs, NJ: Lawrence Erlbaum Associates.

Grey, M., Cameron, M., & Lipman, T. (1995). Psychosocial status of children with diabetes over the first two years. *Diabetes Care, 18*, 1330-1336.

Hamlett, K., Pellegrini, D., & Katz, S. (1992). Childhood chronic illness as a family stressor. *J Pediatr Psychol, 17*(1), 33-47.

Harvey, J., Hobbie, W., Shaw, S., & Bottomley, S. (1999). Providing quality care in childhood cancer survivorship: Learning from the past, looking to the future. *J Pediatr Oncol Nurs, 17*, 268-273.

Hatton, D.L., Canam, C., Thorne, S., & Hughes, A.M. (1995). Parents' perceptions of caring for an infant of toddler with diabetes. *J Adv Nurs, 22*, 569-577.

Hinds, P., Birenbaum, L., Clarke-Steffen, L., Quargnenti, A., Kreissman, S., et al. (1996). Coming to terms: Parents' response to a first cancer recurrence in their child. *Nurs Res, 45*(3), 148-153.

Hobbie, W. & Ogle, S. (2001). Transitional care for young adult survivors of childhood cancer. *Semin Oncol Nurs, 17*, 268-273.

Hobbie, W., Stuber, M., Meeske, K., Wissler, K., Rourke, M., et al. (2000). Symptoms of post-traumatic stress in young adult survivors of childhood cancer. *J Clin Oncol, 18*, 4060-4066.

Hobbs, N., Perrin, J., & Ireys, H. (1985). *Chronically ill children and their families.* San Francisco: Jossey-Bass.

Horner, S.D. (1998). Catching the asthma: Family care for school-aged children with asthma. *J Pediatr Nurs, 13*(6), 356-366.

Institute, N.C. (2002). [online]. Available: http://dccps.nci.nih.gov/ocs/about.html.

Jessop, D.J. & Stein, R.E. (1985). Uncertainty and its relation to the psychological and social correlates of chronic illness in children. *Soc Sci Med, 20*(10), 993-999.

Kazak, A.E., Stuber, M.L., Barakat, L.P., Meeske, K., Guthrie, D., et al. (1998). Predicting posttraumatic stress symptoms in mothers and fathers of survivors of childhood cancers. *J Am Acad Child Adolesc Psychiatry, 37*(8), 823-831.

Keene, N. (2002). 2002's top follow-up clinics for childhood cancer survivors [online]. Available: http://www.patientcenters.com/press/follow-up.clinics.html.

Kessler, R. (2000). Posttraumatic stress disorder: The burden to the individual and society. *J Clin Psychiatry, 61S5*, 4-12.

Knafl, K. Breitmayer, B., Gallo, A., & Zoeller, L. (1992). Parents' views of health care providers: An exploration of the components of a positive working relationship. *Child Health Care, 21*, 90-95.

Knafl, K. & Deatrick, J. (1990). Family management style: Concept analysis and development. *J Pediatr Nurs, 5*(1), 4-14.

Knafl, K. & Deatrick, J. (2002). The challenge of normalization for families of children with chronic conditions. *Pediatr Nurs, 28*, 49-53.

Knafl, K. & Gilliss, C. (2002). Families and chronic illness: A synthesis of current literature. *J Fam Nurs, 8*, 178-198.

Koocher, G.P. (1985). Psychosocial care of the child cured of cancer. *Pediatr Nurs, 11*(2), 91-93.

Kopp, M., Richter, R., Rainer, J., Kopp-Wilfing, P. R., G., & Walter, M. (1995). Differences in family functioning between patients with chronic headache and patients with chronic low back pain. *Pain, 63*(2), 219-224.

Lavigne, J.V. & Faier-Routman, J. (1992). Psychological adjustment to pediatric physical disorders: A meta- analytic review. *J Pediatr Psychol, 17*(2), 133-157.

Leahey, M. & Harper-Jaques, S. (1996). Family-nurse relationships: Core assumptions and clinical implications. *J Child Fam Nurs, 2*(2), 133-151.

LoBato, D., Faust, D., & Spirito, A. (1988). Examining the effects of chronic disease and disability on children's sibling relationships. *J Pediatr Psychol, 13*, 389-407.

Masten, A. (2001). Ordinary magic: Resilience processes in development. *Am Psychol, 56*, 227-238.

McCubbin, H., Thompson, A., & McCubbin, M. (1996). *Family assessment: Resiliency, coping, and adaptation.* Madison, WI: University of Wisconsin Publishers.

McCubbin, M., Balling, K., Possin, P., Frierdich, S., & Byrne, B. (2002). Family resiliency in childhood cancer. *Fam Relat, 51*, 103-111.

McCubbin, M. & Patterson, J. (1983). The family stress process: The double helix ABCX model of adjustment and adaptation. In H. McCubbin, M. Sussman & J. Patterson (Eds.), *Social stress and the family: Advances in family stress theory and research* (pp. 7-38). New York: Haworth.

McLoyd, L. (1998). Socioeconomic disadvantage and child development. *Am Psychol, 53*, 185-204.

Meeske, K., Ruccione, K., Globe, D., & Stuber, M. (2001). Posttraumatic stress, quality of life and psychological distress in young adult survivors of childhood cancer. *Oncol Nurs Forum, 28*, 481-489.

Mishel, M. (1981). The measurement of uncertainty in illness. *Nurs Res, 30*, 258-263.

Mishel, M. (1988). Uncertainty in illness. *Image: Journal of Nursing Scholarship, 20*, 225-232.

Mishel, M. (1990). Reconceptualization of uncertainty in illness theory. *Image: Journal of Nursing Scholarship, 22*, 256-262.

Mishel, M. (1997). *Uncertainty in Illness Scale manual.* Chapel Hill, NC: University of North Carolina.

Mishel, M. (1999). Uncertainty in chronic illness. *Annu Rev Nurs Res, 17*, 269-294.

Mishel, M.H. (1983). Parents' perceptions of uncertainty concerning their hospitalized child. *Nurs Res, 32*, 324-330.

Moore, L. (1998). People like that are only people here: Canonical babbling in Peed Onk. *Birds of America* (pp. 212-250). New York: Knopf.

Morris, J., Blount, R., Cohen, L., Frank, N., Madan-Swain, A., et al. (1997). Family functioning and behavioral adjustment in children with leukemia and their healthy peers. *Child Health Care, 26*(2), 61-75.

National Coalition for Cancer Survivors. The organization. Retrieved June 6, 2003 from http://www.canceradvocacy.org/about/org1.

Nehring, W., Lashley, F., & Malm, K. (2000). Disclosing the diagnosis of pediatric HIV infection: Mothers' views. *J Soc Pediatr Nurs, 5*, 5-15.

Newacheck, P.W. (1998). Prevalence and impact of disabling chronic conditions in childhood. *Am J Public Health, 88*(4), 610-617.

Oeffinger, K., Eshelman, D., Tomlinson, G., & Buchanan, G. (1998). Programs for adults survivors of childhood cancer. *J Clin Oncol, 28*, 481-489.

Park, E.S. & Martinson, I.M. (1998). Socioemotional experiences of Korean families with asthmatic children. *J Child Fam Nurs, 4*, 291-308.

Patterson, J., Jernell, J., Leonard, B., & Titus, J. (1994). Caring for medically fragile children at home: The parent-professional relationship. *J Pediatr Nurs, 9*(2), 98-106.

Perrin, E., Ayoub, C., & Willet, J. (1993). In the eyes of the beholder: Family and maternal influences on perceptions of adjustment of children with a chronic illness. *J Dev Behav Pediatr, 14*(2), 94-105.

Rehm, R.S. & Catanzaro, M.L. (1998). "It's just a fact of life": Family members' perceptions of parental chronic illness. *J Child Fam Nurs, 4*(1), 21-40.

Robinson, C.A. (1993). Managing life with a chronic condition: the story of normalization. *Qual Health Res, 3*(1), 6-28.

Robinson, C.A. (1996). Health care relationships revisited. *J Child Fam Nurs, 2*, 152-173.

Rolland, J. (1984). Toward a psychosocial typology of chronic and life threatening illness. *Fam Syst Med., 2*, 245-262.

Rolland, J. (1994). *Families, illness, and disability. An integrative treatment model.* New York: Basic Books.

Santacroce, S. (2000). Support from health care providers and parental uncertainty during the diagnosis of perinatally-acquired HIV infection. *J Assoc Nurses AIDS Care, 22*, 63-75.

Santacroce, S. (2001). Measurement of parental uncertainty during the diagnosis phase of life- threatening illness in a child. *J Pediatr Oncol Nurs, 19*, 104-111.

Santacroce, S. (2002). Uncertainty, anxiety, and symptoms of posttraumatic stress in parents of children recently diagnosed with cancer. *J Pediatr Oncol Nurs, 19*, 104-111.

Santacroce, S. (2003). Parental uncertainty and symptoms of posttraumatic stress in serious childhood illness. *J Nurs Scholarship, 35*, 45-51.

Santacroce, S., Deatrick, J., & Ledlie, S. (2002). Redefining treatment: How biological mothers manage their children's treatment for perinatally acquired HIV. *Aids Care: Psychological and Socio-Medical Aspects of AIDS/HIV, 14*, 247-260.

Sawyer, E.H. (1992). Family functioning when children have cystic fibrosis. *J Child Fam Nurs, 7*(5), 304-311.

Sharkey, T. (1995). The effects of uncertainty in families with children who are chronically ill. *Home Health Nurse, 13*(4), 37-42.

Sparacino, P.S., Tong, E.M., Messias, D.K., Foote, D., Chesla, C.A., & Gilliss, C.L. (1997). The dilemmas of parents of adolescents and young adults with congenital heart disease. *Heart Lung, 26*, 187-195.

Stein, R.E. & Jessop, D. (1982). A non-categorical approach to chronic childhood illness. *Public Health Rep, 97*, 354-362.

Stewart, J. & Mishel, M. (2000). Uncertainty in childhood illness: A synthesis of the parent and child literature. *Scholarly Inquiry for Nursing Practice: An International Journal, 14*, 299-319.

Survivors, National Coalition for Cancer Survivorship (NCCS) (2002). Available online at http://www.canceradvocacy.org.

Thompson, R., Armstrong, F., Kronenberger, W., Scott, D., McCabe, M., et al. (1999). Family functioning, neurocognitive functioning, and behavior problems in children with sickle cell disease. *J Pediatr Psychol, 24*(6), 491-498.

Wallander, J. & Varni, J. (1998). Effects of pediatric chronic physical disorders on child and family adjustment. *J Child Psychol Psychiatr, 39*, 29-46.

Walsh, F. (2002). A family resilience framework: Innovative practice applications. *Fam Relat, 51*, 130-137.

Wright, L. & Leahey, M. (2000). *Nurses and families: A guide to family assessment and intervention* (3rd ed.). Philadelphia: F.A. Davis.

Wright, L., Watson, W., & Bell, J. (1996). *Beliefs: The heart of healing in families and illness.* New York: Basic Books.

Youngblut, J.M., Brennan, P., & Swegart, L. (1994). Families with medically fragile children: An exploratory study. *Pediatr Nurs, 20*(5), 463-468.

4 Family Culture and Chronic Conditions

Roberta S. Rehm

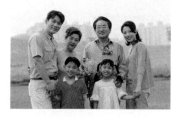

Historic Roots of Diversity

Because America has a long and complex multicultural heritage, it is important for health care providers to understand the roles that culture plays in modern US society in order to provide sensitive and appropriate care for children and families from diverse cultural backgrounds. The components of cultural identity are complex and vary even among people of the same ethnic, racial, or religious group. This chapter explores the interaction of culture and health care and discusses the cultural implications for providing care to children with chronic conditions and their families.

North American Multicultural Heritage

The early seventeenth century English Pilgrims are the best known of the early permanent immigrants to the United States, but explorers, refugees, and immigrants seeking a better life began arriving on North American lands long before the Pilgrims. Scientists believe that humans began migrating to North America from Asia across the Bering land bridge perhaps 12,000 years ago and may be ancestors of some of the peoples now called Native Americans or American Indians (Jordan, 2001). Although the exact history of the earliest settlers varies according to each tribe's origination myths, it is certain that migration has always been an important factor in US history. Spanish conquistadors began exploring what would become the American Southwest in the early sixteenth century. They led the first permanent colonial era settlers, who arrived in New Mexico in 1598. This group of 800 colonists consisted mostly of natives of Spain or Portugal but also included Mexican Indians and Africans who were servants to the soldiers and settlers (Preston, 1998).

The foreign-born portion of the US population reached its peak at 14.7% in 1910. In 2000, foreign-born US residents constituted 10.4% of the total population, or 28.4 million people (Lollock, 2001). Europeans made up the largest percentage of immigrants to the United States from 1820 (when formal immigration records began) until 1970. Since then the proportion of Hispanic and Asian immigrants has grown significantly. In 2000, 15.3% of immigrants came from Europe; 25.5% from Asia; and 51% from Latin America. Of the 51% Latin American immigrants, 34.5% came from Mexico and Central America, 9.9% from the Caribbean, and 6% from South America. Besides these legal entrants, about 275,000 immigrants illegally enter the United States each year. Although this number has dropped since the early 1990s, about 5 million undocumented immigrants still reside in the United States (US Immigration and Naturalization Service, 2001). In the past decade, the number of children in immigrant families has grown seven times faster than the number in families born in the United States; moreover, immigrant children are less likely to have a regular source of health care and less likely to have health insurance than native-born children (Guendelman et al, 2001).

Dynamic Nature of Culture

These trends in immigration reflect the changing face of our society and the dynamic nature of American culture. It was once presumed that most immigrants would give up traditional values, languages, and ways of life to join the "melting pot" of US society, but scholars now recognize that the melting pot is an American myth. Chandler & colleagues (1999) found, however, that over a 20-year period there was a convergence of values in many areas of life between whites and Mexican Americans, perhaps reflecting mutual influence and changes in American society as a whole. In reality the United States is a multicultural nation with an immensely heterogeneous population. There are many—not one—American cultures, and no one set of values and practices clearly defines the United States. Increasing migration around the world in the last decade has contributed to the heterogeneity of many nations. Women and children now constitute the largest portion of transnational migrants around the world (McGuire, 1998).

Culture can be characterized in terms of customs and behaviors exhibited in people's everyday lives, or it can be defined in complex terms that account for tradition, history, recurrent patterns, and common values (Giger & Davidhizar, 1999; O'Hagan, 1999; Roper & Shapira, 2000). Important definitions of cultural terms are found in Table 4-1. Definitions of culture must be fluid enough to recognize that although all cultural groups have commonalties, there is a great deal of intracultural variation.

Cultural identity can influence health and lifestyles affecting health. Airhihenbuwa et al (2000) found that people with a strong identity as black or bicultural were likely to make positive health choices such as lower fat diets and not smoking. Racial identity and ethnic identity form strong components of culture, but many people may identify more with cultural subgroups based on less obvious factors than ethnic or racial identity (Adams & Markus, 2001). Among the shared understandings that constitute cultural subgroups are those based on factors such as religious beliefs or affiliation (e.g., fundamentalist Christian, Sunni Muslim), physical ability (e.g., mobility impairment, athletic nature), sexual preference or identity (e.g., heterosexual, lesbian), occupation (e.g., plumber, accountant), educational attainment (e.g., illiterate, college student),

TABLE 4-1

Definitions of Cultural Terms

Culture	A dynamic and negotiated social construction arising from interaction and resulting in shared understandings among people in contact with one another
Race	Originally, it was human biologic variation, but racial mixing has given the term little biologic significance; race retains social and political significance and may reflect individual or group identity factors
Ethnicity	A socially, culturally, and/or politically constructed group of individuals that holds a set of characteristics in common; often based on language, national origin, and/or religion
Racism	An oppressive system of racial relations justified by an ideology in which one racial group benefits from dominating another and defines itself and others through this domination
Institutional racism	Intentional or unintentional manipulation or tolerance of institutional policies that unfairly restrict the opportunities of particular groups
Ethnocentrism	The belief that one's own ways are the best or preferred way to think, believe, or behave
Prejudice	Preconceived ideas or opinions about an individual or group based solely on factors such as race, gender, or physical ability
Discrimination	Different treatment, including restricted opportunities or choices, of people because of factors such as race, class, or physical ability

socioeconomic status (e.g., inherited wealth, homeless), and women's issues (e.g., feminism, maternal status) (Betancourt et al, 2002).

Religious and Spiritual Influences

Religious and spiritual beliefs are among the most powerful forces that shape human experience. Health care providers for children can incorporate exploration of families' spiritual beliefs into health maintenance visits (McEvoy, 2000), although it must be recognized that many families are not overtly religious and may not characterize themselves as religious or spiritual at all (Draper & McSherry, 2002). Specific belief systems vary widely and are even sometimes directly contradictory, yet religious faith and spiritual beliefs often provide a sense of comfort, strength, and direction for families coping with concerns about health and illness (Coyle, 2002; Rehm, 1999). Spirituality is a concept that includes practices and beliefs that give meaning to life and help an individual to cultivate inner strength to meet the challenges of daily life (Andrews & Hanson, 1999). Spirituality may be expressed in an organized religious setting with formal rituals of prayer and worship or more independently with individual practices. Both organized religious belief systems and spirituality that arises from life experiences may provide a set of values by which life can be lived.

Chronic conditions of childhood may present particular challenges for families, especially in the face of children's suffering, the need for ongoing care, and the possibility of disability or death. Many families seek an explanation for these difficulties in religious beliefs; others use their beliefs to find solace or strength to face the future. One study found that Mexican-American parents recognized three key influences

in determining the outcome of their child's chronic condition: God, family, and health care providers (Rehm, 1999). Although these parents gave the ultimate authority to God, they felt that it was important to take excellent care of the child themselves and to seek the best possible professional care in order to ensure the greatest chance for survival and healing.

In rare instances, families' religious tenets bring them into conflict with health care providers (e.g., when beliefs preclude certain forms of medical care, such as blood transfusion, or lead to preferences for prayer or other healing rituals over biomedical treatment). In such cases, an open dialogue must be maintained with families, and legal and ethical concerns must be formally balanced. When negotiation does not reach a solution acceptable to both the family and the care provider, the courts may be consulted. Because the dominant value in the United States usually includes preservation of a child's life, families are sometimes forced to accept care that is against their wishes and belief systems (Furrow et al, 2001). Health care providers must recognize the profound effect of such a situation and work to preserve respectful relationships with the family to ensure ongoing care for the child and to try to avoid future legal conflicts if possible.

Socioeconomic Status and Health

Around the world, economic inequalities and the gap between the rich and the poor are growing, a fact reflected in widening disparities in health status (Braveman & Tarimo, 2000). US children are profoundly affected by poverty. One in six children was poor in the year 2000 (Children's Defense Fund, 2001). Socioeconomic status exerts a profound influence—sometimes even more than ethnic or racial characteristics—on health and well-being. Children from economically secure homes are healthier, do better in school, are more likely to graduate from high school and less likely to commit criminal acts, and earn more money as adults than those from poverty-stricken homes (Zedlewski, 2002). There is a well-established link between poverty and the risk for childhood disability. Poor children are also more likely to have learning difficulties and to be receiving special education services (Fujiura & Yamaki, 2000).

Welfare reform legislation, which changed eligibility for income support for children and families, and a generally robust US economy in the 1990s encouraged many mothers and children to leave welfare programs in recent years. More recent downturns in the national economy have focused attention on the still-marginal economic status of many families with one or more employed adults. Families with low-wage jobs often do not receive benefits, such as health insurance, and may not earn enough income to leave poverty behind (Zedlewski, 2002).

Although the majority of poor Americans are white, people of color are disproportionately burdened by poverty and health problems. Black and Hispanic children are significantly less likely than white children to have a usual source of health care (Weinick & Krauss, 2000). Black, Hispanic, and Native American children are poorer, are less healthy, and have less well-educated parents than white children (Flores et al, 1999). Among barriers to access to care are language problems, especially when parents do not speak English, long waiting times for care, lack of insurance or money to pay for care, and transportation problems (Flores et al, 1998).

Cultural Power Struggles and the Impact of Globalization

Perhaps because of the nation's long association with European immigrants and their descendants, political and decision-making power has traditionally been held by white European Americans. Although this group continues to command the greatest degree of political clout, some changes have occurred in some cities and states where other cultural groups have gathered in large numbers over a long time. Examples of changing political power are found in the growing number of black mayors of large cities and in places such as San Francisco, which has many Asian politicians, and New Mexico, where Latinos and Hispanics play a large role in municipal and legislative activities. Of foreign-born US residents, 37.4% have become naturalized US citizens—a percentage that tends to increase with length of residence (Schmidley, 2001). Over time, most residents of the United States adopt English for official and public transactions, although many people continue to speak other languages in their homes and communities.

There is growing recognition that people around the world are interdependent and that issues related to health, environmental, and economic well-being readily cross national borders. Austin (2001) calls for a reexamination of nursing ethics in an era of globalization to incorporate the impact of such transnational, cross-cultural issues. Ethics may assume great importance to practitioners if they find themselves caught in a dilemma between the imperative to provide care for children with special needs and regulations affecting access to care, particularly eligibility for reimbursement of medical expenses. This ethical quandary may be particularly acute when caring for undocumented immigrants, when the requirement to enforce official rules and policies is pitted against personal or professional values to provide care to all in need (Quill et al, 1999; Ruiz-Beltran & Kamau, 2001).

Ethnocentrism and Racism

Ethnocentrism and racism (see definitions in Table 4-1) arise when those in privileged or powerful positions fail to recognize nondominant viewpoints as legitimate or are prejudiced against those from other racial and ethnic groups. These forms of discrimination can be enacted by individuals or become institutionalized and reflective of wider societal attitudes. Health care providers are sometimes ethnocentric in expecting children and families to accept advice or treatment based on their own values instead of those of the family. For example, children and parents are sometimes given diagnostic information and asked to make critical decisions without being able to first consult members of the extended family. This is an untenable position for families from cultures in which decision making is not necessarily centered in the nuclear family.

Technologic advances can also create ethical dilemmas, including who will have access to new, expensive forms of treatment and how decisions should be made about when to use these therapies. This is especially difficult for nurses when families make choices that differ from those of providers

(Coverston & Rogers, 2000). Advances in knowledge about genetic conditions pose challenges for families and providers in genetic testing and counseling. There is a great need for culturally sensitive genetic counseling, but Wang (2001) points out that it is not enough to rely on culture-specific group norms to ensure that the counseling needs of all families are met. Providers need to incorporate multicultural competencies into education, research, and practice. Such competencies include "clarifying one's own racial and cultural identities, developing self-acceptance, and having the ability to respectfully relate and function with people from all racial-cultural groups" (Wang, 2001, p. 212).

Barbee (1993) describes three forms of racism that are common among health care providers in the United States: denial, color-blind perspectives, and aversive racism. Barbee posits that denial arises from attributes of the health professions (i.e., a preference for homogeneity and a need to avoid conflict), as well as an idealistic mission to serve all persons, which has allowed providers to avoid acknowledging and examining racism within the profession. Idealism may also lead to a color-blind perspective, which occurs when providers assert that they treat all people the same regardless of race or ethnicity and can lead to a lack of recognition and respect for cultural differences, which may then be labeled as deviance. Aversive racism occurs when clinicians do not acknowledge the conflict between an egalitarian value system and negative feelings and beliefs toward other cultural groups. Because aversive racists may believe they are not prejudiced, discrimination becomes subtle and providers experience great ambivalence. Health care professionals can and must learn to recognize ethnocentrism and racism and enhance their sensitivity to all clients by working to establish personal and institutional cultural competence.

Intracultural Variation and Diversity

Although it is helpful to learn about the common history, values, and practices of particular cultural groups, it can never be presumed that any particular individual or family is fully represented by these descriptions. Written descriptions of broad cultural groups are offered by authors in order to facilitate the acquisition of knowledge of other cultures; but these depictions often present the most conservative cultural viewpoint, which stands in greatest contrast to that presumed to be "typically" American. These general descriptions rarely account for the dynamic nature of culture, in which traditional values and ways of life are incorporated into modern circumstances and familial needs (Dunn, 2002). There is great diversity within particular ethnic, racial, and religious populations; and many people belong to several subcultures while identifying themselves with one major cultural group (Mills, 2001).

Acculturation and Biculturalism

Acculturation is the process whereby one group of people adapts to living with another, which often includes learning the dominant group's language as well as adopting certain behaviors and practices (Birman & Trickett, 2001). Acculturation can be bidirectional (i.e., both groups influence each other), although the most established culture is likely to remain dominant and to wield greater influence than less-powerful subgroups (e.g., ethnic foods, rituals, and holidays have become popular and are widely enjoyed in the United States without changing the political dominance of powerful groups in most locales).

In individuals exposed to two cultures or languages over long periods, it is common to see biculturalism and bilingualism enabling them to function well in both cultures. For example, Mills (2001) studied third-generation Asian children and found that they adopted multiple identities, based on both their current circumstances in the modern Western world and family traditions. They valued traditional familial languages and customs for maintaining a sense of their heritage and strengthening family and community bonds. Wald & Knutson (2000) found that deaf adolescents who had received cochlear implants had very similar identity beliefs to deaf children who had not received the implants. Although both groups expressed approval of bicultural identity statements, children receiving implants were more likely to say that emulating the hearing majority was a desirable goal. Biculturalism can be helpful to children and families, allowing them to meet the demands of the dominant culture while retaining aspects of their cultural heritage (e.g., language, rituals, family relationships). Biculturalism may cause strain, however, when family members have different levels of acculturation and varying expectations about family roles and obligations.

Potential Differences in the Values of Health Care Providers and Families

Throughout the world, the family is the basic unit of society; however, different societies use family members in various ways to fulfill their basic functions of protecting, nurturing, and educating children. Parenting stress related to children's chronic conditions has been recognized as a cross-cultural phenomenon in such diverse nations as the United States, Israel, Japan, and Jordan (Krulik et al, 1999). In the United States—unlike many parts of the world—it is common for the nuclear family (i.e., parents and their children) to live apart from other family members; therefore presumptions of nuclear family autonomy are widespread among health care providers. Hospital policies may fail to recognize the wide variety of existing family constellations and the interdependence of extended family members that are common throughout the world, as well as in many subcultures in the United States. Many health care providers are harried and distressed when large family groups arrive to visit in small hospital rooms or when family members besides parents seek information about hospitalized children.

When extended family interdependence is customary, decisions about a child's health and well-being often reach far beyond the parents. Parents may wish to consult with, or even rely on, a variety of important people (e.g., grandparents, family or community elders, religious leaders or counselors, native healers) when making critical decisions. When possible, parents should be given time and opportunities for these important consultations; and when the situation is critical or immediate decisions are crucial, families should be encouraged to keep vigil with important members present or nearby (Kinsman et al, 1996).

Although there is no one "American" value system in the multicultural United States, there are many values held widely among particular groups of people, including health care providers, who often share many common traits (e.g., most are white, middle class, and relatively well educated). Some values commonly held by providers (e.g., gender equality) may contrast with those of certain families. When providing care for people who live by contrasting values of male superiority or family protection, professionals may find themselves in conflict with those they seek to serve (Nelson et al, 2001). One way to deal with such potential conflicts is to use cultural relativism, in which values and behaviors are judged only from the context of the client's cultural system (Baker, 1997). Many caregivers are comfortable with a large degree of cultural relativism and can use this principle to avoid ethnocentrism in most clinical encounters; however, providers sometimes find that there are problematic situations or behaviors that cross their "bottom line" belief systems so that they cannot espouse tolerance and understanding. Examples might include spousal dominance that becomes physical abuse or certain rituals that cause pain or physical complications (e.g., female genital excision, infibulation).

Underlying the principles of cultural competence is the goal of achieving a level of cultural relativism that allows care to be both congruent with a client's cultural beliefs and understanding of familial viewpoints and decisions from the family's perspective. Nevertheless, Baker (1997) points out that clinicians are not required to abandon their own principles. Rather, they have an obligation to talk with families, to try to understand the clients' viewpoints and prejudices, and to critically examine their own biases. In such a dialogue, neither the caregiver nor the client may change stances, but each may understand the other better. Where good communication and constructive relationships continue, change may eventually result.

Cultural Competence

Culturally competent health care is sensitive to the needs, backgrounds, and wishes of children with chronic conditions and their families. To be truly culturally competent requires care providers to acquire knowledge about themselves and others; to adopt attitudes of tolerance, curiosity, patience, and appreciation of difference; and to practice interpersonal skills that foster good communication and trust. The persistence of disparities in health and access to health care is associated with a lack of cultural competence among providers and in health care systems (Betancourt et al, 2002).

Hallmarks of culturally competent caregiving and caregiving systems are described in Boxes 4-1 and 4-2. The information given there reiterates that culturally competent care is only achieved when caregivers and institutions form individual relationships with families. In a study of black, Hispanic, and white families interviewed about improving services for children with chronic conditions, the authors stated, "Surprisingly, there were no distinctive differences in families' recommendations based on ethnicity alone. Participants stressed the importance of individualizing care rather than providing culturally

BOX 4-1

Hallmarks of Culturally Sensitive Caregiving

An asset model based on recognizing cultural differences in child rearing, family strengths, and culturally based coping methods should be used:
Information gathering: health records, cultural reading, family interviews.
Family strengths serve as the basis for planning care for child.

Families are directly involved in the family treatment and service plan:
Family decision makers are consulted.
Family helps to prioritize goals of care.
Family's orientation to care providers as authority figures or joint decision makers is determined before care is planned.

Family goals permit intracultural variation on a case-by-case basis:
Standard care plans are altered as needed or desired.
Alternative modes of care are incorporated as possible.

Self-sufficiency of the family is encouraged by promotion of self-esteem, cultural identification, and skill building to negotiate complicated medical systems:
Importance of family decision makers and caregivers is acknowledged.
Family strengths are recognized and praised.
Community resources are used.

Individual family/cultural values are respected:
Parent-child interaction patterns are taught in a culturally appropriate manner.
Differences between family and caregiver goals are negotiated with goodwill, patience, and a willingness to compromise.

Data from Adams, E.V. (1990). *Policy-planning for culturally comprehensive special services: Bureau of Maternal and Child Health,* Washington, DC: U.S. Department of Health and Human Services; Bernstein, H.K. & Stettner-Eaton, B. (1994). Cultural inclusion in part H: system development. *Infant-Toddler Intervention* 4(1):43-50; Betancourt, J.R. et al. (2002). *Cultural competence in health care: emerging frameworks and practical approaches (field report).* New York: The Commonwealth Fund; Dunn, A.M. (2002). Cultural competence and the primary care provider. *J Pediatr Health Care* 16:105-111.

BOX 4-2

Hallmarks of Culturally Sensitive Caregiving Systems

Primary care providers and caregiving systems seek community participation in all stages of program design, development, implementation, and evaluation, including outreach, policy making, and problem solving.
Formal and informal community leaders (e.g., church leaders, traditional healers, elders) are involved in defining culturally appropriate care.
Community outreach to families is ongoing and culturally appropriate, involving bilingual, bicultural providers, and/or community members when possible.

Intake systems are sensitive to family and cultural values:
Family privacy and previous experiences leading to mistrust must be respected.

Team members must have ongoing, culturally appropriate training.

Educational materials, media, evaluation, and monitoring instruments are field-tested for cultural appropriateness and congruency in language content and emotional meaning.

Programs are continuously evaluated to ensure cultural appropriateness and program effectiveness:
The child's progress is monitored by the family, the program, and external evaluators.
Family perceptions of interventions are sought and used in program revisions.

Data from Adams, E.V. (1990). *Policy-planning for culturally comprehensive special services: Bureau of Maternal and Child Health,* Washington, DC: U.S. Department of Health and Human Services; Bernstein, H.K. & Stettner-Eaton, B. (1994). Cultural inclusion in part H: system development. *Infant-Toddler Intervention* 4(1):43-50; Betancourt, J.R. et al. (2002). *Cultural competence in health care: emerging frameworks and practical approaches (field report).* New York: The Commonwealth Fund; Dunn, A.M. (2002). Cultural competence and the primary care provider. *J Pediatr Health Care* 16:105-111.

specific care for particular ethnic groups" (Garwick et al, 1998, p. 446).

Providers seeking cultural competence must explore their own contribution to enhancing or impeding cross-cultural interactions (i.e., their own values, beliefs, and communication patterns). Unconscious prejudices or ethnocentrism may be reflected in strained cross-cultural interactions and require thoughtful self-reflection to identify and rectify. The cross-cultural context of encounters among individuals, providers, and the health care system includes both societal factors (e.g., economic, political, and policy influences) and the immediate environment of the clinical setting (e.g., language congruency, privacy, and the acuity of the client's health needs) (Dunn, 2002).

Cultural competence is a complex phenomenon that requires knowledge of self and others; an open-minded and tolerant attitude toward human differences; and skills in critical thinking, communication, and assessment of the outcomes of cross-cultural interactions. An ongoing effort is generally required to develop cultural competence over time. A recent field report recommended that organizations could better achieve cultural competence by encouraging a more diverse workforce, by involvement of community members in planning and quality improvement programs, and by promotion of underrepresented minorities into positions of leadership (Betancourt et al, 2002). The same report urged health care systems to remove barriers to care, such as a lack of interpreters and culturally or

linguistically inappropriate educational materials. The authors urged education for clinical personnel on topics such as racial/ethnic disparities in health, assessment of community members' health beliefs and behaviors, and methods to help diverse clients develop self-advocacy skills while negotiating complex care systems.

Cultural Variations in the Impact of Childhood Chronic Conditions

A variety of chronic conditions have been reported to occur more frequently in certain ethnic or racial groups (Table 4-2). Recent immigrants must be assessed for conditions that are prevalent in their region of origin, and all children with chronic conditions need comprehensive family and developmental assessment, as well as well-child care in addition to care for their chronic condition. It is important to recognize that definitions of chronic conditions may vary and some cultures may consider minor differences in health or ability as acceptable variants of normal.

Children who have or are at increased risk for chronic physical, developmental, behavioral, or emotional conditions, and also require health and related services beyond those generally required for children, are estimated to make up 18% of US children less than 18 years of age (i.e., about 12.6 million children) (Newacheck et al, 2000). An epidemiologic profile of these children found that 18.6% are white, 19.8% are black, 15% are Hispanic, and 13% fall into other categories (Newacheck et al, 1998). Boys were about one third more likely to have a special

TABLE 4-2
Conditions Found More Frequently in Minority or Immigrant Populations

Ethnic Groups	Condition	Screening Tests	Age of Child
All adolescents	HIV infection	Culture, antibody, or antigen	13-21 yr
All immigrants	Tuberculosis	PPD	Newborn to adult
	PKU	Guthrie	Newborn to adult
	Iron deficiency anemia	Hgb/Hct	>6 mo
All immigrants and high-risk teens	STDs	Examination/laboratory serology	High-risk
All immigrants	Vitamin A deficiency	Serum test for vitamin A deficiency	All children
Asian	Anencephaly	Imaging studies	Newborn
	VSD, PDA	Examination, ECG, echocardiogram	Newborn, child
	Down syndrome	Amniocentesis, MSAFP, chromosome analysis	Fetus, newborn
	Cleft lip	Examination	Newborn
	Congenital hip	Examination, radiograph	Newborn
Black	Sickle cell disease	Hgb electrophoresis	All ages
Black, Mediterranean, Jewish, Thai, Filipino/Chinese	G6PD	Assay for enzyme	Newborn
Black	Prematurity	Early prenatal care	Fetus, newborn
	Perinatal drugs	Toxicology screen	Newborn
	Alcohol/drugs	Toxicology screen	Adolescent
	Microcephaly	Examination, imaging	Newborn
	PDA and pulmonary artery stenosis	Examination, radiograph, ECG	Child
	Low birth weight	Growth chart	Fetus, newborn
	High infant mortality	Prenatal care	Fetus, newborn
French Canadian	Tyrosinemia (1)	Serum tyrosine	High-risk newborn
Filipino	Gout	Serum uric acid	Symptomatic
Hispanic/all races and ethnic groups	Prematurity/LBW	Examination, growth chart	All children and adolescents
	Obesity, low SES		All children and adolescents
Jewish	Tay-Sachs disease	Amniocentesis, chromosome analysis	Fetus, newborn child
Mediterranean	Thalassemia	Hgb electrophoresis	All children
Native American (including Eskimos)	Low birth weight	Prenatal care	Fetus / Neonate
	SIDS	Apnea monitor	Infant
	Persistent otitis	Otoscopy, tympanometry	Infant/school age
	Juvenile diabetes	Blood glucose	School age/teenager
	Fetal alcohol syndrome	Toxicology, examination	All ages
	Alcohol/inhalants	Drug screens	Adolescent
	PDA, valve stenosis/atresia	Examination, radiograph, ECG	Neonate/child
	Cleft lip	Examination, amniocentesis	Newborn
	Hydrocephalus	Amniocentesis, examination	Newborn
	Congenital hip	Examination	Infant
Southeast Asian, Pacific Islander, and Haitian	Parasites/diarrhea	Corneal scars, stool for O & P, peripheral eosinophilia	All children
	Malaria	Blood smear/parasitemia	All ages
	Hepatitis	Hepatitis surface antigen	All ages
	Hemoglobinopathy	CBC with RBC indices	Any child
White	Cystic fibrosis	Sweat test	School age
	Clubfoot	Examination	Newborn
	Congenital hip	Examination, radiograph	Newborn
	Hypospadias	Examination	Newborn
	Asthma	Examination, radiograph	Postnewborn
	Allergic phenomena	Examination, CBC/diff	Infant, toddler, school age
	Otitis media		
British	Neural tube defect	MSAFP amniocentesis	Fetus, newborn

HIV, Human immunodeficiency virus; *PPD*, purified protein derivative (tuberculin); *PKU*, phenylketonuria; *Hgb/Hct*, hemoglobin/hematocrit; *STD*, sexually transmitted disease; *VSD*, ventricular septal defect; *PDA*, patent ductus arteriosus; *ECG*, electrocardiogram; *MSAFP*, maternal serum alpha-fetal protein; *G6PD*, glucose-6-phosphate dehydrogenase; *LBW*, low birth weight; *SES*, socio-economic status; *SIDS*, sudden infant death syndrome; *O & P*, ova and parasites; *CBC*, complete blood count; *RBC*, red blood cell; *diff*, differential.

Data from Acton, K.J., Burrows, N.R., Moore, K., Querec, L., & Geiss, L.S., et al. (2002). Trends in diabetes prevalence among American Indian and Alaska Native children, adolescents, and young adults. *American Journal of Public Health, 92*(9), 1485-1490; Behrman, R.E., Kliegman, R.M., & Jenson, H.B. (2001). *Nelson textbook of pediatrics* (16th ed.). Philadelphia: W.B. Saunders; Centers for Disease Control and Prevention. (2001). *HIV/AIDS Surveillance Report 2001, 13*(2); Department of Health and Human Services. (2000). *Breastfeeding: HHS blueprint for action on breastfeeding.* Office of Women's Health, Washington, DC: HHS; Hoekelman, R.A., Adam, H.M., Nelson, N.M., Weitzman, M.L., Wilson, M.H. (2001). *Primary pediatric care* (4th ed.). St Louis: Mosby; Newacheck, P.W., Stoddard, J.J., & McManus, M. (1993). Ethnocultural variations in the prevalence and impact of childhood chronic conditions. *Pediatrics 91*, 1031-1039; Newacheck, P.W., Strickland, B., Shonkoff, J.P., Perrin, J.M., & McPherson, M. (1998). An epidemiological profile of children with special health needs. *Pediatrics 102*, 117-123; Ogden, C.L., Flegal, K.M., Carroll, M.D., Johnson, C.L. (2002). Prevalence and trends in overweight among U.S. children and adolescents. *JAMA 288*, 1728-1732.

health need than girls; and children whose family incomes were at or below the federal poverty level were also about one third more likely to have special needs than those with higher income levels. Children from single-parent families are about 40% more likely to have special health care needs than those from two-parent families.

In a large epidemiologic study, children with special health care needs who are also from ethnic and racial minorities were more likely than white children to be without a usual source of health care, to lack health insurance, and to be unable to get needed medical care (Newacheck et al, 2002). These gaps were particularly frequent and large for Hispanic children. These findings indicate that access to health care varies by race and ethnicity and is diminished for children of color with chronic conditions. As increasing numbers of children with chronic conditions are enrolled in managed care programs (i.e., through Medicaid, Supplemental Security Income (SSI), SSI/Disability, or private insurance plans [see Chapter 7]), it will be important to monitor access and use of care to ensure appropriate services are available for both well-child and sick care.

Communications

At the heart of all successful relationships is good communication, although the parameters of "good" may vary among different cultural groups. For example, cultural factors (e.g., respect for authority, differences in social class) among families and providers may influence a family's attitude about accepting advice from health care providers or willingness to share reservations or objections to treatment plans. Some families may consider care providers to be consultants whose advice can be considered and either accepted or discarded, but others may consider caregivers to be authority figures whose advice—accepted or not—should never be openly questioned. Therefore follow-ups and ongoing dialogue are necessary to ensure that mutually acceptable care and outcomes are established (Luckman, 1999).

Besides words, communication is established through body language, touch, eye contact, and other nonverbal indicators. To convey respect and establish comfort, health care providers must be good observers and responsive to cues from children and families. Many care providers use direct, to-the-point communication; full eye contact; and firm handshakes, which are common courtesies for many people but may be aggressive or rude gestures to individuals used to indirect approaches and a lack of physical contact among strangers (Giger & Davidhizar, 1999).

The subtleties of effective communication are particularly complicated when interpreters are necessary. Children or friends of the family should not be used as interpreters because their presence may inhibit parents from a frank discussion of sensitive issues. Family members who can usually communicate adequately in English may find themselves tongue-tied or unable to understand complex medical concepts and vocabulary during times of crisis or stress (Rehm, in press). Moreover, parents may desire interpretation to their native language to fully understand explanations related to a child's chronic condition. It is important that interpreters be highly skilled communicators in both languages and cultures and that they convey more than simple, word-for-word translations of dialogue in clinical settings so that the actual meaning of the message is accurately portrayed (Luckman, 1999). When an interpreter is used, it is important to speak in short units of speech; to use simple, nontechnical language; to speak to family members directly—not just to the interpreter; and to listen to the client and family and check their understanding often by asking them to restate the message in their own words.

Variations in Perceptions of Causality and Meaning of Chronic Conditions

Perceptions about the cause and meaning of disability and chronic conditions of childhood vary widely among families. Some of these variations are associated with cultural or religious beliefs or may be related to parental educational levels and past experiences. Groce & Zola (1993) point out three important issues that influence interactions of children with chronic conditions, their families, and health care providers: culturally perceived causes of disability or illness, expectations for survival, and expectations of social roles for children and adults with chronic conditions. These issues are all influenced by multiple social factors, including traditional community- and family-belief systems, educational levels, financial and social support networks, exposure and access to modern health care and community support services, and levels of acculturation to dominant values within the medical and social service sectors of the United States.

Families with belief systems that consider social factors and spiritual influences, as well as pathophysiologic associations, may attribute a child's condition to multiple factors, including environmental, interpersonal, and genetic influences. Chronic conditions may be stigmatizing if thought to result from unacceptable behavior, inherent weaknesses, or external threats that could endanger the rest of the family or community (e.g., hexes, spirit possession) (Joachim & Acorn, 2000). Children with such conditions may be kept at home and out of view to protect either the family from shame or the child from potentially disapproving or threatening community restrictions.

In many communities, however, families caring for children with chronic conditions are admired and offered ongoing support. Belief in causative factors beyond those generally recognized by biomedicine does not often interfere with acceptance and use of modern medical diagnosis and treatment. For example, Mexican-American parents recognized both biomedical and sociocultural causes for their children's disabilities (Mardiros, 1989). Within the biomedical domain, parents described pregnancy problems, iatrogenic causes, substance abuse, genetic factors, and toxic exposures. Sociocultural causation included both familial and personal domains (e.g., difficulties within the marriage, spousal abuse, prior attitudes, past transgressions). Parents in this study placed responsibility for naming the illness with physicians and—regardless of their own predominant view of causation—recognized the necessity of a formal medical label in order to access desired services for their child.

Expectations for the survival of infants and children influence the kinds of familial and community resources that parents seek and provide for their children with chronic conditions. Residents or recent immigrants from parts of the world that are less technologically oriented than the US medical system may be unaware of recent advances in medical care that facilitate survival for many children who would ordinarily die or be profoundly disabled without the surgical, pharmacologic, and mechanical supports routinely available here. Moreover, there may be philosophic and ethical traditions that do not necessarily value survival in the face of stigmatizing factors, such as altered appearance or disability (Scheper-Hughes, 1990). Societies that condone infanticide or neglect of children with physical or developmental impairments are increasingly rare throughout the world because of improved access to sophisticated services and governmental policies that disapprove of such practices. Nevertheless, expectations for children with chronic conditions vary widely and require ongoing education in the face of changing life circumstances, available support services, and official policies.

Family- and community-sanctioned roles for children and adults with chronic conditions help to determine the kinds of educational, health, and other resources that are expended on such individuals. The official US policy (i.e., in the form of laws such as the Americans with Disabilities Act [ADA] and the Individuals with Disabilities Education Act [IDEA]) explicitly entitles children and adults with disabling conditions to the same educational, occupational, and social opportunities as those without such conditions (see Chapter 5). These laws reflect the widely held US beliefs that most people should be independent and self-supporting and therefore are entitled to education and opportunities to ensure such measures of success. These expectations are often modified depending on individual circumstances, but the belief that each person should strive for the highest possible level of independence remains and may be seen, for example, in the widespread practice of group-home living for individuals who cannot live alone. This value is not universally held, however, and notions of independence may not be the highest priority of families who value interdependence of family members and do not perceive ongoing home care as excessively burdensome.

Alternative Therapies

Much of the literature on health care of children from non-US cultures describes exotic folk-healing practices and rituals (Rehm, in press). Many systems of health care and beliefs other than those of Western biomedicine exist throughout the world. Two of the best known are Chinese medicine, which uses herbs and acupuncture, and religious rituals (e.g., prayer, healing touch) that are common to many spiritual systems. In most cases, there is little conflict between biomedical care and traditional practices, and provider support of the alternative therapies favored by a family may foster the growth of trust (Luckman, 1999). Even if the suggestions of primary care providers are found to be acceptable, a family's current practices must be determined, and planned treatments besides those proposed by primary care providers must be recognized. It may be important to determine the effects of herbs or other pharmacologic agents to assess drug interactions and safety, but folk healers are often willing to cooperate with health care providers; and a blending of rituals and healing techniques can be both medically effective and helpful to the family. Pediatric

care providers may facilitate joint practices when blessing ceremonies are conducted before an invasive procedure (e.g., Mormons) or amulets are worn by children for protection (e.g., some American Indians).

Cultural Assessment

Cultural competence requires that children with chronic conditions and their families are assessed to determine their cultural identities and any particular beliefs or needs that should be incorporated into care plans. There are many excellent, in-depth cultural assessment tools (Andrews & Boyle, 1999; Giger & Davidhizar, 1999). Cross-cultural assessment of a family with a child with a chronic condition is described in Table 4-3. These tools are particularly helpful when care providers see families repeatedly over time because the many questions can be incorporated into several interviews. Many times, however, care providers are uncertain if they will see families repeatedly or the nature of the contact is time limited and problem focused. In such cases, it is helpful to distill a few key questions from these larger tools and focus attention on the aspects of assessment that are most relevant to the current encounter.

Key Questions for Brief Encounters in the Primary Care Setting

In the primary care setting, it is helpful to supplement the general client and family history with key questions, such as the following: (1) Would you be more comfortable with a translator present? (2) Who are your child's primary caregivers at home? (3) Is there anyone else who needs to know the treatment plan and have the opportunity to ask questions? (4) What kinds of home remedies have you been using for your child, and what others might you use for this situation? (5) Are you satisfied with the care plan made at this visit, and is there anything that you anticipate might interfere with your ability to carry it out?

In an acute situation or when it is necessary to make major decisions or changes in the care plan, it is important to add the following questions about the family's decision-making procedures: (1) Who are the appropriate people to make this decision for your child? (2) Do you want/need to bring in other family members or authority figures to receive information and help you make this decision?

It may be useful to get to know the family with these key questions and incorporate the answers into a larger assessment that can be left in the chart and completed over time. Primary care providers can bring in additional questions relating to the reason for the visit (e.g., questions about medication acceptability and use, dietary preferences and restrictions, or developmental goals). Many questions asked by clinicians as part of the routine history and physical clearly have cultural relevance, and once practitioners are sensitive to that fact, cultural assessment can be incorporated into all encounters and does not have to take up large blocks of time. A clinician's respect, nonjudgmental attitude, and sincere interest and curiosity about clients are likely to foster trust and open communication. It is important to assure clients that their input is valuable and to verify that the plan of care is acceptable to them.

TABLE 4-3

Cross-Cultural Assessment of a Family with a Child with a Chronic Condition

Family demographics	Who lives in your family (i.e., members, ages, genders)?
	What kind of work do members of the household do?
	What is your family's socioeconomic status?
	What kind of health insurance coverage do you have?
	Which family members are covered?
	Which child are you seeking care for today?
	What chronic conditions or symptoms does the child have?
	How would you describe the problems that have brought you here today?
	Who is the primary caretaker in your family?
Orientation	Where were the members of the family born?
	What is the ethnic background of the family members?
	How many years have family members lived in the United States? (NOTE: Only ask if appropriate.)
	In your family is it important to be on time for an appointment or to get to an appointment based on everyone's schedule for that day?
	Why do you think your child has (the above-named) chronic condition (e.g., punishment for a parent's past behavior such as conceiving a child out of wedlock, the result of a genetic problem, or a gift given because of the family's patience and love)?
Communication	What language(s) and dialect(s) are spoken at home?
	Who reads English in the family? If no one reads English, in what language would you prefer printed materials?
	Do parents and children make eye contact when spoken to, or do they look down?
	To whom should questions be addressed?
	What can be asked of the child directly? (NOTE: Avoid using the child as a translator because of the strain this imposes.)
Family relationships	Besides the immediate household, who else makes up the members of this family?
	Who makes the decisions in this family (e.g., mother-in-law, father, both partners, other family or friends, group decision)?
	Who cares for the child and the child's medical needs?
	What are the housing arrangements (e.g., space, number of rooms, members living in the home)?
	What is the child's or family's usual daily routine like?
	To whom do you turn when you need help with or have questions about your child?
Beliefs about health	What is the present health status of family members?
	What illnesses or conditions are present in the current family members?
	What illnesses or conditions were present in deceased family members?
	How often and for what reasons have family members used Western medicine in the past?
	What complementary therapies are used by your family routinely and specifically for the child (e.g., acupuncture, healers, prayer, massage)?
	What do you do when your child is in pain?
	Who takes care of the child if the child is hospitalized?
	Is it important to keep the child at home or to use institutional placement?
	What do you think will help clear up the problem?
	Are there things that help your child get better that the physicians should know?
	What problems has your child's illness caused your family?
Education	How much schooling have members of the family completed?
	What ways are the best for you to learn about your child's condition (e.g., pamphlets, videos, direct patient teaching, home visits, return demonstrations)?
	From whom are you most comfortable learning about your child's condition (e.g., physician, nurse, social worker, home health aide, other family members)?
Religion	What religion(s) are practiced in your family?
	What religious things do you do to help your child (e.g., pray, meditate, attend a support group, practice the laying on of hands)?
	What things does your religion say you should *not* do for this child (e.g., have blood transfusions, allow strangers or dangerous circumstances to affect child)?
Nutrition	When are usual mealtimes for your family?
	With whom does the child eat?
	What foods does the child usually eat?
	What special foods does the child eat when the child is sick?
	What foods do you *not* give the child and when?

From Andrews, M.M. & Boyle, J.S. (1999). *Transcultural concepts in nursing care*, (3rd ed.). Philadelphia: W.B. Saunders; Davis, B. & Voegtle, K. (1994). *Culturally competent health care for adolescents*. Chicago, American Medical Association. Modified with permission.

Research and Culture

Investigators have extensively described the effect of chronic conditions on children and their family members in both qualitative and quantitative studies (see Chapters 2 and 3). Despite this extensive research foundation, it is often difficult to find data-based information on the experiences of particular cultural groups with specific chronic conditions. Sterling et al (1997) reviewed the literature on black families with children with chronic illnesses and concluded that although these children are often included in research studies, their numbers are often small, and so the information related to blacks is subsumed into the findings of the larger study. These authors also found that blacks are not studied within the context of their own culture.

Despite current regulations that require the inclusion of across-the-life-span and ethnically diverse samples in government-funded studies, children, women, and nondominant ethnic groups continue to be underrepresented in many forms of research studies, particularly clinical trials. Although these regulations help to ensure that all US residents are represented in research, few studies focusing on particular cultural groups, which could help to overcome oft-repeated stereotypes, are conducted. Perhaps these studies are rare because there is an assumption that such research is best conducted by members of a particular culture. If this assumption is accepted, then important questions about particular cultural groups may never be answered because cultural minority groups are vastly underrepresented among the ranks of scholars. Therefore cross-cultural research is necessary but inherently difficult because of the potential for ethnocentrism and cultural misunderstandings. Ethnography is one method that researchers have successfully modified over the years to be less ethnocentric in its approach to research with diverse or cross-cultural samples both in the United States and abroad (Roper & Shapira, 2000).

Ethnocentrism may arise in research studies when investigators assume that findings in one group of people are necessarily applicable across the board, especially if the context or other relevant variables are not considered. For example, Stevens et al (1999) described the need to consider cultural values in development of a questionnaire to assess knowledge, attitudes, and behavior in American Indian children. Researchers found it necessary to consider children's culturally influenced reluctance to think or speak negatively (to avoid shaping reality in a negative direction) and the cultural tradition of avoiding comparisons among individuals, including ranking or rating themselves against others. Another example occurred in a study of Jamaican infants, when higher levels of maternal education and a more nurturing home environment were found to overcome the potentially harmful effects of heavy marijuana use. These infants were more alert, self-regulating, and less irritable when compared with a non–drug-using but poorer peer group (Dreher et al, 1994).

Studies of disadvantaged cultural populations must recognize the effects of racial, class, and other forms of discrimination, as well as seek solutions to health problems through interventions beyond those aimed at individuals who do not conform to generally accepted healthy behaviors. Researchers have demonstrated the effects of poverty and social class on health (Zedlewski, 2002) but seldom acknowledge other societal factors, such as repeated discrimination, exposure to high levels of pollutants and violence, and lack of opportunity for educational or occupational advancement. Interventions that address these factors, as well as those most commonly aimed at individual behavior changes, are necessary.

Prejudice against children with chronic conditions has received relatively little attention from researchers. However, 35% of 365 parents of school-aged children with chronic illnesses reported discrimination, particularly in school settings and from peers (Turner-Henson et al, 1994). More recently, the potential for discrimination against people with genetic conditions has been recognized by clinicians and researchers managing information gleaned from the Human Genome Project, and protection of patient privacy is an emerging area of

interest and concern (Friedrich, 2002). Stigma of both visible and invisible chronic conditions has been well recognized (Joachim & Acorn, 2000) and may affect decisions of parents and children about disclosure of chronic conditions. For example, children with human immunodeficiency virus (HIV) and their parents described stigma as an important factor in determining to whom and under which circumstances they disclosed the children's HIV status to neighbors and school personnel (Rehm & Franck, 2000). These results, coupled with findings that children from ethnic minority groups with chronic conditions use fewer physician services, have more hospitalizations, and are more likely to lack a usual source of care (Newacheck et al, 2002), suggest that social factors and poverty are important areas for future investigation.

Summary

As the United States becomes more culturally diverse, health care providers must develop cultural competence to ensure that sensitive and effective care is delivered. Cultural competence will help to prevent racism and ethnocentrism in practice and research by helping providers to assess their own cultural viewpoints and biases while learning about the issues and needs of children and their families. Care should be congruent with the cultural beliefs and practices of clients whenever possible, and increasing cultural competence will enhance effective communication and facilitate respect and appreciation for the range of human diversity. Researchers must investigate culturally relevant questions and test interventions in a wide variety of populations in order to develop the baseline knowledge that will provide clinicians with a sound foundation on which to develop primary care practices that are culturally competent.

REFERENCES

Adams, G. & Markus, H.R. (2001). Culture as patterns: An alternative approach to the problem of reification. *Cult Psychol*, 7, 283-696.

Airhihenbuwa, C.O., Kumanyika, S.K., TenHave, T.R., & Morssink, C.B. (2000). Cultural identity and health lifestyles among African Americans: A new direction for health intervention research. *Ethn Dis, 10*, 148-164.

Andrews, M.M. & Boyle, J.S. (1999). *Transcultural concepts in nursing care* (3rd ed.). Philadelphia: J.P. Lippincott.

Austin, W. (2001). Nursing ethics in an era of globalization. *Adv Nurs Sci, 24*(2), 1-18.

Baker, C. (1997). Cultural relativism and cultural diversity: implications for nursing practice, *ANS Adv Nurs Sci 20*, 3-11.

Barbee, E.L. (1993). Racism in U.S. nursing. *Med Anthropol Q 7*, 346-362.

Betancourt, J.R., Green, A.R., & Carillo, E. (2002). *Cultural competence in health care: Emerging frameworks and practical approaches* (Field Report). New York: The Commonwealth Fund.

Birman, D. & Trickett, E.J. (2001). Cultural transitions in first-generation immigrants. *J Cross Cult Psychol, 32*, 456-477.

Braveman, P. & Tarimo, E. (2000). Social inequalities in health within countries: Not only an issue for affluent nations. *Soc Sci Med, 54*, 1621-1635.

Chandler, C.R., Tsai, Y-M., & Wharton, R. (1999). Twenty years after: Replicating a study of Anglo and Mexican-American cultural values. *Soc Sci J, 36*, 353-367.

Children's Defense Fund. (2001). Overall child poverty rate dropped in 2000 but poverty rose for children in full-time working families [online]. Available: www.childrensdefense.org/release010925.htm.

Coverston, C. & Rogers, S. (2000). Winding roads and faded signs: Ethical decision making a post modern world. *J Perinat Neonat Nurs, 14*(2), 1-11.

Coyle, J. (2002). Spirituality and health: Towards a framework for exploring the relationship between spirituality and health. *J Adv Nurs, 37*, 589-597.

Draper, P. & McSherry, W. (2002). A critical view of spirituality and spiritual assessment. *J Adv Nurs, 39*(1), 1-2.

Dreher, M., Nugent, J.K., & Hudgins R. (1994). Prenatal marijuana exposure and neonatal outcomes in Jamaica: an ethnographic study. *Pediatrics, 93*, 254-260.

Dunn, A.M. (2002). Culture competence and the primary care provider. *J Pediatric Health Care, 16*(3), 105-111.

Flores, G., Bauchner, H., Feinstein, A.R., & Nguyen, U.S. (1999). The impact of ethnicity, family income, and parental education on children's health and use of health services. *Am J Public Health, 89*, 1066-1071.

Flores, G., Abreu, M., Olivar, M.A., & Kastner, B. (1998). Access barriers to health care for Latino children. *Arch Pediatr Adolesc Med, 152*, 1119-25.

Friedrich, M.J. (2002). Preserving privacy, preventing discrimination becomes the province of genetics experts. *JAMA, 288*, 815-819.

Fujiura, G.T. & Yamaki, K. (2000). Trends in demography of childhood poverty and disability. *Exceptional Children, 66*, 187-199

Furrow, B.R., Greaney T.L., Johnson, S.H., Jost, T., & Jost, T.S. (2001). *Bioethics: Health care law and ethics* (4th ed.). St. Paul, MN: West Publishing Co.

Garwick, A.W., Kohrman, C., Wolman, C., & Blum, R.W. (1998). Families' recommendations for improving services for children with chronic conditions. *Arch Pediatr Adolesc Med, 152*, 440-448.

Giger, J.N. & Davidhizar, R.E. (1999). *Transcultural Nursing: Assessment & Intervention* (3rd ed.). St. Louis: Mosby.

Groce, N.E. & Zola, I.K. (1993). Multiculturalism, chronic illness, and disability. *Pediatrics Supp. 191*, 1048-1055.

Guendelman, S., Schauffler, H.H., & Pearl, M. (2001). Unfriendly shores: How immigrants children fare in the U.S. health system. *Health Affairs, 20*(1), 257-266.

Joachim, G. & Acorn, S. (2000). Stigma of visible and invisible chronic conditions. *J Advanced Nurs, 32*, 243-248.

Jordan, D.K. (2001). Prehistoric Beringia: Homeland of the peoples of the Americas [online]. Available: http://weber.ucsd.edu/~dkjordan/arch/beringia.html.

Kinsman, S.B., Sally, M., & Fox, K. (1996). Multicultural issues in pediatric practice. *Pediatr Rev 17*, 349-354.

Krulik, T., Turner-Henson, A., kanematsu, Y., Al-Maaitah, R., & Swan, J. et al. (1999). Parenting stress and mothers of young children with chronic illness: A cross-cultural study. *J Pediatr Nurs, 14*, 130-140.

Lollock, L. (2001). The foreign born population in the United States: March 2000. *Current Population Reports, P20-534*. Washington DC: U.S. Census Bureau.

Luckman, J. (1999). *Trancultural communication in Nursing*. Albany, NY: Delmar Publishers.

Mardiros, M. (1989). Conceptions of childhood disability among Mexican-American parents. *Med Anthropol, 12*, 55-68.

McEvoy, M. (2000). An added dimension to pediatric health maintenance visit: The spiritual history. *J Pediatr Health Care, 14*, 216-220.

McGuire, S. (1998). Global migration and health: ecofeminist perspectives, ANS. *Adv Nurs Sci, 21*(2), 1-16.

Mills, J. (2001). Being bilingual: Perspectives of third generation Asian children on language, culture, and identity. *Int J Bilingual Ed and Bilingualism, 4*, 383-402.

Nelson, G., Prilleltensky, I., & MacGillivary, H. (2001). Building value-based partnerships: Toward Solidarity with oppressed groups. *Am J Community Psychol, 29*, 649-677.

Newacheck P.W., Hung Y.Y., & Wright K.K. (2002). Racial and ethnic disparities in access to care for children with special health care needs. *Ambul Pediatr, 2*(4), 247-254.

Newacheck, P.W., McManus, M., Fox, H.B., Hung, Y.Y., & Halfon, N. (2000). Access to health care for children with special health care needs. *Pediatrics, 105*, 760-766.

Newacheck, P.W., Strickland, B., Shonkoff, J.P., Perrin, J.M., McPherson, M., et al. (1998). An epidemiologic profile of children with special health care needs. *Pediatrics, 102*, 117-123.

O'Hagan, K. (1999). Culture, cultural identity, and cultural sensitivity in child and family social work. *Child and Family Social Work, 4*, 269-281.

Preston, C. (1998). *The royal road: El Camino Real from Mexico City to Santa Fe*. Albuquerque: University of New Mexico Press.

Quill, B.E. Aday, L.A., Hacker, C.S., & Reagan, J.K. (1999). Policy incongruence and public health professionals' dissonance: The case of immigrants and welfare policy. *J Immigrant Health, 1*(1), 9-18.

Rehm, R.S. (in press). Cultural Intersections in the Care of Mexican American Children with Chronic Conditions. *Pediatr Nurs*.

Rehm, R.S. (1999). Religious faith in Mexican American families living with chronic childhood illness. *Image J Nurs Sch, 31*, 33-38.

Rehm, R.S. & Franck, L.S. (2000). Long term goals and normalization strategies of children and families affected by HIV/AIDS. *Adv Nurs Sci, 23*(1), 69-82.

Roper, J.M. & Shapira, J. (2000). *Ethnography in nursing research*. Thousand Oaks, CA: Sage Publications.

Ruiz-Beltran, M. & Kamau, J.K. (2001). The socio-economic and cultural impediments to well-being along the U.S.-Mexico border. *J Community Health, 26*, 123-132.

Scheper-Hughes, N. (1990). Difference and danger: the cultural dynamics of childhood stigma, rejection, and rescue. *Cleft Palate J, 27*, 301-310.

Schmidley, A.D. (2001). Profile of the foreign born population in the United States: 2000. *U.S. Census Bureau, Current Population Reports, Series P23-206*. Washington DC: U.S. Government Printing Office.

Sterling, Y.M., Peterson, J., & Weekes, D. (1997). African-American families with chronically ill children: oversights and insights. *J Pediatr Nurs, 12*, 292-300.

Stevens, J., Cornell, C.E., Story, M., French, S.A., Levin, S., Becenti, A., Gittelsohn, J., Going, S.B., & Reid, R. (1999). Development of a questionnaire to assess knowledge, attitudes, and behaviors in American Indian children. *Am J Clin Nutr, 69* (Suppl.), 773S-815.

Turner-Henson, A., Holaday, B., Corser, N., Ogletree, G., & Swan, J.H. (1994). The experiences of discrimination: challenges for chronically ill children. *Pediatr Nurs, 20*, 571-577.

U.S. Immigration and Naturalization Service. (2001). Illegal alien resident population [online]. Available: http://www.ins.usdoj.gov/grapgics/aboutins/statistics/illegalalien/illegal.pdf.

Wald, R.L. & Knutson, J.F. (2000). Deaf cultural identity of adolescents with and without cochlear implants. *Ann Oltol Rhinol Laryngol, 185* (Suppl.), 87-89.

Wang, V.O. (2001). Multicultural genetic counseling: Then, now and in the 21st century. *Am J Med Gen, 106*, 208-215.

Weinick, R.M. & Krauss, N.A. (2000). Racial/ethnic differences in children's access to care. *Am J Public Health, 90*, 1771-1774.

Zedlewski, S.R. (2002). Family economic resources in the post-reform era. *Future Child, 12* (1), 120-145.

5 School and the Child with a Chronic Condition

Patricia Jackson Allen and Judith A. Vessey

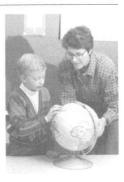

Role of School in a Child's Life

The role of school should not be underestimated in a child's life. School provides opportunities for social, emotional, and cognitive development. In addition to the family, school is the major context in which children develop their sense of self and understanding of their place in relation to peers. More importantly, most children genuinely enjoy school, despite their protestations. This enjoyment of school may be particularly true for children with chronic conditions because they may have fewer opportunities to socialize outside the school setting. Another positive benefit of including children with chronic conditions in school activities is that nondisabled children can develop attitudes of acceptance and respect for their peers with special needs.

Integrating children with chronic needs into the school setting, however, is not without problems. These children and their families may experience community resistance and resentment. Moreover, many schools have inadequate resources to educate these children, despite the fact that educational services are mandated by law. Parents' fears, guilt, and values need to be carefully assessed because these play critical roles in their children's school success. This chapter will initially examine the legislative mandates for education of children with disabilities or chronic conditions that alter their ability to fully participate in the standard educational experience and then explore ways primary care providers can facilitate a child's school experience.

Laws on Education of Children with Chronic Conditions

Legislative and judicial rulings over the past 25 years have dramatically changed the role of public educational institutions in providing services to children with chronic conditions (Box 5-1). The change in public policy actually started with the civil rights movement when the landmark decision of *Brown v. Board of Education* (1954) banned segregated schools and affirmed education as a right of all US citizens. The principle of "separate is not equal" was used almost 20 years later in *Pennsylvania Association for Retarded Citizens v. Pennsylvania* (1972) to challenge the state's right to exclude children with mental retardation from public education (Burns and Thornan, 1993; National Council on Disability, 2000). That same year the Supreme Court ruled that a free, public education must be provided to all school-aged children regardless of disability or degree of impairment (*Mills v. Board of Education of the District of Columbia*, 1972). This landmark Supreme Court decision paved the way for the federal government to enact legislation supporting public education for all children regardless of health or ability.

In 1975 Congress passed Public Law 94-142, the Education for All Handicapped Children Act, as an educational bill of rights for children 5 to 18 years of age (Box 5-2). Public Law 94-142 entitled children to a "free and appropriate public education (FAPE)" including "special education and related services provided at public expense, under public supervision and direction, without charge, which meet the standards of the state educational agency, and are provided in uniformity with the Individualized Educational Program (IEP)" (PL 94-142, 1975a).

Public Law 94-142 was amended in 1986 by Public Law 99-457, which included The Handicapped Infants and Toddlers Program, Part H, of the amended law. Public Law 99-457 extended services to children from birth to 21 years of age and required interagency and interdisciplinary collaboration, development of a child identification system, a care manager designated for the family, and the implementation of an individualized family service plan (IFSP) for children from birth through 2 years, analogous to the IEP for older children (PL 99-457, 1986). This amendment dramatically increased the school systems' role in providing services to infants and young children. In 1990 and 1991, these laws were further amended under the Individuals with Disabilities Education Act (IDEA), Public Law 101-476 (PL 101-476, 1990), and Public Law 102-119, the IDEA Revisions (PL 102-119, 1991).

IDEA'97

In May 1997, Congress passed legislation reauthorizing and amending IDEA again (Public Law 105-17). IDEA'97 is a complex statute divided into four parts: Part A contains general provisions, purpose, goals, and definitions; Part B, "Assistance for Education of All Children with Disabilities," describes how the federal government provides assistance to states for the education of children with disabilities from ages 3 to 21 years, how state agencies must supervise and monitor the statute, and the basic rights and responsibilities of children with disabilities and their parents or guardians; Part C, "Infants and Toddlers with Disabilities," describes the program for children from birth to age 3 years; and Part D, "National Activities to Improve Education of Children with Disabilities," authorizes programs to improve teacher preparation and credentialing in the education of children with disabilities.

IDEA'97 reaffirmed the language regarding the importance of educating children in the least restrictive environment (LRE), including a new emphasis on participation in the

---

BOX 5-1

Major Legislative Rulings on Education for Children with Disabilities or Chronic Conditions

Brown v. Board of Education, 1954
The Civil Rights Act, Rehabilitation Act, Section 504: Public Law 93-112, 1973
The Education for All Handicapped Children Act: Public Law 94-142, 1975; amended by The Education of Handicapped Amendments: Public Law 99-457, 1986; became Public Law 102-119
The Technology Related Assistance for Individuals with Disabilities Act: Public Law 100-407, 1988
Individuals with Disabilities Education Act (IDEA): Public Law 101-476, 1990; amended by IDEA Revisions of 1991: Public Law 102-119, 1991
Americans with Disabilities Act: Public Law 101-336, 1990
The School to Work Transition Act: Public Law 103-239, 1994
Individuals with Disabilities Education Act Amendments of 1997: Public Law 105-17, 1997
Cedar Rapids v. Garrett F., no. 96-1793, 1999
Reauthorization of IDEA 1997, 2003

BOX 5-2

Goals of Public Law 94-142

Public Law 94-142, The Education for All Handicapped Children Act of 1975, provides the following:
1. A free and appropriate education for all children (FAPE)
2. An education in the least restrictive environment (LRE) based on individual needs
3. An assessment of needs that is racially and culturally unbiased and given in the individual's native language or mode of communication
4. An individualized education program (IEP) prepared by a team of professionals that includes parents
5. Due process and a procedure for complaints to ensure the rights of the individual

---

curriculum of general education, the rights of parents to be involved in educational decisions affecting their children, including eligibility and placement, the importance of functional behavioral assessments and strategies to promote positive behavior, and the requirement that states develop performance goals and outcome measurements for children with disabilities as part of school reform issues and district-wide assessments (Lipton, 1997; National Council on Disability, 2000; Siegel, 2001). This legislation clarified that states are required to identify, locate, and evaluate all children with disabilities residing in the state, including children in private schools. This directive is referred to as "child find."

IDEA'97 also expanded covered related services. The term "related services" was initially part of the 1975 Education for All Handicapped Children Act and included "transportation and other developmental, corrective, and supportive services, including speech pathology and audiology, psychologic devices, physical and occupational therapy, recreation, early identification and assessment of disabilities in children, counseling services, and medical services for diagnostic or evaluative purposes." The term also includes school health services, extended school year and school day services, social work services in schools, and parent counseling and training (PL 94-142, 1975b). IDEA'97 expanded related services to include

orientation and mobility services, transition services, and supplemental aids and supports needed to enable children with disabilities to be educated with nondisabled children to the most appropriate extent (Committee on Children with Disabilities, 2000; National Information Center for Children and Youth with Disabilities [NICHCY], 2001; PL 105-17, 1997). In 1999 in *Cedar Rapids v. Garret F.,* the Supreme Court reaffirmed the requirement of schools to provide special education and related services to all children with disabilities, even if this required one-on-one, full-time registered nursing services for a child with complex medical needs (Supreme Court Decision No. 96-1793).

Eligibility for Special Education Services under IDEA

Not all children with chronic health conditions are eligible for special education services under IDEA. Public Law 94-142 (The Education for All Handicapped Children Act, 1975) and IDEA 1990 and 1997 designated only certain health conditions as handicapping, thereby making a child eligible for special education and related services. The list of conditions (Box 5-3) was expanded to include autism and traumatic brain injury in 1990, and IDEA'97 was further amended in 1999 to add attention deficit disorder (ADD) and attention deficit hyperactivity disorder (ADHD) to the list of conditions covered under "Other Health Impairments" (Lipton, 1999).

Table 5-1 shows the number of children 6 to 21 years of age receiving special education services in each category from 1996 to 2001. The numbers indicate an annual increase in children receiving special education services under IDEA in every category except visual impairments. A further breakdown by age for the 2000-2001 school year indicates the dramatic increase in numbers of children receiving services at school entry, age 6 years (Table 5-2). This would appear to indicate the "child find" process does not work well in identifying children before regular school entry, missing years of potentially beneficial early interventions before age 6 years.

To receive special education services a preplacement evaluation must be conducted to determine eligibility. This individual initial evaluation can be requested by the parent or guardian or by a public agency (school, preschool center, residential placement agency, etc.) with written approval of the parent or guardian. In order for a child to be eligible for special education services, including an individualized education program (IEP), the child must have a condition that is covered under one of the mandated categories (Box 5-3) and/or test at or below a designated level of performance (i.e., often 1.5 to 2.0 standard deviations below the norm in specific or multiple areas of function) as a result of his or her disability. Input from the parents or guardians, teachers, and other professionals with knowledge of the child's condition is included in the evaluation process. The law requires that testing evaluations be free and the child be evaluated in all areas related to his or her suspected disability, that is, health, vision, hearing, social and emotional status, general intelligence, academic performance, communication ability, and motor abilities (Siegel, 2001). Previously performed evaluations as part of the child's health care can also be submitted for review during this preplacement phase and are often helpful in documenting the child's abilities and disabilities. This

BOX 5-3

Conditions Identified as Disabilities in Children Under the Individuals with Disabilities Education Act (1997)

Disabilities as Defined for Children 5 to 21 Years of Age

Autism: A developmental disability significantly affecting verbal and nonverbal communication and social interaction

Deaf-Blindness: Children with both deafness and blindness; communication with others is severely impaired

Deafness: Children with a hearing deficiency that impairs processing of linguistic information through hearing with or without amplification

Hearing Impairment: Permanent or fluctuating hearing loss that adversely affects the child's educational process

Mental Retardation: Significant subaverage general intelligence existing with deficits in adaptive behavior

Multiple Disabilities: Concomitant impairments other than deaf-blindness resulting in severe educational problems that cannot be addressed in a special education program solely for one impairment

Orthopedic Impairments: Severe orthopedic impairments that adversely affect the child's educational performance

Other Health Impairments: Limited strength, vitality, or alertness caused by chronic or acute health problems that affect the child's educational performance, such as a heart condition, tubereulosis, rheumatic fever, nephritis, asthma, sickle cell anemia, hemophilia, epilepsy, leukemia, diabetes, attention deficit disorder (ADD), attention deficit hyperactivity disorder (ADHD)

Serious Emotional Disturbance: A child who exhibits over a prolonged period of time one or more of the following characteristics: an inability to learn that cannot be explained by intellectual, sensory, or health factors; an inability to build or maintain satisfactory interpersonal relationships; inappropriate behavior or feelings; depression or unhappiness; and a tendency to develop physical symptoms or fears associated with personal or school problems

Specific Learning Disability: A disorder in one or more of the psychologic processes involved in understanding or using spoken or written language; term does not apply to children who have learning problems primarily caused by other disabilities listed here or environmental, cultural, or economic disadvantages

Speech or Language Impairment: A communication disorder caused by impaired articulation, problems with language development, or voice impairment that adversely affects a child's educational performance

Traumatic Brain Injury: Acquired injury to the brain resulting in total or partial functional and/or psychosocial impairment

Visual Impairments (including blindness): Visual impairments, including ones that can be corrected, that adversely affect a child's educational performance

Disabilities as Defined for Children 3 to 5 Years of Age

Children experiencing developmental delays, as defined by the state, in one or more of the following developmental areas: physical, cognitive, communication, social, emotional, or adaptive

Children meeting these requirements are eligible for services from their school district at age 3 years

Disabilities as Defined for Infants and Toddlers

Infants and toddlers from birth to age 2 years who (1) experience delay in cognitive, physical, communicative, social/emotional, or adaptive development; (2) are diagnosed with a physical or mental condition that has a high probability of resulting in developmental delay; or (3) are at risk of having developmental delays if early intervention services are not provided

From Publication 99-457, Individuals with Disabilities Education Act (IDEA), Part B.

TABLE 5-1

Number of Children Ages 6-21 Yr Served under IDEA, Part B, by Disability during 1996-2001

	1996-1997	1997-1998	1998-1999	1999-2000	2000-2001
Specific learning disabilities	2,674,407	2,754,484	2,815,610	2,867,794	2,887,217
Speech or language impairment	1,048,741	1,063,561	1,074,148	1,087,262	1,093,808
Mental retardation	593,602	603,331	610,677	614,283	612,978
Emotional disturbance	446,279	454,441	462,764	469,759	473,663
Multiple disabilities	99,440	107,253	107,811	112,999	122,559
Hearing impairment	68,773	69,783	70,876	71,400	70,767
Orthopedic impairment	66,342	67,417	69,436	71,417	73,057
Other health impairments	161,362	191,141	221,818	255,349	291,850
Visual impairments	25,762	26,031	26,096	26,385	25,975
Autism	34,375	42,517	54,064	66,043	78,749
Deaf-blindness	1,216	1,320	1,612	1,672	1,320
Traumatic brain injury	10,473	11,914	12,976	13,862	14,844
Developmental delay		3,792	11,907	19,263	28,935
All disabilities	5,230,772	5,396,985	5,539,795	5,677,488	5,775,722

From data based on the December 1, 2000 count, updated as of August 30, 2001. In U.S. Department of Education, Office of Special Education Programs, Data Analysis System (DANS): Number of children served under IDEA, part B by disability and age group, during school years 1991-92 through 2000-01, 2001d; U.S. Department of Education, Office of Special Education Programs, Data Analysis System (DANS): Number of children served under IDEA by disability and age group, during school years 1996-97 through 2000-01: age groups 0-2, 3-5, 3-21, 2001e.

TABLE 5-2

Numbers of Children Served under IDEA, Part B, by Disability and Age during 2000-2001 School Year

Disability	3-5 Yr Old	6-11 Yr Old	12-17 Yr Old	18-22 Yr Old
Specific learning disability	20,022	310,587	1,335,165	138,745
Speech or language impairment	20,022	958,916	129,947	4,958
Mental retardation	25,640	232,677	312,788	69,463
Emotional disturbance	8,508	169,420	287,398	25,482
Multiple disabilities	12,662	54,598	52,328	16,076
Hearing impairment	8,259	33,324	32,768	4,697
Orthopedic impairment	10,683	36,954	32,119	4,909
Other health impairments	13,355	139,617	142,853	9,390
Visual impairment	3,487	12,144	11,889	1,961
Autism	15,590	51,868	22,298	4,818
Deaf-blindness	208	568	519	233
Traumatic brain injury	891	5,444	7,716	1,690
Developmental delay	149,535	28,935	N/A	N/A
All disabilities	599,678	2,811,171	2,685,158	282,422

From data based on the December 1, 2000 count, updated as of August 30, 2001. In US Department of Education, Office of Special Education Programs, Data Analysis System (DANS): Number of children served under IDEA, part B by disability and age, during the 2000-01 school year, 20001c; US Department of Education, Office of Special Education Programs, Data Analysis System (DANS): Number of children served under IDEA by disability and age group, during school years 1996-97 through 2000-01: age groups 0-2, 3-5, 3-21, 2001e. Modified with permission.

preplacement evaluation must be sufficiently comprehensive to determine eligibility and what, if any, related services will be needed by the child. The findings from this evaluation process serve as the foundation for the child's IEP. When the preplacement evaluation is initiated, by law, the parents or guardians must be given information about IDEA, special education services, related services, their rights as parents, and the appeal process. IDEA requires procedural safeguards be established to protect the rights of parents or guardians and the child. The school system has 80 workdays to complete the preplacement evaluation process (Figure 5-1).

Implementation of a Free and Appropriate Public Education (FAPE)

If the child is determined to be eligible for special education an IEP meeting will be called to establish measurable annual goals, short-term objectives, frequency and duration of services, the special education and related services and supplemental aids or assistive technology devices required, strategies to address behavior if behavior impedes learning, and educational placement (NICHCY, 2000) (Box 5-4). Special education instruction is required to adapt the content, methodology, or delivery of instruction to meet the unique needs of children resulting from their disability. The goal is to ensure the child's access to the general curriculum so the education meets the educational standards applied to all children (NICHCY, 2000). The IEP determines how the child will receive a "free and appropriate public education (FAPE)" to meet the learning needs as a result of the child's disability. Box 5-5 lists the people required by law to be part of the IEP team, and Box 5-6 lists the components of an IEP. The IEP is reviewed annually to determine continued relevance, and a complete reevaluation assessment must be done every 3 years. Appendix A, "Individualized Education Programs," of the regulations for IDEA reviews the IEP process in a question-answer format that assists parents' and providers' understanding and development

BOX 5-4

Content Included in an IEP Document

Present level of educational performance: Current performance in school setting and how disability affects involvement in the general curriculum.

Annual goals: Reasonable measurable goals with identified objectives for meeting those goals. The goals should support the child's involvement and progression in the general curriculum.

Special education and related services to be provided including assistive technology devices: All services required to meet the educational goals including supplemental aids (e.g., communication devices) must be identified.

Participation with nondisabled children: Any time the child is not included in regular education programs with nondisabled children must be identified and explained.

Participation in state and district-wide assessments: Modification needed for accomplishing state and district general education testing need to be listed. If the child cannot participate in these standard tests then alternative testing must be planned.

Dates and location of services: When, how often, where, and for how long services will be provided must be stated.

Transition services needed: If the child is 14 years or older the IEP must list services provided to assist student transition to adult services.

Transition services: Children 16 years and older must have transition services and linkages with community agencies for additional services identified.

Measuring progress: Means of measuring progress toward goals and means of informing parents/guardians of progress must be established.

From National Information Center for Children and Youth with Disabilities: Briefing paper: questions often asked by parents about special education services, ed 4, September 1999.

of an appropriate IEP. This document can be obtained on the National Information Center for Children and Youth with Disabilities (NICHCY) Web site (http://www.nichcy.org/pub).

Least Restrictive Environment. Special education services can be provided in a regular classroom, special classroom or facility, home, private nonprofit preschool, private school, college,

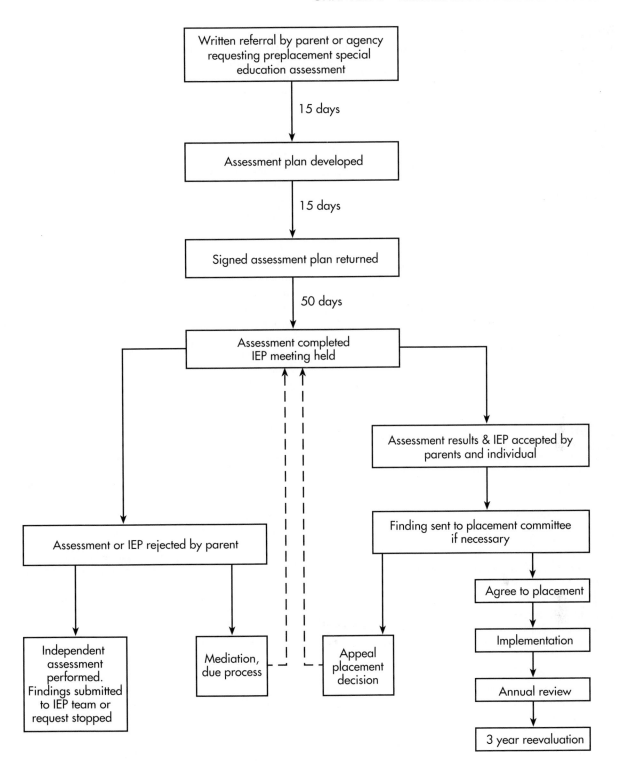

FIGURE 5-1 Preplacement and placement procedure for individualized educational program (IEP).

hospital, and even state prison. Children eligible for services who attend private schools are still eligible through the public school system, but parents will need to bring them to public schools for services.

"Inclusion" is the term used when a child receiving special education services is in a regular daycare, preschool, or school program. This environment is seen as the least restrictive, providing the child the fullest educational potential (Figure 5-2).

Most children in special education are in regular classes. They receive special education services (e.g., speech, physical, or occupational therapy) in the classroom or are removed briefly for services and then return to the classroom when the intervention is completed (Table 5-3). IDEA'97 strengthened the language supporting inclusion and participation of children receiving special education services in the general education curriculum.

Children with severe disabilities or who are medically fragile will require services in special classrooms often found within regular school settings; in special schools, institutions, or hospitals; or at home (if the individual is unable to attend other facilities). Special day classes usually fall into four cate-

gories and serve children with various severe disabilities (Table 5-4). Even profoundly handicapped children are required by law to receive educational services for a designated period of time each week. Depending on the size of the school district and the population served, these special classes may be available in the child's actual school district or in adjoining school districts that contract out services. In some situations, school districts contract special education services to private institutions or programs (Table 5-5).

Some children with disabilities have behaviors that interfere with the educational process. Although IDEA'97 mandates that the IEP address behavior problems proactively through the use of functional behavior assessments and positive behavior strategies, interventions, and supports (Lipton, 1999), IDEA'97 also established a process for school suspensions for children in special education consistent with suspension policies for nondisabled students. These new regulations, summarized in Box 5-7, have some disability rights groups concerned that disabled students with difficult behavior as part of their disability will be disciplined inappropriately and removed from their general education placement and placed in a more restrictive environment (Lipton, 1999; National Council on Disability, 2000; Silverstein, 1999).

BOX 5-5

IEP Team as Required under the Individuals with Disabilities Education Act Amendments of 1997

The parents of the child
At least one regular teacher of the child
At least one special education teacher or provider of the child
A representative of the school district who is:
    Qualified to provide or supervise the provision of special education
    Knowledgeable about the general curriculum
    Knowledgeable about the availability of the district's resources
An individual who can interpret the instructional implications of the evaluation results
At the discretion of the parent or the school district, others who have knowledge or special expertise regarding the child, such as a health care provider
When appropriate, the child or youth with the disability

From Lipton, D.J. *Individuals with Disabilities Education Act Amendments of 1997,* Disability Rights Education and Defense Fund, Inc. 1997. Modified with permission.

BOX 5-6

Components of an IEP

IEP forms vary from school district to school district but should all include the following information:

Present Level of Performance
☐ Describes student in positive way?
☐ Reflects parent concerns?
☐ *Include strengths and needs?
☐ State results of most recent evaluations?
☐ Describe how disability affects involvement in general education program?

Transition
☐ *Before age 14, what needs to happen to prepare for future?
☐ *At age 14, a statement of classes needed to prepare for future?
☐ *By age 16, specific transition services, related services needs, and other agencies to be included?
☐ *Before age 18, what rights will transfer to the student?

Annual Goals and Objectives/Benchmarks
☐ Are they meaningful and attainable within 1 school year?
☐ *Do they allow student to be involved in and progress in the general class program?
☐ Are they clear on *what* student will do and *how, where,* and *when* he or she will do it?
☐ *Do they include positive behavioral supports, if needed?
☐ *Is it clear how progress will be measured?
☐ *Is it clear how parent will be informed of progress?

Related Services, Supplementary Aids, and Supports Necessary
☐ To help the child reach annual goals?
☐ *To progress in the general education program?
☐ *To participate with other students—disabled and nondisabled?
☐ *Specifics listed: start/finish dates? frequency? location, length of time for services?

☐ *Modifications for participation in standardized tests *or*
☐ *A statement of why a particular test is not appropriate and what will be used instead?

Placement
☐ Is placement decided *after* goals, objectives, and supports are agreed upon?
☐ Is placement in the *least restrictive environment*?
☐ *If student is *not* participating in all general education activities, is there an explanation why not?
☐ *Is IEP coordinated with general classroom schedules, activities, and programs?

Instruction and Adaptations
☐ Who does what?
    Special education teacher?
    General education teacher?
    Parents?
    Student?
    Specialists?
    Aides or others?
☐ For the child whose behavior impedes learning does the IEP address appropriate strategics, including positive behavioral interventions?
☐ Are communication needs addressed?
    Limited English proficiency
    Other communication deficits?
☐ When, where, and how often will IEP be carried out?
    Seating preferences?
    Individual or small group instruction as needed?
    Extra time to complete assignments?
    Assistive technology needs?
☐ When and how will progress be reviewed?
☐ How will necessary changes to the IEP be made?

From IEP Checklist Parents Educational Advocacy Training Center 20(2):16–17, 1998; NICHLY New Digest Questions and answers about IDEA, ND21, ed 2, Jan 2000.
*Changes in IEP regulations caused by Public Law 105-17, 1997, Individuals with Disabilities Education Act Amendments of 1997.

TABLE 5-3

Number of Children Ages 6-21 Yr Who Received Special Education Services outside the Regular Class

Year	Total Students in Special Education	<21% of Services Outside Regular Class	21%-60% of Services Outside Regular Class	>60% of Services Outside Regular Class
1995-1996	4,821,557	2,286,505 (47%)	1,445,966 (30%)	1,089,086 (23%)
1996-1997	4,991,225	2,387,926 (48%)	1,487,080 (30%)	1,116,219 (22%)
1997-1998	5,150,860	2,494,209 (48%)	1,560,287 (30%)	1,096,364 (22%)
1998-1999	5,316,213	2,628,322 (49%)	1,575,988 (30%)	1,111,903 (21%)
1999-2000	5,434,707	2,681,082 (49%)	1,605,028 (30%)	1,148,597 (21%)

From data based on the December 1, 1999 count, updated as of August 30, 2001. In U.S. Department of Education, Office of Special Education Programs, Data Analysis System (DANS): Number of children served in different educational environments under IDEA, part B by age group, during school years 1990-91 through 1999-2000: age group 6-21, 2001b. Modified with permission.

TABLE 5-4

Categories of Special Day Classes

Special Day Classes	Diagnostic Category
Learning handicapped (LH)	Severely learning disabled
	Educably mentally handicapped
	Mildly mentally handicapped
Communicatively handicapped (CH)	Severe disorder of language
	Hearing handicapped
	Language delayed
	Severely learning disabled
Physically handicapped (PH)	Orthopedically handicapped
	Physically handicapped/disabled
	Multihandicapped
	Visually impaired/handicapped or disabled
Severely handicapped (SH)	Profoundly mentally handicapped
	Severely mentally handicapped
	Moderately mentally handicapped
	Severely emotionally disturbed
	Autistic
	Multihandicapped

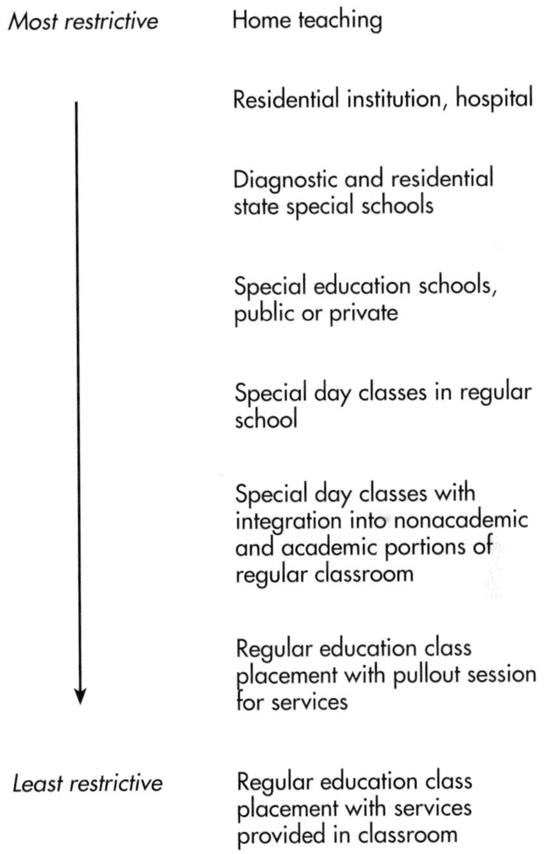

Most restrictive

Home teaching

Residential institution, hospital

Diagnostic and residential state special schools

Special education schools, public or private

Special day classes in regular school

Special day classes with integration into nonacademic and academic portions of regular classroom

Regular education class placement with pullout session for services

Least restrictive

Regular education class placement with services provided in classroom

FIGURE 5-2 Most to least restrictive environments for educational services.

Assistive Technology Devices. Part of the IEP for each child in special education should address the child's need for assistive technology devices, defined as any item, piece of equipment, or product system that is used to increase, maintain, or improve the functional capabilities of a child with disability (PL 100-407, 1988). Assistive technology devices can be simple items commercially avail-able off the shelf, such as a magnifying glass, or complex communication devices, such as a laser-operated computer to establish communication with a severely physically disabled but cognitively intact child (NICHCY, 2000; Support for Families of Children with Disabilities, 2002). Assistive technology devices have become more widely available, and the possibilities for augmenting a child's learning experience with computers, the Internet, and virtual reality seem endless. The financial cost of many of these devices limits their current use and places a severe financial strain on already underfunded school systems.

Problems with Implementation of IDEA'97

Lack of Adequate Funding. The intent of IDEA'97 is honorable, and it is an improvement over previous inequities and lack of services for children with disabilities. Problems exist, however, with funding, eligibility, responsibility for services, and the actual provision of services to the targeted child (Consortium for Citizens with Disabilities, 2002b; Thomas,

TABLE 5-5

Number of Children Ages 6-21 Yr Served in Different Educational Environments under IDEA, Part B, by Year from 1995-2000

Year	Total Children Receiving Services	Children in Public Separate Facility	Children in Private Separate Facility	Children in Public Residential Facility	Children in Private Residential Facility	Home/Hospital Environments
1995-1996	5,042,299	108,234	50,471	21,253	12,856	27,928
1996-1997	5,213,291	107,309	52,012	20,971	13,623	28,151
1997-1998	5,373,016	99,385	55,993	21,462	16,031	29,285
1998-1999	5,541,325	102,876	58,466	21,511	15,941	26,318
1999-2000	5,665,295	106,542	57,723	22,229	17,056	27,038

From data based on the December 1, 1999 count, updated as of August 30, 2001. In. US Department of Education, Office of Special Education Programs, Data Analysis System (DAS): Number of children served in different educational environments under IDEA, part B by age group, during school years 1990-91 through 1999-2000: age group 6-21, 2001b. Modified with permission.

BOX 5-7

Major Discipline Provisions of the 1999 IDEA Regulations

1. School personnel may remove a child with disability from the IEP-designated school placement for up to 10 school days for disruptive behavior or disciplinary reasons. Short-term removals are permissible when consistent with treatment for nondisabled children.
2. If the IEP team concludes the behavior of the child was not a manifestation of the child's disability the child can be disciplined in the same manner as nondisabled children except that appropriate educational services must be provided to meet IEP goals and advancement in the general curriculum.
3. If the behavior of the child was not a manifestation of the child's disability, then the child can be disciplined in the same manner as nondisabled children except that appropriate educational services must be provided to meet IEP goals and advancement in the general curriculum.
4. School personnel can unilaterally remove a child with disability from school for up to 45 days at a time for bringing a weapon to school or use or possession of an illegal drug.
5. If school personnel believe that a child with disability is substantially likely to injure self or others in the child's regular IEP-approved placement they can seek removal to an interim alternative education setting for up to 45 days via an impartial hearing officer. Subsequent extensions for additional 45 days can be requested. Alternative placements should provide educational services that enable the child to progress in the general curriculum, meet goals of their current IEP, and address the child's behavior.

From Silverstein, R. Overview of the major disciplinary provisions in the 1999 IDEA regulations. Center for the Study and Advancement of Disability Policy at the George Washington University School of Public Health and Health Services, March 18, 1999. Modified with permission.

2002). Lack of adequate funding to support public education and services for children with special needs is the basis for most controversies. Federal programs mandate services but do not adequately provide the financial resources to supply these services to all children who would benefit from them. For example, federal aid only funds an estimated 8% of special education costs (Terman et al, 1996). Although the range varies widely, on average the states pay 56% of the costs, and local school districts are responsible for the remainder. This results in poor communities having fewer financial resources to commit to special education services even though there may be more children needing services because of the risks associated with poverty.

Eligibility Restrictions. Because Public Law 94-142 (the Education for All Handicapped Children Act) and Public Law 99-457 (IDEA) identified only certain chronic health conditions as handicapping and as making a child eligible for special education and related services, children with milder handicaps or chronic conditions that do not result in significant disability in a given functional area (e.g., speech, learning, motor function, cognition) are not eligible for special education even though they would benefit from additional support in their educational program. States are mandated to provide the services to "eligible" children—not to all children who would benefit, setting up a complex mechanism for establishing eligibility. This often results in an adversarial relationship between the parents seeking services for their children and the educational departments of school systems functioning under severe budgetary constraints. States that actively embrace the call for early case findings and intervention actually increase their financial obligations without receiving additional money from the federal government.

Schools' Responsibility for Medical Services. Because educational systems are responsible for "related services," which include medical services and therapies needed by a child during the school day (e.g., tracheostomy suctioning, gavage feedings, intermittent catheterization, medication administration), the educational systems have become the overseers and deliverers of medical care, quite often independent of the primary or specialty care providers. All services that can be provided by someone with less training than a physi-cian are the responsibility of the school district (Martin et al, 1996).

Public Law 94-142 identified "a qualified school nurse or other qualified person" as the appropriate person to provide school health services (PL 94-142, 1975c). As the complexity of health conditions increases, the number of school nurses has increased only slightly. One recent study found that less than one half the schools surveyed had a registered nurse or licensed practical nurse for 30 hours per week and many were without any school nurse visit on a daily basis (Brener et al, 2001). As children with chronic conditions live longer and medical technology enables them to participate in school, concern has surfaced about the qualifications of school personnel to provide services to children with special needs (Esperat et al, 1999; McCarthy et al, 1996). Procedures such as tracheotomy care, ileostomy care, gavage feedings, and intermittent clean catheterization are all done routinely in school settings, often by unlicensed health care personnel (Harrison et al, 1995; Krier, 1993). Krier (1993) found that educators were performing medical procedures, such as medication administration (35%), tube feeding (12%), ostomy care (5%), catheter care (2%), and tracheostomy care (1%). Of the educational staff, 68% felt unprepared to care for medically fragile children, and only 30% had any training in health care procedures including first aid or CPR (Krier, 1993).

School districts that identify therapeutic interventions for children with special needs in the IEP process are generally required to pay for these services, although Medicaid fee-for-service or other public funding can often be billed. For children covered by Medicaid managed care, coverage varies substantially among plans (Fox and McManus, 1998). Private insurance will not usually cover services provided in the school setting. School systems are also financially responsible for providing the necessary equipment to support the child's educational program but can attempt to obtain reimbursement or funding from other sources, such as Crippled Children Services, Medicaid, the state children's insurance plans (SCHIPs), or other private health insurance plans (see Chapter 8).

Reauthorization of IDEA

The Individuals with Disabilities Act is up for reauthorization in 2003. Two recent reports (Finn et al, 2001; President's Commission on Excellence in Special Education, 2002) recommend major changes in the law. Disability rights organizations have expressed concern over proposed changes that they believe will limit services to children, limit due process for families, and release special education funds into the general fund for education (Consortium for Citizens with Disabilities, 2002a, 2002b; Disability Rights Education and Defense Fund, 2002). The National Council on Disability (2000) released their own report, "Back to School on Civil Rights," stating that federal efforts to enforce the IDEA have been inconsistent and ineffective, resulting in parents having to invoke formal complaint procedures and request due process hearings to obtain the services and supports their children are entitled to under law. Shortages of qualified personnel to teach children in special education persist (Consortium for Citizens with Disabilities, 2002b).

504 Accommodation Plans

All children in special education are also protected under Section 504 of the Rehabilitation Act (PL 93-112, 1973). In addition, students whose chronic conditions are not listed under the categories of conditions mandated for special education services under IDEA may still be eligible for services under Section 504. Section 504 of the 1973 Rehabilitation Act was modeled after previous laws that banned discrimination based on race, ethnic origin, and gender. This was the first time people with disabilities were seen as a class—a minority group deserving basic civil rights protection in employment, education, housing, and access to society (Golden et al, 1993). As applied to the schools, the language broadly prohibits the denial of public education participation because of a child's disability. It requires that the educational needs of the disabled child must be met and strategies for classroom adaptation be implemented so he or she can be educated as adequately as the nondisabled child in the least restrictive environment (Richards, 2000). Funds to support accommodations in education under Section 504 must come from the general education funds, not the funds earmarked for IDEA. Section 504 requires parental notice regarding identification, evaluation, and placement, but approval is not required. Periodic reevaluations are required, but Section 504 does not specify any timelines. Section 504 regulations have been used successfully to assist children with disabilities or chronic health conditions not covered under IDEA to receive services, including related services and assistive technologic devices, that enable them to participate more fully in the public school program. The Federal Office of Civil Rights has jurisdiction over implementation of Section 504, and conflicts between parents and school districts are mediated through this office.

Americans with Disabilities (ADA) Act of 1990

The Americans with Disabilities Act (ADA) (PL 101-336, 1990) prohibits discrimination against an individual with a disability in employment, all government facilities and services, including public schools, public accommodations, telecommunications, and transportation. The ADA was based on the 1964 Civil Rights Act, which prohibited employment and accommodation discrimination by the private sector against women and racial and ethnic minorities. Before the ADA, no federal law prohibited discrimination against people with disabilities in the private sector. This law has minimal effect on school programs but has been extremely helpful in facilitating the transition of youths with disabilities into employment positions and independent housing. ADA defined disability broadly using definition constructs first used under Section 504 (Box 5-8). Recent Supreme Court decisions have indicated that the disability must not only be present but also be limiting the person's major life activities for the individual to be protected under the ADA. If a person's disability (i.e., severe myopia or severe hypertension) can be mitigated by corrective lenses or medication, then that individual is no longer protected under ADA (*Sutton v. United Airlines, Inc,* 119 S. Ct 2139, 1999; *Murphy v. United Parcel Service, Inc,* 119 S. Ct. 2133, 1999) (Mayerson and Mayer, 2000).

BOX 5-8

Americans with Disabilities Act (ADA) 1990 Definition of Disability

An individual with a disability is a person who:
1. Has a physical or mental impairment that substantially limits one or more of the major life activities of the individual,
2. Has a record of being impaired, or
3. Is regarded as having such an impairment

Role of Health Professionals in Determining Special Education Services

Primary Care Provider

The primary care provider's role starts with early identification and assessment of children with disabilities, as well as "children at risk" for disabilities as part of the mandated "child find" regulations of IDEA. If the primary care provider identifies a child at risk, the family should be referred to the school district's special education office to determine the appropriate public agency to evaluate the child. Children in the birth–to–2 year age range may be evaluated through a variety of agencies depending on the state's implementation strategy for Part C of IDEA. Multiple services and assistive technology devices are available to infants and toddlers with disabilities through this program (Table 5-6). Over a quarter of a million children received services in 2000 to 2001 through Part C of IDEA (US Department of Education, 2001a).

In order to initiate the IEP process, the parents or caretakers must request a special education assessment in writing. The primary care provider can provide the parents with a sample letter to initiate this process and inform them of their rights and their child's rights under IDEA (Box 5-9). A written letter by the primary care provider describing the child's diagnosis, known limitations, available test results, need for medical treatments, and so on can be critical because it provides medical documentation to support the request and can guide the comprehensiveness of the evaluation. The IEP assessment plan is determined by this initial request, so it is important to identify all areas of delay or potential risk.

The primary care provider can be part of the comprehensive multidisciplinary assessment process by providing health records and physical findings, with parental consent, to the IEP team (Committee on Children with Disabilities, 1999). The primary care provider may participate in additional assessments or referrals to other specialists. Although the IEP team is responsible for explaining the assessment findings to the parents and child, the primary care provider may be able to offer additional insight or interpretation.

The primary care provider can be very helpful in reviewing the plan with the family to determine its appropriateness for the child (Committee on Children with Disabilities, 1999, 2000, 2001) (Box 5-10). If the provider and family think that the plan is not sufficient to meet the child's developmental and cognitive needs, then it can be rejected and additional recommendations made to the IEP team. Recommendations supported by assessment findings or relevant literature are more likely to be accepted and incorporated into the plan. The primary care provider should act as an advocate for the parents and child when there is evidence of inappropriate or incomplete planning by the IEP team.

TABLE 5-6

Early Intervention Services for Infants and Toddlers Birth through 2 Yr, United States

Total 2000	% of Population
230,418	1.99

Services Provided 1999	Number of Children/Families Receiving Services
Assistive technology	8,901
Audiology	13,772
Family counseling/home visits	53,764
Health services	19,807
Medical services	17,809
Nursing services	14,399
Nutrition services	10,640
Occupational therapy	61,041
Physical therapy	65,355
Psychologic services	5,744
Respite care	7,890
Social work services	16,460
Special instruction	96,168
Speech/language pathology	93,590
Transportation	25,555
Vision services	6,921
Other early intervention services	70,581

Number of Infants and Toddlers Birth through 2 Yr Receiving Services under IDEA by Year 1996-2001				
1996-1997	1997-1998	1998-1999	1999-2000	2000-2001
186,527	196,337	189,462	206,111	230,853

From data based on the December 1, 2000 count, updated as of August 30, 2001. In US Department of Education, Office of Special Education Programs, Data Analysis System (DANS): Early intervention services on IFSPs provided to infants, toddlers, and their families in accord with part C, December 1, 1999, 2001a; US Department of Education, Office of Special Education Programs, Data Analysis System (DANS): Number of infants and toddlers receiving early intervention services, December 1, 2000, 2001f.

BOX 5-9

Sample Letter to Begin Special Education Assessment Process

Date: _____

To: Principal of Child's School or Director of Special Education Services
    School Address

Re: Student Name, Current Grade, School, and Teacher

I am writing to formally request my child be evaluated through the special education process because of his or her difficulty with _____.
I have discussed my concerns with his or her teacher. I request that the initial plan for assessment for eligibility be sent to me within 10 days so that I may review and approve if appropriate. I understand the school district has 80 days to complete the assessment process. Please keep me informed of scheduled assessments or evaluation of my child once I have approved the plan. Please send me information on the special education programs, eligibility, parental rights and due process, and the IEP process.

Thank you very much for assisting in this evaluation of my child. I look forward to working with you and your staff.

Sincerely,

Signature

Parent or guardian name

Relationship to child

Address

Phone numbers

E-mail address

From Siegel LM: The complete IEP guide: how to advocate for your special ed child, Berkeley, Calif, 2001, Nolo.com, Inc. Modified with permission.

Questions to Ask When Evaluating the Appropriateness of an IEP Plan

1. What does the child know about the condition? How much of the care is the child responsible for? What help will he or she require?
2. Is the child's general health stable, improving, or worsening? Is the child terminally ill?
3. Are any classes or school activities contraindicated by the child's condition? Is the child placed in the least restrictive environment?
4. Is preferential seating in the classroom recommended? Are assistive devices required?
5. What modifications in diet exist? Does the child require any assistance in feeding?
6. What physical restrictions and exercise limitations exist? How are they best managed at school? Can the child access all school services? Is fatigue a problem?
7. What medications and/or treatments does the child receive during the school day? Can dosage times or treatments be modified around school hours?
8. Does the child require counseling, special therapies (e.g., occupational, physical, speech), adaptive equipment, protective devices, or transportation?
9. Does the child need assistance with any activities of daily living (i.e., toileting)?
10. What precautions, first aid interventions, and emergency procedures should school personnel be able to implement? Does the child wear a medic-alert bracelet?

Ongoing involvement of the primary care provider will facilitate a child's adjustment to school. Although the school district is the lead agency for services provided in the school setting, school personnel often welcome input from the child's primary care provider in coordinating health care information and services among specialty clinics, the school, and the child and family. If the school district has a nurse assigned to oversee health care services for children with chronic conditions, the primary care provider should establish a link with that individual.

Before initiating discussion with the school, it is important for primary care providers to seek the permission of the child and the family before releasing medical information to the school district or carrying on any dialogue with school personnel and adhere to HIPAA (Health Insurance Portability and Accountability Act) regulations (see Chapter 8) and FERPA (Family Educational Rights and Privacy Act) guidelines. Although this will not be a problem for most families, establishing open communication with the school district may need to be explored. Students may be hesitant to disclose information because they view their condition as a privacy issue (Betz and Redcay, 2002). If a condition is mild and not visible, families may not want information about the condition conveyed to school personnel to prevent their child being labeled as "different." In other cases, parents or students genuinely fear ostracism or reprisal from the school community. Regardless, some students find dealing with the assumptions others hold about their condition more bothersome than the condition itself (Thies, 1999).

The family's wishes should be respected if at all possible. When withholding information about a child places that child at risk, however, the family must be counseled about the risks and benefits of disclosure, and appropriate legal action must be taken. For example, withholding information about an adolescent with uncontrolled epilepsy who is enrolling in driver's education is both dangerous and illegal.

School Nurse

The school nurse has an important leadership role in the provision of school health services for children with chronic conditions (Committee on School Health, 2001; Wolfe and Selekman, 2002). The school nurse must assess the student's health, identify health problems needing to be addressed at school to enable the student to fully participate in the educational process, and develop a plan to address these issues. When children with chronic conditions require medical interventions in school an individualized health plan (IHP), analogous to the IEP for educational services, must be written and approved by the parents and school officials. The school nurse obtains information from the parents, from the student, and, with parent/student permission, from other health care providers responsible for the child's medical care and establishes goals and objectives for medical care and therapies in the school setting. The nurse oversees the acute, chronic, episodic, and emergency health care of all students in the assigned school. The nurse is also responsible for either direct nursing services or the training and supervision of unlicensed assistive personnel who often perform the medical interventions or therapies required by the IHP because of the limited number of professional school nurses in schools (Wolfe & Selekman, 2002).

The school nurse is in an ideal position to coordinate care with the primary care provider, specialists, and local public health and social services agencies. The nurse has the opportunity to see the child on a daily basis and can identify changes in health status, the effectiveness of newly prescribed interventions or medications, and the effectiveness of the IEP-related services and assistive technologic devices in meeting the educational goals for the child. Potential problems and strategies can be proactively identified and implemented, or changes in the child's condition can be easily communicated (Guilday, 2000).

Facilitating the School Experience

An important developmental task of children at least 5 years old is to move beyond the family sphere into the school community, where academic achievement, regular attendance, and social competence are major goals. Information regarding a student's academic performance, social skills, support networks, capabilities in performing daily living skills, and stamina for handling the demands of the school day needs to be assessed and acted on to best help children cope with the limitations that may be encountered in school while helping them maintain independence.

Factors Affecting Academic Performance

A successful school life is in part a function of academic performance. Youth with chronic conditions experience more academic difficulty than their peers (Thies, 1999). Disease severity, although one component, is not directly linked to academic performance. A nexus of factors, including school attendance, condition management, a child's sense of self, teacher and family expectations, and components of the school environment, facilitates or limits academic success.

School Absenteeism. The relationships among disease and chronicity, absenteeism, and school performance are complex. Illness alone is rarely a suitable excuse for academic difficulty and school failure. However, academic achievement is associated with attendance and absenteeism is significantly higher among children with chronic conditions (Newacheck & Halfon, 1998). Of students with chronic illnesses, 45% report falling behind in their school work and 35% of high school students report failing grades (Thies, 1999). Disease processes (e.g., AIDS dementia, poor oxygen diffusion, repeated hypoglycemia), side effects from various interventions (e.g., long-term steroid use, cranial radiation), and fatigue all may affect academic performance (Thies, 1999). The coexistence of psychosocial problems such as anxiety, depression, or family difficulties further exacerbates the student's potential for poor academic performance (Collins & LeClere, 1996).

The pattern of absences is more predictive of poor academic performance than the number of days missed, with frequent short-term interruptions more disruptive than a single, longer absence. Exacerbations in the child's condition, treatment side effects, fatigue, health care appointments, and family dysfunction are the primary reasons for absenteeism. Repeated absenteeism not only affects academic performance but also may create a downward spiral in a child's self-concept, peer relations, and subsequent family functioning. These consequences are difficult to reverse.

Families and professionals need to work together to reduce absenteeism. Parents must clearly communicate their expectations about school to their children and facilitate their attendance. Whenever possible, health care visits should be scheduled around school hours. If this is impossible, several appointments should be scheduled on one day so that the child does not have to miss several half days of class. Because parental guilt and anxiety can foster school resistance or school phobia and subsequent absenteeism, the primary care provider must address this issue.

If a prolonged absence is anticipated, parents must arrange for home instruction. School policies vary, and delays as a result of child ineligibility, poor coordination of services, or unavailable teachers may be encountered before homebound education is initiated. If schools are not approached before the requisite length of absenteeism (i.e., usually 2 to 4 weeks) is met, additional delays are likely to be encountered before services are arranged. Most schools are willing to work with families in maintaining their child's education by providing homework assignments, communicating with hospital-based teachers, helping parents become informal tutors, and arranging for tutorial services to begin as soon as the child is eligible. If hospitalizations are frequent or prolonged absences are anticipated, a specific objective should be included in the child's IEP to plan for uninterrupted schooling.

Mobility Issues. Limited mobility is an issue for many students with chronic conditions. Mobility is affected by physical impairments, diminished strength, and fatigue. Regardless of the cause, limited mobility can affect students' ability to achieve and compete. Physical changes can limit some children from participating fully in physical education, recess, sports, and afternoon activities. In the worst case scenario, limited mobility will hinder children from participating in critical learning activities.

If mobility is a problem, it must be discussed and appropriate adaptations planned for and addressed in the student's IEP meetings. Two major approaches are used to facilitate a child's mobility: structuring the environment and improving mobility. School districts have eliminated many physical obstacles in compliance with the Americans with Disabilities Act, but individual schools may be more difficult to navigate than others. When choosing a school is an option, its physical layout (e.g., number of floors, width of hallways, presence of elevators, location of bathrooms) needs to be considered. Providing the child with two sets of books, one for the classroom and one for home, eliminates the problem of transporting them. Scheduling classes close to one another and a study hall or lunch after physical education class gives the student more time to change and to avoid tardiness for the next class.

The student's mobility will be improved and normalization promoted if appropriate assistive devices are used. For example, an adolescent in a large high school may prefer to use a wheelchair when traveling long distances between classes rather than limiting the class schedule to classes that are near each other. Adaptive aids can help children write, reach books on library shelves, or respond to questions in the classroom. For students who drive, access to handicapped parking needs to be ensured.

Fatigue. Fatigue is an integral part of many chronic conditions that is sometimes a symptom of the disease (e.g., in heart disease) and other times associated with time-consuming therapies (e.g., with cystic fibrosis) or a side effect of medications (e.g., those given for epilepsy). Fatigue may also occur as a result of induced physiologic changes, such as in children undergoing chemotherapy.

Strategies for reducing fatigue focus on structuring a child's educational experience in a way that is not physically taxing. For example, the child could be encouraged to use a tape recorder for note taking, serve as scorekeeper rather than participating in vigorous activity during physical education, or be assigned easy classroom chores such as sharpening pencils with an electric sharpener. Choosing classes in close proximity is particularly important in large schools or those with several buildings. Scheduling a study hall period immediately after lunch gives the child an opportunity to nap (ideally in a different setting) without missing instructional time. Another strategy is arranging the student's schedule so that the most important classes are either in the morning or in the afternoon; that way if only half-day sessions are possible, the student can still learn the important content. The homework demands of various courses should also be taken into account when planning a child's schedule. It is better to defer one class than to have children take on a rigorous schedule that sets them up for failure. Selected courses may be taken during summer school to lighten a child's academic load. Ideally, this is proactively included in a child's academic plan because many schools have limited summer offerings. Students and families must be helped in setting reasonable expectations around participation in school activities.

Medications and Treatments. If medications are required during the school day, the general guidelines and criteria of each state and school district must be followed: (1) a legal prescriber must authorize the medication, (2) parents must give written permission for medication to be given, (3) the medication should be properly labeled, (4) the medication must be stored in a locked area, and (5) the school must document that the medication was administered. In order to ensure smooth coordination among providers, the school, and the family, orders for any over-the-counter medications also need to be given. When it is desired that children carry their own medications, such as with asthma inhalers, this must be cleared with the school district. If it is likely that a student will need to take medications ordered on an as-needed basis, clearly defined protocols should be made for their administration (Reutzel & Patel, 2001).

Medications that can interfere with learning need to be prescribed judiciously. Steroids, a mainstay with many chronic conditions, can lead to dysthymia, anxiety, sleep disturbances, weight gain, and other distressing symptoms that may interfere with academic performance and social acceptance (Thies, 1999). Other medications, including some analgesics, anticonvulsants, antidepressants, and antipsychotics, also affect academic performance. When monitoring a drug's efficacy in managing a specific condition, its side effects on learning must be assessed.

Whenever possible, clinicians should alter treatment protocols to occur around school schedules for several pragmatic reasons. The child with a chronic condition wants to be considered normal. Requiring the child to go to the nurse for medications may be met with resistance, particularly in this era of "safe and drug-free schools." Schools that have such programs unwittingly place the student with a chronic condition at risk for nonadherence. School nurses can adopt unobtrusive methods, such as instant messaging or vibrating beepers, to remind students about coming to take their medications.

Even in the best of circumstances, there may not be adequate time or qualified personnel within the school to administer medications or oversee treatments. As children enter adolescence, it is often appropriate to explore ways to help them develop self-care behaviors (e.g., self-medication, intermittent clean catheterizations, testing blood glucose levels). Such activities will help children become more autonomous, an important developmental goal.

Promoting the Child's Self-Concept

Developing a healthy self-concept is paramount if children with chronic conditions are to succeed in school and later activities. Many normative school activities (e.g., instruction in nutrition or sexuality) teach children health-promoting behaviors that can help build healthy self-concepts. Helping these children develop wholesome relationships and share their talents with other children is also beneficial; children who excel in a specific academic area or participate in sports and other extracurricular activities are more likely to be successful. Participating in these activities not only helps build self-esteem but

also enhances other spheres of development (Ryan-Wenger, 1996).

Unfortunately, developing the self-esteem of children with chronic conditions in the school setting is not without difficulty. These children face unique stressors associated with their condition that are further exacerbated by insensitive policies or a lack of privacy when taking medications or performing management tasks. They are more likely to be teased; many may experience bullying or even ostracism (Cavendish & Salomone, 2001; Kef, 2002).

Helping youth with chronic conditions develop a social support network will positively influence their psychosocial adjustment and self-esteem (Kef, 2002). Opportunities must be created for these youth to interact with nonaffected peers in nonacademic settings, including sports teams, clubs, and other extracurricular activities. They benefit from interventions to strengthen the coping abilities that help them deal constructively with the peer rejection, loneliness, or isolation resulting from such discriminatory practices (Turner-Henson et al, 1994). Incorporating social skills training into the child's educational plan is one way to help the child and family become more confident in their interactions with others and their use of appropriate behaviors when dealing with discrimination. School personnel can assist by dealing with inappropriate behavior of other students and developing an awareness of what it is like to have a chronic condition.

Students' self-concepts are enhanced when they can successfully communicate information about their condition and its management to their friends and school personnel, thus creating a supportive environment and enhancing their own safety and security (Christian & D'Auria, 1999). This is especially important for adolescents who are increasingly independent of their parents. The primary care provider can role-play situations with students, such as determining what friends they may trust and how to communicate selected information.

Parents, teachers, and school professionals need to acknowledge that children with chronic conditions experience the same developmental stressors as their peers and therefore need to be treated similarly and taught the same coping skills. Using a variety of techniques to help these children normalize their school experience will be beneficial to developing their self-concept (Ryan-Wenger, 1996).

Ensuring Safety

School systems are responsible for ensuring students with chronic conditions are in a safe environment. Because many chronic conditions or their treatments place children at greater risk for infection, illness, or injury, each student's risks must be assessed individually. For example, students with asthma may have varying classroom triggers ranging from chalkboard dust, to cleaning fluids, to fumes associated with science laboratory classes, plants, or class pets (Epstien, 2001). Impaired sensory function (e.g., cataracts, diminished vision) and lowered immunity may result from long-term use of steroids and so on.

The school's policy on notifying parents of possible exposure to communicable diseases must be clarified. Depending on the child's chronic condition, specific areas of concern may include strep throat, measles, mumps, meningitis, hepatitis

A and B, salmonella, or shigella infections. Latex allergy is another potential threat for students with chronic conditions. Although students with myelodysplasia are the most likely to be affected (see Chapter 33), any child with repeated exposure to latex is at greater risk.

For children on life-sustaining equipment such as ventilators, electrical adaptive equipment must be periodically inspected with a reserve generator made available. Adaptations in playground equipment should be made on a case-by-case basis. Disability may hinder participation in sports; appropriate safety equipment must be used under adult supervision. Strengthening exercises also help prevent injury. Provisions for transporting a student with a physical disability during emergencies such as fires and earthquakes need to be determined and disseminated to all school personnel.

Under PL 105-17, school buses may transport children with special needs as young as 3 years of age for related services. School buses need to be retrofitted with appropriate safety devices that meet federal motor vehicle safety standards. In addition, buses should be equipped with forward-facing seats with dynamically tested restraints and four-point tie-down devices for wheelchairs that allow the passenger to face forward. Certified transit wheelchairs should be used whenever possible; lap boards should be removed and stored separately. Strollers are not permitted. Students under 50 pounds should be restrained with safety vests. Oxygen, suctioning equipment, or other specialized equipment needs to be stored appropriately and labeled. An aide or nurse should accompany selected children. Written emergency evacuation plans should be in place with drills held yearly (Committee on Injury and Poison Prevention, 2001).

School Reentry

Primary care providers should actively participate in school reintegration programs for youth who have had prolonged absences or dropped out (Betz and Redcay, 2002). Those returning to school with new disfigurements are especially at risk. A positive experience of reentry can provide children with a sense of accomplishment and social acceptance, strengthen faltering self-esteem, and lessen maladaptive emotional responses to their condition (Thies & McAllister, 2001). Primary care providers can help promote a smooth transition for such children by proactively engaging the child, family members, and school personnel in discussing and determining strategies to facilitate school reentry. The two primary goals are to help the child and family anticipate situations they may encounter and to prepare teachers and classmates for the child's return.

One helpful approach to preparing the child for reentry is role playing, wherein the primary care provider plays the role of a classmate and children play themselves. The purpose is to act out a variety of scenarios that may occur during the first day back at school so that the child can develop answers to potentially embarrassing questions or situations that may arise. Another useful strategy is to ask close friends to accompany the child and serve as a buffer on the return to school. Parents may also bring the child for several drop-in visits or sponsor a welcome back class party designed to promote peer acceptance.

A variety of approaches can be used to help teachers and classmates adjust. A child may be encouraged to write a letter or record a videotape for classmates about the experience of being in the hospital or undergoing treatment, which is then shared with teachers or classmates several days before the child's return. Providing visual images of a child—either on videotape or in photographs—allows time for "sanctioned staring" or for classmates to ask questions or express their concerns without fear of recrimination. This is particularly important if the child has undergone major physical changes (e.g., alopecia secondary to chemotherapy, scarring from burns). Role playing is another helpful strategy. Two classmates can act out the scenario, with the teacher or the primary care provider guiding the experience. Science projects, literature assignments, and video presentations can be used by teachers to promote understanding and acceptance within the child's peer group. Careful advance planning will improve the likelihood of a successful return to school for the child.

The decision to repeat a grade must be made with great care. This setback can cause feelings of shame, inadequacy, and inferiority; but the decision to remain in the same grade may also enhance feelings of success because the work requirements may be easier. New classmates provide a second chance to form friendships.

School and the Terminally Ill Student

School is an appropriate activity for many children who are terminally ill because it provides opportunities for socialization and personal achievement. Depriving a child of such opportunities may cause increased stress. For children to have a successful school experience, several issues must be considered. First, the developmental level of the child and peer group must be considered in deciding on how the "who, what, where, and how" information about the child's condition is shared with the child, peers, school personnel, and other parents. Second, flexibility in planning the child's educational program is necessary if the condition deteriorates. Third, efforts to help the child maintain a positive self-concept and body image are important but may be difficult when a child begins to lose weight, cough productively, or have skin changes. Fourth, academic programming needs to be tailored for the child. For example, an adolescent enrolled in a college preparatory curriculum needs to be helped to develop achievable objectives rather than giving up all hope for the future. Finally, children who are dying often need to exhibit more control over their lives and environments. Whenever possible, efforts must be made to help children reach the goals that they have set for themselves.

It is not enough to focus attention only on the dying child and the family because many children have not had to confront death and dying and do not know how to act or the appropriate thing to say. Many of the strategies suggested in the section of this chapter on school reentry are appropriate for helping students deal with the death of a peer.

The effect that a dying child has on school personnel must be considered. The attitudes of school personnel toward illness and death, as well as their ability to individualize instruction, their concern or need to protect the dying child, and their fear of an emergency arising in the classroom, can influence their effectiveness. Flexibility and realistic expectations are needed if the school experience is to be successful for a child who is terminally ill.

Do Not Resuscitate Orders

Comprehensive planning for end-of-life care for a child with a terminal condition may include promulgating the family's wishes that the child not be resuscitated if a cardiac arrest occurs. A comprehensive approach to responding to do not resuscitate (DNR) orders in the school requires school personnel to develop a protocol to follow when a child with a DNR order attends school.

In 1994 the National Education Association (NEA) developed guidelines for DNR orders in school provided that a school district and state honor DNR orders in school (NEA, 1994, 2000). The NEA has suggested the following minimum conditions if a school board is to honor DNR: (1) the request should be submitted in writing and be accompanied by a written order signed by the student's physician; (2) the school should establish a team to consider the request and all available alternatives and, if no other alternative exists, to develop a medical emergency plan; (3) staff should receive training; and (4) staff and students should receive counseling. In its statement, the NEA delineated the following elements of the medical emergency plan: (1) the student's teacher specifies his or her actions if the student experiences a cardiac arrest or other life-threatening emergency; (2) other school employees who supervise the student receive briefing sessions; (3) the student wears an identification bracelet indicating the DNR order; (4) the parents execute a contract with the local emergency medical service and send a copy to the superintendent; and (5) the team reviews the plan annually.

In 2000 the Committee on School Health and Committee on Bioethics (2000) of the American Academy of Pediatrics released a joint policy statement on DNR orders in schools. This document is similar to that of the NEA, stressing the need for proactive planning among health and school professionals, family members, and, when possible, the student. It goes further, however, in recommending that pediatricians review the plan with the board of education and its legal counsel. The plan should also be updated every 6 months rather than yearly.

Last, individual states have DNR policies and laws that govern the actions of emergency medical personnel actions when treating students (Miller-Thiel, 1998). These regulations are quite varied, and practitioners are encouraged to determine specific regulations for their state. Schools should develop protocols for responding to DNR orders in accordance with NEA guidelines, American Academy of Pediatrics (AAP) policy, and state regulations and in a spirit of collaboration, respect, and sensitivity. Parents, educators, support personnel, and members of the health care team must be committed to a process that is flexible and responsive to the changing needs of the child. Essential to this process are ongoing forums where parents and educators can discuss their concerns, share their values and preferences about how certain situations should be handled, and define or revise plans. Within these discussions, it is crucial to define the range of possible scenarios that are likely to occur for the child and to build contingency plans for how they should be handled.

Summary

Primary care providers must not lose sight of the fact that schools provide opportunities for social, emotional, and cognitive development. A team approach based on the principles of family-centered schools helps guarantee that student's educational and health care needs are met (Thies & McAllister, 2001). School success for the child with a chronic condition is predicated on successful communication and information dissemination across respective parties (Esperat et al, 1999). Primary care providers may assume the role of coordinator by bringing together the child, parents, peers, and school personnel and fostering open communication. Providing in-service training to school personnel and using a "referral pad" that lists contact information for the provider's office, federal and state agencies, organizations, mentor programs, and support groups are ways to foster communication (Betz & Redcay, 2002; Esperat et al, 1999). Innovative school health programs based on delivering primary care in the school and linking it to the school program should be encouraged.

RESOURCES

National Information Center for Children and Youth with Disabilities
PO Box 1492
Washington, DC 20013
(800) 695-0285, (202) 884-8200
E-mail: nichcy@aed.org
Web site: www.nichcy.org

Consortium for Citizens with Disabilities
1331 H St NW
Suite 300
Washington, DC 20005
(202) 783-2229
www.c-c-d.org

Disability Rights Education and Defense Fund (DREDF)
2212 6th St
Berkeley, CA 94710
(510) 644-2555
www.dredf.org

US Department of Education
Office of Special Education and Rehabilitation Services
330 C St, SW
Washington, DC 20202
(202) 205-5507
www.ed.gov/offices/OSER

US Department of Education
Office of Civil Rights
330 C St, SW
Washington, DC 20202
(202) 205-5413
www.ed.gov/offices/OCR

Federation for Children with Special Needs Parents Training and Information Centers (PTI)
Each state has a PTI office.
Federation for Children with Special Needs (central office)
95 Berkeley St, Suite 104
Boston, MA 02116
(617) 482-2915
www.fcsn.org

Children with Disabilities
Web site: www.childrenwithdisabilities.ncjrs.org
Internet portal with links to federal, state, and local resources

The IDEA Practices
www.ideapractices.org
Provides information for professionals and families on IDEA

National Association of School Nurses
www.nasn.org
Provides information on policy statements, local chapters, and link to the Journal of School Nursing

National Association of State Boards of Education
www.nasbe.org/healthyschools
State level policy guides, publications, and annotated links to general school and health Web sites

Centers for Disease Control and Prevention, Division of Adolescent and School Health
www.cdc.gov/nccdphp/dash
Provides information on the coordination of school health programs and important long-term studies on children, youth, and school health

US Department of Education, Office of Special Education
Individuals with Disabilities Education Act (IDEA). Data collects information on student enrollment in special education by age, race, program, and state. Information from the Data Analysis System (DANS) of the U.S. Department of Education, Office of Special Education.
www.Ideadata.org.

American Diabetes Association
www.diabetes.org/advocacy
ADA is dedicated to eliminating discrimination against people with diabetes. ADA has been involved in numerous discrimination cases. ADA does not recommend specific attorneys but is able to provide general information and assistance.

REFERENCES

Betz, C.L. & Redcay, G. (2002). Lessons learned from providing transition services to adolescents with special health care needs. *Issues Compr Pediatr Nurs, 25,* 129-149.

Brener, N., Burstein, G., Dushaw, M., Vernon, M., Wheeler, L., & Robinson, J. (2001). Health services: Results from the school health policies and programs study-2000. *J Sch Health, 71*(7), 294-304.

Brown v. Board of Education. (1954). U.S. Supreme Court 347, US 483.

Burns, M. & Thornan, C.B. (1993). Broadening the scope of nursing practice: federal programs for children. *Pediatr Nurs, 19*(6), 546-552.

Cavendish, R. & Salomone, C. (2001). Bullying and sexual harassment in the school setting. *J Sch Nurs, 17,* 25-31.

Christian, B.J. & D'Auria, J.P. (1999). Gaining freedom: Self-responsibility in adolescents with diabetes. *Pediatr Nurs, 25,* 255-260, 266.

Collins, J.G. & LeClere, F.B. (1996). Health and selected socioeconomic characteristics of the family. *Vital Health Stat, 10,* 195(i-vi), 1-85.

Committee on Children With Disabilities. (1999). The pediatrician's role in development and implementation of an Individual Education Plan (IEP) and/or an Individual Family Service Plan (IFSP). *Pediatrics, 104*(1), 124-127.

Committee on Children With Disabilities. (2000). Provision of educationally-related services for children and adolescents with chronic diseases and disabling conditions. *Pediatrics, 105*(2), 448-451.

Committee on Children With Disabilities. (2001). Role of the pediatrician in family-centered early intervention services. *Pediatrics, 107*(5), 1155-1157.

Committee on Injury and Poison Prevention. (2001). School bus transportation of children with special needs. *Pediatrics, 108,* 516-518.

Committee on School Health. (2001). The role of the school nurse in providing school health services. *Pediatrics, 108*(5), 1231-1232.

Committee on School Health and Committee on Bioethics. (2000). Do not resuscitate orders in schools (RE9842). *Pediatrics, 105,* 878-879.

Consortium for Citizens with Disabilities. (2002a). *Consortium for citizens with disabilities education task force: Comments on the recommendations of the President's commission of excellence in special education.* Washington, DC: Consortium for Citizens with Disabilities.

Consortium for Citizens with Disabilities. (2002b). *CCD responds to "rethinking special education".* Washington, DC: Consortium for Citizens with Disabilities [online]. Available: http://www.c-c-d.org/Fordhamresponse.htm.

Disability Rights Education & Defense Fund (DREDF). (2002). *President's commission on excellence in special education: Final report. IDEA Rapid Response Network (RRN): News Briefing,* #12, July 8, 2002 [online]. Available: http://www.dredf.org/rrn/briefing12.html.

Epstien, B.L. (2001). Childhood asthma and indoor allergens: The classroom may be a culprit. *J Sch Nurs, 17,* 253-257.

Esperat, M.C., Moss, P.J., Roberts, K.A., Kerr, L., & Green, A.E. (1999). Special needs children in the public schools: Perceptions of school nurses and school teachers. *Issues Compr Pediatr Nurs, 22,* 167-182.

Finn, C. E., Rotherham, A.J., & Hokanson, C.R. (Eds.). (2001). *Rethinking special education in a new century.* Washington, DC: Thomas B. Fordham Foundation and the Progressive Policy Institute.

Fox, H.B. & McManus, M.A. (1998). Improving state Medicaid contracts and plan practices for children with special needs. *Future Child, 8*(2),105-118.

Golden, M., Kilb, L., & Mayerson, A. (1993). *Americans with disabilities act: An implementation guide.* Berkeley, CA: The Disability Rights Education and Defense Fund, Inc. (DREDF).

Guilday, P. (2000). School nursing practice today: Implications for the future. *J Sch Nurs, 16,* 25-31.

Harrison, B.S., Faircloth, J.W., & Yaryan, L. (1995). The impact of legislation and litigation on the role of the school nurse. *Nurs Outlook, 43,* 57-61.

Kef, S. (2002). Psychosocial adjustment and the meaning of social support for visually impaired adolescents. *Journal of Visual Impairment & Blindness, 96,* 222-37.

Krier, J.J. (1993). Involvement of educational staff in the healthcare of medically fragile children. *Pediatr Nurs, 19*(3), 251-254.

Lipton, D. (1999). *The final IDEA regulations have arrived!* Support for Families of Children with Disabilities Newsletter.

Lipton, D.J. (1997). *Individuals with disabilities education act amendments of 1997.* Berkeley, CA: 1997 Disability Rights Education and Defense Fund, Inc.

Martin, E.W., Martin, R., & Terman, J.D. (1996). The legislative and litigation history of special education. *Future Child, 6*(1), 25-39.

Mayerson, A.B. & Mayer, K.S. (2002). *Defining disability in the aftermath of Sutton: Where do we go from here?* Berkeley, CA: Disability Rights Education & Defense Fund (DREDF) [online]. Available: http://64.143.22.161/articles/mayerson.html.

McCarthy, A.M., Williams, J.K., & Eidahl, L. (1996). Children with chronic conditions: educators' views. *J Pediatr Health Care, 10,* 272-279.

Miller-Thiel, J. (1998). Do not resuscitate (DNR): state policies for at home and in school. *Pediatr Nurs, 24,* 599-601.

Mills v. Board of Education of the District of Columbia. (1972). U.S. Court of Appeals 348F, Supp. 866.

National Council on Disability (NCD). (2000). *Back to school on civil rights, January 25, 2000* [online]. Available: http://www.ncd.gov/newsroom/publications/backtoschool_1.html.

National Education Association. (2000). *Providing safe health care: The role of educational support personnel* [online]. Available: http://www.nea.org/esphome/nearesources/safecare.html.

National Education Association Executive Committee. (1994). *Policy on do not resuscitate orders.* Washington, DC: The Association.

National Information Center for Children and Youth with Disabilities (NICHCY). (1999). Questions often asked by parents about special education services. Briefing paper: LG1 (4th Ed.). Washington, DC: NICHCY.

National Information Center for Children and Youth with Disabilities (NICHCY). (2000). Questions and answers about IDEA. News Digest: ND21 (2nd Ed.). Washington, DC: NICHCY.

National Information Center for Children and Youth with Disabilities (NICHCY). (2001). Related Services. News Digest: ND16 (2nd Ed.). Washington, DC: NICHCY.

Newacheck, P.W. & Halfon, N. (1998). Prevalence and impact of disabling chronic conditions in childhood. *Am J Public Health, 88,* 610-617.

Pennsylvania Association for Retarded Citizens v. Pennsylvania. (1972). U.S. Court of Appeals, 343 F.

President's Commission on Excellence in Special Education. (2002). *Report. A new era: Revitalizing special education for children and their families* [online]. Available: http://www.ed.gov/inits/commissionsboards/whspecialeducation/reports/index.html.

Public Law 93-112. (1973). The Vocational Rehabilitation Act, 29 USC, Section 504, 45CFR. Washington, DC: US Government Printing Office.

Public Law 94-142. (1975a). The Education for All Handicapped Children Act 20 USC, Sec 11, 404 (18). Washington, DC: U.S. Government Printing Office.

Public Law 94-142. (1975b). The Education of the Handicapped Act, 20 USC, Sec 121a, 13(4). Washington, DC: U.S. Government Printing Office.

Public Law 94-142. (1975c). The Education of the Handicapped Children Act, 20 USC, Sec 121a, 13[10], Washington, DC, 1975c, U.S. Government Printing Office.

Public Law 99-457. (1986). The Education of the Handicapped Act Children Amendments of 1986. Washington, DC: U.S. Government Printing Office.

Public Law 100-407. (1988). Technology-Related Assistance for Individuals with Disabilities Act of 1988. Washington, DC: U.S. Government Printing Office.

Public Law 101-336. (1990). Americans with Disabilities Act of 1990, 42 USC 12101 et seq. Washington, DC: U.S. Government Printing Office.

Public Law 101-476. (1990). The Individuals with Disabilities Education Act of 1990, Washington, DC: U.S. Government Printing Office.

Public Law 102-119. (1991). The Individuals with Disabilities Education Act Revisions of 1991. Washington, DC: U.S. Government Printing Office.

Public Law 105-17. (1997). Individuals with Disabilities Education Act Amendments of 1997, Codified at 20 USC 1401 et seq. Washington, DC: U.S. Government Printing Office.

Reutzel, T.J. & Patel, R. (2001). Medication management problems reported by subscribers to a school nurse listserv. *J Sch Nurs, 17,* 131-139.

Richards, D.M. (2000). *An overview of §504.* Austin, TX: Richards Lindsay & Martin, L.L.P.

Ryan-Wenger, N. A, (1996). Children, coping, and the stress of illness: A synthesis of the research. *J Soc Pediatr Nurs, 1,* 126-138.

Shalit, R. (1997). Defining disability down. *The New Republic,* 16-22.

Siegel, L.M. (2001). *The complete IEP Guide: How to advocate for your special ed child* (2ⁿᵈ Ed.). Berkeley, CA: Consolidated Printers, Inc.

Silverstein, R. (1999, March 18). Overview of the major discipline provisions in the 1999 IDEA regulations. Washington, DC: Center for the Study and Advancement of Disability Policy at the George Washington University School of Public Health and Health Services [online]. Available: http://www.c-c-d.org/discipline.html.

Support for Families of Children with Disabilities. (2002). Support for Families Newsletter.

Terman, D.L., Larner, M.B., Stevenson, C.S., & Behrman, R.E. (1996). Special education for students with disabilities: analysis and recommendations. *Future Child, 6*(1), 4-24.

Thies, K.M. (1999). Identifying the educational implications of chronic illness in school children. *J Sch Health, 69,* 392-397.

Thies, K.M. & McAllister, J.W. (2001). The Health and Education Leadership Project: A school initiative for children and adloescents with chronic health conditions. *J Sch Health, 71,* 167-172.

Thomas, K. (2002). Parents: Special education services can come slowly. *USA Today,* June 17, 2002 [online]. Available: http://www.usatoday.com/news/education/2002-06-17-special-needs.htm.

U.S. Department of Education, Office of Special Education Programs, Data Analysis System (DANS). (2001a). *Number of children served in different educational environments under IDEA, part B by age group, during school years 1990-91 through 1999-2000: Age group 6-21* [online]. Available: http://www.ideadata.org/tables24th\ar_ab7.htm.

U.S. Department of Education, Office of Special Education Programs, Data Analysis System (DANS). (2001b). *Number of children served under IDEA, part B by disability and age group, during school years 1991-92 through 2000-01* [online]. Available: http://www.ideadata.org/tables24th\ar_aa9.htm

U.S. Department of Education, Office of Special Education Programs, Data Analysis System (DANS). (2001c). *Number of children served under IDEA, part B by disability and age, during the 2000-01 school year* [online]. Available: http://www.ideadata.org/tables24th\ar_aa7.htm.

U.S. Department of Education, Office of Special Education Programs, Data Analysis System (DANS). (2001d). *Number of infants and toddlers receiving early intervention services, December 1, 2000* [online]. Available: http://www.ideadata.org/tables24th\ar_ah1.htm.

U.S. Department of Education, Office of Special Education Programs, Data Analysis System (DANS). (2001e). *Early intervention services on IFSPs provided to infants, toddlers, and their families in accord with part C, December 1, 1999* [online]. Available: http://www.ideadata.org/tables24th\ar_ah3.htm.

U.S. Department of Education, Office of Special Education Programs, Data Analysis System (DANS). *Number of children served under IDEA by disability and age group, during school years 1991-2 through 2000-01: Age groups 0-2, 3-5, 3-21* (2001f, August 30). Retrieved August 25, 2002 from http://www.ideadata.org/tables24th\ar_aa9.htm.

Wolfe, L.C. & Selekman, J. (2002). School nurses: What it was and what it is. *Pediatr Nurs, 28*(4), 403-407.

6 Ethics and the Child with a Chronic Condition

Teresa A. Savage and Cynda Hylton Rushton

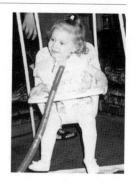

Decision Making Along the Course of Chronic Conditions

The course of a chronic condition is likely to include diagnosis and treatment; periods of recovery, exacerbations, stability, or instability; and in some cases, deterioration and death. These phases are often punctuated by recurring ethical questions, including the following: (1) defining what constitutes a life worth living, (2) recognizing the threshold for certainty in diagnosis and treatment, (3) choosing a decision maker to decide about treatment or nontreatment, (4) determining the role of minors in making treatment decisions, (5) deciding whether to pursue experimental or innovative therapies, and (6) knowing how to resolve conflicts. The range of chronic conditions in childhood and adolescence is paralleled by the range of values held by people with chronic conditions or caregivers of those with chronic conditions. Competing ethical obligations can create a set of problematic situations for children, families, and health care providers.

The Ethical Domain

Ethics is concerned with "what ought to be" and how individuals think about and discuss "what ought to be." Ethics is concerned with the behavior, choices, and character of individuals and groups. Ethical questions arise alongside—but differ from—fundamental social, legal, political, professional, and scientific questions. For example, public policies and laws (e.g., the death penalty) set boundaries for human behavior but do not necessarily correspond to an individual's sense of "what ought to be." It is within this context that ethical discourse occurs.

There are many ways of discerning the ethical dimensions of an issue or quandary. The process of discernment is complex and influenced by emotions, scientific facts, values, interpersonal relationships, culture, religion, the essence of who we are, and myriad situational factors—all of which converge to shape the way ethical questions are framed.

Ethical questions arise because an individual is unsure of the right thing to do or the proper outcome to pursue. For example, primary care providers may be concerned about whether to offer an experimental treatment protocol to a family when the likelihood of altering the natural course of the child's condition is remote and pursuing such treatment will require the family to pay out-of-pocket. Ethical questions may also arise because there are genuine value conflicts about the right thing to do or the proper outcomes to pursue. For example, primary care providers and families may disagree about whether it is justified to continue aggressive treatment for a child with end-stage cystic fibrosis. The providers may reason that continued treatment is burdensome and will prolong death; in contrast, the parents may believe that extending life is the appropriate goal to be pursued—despite the burden endured by the child. In both instances, careful consideration of the judgments and the justifications that are used to defend one's position and behavior is warranted.

Ethical deliberation involves the process of discerning, analyzing, and articulating ethically defensible positions and then acting on them. Ethical thinking provides a reasoned account of an ethical position and helps one move beyond intuition or emotions. The goal of ethical deliberation is not to achieve absolute certainty about what is right but to achieve reliability and coherence in behavior, choices, character, process, and outcomes.

Ethical theories and principles provide a foundation for ethical analysis and deliberation (Box 6-1), as well as a guide for organizing and understanding ethically relevant information in a dilemma or conflict situation. These theories and principles also suggest directions and avenues for resolving competing claims and supply reasons that justify moral action. Ethical principles are universal in nature but are not absolute. Each case involves particular principles and values integral to the decision-making process. One must balance the claims generated from competing principles relevant to a particular case. Moreover, factors such as family dynamics, the nature of relationships, contextual features, integrity, and faithfulness to commitments are also morally relevant to the decision-making process. Even when one chooses a morally justifiable course of action, there are always unmet obligations when resolving ethical dilemmas (i.e., a "moral remainder").

Ethical theories and principles must be applied systematically within the decision-making process. Ethical analysis is enhanced when a framework that provides a systematic process of decision making is used and mistakes are avoided by using only logic and reason (Box 6-2). In addition, because some decisions (e.g., those to withhold or withdraw certain therapies) help to determine the timing and consequences of death, other important social, ethical, and religious values come into play.

A Moral Framework for Decision Making

A specific framework provides a mechanism for individuals, families, and providers dealing with the ethical dimensions of difficult situations. For adults, a morally defensible framework for decision making is relatively straightforward and widely accepted (President's Commission for the Study of Ethical

BOX 6-1
Normative Ethical Theories and Principles

ETHICAL THEORIES
Teleological theories—Determine an action to be right or wrong based on the consequences the action produces. For example, in utilitarianism the principle of utility (i.e., maximizing the good or minimizing harm) is the central criterion for action.
Deontological theories—Focus on doing one's duty. The intrinsic quality of the act itself or its conformity to a rule—not its consequences—determines whether an act is right or wrong.

SELECTED ETHICAL PRINCIPLES
Beneficence—The duty to do good; to promote the welfare of the individual.
Nonmaleficence—The duty not to harm or burden.
Medical Harm
Pain
New Therapies
Maltreatment
Autonomy—Self-determination.
Respect for Persons—Recognizing another person as sharing a common human destiny.
Informed Consent
Justice—Fairness. Distributive justice refers to the equitable distribution of benefits and burdens under conditions of scarcity and competition.
Macroallocation
Microallocation
Beneficence and Justice

DERIVATIVE PRINCIPLES
Veracity—The duty to tell the truth
Fidelity—The duty to keep one's promise or word

Beauchamp T.L. & Childress J.F. (2001). *Principles of biomedical ethics*, ed 5, New York: Oxford University Press. Modified with permission.

BOX 6-2
Process to Facilitate Ethical Decision-Making

1. Identify the ethical problem(s); distinguish from clinical, administrative or legal problems.
2. Identify the key players (including the patient) and what their roles are; identify your role.
3. Identify the ethical issue(s); describe/define them in terms of principles, values of key players, and potential conflicts.
4. Identify the preferences of the key players regarding the decision to be made.
5. Identify the decision-maker(s).
6. Identify options, the range of permissible actions for this situation and the ethical ramifications of each action.
7. Make decision/facilitate decision/abide by decision.
8. Evaluate the decision-making process and your role in the process.
9. Consider what you would do differently in the future and why.

BOX 6-3
A Moral Framework for Decision Making

Beneficence
Balancing benefit and burden

Respect for Persons
Informed consent

Justice
Macroallocation and microallocation of resources
Individual vs. society needs

An Ethic of Care

Problems in Medicine and Biomedical and Behavioral Research, 1983) (Box 6-3). Consistent with the western view of autonomy, treatment options should promote the well-being of the individual according to that individual's understanding of well-being. When individuals lack the capacity to make choices for themselves, someone else must represent their particular values and preferences. Ethical decision making is a process with multiple contributors; it is a combination of the health provider's expertise on the available choices and the individual's or surrogate's expertise on which choices best promote that individual's life goals and values. This decision-making process is also influenced by the family system, culture, religious and spiritual affiliations, and personal values and preferences (Blustein, 1998; Jonsen et al, 1998).

For children, ethical decision making is more complex because most lack the capacity to make informed, independent decisions. Children have not formulated the life goals and values on which to base such decisions. Although the capacity to be involved in decision making varies according to a child's level of maturity, it is generally assumed that children need surrogate decision makers (Committee on Bioethics, 1994). A growing body of research supports the involvement of children in their health care decisions (Angst & Deatrick, 1999; Beidler & Dickey, 2001). Decisions made on behalf of children lack a key feature of the moral framework for adults: an

individual's unique assessment of his or her own well-being. Despite this, minors can be involved in meaningful ways in decisions about their own health care (see the section later in this chapter on respect for persons). The moral principles involved in adult decision making do, however, provide a valuable framework for making decisions on behalf of children (Ross, 1997; Savage, 1997). It is often useful to use ethical principles as an organizational framework for addressing ethical issues in decision making for children.

Beneficence

The primary principles involved in decision making are beneficence (i.e., doing good) and its corollary, nonmaleficence (i.e., avoiding or minimizing harm). Treatment options should include those that benefit the infant or child and clearly outweigh the associated burdens and harms. This "best interest" standard is often used as a hallmark when making decisions for children; it establishes a presumption in favor of life because existence is usually required for other interests to be advanced. Generally, life should be saved when possible. When life cannot be saved or the chance of survival is minimal, however, burdensome treatment should not be provided and palliative care should be considered (Hynson & Sawyer, 2001).

Burdens for children with chronic conditions include repeated pain and suffering associated with invasive procedures, symptoms, or disability, as well as emotional distress caused by fear, immobilization, prolonged hospitalization, or isolation from family and friends. Decisions about a child whose chances of dying are great might reasonably focus on the comfort associated with dying instead of on therapies to prolong life.

An additional standard, the "relational potential" standard, has also been suggested as an adjunct to the "best interest" standard when balancing the benefits and burdens of various courses of action (McCormick, 1974). This standard focuses on the child's cognitive and intellectual capacities, the degree of neurologic impairment, the prognosis of reversing the neurologic condition, and whether the outcome of the condition can be altered through treatment or therapy. For example, infants or children who are permanently unconscious have no capacity to feel either pleasure or pain, so their "interests" are limited to prolonging biologic life. Because such children cannot be burdened in the usual sense and most of the reasons for treatment (e.g., better function, fewer symptoms, the opportunity for human relationships or greater opportunity to achieve life's goals) are gone, many would argue that treatment is not obligatory (Fost, 1999). The Baby Doe regulations (PL 98-457, 1984), for example, regard permanent unconsciousness as a condition that does not require life-sustaining treatment; yet there are a wide range of views on the degree of neurologic impairment that justifies limiting or foregoing treatment. In addition, Saigal and colleagues (1996, 1999) have attempted to learn the perspectives of former "preemies" (now adolescents) on their present quality of life. Their insights debunk conventional thinking about the relationship of function with perceived quality of life.

The challenge for children, parents, and health care providers is to understand the unique meaning of the concepts of health, sickness, disability, suffering, care, and death for a child in a particular situation. The meaning that these concepts give to an individual's life is influenced by that individual's values, interests, aims, rights, and duties. A holistic understanding of a child's life, a recognition of important values that give direction to treatment decisions, and the tenor of the professional-client relationship evolve and change over time; therefore discovering the threshold for balancing benefits and burdens in a certain case may change as the child's condition changes. For example, the initial goals for a newborn with multiple congenital anomalies resulting in neurologic impairment and severe physical disability may be to understand the extent of the child's condition and to preserve life. In this instance, parents and professionals may agree to tolerate a high degree of burden to the child in order to diminish the uncertainty surrounding diagnosis and prognosis. However, 2 years later after the diagnosis and prognosis have been clarified, parents and professionals may have a different view of how much burden the child must tolerate to sustain life, especially when continued treatment will not alter the prognosis and may impose significant burdens.

Beneficence is promoted by helping the child and family construct a meaningful life by balancing the burdens of the condition with the positive dimensions of living. Beneficence is expressed by identifying individualized care outcomes that enhance the child's well-being (e.g., adequately managing symptoms, accommodating to limitations imposed by the chronic condition, maximizing functional capacities). Therefore treatment interventions must be designed to contribute to the individualized goals that enhance quality of life and promote the child's sense of integrity despite the limitations related to the condition.

Parents and professionals must openly discuss the uncertainty in diagnosis and prognosis and explore the extent of certainty necessary for both parental and professional decision making. At times, the need for greater certainty of either parents or professionals may result in burdensome diagnostic evaluations that do not contribute to the child's well-being or outcome. Alternatively, parents may accept uncertainty when professionals are compelled to seek further evidence to support their recommendations. The dynamic nature of the condition's course may create special challenges for caregivers and parents. Ideally, a shared vision and a common understanding of the balance of benefit and burden that is acceptable for a certain child are created.

Nonmaleficence

Health care providers have a duty to prevent or remove harms, yet the interventions they pursue to benefit a child sometimes cause harm. Certain medical interventions are painful and uncomfortable and can cause permanent injury or disability. These unintended harms may be justified if they are proportional to the overall benefit that the child will derive from the treatment. Unintended harms can occur with or without negligence. For instance, interacting with the health care system puts children at risk of iatrogenic harm, failure to adequately assess and treat pain can lead to increased suffering, or certain complementary and alternative medical (CAM) therapies intended to help may pose the risk of harm when their side effects are unknown. In extreme cases children with chronic conditions may receive intentional injuries because of maltreatment. Each of these categories of potential harm will be discussed further.

Medical Harms. Health care providers strive to prevent harm. With technologic interventions that support and improve health, there are often trade-offs in terms of comfort, side effects, restrictions of mobility, and, unfortunately, iatrogenicity. In the decision to accept treatment, parents and children (when developmentally appropriate) weigh the potential benefits against the known or potential harms that can occur with treatment. Chemotherapy usually causes side effects of temporary immunosuppression, gastrointestinal disturbances, hair loss, and fatigue and more permanent complications of peripheral neuropathy or sensorineural hearing loss. Even with careful symptom management, some children cannot escape the side effects. However, for many families, the potential benefit of cure (beneficence) over the burdens of treatment justifies the harm.

Other harms can befall children with chronic conditions who interact with health care professionals. Infiltrations of intravenous fluids, burns, nosocomial infections, and fractures are among the complications that can occur in an inpatient setting. The most common harm that occurs in pediatrics is medication error (Kaushal et al, 2001). These investigators found the majority of errors occurred in the neonatal intensive care unit. Children have less physiologic ability to sustain a medication error, yet there were often more opportunities for error. More calculations are required in ordering, dispensing, and administering medication to children than adults, increasing the likelihood of error at each juncture. Progress has been made in computerizing orders and altering how medications are administered, but the safety of children depends on the vigilance of the care providers.

Pain Assessment and Management. It is unequivocally substantiated that children have pain associated with disease and/or treatments. In 2001, standards for assessing and managing pain were required by the Joint Commission on Accreditation of Healthcare Organizations (2001) under the category of "Rights, Responsibilities and Ethics." The standard requires systematic assessment and monitoring of the child's response to treatment. Unless the pain provides a therapeutic, necessary use (aid in diagnosis or progression of symptoms), it should be treated, and then it should be reduced to the lowest possible level. When a child's pain is not treated adequately, the child experiences unjustified harms. Concern about oversedation or the dismissal of the child's self-report contributes to the undertreating of pain in children. Nonverbal children, very young children, or children with significant disabilities are especially vulnerable, and the health care providers must depend on the parents' interpretation of the child's behavior to assess pain and pain relief (Carter et al, 2002). Health care providers have a duty to stay abreast of assessment techniques and interventions for relieving pain in children (American Academy of Pediatrics and American Pain Society, 2001).

New Therapies. The introduction of new therapies for children with chronic conditions often raises ethical concerns. There are two categories of new therapies—complementary and alternative therapies and experimental therapies. Complementary and alternative medicine (CAM) has become increasingly popular. Micozzi (2001, pp. xxiii-xxv) identifies three major areas: alternative medical therapies, such as homeopathy and naturopathy; complementary medicine, such as psychoneuroimmunology, mind-body interventions, humor, or expressive and creative arts therapies; and traditional medical systems, such as yoga, Chinese medicine, and curanderismo. Koop (2001) cites that 80% of the population of the world depends on these therapies, so it behooves practitioners to be familiar with them. The ethical issues revolve around the safety of the therapies (Silva & Ludwick, 2002). For parents to make an informed decision about the use of CAM, they need information. Health care providers can assist the parents in finding reliable information on CAM, although there has been limited research. As with all decisions that parents make, the health care providers strive to ensure that parents have as much available information as possible to make their decision. The parents' choice of CAM may reflect their values stemming from their culture. Unless providers believe that the use of CAM represents a real danger to the health of the child, parents are given wide latitude in their use of CAM. The health care provider and the parents together can evaluate the available data, analyze the possible risks and benefits, and come to a decision in the best interests of the child. Nickel & Gerlach (2001) suggest a model

for communication between providers and parents that evaluates CAM on efficacy, safety, and costs.

Another view of "new" therapies is the use of experimental treatments or procedures in children. In addition, the National Institutes of Health (NIH) issued a mandate to include children in all federally funded research unless it was inappropriate, but the investigator must justify excluding children (NIH, 1998). Although research on children can be extremely crucial in discovering efficacious treatments, the NIH mandate is controversial. The Food and Drug Administration issued a Pediatric Rule requiring pharmaceutical companies to conduct clinical trials in children, but this rule was overturned by a federal court in late 2002 (Albert, 2002). Researchers must be aware of the different approaches that are necessary when conducting research in children (Broome, 1998).

Before children are included in clinical research, investigators must get approval from their institutional review board (IRB) to conduct their study in a particular institution. The IRB follows federal regulations for children, which stipulate four conditions under which a child may be included in a study. Briefly, those conditions are when the research (1) poses minimal risk to the child; (2) poses greater than minimal risk but there is the possibility of direct benefit to the child; (3) poses greater than minimal risk, there is no direct benefit, but the research should generate generalizable knowledge about the disorder or condition; and (4) would not otherwise be approved but "presents an opportunity to prevent, or alleviate a serious problem affecting the health or welfare of children" (US Department of Health and Human Services, 1991). Many, if not all, oncology treatments for children are through enrollment of the child in a national clinical trial. Parents must understand the nature of the research, risks, benefits, and alternatives. Again, the ethical imperative is to foster a complete and thorough understanding of the information for parents to make an informed decision. For children developmentally capable of giving assent, obtaining the child's assent is required, unless the study offers the prospect of a direct benefit.

It is important for health care providers to be aware of the "therapeutic misconception" that parents may have. Although they are told that the child will be randomized into the standard therapy or the experimental therapy, parents may believe that the inclusion of the child in a study is for the child's good. Although it is hoped that the child will benefit from inclusion, clinical equipoise exists; that is, it is not known which treatment, the standard therapy or the experimental therapy, is better. It is ethical therefore to randomize the child into one of the two groups. However, the purpose of the study is to determine the better treatment, thereby helping children in the future, but not guaranteeing the children in the study will be helped.

Primary care providers, children, and families must consider the balance of benefit and burden of both CAM and experimental therapies. To address these challenging situations, parents and caregivers should engage in ongoing, open discussions about poorly tested therapies or experimental treatments. For example, when an innovative surgical procedure is considered for a young child with an orthopedic deformity, the health care provider must disclose the uncertainty surrounding its effectiveness.

Maltreatment

Children with chronic conditions are 1.7 to 2.2 times more likely to be abused or neglected (Committee on Child Abuse and Neglect and Committee on Children with Disabilities, 2001). Many of the same factors that contribute to maltreatment of children without chronic conditions are also present in families of children with chronic conditions, such as dysfunctional families, high levels of stress in the parents, low socioeconomic status (SES), and lower educational level of parents (Goldson, 2001). However, maltreatment of children crosses all SES and educational levels; it is likely that poor, uneducated parents are reported for suspected or actual abuse and neglect more often than parents of higher SES and educational levels. It is also likely that fatalities caused by maltreatment are underrecognized (Crume et al, 2002). Primary care providers should be aware of the increased risk and assess families for parenting stress. Recognition and early intervention may reduce the incidence of maltreatment. Advocacy in the political arena for improved services for families of children with disabilities or chronic conditions may also aid in reducing the parental stresses contributing to maltreatment.

Autonomy

A child's autonomy, or self-determination, develops as the child matures. Before the child becoming an independent decision maker, parents make decisions for their children. Underlying the principle of autonomy is respect for persons.

Respect for Persons

A fourth principle involved in decision making is respect for persons. Respect for persons means respecting another person as sharing a common human destiny (Curtin, 1986). Adult decisions focus on the unique life goals and values of the individual out of respect for that individual and the integrity of each life. The uniquely human freedom of each person to create a meaningful life is highly valued. Even though children are neither autonomous nor self-determining, respect is still required because their lives also have unique meaning. To treat individuals with respect is to acknowledge and value who they are outside of a medical context, rather than to only treat them in accordance with how professional goals and values are advanced. Most children live in families that provide nurturance and care. The relationships that arise within families are inherently valuable to the well-being of children. To respect a child is to acknowledge the importance of the child's world and the relationships that are central to it. Unilateral decision making by health care professionals based solely on "medical indications" denies a child fullness of life and relationships that are also benefiting and sustaining.

A central problem associated with parental or other surrogate decisions is the inherent difficulty of judging the quality of a child's life and the benefits and burdens that are experienced. The child, family members, and health care providers may attach different meanings to the child's life. Although life is regarded as valuable, professionals and surrogate decision makers cannot consider the prolongation of life exclusively. Decisions need to benefit and respect the child as an individual but recognize that the child relies on the family for nurturance and physical care. The values that parents place on their parenting roles may make it difficult for them to separate the benefits and burdens of parenting a child with special needs from the benefits and burdens that the child experiences. These decisions are even more complex for primary care providers as they attempt to discern what is best for the child in the context of the family. The choice of interventions can positively or negatively affect the comfort or ease with which a child lives.

Respect for others is enhanced and evidenced by nonjudgmental attitudes and behaviors. It is important to stress that being nonjudgmental does not mean relinquishing values or being blind or indifferent to personal principles. Instead, the goal is openness to different ways of viewing and acting on personal commitments and life circumstances. An essential dimension of nonjudgmental behavior is not imposing personal judgments on others.

Informed Consent. The standard of informed consent is derived from the principle of respect for persons. Autonomy (i.e., self-determination) is the central moral value expressed through the process of informed consent. Legally, informed consent requires disclosure, comprehension, and voluntary agreement or consent by the competent individual or surrogate. To every possible extent, relevant information about diagnosis and treatment—including a description of the nature and purpose of the treatment or procedure, the benefits and risks, the problems related to recovery, the likelihood of success, and alternative treatments—must be discussed with the surrogate and the child (Ross, 1997; Savage, 1997). The person giving consent (i.e., usually a parent) must be able to understand relevant information, to reason and deliberate according to his or her values and preferences and the perceived values and preferences of the child, and to communicate the choices to others. Finally, consent must be given voluntarily without coercion. The informed consent process must be evaluated as the child matures and altered as necessary to include the child's expressed decisions or concerns.

Veracity and Fidelity

As part of respect for persons, the health care provider has a duty to be truthful and faithful. In caring for children, the health care provider may feel a conflict in loyalties; sometimes the provider feels a conflict between being truthful with the child and following the request of the parents. For example, a conflict may arise when total parental nutrition (TPN) is being recommended for a 14-year-old girl with Crohn's disease. Her parents have requested that she not be told her diagnosis or the length of time she is expected to need TPN. The health care team expresses their desire to engage the child in decisions affecting her care, but the parents are steadfast in demanding she not be told. In another example, a child who has sustained a spinal cord injury is told by his parents that his paralysis is not permanent. Despite his direct questions, his parents tell him that his condition is temporary and he will walk again "soon." Although the relationships between providers and parents can become tense, open, honest communication and transparency in decision making can facilitate decisions in the child's best interests. If a mutually acceptable approach to veracity cannot be reached, health care providers have the option of negotiating a smooth transfer of care to another appropriate health care provider when they believe they cannot, in good conscience, participate in a child's care. However, the transfer is not always feasible or desirable.

Justice

Justice pertains to fair and equal treatment of others. Therefore justice also refers to an individual's access to an adequate level of health care and the distribution of available health care resources. Caregivers promote the principle of justice by being fair in providing care and attending to children and their families. For example, the *Code of Ethics for Nurses* focuses on delivery of care with respect for human dignity, which is not to be defined in terms of personal attributes, socioeconomic status, or the nature of an illness (American Nurses Association, 2001). This provision requires that a criterion (e.g., age, gender, wealth, religious beliefs, social unacceptability) should not be a factor in deciding between individuals competing for the same treatment. This provision strives for genuine impartiality, equal respect for all persons, and refusal to create a hierarchy of individual worth. Prejudicial treatment on the basis of personal or other attributes is a violation of a moral norm and ideal precious to the health care professions for generations.

Consistent with the ethical obligations of justice, children with chronic conditions are legally protected from discriminatory treatment by state and federal laws. Section 504 of the Rehabilitation Act of 1973 (PL 93-112, 1973) grants protection from discrimination based on disability, whereas the Individuals with Disabilities Education Act (IDEA) (PL 101-476, 1990) and its amendments (PL 105-17) guarantee access for children with disabilities to education by establishing a federal grant program to help states provide a free and appropriate public education to all children in need of special education (see Chapter 5). The Americans with Disabilities Act (ADA) (1990) gives civil rights protection to individuals with disabilities by guaranteeing equal opportunity to public accommodations, employment, transportation, state and local government services, and telecommunications. Such laws create important obligations for both parents and health care providers and must be considered within the ethical analysis of troubling cases.

Macroallocations of Justice. Health policies for children with chronic conditions address some of the concerns encompassed in the principle of justice. These policies include strategies to avoid discrimination, stigmatization, and the exploitation of dependence. Strategies to support health insurance reform, delivery of family-centered service, access to employment and educational opportunities, as well as the community's role in supporting children and their families, are consistent with a justice perspective.

Issues involving the just distribution of health care resources arise at two levels. The macroallocation level refers to the share of societal resources allocated to specific societal goods, such as health care. Resources allocated to support the health, development, and education of children with chronic conditions reflect society's values and willingness to recognize and address the unique circumstances and needs of these children. Unfortunately, health care coverage for children rarely includes habilitation-rehabilitation services, and access to long-term care and other services (e.g., home nursing, some durable and nondurable equipment, and/or services for children without clear diagnoses) is usually limited. Eligibility is often restricted and based on income or physical, mental, or emotional disabilities. In addition, by not establishing uniform eligibility requirements for Medicaid or the state children's health insurance programs (SCHIPs) from state to state, children who depend on either of these insurance plans for support services and care in one state may not be able to obtain the same services if they move to another state (see Chapter 8). These issues reflect some of the challenges of devising a national health policy that supports the interests of children with chronic conditions.

Within health care, macroallocation refers to division of a resource (e.g., money) among various services (e.g., transplantation programs, critical care, outpatient services) (Beauchamp & Childress, 2001). This issue is particularly relevant at the institutional level, where costs and priorities for allocating scarce resources are determined. In an era of cost containment and downsizing, institutions and programs providing specialized services to children with chronic conditions are particularly vulnerable. For example, providers may reason that the expenditures for specialized services for children with organ transplants consume a disproportionate share of the overall budget for pediatric care. They may conclude that more children can be helped if money is spent on preventive services. Such reasoning focuses on the consequences of actions by evaluating their utility based on how they can maximize the benefits and outcomes for the greatest number of children. Focusing on a single criterion, such as utility, may not account for other important moral values (e.g., protection of vulnerable populations, existing obligations toward those in the greatest need of services).

Microallocation of Justice. The term "microallocation" is applied at the individual level; these decisions involve determining the distribution of a specific resource. In general, the professional's main concern is for the individual, but the needs of others may impinge on an individual's care—especially during periods of shortages of human and material resources. Health care providers participate in microallocation decisions when determining which child needs the greatest amount of care, thereby limiting care to others perceived as less needy. Microallocation issues arise when resources are limited and there is not enough of a resource to provide for all who need it.

Beneficence and Justice. The ethical principles of beneficence and justice are central to issues of resource allocation and rationing. The principle of beneficence requires health care providers to help others and promote good. This principle is evident on two levels: the societal level and the individual level (Beauchamp & Childress, 2001). Each level includes different considerations about allocating limited resources. To realize beneficence at the societal level, resources are allocated based on the needs of society. From a utilitarian perspective, the greatest good for the entire community is considered. The focus shifts from crisis care and doing good for the individual to preventive care and actions that benefit society. This shift is particularly important for children with chronic conditions because greater emphasis on prevention may diminish the specialized services designed to meet their needs. As resources become scarce, difficult decisions must be made to balance the needs of individuals—

especially those with chronic conditions—with the needs of society.

On the individual level, health care providers fulfill the duty of beneficence by allocating resources based on individual needs. Scarce resources are distributed to those with immediate needs without regard for the needs of other potential clients or the community at large. For example, when an infant is born with spina bifida, a cadre of medical, developmental, educational, and social resources is mobilized regardless of socioeconomic status, cultural or religious heritage, or ability to pay. This initial commitment to provide equitable and fair services for all families may not be sustained. Cost constraints, lack of available resources, and accessibility of resources may limit services for some children as they mature.

An Ethic of Care

Traditional ethical reasoning requires providers to ascertain the rights of the individual and weigh the ethical principles in order to resolve conflicting obligations. Applying ethical principles alone cannot resolve the clinical quandaries that arise during the care of a child with a chronic condition. The language and method used to analyze a particular case can either clarify or confound the situation. When the rights of children are held in opposition to the rights of their parents, for example, an adversarial tension can be established that may polarize discussion. In contrast, if it is recognized that most parents are motivated to promote their child's interests, such polarity may be avoided. Considering other aspects of the moral life (e.g., virtue, individual experience) may reduce adversarial tensions between the rights of children and their parents and allow for a more comprehensive appreciation of the attitudes, values, and moral commitments of decision makers within the context of family relationships. This perspective is often referred to as an ethic of care.

From the care perspective, the resolution of ethical quandaries is focused on the child's needs in the context of the family's and the provider's corresponding responsibilities within the provider-client relationship. Primary care providers can focus on the special circumstances and context of the specific situation in which moral action occurs instead of merely considering the individual's interests and preferences in isolation. Becker & Grunwald (2000) identify contextual dynamics of ethical decision making in the neonatal intensive care unit, but their sociologic observations resonate with other health care settings that care for children with chronic conditions. Such a model supports efforts to help children and their families find unique meaning or purpose in living or dying and realize goals that promote a meaningful life or death.

From this vantage point, the values and expectations involved in certain roles and relationships are primary. Therefore being an advocate for a child with a chronic condition involves appreciating the relationships significant to the child and understanding how those relationships affect care. Children with chronic conditions develop an intricate web of relationships that support and sustain them throughout their lives. In keeping with a family-centered philosophy of care, families are viewed as essential partners in the treatment and care of a child. Professionals must recognize and respect these interconnections as central to the well-being of a child. A care perspective

also emphasizes the interrelationships of the members of the health care team. Therefore it recognizes that nurses, physicians, and other caregivers work collaboratively to advance the interests and goals of children with chronic conditions.

Ethical principles (e.g., beneficence, nonmaleficence, autonomy, respect for persons, veracity, fidelity, justice) and an ethic of care provide a framework for approaching ethical questions that occur in clinical practice. It must also be acknowledged that although these are the most common, they may not be the only principles that are relevant to a particular case. The challenge for primary care providers is to discern how these and other principles can help illuminate the ethical issues and guide the resolution of competing obligations.

The Process of Decision Making

Shared Decision Making

Traditionally, a model of shared decision making is based on the assumption that decisions are shared among children (if capable), parents, and professionals (Box 6-4). Treatment decisions must represent a combination of the individuals' expertise in order to select choices that best promote the life goals and values of the child. Parents do not have the expertise to act as surrogate health care professionals, and health care professionals cannot replace the expertise of parents. Shared decision making means that parents and professionals should agree about general treatment goals, but professionals should make decisions about which treatment modalities are necessary to advance the agreed-on goals.

Endorsement of a model of shared decision making ideally means that parents and children (if capable) engage fully in the process by understanding the range of treatment possibilities and the consequences of each and sharing their goals, values, and aspirations in a meaningful way. Such a model goes beyond the legal requirements for disclosure, comprehension, and voluntary consent (Gale & Franck, 1998). Although professionals theoretically embrace the ideal of shared decision making as the desired model of parent-professional decision making, it is rarely accomplished in reality (Gale & Franck, 1998).

Role of Parents in Treatment Decision Making

Based on the moral framework of shared decision making described here, someone must represent the interests of the child. There is a strong presumption that parents should make judgments about the best interest of the child (Gale & Franck, 1998). Parents are appropriate surrogates because their strong bonds of affection and commitment are likely to yield the

---

BOX 6-4
Shared Decision Making

Role of parents
Limits of parental authority
Role of minors
Legal issues in role of minors
Reality of shared decision making

greatest concern for the well-being of their children. Parents are expected to protect their children from harm and to do as much good for them as possible.

There is a direct connection between the well-being of parents and children; the identities of each are inextricably linked. For example, a woman who defines herself as a mother regards her own welfare partly in terms of the welfare of her child. Harm to the child constitutes personal harm to the mother. Such relationships are valuable to both parents and children, and society needs to limit its interference in this private realm (Caplan & Cohen, 1987). Further, parents are identified as primary decision makers because of the importance of the family institution. Families play an essential role in maintaining the integrity of society. Children learn values of cooperation and commitment within the family context that can then be generalized to other members of society.

Parents must be involved in treatment decisions for their infants and children because there are lifelong consequences of these decisions. Parents will be responsible for the ongoing physical, emotional, medical, and financial care of the infant or child who survives with serious disabilities (Savage, 1998) and will also live with the consequences of those decisions. Long after health care professionals have forgotten a case, the family will remember and have incorporated such momentous decisions into the fabric of their lives.

Limits of Parental Authority

Children are not only members of their immediate families but also members of the broader community. A moral community shares an interest in the life and well-being of each member. There are certain community standards of best interest (e.g., preservation of life) that may override a family's interpretation of a child's best interest. Although there are compelling reasons to support the decision-making authority of parents, such authority is not absolute. The interests of the parents and the family must take a high priority but should not override the fundamental respect for the best interest of the infant or child. Ideally the family and providers engage in a partnership to include the child in decision making as appropriate (Dixon-Woods et al, 1999).

Even when parents and professionals presume shared responsibility to promote the well-being of a child, there are times when parents should be disqualified as primary decision makers. This disqualification may be the result of incapacity or choosing a course of action that is clearly against the child's best interest (President's Commission for the Study of Ethical Problems in Medicine and Biomedical and Behavioral Research, 1983). If a parent has a known psychiatric condition and is behaving irrationally or has a documented history of child abuse or neglect, the primary care provider may question parental capacity to advocate on behalf of the child. If there is a dispute about parental intentions or capacity to function as decision makers, it is incumbent that those who substitute another decision maker provide convincing evidence why the parents should be disqualified. For example, even though respect for religious beliefs is an important community value, so is the value of life. Although adults who are Jehovah's Witnesses can choose to forgo a lifesaving blood transfusion for themselves, they are often not permitted to make a similar decision for their children. Moreover, children are entitled to grow up and make independent assessments of their own religious beliefs.

In such circumstances health care providers must advocate for children and uphold the community standard of best interest. There will always be cases in which such assumptions are challenged; but these are likely to be few. Those who challenge parental motives and commitments must prove that parents should be disqualified as decision makers instead of having parents prove that their motives and commitments are authentic. Safeguards to protect the interests of children, families, and professionals will continue to be necessary and prudent. Assessing when community standards should outweigh a family determination is extremely difficult.

Whether the disqualification of parents always requires court intervention is the source of much debate (President's Commission for the Study of Ethical Problems in Medicine and Biomedical and Behavioral Research, 1983; Traugott & Alpers, 1997). When parents are disqualified, a surrogate decision maker should know all relevant facts and be able to perceive and represent the feelings and interests of those involved. Surrogate decision makers should also be free of serious conflicts of interest that may bias a decision. A court-appointed guardian ad litem often serves as a surrogate decision maker. In special circumstances, such as obtaining permission for withholding resuscitation for a child with significant disabilities who is a ward of the state, it is difficult to identify a single surrogate. The personnel in the child welfare agency may not know the child well, the foster parents may not know the child well, and the natural parents may not have any contact with the child. In these instances, ethics consultation may aid in identifying key people and designing a process for arriving at a decision in the best interests of the child (Savage & Michalik, 2002).

Role of Minors in Treatment Decision Making

Professionals who care for children and adolescents with chronic conditions are increasingly concerned about the role minors play in making decisions about their health care. Many adolescents experience catastrophic physical and mental health problems associated with severe disabilities, malignancies, or cardiac, pulmonary, and hepatic organ disease without having the legal right to decide about their treatments.

As client advocates, primary care providers must be concerned with how to promote the interests of adolescents in decisions regarding their health care. The concerns of adolescents escalate when parents and primary care providers seem to disregard the adolescent's previously expressed preferences or embark on a course of treatment that is inconsistent with the adolescent's life goals and values. Many health professionals are questioning the adequacy of current decision-making models and searching for creative solutions, perhaps through the advent of advance directives for minors.

From a moral viewpoint, minors with decision-making capacities have a legitimate claim to be involved in decisions about their health care. This claim is based on a respect for persons that recognizes that adolescents and young adults can be self-determining and therefore should have a voice in their care and the extent of medical interventions provided. Such respect for them as individuals and members of families and society compels primary care providers to take their preferences seriously when treatment decisions are made. Moreover, adolescents' interpretations of the benefits and burdens of treatment should be considered.

The standards for determining the decision-making capacity of minors are the same as those for adults: (1) the ability to comprehend essential information about their diagnosis and prognosis, (2) the ability to reason about their choices in accordance with their values and life goals, and (3) the ability to make a voluntary informed decision, which includes being able to recognize the consequences of various courses of action (American Academy of Pediatrics Committee on Bioethics, 1994; Awong, 1998; Midwest Bioethics Center Task Force on Health Care Rights for Minors, 1995). Based on our knowledge of conceptual development, most children do not reach this level of maturity until they are 11 or 12 years of age (Grisso & Vierling, 1978; White, 1994), although there is wide variation. These standards are straightforward, but applying them in clinical practice requires clinicians to be skilled in systematically assessing and documenting the decision-making capacity of minors.

Despite the importance of self-determination and well-being in justifying the participation of minors in treatment decisions, there is another competing value at stake: the interests of parents in making decisions for their minor children. It has traditionally been assumed that minors require surrogates to make decisions for them. Parents are generally identified as the appropriate surrogates for their children and have been afforded considerable discretion in making treatment decisions.

Currently, treatment decisions for adolescents are made through a joint determination by the physician and/or health care team and the parent or guardian for the child. Joint decisions to withhold or withdraw therapeutic interventions are difficult for both parents and health care providers to formulate. Parents may seek any possible intervention to prolong their child's life, regardless of the burden to be endured. Alternatively, they may wish to relieve their child's suffering by forgoing certain life-sustaining treatments. The physician and/or health care team and the parent or guardian may have different agendas for either continuing or initiating certain therapeutic interventions or instead forgoing certain interventions; yet both groups may interpret their decisions as being in the best interest of the child. Despite their assessments, neither group may truly understand the adolescent's perspective. In many cases, the adolescent may already understand the pain and consequences of the treatment options, including the finality of death. Unfortunately, parents and health care providers may hesitate to consider adolescents as legitimate decision makers about medical treatment.

As the model of decision making enlarges to include a definitive role for minors with decision-making capacity, health care providers must recognize that such a departure will also challenge the traditional process of decision making and may create conflicts between minors and their parents. The potential for such moral and legal conflicts will necessitate the determination of a mechanism for resolving disputes. Researchers combined information from three studies on decision making in pediatric oncology, published literature, and professional associations' positions to posit evidence-based practice guidelines

for end-of-life decision making by adolescents, their parents, and health care providers (Hinds et al, 2001). These guidelines may be useful outside the oncology setting as well.

Legal Viewpoint on the Role of Minors in Decision Making. The legal system has determined that adolescents in certain circumstances have specific rights and responsibilities associated with their decision-making capabilities for health care. Emancipated minors are children under 18 years of age who are in the armed forces or are financially self-supporting and live away from home (Traugott & Alpers, 1997). Most states have legislation recognizing the rights and responsibilities of emancipated minors. Emancipation is rarely determined by the courts and is generally implied through factors such as marital status, pregnancy or parenthood, and financial self-sufficiency. Emancipated minors do not need parental consent for medical treatment and have rights similar to adults in refusing medical treatment (Traugott & Alpers, 1997).

The courts have also classified some adolescents as mature minors in relation to their decision-making capacity for seeking and accepting health care interventions. Mature minors are at least 15 years of age and thought to have the capacity to understand the nature and risk of medical interventions. Adolescents classified as mature minors may consent to treatment that benefits them and does not involve any substantial risk. Derish & Vanden Heuvel (2000) present the various arguments, pro and con, for the mature minor's right to refuse life-sustaining treatment.

State statutes generally support a minor's (i.e., 14- to 17-year-old's) rights to consent to ordinary medical care. For example, some state statutes support the right of minors to consent to specific medical treatment (e.g., contraceptive therapies) without parental notification and consent; the right to consent to abortion, however, is complex and varied. The Omnibus Reconciliation Act of 1990, which is also called the Patient Self-Determination Act (PSDA) of 1990, supports the right of adults (i.e., at least 18 years old) admitted to health care facilities to accept or refuse medical treatment. This age limit is based on the belief that only adults have the capacity and the right to determine what should be done to their bodies—even if executing this right means implementing their right to die. It is crucial, however, that health care providers do not ignore the plight of thousands of adolescents (i.e., 12- to 17-year-olds) who face similar catastrophic and terminal conditions but are not given this legal right.

Although the PSDA was created for adults, the spirit of the PSDA provides an opportunity to examine the potential role of minors in their treatment decisions and ultimately their right to determine the circumstances of their death. It is likely that many young children and adolescents have the capacity to help make their own treatment decisions and determine what is in their best interest. There has been minimal guidance from the courts or from legislation on a minor's right to refuse lifesaving medical care. In the few decisions that have been rendered, the application of the mature minor status was used to support the minor's decision-making capacity to refuse treatment and understand the consequences of this decision. Unfortunately, because there are minimal and vague legal guidelines available to support a minor's rights to refuse treatment, health care providers are reluctant to intervene and support the minor's decision to withhold treatment—especially if this opposes the parents' wishes.

Involving minors in decision making about treatment requires families and professionals to create a system that supports the participation of minors. Such a system must include comprehensive guidelines for assessment, intervention, and ongoing revision (McCabe et al, 1996).

Making Shared Decisions a Reality

Regardless of the child's age, the family's composition, or professionals' involvement, resolution of ethical concerns is supported by an authentic model of shared decision making that accommodates the diverse ways children and families choose to participate. To resolve ethical concerns, it is necessary to move beyond a procedural model of informed consent to an authentic partnership where parents, the child, and professionals create an alliance that promotes the child's interests. The foundation for this alliance is a mutual understanding of each other's aspirations and goals, perspectives on what makes life meaningful for the child, and concepts of benefit and burden. In addition, parents need to share their goals, values, and definition of being good parents; and professionals must share their uncertainties and boundaries of their professional responsibility.

Shared decision making requires a vision that results from collaboration and open, effective communication using language without technical terminology and jargon. One reason success in achieving shared decision making fails is that professionals may focus primarily on the decision itself, instead of on the process. Parents also may have difficulty separating emotions from facts. A revised model of shared decision making would focus more on the context of the situation—especially the relational dimensions, the parents' unique concept of good parenting, and the factors that mediate decision making—rather than on the decision itself.

Professionals must begin to appreciate the parents' perspective in decision making and not try to force them into a traditional, rational, stepwise model that is incongruent with their perspective. Therefore the goals of the parent-professional relationship, the outcomes of the process, and the process itself must be closely scrutinized. For example, if the goal of the relationship with families is to get them to see the world in the same way as the professional, then dissenting views cannot be articulated or respected. Parents should be engaged early in a variety of choices about their child's care so that their involvement is not reserved for required consents for treatment or decisions about life-sustaining treatment. Parents need and want professionals to be partners in the care of their child—regardless of the outcome—and want professionals to help them be good parents in the process. Therefore sharing in decision making must begin early in the management of the condition.

Authentic shared decision making does not mean that differences will not exist or that everyone will come to the same conclusion about when and how to advance the child's interests. Nor does it mean that all participants will have the same skills, abilities, or preferences. Shared decision making is a process in which differences are discussed, differing opinions are valued, and the quality of care ultimately provided to the child and family is enhanced.

Transition to Adulthood

In most states, people 18 years of age and older are legally responsible for giving or refusing consent for medical treatment. People with chronic conditions often continue to be treated by pediatric subspecialists into their 20s and 30s because children with these disorders (e.g., spina bifida) in the past did not survive into adulthood. Unfortunately, some pediatric health care providers operate under a child-focused model of decision making and do not transition to an adult model when young adults are legally able and willing to serve as primary decision makers. Many transition programs are in place or being developed, but those are not without ethical problems (Callahan et al, 2001). Ideally, the adolescent or young adult would have increasingly participated in decision making as developmentally appropriate. However, in some families, children with chronic conditions are prevented from participation because their parents see them as too immature and unable to make rational decisions. The child's lack of experience makes their parents' impression a self-fulfilling prophecy. Lacking the experience, the child is unable to participate or fears participating in decision making. The health care team can educate parents to identify and foster the capabilities for decision making in their child: understanding information, manipulating information, appreciating the impact of the decision on one's own situation, and making a choice (Grisso & Appelbaum, 1998).

Many older adolescents and young adults demonstrate a sophisticated level of understanding of their conditions and treatment. Members of the health care team can honor the autonomy of older adolescents and young adults by preparing them to participate in decisions and acting on their choices after the informed consent process (Awong, 1998; Dixon-Woods et al, 1999; Traugott & Alpers, 1997). There are other older adolescents or young adults who—because of cognitive co-morbidity or immaturity—do not have the capacity to make decisions. Although they may be legally competent because they have not been declared incompetent by the courts, their ability to reason may be legitimately questioned. An assessment of their decision-making capacity, specific to the decision, should be undertaken and documented. Traditionally, parents or guardians have retained decision-making authority in such circumstances. Clinicians must work to foster decision making within the family context. To avoid confusion, parents should be counseled to seek legal guardianship for adult sons or daughters who lack decision-making capacity. Unfortunately, the cost of doing so is prohibitive for some families. Persons who lack the capacity to make decisions (e.g., those with severe mental retardation) should be respectfully allowed to participate in the decision-making process. As with young children, every child should be afforded the opportunity to be prepared for medical interventions, to receive developmentally appropriate explanations, and to express preferences. The more important the decision in the life of the person, the greater the care in assessing that person's decision-making capacity pertinent to the specific decision should be. Health care providers must be familiar with their institution's policies on surrogate decision making for adults who lack decisional capacity.

The Olmstead decision (*Olmstead v. L.C.,* No. 98-536, US Supreme Court, June 22, 1999) bolstered the move toward independent and assisted living. Young adults who previously would have remained at home or been placed in residential facilities may choose the most integrated setting possible vs. the most restrictive. The public entity, such as a state-supported institution, must facilitate placement in the most integrated setting appropriate to the needs of qualified individuals with disabilities. In the transition program, the health care provider who is knowledgeable about the Olmstead decision can assist in removing barriers so often faced by young adults with chronic disabling conditions.

Strategies for Ethical Decision Making

Increased Knowledge of Ethics, Laws, and Policies

Professionals can enhance their effectiveness in resolving ethical conflicts by seeking opportunities to enhance their knowledge of and skills in ethical analysis, as well as by identifying resources to assist them in resolving dilemmas. Further, knowledge of legal, public, and professional policies is advantageous. In particular, primary care providers who care for children with chronic conditions should be aware of pertinent state statutes and case laws that may affect their health care. Primary care providers must be particularly aware of institutional policies on discontinuing life-sustaining treatment, if such policies exist, and participate in developing them if they do not. Institutional policies that permit information to be withheld from parents or effectively deny parental access to divergent medical opinions should also be examined and challenged.

Proactive Dialogue, Assessment, and Planning

Children with chronic conditions and their families often have a high level of personal interaction with primary care providers. Because many chronic conditions persist over a lifetime, there are many natural opportunities to examine, revise, or abandon various goals or dimensions of the treatment plan. With proactive planning, it is also possible and desirable to anticipate the ethical conflicts that accompany the treatment plan. Ongoing dialogue about the treatment plan is essential for optimal planning and must not be reserved for crisis situations associated with acute episodes or illness, deteriorating conditions, or death.

Many children with chronic conditions and their families and providers will confront difficult decisions about treatment that will create significant moral tension. Questions about parental acceptance of psychoactive medications to treat children with attention deficit hyperactivity disorder or to try an experimental protocol for treating cancer may arise. Such morally difficult decisions are best made when there is adequate time for education, discussion, and reflection. Therefore ethical issues should be anticipated and discussions begun early.

Genetic Testing: Privacy and Confidentiality

With the Human Genome Project completed, ethical questions regarding the use of genetic testing and—it is hoped—successful techniques for preventing or curing genetic disorders arise. Genetic testing has long been accepted in newborn testing for the purposes of early identification for treatment. Technology has advanced to be able to identify many genetic disorders. Parents

may be offered the opportunity to have genetic testing for themselves and their child in an attempt to diagnose their child's condition. When signs and symptoms indicate that a child may have a genetic disorder, even if a cure is not available, the family may benefit by knowing the diagnosis, planning for the child's future needs, and learning the probability of future children being affected. Although parents may have an intense desire to discover their child's diagnosis, they may fear that their child will be stigmatized and discriminated against by insurance, school, and eventually employment. Hall and Rich's (2000) study of genetic counselors revealed that the fear of discrimination by insurers is not a major barrier to genetic testing.

There is disagreement between genetic counselors and insurers as to the need for federal antidiscrimination legislation: the counselors favor legislation, and the insurers oppose any legislation. No federal legislation has been passed to date to prevent discrimination, but individual states have enacted legislation. (Go to www.genome.gov/10002338 for a list of current state legislation.) Federal legislation to prevent exclusion from health care coverage and discrimination in employment has been proposed, but it is not known if the final laws will be sufficient (Beckwith & Alper, 1998; Rothstein, 1998).

Although the technique of obtaining a blood test or a buccal smear or performing a skin biopsy in the office may seem rather benign, the ramifications of the findings can have profound consequences on the child's and family's future. Primary care providers can guard the privacy and confidentiality of a child's medical information by developing and implementing institutional policies on informed consent for genetic testing, special disposition of test results, and special procedures for releasing medical records containing test results (i.e., to school [National Task Force on Confidential Student Health Information, 2000], insurers, and others). Many institutions currently have special procedures for tests (e.g., human immunodeficiency virus [HIV]) that protect a client from unwarranted disclosure of information. However, the Health Insurance Portability and Accountability Act of 1996 (HIPAA) (2002), effective April 2003, contains no special provisions protecting genetic information.

Presymptomatic genetic testing for adult-onset conditions (e.g., Huntington's disease, breast cancer) is not recommended for children (American Academy of Pediatrics Committee on Bioethics, 2001; American Society of Human Genetics and American College of Medical Genetics, 1995; Ross & Moon, 2000). Kodish (1999, p. 390) proposes the "rule of earliest onset" as a guide for testing children for cancer genes. If it is highly unlikely the child will develop cancer for which there is a genetic marker before the age of 18 years, testing for that marker is not recommended before 18 years of age. Another author argues in favor of predictive testing at the discretion of the parents for late childhood–onset disorders but is opposed to government-sponsored predictive screenings that "do not fulfill public health screening criteria" (Ross, 2002, p. 225).

Testing one member of the family can yield information about other members. Families need to be aware of the ramifications of testing. Genetic counselors are skilled in assisting families in making decisions to share or withhold information about a tested relative. Sometimes it is necessary to test relatives. Again genetic counselors assist families in understanding the extent to which other family members need to be involved to yield useful information. Guidelines in protecting privacy of family members for genetics research may also prove useful for protecting privacy for nonresearch testing (Botkin, 2001; Chen et al, 2001). Doukas & Berg (2001) propose a family covenant model in working with families who have genetic testing. The family covenant recognizes the family as a unit and its members in the context of the family. With genetic knowledge increasing exponentially, professionals working with children with chronic conditions and their families should stay abreast of genetic advances and applicable laws. Programs such as the ethical, legal, and social implications (ELSI) branch of the National Human Genome Research Institute provide leadership in this area (www.genome.gov). A special supplement to the *Journal of Law, Medicine, & Ethics 29*(2), 2001 is entirely devoted to a decade of ELSI research. Professional organizations may also provide information and advocacy on advances in genetics.

Anderson (2002) predicts in this decade there will be enormous advances in gene therapy, despite the setback with the death of an 18-year-old research subject in the late 1990s. Jesse Gelsinger was a young man with ornithine transcarbamoylase deficiency syndrome, a metabolic disorder that leads to an excessive buildup of ammonia. In an article written by his father, Jesse's enrollment in a clinical trial for "gene therapy" was described (Gelsinger, 2000). Although Jesse did not meet inclusion criteria for the clinical trial, he was included, and his father maintains that although they were told that the research would provide *no direct benefit* to Jesse, the risks were not fully disclosed. He died as a result of being injected with a viral vector intended to transport a gene to correct the enzyme deficiency. His father learned of the breaches in the research protocol and of the substantial financial interests the investigators had in the company sponsoring the clinical trial. Gene research at the University of Pennsylvania was suspended, and the father brought suit against the university, the investigators, and others, later settling out of court. A call for improved oversight of gene therapy trials was issued by public watchdog groups.

Hundreds of gene transfer protocols are underway or will be underway for conditions such as cystic fibrosis, hemophilia, muscular dystrophy, Fanconi anemia, Gaucher disease, and Canavan disease. As with any clinical trial, parents need as much information as possible to make an informed decision, and the child, if capable, should be included in the discussions. Additional ethical issues surrounding genetic advances, such as their availability and limitations (Scheuerle, 2001), will need to be addressed in the future. The use of stem cells shows promise, but use of embryonic stem cells remains controversial (Geron Ethics Advisory Board, 1999; Kaji & Leiden, 2001).

Strategies for Dealing with Conflict

Even when communication among children, parents, and professionals is optimal, conflicts arise. In fact, good communication may illuminate points of real ethical dispute. Participants often prioritize values differently and employ different processes to reach morally defensible conclusions. Therefore activities that promote multidisciplinary sharing, analysis, and decision making in an atmosphere of openness, objectivity, and diversity can lead to more tolerance of others' views.

When moral disagreements occur, strategies for resolution include the following: (1) obtaining the most current factual information on points of controversy; (2) reaching a consensus about the language used for concepts or definitions; (3) agreeing on a framework of moral principles to guide discussions; and (4) engaging in a balanced discussion of the positive and negative aspects of a viewpoint.

Institutions can review difficult or disputed cases through institutional ethics committees and other means of efficiently accessing legal, governmental, and consultative services. An internal review process can serve several purposes, including (1) verifying the facts of the case, (2) confirming the propriety of decisions, (3) resolving disputes, or (4) making referrals to public agencies when appropriate. Institutional ethics committees are often consultants to staff and families experiencing ethical conflict. Multidisciplinary membership (i.e., including a parent) provides a broad representation of different viewpoints. In general, these committees are primarily consultative without any binding authority. The opportunity for uninvolved parties to assist in reviewing difficult cases, however, can provide constructive recommendations for resolution. Ethics committees or the use of ethics consultants is increasing in home health agencies, nursing homes, and community health facilities.

Mechanisms to resolve conflicts between minors and their parents must be developed as the process of involving minors in treatment decisions unfolds. Based on a model of family-centered care, mechanisms supporting individual self-determination within the context of the family system are necessary. Strategies will also be needed to support families as they allow their minor children to be more involved in decision making. Mechanisms for examining the decision-making patterns of families and the roles of children and parents in other types of decisions within the family are also necessary. Finally, strategies to prepare minors to participate in decisions about health care through community and/or school educational programs and as part of routine health care encounters are important prerequisites (Dixon-Woods et al, 1999).

Summary

The resolution of ethical conflicts requires that health care professionals recognize there is a moral problem, use a systematic process of moral reasoning, and take action. As a prerequisite to such analysis, primary care providers who care for children with chronic conditions and their families must examine their own values about the content and structure of treatment decisions. Such clarification is necessary to ensure that the ideal of authentic shared decision making becomes a reality.

RESOURCES

Alliance of Genetic Support Groups, Inc
www.medhelp.org/geneticalliance/
American Nurses Association*
www.nursingworld.org

---

*State nurses association sites can be accessed here as well as through the SNA Gateway.

American Society for Bioethics and Humanities
www.asbh.org

Bioethics Online Service, Medical College of Wisconsin
www.mcw.edu/bioethics

Center for Bioethics, University of Pennsylvania Medical Center
www.med.upenn.edu/bioethic

Center for Clinical Ethics and Humanities in Health Care, University of Buffalo
www.wings.buffalo.edu/faculty/research/bioethics

Council for Responsible Genetics
www.gene-watch.org

Eubios Ethics Institute
www.biol.tsukuba.ac.jp/;macer/index.html

International Society of Nurses in Genetics (ISONG)
www.nursing.creighton.edu/isong

Kennedy Institute of Genetics, Georgetown University
www.adminweb.georgetown.edu/kennedy/

MacLean Center for Clinical Ethics at University of Chicago
http://CCME-mac4.bsd.uchicago.edu/ccme.html

National Bioethics Advisory Commission
bioethics.georgetown.edu/nbac

National Human Genome Research Institute
www.genome.gov

National Library of Medicine
www.nlm.nih.gov/

National Reference Center for Bioethics line
guweb.georgetown.edu/research/nrcbl/nrcbl.htm

REFERENCES

Albert, T. Federal court overturns FDA pediatric drug testing rule [online]. Available:
    http://www.ama-assn.org/sci-pubs/amnews/pick_02/gvsc1118.htm.
American Academy of Pediatrics & American Pain Society. (2001). The assessment and management of acute pain in infants, children and adolescents. *Pediatrics, 108*(3), 793-797.
American Academy of Pediatrics Committee on Bioethics. (2001). Ethical issues with genetic testing in pediatrics. *Pediatrics, 107*(6), 1451-1455.
American Academy of Pediatrics Committee on Bioethics. (1994). Guidelines on forgoing life sustaining medical treatment. *Pediatrics, 3*, 533-535.
American Nurses Association. (2001). *Code of ethics for nurses with interpretive statements.* Washington, DC: The Association.
American Society of Human Genetics & American College of Medicine Genetics. (1995). Point to consider: ethical, legal, and psychosocial implications of genetic testing in children and adolescents. *Am J Hum Genet, 57*, 1233-1241.
Americans with Disabilities Act of 1990. (1990). 42 USC 12101 et seq.
Anderson, W.F. (2002). The current status of clinical gene therapy. *Hum Gene Ther, 13*,1261-1262.
Angst, D.B. & Deatrick, J.A. (1999). Involvement in health care decisions: Parents and children with chronic illness. *J of Fam Nurs, 2*, 174-194.
Awong, L. (1998). When an adolescent wants to forgo therapy. *Am J Nurs, 98*(7), 67-68.
Beauchamp, T.L. & Childress, J.F. (2001). *Principles of biomedical ethics* (3rd ed.). New York: Oxford University Press.
Becker, P.T. & Grunwald, P.C. (2000). Contextual dynamics of ethical decision making in the NICU. *J Perinat Neonatal Nurs, 14*(2), 58-72.
Beckwith, J. & Alper, J.S. (1998). Reconsidering genetic anti-discrimination legislation. *J Law Med Ethics 26*, 205-210.
Beidler, S.M. & Dickey, S.B. (2001). Children's competence to participate in healthcare decisions. *JONA's Healthc Law Ethics Regul, 3*, 80-87.

Blustein, J. (1998). The family in medical decision making. In J F. Monagle, D. C. Thomasma (Eds), *Health care ethics: Critical issues for the 21st century* (pp. 81-91). Gaithersburg, MD: Aspen Systems.
Botkin, J. (2001). Protecting the privacy of family members in survey and pedigree research. *JAMA, 285*, 207-211.
Broome, M.E. (1998). Researching the world of children. *Annu Rev Nurs Res, 47*(6), 305-306.
Callahan, S.T., Winitzer, R.F. & Keenan, P. (2001). Transition from pediatric to adult-oriented health care: a challenge for patients with chronic disease. *Curr Opin Pediatr, 13*(4), 310-316.
Caplan, A. & Cohen, C. (1987). *Ethics and the care of imperiled newborns: a report by the Hastings Center's research project on ethics and the care of imperiled newborns.* New York: The Hastings Center.
Carter, B., McArthur, E., & Cunliffe, M. (2002). Dealing with uncertainty: Parental assessment of pain in their children with profound special needs. *J Adv Nurs, 38*, 449-457.
Chen, D.T., Worrall, B.B., & Meschia, J.F. (2001). Protecting the privacy of family members in research. *JAMA, 285*, 1960-1963.
Committee on Bioethics. (1994). Guidelines for forgoing life-sustaining medical treatment. *Pediatrics, 93*(3), 532-536.
Committee on Child Abuse and Neglect and Committee on Children with Disabilities. (2001). Assessment of maltreatment of children with disabilities. *Pediatrics, 108*, 508-512.
Crume, T.L., DiGuiseppi, C., Byers, T., Sirotnak, A.P., & Garrett, C.J. (2002). Underascertainment of child maltreatment fatalities by death certificates, 1990-1998. *Pediatrics, 110*, e18.
Curtin, L. (1986). The nurse as advocate: a philosophical foundation for nursing. In P.I. Chinn (Ed.), *Ethical issues in nursing.* Gaithersburg, MD: Aspen Systems.
Derish, M.T., & Vanden Heuvel, K. (2000). Mature minors should have the right to refuse life-sustaining medical treatment. *J Law Med Ethics, 28*, 109-124.
Dixon-Woods, M., Young, B., & Heney, D. (1999). Partnerships with children. *Br Med J, 319*(7212), 778-780.
Doukas, D.J., & Berg, J.W. (2001). The family covenant and genetic testing. *Am J Bioeth, 1*(3), 2-10.
Duckett et al: Ethics education project, 1986, Minneapolis, Univ. of Minnesota School of Nursing.
Fost, N. (1999). Decisions regarding treatment of seriously ill newborns. *JAMA, 281*(21), 2041-2043.
Gale, G. & Franck, L.S. (1998). Neonatology: toward a standard of care for parents of infants in the neonatal intensive care unit. *Crit Care Nurs 18*(5), 66-74.
Gelsinger, P. (2000). Jesse's intent. *Guinea Pig Zero, 8*, 7-17.
Geron Ethics Advisory Board. (1999). Research with human embryonic stem cells: ethical considerations. *Hastings Center Report, 29*(2), 31-36.
Goldson, E. (2001). Maltreatment among children with disabilities. *Inf Young Children, 13*(4), 44-54.
Grisso, T., & Appelbaum, P.S. (1998). *Assessing competence to consent to treatment.* New York: Oxford University Press.
Grisso, T. & Vierling, L. (1978). Minors' consent to treatment: a developmental perspective, *Prof Psychol, 9*, 412-427.
Hall, M.A., & Rich, S.S. (2000). Genetic privacy laws and patients' fear of discrimination by health insurers: The view from genetic counselors. *J Law Med Ethics, 28*, 245-257.
Health Information Portability and Accountability Act (HIPAA) [online]. Available : http://www.hhs.gov/ocr/hipaa/.
Hinds, P.S., Oakes, L., Furman, W., Quargnenti, A., Olson, M.S., et al. (2001). End-of-life decision making by adolescents, parents, and healthcare providers in pediatric oncology: Research to evidence-based practice guidelines. *Cancer Nurs, 24*(2), 122-134.
Hynson, J.L., & Sawyer, S.M. (2001). Paediatric palliative care: Distinctive needs and emerging issues. *J Paediatr Child Health, 37*(4), 323-325.
Joint Commission on Accreditation of Healthcare Organizations. (2001). *Comprehensive accreditation manual for hospitals: the official handbook.* Oakbrook Terrace, IL: Author.
Jonsen, A.R., Siegler, M., & Winslade, W.J. (1998). *Clinical ethics.* (4th ed.). New York: McGraw-Hill.
Kaji, E.H., & Leiden, J.M. (2001). Gene and stem cell therapies. *JAMA, 285*, 545-550.
Kaushal, R., Bates, D.W., Landrigan, C., McKenna, K.J., et al. (2001). Medication errors and adverse drug events in pediatric inpatients. *JAMA, 285*(16), 2114-2120.
Kodish, E. (1999). Testing children for cancer genes: The rule of earliest onset. *J Pediatr, 135*(3), 390-395.

Koop, C.E. (2001). The art and science of medicine. In M.S. Micozzi (Ed.), *The fundamentals of complementary and alternative medicine,* (2nd ed., p. xi). New York: Churchill Livingstone.

McCabe, M.A., Rushton, C.H., Glover, J., Murray, M.G., & Leikin, S. (1996). Implications of the patient self-determination act: guidelines for involving adolescents in medical decision-making, *J Adolesc Health, 19*(5), 319-324.

McCormick, R. (1974). To save or let die: the dilemma of modern medicine. *JAMA 229*(2), 172-176.

Micozzi, M.S. (2001). *Fundamentals of complementary and alternative medicine* (2nd ed.). New York: Churchill Livingstone.

Midwest Bioethics Center Task Force on Health Care Rights for Minors. (1995). Health care treatment decision-making guidelines for minors. *Bioethics Forum, 11*(4), A1-A16.

National Institutes of Health: Policy and guidelines on the inclusion of children as participants in research involving human subjects [online]. Available: http://grants1.nih.gov/grants/guide/notice-files/not98-024.html.

National Task Force on Confidential Student Health Information. (2000). *Guidelines for protecting confidential student health information.* Kent, OH: American School Health Association.

Nickel, R.D. & Gerlach, E.K. (2001). The use of complementary and alternative therapies by the families of children with chronic conditions and disabilities. *Inf Young Children, 14*(1), 67-78.

Olmstead v. L. C. (98-536) U. S. Supreme Court, decided June 22, 1999. [online]. Available: http://supct.law.cornell.edu/supct/html/98-536.ZO.html.

Omnibus Reconciliation Act (Patient Self-Determination Act [PSDA]), Title IV, Section 4206, h12456-h12457, Congressional Record, October 26, 1990.

President's Commission for the Study of Ethical Problems in Medicine and Biomedical and Behavioral Research: Deciding to forgo life-sustaining treatment. (1983). Washington, DC: U.S. Government Printing Office.

Public Law 93-112, Section 504 of the Rehabilitation Act of 1973. (1973). Washington, DC: U.S. Government Printing Office.

Public Law 98-457, The Child Abuse Amendments 42 U.S. Code, 101, Interpretative guidelines (45 CFR Part 1 1340.15 et eq.). (1984). Washington, DC: U.S. Government Printing Office.

Public Law 101-476, Individuals with Disabilities Education Act (IDEA). (1990). Washington, DC: U.S. Government Printing Office.

Public Law 105-17 [online]. Available: http://www.ed.gov/offices/OSERS/Policy/IDEA/the_law.html.

Ross, L.F. (1997). Health care decision making by children: is it in their best interest? *Hastings Cent Rep, 27*(6).

Ross, L.F. (2002). Predictive genetic testing for conditions that present in childhood. *Kennedy Inst Ethics J, 12*(3), 225-244.

Ross, L.F. & Moon, M.R. (2000). Ethical issues in genetic testing of children. *Arch Pediatr Adolesc Med, 154*(9), 873-879.

Rothstein, M.A. (1998). Genetic privacy and confidentiality: why they are so hard to protect. *J Law, Med Ethics, 26,*198-204.

Saigal, S., Feeny, D., Rosenbaum ,P., Furlong, W., Burrows, E., & Stoskopf, B. (1996). Self-perceived health status and health-related quality of life of extremely low-birth-weight infants at adolescence. *JAMA, 276,* 453-459.

Saigal, S., Stoskopf, B.L., & Feeny, D. (1999). Differences in preferences for neonatal outcomes among health care professionals, parents, and adolescents. *JAMA, 281,* 1991-1997.

Savage, T.A. (1998). Children with severe and profound disabilities and the issue of social justice. *Adv Pract Nurs Quart 4*(2), 53-58.

Savage, T.A. (1997). Ethical decision-making for children. *Crit Care Nurs Clin North Am, 9*(1), 97-105.

Savage, T.A. & Michalik, D.R. (2002). Finding agreement to limit life-sustaining treatment for children who are in state custody. *Curr Pract Pediatr Nurs, 27,* 594-597.

Scheuerle, A. (2001). Limits of the genetic revolution. *Arch Pediatr Adolesc Med, 155,* 1204-1209.

Silva, M.C. & Ludwick, R. Ethical issues in complementary/alternative therapies. *Online J Issues Nurs* [online]. Available: http://nursingworld.org/ojin/ethicol/ethics_7.htm.

Traugott, I. & Alpers, A. (1997). In their own hands: Adolescents' refusals of medical treatment. *Arch Pediatr Adolesc Med, 151*(9), 922-927.

U.S. Department of Health and Human Services. (1991). 45 CFR 46 Subpart B. 46.404-407.

White, B.C. (1994). *Competence to consent.* Washington DC: Georgetown University Press.

7 Care Coordination

Barbara J. Kruger

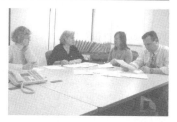

Definition and Background

Care coordination is the process of arranging and integrating the delivery of health and related services across providers and service systems, over time, for families and their children with special health care needs (CSHCN). Care coordination and case management are described as separate end points on a continuum of services according to a multistate study of Medicaid managed care programs (Rosenbach and Young, 2000). In these programs, care coordination was based on a social service model whose goal was to facilitate access to quality care across a broad range of programs in the community for vulnerable populations. Case management, in contrast, was focused on containing costs within a medical model of service delivery for high users of costly services. More significantly, "care coordination" is the term families of CSHCN prefer.

The most commonly disseminated definitions or descriptions of care coordination specific to CSHCN are promoted by the Maternal and Child Health Bureau (MCHB) within the Department of Health and Human Services and the American Academy of Pediatrics (Box 7-1). They focus on the process of connecting both child and family to resources to achieve positive health outcomes. Definitions of case management also exist from the American Nurses Association (Bower, 1992) and the international, interdisciplinary Case Management Society of America (2002) that include all populations. The commonalties among all these processes of care coordination and case management include the identification of short-term client outcomes (meet planned health needs, ensure access to services), long-term client outcomes (positive health status, self-management, empowerment), and system outcomes (improved quality and cost-effective use of resources).

Care coordination occurs on behalf of a client or family and is the *individual* response to service system fragmentation (Hughes et al, 1996). This is distinct from a service *system* response to fragmentation that seeks to integrate services through pooling funding sources, creating single points of entry for a group of programs, and otherwise improve the infrastructure under which health care services are provided. A service system response in primary care practices might include improving office procedures and establishing contracts for community services, whereas an individual response would be to designate a team to coordinate care for a group of children. Both individual and system approaches are considered necessary to ensure that services are coordinated for CSHCN and their families.

Care coordination for CSHCN has a historic basis in community health nursing and social work and has also been discussed as an essential role for pediatricians for many decades. School nurses report involvement with care coordination for this population (Lowe and Miller, 1998), and nurse practitioners are particularly involved in coordinating care of children accessing hospital-based chronic illness or specialty programs (Horst et al, 2000). The advanced practice skills of primary care clinicians are well suited toward coordinating the overall health needs of CSHCN and other special populations in community settings (Davidson, 1999; Lindeke et al, 2001; Taylor, 1999).

A number of circumstances are influencing the development of models and financing mechanisms for care coordination to families of CSHCN within primary care settings. Some of these factors discussed in this chapter are the historic advocacy of federal and state maternal and child health services under Title V and *Healthy People 2010*, family access to a myriad of fragmented services, the shift in health care services delivery, and an emerging model of primary care delivery called the "medical home." Primary care providers are particularly well situated to collaborate with families and community partners to improve child and family outcomes by developing community-based coordinated systems of care and ensuring that families receive the individualized care needed to promote optimal well-being for their children with special needs.

Why Care Coordination for CSHCN?
Title V–CSHCN

Care coordination services for families of CSHCN have been an important component of most state Title V programs for decades. Title V, known as the Maternal and Child Health Block Grant, has been authorizing federal funds to states for maternal and child health services, including children with special health care needs, since 1935 (see Chapter 8). A revision to this federal mandate in 1989 resulted in changes that continue to influence service delivery to CSHCN (Kruger, 2001). One significant change was the emphasis on creating systems of care for *all* children with special needs, not just those enrolled in state programs. States are required, under Title V, to provide and promote family-centered, culturally competent, community-based, coordinated care and to facilitate the development of systems of care in communities where families and children live (US Department of Health and Human Services [US DHHS], 1998).

In 1984, a majority of state Title V–CSHCN programs reported that coordinating client services was an important mission of their agency and an activity that they did not spend enough time doing (Ireys and Eichler, 1988). Almost 2 decades

Definitions of Care Coordination for CSHCN

The Maternal and Child Health Bureau (MCHB): ". . . the effective and efficient organization and utilization of resources to assure access to necessary comprehensive services for children with special health care needs and their families" (Omnibus Reconciliation Act, 1989).

The American Academy of Pediatrics (AAP): ". . . a process that links children with special health care needs and their families to services and resources in a coordinated effort to maximize the potential of the children and provide them with optimal health care" (American Academy of Pediatrics, 1999a, p. 978).

Healthy People 2010 action plan

Goal 1: Families of children with special heath care needs will partner in decision making at all levels and will be satisfied with the services they receive.

Goal 2: All children with special health care needs will receive coordinated, ongoing, comprehensive care within a medical home.

Goal 3: All families of children with special health care needs will have adequate private and/or public insurance to pay for the services they need.

Goal 4: All children will be screened early and continuously for special health care needs.

Goal 5: Community-based service systems will be organized so families can use them easily.

Goal 6: All youth with special health care needs will receive the services necessary to make transitions to all aspects of adult life, including adult health care, work, and independence.

From U.S. Department of Health and Human Services: All aboard the 2010 Express: a 10-year action plan to achieve community-based service systems for children and youth with special health care needs and their families, Washington, DC, 2001, Author.

later, only 18 states report that care coordination services are available to *all* CSHCN in their state (Zimmerman et al, 2000). State Title V–CSHCN needs assessments to continue to validate that care coordination services are a priority for families (Reiss, 2000), and approximately 60% of state programs are actively working on expanding eligibility and initiatives to ensure care coordination services to families of CSHCN (Zimmerman et al, 2000). National advocacy groups are involved in identifying goals for Title V–CSHCN programs and guide the development of systems of care in the community as well as individual care coordination services (Association of Maternal and Child Health Programs, 2002).

Healthy People 2010

The nation's prevention agenda, known as *Healthy People 2010,* reinforces the 1989 legislative mandate by including objectives to build systems of care in communities and increase the proportion of states that have community-based systems of care for CSHCN (US DHHS, 2000). The two goals of *Healthy People 2010* are (1) to increase quality and years of healthy life and (2) to decrease health disparities. The Maternal and Child Health Bureau (MCHB) released a 10-year action plan to address *Healthy People 2010* goals and objectives for CSHCN. This plan identifies six core goals (Box 7-2) to guide the achievement of the *Healthy People 2010* objectives for CSHCN (McPherson and Honberg, 2002). Selected strategies derived from these six goals directly relate to coordination of care. These include developing models of coordination among primary care, specialty, and community providers; implementing medical homes; improving pediatric-adult medical transitions for young adults; supporting telehealth initiatives; and developing financial models for reimbursement for care coordination (US DHHS, 2001). Goal three clearly states that all children with special heath care needs will receive coordinated, ongoing, comprehensive care within a medical home, which is at the community-based primary care level. To ensure that states are working on this goal the MCH Block Grant requires that all state Title V–CSHCN programs annually report the percent of CSHCN who receive coordinated care within a medical home. Collectively, the Title V legislative mandate, integration into *Healthy People 2010*, and an MCHB action plan and accountability requirement are the driving forces to ensure that goals are met.

Accessing Services

CSHCN use a greater volume and variety of services than do children generally, which is normative for this population (see Chapter 1). High service use means that families are in frequent contact with medical, allied health, and community providers seeking services and making arrangements (phoning, funding, transportation, time off from work) for appointments to receive services. Data from a parent-to-parent information and referral program, which tracked the reasons for phone inquiries over 10 years from families of CSHCN, and from providers for families demonstrate the breadth of services that families seek (State of New Hampshire, 2002) (Table 7-1). Matching family needs to program services is a challenge for families and providers unfamiliar with available resources. It is estimated that during the past 30 years more than 500 publicly funded programs for children and families have been developed (Grason and Guyer, 1995; National Governors Association, 1996). Most of these programs are categorical, separately funded, with specific condition and/or financial eligibility criteria, and with a defined scope of services that may include care coordinators. A possible need to coordinate multiple coordinators is one by-product of system fragmentation.

Access to particular services for CSHCN may be hampered by application and eligibility procedures, waiting lists, appeal processes, and multiple applications to individual programs. For example, a family with a young child may complete an application to early intervention, Title V–CSHCN; Medicaid or a state children's health insurance program (SCHIP); nutrition services through the women, infants, and children (WIC) program, the primary care office, or a clinic; and a family support program through mental health—all in different agencies, in different places across town. Even if families are currently deemed eligible for services they may be required to reapply the following year to maintain their eligibility. Although some agencies make efforts to collaborate and integrate services to eliminate duplicative paperwork, that is the exception rather than the norm.

TABLE 7-1

Resources Sought by Families of CSHCN

Financial Assistance	Health and Medical	Education and Development	Family Support
Charitable foundations	Dental care	Adult day programs	Adoptive services
Food and fuel assistance	Durable medical and technology vendors	Assisted living	Behavior management
Food, housing, clothing	Local and regional subspecialty care	Assistive technology	Child and family services
Health care plans	Local and specialty hospitals	Developmental services	Counseling
Home and automobile adaptations	Mental health and behavioral	Early intervention	Daycare and after-school care
Home- and Community-based homeless shelters	Pharmacy and supplies	Employment, ready to work	Disability rights and advocacy
Medicaid	Prehospital EMS planning	Group home	Disability-specific group
State children's health insurance	Primary care	Head Start	Divorce and custody
Supplemental Security Income	Rehabilitative services	Preschool	Faith community
TANF/city welfare	Skilled nursing/home health	School health	Father, sibling groups
Title V–CSHCN	Transition services	Sheltered workshop	Legal aid
Transportation	WIC nutrition	Special education	Library resource center
Waivers		Transition services	Parent information center
		Vocational education	Parenting
			Parent-to-parent support
			Personal care attendant
			Recreation/camp
			Very Special Arts

From State of New Hampshire: *Information and referral report, 1991-2001*, Concord, NH, 2002, Special Medical Services Bureau, Office of Health Planning and Medicaid. *TANF,* Temporary Assistance for Needy Families; *EMS,* emergency medical service; *WIC,* Women, Infants, and Children (program).

Denial for services creates more work for those families who know about the appeal process and have the perseverance to proceed. For example, grandparents who are primary caregivers of children with special needs were reported to have a difficult time meeting eligibility criteria and were denied benefits such as Supplemental Security Income, Medicaid, or special education for their grandchildren (McCallion et al, 2000). Care coordinators who accompanied grandparents to appeal denials for services had to refer 25% of the cases to legal aid before the grandchild could receive the service. In another example, preadoptive families of CSHCN enrolled in a support program (child welfare) were aware of medical and educational services but reported that they were not able to receive or pay for them (Kramer and Houston, 1999). Members of the adoption team staff were able to assist families to proactively meet most of their identified needs. The advocacy role of the care coordinator is especially evident when helping families access services.

Families gain experience navigating the service system through their contact with a variety of knowledgeable providers, other parents, and trial and error. The need to navigate the system and coordinate care is described by families in countries with universal health care (Baine et al, 1995; Ray, 1997; Sloper and Turner, 1992) as well as the United States. The Family Partners Project, a national survey, reported that families often function as their child's care coordinator. Only 50% of families with CSHCN in this study identified having a person designated as a care coordinator, whereas 70% of families of children who were technology dependent (TD) reported having a care coordinator (Krauss et al, 2000, 2001). The parents of children who were TD and who also provided in-home care spent an additional 5 or more hours per week coordinating care for their child. Care coordinators helped families to identify community-based services (63%), coordinate care

among different providers and services (56%), find resources to pay for services/equipment (47%), help access public programs (43%), and help understand their child's health insurance plan benefits (39%).

Coordinating care requires persistence, skill, time, and energy and is an additional responsibility that caregivers assume. The national focus on health disparities has emphasized the influence of race, ethnicity, language, and culture as factors in mediating access to care for vulnerable populations (Halfon et al, 1995; Weinick and Krauss, 2000). CSHCN are reported to more likely be living in single-parent families where incomes are below the poverty level and the education level of the head of household is low (Newacheck et al, 1998). Responsive care coordination strategies must provide understandable information and direction, assistance with negotiating eligibility processes, and education on how to access resources for a broad range of families.

Shift in Health Care Services for CSHCN

The decade of the 1990s and the advent of managed care precipitated a shift from hospital tertiary care or specialty services to community-based primary health care. Historically, children with special needs have been higher users of specialty medical services than primary care services (Perrin and Ireys, 1984). Further, children attending specialty clinics were reported to not always have a source of primary care (Palfrey et al, 1980). Pediatric primary care was a luxury for some families whose health insurance only partially covered acute care and rarely covered preventive care. With managed care, families have greater opportunities to access comprehensive pediatric primary care. However, concerns have been raised about how CSHCN fare under managed care programs, which may limit access to the variety of services and subspecialists these children may need, disrupt family–specialty provider relationships, and/or substitute adult subspecialists for pediatric subspecialists (Grossman et al, 1999; Mele and Flowers, 2000; Simpson and Fraser, 1999; Szilagyi, 1998).

The replacement of fee-for-service indemnity insurance with managed care plans has meant that some families have forfeited the services of established multidisciplinary specialty teams while not necessarily acquiring a primary care provider. Kaufman et al (1994) reported that 3 years after disbanding a team clinic for children with myelomeningocele, one half of the clients responded that they had no orthopedic or urologic follow-up, two thirds reported no neurologic or pediatric follow-up, and one third did not identify a pediatric primary care provider. Clients from the disbanded multidisciplinary specialty clinic also were observed to undergo fewer proactive surgical procedures and more preventable and serious surgical procedures compared to another site. The role of the coordinator, central to a multidisciplinary team, was not assumed by the community primary care provider nor by the family. Dosa and colleagues (2001) examined unscheduled admissions to the intensive care unit (ICU) over a 1-year period among children with chronic illness who presented with severe acute illness. One third of potentially preventable hospital admissions occurred more frequently among children with chronic illness (38%) who were not technology dependent compared with children who were technology dependent (19%). Family and health care system factors were associated with the preventable admissions. Family factors included stress and delay in seeking care. Health system factors were related to inadequate coordination of care and failure to provide particular services.

The federal government has been incrementally assisting families to improve access to health care through health insurance financing programs such as Medicaid and SCHIP (see Chapter 8). More CSHCN are enrolled in Medicaid vs. employer-insured plans (Shatin et al, 1998). These children now receive a majority of their care from primary care providers (Kuhlthau et al, 2001). Although care coordination services are generally included within Medicaid and SCHIP programs as safeguards, they are still not universally available in all public and private health financing plans for CSHCN (Hill et al, 1999; Kaye et al, 2000; Schwalberg et al, 2000). The Family Partners Project reported that the funding source of care coordination services included more public programs such as state Title V–CSHCN (30%), other state programs (28%), and other community sources (27%) compared with only 11% funded by private health insurance plans (Krauss et al, 2000). The primary health care system is designed to meet the occasional acute illness and health promotion needs of the majority of children without special needs who do not require ongoing care coordination. The ability of primary care to manage long-term chronic conditions of children in conjunction with the ongoing information and support needs of their families is perceived to be inadequate.

The Primary Care "Medical Home"

The *medical home* is the primary care model being proposed for CSHCN and their families nationally. This initiative is led by the American Academy of Pediatrics in partnership with the Maternal and Child Health Bureau (MCHB), the advocacy organization Family Voices, and the March of Dimes. The medical home is defined as a pediatric primary care approach that is delivered or directed by primary care physicians (American Academy of Pediatrics [AAP] and Medical Home Initiatives for Children with Special Needs Project Advisory Committee, 2002). The values and principles associated with the medical home approach include care that is accessible, continuous, comprehensive, family centered, coordinated, compassionate, and culturally effective. Care is coordinated when an individualized plan of care exists that includes information, tracking, evaluation, documentation in a retrievable format, and communication among family, child, and providers. There is an emphasis on the role of the physician, identified as a pediatrician, pediatric medical subspecialist, pediatric surgical specialist, or family practitioner, as the primary medical home provider. However, in these emerging models, the role of care coordinator has been assumed by nurses, nurse practitioners, social workers, and paraprofessionals and is sometimes shared with parent consultants.

The medical home was initially proposed in the 1980s as an integrated community approach to address prevention of child abuse and neglect and later to extend preventive early intervention services to vulnerable families (Sia, 1992). The revision of the Title V–CSHCN mandate in 1989 provided the impetus to move the care of CSHCN to the community and primary care. The medical home became incorporated into a description of this federal mandate for physicians, encouraging their participation in the care of these children (Brewer et al, 1989). Pediatricians were encouraged to work with parents, fellow professionals, and community teams in the best interest of coordinating care. More recently there has been interest within pediatrics for delineating roles in interdisciplinary team assessments (AAP and Committee on Children with Disabilities, 1999b), care coordination (AAP and Committee on Children with Disabilities, 1999a), and a role for the school nurse, particularly as it relates to CSHCN (AAP and Committee on School Health, 2001).

There are challenges to making the medical home a reality in primary care practices, particularly since specialists more than primary care providers have traditionally met family needs related to care coordination (Scholle and Kelleher, 1995). Less than one half of families received care coordination from their physician compared with the two thirds who expressed a need for this service (Perrin et al, 2000). Pediatricians who were highly committed to providing services to CSHCN reported very low satisfaction with the time available to care for CSHCN, assisting with coordinating school services, and transitioning adolescents to adult services (Davidson et al, 2002).

MCHB support of demonstration programs across the United States has developed practical tools to guide primary care practices in the development of a medical home (see Resources). Common among these projects is an emphasis on creating a supportive office environment designed by health care providers, parents, and office staff (Cooley et al, 1995). The Center for Medical Home Improvement (2001) provides a validated measurement tool to assess how well primary care settings provide care to CSHCN ("medical homeness") as an initial step toward improving the quality of care within a practice. The domains measured within this tool reflect the needs of families and include organizational capacity, chronic condition management, care coordination, community outreach, data management, and quality improvement. A complementary index also identifies "medical homeness" from the family perspective. This comparative assessment sets the stage for a team (primary care provider, parents, care coordinator, office staff) to begin identifying goals, objectives, and strategies to improve the quality of care.

The development of the Model for Effective Chronic Illness Care, supported by the Robert Wood Johnson Foundation, also addresses the need to move beyond managing acute or episodic care for all populations who have chronic illness (Wagner et al, 2002). Components of the chronic care model identified through literature and expert review and analysis of 72 successful programs focus on the organization of services within the health care system. The elements identified as influencing quality of care are client self-management support, design of the delivery system or environment, support from specialists and experts or practice guidelines, and availability of data information systems. Health care system components are then viewed within the context of the policies and resources of the surrounding community with an intent to encourage informed clients and proactive practitioners.

These health care delivery system redesign models consider the context of the office practice and larger community and include care coordination as an integral component of service delivery to families and individuals. In fact, 82% of programs reviewed by Wagner and colleagues (2002) identified registered nurses, social workers, and nurse practitioners as providing coordination that was either integrated with primary care or delivered as a carve-out (separate from health care delivery). However, many programs were reported to focus narrowly on utilization review and the process of care coordination was not always well defined.

The Care Coordination Process

Care coordination (Box 7-3) is a *proactive process* that plans, implements, and evaluates the delivery of comprehensive health care to the child *and* support services to the family *in conjunction* with the family and community providers. Whereas the clinical service is directed toward the child, care coordination is directed toward the family unit. This is an important distinction because it broadens child health service delivery to include a full range of community services for child and family and moves beyond medical management.

The process of care coordination includes assessment, individualized family service care planning, plan implementation, monitoring, evaluation, and transition to adult services. This process is organized according to the domains of health, environment/access, school, financial, psycho-social-cultural, and community resources and is reflected in the sample documentation forms in Figure 7-1. These domains were derived from public health care coordination practice (State of New Hampshire, 1993) and provide a generic overview of some of the details of the care coordination process. It is recognized that

---

> **BOX 7-3**
> ## Care Coordination Process
>
> **Guiding framework**
> **Family identification and engagement**
> **Family assessment**
>   Health records review
>   Environmental modifications
>   School placement
>   Finances
>   Psychosocial and cultural assessment
>   Community resources
>   Family strengths
> **Family service plan**
>   Coordinator selection
>   Plan development
> **Plan implementation**
>   Resource information
>   Facilitating referrals
>   Arranging services
>   Teaching
>   Information exchange
> **Monitoring, transition, and evaluation**

---

agency structure and the disciplinary orientation of the care coordinator influence the extent to which care coordination and clinical interventions are integrated.

Guiding Framework

Dunst and Trivette (1994, p 187) conceptualized case management as ". . . a particular set of functions for linking what is needed with what resources are provided." Resources are conceptualized as informal supports, such as family and friends who are close to the family, and formal supports, such as professional services that are more distant to the family. The idea is that professionals should ensure that a variety of supports are mobilized for families rather than replace the family informal support network (Dunst et al, 1988). Informal and formal supports are thought to interact with each other to strengthen family functioning and help families gain mastery depending on how coordinators work with families. This model suggests that the creation of opportunities (empowerment) for families to meet their needs is related to how families are involved in identifying needs and acquiring resources with a particular emphasis on family-centered care.

Family-centered care is a standard of care in many programs for CSHCN promulgated by its incorporation in the 1989 Title V–CSHCN legislative revision. How families are viewed, approached, and helped influences how programs are planned, implemented, and evaluated. The principles of family-centered care emphasize the family as experts about their child with whom providers collaborate, share unbiased information, show respect, and approach from an individualized and strengths-based perspective (Shelton and Stepanek, 1994). This "belief" framework is integral to the practice of care coordination (Patterson and Hovey, 2000). Identifying a conceptual model to guide family care coordination practice provides a road map for program design.

NAME _____   DATE _____

DOB _____ GENDER   F   M   AGE _____

MEDICAL CONDITION _____

_____

PHONE   HOME _____ MESSAGE_____ WORK_____

     CAREGIVER_____ MOTHER_____ FATHER_____

     LANGUAGE SPOKEN AT HOME_____

ANTICIPATED TRANSITIONS   ☐ HOSPITAL-HOME   ☐ PEDIATRIC TO ADULT CARE

          ☐ BETWEEN HEALTH PLANS   ☐ BETWEEN PCP'S

PROVIDERS	CONTACT NAME & ADDRESS	PHONE	RECORDS ✓
PRIMARY CARE			
SPECIALIST			
SPECIALIST			
DENTIST			
SCHOOL NURSE			
SCHOOL TEACHER			
SCHOOL OTHER			
DEVELOPMENT PROG			
AFTER-SCHOOL PROGR			
DAY CARE			
HEALTH PLAN			
TITLE V PROGRAM			
COMMUNITY SUPPORT			

INTAKE

FIGURE 7-1 Sample care coordination record. (Adapted from state of New Hampshire Special Medical Services Bureau, Office of Health Planning and Medicaid, Title V–CSHCN program.)

Continued

HOW CAN WE HELP?

Please let us know how we may help you help your child and family
Check ✓ the items you would like information or referral

Information about
- ❒ Child's health condition
- ❒ Nutrition/Feeding
- ❒ Development
- ❒ Behavior

Finding or Getting Medical and Dental Care
- ❒ Specialty medical services
- ❒ Medicines / special foods
- ❒ Dentist
- ❒ Help pay for special needs care
- ❒ Special equipment or supplies
- ❒ Therapy

Help with Child / Home Care
- ❒ Finding and funding child care
- ❒ Managing daily needs of child
- ❒ Having an emergency plan
- ❒ Finding respite care
- ❒ Making physical changes in home/care
- ❒ Teaching others how to care for child

Help Talking about our Child with
- ❒ Our children, friends, or family
- ❒ Other parents with similar concerns
- ❒ Health providers
- ❒ Teachers / school personnel

Help Planning for the Future
- ❒ Future health care needs
- ❒ Determining placement
- ❒ Transition to adult services
- ❒ Special / vocational education

Find or Get Community Services for our Child and Family

- ❒ Supplemental Security Income (SSI)
- ❒ Transportation to doctor or other special visits

- ❒ Social/Recreation opportunities/Summer Camp

- ❒ Support for parents, father, siblings, child with special needs
- ❒ Family counseling
- ❒ Legal Assistance or disability advocacy

- ❒ Food or nutrition program
- ❒ Clothing
- ❒ Housing
- ❒ Fuel Assistance

Other ways we can help?_____

CHILD _____ COORDINATOR _____ DATE _____

INTAKE

FIGURE 7-1, cont'd.

CATEGORY	CONTENT	CONCERNS	CHILD & FAMILY STRENGTHS
HEALTH	Family, prenatal, birth, newborn, child health history; immunizations, nutrition, medications, specialty care, hospitalization, treatment goals, family experience with health system, health of other family members		
ENVIRONMENT & ACCESS	Self-care, activities of daily living, adaptive equipment, home safety, modification, emergency home and transportation plan, home care-giving demands		
SCHOOL	Early intervention or special education program, educational coding, existence of individualized family service plan or individual education plan, daycare/school personnel education needs		
FINANCES	Primary and secondary health insurance plan(s), family understanding of benefits and terms, family income and resources		
PSYCHO-SOCIAL-CULTURAL	Support network for caregivers, parents, child, sibs; family attitude/outlook related to child's condition; cultural beliefs and practices, interpreters; leisure activities; coping and problem-solving strategies		
COMMUNITY RESOURCES	Resources used, knowledge of resources, help-seeking behaviors, prior success accessing resources		

CHILD_____COORDINATOR_____DATE_____

ASSESSMENT

FIGURE 7-1, cont'd.   *Continued*

Family Identification and Engagement

Family case finding generally occurs as children come into contact with providers. Further, some families may need to be actively recruited since they are unlikely to know and therefore inquire about these services. Identifying the child with a special need is generally the first step to identifying families who need care coordination.

The CSHCN Screener (Box 7-4) is a noncategorical, five-item questionnaire developed by the Child and Adolescent Health Measurement Initiative for the purpose of quality assessment and population-based survey (Bethell et al, 2002; Foundation for Accountability, 2002a). Although it was not specifically intended to screen individual children it can be self-administered by parents and/or used as a reference for the development of a screening tool (Silva et al, 2000).

Primary care staff can apply screening criteria to query administrative databases, perform record audits, or screen individual families during office visits. A software application that uses medical conditions reported in claims data to identify CSHCN shows promise for application to health plan databases (Neff et al, 2002). Using claims data to identify children who are high users of services, especially hospital and emergency

visits, may be a useful strategy to target an initial cohort of children. It is likely that a combination of methods will need to be used in order to find CSHCN. Once children are found, consideration should be given to tagging the child's medical record and computer file for future retrieval.

Once children are identified the next step is to determine which families need or want professional care coordination services. Medical episodes usually generate paperwork, which can alert providers to an opportunity to engage the family. Families may be amenable to discussing care coordination when the child's condition is in the foreground (hospitalization, emergency visit, referral, diagnosis, office visit) or when the family actively requests information and services. These opportunities allow primary care providers to explore related needs. In addition, transitions between early childhood and special education services at ages 3 years or 6 years and again from adolescent to adult services are times when families may require professional assistance.

Family Assessment

The most skilled rather than the least skilled professional should perform the assessment since it is the foundation on

CATEGORY	SHORT - TERM OUTCOME		ACTION	REVIEW DATE	RP
HEALTH		1			
		2			
		3			
ENVIRONMENT & ACCESS		1			
		2			
		3			
SCHOOL		1			
		2			
		3			
FINANCES		1			
		2			
		3			
PSYCHO-SOCIAL-CULTURAL		1			
		2			
		3			
COMMUNITY RESOURCES		1			
		2			
		3			

RP = responsible person

CHILD_____ COORDINATOR_____ DATE_____

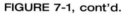

SERVICE PLAN

FIGURE 7-1, cont'd.

which service planning and implementation depend. Family assessment moves beyond the immediate clinical needs of the child and focuses on current and long-range planning for the family. The purpose of the family assessment is to elicit concerns and needs, identify strengths, explore sources of support, and identify potential resources. Assessment is an ongoing process that may occur before, during, or after the child record collection process and over a number of home, office, and telephone encounters over time. Preference is given to visiting the family at home or a comfortable environment that is conducive to discussion and relationship building.

Communication with providers is an essential component of the care coordination process. Families should be asked to sign release of information forms to facilitate health and education record requests and telephone communication. A provider list should be included in the child record and include the names and contact information for primary care, specialists/sub-specialists, tertiary center services, habilitative/rehabilitative services, education (early intervention or special education), dental, community support (transportation, recreation, parent-

support programs, developmental, etc.), care coordinators, and health insurance plan. Prototype family notebooks to record provider information and child service visits are available from programs such as the Institute for Child Health Policy, Division of Specialized Care for Children at the University of Illinois at Chicago, and Los Angeles Medical Home Project (see Resources). Families should be encouraged to maintain their child's medical record/notebook and share updates with providers. See sample *Care Coordination Record*, Figure 7-1.

Health Record Review. A chronologic review of medical and allied health records provides information about the progression of the child's condition and can uncover gaps and breaks in continuity and help anticipate needs. Child diagnostic, consult, treatment, and hospital discharge records should be collected to facilitate this review. Families should be asked about any mental health, psychologic, or behavioral consultations.

Caregiver experience with health care providers, particularly their satisfaction or reason for dissatisfaction, is an important

CATEGORY	DATE	PROGRESS NOTE	CONTACT CODE
HEALTH			
ENVIRONMENT & ACCESS			
SCHOOL			
FINANCES			
PSYCHO-SOCIAL-CULTURAL			
COMMUNITY RESOURCES			

Contact Code	TC = Telephone Call	HV = Home Visit	OV = Office Visit	FC = Family Conference
	AV = Agency Visit	EM = E-mail	TH = Tele-Health	M = Mail

CHILD_____COORDINATOR_____DATE_____

PROGRESS NOTE

FIGURE 7-1, cont'd.

predisposing factor to explore since it may influence the future use of health care services (Andersen, 1995). How families have learned to get what they need from the health care system can demonstrate family strengths and reveal a need for communication and advocacy skill development. Assessment of family understanding of the child's condition, treatment goals, use of alternative therapies, and caregiving knowledge and skill should also be completed. This includes knowledge about medications, dietary supplements, and child self-care.

Environmental Modifications. Home care, modifications in the environment, and equipment needs may be extensive depending on the child's condition. The family home should be assessed for adaptive modifications or wheelchair access (safety rails, doorways, ramps) and safety. Children who are technology dependent require home backup electrical supply, an in-home and transportation emergency transportation plan, and caregiver training. This is generally done before hospital discharge by a specialized transition team. Realistically, not all

the planning is completed and skilled nursing and respite care plans may become disrupted once the child is home. Access to a vehicle, a van to accommodate a wheelchair, or transport for children who are ventilator dependent must be considered.

Assessing the level of assistance (total or partial) and equipment aids that children require for feeding, bathing, transferring, bowel and bladder functions, and dressing provides an indication of time and financial demands on caregivers. Preparing a special diet or implementing a toileting program requires a plan, consistency, and funding for food or supplies. Determining child self-responsibility and independence should consider opportunities for practicing skills in the context of competing family demands.

School Placement. Children who are enrolled in early intervention and special education programs should already have an individualized service plan (see Chapter 5). Special education and early intervention services provide related services such as speech, occupational, and physical therapy as well as communication and interpreter services, nutrition, developmental

---

BOX 7-4

Children with Special Health Care Needs (CSHCN) Screener

All three parts of at least one screener question (or, in the case of question 5, the two parts) must be answered "yes" in order for a child to meet CSHCN screener criteria for having a special health care need.

1. Does your child currently need or use **medicine prescribed by a doctor** (other than vitamins)?
   - ☐ Yes → Go to Question 1a
   - ☐ No → Go to Question 2
   1a. Is this because of ANY medical, behavioral, or other health condition?
      - ☐ Yes → Go to Question 1b
      - ☐ No → Go to Question 2
   1b. Is this a condition that has lasted or is expected to last for *at least* 12 months?
      - ☐ Yes
      - ☐ No

2. Does your child need or use more **medical care, mental health, or educational services** than are usual for most children of the same age?
   - ☐ Yes → Go to Question 2a
   - ☐ No → Go to Question 3
   2a. Is this because of ANY medical, behavioral, or other health condition?
      - ☐ Yes → Go to Question 2b
      - ☐ No → Go to Question 3
   2b. Is this a condition that has lasted or is expected to last for *at least* 12 months?
      - ☐ Yes
      - ☐ No

3. Is your child **limited or prevented** in any way in his or her ability to do the things most children of the same age can do?
   - ☐ Yes → Go to Question 3a
   - ☐ No → Go to Question 4

   3a. Is this because of ANY medical, behavioral, or other health condition?
      - ☐ Yes → Go to Question 3b
      - ☐ No → Go to Question 4
   3b. Is this a condition that has lasted or is expected to last for *at least* 12 months?
      - ☐ Yes
      - ☐ No

4. Does your child need or get **special therapy**, such as physical, occupational, or speech therapy?
   - ☐ Yes → Go to Question 4a
   - ☐ No → Go to Question 5
   4a. Is this because of ANY medical, behavioral, or other health condition?
      - ☐ Yes → Go to Question 4b
      - ☐ No → Go to Question 5
   4b. Is this a condition that has lasted or is expected to last for *at least* 12 months?
      - ☐ Yes
      - ☐ No

5. Does your child have any kind of emotional, developmental, or behavioral problem for which he or she needs or gets **treatment or counseling?**
   - ☐ Yes → Go to Question 5a
   - ☐ No
   5a. Has this problem lasted or is it expected to last for *at least* 12 months?
      - ☐ Yes
      - ☐ No

From Bethell, C.D. et al. (2002). Identifying children with special health care needs: development and evaluation of a short screening instrument, *Ambulatory Pediatrics* 2:38-48. Reprinted with permission. Address correspondence to Christina Bethell, PhD, FACCT—The Foundation for Accountability, 1200 NW Naito Parkway, Suite 470, Portland, OR 97209, cbethell@facct.org.

---

testing and intervention, and other specialized instruction. Assessment should include and build on information already collected and not duplicate or compete for established family-provider relationships. Information from these service plans can be shared by families, or the plans can be requested with family permission.

Assessing family use of daycare, preschool, Head Start, after-school, and school programs may uncover unmet needs for these services as well as needs to educate school staff about the child's individual caregiving needs and preferences for self-care. Parents frequently educate school personnel about their child, the condition, and daytime treatment. Even though parents are the experts about their child, they may require support and assistance from health care providers and professional parent advocates. Determining the nature of the family relationship with school personnel and establishing a link with the school nurse are important functions of the primary care provider (see Chapter 5).

Finances. Having a source of health insurance is critical for CSHCN to obtain primary and specialty medical services, and it is frequently insufficient to meet needs. Some families have both a private source of health insurance as well as a public plan such as Medicaid. Families may have out-of-pocket costs for durable medical equipment, disposable medical supplies, dental care, nutritional supplements, and other services not reimbursed through their health insurance plan. The Family

Partners Project (Krauss et al, 2000) reported that over one half of families spent more than $1000 and 10% spent more than $5000 in out-of-pocket expenses during the past year for their child. Slightly more than one half of the parents also reported that they stopped working or reduced their employment hours to care for their child. A triple effect of providing in-home care, decrease in employment, and financial hardship was reported by 29% of these families.

Assessing family financial concerns includes identification of a health insurance plan or plans; family understanding of terms, benefits, and how to access benefits and appeal denials; amount of out-of-pocket expenses; and other family financial obligations, including alimony and child support. Family awareness about other sources of funding, such as supplemental security income (SSI), charitable organizations and equipment exchange, rental banks, negotiating payment with vendors, and optimizing tax deductions is also an area that should be assessed. In many states, Title V–CSCHN programs may offer flexible funds for services not reimbursable by traditional health plans and/or be able to direct families to sources of financial assistance. See Resources section at the end of this chapter for a link to state Title V programs.

Psycho-Social-Cultural Assessment. The impact (demands and joys) of life with a child with special needs on the immediate and extended family has been described extensively in the professional and lay literatures. Listening to families describe their personal story provides information about the lens they use to view their life situation and how they manage and adapt. Families may depend on each other and their immediate social network for a variety of supports. Assessment of this network would include mapping the relationships and types of support the family (child with special needs, siblings, parents, etc.) receives. This may be material support, such as personal care attendant, babysitting, or grocery shopping; emotional support, such as someone to talk to; or affirming support, such as someone who recognizes the effort of the primary caregiver. Some families may need assistance to mobilize or organize their informal support networks, whereas others may not be aware of the availability of local parent organizations. Parents report dissatisfaction when primary care providers do not connect them with support groups (Ireys and Perry, 1999). In addition, cultural and spiritual beliefs have implications for the way families frame the context of the child's condition, incorporate alternative methods of healing, and carry out prescribed medical treatment and need to be assessed (see Chapter 4).

Child involvement in special YMCA programs, centers for independent living, Special Olympics, summer camp, and special arts activities provides recreation, socialization, and friendships. It consequently may also provide the family with respite periods. Caregiver and sibling opportunities to pursue their own interests should be explored because it provides insight into how the family balances demands of caregiving.

Community Resources. Considering the voluminous amount of information that exists on the Internet and within regional human resources directories it is paradoxical that the literature continues to report that family information needs are not adequately met by health care providers. Parents expect to receive information about their child's condition and resources from their health care provider and express frustration when this does not happen (Garwick et al, 1998). Further, parents identified a variety of information and resources they needed that were underestimated by health care providers (Perrin et al, 2000). Assessment should determine family awareness of resources, determine services used in the past and why no longer used, and anticipate what resources families may want to consider in the future. Self-administered family checklists may help families to consider their needs, but they also raise family expectations that someone will help them to address these concerns.

Family Strengths. Family strengths are intrafamily resources, such as cognitive, attitudinal, and behavioral characteristics that help enhance family functioning and well-being and help balance the discussion centered on problems and needs (Dunst et al, 1994). All families, as well as children with special needs, have strengths that are reflected in values, competencies, and interaction patterns. For example, family traditions, ability to identify resources, and expressing appreciation to other family members are examples of strengths. Although family strength, hardiness, and family functioning self-report tools exist (Dunst et al, 1994), providers can also observe and interview families about how they manage their child's care and other life events. Coordinators should observe the home environment and family interactions, listen to the family's story,

ask them to identify their strengths, or help them to recognize these.

The Family Service Plan

The assessment information must be summarized and include family strengths and areas of concern to effectively guide care planning. Members who should participate in plan development are the child, caregivers or parents, primary care provider, care coordinator, health plan representative, and related providers. The family service plan is a written document developed by the team as a result of conferencing or discussion. Discussion includes analysis of the assessment and identification of concerns, strengths, outcomes, and related actions. The plan's language should reflect the words of the family as much as possible. If the family cannot be present at the conference then the coordinator should meet with the family to discuss and revise the plan. Families should sign the plan to confirm their agreement.

The written plan becomes a guide for all providers who serve the child and family. It should include the frequency and location of direct care services provided to child and family, the funding sources, roles and responsibilities of all providers, agency and provider contact information, and a schedule or timeline for periodic review and follow-up. The inclusion of community representatives is important since action plans may be implemented by more than one person, other resources may be identified, and communication is enhanced.

Coordinator Selection. One coordinator should be identified, ideally, based on the best match with family needs and family choice, to assume responsibility for working with the family and all providers to ensure implementation. Coordinator selection depends on the child's level of care need, family's knowledge and skill to manage caregiving, family's ability to acquire resources, and family's time and desire to take on added roles and responsibilities. Certain responsibilities may be shared among members of the team such that the primary care provider assumes the central role for medical or disease management while other team members assume activities related to the coordination of services outside the direct care setting. It is important that one person be clearly identified to the family and all other providers as the lead synthesizer. The family's role may range from assuming major responsibility to no responsibility for coordination. Family-centered care predicates that receiving professional care coordination is a choice made by the family.

Coordinators can be assigned based on complexity of family need. Hill and colleagues (1996) describe level I services as those directed to families who may need assistance to identify services. Coordinator functions at this level are focused on information and referral that can be managed through telephone contact by a paraprofessional. Level II services are targeted to families at risk because of psychosocial and environmental factors or with children who are medically involved and need assistance coordinating multiple services. This level of family and child need will more likely require the involvement of a health care professional. Level III coordination services are focused on families of children who are medically fragile or at high risk because of psychosocial and environmental factors. These families will require continuous specialized professional assistance.

Service Plan Implementation

The most common family service plan implementation activities include providing information about resources, facilitating referral, arranging services, teaching, and information exchange among all providers and family. Successful implementation of the mutually agreed on family service plan depends on interpersonal and communication skills of the coordinator. During this period, the work of the coordinator becomes intense as family contact is maintained, referrals are made, and direct services are provided. The less integrated or the more varied the services, the more the coordinator must cross agency boundaries and enlist cooperation and ensure that information is being shared and services provided. Through implementation, coordination weaves disengaged providers and services together into a cohesive arrangement that meets current family needs and anticipates future ones.

Resource Information. Care coordinators, over time, develop a network of relationships with community agencies and become adept at using that network to seek out additional resources at local, state, and national levels. Numerous generic and disability-specific organizations and parent information and support agencies exist on federal, state, and local levels that generate resource directories and parent literature. Many Title V–CSHCN programs have parent consultants whose role is connecting families to other parents and support agencies. An office parent consultant is an invaluable asset in connecting families to sources of literature, agencies, and resources.

Facilitating Referrals. Facilitating referrals to numerous services and following up on their completion is a time-consuming activity. Recent studies suggest that referrals made to specialists are not well tracked. Fewer than one half of referring pediatricians scheduled the appointment with the specialist, and only 54% to 62% either sent information about the client to the specialist or were aware that the client made the visit (Forrest et al, 1999). Pediatricians who make referrals on the basis of telephone conversation with the family, in contrast to office visits, are even less aware of referral completion (Glade et al, 2002). Health plan policies may require that families arrange specialty consultation themselves and may restrict primary care and specialist communication.

The referral process consists of identifying families' desire and ability to make the connection with the agency, anticipating barriers that interfere with completion of the referral, and facilitating completion. Experienced coordinators can provide families with contact names and specific services to request and may phone the agency ahead of the family to pave the way. Referrals can fall through because the family received the wrong phone number, lost the phone number, did not receive a call back from the agency, received a discourteous response, does not have transportation, or changed their mind about seeking the referral. Hierarchic telephone trees and eligibility paperwork processes can be daunting for some families. Accompanying the family to an agency, such as social services, may be necessary to help families to acquire resources. Talking families through the request process and role-playing scenarios help families to develop skills and self-efficacy. Eliminating barriers or creating detours depends on communication, negotiation, and advocacy skills. Completion of the referral process occurs when the family receives the service, the report of the consultation or visit is recorded and filed in the medical record, and the results have been communicated and integrated into the ongoing assessment and family care plan.

Arranging Services. Arranging for services is an extension of the referral process and means doing whatever it takes to connect the family with a resource or provider in a way that they can use the service easily. At the minimum, it may include scheduling multiple appointments in a medical center on one day to minimize travel time and loss of employment and school time. For families who have transportation difficulties, this means finding them a ride through a local community service or another family or teaching them how to use their health care plan to access transportation. Sometimes, families cannot decipher what services are allowable under their health plan, do not remember what they were told, or were never told about their benefits and how to access them.

Identifying funding sources for durable medical equipment or supplies not reimbursable by the health plan or brokering for authorization of payment can result in multiple phone calls and delays. The coordinator may convene a meeting of representatives from public and private agencies, who individually deny a request to fund a service, to explain the overall plan of care and negotiate interagency cooperation such that family needs can be met. Helping families to appeal denials by drafting letters for a clinician's signature or explaining the family situation is a customary function. Knowing which services are subsidized by charitable organizations, grants, special projects, and so on depends on the extent of the coordinator's professional network and experience and the availability of an updated resource directory.

Coordinators may also need to arrange in-home services. An example is creating an emergency medical services plan for home care or transfer to the hospital or evacuation to a special needs shelter in the event of disaster for a child dependent on technology. These plans identify roles and responsibilities among the family, primary care provider, visiting nurse, hospital, police, fire department and emergency medical services personnel. If the family residence is located on a road that is impassable, a government road commission representative may be included to address road improvement. In addition, connections with the city agency responsible for special needs population evacuation and placement, usually the health department, are needed. The county or city emergency response plan assigns responsibility to a combination of agencies for medical services, shelter placement, and special transportation to ensure that residents who require these services are identified and entered into a database.

Finally, coordinators may need to assist families to mobilize a system of supports, such as respite, routine, occasional, or emergency child care or recreation and social support. Families not established in the community or unable to rely on friends or family require help acquiring these services. It can be frustrating when these resources either do not exist in or are in limited supply. Mobilizing respite services, for example, may mean piecing together providers from a variety of sources (extended family, neighbors, church volunteers, nursing students and agencies) and educating them to provide this service.

Teaching. Teaching includes individualized health content for the child and family, parent-professional relationship building, parental advocacy skill development, and education for community providers. The content to be taught and the professional responsible for teaching should be identified in the family service plan. Education about the child's condition and treatment plan, specific therapeutic skills, or child self-management skills is a clinical activity performed by the primary care provider but can be reinforced by a nurse care coordinator, visiting nurse, or therapists. Interpreting diagnostic testing and subspecialty consultant reports, in language understand-able to families and community providers, is also an important function.

Families consistently express the need for anticipating their child's future health care and related needs. Although projecting a medical condition's progress may be difficult, families want to know what to expect in the future, particularly when primary caregivers become ill or old. Families can be connected with parent support organizations and other agencies that provide advocacy and financial planning. Parent consultants should also be enlisted to teach families how to communicate with health care professionals and how to effectively advocate for their child.

Educating community providers, especially nonmedical personnel, is an important outreach activity. This may include interpreting medical information to school personnel; teaching about the chronic illness or rare disorder and explaining ramifications in relationship to special diets, additional mealtimes, physical activity, or adaptive physical education; and promoting independent self-care.

Information Exchange. Promoting information exchange among the family and care providers is essential if care is to be coordinated. The ability to assist parties in granting permission to release and share information is needed. Each contact among parties generates a report or documentation that must be obtained and integrated into the child and family plan and progress notes. The more providers involved with the child and family, the greater the need for communication to ensure that everyone is working in concert with each other. Building positive relationships among family and all providers enables coordination. Developing systems between the primary care office and other agencies (fax notification of an emergency room visit, hospital admission or discharge, or a provider visit) helps to improve communication. Families with young children and adolescents should be enlisted to maintain and share their health records and notebooks.

Monitoring

Monitoring is the periodic review and documentation of whether, and when, services were implemented and results of referrals. This requires maintaining and nurturing relationships with the family and providers. Frequent contact with the family also allows for increased opportunities to reassess family priorities, anticipate needs, and revise plans. A "tickler" or reminder system (manual or computer generated) should be implemented to ensure that the coordinator is able to track completion of planned services. Monitoring in a primary care setting may be integrated with office visits, thereby decreasing the frequency of telephone contacts.

The monitoring system should "catch" families when they do not return for scheduled office visits or complete referrals

or when telephone contact is disrupted and mail is returned. Families who have not returned for visits and who send a request to transfer medical records should be identifiable within the system. Follow-up should become customary practice, such as extra attention from the coordinator through written reminders and telephone calls to home or work. Financial stress may cause families to move in with relatives and temporarily lose contact with providers. Service providers involved with the family, particularly school and public health nurses, should be enlisted to help locate families who have not returned for appointments. Follow-up is not optional for CSHCN since they eventually surface somewhere in the health care system. The anticipatory nature of care coordination is to guide CSHCN back to proactive primary and specialty care rather than reactive and episodic emergency care.

Need for Care Coordination during Transition Periods

Services that focus on particular age-groups (e.g., birth to 3 years) or specific functions (e.g., transition from hospital) are time limited. Although coordination services may be terminated by one agency, families should be transitioned to other community-based agencies. For example, termination from hospital-to-home programs requires transferring care coordination to community providers to ensure that no disruption in support and services occurs. Transitioning to adult health services from pediatric care is a critical need for adolescents with special needs (see Chapter 9). Transitioning between health plans, and perhaps primary care providers, may be especially problematic. Whether this occurs within the same town or across state lines, there should be communication between primary care settings to ensure continuity of care. Title V–CSHCN programs and family information and referral centers are valuable sources of information to families who relocate to a new area.

Families may not require the same intensity of care coordination all the time, since needs will fluctuate with changes in the child's condition, growth and development, and so on. Consequently, families may enter and exit the care coordination process as they need it, alternating between high- and low-intensity periods. Discharge or termination from care coordination is relative. The benefit of primary care coordination is that it does not depend on categorical eligibility and can be consistently available.

Evaluation of Care Coordination

Evaluation should be completed with the child and family on a previously agreed to schedule and include documentation of the achieved outcomes, implementation constraints, and facilitators and revision of the family service plan. Consideration should be given to measuring family perceived benefits of care coordination. For example, families in the CHOICES project (Shriners Hospitals) reported that care coordination for children resulted in fewer trips to the doctor (43%), improvement in function (36%), more use of community-based services (35%), fewer complications (29%), and fewer hospitalizations (22%) (Presler, 1998). Meanwhile, benefits to the family were ease in obtaining equipment and supplies (49%), better understanding of services and agencies (48%), help from people who cared (45%), and saving time finding health care and worrying less (41%).

The Clinical Value Compass (Nelson et al, 1996) is a model that has potential applicability for organizing the indicators and measures related to care coordination interventions (Figure 7-2). It combines structure, process, and outcome measures within the points of the compass, which represent satisfaction, functional status and well-being, clinical status, and health care utilization and cost. The components have been applied to evaluation of managed health care plans (Lind, 2001), primary care in small office settings (Center for Medical Home Improvement, 2001), and the Model of Chronic Illness Care (Wagner et al, 2002). Data could be collected from multiple sources, such as administration/claims, medical records, and family and provider interviews or surveys.

Satisfaction with care coordination focuses on the amount and type of information and services received, family ease in obtaining and using services, family communication with providers, and relationship with coordinator and primary care team. Tools are in the process of being tested and have future applicability for measuring satisfaction at the primary and specialty provider level of care (Cassady et al, 2000; Ireys and Perry, 1999; Seid et al, 2001). It is important to consider the fit between the objectives of care coordination and the tool.

Functional measures could consider the level of family involvement in health care decision making, ease in accessing services, and communication with providers. Some of these measures are incorporated into the Consumer Assessment of Health Plan Survey (CAHPS) 2.0H Child Questionnaire with CSHCN module being implemented by the National Committee on Quality Assurance (Foundation for Accountability, 2002b). This survey will measure family experience related to their children's health care within managed care plans for national comparison. Measures of quality of life or family functioning sensitive to care coordination and resource use have not been developed. This information can be obtained qualitatively by asking families their own perception about how care coordination has affected them. One measure to be considered is the number of family work or child school days missed.

Clinical indicators related to care coordination interventions could include increased knowledge of resources, ability to acquire or access resources, and improved knowledge of

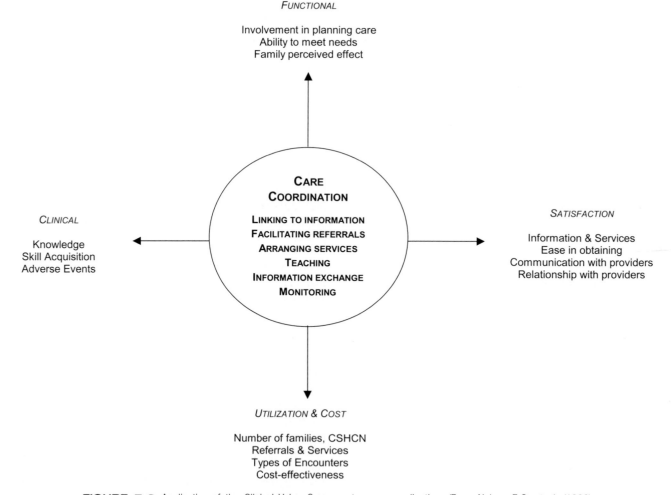

FIGURE 7-2 Application of the Clinical Value Compass to care coordination. (From Nelson E.G. et al. (1996). Improving health care, Part I: The clinical value compass. *Joint Commission Journal of Quality Improvement, 22*(4), 243-258.) Modified with permission.

condition and treatment goals. Since each care plan is individualized for the family this could be measured by the degree of change either reported by the family or observed. Clinical indicators can also consider the number of missed primary care visits and families "lost" to follow-up as well as the number of adverse events, such as unplanned hospital and emergency room visits.

Utilization measures might be the number of families and children served compared with total CSHCN population, number and type of services used, number and type of referrals made and completed, and number and type of visits made with families and providers. The economic costs of health care service utilization, including time, are an important outcome to measure. For example, the Maryland Rare and Expensive Case Management (REM), a component of Maryland's Medicaid managed care program, reported that case management helped to lower total and acute care costs (hospital) of health care while displacing some of those savings to nonacute care community services and pharmacy (Pandey et al, 2000). Economic or cost-effectiveness analysis (in contrast to cost-benefit) is proposed by Tahan (2001) as a method for comparing care coordination with traditional client services delivery models.

Evaluation must also consider the community and the extent to which services are available and accessible to all families. Networking with community providers allows for joint identification and problem solving of community capacity to meet family needs. A community coalition could design strategies to address gaps in local service delivery and provide feedback to policy makers.

Methods

Coordinators use all opportunities to remain connected with families. Home visits may be made jointly with other disciplines, and family care or school conferences may be initiated by any community provider. Telephone calls, office contacts, and accompanying families to health care and community agency visits are ways in which the coordinator maintains contact with the family and facilitates implementation and monitoring of the family service plan. Telehealth, the use of electronic technology, has been described as a method to provide follow-up health care and support services to families who live in rural areas (Farmer and Muhlenbruck, 2001).

Partnering with other professionals is an important strategy to consider. Coordinators in a primary care office may have limited opportunities for outreach. Meanwhile, families with long-standing multiple issues complicated by poverty may present challenges for health care professionals who are not accustomed to working with vulnerable populations (Aday, 2001). Collaborating with community partners such as social workers and public (community) health nurses may benefit family and provider relationship development as well as promote the health of the child and family.

Summary

Care coordination is a proactive, goal-directed process, individualized with and for families of CSHCN, for the purpose of meeting identified child and family needs and ensuring access to resources, thereby improving health outcomes and the cost-effective use of health services. The process of care coordination includes assessment, family service planning, implementation, monitoring, evaluation, and transition. Key functions of the process are the identification of CSHCN within primary care settings, child and family assessment, establishment and maintenance of a community resource network, information and referral, arranging for services, child and family education, and information exchange among family and involved professionals.

The medical home is an emerging model that is being promoted for implementation in primary care settings. Primary care practices will need to organize office systems and engage the help of parents and staff to transform them into medical homes. Bridging the gap between family expectations and what primary care providers deliver will require improvements in relationship building, continuing professional education, and system changes. Provider knowledge about resources, time and financial constraints, and evaluation are areas that will need to be addressed if care coordination services are to become an integrated standard of care. Meanwhile, collaboration and partnerships among all providers are essential if community-based systems of care for families of CSHCN are to be realized.

RESOURCES

Center for Medical Home Improvement, Hood Center for Children and Families, Children's Hospital at Dartmouth–Hitchcock Medical Center
http://www.medicalhomeimprovement.org/
Provides a medical home improvement kit, including the medical home measurement tool, describing their quality improvement approach to developing a medical home

Division of Specialized Care for Children (DSCC) at the University of Illinois at Chicago
http://internet.dscc.uic.edu/dsccroot/providers/providers.asp
http://internet.dscc.uic.edu/forms/medicalhome/

MedHomeCMEMonograph.pdf
Provides a continuing medical education monograph for providers who want to be approved and receive reimbursement for providing a medical home example of a family coordinated care record
http://internet.dscc.uic.edu/dscctext/parents/parents.asp

The Exceptional Parent Magazine
http://www.exceptionalparent.com/
Information for parents and professionals with practical advice, resource information, and parent matching opportunities; recommended for office waiting rooms

Family Voices, a national family advocacy organization with links to state family coordinators and resources
http://www.familyvoices.org/

The Los Angeles Medical Home Project for Children with Special Health Care Needs
http://www.medicalhomela.org/
Provides user-friendly resources for families, providers, and training materials, as well as a family notebook called "All about Me"

Medical home Hawaii. Medical Home Reaching the Next Level: Culturally Effective Service and Training Partnerships to Benefit Children and Families
http://www.medicalhomehi.com

National Center for Medical Home Initiatives for Children with Special Health Needs
http://www.medicalhomeinfo.org/index.html

Provides information related to all activities of the national center, including the "Every Child Deserves a Medical Home" training program, screening initiatives, and technical assistance

The Pediatric Alliance for Coordinated Care (PACC), Children's Hospital Boston, sponsored by the Institute for Community
http://www.communityinclusion.org/publications/compcare.html
Provides an operations manual for implementing a medical home

REFERENCES

Aday, L.A. (2001). *At risk in America: The health and health care needs of vulnerable populations in the United States* (2nd ed.). San Francisco: Jossey-Bass.

American Academy of Pediatrics & Committee on Children With Disabilities. (1999a). The pediatrician's role in development and implementation of an Individual Education Plan (IEP) and/or an Individual Family Service Plan (IFSP). *Pediatrics, 104,* 124-127.

American Academy of Pediatrics & Committee on Children With Disabilities. (1999b). Care coordination: integrating health and related systems of care for children with special health care needs. *Pediatrics, 104,* 978-981.

American Academy of Pediatrics & Committee on School Health. (2001). The role of the school nurse in providing school health services. *Pediatrics, 108,* 1231-1232.

American Academy of Pediatrics & Medical Home Initiatives for Children with Special Needs Project Advisory Committee. (2002). The medical home. *Pediatrics, 110,* 184-186.

Andersen, R. M. (1995). Revisiting the behavioral model and access to medical care: does it matter? *J Health Soc Behav, 36,* 1-10.

Association of Maternal and Child Health Programs. (2000). *Care coordination for children with special health care needs and their families in the new millennium, Principles, goals and recommendations developed by the AMCHP working group on care coordination.* Washington, DC: Assoc. MCH Programs.

Association of Maternal and Child Health Programs. (2002). *Meeting the needs of families: Critical elements of comprehensive care coordination in Title V children with special health care needs programs.* Washington, DC: Assoc. MCH Programs.

Baine, S., Rosenbaum, P., & King, S. (1995). Chronic childhood illnesses: what aspects of caregiving do parents value? *Child Care Health Dev, 21,* 291-304.

Bethell, C.D., Read, D., Stein, R.E., Blumberg, S.J., Wells, N., et al. (2002). Identifying children with special health care needs: Development and evaluation of a short screening instrument. *Ambul Pediatr, 2,* 38-47.

Bower, K.A. (1992). *Case management by nurses.* Kansas City, MO: American Nurses Pub.

Brewer, E.J., Jr., McPherson, M., Magrab, P.R., & Hutchins, V.L. (1989). Family-centered, community-based, coordinated care for children with special health care needs. *Pediatrics, 83,* 1055-1060.

Case Management Society of America. (2002). *CMSA standards of practice for case management.* 8201 Cantrell Road, Suite 230, Little Rock, AR 72227.

Cassady, C.E., Starfield, B., Hurtado, M.P., Berk, R.A., Nanda, J.P., et al. (2000). Measuring consumer experiences with primary care. *Pediatrics, 105,* 998-1003.

Center for Medical Home Improvement. (2001). *The CMHI medical home improvement kit.* Hood Center for Children & Families, Children's Hospital at Dartmouth-Hitchcock Medical Center [online]. Available: http://www.medicalhomeimprovement.org.

Cooley, W.C., Olson, A.L., & McAllister, J. (1995). Improving primary health services to children with chronic illnesses. *CATCH Quarterly, 3,* 2-3, 8.

Davidson, E.J., Silva, T.J., Sofis, L.A., Ganz, M.L., & Palfrey, J.S. (2002). The doctor's dilemma: Challenges for the primary care physician caring for the child with special health care needs. *Ambul Pediatr, 2,* 218-223.

Davidson, J.U. (1999). Blending case management and quality outcomes management into the family nurse practitioner role. *Nurs Adm Q, 24,* 66-74.

Dosa, N.P., Boeing, N.M., Ms, N., & Kanter, R.K. (2001). Excess risk of severe acute illness in children with chronic health conditions. *Pediatrics, 107,* 499-504.

Dunst, C.J. & Trivette, C.M. (1994). Empowering case management practices: A family-centered perspective. In C.J. Dunst, C.M. Trivette, & A.G. Deal (Eds.), *Supporting and strengthening families, Volume 1: Methods, strategies and practices* (pp. 187-211). Cambridge, MA: Brookline Books.

Dunst, C.J., Trivette, C.M., & Deal, A.G. (1988). *Enabling and empowering families: Principles and guidelines for practice.* Cambridge, MA: Brookline Books.

Dunst, C.J., Trivette, C.M., & Mott, D.W. (1994). Strengths-based family-centered intervention practices. In C.J. Dunst, C.M. Trivette, & A.G. Deal (Eds.), *Supporting and strengthening families, Volume 1: Methods, strategies and practices* (pp. 115-131). Cambridge, MA: Brookline Books.

Farmer, J.E. & Muhlenbruck, L. (2001). Telehealth for children with special health care needs: Promoting comprehensive systems of care. *Clin Pediatr, 40,* 93-8.

Forrest, C.B., Glade, G.B., Starfield, B., Baker, A.E., Kang, M., et al. (1999). Gatekeeping and referral of children and adolescents to specialty care. *Pediatrics, 104,* 28-34.

Foundation for Accountability. (2002a). *The children with special health care needs (CSHCN) Screener* [online]. Available: http://www.facct.org/facct/doclibFiles/documentFile_446.pdf.

Foundation for Accountability. (2002b). *Consumer assessment of health plans (CAHPS)* [online]. Available: http://www.facct.org/cahmiweb/chronic/CAHPS/lwicahps.htm.

Garwick, A.W., Patterson, J.M., Bennett, F.C., & Blum, R.W. (1998). Parents' perceptions of helpful vs unhelpful types of support in managing the care of preadolescents with chronic conditions. *Arch Pediatr Adolesc Med, 152,* 665-671.

Glade, G.B., Forrest, C.B., Starfield, B., Baker, A.E., Bocian, A.B., & Wasserman, R.C. (2002). *Ambul Pediatr, 2,* 93-98.

Grason, H. & Guyer, B. (1995). Rethinking the organization of children's programs: lessons from the elderly. *Milbank Q, 73,* 565-597.

Grossman, L.K., Rich, L.N., Michelson, S., & Hagerty, G. (1999). Managed care for children with special health care needs: The ABC program. *Clin Pediatr, 38*(3), 153-160.

Halfon, N., Inkelas, M., & Wood, D. (1995). Nonfinancial barriers to care for children and youth. *Annu Rev Public Health, 16,* 447-472.

Hill, I., Shwalberg, R., Zimmerman B., Tilson, W. (1999). *Achieving service integration for children with special heath care needs: An assessment of alternative Medicaid managed care models: Volumes 1 and 2* [online]. Available: http://www.hsrnet.com/pubs/ pub09.htm.

Hill, I. Zimmerman, B., & Siderits, P. (1996). *Integrating case management services in a managed care environment* [online]. Available: http://www.hsrnet.com/pubs/ pub01.htm.

Horst, L., Werner, R.R., & Werner, C.L. (2000). Case management for children and families. *J Child Fam.Nurs, 3,* 5-14.

Hughes, D.C., Halfon, N., Brindis, C.D., & Newacheck, P.W. (1996). Improving children's access to health care: the role of decategorization. *Bull NY Acad Med, 73,* 237-254.

Ireys, H.T. & Eichler, R.J. (1988). Program priorities of crippled children's agencies: a survey. *Public Health Rep, 103,* 77-83.

Ireys, H.T. & Perry, J.J. (1999). Development and evaluation of a satisfaction scale for parents of children with special health care needs. *Pediatrics, 104,* 1182-1191.

Kaufman, B.A., Terbrock, A., Winters, N., Ito, J., Klosterman, A., et al. (1994). Disbanding a multidisciplinary clinic: effects on the health care of myelomeningocele patients. *Pediatr Neurosurg, 21,* 36-44.

Kaye, N., Curtis D., & Booth, M. (2000). Certain children with special health care needs: An assessment of state activities and their relationship to HCFA's interim criteria [online]. Available: http://cms.hhs.gov/states/letters/needsrpt.pdf.

Kramer, L. & Houston, D. (1999). Hope for the children: A community-based approach to supporting families who adopt children with special needs. *Child Welfare, 78,* 611-635.

Krauss, M.W., Gulley, S., Leiter, V., Minihan, P., & Sciegaj, M. (2000). *The Family Partners Project: Report on a national survey of the health care experiences of families of children with special health care needs.* Waltham, MA: Heller School, Brandeis Univ.

Krauss, M.W., Wells, N., Gulley, S., & Anderson, B. (2001). Navigating systems of care: Results from a national survey of families with children with special health care needs. *Children's Services: Social Policy, Research, and Practice, 4,* 165-187.

Kruger, B.J. (2001). Title V-CSHCN: A closer look at the shaping of the national agenda for children with special health care needs. *Policy, Politics, & Nursing Practice, 2,* 320-329.

Kuhlthau, K., Ferris, T.G., Beal, A.C., Gortmaker, S.L., & Perrin, J.M. (2001). Who cares for medicaid-enrolled children with chronic conditions? *Pediatrics, 108,* 906-912.

Lind, P.H. (2001). Applying systems thinking to quality patient care delivery. In E.L. Cohen & T.G. Cesta (Eds.). *Nursing case management: From essential to advanced practice applications* (3rd ed., pp. 37-48). St. Louis: Mosby.

Lindeke, L.L., Krajicek, M., & Patterson, D.L. (2001). PNP roles and interventions with children with special needs and their families. *J Pediatr Health Care, 15*, 138-143.

Lowe, J. & Miller, W. (1998). A 1996 NASN research award winner. Health services provided by school nurses for students with chronic health problems. *J School Nurs, 14*, 4-16.

McCallion, P., Janicki, M.P., Grant-Griffin, L., & Kolomer, S. (2000). Grandparent Carers II: Service needs and service provision issues. *J Gerontological Social Work, 33*, 57-84.

McPherson, M. & Honberg, L. (2002). Identification of children with special health care needs: a cornerstone to achieving healthy people 2010. *Ambul Pediatr, 2*, 22-23.

Mele, N.C. & Flowers, J.S. (2000). Medicaid managed care and children with special health care needs: a case study analysis of demonstration waivers in three states. *J Pediatr Nurs, 15*, 63-72.

National Governors Association. (1996). Maximizing the flexibility of categorical funding for children's health services. *Issue Brief* [online]. Available: http://www.nga.org/nga/1,1169,C_REPORTS,00.html.

Neff, J.M., Sharp, V.L., Muldoon, H., Graham, J., Popalisky, J., et al. (2002). Identifying and classifying children with chronic conditions using administrative data with the clinical risk group classification system. *Ambul Pediatr, 2*, 71-79.

Nelson, E.G., Mohr, J.J., Batalden, P.B., & Plume, S.K. (1996). Improving health care, Part 1: The clinical value compass. *Joint Commission Journal of Quality Improvement, 22*(4), 243-258.

Newacheck, P.W., Strickland, B., Shonkoff, J.P., Perrin, J.M., McPherson, M., et al. (1998). An epidemiologic profile of children with special health care needs. *Pediatrics, 102*, 117-123.

Omnibus Reconciliation Act. (1989). Omnibus Reconciliation Act of 1989. Title V, 501.

Palfrey, J.S., Levy, J.C., & Gilbert, K.L. (1980). Use of primary care facilities by patients attending specialty clinics. *Pediatrics, 65*, 567-572.

Pandey, S.K., Mussman, M.G., Moore, H.W., Folkemer, J.G., & Kaelin, J.J. (2000). An assessment of Maryland Medicaid's rare and expensive case management program. *Eval Health Prof, 23*, 457-479.

Patterson, J.M. & Hovey, D.L. (2000). Family-centered care for children with special health needs: Rhetoric or reality. *Families, Systems & Health, 18*, 237-251.

Perrin, E.C., Lewkowicz, C., & Young, M.H. (2000). Shared vision: concordance among fathers, mothers, and pediatricians about unmet needs of children with chronic health conditions. *Pediatrics, 105*, 277-285.

Perrin, J.M. & Ireys, H.T. (1984). The organization of services for chronically ill children and their families. *Pediatr Clin North Am, 31*, 235-257.

Presler, B. (1998). Care coordination for children with special health care needs. *Orthop Nurs, 17*, 45-51.

Ray, L. (1997). *Promoting the health of families raising a child with a chronic condition: Directions for outcomes research.* DAI, 58, no. 08B, (UMI No. 9807018).

Reiss, J.G. (2000). *Status report: MCH Title V block grant needs assessment* [online]. Available: http://cshcnleaders.ichp.edu/triregionals2000/KansasCityAgenda.htm.

Rosenbach, M. & Young, C. (2000). *Care coordination and Medicaid managed care: Emerging issues for states and managed care organizations.* Princeton, NJ: Mathematica Policy Research, Inc.

Scholle, S.H. & Kelleher, K.J. (1995). Children with chronic medical conditions: looking for a medical home. *Ambul Child Health, 1*, 130-138.

Schwalberg, R., Mathis, S.A., & Hill, I. (2000). *New opportunities, new approaches: Serving children with special health care needs under*

SCHIP, Vol. 1 [online]. Available: http://www.jhsph.edu/centers/cshcn/volume1.pdf.

Seid, M., Varni, J.W., Bermudez, L.O., Zivkovic, M., Far, M.D., et al. (2001). Parents' perceptions of primary care: Measuring parents' experiences of pediatric primary car quality. *Pediatrics, 108*, 2, 264-270.

Shatin, D., Levin, R., Ireys, H.T., & Haller, V. (1998). Health care utilization by children with chronic illnesses: a comparison of Medicaid and employer-insured managed care. *Pediatrics, 102*, E44.

Shelton, T.L. & Stepanek, J.S. (1994). *Family-centered care for children needing specialized health and developmental services.* Association for the Care of Children's Health, 7910 Woodmont Avenue, Suite 300, Bethesda, Maryland 20814, 301-654-6549.

Sia, C.C. (1992). Abraham Jacobi Award address, April 14, 1992 the medical home: pediatric practice and child advocacy in the 1990s. *Pediatrics, 90*, 419-423.

Silva, T.J., Sofis, L.A., & Palfrey, J.S. (2000). *Practicing comprehensive care: A physician's operations manual for implementing a medical home for children with special health care needs.* Boston: Institute for Community Inclusion/UAP Boston.

Simpson, L. & Fraser, I. (1999). Children and managed care: What research can, can't, and should tell us about impact. *Med Care Res Rev, 56*(2), 13-36.

Sloper, P. & Turner, S. (1992). Service needs of families of children with severe physical disability. *Child Care Health Dev, 18*, 259-282.

State of New Hampshire. (1993). *Care coordination services manual.* Concord, NH: Special Medical Services Bureau, Office of Health Planning and Medicaid.

State of New Hampshire. (2002). *Information and referral report, 1991-2001.* Concord, NH: Special Medical Services Bureau, Office of Health Planning and Medicaid.

Szilagyi, P.G. (1998). Managed care for children: Effect on access to care and utilization of health services. *Future Child, 8*(2), 39-59.

Tahan, H.S. (2001). Case management evaluation: The use of the cost-effectiveness analysis method. In E.L. Cohen & T.G. Cesta (Eds.). *Nursing case management: From essential to advanced practice applications* (3rd ed., p. 503-524). St. Louis: Mosby.

Taylor, P. (1999). Comprehensive nursing case management: An advanced practice model. *Nursing Case Management, 4*, 2-10.

U.S. Department of Health and Human Services. (1998). *Implementing Title V CSHCN programs: A resource manual for state programs.* Washington, DC: U.S. DHHS.

U.S. Department of Health and Human Services. (2000). *Healthy people 2010.* [online]. Available: http://www.health.gov/healthypeople/document/html/volume2/16mich.htm.

U.S. Department of Health and Human Services. (2001). *All aboard the 2010 express: A 10-year action plan to achieve community-based service systems for children and youth with special health care needs and their families.* Washington, D.C.: U.S. DHHS.

Wagner, E.H., Davis, C., Schaefer, J., Von Korff, M., & Austin, B. (2002). A survey of leading chronic disease management programs: Are they consistent with the literature? *Journ Nurs Care Qual, 16*, 67-80.

Weinick, R.M. & Krauss, N.A. (2000). Racial/ethnic differences in children's access to care. *Am J Public Health, 90*, 1771-1774.

Zimmerman, B., Schwalberg, R., Gallagher, J., Harkins, M., & Sines, E. (2000). *Title V roles in coordinating care for children with special health care needs.* Retrieved, August, 1, 2000 from http://www.jhsph.edu/centers/cshcn/final.pdf.

8 Financing Health Care for Children with Chronic Conditions

Judith A. Vessey

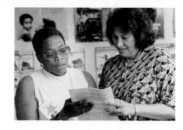

USING the Maternal and Child Health Bureau's definition, it is estimated that approximately 18% of children have special health care needs with only 89% of this cohort having some type of health insurance (Newacheck et al, 2000). Those with health insurance were more likely than the uncovered cohort to report regular care (96.9% vs. 79.2%) (Newacheck et al, 2000). Children without coverage have many unmet health care needs and experience significant delays in receiving care, resulting in poorer health and social outcomes. Financing health care is essential, but expensive, for children with chronic conditions. Children with relatively minor health care needs may have double to triple the health care expenditures of healthy children. Within the population of children with chronic conditions, care for those with a catastrophic condition costs up to 26 times that of those with a single minor condition, a difference of $3451 vs. $130 per year (Ireys et al, 2002). It is estimated that the 5% of children with significant health care needs account for approximately 35% of pediatric health care expenditures (Committee on Children with Disabilities, 1998).

Sources of Funding

Today in the United States, care for children with chronic conditions is financed by complex methods that are generally categorized as follows: (1) private, employer-sponsored health insurance; (2) private, personal policies; (3) public programs (e.g., Medicaid, the State Children's Health Insurance Program [SCHIP], and other federal and state categorical programs); (4) private, philanthropic sources; and (5) the family's own funds (Stein, 1997). A child's health care may be supported by one or a combination of these methods. The source of financial coverage depends on a number of factors, including the type of health condition, the family's socioeconomic status, the state and county of residence, the availability of a voluntary organization for the specific condition, and the availability of health care and legal personnel to advocate for the child's rights for specific sources of financial assistance.

Both private and public sources of funding for the general population continue to undergo reforms to control costs of care while improving access to and quality of care. The range of available health plan options is depicted in Figure 8-1. These reforms have had mixed results but are of particular interest to families and primary care providers of children with chronic conditions because they may be insensitive to the interests of children—especially those with chronic conditions (Garwick et al, 1998).

Major Financing Structures of Insurance

Indemnity, Fee-for-Service Plans

Historically, private and government insurance were *fee-for-service,* indemnity plans (Box 8-1 gives definitions of italicized words). Fee-for-service, indemnity plans are insurance schemes that are separate from care-delivery systems and are determined by a variety of market forces, including custom, altruism, profit, and administrative costs. Well-known examples are the traditional major nonprofit associations, such as Blue Cross/Blue Shield; commercial health insurance offered by profit-making organizations; and traditional Medicaid. Benefits that are likely to be covered by fee-for-service plans are hospital room and board, miscellaneous hospital expenses, surgery, physicians' nonsurgical services rendered in a hospital, and outpatient diagnostic radiographic examinations and laboratory expenses. Room and board in an extended care facility may be included when there is proof that continued medical—as opposed to custodial—care is required. Medicaid also covers a variety of ambulatory care and outpatient expenses, but such coverage is highly variable in private fee-for-service plans. Today, pure fee-for-service indemnity plans are costly and rare.

Managed Care Plans

Managed care plans were initiated in the 1920s and 1930s but remained relatively unknown until 1973, with the passage of the HMO Act (Kongstvedt, 2001), which required companies of more than 25 individuals to offer such a plan as an alternative to indemnity insurance should they be approached by an *HMO (health maintenance organization)* agent. HMOs and other managed care entities became a major market force in the 1990s when the gross domestic product (GDP) for health care goods and services began to approach 14%, up from 5.1% in 1960 and 8.9% in 1980, with projected increases of 11% annually. Managed care was seen as a viable alternative to curtailing spiraling costs. Currently, it is estimated that 176.4 million lives are covered by managed care plans (Kongstvedt, 2001).

Managed care is an integrated system of health insurance, financing, and service delivery functions that attempts to control and coordinate its enrolled members' use of health services in order to contain health expenditures, eliminate inappropriate care, and improve quality. In the classic managed care arrangement, the insured individual or family has access to selected providers who have agreed to furnish a defined set of health care services at a fee that is lower than usual. This is typically done through *prospective payment* and *capitation.*

There are many types of managed care plans, including HMOs, *preferred provider organizations (PPOs)*, and *point-of-service (POS) plans.* There also are different models of HMOs, such as (1) the *staff model,* (2) the *group model,* (3) the *network model,* and (4) the *independent practice association (IPA),* to name but a few. Although services provided by managed care organizations (MCOs) are similar to those offered in fee-for-service plans, MCOs include preventive health services as a

covered benefit because they have a strong financial incentive to keep their enrollees healthy. MCOs may also offer better care coordination for common chronic conditions (e.g., asthma) that are in the MCO's best interest to manage effectively (Committee on Children with Disabilities, 1998).

Traditional managed care plans operate by providing the insured with a list of providers enrolled with their plan. The insured chooses a primary care provider to go to for all routine care and has little or no *out-of-pocket expenses.* To go outside the plan for care, the insured must pay a significantly higher share of the cost. The primary care provider may also suffer financially by referring the insured to more costly specialty services, especially those that are "out of plan." MCOs may restrict access to specialty health care in the interest of controlling overall health plan costs. MCOs restrict access to pediatric specialty care by limiting referrals to selected specialty providers, requiring the family to bear a higher share of the total cost of out-of-plan services, and/or penalizing the primary care provider for referrals to out-of-plan specialists or subspecialists. In most capitation arrangements, the primary care provider is penalized by deducting the cost of specialty care from the overall profit of the plan or the fees paid to the provider, and

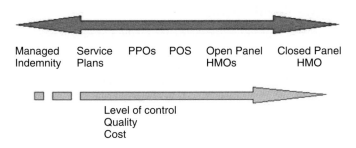

| Managed Indemnity | Service Plans | PPOs | POS | Open Panel HMOs | Closed Panel HMO |

Level of control
Quality
Cost

FIGURE 8-1 Continuum of managed care in relationship to control, quality, and cost.

BOX 8-1

Glossary of Italicized Words

Adverse selection: When a larger proportion in individuals with poorer health status enroll in specific plans or select specific options. Plans with a subpopulation of higher-than-average costs are adversely selected.

Capitation: A method of payment wherein a fixed amount per enrollee per month is paid to the provider to cover a specified set of services regardless of the actual services rendered.

Case management: A system of improving the quality of care while managing costs by monitoring and coordinating the delivery of health services to individuals with complex health problems.

Co-insurance: A method of cost sharing in which the insurer and insured party share payment for an approved charge of covered services according to a predetermined specified ratio after payment of the deductible.

Co-payment: A method of cost sharing in which the insured party pays part of the amount due on receiving services and the insurer pays the remaining portion.

Deductible: A method of cost sharing in which the insured party pays a predetermined amount with the insurance covering the balance.

ERISA: The Employee Retirement Income Security Act, which exempts self-insured health plans from state laws governing health insurance.

Exclusions: Populations or services that are not covered by an insurance plan.

Fee-for-service: Plans in which the payer (i.e., either patients or insurers) agrees to pay the fee set by the provider after the service is provided.

Gatekeeper: An MCO employee who authorizes patient referrals for specialty care.

Health maintenance organization (HMO): A managed care plan that integrates financing and delivery of a comprehensive set of health services to an enrolled population.

Group model HMO: An HMO that pays a medical group a negotiated, per capita rate that the group distributes among its providers, often as salary.

Independent practice association (IPA): An HMO that contracts with individual providers to provide services to enrollees as a negotiated per capita or fee-for-service rate. Providers may see other patients besides those enrolled in the HMO plan.

Network model HMO: An HMO that contracts with several medical groups, often at a capitated rate.

Staff model HMO: An HMO where providers practice solely as employees and provide services exclusively to HMO plan enrollees.

HEDIS: A standardized set of measures used in evaluating health plan performance.

Integrated service networks (ISNs): Organizations that are accountable for the costs and outcomes associated with delivering a full continuum of health care services to a defined population. All necessary health services are provided for a fixed payment.

Out-of-pocket expense: Payments made by an individual for medical services, which may include direct payments to providers, deductibles, co-insurance, and for services not covered by the plan and/or charges in excess of the plan's limits.

Outliers: Cases with extremely long lengths of stay or extraordinarily high costs.

Point-of-service (POS) plan: A managed care plan that combines features of both prepaid and fee-for-service insurance. Enrollees decide whether to use network or nonnetwork providers, generally with sizable co-payments for selecting the latter.

Population carve-outs: A population carve-out provides health care to a designated population that is targeted or defined by a specific health condition.

Preexisting condition exclusion: A practice of some health insurers to deny coverage to individuals for a certain period for health conditions that already exist when coverage is initiated.

Preferred provider organizations (PPOs): A health plan with a network of providers whose services are available to enrollees at lower cost than services of nonnetwork providers.

Prospective payment: A method of paying health care providers in which rates are established in advance. Providers are paid these rates regardless of the costs they actually incur.

Service carve-outs: A set of specific services provided outside a mainstream plan.

Stop-loss provision: The amount that the enrollee must pay out-of-pocket in a calendar year before the plan pays 100% of further covered charge.

either way of imposing restrictions may not be in the best interests of a child with a chronic condition. Because most MCOs restrict participating providers, the child's primary care provider or specialist may not be as knowledgeable about either the diagnosis or treatment of rare conditions as a pediatrician or pediatric specialist. The child may be at further risk by not having easy access to approved ancillary health care services (e.g., physical therapy, in-home care) that may greatly enhance the quality of life for the child and family.

Managed care plans may use *service carve-outs* as a way of providing care to a historically difficult and expensive group of beneficiaries who are often referred to as *outliers.* Care for children with selected pediatric conditions, primarily those that are behavioral in nature, is handled under a separate managed health care contract that is often held by a different agency. Although carve-outs should theoretically provide higher levels of specialty care to populations formerly denied access to managed care (e.g., *population carve-outs*), they actually may further fragment care.

Hybrid Plans

In recent years, consumer and provider backlashes against the restrictions imposed by traditional managed care plans have led to significant changes (Lesser & Ginsburg, 2000). Consumers were concerned that under managed care, providers would put their financial considerations (e.g., capitation) and practice obligations *(gate keeping)* ahead of client well-being while providers reacted negatively to provider profiling, utilization management, and other cost containment measures. In order to restore consumer confidence, numerous state consumer (patient) protection laws have been passed with federal legislation, including the Patient's Bill of Rights, which is under review. Managed care plans responded by offering broader provider networks, curtailing preauthorization and concurrent utilization management controls, and reducing reliance on capitation and other measures designed to improve cost containment (Reed & Trude, 2002). Meanwhile, indemnity plans have adopted some cost containment measures (e.g., discounted, negotiated rates) in order to stay competitive. Today, most health plans are hybrids.

Selecting a Plan

Parents of children with chronic conditions must carefully consider their health insurance options to choose the best coverage for their particular needs. Table 8-1 provides a guide for families to use in evaluating plans. When choosing a plan, advice offered by the Committee on Children with Disabilities of the American Academy of Pediatrics (1998) should be considered: children with chronic conditions differ from adults with similar conditions. The changing dynamics of children's development combined with the situational stressors of serious illness or disability can significantly, and irreversibly, affect a child's developmental attainment. Moreover, the epidemiology of chronic conditions in pediatric populations is quite different from in adult populations. Children with chronic conditions are best served by knowledgeable pediatric clinicians. Families need to select a plan that is sufficiently flexible to support such care, which includes providing a medical home for the child (see Chapter 7) and access to pediatric specialists and subspecialists.

Once the policy is obtained through employment or government agencies, attention must be given to filling out claims accurately and filing them promptly, working with a claims agent and care coordinator who understand the family's problems, and following up rejected claims with convincing evidence of the treatment or piece of equipment's importance to the child's well-being. The primary care provider can help the parents by supporting their legitimate health plan claims and completing forms accurately and promptly.

Private Health Insurance

Private insurance remains the major method of financing health care in the United States, although small decreases in the percent of expenditures, as well as in the number of people covered, have been realized during the last decade. The role of private health insurance in paying the costs of care for children with chronic conditions is substantial but difficult to comprehend because of the variation in patterns of coverage and scope of benefits. Private health insurance is generally categorized by the method of reimbursement. Historically, most of these plans were indemnity, fee-for-service, but over the last decade managed care has become the dominant organizational form (Kongstvedt, 2001). A continuum of arrangements, varying by the onset of prepayment required and restriction to selected providers, is now available to consumers.

Indemnity, Fee-for-Service Plans

Despite the decreased availability of private fee-for-service arrangements, families of children with chronic conditions may prefer this type of coverage. Ferris and colleagues (2001) demonstrated that despite virtually identical coverage but higher costs, families strongly preferred indemnity plans over managed care plans with gate keeping because they perceived fewer restrictions on choice of providers and care facilities.

In fee-for-service arrangements, the insured person usually pays an annual fee or deductible, usually $100 to $300 per individual or $500 per family, before insurance benefits are realized. The insured individual may also pay *co-insurance,* which is approximately 20% of physician, hospital, and other related fees. There is usually also a *stop-loss provision,* as well as a maximum lifetime benefit. Providers of care are reimbursed for services rendered based on schedules of usual and customary charges (Health Insurance Association of America [HIAA], 2002). In general, coverage is good for medical supplies and equipment. Most plans have only minimal coverage for preventive services or therapies (e.g., speech, occupational, physical; nutrition support; home care). Mental health services also may be covered with limitations on the number of visits and the type of provider.

The problems faced by families who depend on fee-for-service private health insurance to finance care for a child with a chronic condition are evident by looking at the *exclusions* and limitations of the health care policies. The insurer usually does not pay for *preexisting conditions.* Thus if a family was not adequately covered before their child acquired the chronic condition, a fee-for-service plan will not often cover the medical expenses related to the chronic condition. Other

TABLE 8-1
Plan Features to Evaluate

Pediatric Services Covered	Extent of Coverage	In-Plan Cost Sharing	Out-of-Plan Cost Sharing
PEDIATRIC PREVENTIVE CARE SERVICES			
Well child and adolescent visits, including developmental screening			
Immunizations			
Vision and hearing			
Dental care			
Health education			
PEDIATRIC PRIMARY AND OTHER SERVICES			
Physician services			
Hospital services			
Emergency services			
Surgical care			
Prescription medications			
Lab and radiographic services			
PEDIATRIC CHRONIC CARE SERVICES			
Medical subspecialists and surgical specialty services			
Occupational, physical, speech, and respiratory therapy services			
Mental health and chemical dependency services			
Durable medical equipment, supplies and assertive technology devices			
Home health care			
Nutrition services and products			
Care coordination services			
Other			

**COST-SHARING PROVISIONS
AND CATASTROPHIC PROTECTIONS**

	Amount
Annual premium	
Annual deductible	
Annual out-of-pocket cost limit	
Lifetime out-of-pocket cost limit	

PEDIATRIC PROVIDER NETWORK CAPACITY

	Yes	No
Are pediatricians included as primary care clinicians?		
Does the plan recruit physicians and other health professionals with expertise in the care of children with chronic conditions?		
Does the plan make exceptions to allow specialists to serve as primary care clinicians for certain children with complex conditions?		
Does the plan allow for shared management of children with chronic conditions between primary care physicians and subspecialists?		
If the primary or specialty care provider of a child with a chronic condition is not in the plan's network, are exceptions made to reimburse the physician to ensure continuity of care?		
Does the plan rely on pediatric—not adult—subspecialists to care for children with chronic conditions?		
Does the plan have an up-to-date inventory that lists and describes pediatric professionals within the plan who are experts in the care of children with chronic conditions?		

From Institute for Child Health Policy, Gainesville, FL; Web site: http://www.ichp.edu/managed/materials/purchaser/pedserv.html. Reprinted with permission.   *Continued*

TABLE 8-1

Plan Features to Evaluate—cont'd

Pediatric Services Covered	Extent of Coverage	In-Plan Cost Sharing	Out-of-Plan Cost Sharing
Does the plan include or contract with the following primary care pediatricians, pediatric medical subspecialists, and pediatric surgical specialists in the following areas? (If not, what alternative arrangements are used to ensure access to these pediatric subspecialists?)		**Yes**	**No**
Adolescent medicine			
Allergy/immunology			
Anesthesiology			
Cardiology			
Child and adolescent psychiatry			
Critical care			
Dermatology			
Development/behavioral medicine			
Emergency medicine			
Endocrinology			
Gastroenterology			
Genetics			
Hematology/oncology			
Infectious disease			
Neonatology/perinatology			
Nephrology			
Neurosurgery			
Ophthalmology			
Oral surgery			
Orthopedics			
Otolaryngology			
Pediatric surgery			
Plastic surgery			
Pulmonology			
Radiology			
Rheumatology			
Urology			
Does the plan include or contract with the following other pediatric specialty health professionals and facilities? (If not, what alternative arrangements are used to ensure access to these other pediatric specialty providers?)			
Nurses with pediatric expertise			
Child and adolescent psychologists			
Social workers with pediatric expertise			
Physical therapists with pediatric expertise			
Occupational therapists with pediatric expertise			
Speech therapists with pediatric expertise			
Respiratory therapists with pediatric expertise			
Home health providers with pediatric expertise			
Nutritionists with pediatric expertise			
Genetic screening and counseling services			
Care managers with pediatric expertise			
Dentists or orthodontists with pediatric expertise			
Hospitals and/or medical centers specializing in the care of children			
Does the plan encourage coordination and integration of physical and mental health services for children with chronic conditions?			
Does the plan include state-designated pediatric centers of care (e.g., perinatal, hemophilia, trauma, transplant care)?			
Are multidisciplinary teams available for the care of children with chronic conditions through the following:			
Contracts with hospital outpatient departments that specialize in the care of children?			
Contracts with specialty pediatric clinics?			
Contracts with developmental centers?			
Other arrangements?			
Do durable medical equipment vendors have the capacity to individualize and customize equipment for children?			
Are the plan's utilization review and appeals processes performed by appropriate pediatric specialists and subspecialists?			

common exclusions are payments for preventive health care, rehabilitation services and equipment, and expenses associated with the birth of an infant up to the first 30 days of life. Coverage for health needs defined as nonmedical (e.g., special education, transportation to health care facilities, home renovations needed to care for a child with a chronic condition) are rarely included in fee-for-service plans.

Separate from general health insurance policies are major medical expense policies (e.g., catastrophic coverage) that provide additional protection. They cover a broad range of catastrophic medical expenses above a certain and generally very high (e.g., $15,000 or more) deductible. These policies generally have a maximum lifetime limit high enough to cover the costs of catastrophic illness. The cost of major medical insurance is controlled by sizable deductible fees and co-insurance fees for medical expenses that exceed the deductible. They are generally most helpful in catastrophic situations when a person's basic coverage is either a hospital-surgical policy or a major medical policy with a lower-than-adequate lifetime limit (HIAA, 2002). Major medical plans are not necessarily advantageous for children with chronic conditions because their health care needs do not fit into the designated structure of catastrophic coverage plans.

Managed Care Plans

It is hard to evaluate the effectiveness of private managed care plans in providing care for children with chronic conditions because of their structural diversity and rapid evolution. The majority of MCOs, however, avoid *adverse selection* and do not actively enroll children with special needs or develop programs for them; *population and service carve-outs* are common (Ireys et al, 1996). Most plans do not actively restrict the enrollment of such children, but there is little incentive for them to do so. Many primary care providers also may be reluctant to care for children with special health care needs if capitation and other contractual arrangements with the MCO provide a disincentive for doing so (Smucker, 2001).

Of the various types of private managed care plans, HMOs have the potential to provide more comprehensive services to children with chronic conditions because they may include (1) comprehensive outpatient services, including basic mental health care; (2) coverage for ancillary therapies; (3) home health services; (4) coverage for durable medical equipment, supplies, and prescription drugs; and (5) access to pediatricians and pediatric subspecialists, pediatric nurse practitioners, psychologists, nutritionists, and social service workers with expertise in various problems of living with a chronic condition (Fox et al, 1993). Other advantages are that preexisting conditions are generally not excluded, *co-payments* are small, and there may be no *deductible* or *co-insurance* provision.

Conversely, gatekeeper activities that restrict access to the best providers for a child's condition are a serious limitation of HMO plans (Smucker, 2001). Moreover, a large number of services are excluded when a child goes out-of-plan, which may be very costly to the family. Out-of-pocket expenses can become a substantial burden, especially because many plans do not have a *stop-loss provision* (Fox et al, 1993). Although care coordination or *case management* services are included, they may be ineffective in providing higher quality care because of the other limitations.

Self-Insured Plans

Self-insured plans, whether they are fee-for-service or managed care, are not governed by the same laws as other private health insurance plans. They may offer even fewer benefits to children than other private insurance plans that are subject to the statutory and common law doctrines regulating insurance. Self-insured plans are governed by the Employee Retirement Income Security Act of 1974 (*ERISA*), which makes them exempt from state and federal insurance regulations and allows employers to establish, modify, and cancel employee medical benefits without state or federal interference (Kongstvedt, 2001). The children of employees on self-insured plans can be left without coverage for costly conditions, and their families have little legal recourse. ERISA protections are currently being challenged in a number of legal proceedings.

HIPAA

The Health Insurance Portability and Accountability Act, more commonly known as HIPAA, was passed in 1996 to provide additional protections for families with private health insurance. Of specific note for children with chronic conditions and their families, HIPAA limits group health plans from discriminating against potential subscribers for previous poor health and limits the use of preexisting condition exclusions. It also guarantees selected small employers and individuals who have lost their job-related coverage the right to purchase health insurance and the ability to renew the coverage, regardless of any health conditions covered by the policy (U.S. Department of Health and Human Services, Centers for Medicare and Medicaid Services [U.S. DHHS, CMS], 2002a, August 5). These are important protections for families with children with chronic conditions. HIPAA is limited, however, in that it does not require selected benefits to be covered in group health plans or control the amount an insurer may charge for coverage. Health plans may seek to opt out of selected HIPAA requirements if they increase the plan cost above 1% and they meet other federal requirements.

Several amendments to HIPAA have been enacted. Of these, the Mental Health Parity Act (MHPA) is the most salient for families of children with chronic conditions (U.S. DHHS, CMS, 2002b, August 5). The MHPA requires parity between mental and medical/surgical health care benefits. Specifically, group health plans cannot place lower annual or lifetime financial limits on mental health benefits than on medical and surgical benefits. MHPA, however, does not require group health plans to offer mental health care coverage nor does it prohibit these plans from having different cost-sharing arrangements, such as higher co-payments or co-insurance requirements, or imposing limits on the number of covered visits.

The full impact of HIPAA has not yet been realized. Early findings indicate that while HIPAA has improved group coverage protections, access to individual coverage has not improved (Pollitz et al, 2000). It also has changed the way health plans are regulated by states and the federal government. Further legal interpretations of this law will determine its eventual impact on the private insurance market and consumer protections.

Government Health Care Programs

There are public health care financing programs for individuals and families who do not have access to employer-based health insurance or cannot afford to purchase private insurance. These programs may be entirely supported by federal money or may be jointly administered and funded by the federal government and the states. States also may have revenue-sharing agreements with counties or other local health jurisdictions to provide financial coverage for health care through public revenue.

The likelihood of being covered by health insurance rises with parental income. Approximately 11.7% of all children and 21.3% of poor children were without coverage, with more coming from single-parent homes (U.S. Bureau of Labor Statistics and Bureau of the Census, 2002). Yet, even with Medicaid expansions and the advent of SCHIP (State Children's Health Insurance Programs) (see p. 129), there have been no net gains in coverage for low-income children since private insurance coverage has sharply decreased (Cunningham & Park, 2000).

Those who do not have health insurance are not necessarily unemployed or living at or below the federal poverty level (FPL). Uninsured workers are usually employed in small businesses or are self-employed. Employed persons may lose health insurance if they or their family member acquires a chronic condition with high medical costs and the employer cancels the coverage. Employers also avoid the high cost of insuring their employees by relying on part-time workers or contracting work out to small firms, neither of which requires employers to offer insurance benefits. Undocumented residents are another group at risk for being uninsured. They may not wish to be identified as working in the United States and therefore may accept positions without health insurance coverage or other work-related benefits.

Medicaid

Medicaid (Title XIX of the Social Security Act) is a federal-state matching entitlement program that pays for medical assistance for selected needy populations. In fiscal year 2000, Medicaid served approximately 18.7 million children, including 1.5 million with chronic conditions who make up more than 48% of the 36 million Medicaid recipients (U.S. DHHS, CMS, 2002c, May 29). Children's share of total Medicaid expenditures, however, is only $17.9 billion (i.e., approximately 15% of total expenditures). Children with special health care needs are more likely than other children to be enrolled in Medicaid (Mele & Flowers, 2000).

Medicaid is the largest public health care program in the United States and is administered by the Centers for Medicare and Medicaid Services (CMS) (formerly the Health Care Financing Administration [HCFA]) within the US Department of Health and Human Services (US DHHS). It was established in 1965 and soon surpassed any other federally funded public health care program serving children. Medicaid guarantees eligible children a comprehensive package of health insurance benefits, which is generally more extensive than those of private insurance plans (Fox et al, 1997).

Medicaid programs vary among states. Within broad federal statutes and policies, each state (1) establishes its own eligibility standards, (2) determines the scope of services, (3) sets payment rates, and (4) administers its own program. The complexity of Medicaid regulations accompanied by the state's latitude in designing programs has resulted in disparity among state plans.

Eligibility.   States have some discretion in determining which groups to cover under their Medicaid programs. Eligibility for federal funds also requires states to provide Medicaid coverage for selected "categorically needy" groups, which include (1) low-income families with children who meet certain eligibility requirements of their state's AFDC (Aid for Dependent Children) in effect on July 16, 1996*; (2) children under 6 years of age and pregnant women whose family income is at or below 133% of the FPL; (3) Supplemental Security Income recipients (in most states); (4) infants born to Medicaid-eligible women; (5) children under 6 years of age and pregnant women whose family income is below 133% of the FPL; (6) recipients of adoption assistance and foster care under Title IV-E of the Social Security Act; (7) selected Medicare recipients; and (8) special protected groups (i.e., typically individuals who lose their cash assistance because of increased work earnings or increased Social Security) for a limited period of time (U.S. DHHS, CMS, 2002, May 23).

States have the option of providing Medicaid coverage to "categorically related" groups including but not limited to (1) infants up to age 1 year and pregnant women whose family income is no more than 185% of the FPL, (2) institutionalized individuals with income and resources below specified limits, (3) children who are receiving care under home- and community-based waivers, (4) targeted low-income children covered under SCHIP (see section on SCHIP later in this chapter), (5) recipients of state supplementary payments, and (6) medically needy persons (U.S. DHHS, CMS, 2002, May 23).

The optional medically needy program gives states the option to extend Medicaid eligibility to persons who would be eligible for Medicaid under other criteria except that their income and/or resources are too high. "Medically needy" eligibility requirements are not as extensive as those for "categorically needy" eligibility. Individuals may qualify immediately or may "spend down" by incurring medical expenses that reduce their income to state-designated levels. If states choose to have a medically needy program, they must include services for medically needy children under age 18 years and pregnant women (U.S. DHHS, CMS, 2002, May 23).

Legal resident aliens who entered the United States after August 22, 1996, are generally restricted from receiving Medicaid for 5 years; refugees, persons seeking asylum, Cuban and Haitian entrants, and several other finite groups are exempt (U.S. DHHS, CMS, 2002, October 22). The eligibility of other groups of legal resident aliens is an option left up to individual states.

It is very important that families of children with chronic conditions and their primary care providers are informed of the

---

*Before 1996, another group automatically eligible for Medicaid were those who met their state's requirements for Aid for Families with Dependent Children (AFDC), but the Temporary Assistance for Needy Families (TANF) program has replaced AFDC in all states. Although most persons covered by TANF will receive Medicaid, it is not required by federal law.

Medicaid service rights and entitlement programs of the state where the child resides. All states that receive funds from the Developmentally Disabled Assistance and Bill of Rights Act of 1978, the Protection and Advocacy for Mentally Ill Individuals Act of 1986, the Protection and Advocacy of Individual Rights Act of 1992, and the Technology-Related Assistance for Individuals with Disabilities Act of 1988 are required to have a protection and advocacy organization to inform persons with disabilities of their rights to payment for health care through Medicaid. Contact may be made through information from the local Medicaid office. In most states, eligibility for Medicaid for individuals and families is determined by the Department of Social Services in each county. Social workers in hospitals, public health, child welfare, and other human services agencies can help families with children with chronic conditions to determine if they are eligible for Medicaid coverage.

Basic Service Provision. A full range of preventive-related and illness-related services are covered by Medicaid. These include inpatient, outpatient, rural health clinic, and federally qualified health center services; prenatal care; vaccines for children; physician, nurse practitioner, and midwife services; family planning services and supplies; laboratory and radiographic services; skilled nursing services or home health care; and the Early Periodic Screening Diagnosis and Treatment Program (EPSDT) for those eligible (U.S. DHHS, CMS, 2002, September 3).

EPSDT. EPSDT is of particular importance to children with chronic conditions. This preventive health program was added to Medicaid in 1972 and amended in the 1989 Omnibus Budget Reconciliation Act, PL 101-329 (1989). The 1989 revisions require states to establish standards for medical, vision, hearing, and dental screenings. Section 1905(r)(5) of the Social Security Act further require states to offer additional screening and services, including a comprehensive health and developmental history, a comprehensive physical examination, appropriate immunizations, needed laboratory tests including lead toxicity screens, and health education. Additional services needed to treat a suspected illness or condition found in the EPSDT screen are to be furnished at other than the mandated scheduled intervals. States must offer these services whether or not such services are covered by the state plan (U.S. DHHS, CMS, 2002, June 4).

Related Child Services. Federal law (PL 101-329, 1989) further stipulates that children enrolled in Medicaid are entitled to *case management*, rehabilitative services, psychologic counseling, and recuperative and long-term residential care as deemed necessary by a primary care provider. States must now include in their Medicaid benefit package all ambulatory health care services offered to Medicaid beneficiaries receiving care in the community and migrant health centers that are funded by the federal Public Health Services Act. The law also encourages the use of pediatric and family nurse practitioner services in rural health clinics by mandating states to cover their services as long as they are practicing within the scope of state law—regardless of whether they are supervised by or associated with a physician. Other provisions of Public Law 101-329 (1989) encourage the referral of mothers eligible for Medicaid and infants at nutritional risk to the Special Supplemental Food Program for Women, Infants, and Children (WIC), which

is funded by the Department of Agriculture (U.S. DHHS, CMS, 2002, June 4).

Medically Needy Services Option. States may choose to include the medically needy population in their plans. If they choose to do so, services that must be included are prenatal care and delivery care; home health services to individuals entitled to nursing facility services, and ambulatory services to children with medical needs. States also may choose to cover any of 34 other approved services; some of the more common are clinic services, rehabilitation and physical therapy services, optometrist services and eyeglasses, prescribed medications and prosthetic devices, dental care, and facility services for the mentally retarded (U.S. DHHS, CMS, 2002, September 3).

Providers who are familiar with Medicaid law can advocate for families who may be denied services to which they are entitled. The provider should also know the local protection and advocacy staff and parent advocacy groups who stay abreast of issues regarding the various laws affecting both private and public health insurance plans and are able to protect the civil, legal, and service rights of children with chronic conditions. Social workers can help primary care providers to remain informed of Medicaid's ever-changing services and eligibility requirements. Receiving Medicaid coverage for health care does not preclude receiving assistance from other federal programs for services and equipment not covered by Medicaid.

Traditional Medicaid. Medicaid was originally fashioned along the same lines as private fee-for-service insurance and designed as a program of inclusion. That is, eligible families were able to seek care from any provider, and then Medicaid reimbursed willing providers at set rates for services. There were nominal participation requirements, and each state oversaw the statutes and regulations of provider participation (Stein, 1997).

During its first 25 years, Medicaid liberalized its eligibility criteria several times. The total number of children served increased as did the percent of medically needy children. For example, in order to meet the needs of children who depend on ventilators, parenteral nutrition, or other technologies and who could not be discharged from the hospital without skilled nursing and other health services, the Medicaid Model Home and Community-Based Waiver (1915[c]) was created. These services were initially authorized in 1981 in the Omnibus Budget Reconciliation Act, Section 2176 (PL 97-35). Today, all states with the exception of Arizona* participate (U.S. DHHS, CMS, 2002, July 16). The purposes of the program are to reduce the cost of care to Medicaid that results from lengthy hospitalizations and to avoid the unnecessary institutionalization of children by providing case management, homemaker services, home modifications, and other therapies.

Qualification for coverage and services for home care varies among states. States may remove parental income and assets as an eligibility consideration or may raise the Medicaid income standard. The eligible conditions may differ, and some states require that the child be discharged from an institution immediately before applying for the waiver. Primary care providers who wish to determine if this program is appropriate

---

*Arizona runs a similar program under its 1115 waiver.

for a Medicaid-eligible or medically needy client and available in their state should request information from the state agency responsible for implementing the Medicaid program. The local Office of Protection and Advocacy will explain a family's rights to have a child cared for under home care Medicaid waiver programs (see next section) and will help the family plead their case when a waiver is denied by the local Medicaid agency.

A major problem faced by traditional Medicaid programs is that provider reimbursement rates are often significantly lower than the prevailing rates in the community. In order to compensate for this, states without Medicaid managed care programs may choose to reimburse obstetricians and pediatricians at rates that are higher than prevailing Medicaid rates. Such reimbursement would ideally enlist enough providers to serve eligible families and encourage them to accept these families into their practices and reduce visits to hospital emergency and/or outpatient departments for needed health care services.

This provision met with limited success, however; states using a fee-for-service Medicaid structure also needed to address spiraling costs. In order to improve access and outcomes while reducing expenditures, states are adopting a managed care structure for administering Medicaid programs.

Medicaid Managed Care. The majority of states are adopting a variety of managed care strategies in their Medicaid programs to conserve funds. These programs have been designed and implemented under several Medicaid waivers authorized by the US Department of Health and Human Services.

1115: Comprehensive Health Care Reform Waiver Research and Demonstration Projects. The majority of Medicaid managed care programs fall under section 1115 waivers (U.S. DHHS, CMS, 2002, July 24). This waiver program was designed by CMS's precursor, the Health Care Financing Administration (HCFA), to allow states to develop innovative solutions to health and welfare problems and expand coverage to additional populations provided that they do not increase the proportion of federal spending. Twenty states have active waiver programs, and others are pending (U.S. DHHS, CMS, 2002, July 24).

1915(b): Freedom of Choice Waivers and 1915(c): Home and Community Based Waivers. 1915(b): Freedom of Choice Waivers allow states to mandate Medicaid beneficiaries to enroll in a Medicaid managed care program. States may use the savings realized to expand services to other Medicaid populations. These waivers are limited to current Medicaid beneficiaries and cannot be used to expand coverage to other populations (U.S. DHHS, CMS, 2002a, May 29). Still other states include 1915(c): Home and Community Based Waivers in their Medicaid packages to provide home- and community-based alternatives to institutional care for children with complex medical needs. Populations of individuals with severe physical disabilities, developmental disabilities, mental retardation, and mental illness may be covered. They offer a wide range of individual supports, including up to 24-hour live-in care and respite care (U.S. DHHS, CMS, 2002, July 16). States may simultaneously utilize the authorities of the 1915(b) and 1915(c) waiver programs in order to provide long-term services in a managed care environment for special populations (U.S. DHHS, CMS, 2002b, May 29).

In 2001, more than 56% of covered lives were enrolled in Medicaid managed care programs. The Medicaid managed care penetration exceeds 90% in six states (Arizona, Colorado, Tennessee, South Dakota, Utah, Washington) whereas two states and one territory (Alabama, Virgin Islands, Wyoming) have none (U.S. DHHS, CMS, 2002c, May 29). These managed care plans are similar to the plans described earlier for private insurance. State Medicaid agencies sign service agreements with MCOs to provide Medicaid services. Like private insurance, states use a variety of managed care products including contracting with commercial HMOs and PPOs, establishing Medicaid-only MCOs, operating prepaid health plans, and providing primary case management MCOs (U.S. DHHS, CMS, 2002c, May 29). These programs must operate against the backdrop of Medicaid and other relevant state and federal laws. The individual or family receiving Medicaid has access to selected MCOs and providers who have agreed to furnish a defined set of health care services using prospective capitated payment, which is paid by the state Medicaid agency.

CMS released the final regulations implementing protections for individuals covered by Medicaid managed care (U.S. DHHS, CMS, 2002, October 1). These final rules provide guidance to states, MCOs, and beneficiaries. They should serve as minimal standards for managed care Medicaid. However, these rules allow states considerable discretion in interpretation of Medicaid provisions (Alker et al, 2002). Because they do not go into effect until August 2003, their impact on services for children with chronic conditions is not known.

If the state plan is well constructed, joining a managed care plan could benefit children with chronic conditions because a more comprehensive range of preventive health services and other therapies may be available and better coordinated than under the traditional Medicaid fee-for-service plan (Fox et al, 1997).

There is evidence, however, that the access to and quality of services for children with special health care needs (CSHCN), a subset of all children with chronic conditions (see Chapter 1), are not fully met by Medicaid managed care products. For example, these managed care organizations may not capture all deserving populations and have difficulty tracking children receiving Title V–funded care coordination services (Kaye et al, 2000). Program or service carve-outs for CSHCN are rare among 1115 waiver programs (Mele & Flowers, 2000). Title V program staff do not necessarily have an active role in helping states develop their waiver programs (Mele & Flowers, 2000) (see Chapter 7; Title V section in this chapter). State policies regarding enrollment and disenrollment may also not be specific to the CSHCN population. Under some state plans, access to specialty providers and services may be restricted because of contract language; special provisions for the CSHCN population are not explicitly considered (Mitchell et al, 2001; Stein, 1997).

Contract constraints also may limit access and services for all children with chronic conditions, whether or not they meet the CSHCN definition. Plans may be underfunded by states; the proportion of physicians who care for Medicaid beneficiaries, now at 85.4%, has decreased annually since 1997 (Cunningham, 2002). When MCOs are underfunded, the capitation rate may be too low to refer a child to pediatric specialty providers outside the plan, and pediatric specialty providers and services may not be available within the plan. Benefit packages offered by HMOs contracted with Medicaid are generally less comprehensive than those under Medicaid fee-for-service plans because many optional services are eliminated (Fox et al, 1997; Kaye et al, 2000). EPSDT may prove to be the major funding source for children with chronic conditions, and especially CSHCN, because of its generous benefits package (Mele & Flowers, 2000). As with private MCOs, Medicaid-contracted MCOs have little incentive to establish a link with community agencies unless mandated in state contracts. Another problematic area is the relationship between Medicaid-contracted MCOs and the responsibility for, and payment of health services provided to, children with special needs by school districts under PL 101-476: IDEA (see Chapter 5). Many MCOs also have little experience providing selected Medicaid-required services (e.g., transportation).

The Medicaid managed care programs of many states are still in development, so their ability to provide care for children with chronic conditions must be monitored in terms of quality, eligibility, cost efficacy, access to care, provider qualifications, and reimbursement levels.

State Children's Health Insurance Programs (SCHIP, CHIP)

SCHIP (PL 105-100: Title XXI of the Social Security Act) enables states to expand insurance coverage to uninsured, low-income children through a program of matching funds. This program was included in the Balanced Budget Act of 1997 in response to the growing percentage of children without health insurance (PL 105-33, 1997). The increased number of uninsured children in part is the result of legislative reform of AFDC, Medicaid, and Supplemental Security Income (SSI) (Perrin, 1997). The goal of SCHIP is for states to provide health care coverage for all uninsured children in families with incomes below 200% of the FPL or 50% above their Medicaid eligibility level—whichever is higher. All states have expanded their children's health insurance programs using Title XXI funds with over two thirds expanding coverage to or beyond 200% of the FPL (Committee on Child Health Financing, 2001).

SCHIP programs vary widely in structure and coverage because the federal government has given states considerable latitude to design their programs in accordance with their political and fiscal climates. All programs, however, provide assistance through the following broad mechanisms: (1) establishing or expanding a separate child health insurance program, (2) expanding the state's Medicaid program, or (3) a combination of the two (PL 105-100, 1997). Medicaid expansion programs must meet federal Medicaid program guidelines and benefits packages (see discussion earlier in this chapter). The federal government has established benchmarks for non–Medicaid-based programs that mirror those of health plans offered to state and/or federal employees (Committee on Child Health Financing, 1998; U.S. DHHS, PL 105-100, 1997). Sixteen states have established new programs, 17 states and the territories have expanded Medicaid, and 17 states have combined new

programmatic efforts with Medicaid (Committee on Child Health Financing, 2001) (Figure 8-2).

It is estimated that 18% of eligible children have a special health care need, so Title XXI legislation has wide-ranging implications for children with chronic conditions (Newacheck et al, 2000). The Maternal Child Health Policy Research Center (Fox et al, 1998) and the Association of Maternal and Child Health Programs (AMCHP) (2000) have analyzed both the legislation and the state plans to assess how SCHIP will service CSHCN in terms of eligibility, benefits, plan design, and cost sharing. The majority of states have retained the same eligibility thresholds for special needs children as for other eligible children, although states may adopt more liberal eligibility requirements for special needs children than for other enrollees (e.g., states may use the Social Security Administration's [1997] definition of "special needs" or choose a more inclusive definition). States also may choose to provide additional benefits to CSHCN by selectively expanding the FPL (i.e., up to the designated maximum), using more liberal methodologies in determining the family's income, and/or shortening the designated period of uninsurance (Fox et al, 1998). Some states have implemented outreach initiatives targeted toward CSHCN (AMCHP, 2000).

CSHCN often require services beyond what are offered by general SCHIP plans. The benchmarks of the benefits set by federal legislation provide limited coverage for the many specialized services required by children with chronic conditions, which is reflected in the majority of non-Medicaid SCHIP programs. Limits are often imposed on services such as ancillary therapies, durable medical equipment, disposable supplies, home health care, and case management, although most programs provide coverage for basic primary care (Fox et al, 1998). Mental health coverage is also highly variable, being expanded by some states and completely excluded by others.

Benefit packages for CSHCN under SCHIP are highly variable; for states with separate SCHIP plans and major CSHCN initiatives, benefits range from less to more generous than what is found in their Medicaid package. States offering generous packages often included services such as nutrition support, transportation, respite care, or behavioral health care (AMCHP, 2001; English, 1998). For states offering restricted benefits, services for therapies (e.g., physical therapy [PT], occupational therapy [OT]), durable medical equipment, and mental health were most likely to be curtailed. Care coordination efforts are also highly variable across state plans. Unfortunately, states with plans to expand only Medicaid generally do not offer special service provisions for CSHCN.

Plan arrangements for providing services vary widely. Medicaid expansion plans mirror the fee-for-service or managed care arrangements of their state's Medicaid program. States with non-Medicaid plans have broad discretion in structuring the insurance plan using fee-for-service or capitation arrangements—with or without carve-outs for selected services. Establishing comprehensive health plans that specifically address these children's needs is another avenue that has been adopted. States may also establish separate requirements in the plan's structure to better address the needs of children with chronic conditions. For example, states enrolling children into MCOs may require participating MCOs to provide mechanisms to

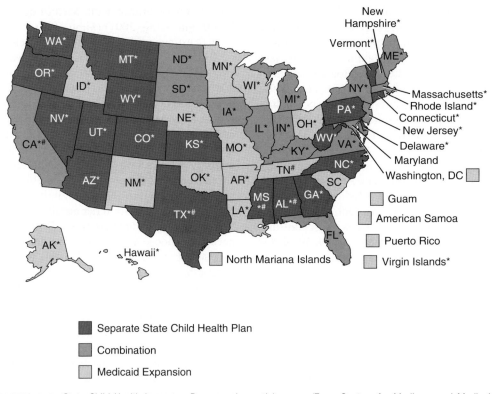

Separate State Child Health Plan

Combination

Medicaid Expansion

FIGURE 8-2 State Child Health Insurance Program plan activity map. (From Centers for Medicare and Medicaid Services: Web site: http://www.cms.gov/schip/chip-map.asp.)
* State Plan Amendment
# State no longer has a Medicaid expansion program as of September 30, 2002, due to the aging out of the children phased into Medicaid program under OBRA '90.

ensure that these children receive the necessary care required (e.g., providing access to pediatric specialty providers, allowing a specialist to be designated as the primary care provider, or guaranteeing out-of-plan access to specialty care). Despite these options, some state plans are silent on the issue of medical necessity. Measures of quality also vary dramatically among plans (Fox et al, 1998).

State plans include a wide variety of cost-sharing requirements, such as premiums, deductibles, co-payments, and/or co-insurance, although the level of cost sharing is restricted in accordance with the family's income level. Because of the child's increased care needs, however, the level of cost sharing required by families of children with chronic conditions is likely to be higher than the cost sharing required by other families. In order to better meet the needs of children with chronic conditions, some states have made adjustments for this in their cost-sharing requirements for populations with special needs. Tracking SCHIP's 5% out-of-pocket limit may also be problematic for families because they are generally required to keep track of these expenditures and seek reimbursement. Despite these limitations, most states have designed plans with modest cost-sharing requirements for CSHCN (Committee on Child Health Financing, 1998; Fox et al, 1998). Although most states have not structured their SCHIPs with special attention to the needs of children with chronic conditions, some have pursued innovative strategies in this area (Fox et al, 1998).

SCHIP is still relatively new, and final legislative rules have not yet been promulgated. Changes in the enrollment eligibility, benefits, and structure of state plans are likely. Because SCHIP is still evolving and each state's program is unique, practitioners are advised to consult specific sources for their state (Felland & Benoit, 2001; Rosenbach et al, 2001).

Supplemental Security Income

The SSI program, which is Title XVI of the Social Security Act, was established by Congress in 1972 for aged, blind, and disabled adults and in 1976 for children under 16 years of age with disabilities. This program is based on the assumption that those with substantial disabilities and little income have increased costs of health care and daily living. Income support is provided to help recipients become as self-sufficient as possible within the limits of their disability. SSI does not pay directly for the health care costs of a child with a chronic condition, but its recipients are generally eligible to receive health care services through Medicaid (i.e., regardless of other state Medicaid eligibility requirements) and food stamps. It can be of great financial help to families to have their children with chronic conditions become eligible for SSI and thus receive Medicaid coverage for costly health care.

Eligible children are those who are US citizens or nationals, have significant disabilities, and live in low-income households. Until 1990, children with disabilities were less likely than adults with disabilities to be eligible for SSI because children's impairments had to meet or equal those on a specified list of conditions designed for adults. This definition of disability for children seeking SSI was contested in the courts. On February 20, 1990, the Supreme Court upheld a lower court ruling that the policy for determining SSI eligibility for children was unfair and inconsistent with the statutory standards of comparable severity, and the regulations were changed. The definition of disability for children was again revisited in the 1996 Personal Responsibility and Work Opportunity Reconciliation Act (PL 104-193). The current definition is as follows: (1) a child must have a physical or mental condition that can be medically proven and results in marked and severe functional limitations; (2) the medically proven physical or mental condition(s) must last or be expected to last at least 12 months or expected to result in death; and (3) a child may not be considered disabled if he or she is working at a job that is considered substantial work (Social Security Administration [SSA], 1997). If a child has one of 15 specific impairments he or she may be found to be "presumptively eligible," allowing payments to begin quickly (Committee on Children with Disabilities, 2001). Examples of these impairments are Down syndrome, total deafness or blindness, terminal cancer with hospice care, leg amputations, AIDS, and birth weight of less than 1200 g and under 6 months of age. Continuing eligibility reviews are done no later than 12 months for low birth weight infants and at least every 3 years for children. At age 18 years, full reevaluation is required.

The SSI program continues to expand dramatically—from 297,000 enrollees in 1989 to 6.4 million enrollees in 2002; with just over 1 million (about 17%) disabled youth under age 18 years (SSA, 2002b). Despite the initial expansion of the program in 1990, selected children have lost their eligibility because of the new definition of disability adopted in 1996. Today, the program limits its support to those children with severe developmental and behavioral problems (Doolittle, 1998). Children with chronic conditions that do not meet the current SSI eligibility requirements may, however, still be eligible for Medicaid or SCHIP depending on their state's eligibility requirements. The eligibility requirements for SSI continue to be debated (Perrin, 1999).

The financial requirements for SSI eligibility are complex (SSA, no date). The first step is to document that the applicant must be beneath the maximum income level. The amount of SSI paid to an individual and the administration of the program vary by state because states have the option of supplementing the payments. SSI rules allow families up to 200% of the FPL to enroll (SSA, no date). Many states administer their own supplementary payments, and the recipients receive this payment separately from that of the federal program. Other states elect to have the federal SSA issue the federal payment and the state supplement in one check; seven states offer no supplementation. Applications for SSI payments are made at district offices of the SSA, where supporting documentation on age, income, and assets is examined (SSA, 2002a).

The second step in determining financial eligibility is to know the cash value of the applicant's resources, which for children involves determining the portions of the parents' income that are available to the child. The regulations must be carefully studied to understand how the amount of available income is calculated. Countable income, which is the amount of parental income determined to be available to the child or any income earned by the child, reduces this amount, and state supplements increase it.

Medicare's End-Stage Renal Disease Program

Medicare is authorized under Title XVIII of the Social Security Act. Children are generally not entitled to any health care benefits under Medicare because it provides health insurance protection for persons over 65 years of age and persons under 65 years of age who are collecting Social Security or Railroad Retirement Benefits. Children with end-stage renal disease, however, may be eligible to receive health care benefits to cover the costs of peritoneal dialysis or hemodialysis and related services in the hospital or home. This program is subject to change as the Center for Medicare and Medicaid Services attempts to streamline services between the agencies and as Medicare continues to adopt a managed care structure.

TRICARE: The Department of Defense Insurance Program

Traditionally, the Department of Defense provided health insurance to active duty personnel and their dependents, retirees, and other eligible individuals through the Civilian Health and Medical Program of the Uniformed Services (CHAMPUS). Military health care, however, has undergone significant reforms as the federal government responds to rising health care costs and the closing of military bases and hospitals. TRICARE is the current health plan offered by the Department of Defense. It provides coverage for essentially the same population as CHAMPUS but is called TRICARE because it offers three managed care plans (U.S. Department of Defense, 2002).

The first option is TRICARE Prime, which is similar to an HMO. The majority of care comes from a military treatment facility and is augmented by the TRICARE contractor's preferred provider network. Provider choice is limited. Although there is no enrollment fee for active duty personnel and their families, other eligible persons pay an annual fee. A primary care manager supervises and coordinates care, and serves as the gatekeeper for specialty referrals. Appointments are guaranteed. There also is a point-of-service option and a reduced catastrophic cap for retirees. A small fee per visit to civilian providers is assessed if the claimant is not from an active duty family. One major disadvantage is that it is not universally available (U.S. Department of Defense, 2002).

The second option is TRICARE Extra. In this preferred provider arrangement, participating individuals do not enroll but choose an authorized civilian network provider who agrees to accept a fee set by CHAMPUS. This option covers a discounted share of costs over TRICARE Standard (see next paragraph) if the client uses services within the network. This plan does not provide a primary care manager; provider choice is limited; and cost sharing through deductibles and co-payment is required. To date, it is not universally available (U.S. Department of Defense, 2002).

The third option is TRICARE Standard, which is a fee-for-service option that is the same as the traditional CHAMPUS plan. This plan is widely available and allows an unrestricted choice of providers. There is no enrollment fee or primary care manager. Significant cost sharing through deductibles, co-payments, and balances for nonparticipating provider charges that exceed the insurance cap is imposed. The scope and structure of these three options vary as widely as their costs. Moreover, eligible individuals may seek additional coverage through TRICARE/CHAMPUS supplemental insurance policies (U.S. Department of Defense, 2002).

The effect of these plans on access to care for military dependents with chronic conditions is not yet known. Military organizations provide families of children with chronic conditions with information, financial assistance, and health care within the military community or through local community, state, and federal agencies. Health benefits advisors located on military bases facilitate access to both military and public programs in coordination with the multidisciplinary medical and social service support from the Army's Exceptional Family Member Program, the Air Force's Children's Programs, and the Navy's Family Support Program. Eligible families with children with chronic conditions must choose the plan that best fits their needs after considering the issues of access to care, quality of care, overall out-of-pocket costs, other nonmilitary insurance coverage, and the need for other services, such as home care, durable medical equipment, drugs and supplies, or physical, occupational, or speech therapy.

Indian Health Service

The Indian Health Service (IHS) is an organization within the Public Health Service of the US Department of Health and Human Services that provides an array of services to more than 557 tribes in 35 states. In conjunction with maximal tribal involvement, one effort is to ensure that a comprehensive health care delivery system is available to American Indians and natives of Alaska. Services include primary and tertiary care, rehabilitation services, health education, school-based services, mental health services, and other community and environmental health programs (U.S. DHHS, Indian Health Service [IHS], 1999). The IHS integrates health services delivered directly through IHS facilities with purchased contract health services (CHSs) from the private sector. CHSs help pay for care when other sources (e.g., private insurance, SCHIP) are not available. Referrals for CHS funds are based on medical priorities and are not available in all instances.

The extent to which children with chronic conditions are well served in this system depends on the staff at the local IHS unit's skill in determining the family's eligibility for third-party payment for health services, making appropriate referrals, and providing culturally sensitive counseling and education. The IHS interacts with other federal and state agencies and public and private institutions to develop ways to deliver health services, stimulate consumer participation, and apply resources. These resources include tribal-operated hospitals and health centers and rural and urban health programs that receive both state and federal funding and are subject to regulations of Medicaid, SCHIP, and private health plans. Information on eligibility and the location and health care programs of the local IHS unit may be obtained from the IHS headquarters in Washington, DC, the west headquarters in Albuquerque, through one of 11 area service offices, or at http://www.ihs.gov.

Maternal and Child Health Services Block Grant: Title V

The Maternal and Child Health Services Block Grant is a federal-state program established under Title V of the Social Security Act of 1935. The purpose of this block grant is to improve the health of mothers and children and is the only federal program solely devoted to this population (AMCHP, 2001). It is administered by the Maternal Child Health Bureau (MCHB), which is a division of the Health Resources Services Administration (HRSA) of the US Department of Health and Human Services. The MCHB's strategic plan for 1998 to 2003 focuses on three overarching goals: (1) to eliminate health disparities in health status outcomes by removing socioeconomic and cultural barriers, (2) to ensure high-quality care through the utilization of evidenced-based research and quality monitoring tools, and (3) to facilitate access to care by improving the MCH health systems infrastructure (U.S. DHHS, HRSA, no date). The Title V MCH Health Services Block Grant, with its 3 billion dollar budget, is the largest of MCHB's seven programs designed to accomplish these goals. In order to meet its diverse mandate, Title V is organized into five divisions, two of which are of particular interest to primary care providers for children with special needs: the Division of Services for Child, Adolescent, and Family Health and the Division of Services for Children with Special Needs.

Title V legislation grew out of increased recognition at the turn of the century that the federal government should bear some responsibility for the well-being of mothers and children and that federal assistance to state health departments would enable the states to provide needed services on the local level. MCHB's predecessor, the Children's Bureau, was established in 1912; and the Maternal and Infancy (Sheppard-Towner) Act of 1920-1929 then set the precedents for federal assistance to states for services for pregnant women and for infants and children with disabilities or conditions that might lead to a disability. Although the Sheppard-Towner Act only survived briefly, states had the opportunity to establish a public health unit for mothers and children, improve birth registration, and increase public health nursing services. These positive experiences with federal support of state public health programs helped to lessen resistance to federal intervention in health care on the part of private practitioners of medicine and enabled passage of Title V (Kruger, 2001). Over time, expansion in the number and variety of categorical services was realized (Stein, 1997).

In 1981, with passage of the Omnibus Reconciliation Act (PL 97-35), specific Title V programs were consolidated and continued as the MCH Services Block Grant. Control was returned to the states, and the federal government's role in organizing health services for mothers and children was diminished (Stein, 1997). The MCH Block Grant, as amended in 1989 (PL 101-329), continues the original purpose of the 1981 act, but efforts at consolidation and state control eroded as Congress began mandating categorical services as a requirement of funding. Provisions to strengthen connections between health services for mothers and children on Medicaid and its EPSDT program were included in these mandates. The 1989 MCH Block Grant legislation also specified connections between the infants' and children's immunization programs of the US Public Health Service, Centers for Disease Control and Prevention

(CDC), and the supplemental feeding program for low-income women, infants, and children (WIC) in the Department of Agriculture. Today, Title V seeks to broaden its scope of services to mothers and children by embracing a "family health" perspective, recognizing that improving the lives of children and mothers is difficult to accomplish in isolation from the larger family unit (Whitehand & Kagan, 2001).

Current goals of the program are as follows:

1. To significantly reduce infant mortality and handicapping conditions
2. To provide and ensure access to comprehensive care for women
3. To promote the health of children by providing primary care and preventive services
4. To increase the number of children who receive health assessments and diagnostic and treatment services
5. To provide family-centered, community-based, coordinated services for children with special health care needs (CSHCN) (HRSA, no date)

Each state's share of the total allocation is based in part on the number of births and the percentage of the nation's low-income children residing in each state and prior grant experience. The states are required to match each $4 of federal funds with $3 in cash or in-kind services. In addition, Title V sets aside 15% of block grant funds to be used for special projects of regional and national significance (SPRANS grants) and more recently funded (fiscal year 2000) community-integrated service systems (CISS) projects (AMCHP, 2001).

CISS projects may help with coordinating eligibility criteria among health and social programs, coordinating the financing of services, improving shared data and information systems, and coordinating services with the medical home (see Chapter 7). Selected SPRANS programs directly impact financing of care for children with chronic conditions, including the following:

- Genetic services
- Hemophilia diagnostic and treatment centers
- Maternal and child health improvement projects

States have some authority to prioritize how they will meet the goals of the program but are required to allocate at least 30% of Title V funds for pediatric primary care services and 30% for children with special health care needs (CSHCN). No more than 10% of the state allocation may be spent on administrative costs (HRSA, no date).

Today, services for CSHCN are primarily coordinated by the Division of Services for Children with Special Health Needs. Their mission is to improve the infrastructure for service delivery, including projects supporting the medical home (see Chapter 7), rather than providing direct care services. This is a significant change from earlier Title V activities. The advent of SCHIP and other developments within the health care system have led Title V programs for CSHCN to move beyond direct service provision to embrace expanded roles focusing on models of service delivery and identifying outcome indicators (Brown, 2000; Kruger, 2001).

HIV/AIDS Bureau

This bureau, which is administered by HRSA, was formed in 1997 by consolidating programs funded under the Ryan White Comprehensive AIDS Resources Emergency Act (CARE). It was amended and reauthorized in 2000. The CARE Act primarily funds local and state primary care and support services to uninsured individuals with HIV/AIDS (human immunodeficiency virus/acquired immunodeficiency syndrome). In addition to the development and operations of community-based primary health care and social service systems, funds are provided to communities for health care provider training, technical assistance to programs, and demonstration projects (U.S. DHHS, HRSA, no date).

Individuals with Disabilities Education Act

The Education for All Handicapped Children Act (PL 94-142, 1975) resulted from legal decisions establishing that children with disabilities had a constitutional right to a publicly funded education in the least restrictive environment. This law and its amendments covered children aged 3 to 21 years. The Education for the Handicapped Amendments of 1986, Public Law 99-457, Part H, extended the benefits of Public Law 94-142 to handicapped children from birth to 2 years of age. This act designated funds for the development of a statewide comprehensive, coordinated, multidisciplinary interagency system to provide early intervention services. The Individuals with Disabilities Education Act (IDEA: PL 101-476, 1990) and its 1997 reauthorization and amendments (PL 105-17, 1997) further expanded the educational mandate for children with chronic conditions. An expanded description of this legislation and its ramifications for health care may be found in Chapter 5. Under IDEA, health services deemed necessary to the educational program must be provided. These services may include speech and hearing therapy, psychologic services, physical and occupational therapy, recreation, counseling, social work, and nursing and medical services. School districts may bill Medicaid or SCHIP for these services if allowable by law.

Future Trends in Financing Health Care for Children with Chronic Conditions

Research indicates families have four basic recommendations for improving services for their children with chronic conditions: (1) improving the quality of services; (2) decreasing barriers to services and programs; (3) improving the training that health care professionals, families, and members of the community receive about chronic conditions and their management; and (4) bettering the quality and availability of community-based services (Garwick et al, 1998). All these recommendations are predicated on two factors: adequate financing and universality of care.

Unfortunately, accessing and financing children's health care—including care of children with chronic conditions—continue to be fragmented. The presence or absence of health insurance is a powerful indicator of children's degree of access to care. Analyses suggest that the disparity in access between uninsured and insured children has worsened over the last decade (Newacheck et al, 1998), despite reform efforts of the way health care is organized, administered, financed, and delivered. Private and public programs and agencies for financing care for children with chronic conditions are examining ways to provide adequate health care while reducing the costs of care.

The immediate future of health care for children with chronic conditions is marked, in part, by health care spending. Although flat during the late 1990s, spending began to rise sharply in 2001 and is projected to do so in the foreseeable future. In response, new federal, state, and private initiatives are being implemented to help provide efficacious care more efficiently and curtail unnecessary expenditures. Because children with special health care needs utilize such a disproportionate amount of health care and health care dollars, these initiatives will directly affect this population.

All health insurance programs—public and private—are becoming increasingly complex as efforts are made to balance the quality and cost of care with access to services. New variations (e.g., capitating specialists, expanding carve-outs, designating specialists as primary care providers) are being tested. Comprehensive coverage by private health insurance companies has been a long-standing problem. The dilemma faced by health care providers and children's advocates is how to support the highest quality of pediatric care in a managed care environment. In order to accomplish this objective, emphasis is placed on the development of *integrated service networks*. These organizations offer tremendous potential for meeting the special health care needs of children. Employers, insurance companies, and the government need to work toward more universal standards of eligibility and access, enhanced program consolidation and coordination, and improved continuity of care (Perrin, 1999).

Depending on the success of the medical home initiative (see Chapter 7), primary care providers may find that they are increasingly limited in their abilities to advocate for quality care for children in their caseloads who have chronic conditions. Families can advocate more effectively for their children by joining together, becoming informed of their rights under the law, and using the legal system for access to care. Adding to the complexity of seeking health care for children with chronic conditions are the inequalities in implementing private and public health care programs among counties both within a state and among states. Access to private insurance is favorable for those who are steadily employed in large businesses or members of strong labor unions that can negotiate comprehensive benefit packages.

Primary care providers must be informed about how families of children with chronic conditions in their caseloads are paying for care and about access to specialty services under the various payment plans so that families realize the benefits for which they are eligible. Referral for help in purchasing appropriate insurance or accessing a federal-state public benefit requires dedication and persistence on the part of the family and primary care provider and is crucial to implementing the care plan.

RESOURCES

Federal Web sites

HIPAA	http://cms.hhs.gov/hipaa/
HIV/AIDS Bureau	www.hab.hrsa.gov
Indian Health Service	www.ihs.gov
Maternal Child Health Bureau	www.mchb.hrsa.gov
Medicaid	http://cms.hhs.gov/medicaid/
SCHIP	http://cms.hhs.gov/schip/
Tricare (military insurance)	www.tricare.osd.mil

Advocacy, Policy, and Professional Organizations

American Association of Health Plans
1129 20th St, NW, Suite 600
Washington, DC 20036
(202) 778-3200
www.aahp.org

Center for Studying Health Systems Change
600 Maryland Ave, SW, Suite 550
Washington, DC 20024-2512
(202) 484-5261
www.hschange.org

Families USA
1334 G St, NW, 3rd floor
Washington, DC 20005
(202) 628-3030
www.familiesusa.org

Health Insurance Association of America
1201 F St, NW, Suite 500
Washington, DC 20004-1204
(202) 824-1600
www.hiaa.org

Health Systems Research, Inc
1200 18th St, NW, Suite 700
Washington, DC 20036
(202) 828-5100
www.hsrnet.com

Kaiser Family Foundation
2400 Sand Hill Rd
Menlo Park, CA 94025
(650) 854-9400
www.kff.org

National Center for Children in Poverty
Mailman School of Public Health
Columbia University
154 Haven Ave
New York, NY 10036
(212) 304-7100
www.nccp.org

REFERENCES

Alker, J., Fish-Parcham, C., & Waxman, J. (2002). *Medicaid managed care. Final regulations issued.* Available: http://www.familiesusa.org/site/DocServer/MMCSept2002.pdf?docID=335.

Association of Maternal and Child Health Programs. (2000). The impact of the State Children's Health Insurance Program (SCHIP) on Title V children with special health care needs programs (updated edition) [Issue Brief].

Association of Maternal and Child Health Programs. (2001). The Maternal and Child Health (MCH) Services Block Grant (Title V of the Social Security Act) [Fact Sheet].

Brown, T. (2000). The impact of the State Children's Health Insurance Program (SCHIP) on Title V children with special health care needs programs (updated edition) [Issue Brief]. Association of Maternal and Child Health Programs; Available: http://www.amchp1.org/news/Impact%20 SCHIP_CSHCN.pdf.

Committee on Child Health Financing. (2001). Implementation principles and strategies for the State Children's Health Insurance Program. *Pediatrics, 107*, 1214-1220.

Committee on Child Health Financing. (1998). Implementation principles and strategies for Title XXI (State Children's Health Insurance Program). *Pediatrics, 101*, 944-948.

Committee on Children with Disabilities. (2001). The continued importance of Supplemental Security Income (SSI) for children and adolescents with disabilities (RE0040). *Pediatrics, 107*, 790-793.

Committee on Children with Disabilities. (1998). Managed care and children with special health care needs: A subject review (RE9814). *Pediatrics, 102,* 657-660.

Cunningham, P.J. (2002). Mounting pressures: Physicians serving Medicaid patients and the uninsured, 1997-2001. *Tracking Report: Results from the Community Tracking Study* (Center for Studying Health System Change), no. 29, 2.

Cunningham, P.J. & Park, M.H. (2000). Recent trends in children's health insurance coverage: No gains for low-income children. *Findings from HSC,* no. 29 [Issue Brief].

Doolittle, D.K. (1998). Welfare reform: Loss of supplemental security income (SSI) for children with disabilities. *JSPN, 3*(1), 33-44.

English, A. (1998). Special populations of children need special attention by CHIP programs. *Youth Law News, 19*(6), 1-8.

Felland, L.E. & Benoit, A.M. (2001). Communities play key role in extending public health insurance to children. *Findings from HSC,* no. 44 [Issue Brief].

Ferris, T.G., Perrin, J.M., Manganello, J.A., Chang, Y., Causino, N., et al. (2001). Switching to gatekeeping: Changes in expenditures and utilization for children. *Pediatrics, 108,* 283-290.

Fox, H.B., Graham, R.R., & McManus, M. (1998). States' CHIP policies and children with special health care needs: The Child Health Insurance Project. Maternal and Child Health Policy Research Center. Available: http://www.mchpolicy.org/ issue4.html.

Fox, H.B., McManus, M.A., Almeida, R.A., & Lesser, C. (1997). Medicaid managed care policies affecting children with disabilities: 1995 and 1996. *Health Care Finance Rev, 18*(4), 23-26.

Fox, H.B., Wicks, L.B., & Newacheck, P.W. (1993). Health maintenance organizations and children with special needs. A suitable match? *Am J Dis Child, 147,* 546-552.

Garwick, A.W., Kohrman, C., Wolman, C., & Blum, R.W. (1998). Families' recommendations for improving services for children with chronic conditions. *Arch Pediatr Adolesc Med, 152,* 440-448.

Health Insurance Association of America. (2002). *Guide to health insurance.* Available: http://www.hiaa.org/consumer/guidehi.cfm.

Ireys, H.T., Grason, H.A., & Guyer, B. (1996). Assuring quality of care for children with special needs in managed care organizations: Roles for pediatricians. *Pediatrics, 98*(2), 178-185.

Ireys, H.T., Humensky, J., Wickstrom, S., Manda, B., & Rheault, P. (2002). *Children with special health care needs in commercial managed care: Patterns and cost.* Available: http://www.mathematica-mpr.com/PDFs/childrenspecial.pdf.

Kaye, N., Curtis, D., & Booth, M. (2000). *Certain children with special health care needs: An assessment of state activities and their relationship to HCFA's interim criteria.* Available: http://www.nashp.org/Files/Certain_Children_w_Special_HC_needs.pdf.

Kongstvedt, P.R. (2001). *Essentials of managed health care* (3rd ed.). Gaithersburg, MD: Aspen.

Kruger, B.J. (2001). Title V-CSHCN: A closer look at the shaping of the national agenda for children with special health care needs. *Policy, Politics, and Nursing Practice, 2,* 321-330.

Lesser, C.S. & Ginsburg, P.B. (2000). Update on the Nation's health care system: 1997-1999. *Health Aff, 19,* 206-216.

Mele, N.C. & Flowers, J.S. (2000). Medicaid managed care and children with special health care needs: A case study analysis of demonstration waivers in three states. *J Pediatr Nurs, 15,* 63-72.

Mitchell, J.B., Khatutsky, G., & Swigonski, N.L. (2001). Impact on the Oregon health plan on children with special health care needs. *Pediatrics, 107,* 736-743.

Newacheck, P.W., McManus, M., Fox, H.B., Hung, Y., & Halfon, N. (2000). Access to health care for children with special health care needs. *Pediatrics, 105,* 760-766.

Newacheck, P.W., et al. (1998). *New estimates of children with special health care needs and implications for the State Children's Health Insurance Program.* Washington, DC: Maternal and Child Health Policy Research Center.

Perrin, J.M. (1997). The implications of welfare reform for developmental and behavioral pediatrics. *J Dev Behav Pediatr, 18*(4), 264-266.

Perrin, J.M. (1999). Universality, inclusion, and continuity: Implications for pediatrics. *Pediatrics, 103*(4), 859-863.

Pollitz, K., Tapay, N., Hadley, E., & Specht, J. (2000). Early experience with 'new federalism' in health insurance regulation. *Health Aff, 19*(4), 7-21.

Public Law 94-142. (1975). Education for all Handicapped Children Act.

Public Law 97-35. (1981). Omnibus Budget Reconciliation Act of 1981, Section 2176.

Public Law 99-457. (1986). Education of the Handicapped Children Act.

Public Law 101-329. (1989). Omnibus Budget Reconciliation Act of 1989, Section 6403.

Public Law 101-476. (1990). Individuals with Disabilities Education Act.

Public Law 104-193. (1996). Personal Responsibility and Work Opportunity Reconciliation Act of 1996.

Public Law 105-17. (1997). Individuals with Disabilities Education Act Amendments of 1997.

Public Law 105-33. (1997). Balanced Budget Act of 1997. Subtitle J—State Children's Health Insurance Program; Establishment of Program (Section 4901).

Public Law 105-100. (1997). State Children's Health Insurance Program, Section 4901, HCFA.

Reed, M.C. & Trude, S. (2002). Who do you trust? Americans' perspectives on health care, 1997-2000. *Center for Health System Change Tracking Report,* no. 3.

Rosenbach, M., Ellwood, M., Czajka, J., Irvin, C., Coupé, W., et al. (2001). *Implementation of the State Children's Health Insurance Program: Momentum is increasing after a modest start. First annual report.* Available: http://www.mathematica-mpr.com/PDFs/schip1.pdf.

Section 504 of the Rehabilitation Act of 1973.

Smucker, J.M. (2001). Managed care and children with special needs. *J Pediatr Health Care, 15,* 3-9.

Social Security Administration. (1997). *The definition of disability for children.* Pub no. 05-11053. Available: http://www. socialsecurity.gov/pubs/11053.html.

Social Security Administration. (2002a). Part 416—Supplemental Security Income for the aged, blind, and disabled; Available: http://www.ssa.gov/OP_Home/cfr20/416/416-0000.htm.

Social Security Administration. *Social Security handbook.* Available: http://www.ssa.gov/OP_Home/handbook/handbook-toc.html.

Social Security Administration. (2002b). *2002 Supplemental Security Income annual report.* Available: http://www.ssa.gov/OACT/SSIR/SSI02/exec_sum.html.

Stein, R.E. (1997). Health care for children: What's right, what's wrong, what's next. New York: United Hospital Fund.

U.S. Bureau of Labor Statistics and Bureau of the Census. (2002). Annual demographic survey. March supplement. Available: http://ferret.bls.census.gov/macro/032002/health/h08_000.htm.

U.S. Department of Defense. (2002). What is Tricare? Available: http://www.tricare.osd.mil.

U.S. Department of Health and Human Services, Centers for Medicare and Medicaid Services. (2002, May 23). *Medicaid eligibility.* Available: http://www.cms.hhs.gov/medicaid/eligibility/criteria.asp.

U.S. Department of Health and Human Services, Centers for Medicare and Medicaid Services. (2002a, May 29). *1915(b) Freedom of choice waivers.* Available: http://www.cms.hhs.gov/medicaid/1915b.default.asp.

U.S. Department of Health and Human Services, Centers for Medicare and Medicaid Services. (2002b, May 29). *Section 1915(b)/(c) waivers programs* [online]. Available: http://www.cms.hhs.gov/medicaid/1915b/1915bc.asp.

U.S. Department of Health and Human Services, Centers for Medicare and Medicaid Services. (2002c, May 29). *Medicaid services.* Available: http://www.cms.hhs.gov/medicaid/managedcare/mmcss01.asp.

U.S. Department of Health and Human Services, Centers for Medicare and Medicaid Services. (2002, June 4). *Medicaid and EPSDT.* Available: http://www.cms.hhs.gov/medicaid/epsdt/default.asp.

U.S. Department of Health and Human Services, Centers for Medicare and Medicaid Services. (2002, July 16). *Home and community-based services 1915(c) waivers.* Available: http://www.cms.hhs.gov.medicaid/1915c.default.asp.

U.S. Department of Health and Human Services, Centers for Medicare and Medicaid Services. (2002, July 24). *1115 Waiver research and demonstration projects.* Available: http://www.cms.hhs.gov/medicaid/1115.

U.S. Department of Health and Human Services, Centers for Medicare and Medicaid Services. (2002a, August 5). *HIPAA insurance reform.* Available: http://www.cms.hhs.gov/hipaa/hipaa1/content/more.asp.

U.S. Department of Health and Human Services, Centers for Medicare and Medicaid Services. (2002b, August 5). *The mental health parity act.* Available: http://www.cms.hhs.gov/hipaa/hipaa1/content/mhpa.asp.

U.S. Department of Health and Human Services, Centers for Medicare and Medicaid Services. (2002, September 3). *Medicaid services.* Available: http://www.cms.hhs.gov/medicaid/mservice.

U.S. Department of Health and Human Services, Centers for Medicare and Medicaid Services. (2002, October 1). *Medicaid managed care. Link to final rules.* Available: http://www.cms.hhs.gov/medicaid/managed care.

U.S. Department of Health and Human Services, Centers for Medicare and Medicaid Services. (2002, October 22). *Immigrant eligibility for Medicaid and SCHIP.* Available: http://www.cms.hhs.gov/immigrants/default.asp.

U.S. Department of Health and Human Services, Health Resources and Services Administration. *About HIV/AIDS Bureau.* Available: http://hab.hrsa.gov/aboutus.htm.

U.S. Department of Health and Human Services, Health Resources and Services Administration. Ryan White CARE Act. Available: http://hab.hrsa.gov/history/purpose.htm.

U.S. Department of Health and Human Services, Health Services and Resources Administration. *Understanding Title V of the Social Security Act.* Washington, DC: Department of Health and Human Services.

U.S. Department of Health and Human Services, Indian Health Service. (1999). *Comprehensive health care program for American Indians and Alaska Natives.* Available: http://www.ihs.gov.

Whitehand, L. & Kagan, J. (2001, September). *Family health: The next generation of MCH?* Available: http://www.amchp1.org/news/FHealthSurveyRpt.pdf.

9 Transitions to Adulthood

Kathleen J. Sawin, Ann W. Cox, and Stephanie G. Metzger

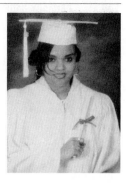

TRANSITION planning for adolescents with chronic conditions is a much more prevalent issue for primary care providers than it has been in the past (American Academy of Pediatrics [AAP], 2002a; Johnson, 1996). Although there have been substantial philosophic developments (AAP 2002a; 2002b; Betz, 2000) and an expansion of resources (see Resources at the end of this chapter) for adolescents, their families, and primary health care providers, the challenges remain essentially unchanged. The life expectancy for youth with chronic conditions has dramatically increased in the last 20 years. Most data suggest that 90% of all children with disabilities now live beyond the age of 20 years. Today more than 2 million young people between the ages of 10 and 18 years (i.e., 3.8% of our population) have some functional limitation caused by chronic and disabling conditions, which is a 100% increase since 1960 (Betz, 2000; Blum & Garber, 1992; Newacheck & Halfon, 1998). Therefore, by the year 2000, more than 1 million young Americans with chronic conditions or disabilities had transitioned to young adulthood.

An expanded civil rights movement has demanded equal life options for individuals with disabilities and chronic conditions (Table 9-1). The most influential event in this movement has been the adoption of the Americans with Disabilities Act (ADA) of 1990. This act was designed to ensure that persons with disabilities have the same rights as those without disabilities: specifically, the right to a free public education and access to public transportation, clinics, restaurants, stores, and recreational facilities. The rights to live in the community and hold a job are hallmarks of the ADA. The thrust of the legislation was to "normalize" life for persons with a disability. Discrimination against those with disabilities or chronic conditions in school, health care, or community living is prohibited. These changes have made the concept of purposeful planned transition a priority for primary care providers.

Outcome data suggest that youth with disabilities are not making the transition to a full adult life in the areas of education, employment, development of meaningful relationships, and independent community living. In a comprehensive longitudinal study of students with and without chronic conditions, school dropout rates for students with chronic conditions in ninth grade were greater than for their unaffected peers—a rate almost doubled in tenth grade and continued at an alarming rate even in twelfth grade (Pledgie et al, 1998). The most recent Harris study indicates that outcomes are improving but still reflect limitations for those with disability. More than one of five people with disabilities failed to complete high school (22%), compared with less than 1 of 10 people without disabilities (9%)—a gap of 13 percentage points (National

Organization on Disability [NOD], 2000). Of those with disabilities who finished high school, the college graduation rates are less than one half (Betz, 1998). The number of students with disabilities who exit high school has increased since 1995 (Table 9-2). Whereas the numbers who graduate with a diploma or certificate of completion have risen 25% and 27%, respectively, the numbers who exit school because they have reached the maximum age have increased 64%. Clearly, progress has been made for some with disabilities more than others (U.S. Department of Education, 2002).

Of all working-age people with disabilities (18 to 64 years), only 3 out of 10 (32%) are employed full-time or part-time, compared with 8 in 10 working-age people without disabilities (81%)—a gap of 49 percentage points. However, among those who are able to work despite their disability or health problem, 56% of people with disabilities are working, and the gap decreases to 25%. Native American youth with chronic conditions have an even more difficult time, with fewer than 30% employed or living independently. Of those unemployed with chronic conditions, 72% indicate that they would prefer to work. In addition, 40% of adults with disabilities have household incomes of $15,000 or less compared with only 16% of those without disabilities (NOD, 2000), and many young adults with disabilities do not live independently after high school (Pledgie et al, 1998).

Youth with disabilities are also at greater risk for other compromising behavioral morbidities. For instance, there is a higher than average prevalence of depression and attempted suicide with this population, reflecting the social isolation experienced by many youth with disabilities (Sawin et al, 1999). Substance abuse rates among persons with disabilities may be twice as high as those for the general population (Wolkstein, 2002), again with a disproportionate rate in minority communities. In addition, segregation, dependency, and nonproductivity occur for many young adults with disability (Healy & Rigby, 1999). These co-morbidity outcomes make it more difficult to obtain an independent and fulfilling adult life.

Unsuccessful transition to adult life has become a concern to health professionals, educators, and community activists, and barriers to optimal transition have been identified. The ultimate goal of transition planning is to provide comprehensive health, education, and vocational services that are seamless, coordinated, developmentally appropriate, and psychosocially sound. Educators and health care providers, directed by the 1997 revision to the Individuals with Disabilities Education Act (IDEA), have begun to initiate transitional planning for youth with chronic conditions during middle school. Whether formal or informal, assessment and counseling interactions must focus

TABLE 9-1

Legislation Affecting the Transition to Adulthood for Youths with Chronic Conditions

American with Disabilities Act of 1990	Prohibits discrimination against persons with disability in employment, public accommodations, and public services
Rehabilitation Act—1992 and 1998 Amendments of the 1973 Act	Strengthens the focus on employment for youths with disabilities, expanded eligibility criteria, and expanded customer choice
Section 504 of Rehabilitation Act	Prohibits discrimination for those with disabilities by any program or agency receiving federal funds; mandates equal opportunity to participate in or receive services from programs or activities and requires accommodations necessary to participate
Individuals with Disabilities Education Act Amendments (IDEA) of 1997 (PL 105-17) and Amendments of 1999	Modified earlier transition-planning requirements by lowering the age that schools must initiate transition planning and services to 14 yr
Carl D Perkins Vocational and Applied Technology Education Act Amendments of 1998 (PL 105-332)	Helps provide vocational and/or technical education programs and services to youths and adults. Funds go to local education agencies and postsecondary institutions to provide educational opportunities for students with disabilities
School to Work Opportunities Act of 1994 with 1998 amendments (PL 103-239)	Support to build high school learning systems to prepare students for further education and careers
Title XIX of the Social Security Act Medicaid Amendments Home and Community-Based Services Waiver (PL 97-35), 1990	Provides funds to support community services that enhance community living options
Community Supported Living Arrangements (CSLA) (PL 101-508), 1990	Promotes development of statewide systems of individual supported living
Supplemental Security Income (SSI) and Social Security Disability Insurance (SSDI)	Provides income benefits for youths (over 18 yr of age) with substantial disabilities and low income. Parental income is not considered. Usually provides Medicaid benefits
Health Insurance Portability and Accountability Act of 1996	Allows health care eligibility coverage to be portable from a previous plan to a new plan
Ticket to Work and Work Incentives Improvement Act of 1999	Provides incentive to states to allow workers with disabilities to purchase Medicaid to maintain employment
New Freedom Initiative 2001	Proposes to reduce barriers to full community integration for people with disabilities

TABLE 9-2

Numbers of Students Ages 14-21 Yr with Disabilities Exiting School by Graduation with High School Diploma, Certificate of Completion, or Reaching Maximum Age during 1995-2000

	1995-96	1996-97	1997-98	1998-99	1999-2000
High school diploma	126,051	134,614	147,942	152,485	159,578
Certificate of completion	26,146	28,614	29,909	29,650	32,719
Maximum age	4,176	4,396	4,607	4,853	6,838

From U.S. Department of Education, Office of Special Education Programs. (2002). *Annual report to Congress. Data analysis system (DANS);* Web site: www.ideadata.org/tables24th\ar_ad3.htm.

on developing skills in adolescents that enhance competency, autonomy, and responsibility, which are all necessary to make transition successful (Blum, 2002). As with the concept of "discharge planning begins with admission," transition planning must begin early in childhood. Attainment of competency requires time for maturation and training and therefore must begin early and build over time. The primary care provider has a significant role to play in the purposeful endeavor of transition.

An emerging issue in primary care during transition and indeed throughout childhood for children and youth with disabilities is the medical home initiative, "Every Child Deserves a Medical Home" (Kelly et al, 2002) (see Chapter 7). The American Academy of Pediatrics (2002b) recently issued a new policy statement regarding medical homes, asserting that children with special health care needs should have accessible, continuous, comprehensive, family-centered, coordinated, compassionate, and culturally effective medical care delivered through a primary provider. This care must transition into adult care.

Adolescence: A Universal Time of Change

The central developmental task during adolescence is achieving a sense of personal identity based on adaptation to a new physical, cognitive, and social self (Orr, 1998). Youth with chronic conditions and disabilities confront obstacles similar to those experienced by all adolescents living and growing up in our complex and pluralistic society, but they encounter additional challenges associated with the demands and restrictions of their conditions. Primary health care providers must be aware of both the typical and condition-based challenges encountered by youth with a chronic illness or disability in order to effectively support their need for autonomy as they transition into adulthood.

Adolescence is one of the most fascinating and complex periods of transitions in an individual's life. It is a time of accelerated growth and change second only to infancy, as well as expanding horizons, self-discovery, and emerging independence. This metamorphosis from childhood to adulthood can extend a full decade and in many ways encompasses a series of multiple transitions from early to late adolescence.

All adolescents, including youth with chronic conditions or disability, must meet the same fundamental requirements if they are to grow up to be healthy, constructive adults. The Carnegie Council on Adolescent Development (1995, pp. 10-11) summarizes these competencies as follows:

- Finding a valued place in a constructive group
- Learning how to form close, durable human relationships
- Feeling a sense of worth as a person
- Achieving a reliable basis for making informed choices
- Knowing how to use the available support systems
- Expressing constructive curiosity and exploratory behavior
- Finding ways of being useful to others
- Believing in a promising future with real opportunities

While striving toward these outcomes, youth experience an array of interconnected challenges that are related to the following: (1) the biologic changes of puberty that result in reproductive capacity and new social roles, (2) the movement toward psychologic and physical independence from parents, and (3) the search for friendship and belonging among peers.

Today's youth are growing up in a climate marked by dramatic changes in American families; less time spent with adults; changing work expectations; earlier reproductive capacity but later marriage and financial independence; dominance of electronic media; and a more diverse, pluralistic society (Carnegie Council on Adolescent Development, 1995). The result is that a series of new morbidities plague adolescents: higher rates of suicide, depression, and reported abuse (Keith, 2001, Schoen et al, 1997); earlier experimentation with drugs (Lynch & Bonnie, 1994); earlier sexual activity (Alan Guttmacher Institute, 2002); inadequate learning (Wirt et al, 2002); and more health-damaging behavior (Kann et al, 2000). Today, younger adolescents exhibit many of the risky behaviors that were once associated with middle and late adolescence.

Youth with chronic conditions or disability find that the integration of their chronic condition or disability with their self-identify only reinforces a sense of being different at a time when sameness is desired. Further, the physiologic changes of maturation may influence the actual management of a chronic condition (e.g., diabetes, asthma), and social role expectations may be inconsistent with cognitive ability (e.g., with mental retardation). The challenges of puberty, autonomy, personal identity, sexuality, education, and vocational choices may all be influenced by physical or mental abilities, pain, medical setbacks, forced dependence, and perceived prognosis. Arnett (2000) proposes that the ages 18 to 25 years are actually an extended time of emerging adulthood. During this time the individual accepts responsibility for one's self, makes independent decisions, and becomes financially independent. In addition, most live independently and many expand their education. Several authors propose adolescents with disabilities may lag behind their peers in these transition activities by several years. It is important to assess continued progress, even if, for some with disabilities, the transition is on a slightly different timetable than is typical for those without disabilities (Healy & Rigby, 1999).

Key developmental parameters of early and mid-to-late adolescence and those of early or emerging adulthood are provided in Table 9-3, along with the associated implications of chronic conditions or disability. These implications are generic in nature because specificities of conditions are addressed in subsequent chapters. The heterogeneity of youth with chronic conditions or disabilities implies that primary providers must take the time to know the individual's and family's uniqueness.

Understanding Transition

Clinicians and researchers studying transition (Cowan & Hetherington, 1991; Meleis et al, 2000; Schumacher & Meleis, 1994; Selder, 1989) propose that transition is a process—not an event. Bridges (1994, p. 5) defines it as "the psychological process people go through to come to terms with the new situation. Change is external, transition is internal." For life changes to be described as transitional, they must involve both a qualitative internal shift (i.e., how people understand and feel about themselves and the world) and an external visibility of this change reflected in a reorganization of personal competence and roles and/or relationships with significant others (Cowan & Hetherington, 1991).

Transitions can be classified as (1) developmental, (2) situational, (3) health and/or illness, and (4) organizational. Schumacher & Meleis (1994) indicated that the process and outcome of transition are powerful determinants of an enhanced sense of subjective well-being, role mastery, and the well-being of relationships, which enables the individual to function with increased confidence and skill in future challenges (Meleis et al, 2000; Schumacher & Meleis, 1994; Younger, 1991). In addition, facilitating and inhibiting conditions are delineated. Meleis and colleagues later expanded the model and identified characteristics of transition. These characteristics were awareness (perception, knowledge, and recognition of the transition), engagement in the process, change, and difference (dealing with feelings of difference), happening over a time span, and often having critical points or events (i.e., moving out of the home) (Meleis et al, 2000).

Lenz (2001) discusses the use of this theory in adolescent transition, including the role of anticipatory guidance and planning in facilitating transition and the negative impact of ignoring the transition. Lenz also discussed the contribution of counseling and developmental frameworks in this specific transition. Developmental theory delineates the issues in adolescent transition, especially the questions about who adolescents will become, including family, employment, and careers. Counseling theory supports the role of the environment, the characteristics of the individual, the role change undertaken, the degree of stress involved in transition, and the need for all these components to be addressed in counseling.

Adolescents with chronic conditions enter into developmental, health and/or illness, and potentially situational transitions. Primary care providers are in an excellent position to assess the factors associated with the quality of the transition experience and the factors that inhibit or facilitate transition and intervene with adolescents and families to optimize outcomes. To do this effectively, primary care providers need to understand the family and individual factors that can moderate the transitional process.

Family Factors Moderating Transition

The family is a constant factor in all transition endeavors working to prepare youth to consider options, set goals, develop the skills to work with service agencies and bureaucracies, find and use community support services, and solve problems to shape their lives and environments (Hallum, 1995). Primary care providers have an opportunity to facilitate parent practices to facilitate independence in youth and reduce stress in the family.

TABLE 9-3

Key Developmental Parameters and Associated Implications of Chronic Conditions

Adolescent Developmental Stage	Typical Developmental Parameters	Chronic Illness/Disability Implications
Early adolescence (generally 11-14 yr of age)	*Rapid physical growth*—particularly sensitive to their changing bodies *Sexual maturation*—initiation of the biologic changes of puberty; new social roles reinforced *Relationships*—shift from family to peer groups as source of security and status; intense need to belong to a group, usually of the same gender *Cognitive*—generally remain in concrete operational thought *Self-concept/esteem*—described in terms of physical features and likes; less tolerant of deviations from the "norm" *Health issues*—nutrition, acne, smoking, alcohol consumption; homicide from firearms has more than doubled in this age-group; increase in reported victims of child abuse and neglect *Career awareness*—typically begin thinking about the future	Certain developmental and disease conditions can alter rate of physical growth. Primary providers need to address these with youth and their families. In some conditions sexual maturation is early and menstruation is accelerated by several years. Anticipate interaction of sex hormones with other medication, and counsel accordingly. Education regarding emerging sexuality and consequences of resultant choices is essential. Social isolation is a critical issue. Encourage peer group activities at and away from home. Teens are eager for information about their development and need accurate information about chronic conditions or disabilities—especially implications for sexuality and fertility. Respectfully deal with their many questions and concerns. At risk for some health consequences. Reported to have higher risk for victimization because of desire to "fit in." Career awareness activities are often overlooked by youths with disabilities. Have high and realistic expectations, and communicate these.
Middle and late adolescence and emerging adulthood (15-25 yr of age)	*Physical growth*—continued physical growth but at a slower rate; strength and endurance increase *Sexuality*—sexual maturation and/or experimentation heightened; sexual development typically completed by 16 yr of age; intimate sexual relationships develop *Relationships*—achieving psychologic independence from parents becomes particularly important; peer relationships become central; although family relationships are changing, they remain important *Cognitive skills*—rapid growth and increasingly comprehend abstractions; movement into formal operational and abstract thinking *Self-concept/esteem*—increasing individuation with some diminishing of peer influence; self is defined by including interpersonal traits and abstract categories *Health issues*—experimentation with alcohol, cigarettes, and illicit drugs increases. Unintentional injury, homicide, and suicide are leading causes of morbidity and mortality. Exposure and/or participation in violence may arise. Females report higher incidence of depression than males. *Career*—planning emphasizes examination of own interests, aptitude abilities, and occupational aptitudes	Physical activity may be limited by certain conditions or disabilities; alternate means of physical activity must be provided. Information on risks associated with sexual activity is needed. Contraception explored, and implications of interactions with other medications are provided. If sexual maturation is delayed, this must be addressed with adolescent. In many settings, because of age and/or physical development, appropriate social skills are expected. Even individuals who are developmentally and/or cognitively disabled must be taught appropriate public behavior. Youth vary in their ability to assume independent activities because of skills, cognition, or the complexity of the condition, but every effort should be made to foster choice in decisions related to health condition. Address strengths, and encourage positive self-concept. There are some particularly dangerous interactions between prescribed medications and other drugs and substances. Additional nutritional education is particularly relevant because youth with limited mobility can be overweight and experience resultant complications. Abuse and victimization are higher in youth with disabilities than nondisabled peers. Emphasis should be on developing self-sufficiency skills, vocational and career decisions, and future planning. Active transition planning in health care, employment, and independent living must begin.

The adolescent transitional years are stressful for all parents—but especially for those whose dependents have severe disabilities. Families with adolescents with disabilities indicate continued protectiveness and worry (Sawin et al, 2002b). Parents of preadolescents whose life expectancies are uncertain or those who have intermittently unpredictable symptoms report greater family/social disruption, emotional strain, and financial burden than parents whose preadolescent with chronic conditions has a more certain future (Garwick et al, 2002).

According to Hallum (1995), families whose adolescents do not become as independent as expected report high levels of stress. The transition to independent living may be delayed by several years for youth with severe disabilities. In such situations, families must advocate for their adolescents to achieve supported living arrangements. Families with youth who have severe physical or cognitive limitations and who plan to remain in the family home face increasing responsibility as school eligibility terminates and family members' daily care responsibilities increase. Often resources to employ other caregivers are limited in the community (Hallum, 1995). These families need support and resource information to connect them with independent living centers and other community programs that offer alternative options and respite care. Families of youth who need continual supervision also must consider developing plans for custody and financial arrangements to ensure ongoing supervision when parents die or are unable to provide care. Medicaid-financed homes and daycare programs for adults with disabilities are scarce; so many parents must continue to care for their adult children at home. Advocates for people with mental retardation have filed class action suits to require states to provide housing and daycare services to these people or risk losing state Medicaid funding (Associated Press, 1999).

Extensive studies of parents and adolescents without disabilities confirm that authoritative parenting produces adolescents who achieve in school, have positive mental health, are more self-reliant, have higher self-esteem and are less likely to participate in antisocial behavior, including delinquency and drugs. Authoritative parents are warm and involved and offer strong support to their adolescents, but at the same time they are firm and consistent in establishing and enforcing guidelines, limits, and developmentally appropriate expectations. In addition, during adolescence they encourage and permit the adolescents to develop their own opinions and beliefs (Steinberg, 2000). Data support similar family characteristics supportive of youth with disabilities (Schultz & Liptak, 1998) with family warmth, family satisfaction, and family activity related positively to outcome (Sawin et al, 2002c; Schultz & Liptak, 2002).

One difference in families of adolescents with disabilities may be the issue of overprotection. In a recent qualitative study exploring the experience of parenting an adolescent with spina bifida, parents of adolescents who had normal intelligence simultaneously reported an interest in supporting independence and a need to protect their adolescents (Sawin et al, 2002b). Similarly, paradoxical findings support the crucial function of families in developing transition skills. Although some adolescents experience social isolation and their family essentially becomes their peer group, data also support the modeling of families. Adolescents who participate in more activities with their families are also more likely to participate in more activities with their friends and participate fully in society (Sawin et al, 2002d).

Participants in a study of "successful" young adults with disabilities reported several family themes associated with effective transitions (Powers et al, 1996). Families (1) treated them as typical children and adolescents, (2) expected them to participate fully in family responsibilities, (3) gave them no preferential treatment, (4) facilitated their participation in leisure activities, (5) focused on their strengths, (6) discussed their disability with them, and (7) assisted them in accommodating challenges. These young adults valued family experiences and discussions that allowed them to develop skills, participate in risk taking, and cope with social rejection. These youth perceived that their family was a safe and nurturing environment where competence was developed.

Providers need to assess family knowledge and family behaviors that facilitate the development of competence. Primary care providers working with families of youth with chronic conditions should begin to talk to parents about strategies that foster effective transition into adulthood when the affected child is still young. Many parents of children with chronic or disabling conditions have difficulty letting go and encouraging independence and may see their children as vulnerable. Early discussions on the importance of fostering autonomous decision-making skills and independence in the activities of daily living may help parents realize the importance of assisting their child to build the necessary skills for a successful transition into adulthood.

Factors Moderating Individual Transition

Cognitive ability, personal philosophy of self-competence, ability to solve problems, degree of autonomy, and peer relationships are all factors that influence an adolescent's ease and success in the transition to adulthood.

Cognitive Ability. Cognition plays a major role in transition planning. Self-sufficiency assumes the cognitive abilities necessary to carry out the education, employment, and management of health care and community living (Sawin et al, 1999). An adolescent's developmental abilities and age need to be considered in individual planning. If cognition is moderately or significantly impaired, families or advocates must increase their participation in the planning and implementation of the transition plan (Sawin et al, 1999). Many people with significant cognitive disabilities, however, can be competent, self-determined individuals (Wehmeyer, 1996). Achieving this goal may require individual skill building, alteration of the environment and interaction patterns, and use of available supports. Youth with cognitive disabilities must be afforded the basic rights that accompany the belief that all people are worthy of respect and dignity (Wehmeyer, 1996). Supportive employment has been shown to facilitate skill building and social outcomes in adolescents and young adults with disabilities (Wehman et al, 1999).

At the age of 18 years all youth obtain the legal right to make decisions about life activities. When cognition is impaired, legal guardianship of a young adult should be considered and pursued by family members. Once the age of majority is reached, medical, school, and financial information, as well as consent to treatment, is not accessible to others without the youth's or guardian's permission. It is important to be clear about access to information and consent of the individual, family, school, primary care provider, and other agencies involved. Youth can determine access to information unless a court finds otherwise. Issues of information sharing should be openly discussed with youth and their families; a plan should be created as youth near the age of 18 years (Sawin et al, 1999).

Self-Competence. All transition programs are built on the assumption that youth are being educated to develop self-competence. Self-competence is thought to be a function of two domains: skills or efficacy and a sense of well-being (Powers et al, 1996) and comprises self-determination, self-advocacy, assertiveness, coping, and self-esteem. Activities, experiences, and programs should be designed to develop self-competence and each of its components (Betz, 2000; Healy & Rigby, 1999).

Problem Solving and Autonomy. Studies of youth with chronic conditions have identified that problem solving and autonomy skills are related to positive health outcomes (Blum et al, 1991; Johnson, 1996; Sawin & Marshall, 1992; Sawin et al, 2002c). Interestingly, many youth with disabilities have limited experience making basic life decisions, much less decisions about health care (Hallum, 1995; Johnson, 1996; Sawin et al, 1996,

2002c). Knowledge about health care, the specific chronic condition, and experience in making decisions are prerequisites for making decisions about health. By practicing decision making in other areas (e.g., what clothes to purchase, how to wear your hair, what to do with friends, how to budget money), youth will gain confidence through experience. Without these basic decision-making skills, choices related to health care are not possible. Because all problem solving is context based, experience is essential to solving potential health care dilemmas. Simple choices (e.g., whether to take medication with applesauce or gelatin) should be given as early as developmentally possible so that there is a gradual movement to making all choices about health care management (Sawin et al, 1999).

Specific interventions to enhance autonomy through skill development have been developed over the last decade (Denniston & Enlow, 1995; Hardin, 1995a, 1995b; Hostler et al, 1989; Igoe, 1994). Evaluations indicated that significant gains in knowledge and autonomy were achieved with these interactive approaches. Two programs (Health PACT, TAKE CHARGE) are the most comprehensive. The first is a prototypic, consumer-oriented, health education program that prepares youth to communicate with health professionals and actively participate in their care (Igoe, 1994). The second is designed to systematically promote self-determination and functional competence by reducing learned helplessness and promoting motivation and self-efficacy expectations. This comprehensive program has components of skill development, the role of mentors, and peer and parental support. Qualitative and quantitative evaluations support the effectiveness of this program to promote self-determination (Powers et al, 1996).

Few research projects have examined the effect of interventions targeting enhanced autonomy of youth with chronic conditions in health or adaptation outcomes, but two are notable: one in the school setting and one in the health care setting. Magyary and Brandt (1996) developed and evaluated a school-based self-management program for youth with chronic health conditions. The intervention involved peer groups, cognitive and/or behavioral intervention, and parental support groups. The evaluation showed that youth in the intervention group had improved self-responsibility with higher therapeutic adherence. Although the youth-reported intervention effects began to fade after several months, parental reports indicated that important effects remained.

Additional data on the effectiveness of adolescent interventions can be expected in the near future from the Healthy and Ready to Work (HRTW; see Resources) programs. Another interesting program is Oregon's empowerment program (see Resources). In addition, a new program funded by the National Institutes of Rehabilitation Research (NIDRR) at the University of Florida, offers to provide us with new insights into the transition experience for those who traverse it. This program has both a research and a program arm (see Resources).

Attitudes, Beliefs, Perceptions, and Peer Relationships. An adolescent's attitudes, beliefs, and perceptions, such as hope, communication self-efficacy, coping, and future expectations, can have a major impact on outcomes. Although problem solving and autonomy are critical skills necessary to develop self-management and independence, attitudes and beliefs have been found to be the strongest predictors of mental health measures, such as depression, behavior problems and health-related quality of life. Indeed, in a recent study of adolescents with spina bifida, attitude was the strongest predictor of developmental competence and quality of life ($r = .56$ to $.62$) but was not a significant predictor of functional status or self-management outcomes. In contrast, decision-making skill and household responsibility had strong relationships ($r = .42$ to $.61$) with functional status and self-management but not with developmental competence and quality of life (Sawin et al, 2002a, 2002d).

Establishing meaningful friendships with others is the hallmark of successful social interaction. Friendships are the basis for the social, emotional, and practical support needed to become truly integrated into society and are one measure of success in community integration. The social skills necessary for successful peer relationships are the ability to read both verbal and nonverbal cues from others, make judgments about those cues, and respond in a socially appropriate manner. Mastering these social skills can be hard for many individuals with learning disabilities or neurodevelopmental deficits. Social expectation for displays of affection, caring, anger, and frustration must be learned in adolescence if not acquired during childhood. Social immaturity, social isolation, restricted social lives, and lack of social skills may all be present in youth with chronic conditions (Healy & Rigby, 1999). Transition plans must aggressively identify mechanisms for integrating youth with chronic conditions with their peers in educational, recreational, sports, and social activities. Adults who have made successful transitions report that peer and inclusion activities are fundamental to achieving independence (Powers et al, 1996).

Sexuality. Sexuality is a basic component of a full, adult life. Developing an identity as a sexual being is a universal developmental task of adolescents and young adults and should not be confused with sexual activity. Youth with chronic conditions are sexual beings with desires and interests similar to those of their unaffected peers, yet society often views and treats them as asexual. This can have disastrous consequences for youth (i.e., from being uneducated about sex and vulnerable to exploitation to feeling they have to prove their sexuality through risky behaviors) (Cox & Sawin, 1999). Adolescents report having limited sources of sexuality information and wanting more sexuality information, both general information and condition-specific information (Sawin et al, 2002d). A survey of parents of youth with chronic conditions identified that 24% to 34% of women with sensory conditions (vision, hearing) dropped out of school on account of pregnancy or childbearing issues.

For a successful transition, sexuality education should start with a focus on the physical changes of puberty integrated with alterations caused by the youth's condition (Blum, 1997; Sawin et al, 2002d). Discussions over time should include abuse and pregnancy prevention, access to reproductive health care, and responsible sexual decision making. Youth, particularly females in this population, are at high risk for sexual and substance abuse (American Academy of Pediatrics, 1996b, 2001; Lollar, 1994; Nosek, 1995; Sobsey, 1994). Early sexuality education is important for youth with chronic conditions because of their high risk for sexual abuse and pregnancy (Spencer et al, 1995).

Unfortunately, issues of sexuality for children and youth with chronic conditions are not routinely addressed by school programs, families, health care providers, or other transition team members (Blum, 1997; Sawin et al, 2002d). Thus issues of sexuality can pose major threats to the transition plan if overlooked (Blum, 1997; Sawin & Horton, 2003; Suris et al, 1996).

Condition-specific information is critical. For example, it is important for youth with spina bifida, who have a very high incidence of latex allergy, to avoid latex condoms. Likewise, women with spinal cord injuries may not be good candidates for oral contraceptives because of their high risk for deep vein thrombosis (Sawin, 1998). Young women with epilepsy treated with select anticonvulsants have an increased risk of fetal anomalies if the type and dose of the medications are not altered before conception. It is also important to realize that seizure medication can interact with some oral contraceptives, decreasing their effectiveness (American Academy of Neurology [AAN], 1998). All young women of childbearing age should be taking a multivitamin with 0.4 mg of folic acid. Because women with spina bifida, epilepsy, and diabetes have an increased risk of bearing an infant with neural tube deficits, it is especially important for these women to take a multivitamin and have preconception counseling (Cox & Sawin, 1999). However, in a recent survey 20% of adolescents in the highest risk category were unaware of this need (Sawin et al, 2002d).

Neurologic deficits (e.g., those from spinal cord injury, spina bifida, or muscular dystrophy and musculoskeletal limitations, such as those associated with severe juvenile rheumatoid arthritis or a high degree of spasticity) may limit some sexual positions or practices (Metzger, 1999; Sawin & Horton, 2003). Alternative strategies for sexual gratification must be openly discussed.

Transition Planning for Health Care
Condition Self-Management

In order to begin the transition to adult health care, adolescents must have a basic understanding and awareness of their condition or disability. Each contact with the adolescent is an opportunity to assess self-care knowledge and to provide further education (AAP, American Academy of Family Practice [AAFP], & American College of Physicians–American Society of Internal Medicine [ACP-ASIM], 2002). Primary care providers need to have a wide range of educational materials in multiple formats and be open to exploring new ways for youth to acquire the knowledge necessary to build self-management skills. The Internet is a powerful source of information that can be used to encourage knowledge acquisition. Adolescent chat lines for specific conditions are increasing and may be accessible sources of support and information for many teens. Web TV is relatively inexpensive and is being used to provide health-related information on a variety of subjects. Adolescents and their parents must be cautioned about the accuracy of information from the Internet and encouraged to discuss what they learn with health care providers. In addition, Internet safety (e.g., privacy) needs to be addressed. Agencies or organizations with a broad focus (e.g., the March of Dimes) can often be a source of program support for other educational

materials. Additional avenues for education include conferences sponsored by disability agencies, health camp experiences, and mentoring by an adult with a similar condition or disability.

The primary care provider must assist adolescents in developing age-appropriate self-care skills for health promotion and condition management (i.e., knowing their condition and its management in detail and knowing how to use the health care system to address their needs).

Developing self-care skills to manage chronic health conditions must begin as early as developmentally feasible and be emphasized as the child approaches adolescence. Self-care skills include all activities of daily living (e.g., dressing, toileting, feeding), use of medical prosthesis or equipment, administration of medication, health promotion activities, prevention of secondary conditions, and how to access health care services. Table 9-4 provides a developmental checklist for acquisition of needed self-care skills.

In addition to the tables presented in this chapter, primary care providers may find four other resources helpful in this endeavor. (1) The California Healthy and Ready to Work Project (Betz, 2000) has created the Developmental Guidelines for Teaching Health Care Self Care Skills to Children. These guidelines address self-care skill development by age category (infant, toddler, school-aged child) and by participant (parent, child). The guidelines delineate for the health care provider competencies in three areas: knowledge of health condition and management, preventive health behaviors, and emergency measures. (2) The CHOICES project (AAP, 2002a; Betz, 2000) has also developed Transition Guidelines by age and focus area. The guidelines identify expected outcomes and useful interventions in five areas: health promotion and disease prevention, health problem management, development and self-care, coping and stress, and family and community support. (3) The autonomy checklist (depts.washington.edu/healthtr/Checklists/home.htm) can be a useful tool for adolescent, family, and provider to evaluate the presence of important autonomy skills. (4) The newly developed outcome tool, the Adolescent Self-Management and Independence Scale (AMIS) (Sawin et al., 2002a) may be used by providers to evaluate outcomes of their intervention programs. This instrument measures outcomes in the area of self-management (i.e., independence in condition and medication knowledge, ordering supplies, making appointments) and independence (i.e., independence in household skills, advocacy activities, arranging for community transportation, managing finances).

Close evaluation of the development of self-care skills is critical. Familiarity with language and procedures may make young and middle adolescents with chronic conditions seem more knowledgeable or sophisticated than they really are. The gradual transfer of responsibility for complex self-care is optimal but can be overwhelming for young adolescents striving to assume total responsibility for managing their condition (Vessey & Miola, 1997). Moreover, it can lead to poor condition outcomes. The driver's license model is a useful analogy for establishing self-care responsibility. That is, youth drive under supervision for a prolonged period. Even after new drivers get a license, many parents often restrict them to familiar routes and provide them with a way of obtaining help in

TABLE 9-4

Developmentally Based Skills Checklist

Stage of Adolescence	Health Promotion and Condition Management	Medications, Supplies, and Other Equipment	Health Care System
Early (11-14 yr)	Knows simple anatomy, physiology, and pathology Able to tell health care provider what's wrong Discusses diagnosis and management plans with parents and providers Knows name(s), dates, and significance of any chronic illness and significant injuries Can perform appropriate first aid Knows CPR Knows any allergies and can outline avoidance and emergency treatment actions Takes responsibility to monitor chronic condition and quickly notify parents of any new developments Manages aspects of chronic condition in predictable or common situations, accessing consultation for family or other resource people in unfamiliar situations If assistance with ADLs needed, can identify needs and preferences and knows the tasks to be carried out by others Has opportunity to develop decision making and has responsibilities at home Knows about basic money management (e.g., function of checking and saving accounts) and manages small personal resources	Knows names of medication taken, dose, reason, expected response Is aware of amount of regularly taken medication remaining in container and alerts parents or caregiver when low Understands the difference between illicit drugs and medications Takes medications for chronic condition correctly Knows use and care of equipment and supplies and can notify parents when problems occur	Knows the difference in kinds of health care providers (e.g., obstetrician vs. optometrist) Knows date of and reason for next health appointment Knows where primary care providers and specialists are located and how to contact them
Middle (15-17 yr)	Knows date of last menstrual period (girls) and keeps record on personal or family calendar (i.e., may be early task for females with early-onset menses) Knows the basics of own health history, including family history Knows year of last tetanus shot Knows about TSE and BSE; performs regularly Manages chronic conditions in less predictable situations; seeks consultation when needed; requires minimal day-to-day supervision Can plan ahead to anticipate problem areas and generate options If assistance with ADL is needed, knows care well enough to direct others in what he or she is unable to do Has increasing responsibility in family Has a savings or checking account and manages it with supervision from parents if needed	Calls pharmacy to reorder own meds or calls own provider about need for refill Knows the difference between generic and proprietary medications Selects own medications for minor illnesses (e.g., URI, headaches) Orders new supplies or equipment with supervision; can reorder these materials independently Arranges for transportation to get medication supplies or for appointments	Makes own health care appointments Knows basic facts of own health insurance; knows limitations and issues for insurance in ordering supplies and/or medications and other equipment
Late and emerging adulthood (18-25 yr)	Manages stable chronic condition independently; uses parents and/or professionals to get advice regarding complex situations but makes management decisions Participates in discussions regarding adult health care options Understands the connection among mind, body, and spirit in health and illness Engages in healthy lifestyle activities; chooses healthful foods; exercises regularly; avoids caffeine, tobacco, illicit substances; gets adequate amount of sleep If assistance for ADL is needed, participates in the hiring, supervision, and termination of attendant caregiver	Independently manages medication, assessment and repair of any equipment, and pays for or arranges payment for medication and/or supplies	Understands the complexities of own health insurance plan Understands effect of change in employment and/or school status on insurance options Keeps updated file of own health records Takes responsibility to initiate contact with providers when transition to new living or educational environment occurs

Data from Hallum, A. (1995). Disability and the transition to adulthood: Issues for the disabled child, the family, and the pediatrician. *Current Problems in Pediatrics, 25*(1), 12-50; Sawin, K. (Ed.). (1998). Health care concerns for women with physical disability and chronic illness. In E. Yougkin & M. Davis (Eds.). *Women's health: A primary care clinical guide* (2ⁿᵈ ed.). Stamford, CT: Appleton & Lange; Sawin, K.J. (1999). Transition planning for youth with chronic conditions: an interdisciplinary process. *N Acad Pract For. 1*(2), 183-196; Vessey, J., & Miola, E.S. (1998). Teaching adolescents self-advocacy skills. *Pediatric Nursing, 23*(1), 53-56.
CPR, Cardiopulmonary resuscitation; *ADL*, activities of daily living; *TSE*, testicular self-examination; *BSE*, breast self-examination; *URI*, upper respiratory infecstion.

unexpected or complex situations. If youth are driving long distances or to unfamiliar territory, parents intervene by providing discussions on how to manage unforeseen occurrences. Parents often reassess the skill of the driver and, if major deficits occur, arrange additional training or supervision. Even when an adolescent with a chronic condition masters a skill, occasional help or a holiday from selected responsibilities helps maintain the commitment necessary for care of a chronic condition (Sawin et al, 1999).

Adolescents unable to care for themselves need to develop the ability to supervise others caring for them. There is little in the literature, however, on how to teach adolescents or families to recruit, train, evaluate, and hold attendants or personal care providers accountable—critical skills for youth in transition who need assistance in activities of daily life. In addition, service animals may be a reasonable resource for youth who are not functionally independent. Several states currently have or are developing Medicaid waiver programs that will give adolescents and their families more control over issues such as attendant care. Such resources and an array of technologic resources must be explored when considering transition planning for adolescents who are not independent in activities of daily living (Sawin et al, 1999).

Health Care Maintenance

The development of a condition-specific health care maintenance plan for adults is an important part of transition planning. Key issues include nutrition, exercise, dental care, safety, injury prevention, substance abuse, and mental health. Although these goals are the same for all adolescents making the transition into adulthood, adaptations and accommodations must be made for individuals with cognitive impairments, impaired mobility, and altered physiologic states. For example, planning for the transition to an adult dental care provider needs to include issues of spasticity, latex allergy, and decreased cognition or behavioral difficulties if any exist.

Youth with chronic conditions are generally at greater risk for substance abuse and mental health issues, and focused attention is appropriate. Having a chronic condition is not a cause of psychiatric illness in either individuals or families. However, youth with chronic conditions and their families do have more psychosocial and adaptive issues that can be severe (Faux, 1998). A person with a disability has a higher risk of abusing alcohol and other drugs than a person without a disability. Rates of abuse in persons with disabilities range from 15% to 30%, which is well above the national average (SARDI, 2002; Wolkstein, 2002; http://www.med.wright.edu/citar/sardi). Most youth with chronic conditions are on two or more prescription medications. The dangers of prescription drug abuse and mixing prescriptions with alcohol or other street drugs are often overlooked by the adolescent, parents, professionals, and friends (Hallum, 1995; Sawin & Horton, 2003). Even when adolescents ask about the possible interaction of their prescribed medication with recreational drugs, the answers are often not readily available. Just having access to a no-nonsense discussion of the potential interactions of street and prescription drugs, as well as the legal consequences of illicit drug use, is often useful to adolescents. When referral is necessary, it must be made to a professional with training and compassion for the struggles and transition needs of youth with chronic or disabling conditions.

The "dual diagnosis" must be addressed in any counseling program (Wolkstein, 2002).

Prevention of Secondary Disabilities

The prevention of secondary disabilities must be a major theme of each health care transition plan. This prevention is accomplished by the following: (1) aggressively addressing health maintenance and condition-specific primary prevention issues, (2) aggressively addressing condition-specific management issues, (3) facilitating the development of a philosophy of self-competence in the adolescent, and (4) identifying condition-specific, high-risk issues and developing a plan for early recognition of the need for treatment and specific management plans (Farley et al, 1994).

Recently the Centers for Disease Control and Prevention (CDC) launched a new center, the National Center for Chronic Disease Prevention and Health Promotion (http://www.cdc.gov/nccdphp/). The purpose of this center is to impact both the prevention of disability and the quality of life of those living with disability. The center, partnering with state health and education agencies, voluntary associations, private organizations, and other federal agencies, will be undertaking a number of initiatives to better understand the causes of these diseases, support programs to promote healthy behaviors, and monitor the health of the nation.

Access to Health Care as an Adult

The majority of adolescents with chronic conditions receive their health care in the pediatric primary care setting. It is the responsibility of the pediatric primary care provider to facilitate the transition from child-centered to adult-centered health care. This responsibility is identified and supported by both the AAP (1996a, 2002a, 2002b) and the Society of Adolescent Medicine (Blum et al, 1993) and jointly by AAP, AAFP, and ACP-ASIM (AAP, AAFP, & ACP-ASIM, 2002). The primary care provider often initiates and facilitates the transition for youth with chronic conditions by helping the adolescent and family to develop competency in condition self-management (i.e., including knowledge and self-care skills, health care maintenance, and prevention of secondary or associated conditions). Studies have demonstrated a host of barriers to effective transition to adult care (Patterson & Lanier, 1999, Reiss & Gibson, 2002; Scal, 2002), including the following:

- Lack of adult care providers and disconnect between the adult and pediatric approaches to care: the adult provider focuses on the medical condition of the adolescent rather than the broader social, developmental, and family concerns of the pediatric system
- Limited experience of adult providers with managing conditions previously only thought to be chronic illness of children
- Protectiveness of pediatric providers
- Bond between pediatric providers and families
- Not beginning early
- Focus of the teen on the here and now
- Structural issues (e.g., age limits to Title V programs; licensing and practice limitations; mission of facilities and charities, such as children's hospitals)
- Organizing, financing, and delivery of care

Health care providers need to initiate and coordinate referral to an adult-focused health care system. The AAP (1996a) and other experts (Reiss & Gibson, 2002) recommend that in "some cases" pediatricians with skills in the health care needed by certain youth may provide care into adulthood. One of the barriers to an effective transition to adult care is the perception among many pediatric primary care providers that there is a lack of knowledgeable, sensitive providers in the adult health care system to care for adult survivors of congenitally acquired conditions (AAP, 2002; Scal, 2002; Viner, 1999). The focus must be on consulting adult specialists to enable them to address the needs of young adults with chronic conditions—not on keeping these individuals in the pediatric health care system (AAP, AAFP, & ACP-ASIM, 2002).

Health Insurance Issues

The quality and amount of health care available to transitioning adolescents may be adversely affected by insurance limitations and a lack of coordinated case management. Insurance coverage becomes an issue as youth transition into adulthood and are no longer covered by their parents' insurance or federal and state programs established for care of children. Youth with disabilities aged 19 to 23 years often lose health insurance (White, 2002). Recently, Fishman (2001) reported data indicating that 20% of young adults with disabilities are uninsured. If an individual has a high health care risk, lack of insurance may be a major barrier to fully independent living. Once a young adult leaves school, parental insurance is usually terminated. The cutoff age for students still in school varies by policy, but almost no coverage exceeds age 25 years. Youth in college can access the student health center for primary care but may need to have another source of inpatient coverage. Most medical plans for college students, however, have a preexisting condition clause that eliminates eligibility for many.

Youth can opt to continue parental insurance through the Consolidated Omnibus Budget Reconciliation Act of 1986 (COBRA insurance program). This program allows youth to retain parental insurance with the same coverage for 18 months, but the cost is high and extended benefits must be applied for within 60 days of loss of group coverage. HIPAA (Health Insurance Portability and Accountability Act of 1996) provisions allow eligibility coverage to be portable from a previous plan to a new plan, thus avoiding the preexisting conditions clause. Youth in some states can join a high-risk insurance plan supplemented by the state, but this option is also costly and usually has no sliding scale for income. Options for individuals to buy into a Medicaid plan on a sliding-fee scale have received federal approval and are now state options (American Academy of Pediatric, 2002a). The Ticket to Work and Work Incentives Improvement Act of 1999 includes incentives to states to allow workers with disabilities to purchase Medicaid to maintain employment as well as an option to workers to maintain Medicare coverage. Families and health care providers must advocate for innovative state insurance options that would support optimal transition outcomes and ensure continued health care.

Further complicating the loss of personal insurance is the termination at a specific age of supplemental benefits available in most states through block grant programs (e.g., Title V programs) for children with special health care needs. Federal block grants give states financial resources to provide specialty clinical services, care coordination, and supplemental fiscal support for families with children with special health care needs. These programs were created as a health care safety net for at-risk children and families and cease at age 21 years. Eligible youth may apply for Supplemental Security Income (SSI) or Social Security Disability Insurance (SSDI), which come with automatic Medicaid benefits in many states. Employment, however, may result in loss of eligibility and termination of financial and medical benefits (see Chapter 8). Youth with disabilities will automatically lose SSI benefits when they turn 18 years old unless they are redetermined to be eligible under the adult SSI criteria. This must occur during the month preceding their eighteenth birthday. Thus youth in transition may lose the medical support available from the state and not be able to access any other type of insurance. Even if insurance is available to youth in transition, the benefits may be severely restricted—especially for therapies important to youth with mobility, communicative, or psychologic challenges. If services are provided, they are often limited in amount and duration (AAP, 1996a), which is a problem that may be accentuated if an individual uses a managed care organization with limited resources and restricted referral options. If these youth are to become independent members of society, new policies and solutions for health insurance need to be developed to address these important insurance issues for youth with special health care needs (White, 2002).

Transition Planning in the School System

Although the focus of transition planning in the health care system is accessing adult health care services, the focus in the school system is preparing individuals for life in the community and meaningful employment (see Chapter 5). The Individuals with Disabilities Education Act (IDEA) is the only federal legislation that requires a planning process to enable students with disabilities to achieve a smooth, gradual, and planned transition to community life. The legislation defines transition services as follows:

. . . a coordinated set of activities for a student, designed with an outcome oriented process that promotes movement from school to post-school activities including secondary education, vocational training, integrated employment (including supported employment), continuing and adult education, adult services, independent living and community participation. A coordinated set of activities shall be based upon the individual student's needs, taking into account the student's experiences, level of employment, post-school adult living objectives and when appropriate, acquisition of daily living skills and a functional vocational evaluation (National Information Center for Children and Youth with Disabilities, 1997).

The transition provisions were set forth in the 1990 reauthorization of IDEA that required schools to develop individualized transition plans (Tips) for students 16 years of age with a chronic condition or disability (see Chapter 5). IDEA'97 (PL 105-17) modifies transition planning by requiring that each student's individual education plan (IEP) contains a statement of transition service needs beginning at age 14 years.

Students with chronic or disabling conditions who are not eligible for special education and therefore do not have an IEP can and should receive transition services under Section 504 of the Rehabilitation Act. Students with chronic health conditions (e.g., diabetes, asthma) often have transition services addressed in their individual health service programs (IHPs). These 504 plans and IHPs should address transition service needs starting at 14 years of age. Neither 504 plans nor IHPs have legal mandates for transition planning, even though it is a recommended practice. Primary care providers may need to advocate for appropriate school-based services for youth who do not have a legal mandate for transition planning in the school.

School nurses have unique opportunities to support high school students through an impending developmental transition and address quality of life as well as disease management issues (Lenz, 2001), yet these nurses are often underutilized. Primary care providers often find requesting the involvement of the school nurse in all IEP or 504 processes facilitates communication among the family, school, and primary care practice. Primary care providers, especially those who have embraced the medical home initiative for children with special health care needs, often participate in the IEP, especially if attendance can be by phone or held in the provider's office (AAP, 2002a). Educational transition teams often overlook the health care issues that must be addressed for successful planning. If health care issues are not adequately addressed, a successful transition into postsecondary education or full-time employment, community living, and self-sufficiency will be jeopardized.

Postsecondary Education

The statistical profile of college students with disabilities reveals that in the 2000 school year, 6.0% of first-time, full-time freshman attending 4-year institutions self-reported disabilities (Henderson, 2001). The percentage of freshmen with disabilities who reported a learning disability more than doubled from 1988, increasing from 15.3% to 32.2% (Henderson, 1995). More than one half of all freshmen with disabilities are students with hidden disabilities (i.e., learning, health, etc.), and freshmen who reported having disabilities were more likely than their nondisabled peers to be older men, from lower-income families, and significantly concerned about financing their college education. Many received financial aid from vocational rehabilitation funds and were more interested in education and technical fields than in business. Many used special support programs offered at colleges and reported having been influenced by a role model or mentor to go to college.

Plans for a transition from high school to college should be reflected in an IEP, IHP, or 504 accommodation plan. Certain schools around the United States are especially noted as having strong support programs for those with chronic conditions (Back to School, 1996). Youth—especially those with severe physical disabilities—may find the extensive educational, health, recreational, and social support services of these universities helpful. Almost all colleges and universities have an office of disabled student services. Contacting this office before applying to determine available services is often useful. Some students are unwilling to identify themselves as having a chronic condition or disability because of the stigma associated with differences in our society. Students should be encouraged to use all services available to them to enhance their potential for success.

As with other college students, financial considerations are important. Early consultation in high school with the Division of Rehabilitation Services can determine if a student is eligible for any educational or support services. Services vary across states, and early consultation is important because staff in all agencies have a heavy caseload. Youth and their parents must be clear about what services are available and then vigorously pursue them.

A major source of information about postsecondary education is the HEATH Resource Center (see Resources), formerly of the American Council on Education, but now located at George Washington University. HEATH is the national clearinghouse on postsecondary education for individuals with disabilities. Support from the US Department of Education enables the center to serve as a resource for exchange of information about educational support services, policies, procedures, adaptations, and opportunities at American campuses, vocational-technical schools, and other postsecondary training entities. In operation since 1984, HEATH offers a multitude of resource papers, monographs, guides, and directories focusing on a broad range of disability-related topics, such as accessibility, career development, classroom and laboratory adaptations, financial aid, independent living, transition resources, training and postsecondary education, vocational education, and rehabilitation. Providers should encourage youth and their families to access this information via the public library or Internet early in the planning process. At a minimum, youth and families need to ask basic questions about a school. Box 9-1 outlines useful questions proposed by HEATH.

Some universities have preenrollment programs for students with severe disabilities—especially those who will need attendant care. The focus of the health providers in these situations is evaluation of the attendant care needs of the student, as well as—and more importantly—the student's independent ability to teach others to provide the necessary care. Each student must determine if health care should be transferred from their home community to either the college health care center or a local specialty provider or if the community provider should be maintained. Access to emergency health care must always be evaluated, and youth should have a copy of all critical health care records with them if they are far from their usual sources of health care.

Vocational Training and the Transition to Work

The 1992 and 1998 Amendments to the Rehabilitation Act of 1973 (PL 102-569) strengthened the role of vocational rehabilitation to work collaboratively with special education in preparing youth for transition into adult life while they are in school. Having already initiated the independent living movement with the 1986 amendments, the Rehabilitation Act of 1992 addressed the needs of youth and young adults for personal assistant services, supported employment opportunities, and a broad range of assistive technology. The 1998 amendments reinforce that employment is the intended outcome of vocational rehabilitation services. Two of the characteristics identified as important in the transition process were preparation and knowledge (Meleis et al, 2000). Most high school students identified as having a disability intend to enter the

BOX 9-1

Useful Questions in Assessing a Postsecondary Education Environment

What are the medical and health needs of this young adult?
Will a plan for health care transition need to be developed?
What factors would be included in the health component of the transition plan?
When should the health transition process be initiated?

How will the chronic illness affect this individual?
How does the chronic illness affect this youth's educational process?
How does the chronic illness affect this individual's living environment?
How does the chronic illness affect activities of daily living?

Disclosure
Should the individual disclose the chronic illness when applying to colleges or other postsecondary training institutions? To whom? When?
What laws are in place to protect the rights of people with disabilities? How do they relate to young adults with chronic illness?

Accommodations
What educational or environmental accommodations or modifications will need to be in place to increase independence?
What accommodations are postsecondary educational institutions required by law to provide?
If this individual needs additional accommodations or modifications, who will pay for them?
How can this individual assess the ability of the postsecondary institution and the surrounding community in meeting his or her needs?

Locating resources
When should financial, medical, and support service resources begin?
Who can assist at the postsecondary site?
Whose responsibility is it?

From Edelman, A. (1995). Maximizing success: transition planning for education after high school for young adults with chronic illness, *Information from HEATH 15*(1):3. Reprinted with permission.

---

workforce on leaving school but face many employment barriers. Wagner and Blackorby (1996) studied data from the National Longitudinal Transition Study of Special Education Students and identified factors that contributed to the outcomes for youth who were in special education. They found that students from low-income households experienced the worst postschool outcomes; students with sensory or motor disabilities benefited the most from special education; and concentrated vocational education (i.e., several courses focusing on a specific area)—as opposed to one course from a variety of concentrations—yielded higher employment and income rates. Even with vocational courses, however, outcomes for employment were still low compared with those of youth not in special education.

The major resource for youth making the transition to work is the Vocational Rehabilitation Service in their state. The changes in the Rehabilitation Act in 1992 and 1998 strengthened the focus on employment and changed the criteria for service. The only criterion is that the adolescent would benefit from employment, and the definition of employment has been broadened to include supported employment (Johnson, 1996). The act also provides technologic resources and personal assistance services if necessary to provide assistance in activities of daily living on or off the job. Even with these resources, however, the transition

to work is often problematic. Early referral to vocational support services and conveying the expectation that work, in some form, is an expected outcome must be the focuses of the home, school, and health care communities.

A supportive workplace is a critical factor for transition-age youth. Butterworth and colleagues (2000) found that multiple context relationships, specific social supports, a personal and team building management style, and interdependent job designs individually and collectively made for a supportive workplace. Providers may need to guide youth and their families to successful first-workplace experiences. However, this time of change may also result in vulnerability and risks that affect health.

Transitioning from Home to Community Living

The transition to independent living is difficult for many youth and young adults with cognitive, physical, and emotional disabilities to achieve because necessary support systems are not readily available. Youth with chronic unstable health conditions find this transition particularly difficult if they have not developed the skills necessary to manage their conditions and solve problems associated with their condition and limited functional capacity.

Several legislative initiatives have given communities the impetus to develop supports for young adults who want to study, work, and live as independently as possible in the community. These initiatives include the Americans with Disabilities Act (ADA) of 1990 (PL 101-336), the 1992 Amendments to the Rehabilitation Act of 1973 (PL 102-569), the Home and Community Based Services (HCBS) waiver, the Community Supported Living Arrangements (CSLA) of 1990 (PL 101-508) amendments to Medicaid, and, most recently, the New Freedom Initiative, launched in February 2001. The latter was created to reduce barriers to full community integration for people with disabilities. These programs are often underfunded, however, and there are often insufficient resources available in the community to meet the needs of youth and adults with disabilities who seek independence.

Two amendments to the Medicaid program have systematically provided funding mechanisms to support community living for young adults with chronic conditions or disabilities (see Chapter 8). The first, the Home and Community Based Services (HCBS) waiver, which was first enacted in 1982, has gained momentum and is rapidly replacing Title XX as the major source of federal funding for community services (White, 2002). Although originally intended to support the movement of individuals from institutional care to residential care, this program now finances case management, homemakers, home health aides, personal care, residential habilitation, day habilitation, respite care, transportation, supported employment, adapted equipment, and home modification. The second amendment, the Community Supported Living Arrangements (CSLA), promotes the development of statewide systems of individualized supported living. This program provides person-centered planning processes and provides individuals with the support needed to enable them to live in their own homes, apartments, or family homes.

The support services available through these two programs are critical for many youth and young adults with disabling conditions making a transition to the community. Individual states may develop other waiver programs. Two new Medicaid waiver templates were recently unveiled (Centers for Medicaid and Medicare, 2002) that streamline the state application process for consumer-directed, community-based services, including purchasing health care services.

If young adults with chronic conditions or disabilities are to be successful living independently, they must have the social skills—including the skills necessary to make appropriate decisions about their health and activities of daily living—as well as the technical skills or assistance to actually meet their daily needs for physical care, communication, and transportation. Most youth with chronic conditions and those with mild degrees of disability negotiate the road to community living much like youth without disabilities. Youth with moderate to severe degrees of functional disability will have more difficulty.

Learning to be as independent as possible with activities of daily living does not mean doing things without help or modification. On the contrary, distinguishing between when and how much assistance is needed is indicative of mature decision making for many young persons with chronic conditions or disabilities. Ideally, the development of self-help skills that began at home and continued throughout school was geared toward the ultimate goal of independent living. These skills include personal hygiene; domestic skills; transportation; safety; financial management including banking, purchasing, and spending; and seeking and developing meaningful leisure activities (Axelson & Jackson, 1997; Hallum, 1995).

Coordination of Transition Planning

Families report not only frustrations with obtaining a co-ordinated transition plan but also confusion about where to turn for assistance (Stevenson et al, 1997; Patterson & Lanier, 1999). Care coordination across all the systems, family, education, employment, community, and health care is complex; and communication among providers, transition team members, and the family is essential for transition into adulthood (see Chapter 7). Families are often the leaders in the transition process, but the primary care provider may facilitate both the process and communication across systems. When an individual's health problems are significant, the primary care provider may need to assume a leadership role in the transition process. In order to facilitate the plan, the primary care provider must know the needs of the adolescent and family; the agencies and team members involved; and the family, school, community, and health care resources available. The AAP has developed several position statements addressing youth with special health care needs and transition issues (AAP, 2001, 2002a, 2002b).

When the family is articulate and knowledgeable and can access resources, the primary care provider may only need to coordinate health information and referrals to community health agencies. Primary care providers may provide health information on a regular basis for school transition team conferences as well as for community experiences such as

"camperships" and athletic teams and also serve as consultants. If there is a significant health component to the transition plan, the primary care provider may actually be the case manager or can be the team leader while a specialty provider is the case manager. In order to achieve a smooth transition to adult health care, similar goals much be present between all transition team members.

As adulthood approaches, primary care providers must encourage youth and their families to address future planning for education, health care, employment, and community living options with referrals to appropriate resources. In preparation for adulthood, the primary health care provider has an obligation to do the following: (1) educate and inform adolescents of their conditions, including future expectations and preventive health care; (2) encourage parents to adopt parenting styles that support the transition to independent adulthood; (3) recognize and plan for opportunities to support young adults' autonomous decision making regarding health care, building on the strengths of the individual; (4) convey a positive attitude about the potential of young adults and provide information to agencies or people who can help them reach their full potential; (5) be knowledgeable about the evolving community system of supports and legal mandates for services; (6) help individuals access appropriate health care services and function as a consultant to adult providers when necessary; (7) advocate at the legislative level for insurance coverage and community services to enable individuals to live as full and healthy adult lives as possible; (8) advocate for appropriate and comprehensive transition services that integrate systems of care and educational, health, community, and family resources; and (9) provide genetic and family planning information and resources.

RESOURCES
Organizations
ABLEDATA
A database of products
http://www.abledata.com

Adolescent Health Transition Project
Provides checklists for ongoing assessment of independence skills depts.
washington.edu/healthtr

Alliance for Technology Access
Provides access to technology for people with disabilities
http://www.ataccess.org

HEATH
Provides specialized educational information
www.heath.gwu.edu

National Information Center for Children and Youth with Disabilities (NICHCY)
Provides information in English and Spanish
www.nichcy.org

National Organization on DisABILITY
www.nod.org

National Organization for Rare Diseases or other illness-specific organizations, such as United Cerebral Palsy
www.rarediseases.org
http://www.ucp.org

National Transition Alliance
www.dssc.org/nta

Parent Training and Information Centers (PTI), Technical Assistance to Parents Program (TAPP), including Parenting Educational Advocacy Training Center Provides links to almost every disability organization
www.peatc.org

TASH
An international advocacy association
http://www.tash.org

University centers on disabilities
Located at major universities and teaching hospitals
http://www.aucd.org

Projects

The Maternal Child Health Bureau (MCHB) has policy briefs and national demonstration projects currently funded. These programs will test new health care transition models that can be replicated throughout the United States. Many have produced or are developing useful materials for primary care providers. Several are Healthy and Ready to Work programs. Providers can contact the MCHB (http://www/mchb.hrsa.gov/chcnmc.html) for information on these programs or contact the programs directly at the following addresses:
California
UCLA-affiliated program at the Southern California Transition Center: "Healthy and Ready to Work"
http://www.cahrtw.org

Iowa
Consortium of Iowa Child Health Specialty Clinics, Iowa UAP, Iowa Creative Employment Options, Adolescent Transition: "Healthy and Ready to Work"
http://www.iowaceo.com

Kentucky
Collaborative public-private effort among the state's Children with Special Health Care Needs (CSHCN), Title V, Early Intervention, Vocational Rehabilitation, and Shriners Hospitals CHOICES (Children's Health Care Options Improved through Collaborative Efforts and Services) Transition Project
choices001@aol.com

Louisiana
The Human Development Center (HDC), Louisiana State University: "Healthy and Ready to Work"
http://www.hdc.lsuhsc.edu/programs/AS/hightoadult/default.htm

Maine
Department of Human Services, Bureau of Health, Division of Community and Main Adolescent Transition Partnership
http://www.ume.maine.edu/~cci/matp/

Massachusetts
Division for Children with Special Health Care Needs (DCSHCN) Initiative for Youth with Disabilities (MIYD)
http://www.state.ma.us/dph/shcn/miyd.htm

Minnesota
PACER Center, a parent training and information center
www.pacer.org

Ohio
Lighthouse Youth Services, Inc with Work and Rehabilitation Center of Greater Cincinnati, Inc, Hamilton County Adolescent Transition Project
http://www.lys.org/

Oregon
Oregon Center for Self Determination
http://cdrc.ohsu.edu/selfdetermination

LAY RESOURCES FOR TEENS AND FAMILIES

Kaufman, M. (1995). Easy for you to say: Questions and answers for teens living with chronic illness or disability. Toronto: Key Porter Books.

Kriegsman, K.H., Zaslow, E.L., & D'Zmura-Rechsteiner, M.A. (1992). Taking charges: Teenagers talk about life and physical disability. Bethesda, MD: Woodbine House.

REFERENCES

Alan Guttmacher Institute. (2002). *Sexuality education.* New York: The Institute.

American Academy of Neurology (AAN). (1998). Practice parameter: Management issues for women with epilepsy. *Neurology, 51,* 944-948.

American Academy of Pediatrics (AAP). (2002a). *Every child deserves a medical home: Component five—transitioning children and youth to adulthood.* Elk Grove Village, IL: Author.

American Academy of Pediatrics (AAP). (2002b). The medical home. *Pediatrics, 110*(1), 184-186.

American Academy of Pediatrics (AAP). (2001). Sexuality education for children and adolescents. *Pediatrics, 108,* 498-502.

American Academy of Pediatrics (AAP). (1996b). Sexuality education of children and adolescents with developmental disabilities. *Pediatrics, 97*(2), 275-278.

American Academy of Pediatrics (AAP), American Academy of Family Practice (AAFP), & American College of Physicians–American Society of Internal Medicine (ACP-ASIM). (2002). A consensus statement on health care transitions for young adults with special health care needs. *Pediatrics, 100*(Suppl 6), 1304-1306.

American Academy of Pediatrics (AAP), Committee on Children with Disabilities and Committee on Adolescence. (1996a). Transition of care provided for adolescents with special health care needs. *Pediatrics, 98*(6), 1203-1206.

Arnett, J.J. (2000). Emerging adulthood. A theory of development from the late teens through the twenties. *American Psychologist, 55,* 469-480.

Associated Press. (1999, March 20). Parents with retarded children file lawsuit over long wait for care. *San Francisco Chronicle.*

Axelson, P. & Jackson, P. (1997). Transition for adolescence to adulthood. In J. Vessey (Ed.). *The child with a learning disorder or ADHD: A manual for school nurses.* Scarborough, ME: National Association of School Nurses.

Back to school. (1996, May/June). *Sports 'n Spokes,* 11-17.

Betz, C.L. (1998). Adolescent transitions: A nursing concern. *Pediatr Nurs, 24*(1), 23-29.

Betz, C.L. (2000). California Healthy and Ready to Work Transition Health Care Guide. *Issues Compr Pediatr Nurs, 23,* 203-244.

Blum, R.W. (Ed). (2002). Improving transition for adolescents with special health care needs from pediatric to adult-centered health care. *Pediatrics, 100*(3, Suppl), 1301-1335.

Blum, R.W. (1997). Sexual health contraceptive needs of adolescents with chronic conditions. *Arch Pediatr Adolesc Med, 15*(3), 290-297.

Blum, R.W., Garell, D., Hodgman, C.H., Jorissen, T.W., Okinow, N.A., et al. (1993). Transitions from child-centered to adult-care systems for adolescents with chronic conditions: A position paper of the Society of Adolescent Medicine. *J Adolesc Health, 14*(7), 570-576.

Blum, R.W. & Garber, J. (1992). Chronically ill youth. In E.R. McAnarney et al. (Eds.). *Textbook of adolescent medicine.* Philadelphia: W.B. Saunders.

Blum, R.W., Resnick, M.D., Nelson, R., & St. Germaine, A. (1991). Family and peer issues among adolescents with spine bifida and cerebral palsy. *Pediatrics, 88,* 280-285.

Bridges, W. (1994). *Transitions—making sense of life's changes.* Reading, MA: Addison-Wesley.

Butterworth, J, Hagner, D., Helm, D., & Whelley, T. (2000). Workplace culture, social interactions, and supports for transition-age young adults. *Mental Retardation, 38*(4), 342-353.

Carnegie Council on Adolescent Development. (1995). *Great transitions: Preparing adolescents for a new century.* New York: Author.

Centers for Medicaid and Medicare. (2002). Web site: http://www.cms.hhs.gov.

Cowan, P.A., & Hetherington, M. (Eds.). (1991). *Family transitions.* Hillsdale, NJ: Lawrence Erlbaum Associates.

Cox, A. & Sawin, K.J. (1999). The school nurse. In S. DeFur & J. Patton (Eds.). *The relationship of school-based services to the transition process.* Austin, TX: Pro-Ed.

Denniston, S., & Enlow, C. (1995). *Making choices: a journal workbook for teens and young adults with spina bifida that provides opportunities for making choices about their lives.* Louisville, KY: Spina Bifida Association of Kentucky's Transition to Independence Project.

Farley, T., Vines, C., McCluer, S., Stefans, V., & Hunter, J. (1994). Secondary disabilities in Arkansans with spina bifida. *Eur J Surg, 40,* 39-40.

Faux, S.A. (1998). Historical overview of responses of children and their families to chronic illness. In M.E. Broome et al. (Eds.). *Children and families in health and illness.* Thousand Oaks, CA: Sage Publications.

Fishman, E. (2001). Aging out of coverage: Young adults with special health needs. *Health Affairs, 20*(6), 254-266.

Garwick, A.W., Patterson, J.M., Meschke, L.L., Bennett, F.C., & Blum, R.W. (2002). The uncertainty of preadolescents' chronic health conditions and family distress. *J Fam Nurs,* 11-31.

Giordano, B.P., Petrila, A., Banion, C.R., & Neuenkirchen, G. (1992). The challenge of transferring responsibility for diabetes management from parent to child. *J Pediatr Health Care, 6*(5, pt 1), 235-239.

Hallum, A. (1995). Disability and the transition to adulthood: Issues for the disabled child, the family, and the pediatrician. *Curr Probl Pediatr, 25*(1), 12-50.

Hardin, P. (1995a). *Becoming the me I want to be: A guide for youth with spina bifida and their parents.* Louisville, KY: Spina Bifida Association of Kentucky's Transition to Independence Project.

Hardin, P. (1995b). *Building skills: A guide for parents and professionals working with young people who have spina bifida.* Louisville, KY: Spina Bifida Association of Kentucky's Transition to Independence Project.

Healy, H. & Rigby, P. (1999). Promoting independence for teens and young adults with physical disabilities. *Can J Occup Ther, 66,* 24-249.

Henderson, C. (2001). *College freshman with disabilities: A biennial statistical profile.* Washington, DC: American Council on Education.

Henderson, C. (1995). *College freshmen with disabilities: A statistical profile.* Washington, DC: HEATH Resource Center.

Hostler, S.L. et al. (1989). Adolescent autonomy project: transition skills for adolescents with physical disabilities. *CAC, 18,* 12-18.

Igoe, J.B. (1994). School nursing. *Nurs Clin North Am, 29*(3), 443-458.

Johnson, C.P. (1996). Transition in adolescents with disabilities. In A. Capute & P. Accardo (Eds.). *Developmental disabilities in infancy and childhood* (2nd ed.). Baltimore, MD: Paul H. Brookes Publishing Co.

Kann, L., Kinchen, S.A., Williams, B.I., Ross, J.G., Lowry, R., et al. (2000). Youth risk behavior surveillance—United States, 1999. *MMWR CDC Surveill Summ, 9,* 49(5), 1-32.

Kaufman, M. (1995). Easy for you to say: Questions and answers for teens living with chronic illness or disability. Toronto: Key Porter Books, Ltd.

Keith, C. (2001). Suicide in teenagers: Assessment, management and prevention. *JAMA, 286,* 3120-3125.

Kelly, A.M., Kratz, B., Bielski, M., & Rinehart, P.A. (2002). Implementing transitions for youth with complex chronic conditions using the medical home model. *Pediatrics, 110*(6, Suppl), 1322-1327.

Lenz, B. (2001). The transition from adolescence to young adulthood: A theoretical perspective. *J Sch Nurs, 17*(6), 300-306.

Lollar, D.J. (Ed.) (1994). *Preventing secondary conditions associated with spina bifida or cerebral palsy.* Washington, DC: Spina Bifida Association of America.

Lynch, B.S. & Bonnie, R.J. (1994). *Growing up tobacco free: Preventing nicotine addiction in children and youth.* Washington, DC: National Academy Press.

Magyary D. & Brandt, P. (1996). A school-based self-management program for youth with chronic health conditions and their parents. *Can J Nurs Res, 28*(4), 57-77.

Meleis, A, Sawyer, L, Im, E. Hilfinger, D., & Schumacher, K. (2000) Experiencing transitions: An emerging middle-range theory. *ANS Adv Nurs Sci, 23*(1), 12-28.

Metzger, S.G. (1999). Individual with disabilities. In E. Youngkin et al. (Eds.). *Pharmacotherapeutics: A primary care clinical guide.* Stamford, CT: Appleton & Lange.

National Information Center for Children and Youth with Disabilities. (1997). The IDEA amendments of 1997. *News Digest, 26.* Washington, DC: Author.

National Organization on Disability (NOD). (2000). *The 2000 N.O.D./Harris Survey of Americans with Disabilities.* Washington, DC: Author. Available: www.NOD.org.

Newacheck, P.W. & Halfon, N. (1998). Prevalence and impact of disabling chronic conditions in childhood. *Am J Public Health, 88*(4), 610-617.

Nosek, M.A. (1995). Sexual abuse of women with physical disabilities. *Phys Med Rehabil, State of the Art Reviews, 9*(2), 487-501.

Orr, D.P. (1998). Helping adolescents toward adulthood. *Contemp Pediatr, 15*(5), 55-76.

Patterson, D.L. & Lanier, C. (1999). Adolescents' health transitions: Focus group study of teens and young adults with special health care needs. *Fam Comm Health, 22*(2), 43-58.

Pledgie, T.K., Tao, Q., & Freed, C. (1998). Documenting the need for transition services at an earlier age. *Work, a Journal of Prevention, Assessment and Rehabilitation, 10*(1), 15-19.

Powers, L.E., Singer, G.H., & Sowers, J.A. (1996). Self-competence and disability. In L. Powers, G. Singer, & J.A. Sowers (Eds.). *On the road to autonomy, promoting self-competence in children and youth with disabilities.* Baltimore: Paul H. Brookes.

Powers, L.E., Singer, G.H., & Todis, B. (1996). Reflections on competence, perspectives on successful adults. In L. Powers, G. Singer, & J.A. Sowers (Eds.). *On the road to autonomy, promoting self-competence in children and youth with disabilities.* Baltimore: Paul H. Brookes.

Powers, L.E. et al. (1996). TAKE CHARGE: A model for promoting self-determination among adolescents with challenges. In L. Powers, G. Singer, & J.A. Sowers (Eds.). *On the road to autonomy, promoting self-competence in children and youth with disabilities.* Baltimore: Paul H. Brookes.

Reiss, J., & Gibson, R. (2002). Health care transition: Destinations unknown. *Pediatrics, 111*(Suppl 6), 1307-1314.

SARDI: Substance abuse and students with a disability. (2002, October/November). *Information from HEATH,* 5-6.

Sawin, K.J. (1998). Health care concerns for women with physical disability and chronic illness. In E. Youngkin & M. Davis (Eds.). *Women's health: A primary care clinical guide* (2nd ed.). Stamford, CT: Appleton and Lange.

Sawin, K.J., Bellin, M., Roux, G., Buran, C.F., Brei, T.J., et al. (2002a). *The experience of parenting an adolescent with spina bifida: Trying to decide where to cut the umbilical cord and how much.* Unpublished manuscript. Virginia Commonwealth University.

Sawin, K.J., Brei, T.J., Buran, C.F., & Fastenau, P.S. (2002b). Factors associated with quality of life in adolescents with spina bifida. *J Holist Nurs, 20*(9), 279-304.

Sawin, K.J, Buran, C.F, Brei, T., & Fastenau, P. (2002c). Sexuality issues in adolescents with a chronic neurological condition. *J Perinat Educ, 11*(1), 22-34.

Sawin, K.J, Buran, C.F., Brei, T.J., & Fastenau, P.S. (2002d). *The development of the Adolescent Self Management and Independence Scale.* Unpublished manuscript. Virginia Commonwealth University.

Sawin, K.J. & Marshall, J. (1992). Developmental competence in adolescents with an acquired disability. *Rehabil Nurs Res J, 1,* 41-50.

Sawin, K.J., Metzger, S., & Pellock, J. (1996). The experience of living with epilepsy from an adolescent and parent's perspective. *Epelilepsia, 37*(Suppl 5), 86.

Sawin, K.J. et al. (1999). Transition planning for youth with chronic conditions: An interdisciplinary process. *National Academies of Practice Forum, 1*(3), 183-186.

Scal, P. (2002). Transition for youth with chronic conditions: Primary care physicians' approaches. *Pediatrics, 110*(Suppl 6), 1315-1321.

Schoen, C., et al. (1997). The Commonwealth Fund survey of the health of adolescent girls. New York: Louis Harris and Associates, Inc.

Schultz, A.W. & Liptak, G.S. (1998). Helping adolescents who have disabilities negotiate transitions to adulthood. *Issues Compr Pediatr Nurs, 21,* 187-201.

Schumacher, K.L. & Meleis, A.I. (1994). Transitions: A central concept in nursing, *IMAGE J Nurs Sch, 26*(2), 119-127.

Selder, F. (1989). Life transition theory: The resolution of uncertainty. *Nurs Health Care, 10,* 437-451.

Sobsey, D. (1994). *Violence and abuse.* Baltimore: Paul H. Brookes.

Spencer, A., Fife, R., & Rabinovich, C. (1995). The school experience of children with arthritis: Coping in the 1990s and transition into adulthood. *Pediatr Clin North Am, 42*(5), 1285-1298.

Steinberg, L. (2000). Family at adolescence: Transition and transformation. *J Adolesc Health, 27;* 170-178.

Stevenson, C.J., Pharoah, P.O., & Stevenson, R. (1997). Cerebral palsy—the transition from youth to adulthood. *Dev Med Child Neurol, 39*(5), 336-342.

Suris, J.C., Resnick, M.D., Cassuto, N., & Blum, R.W. (1996). Sexual behavior of adolescents with chronic disease and disability. *J Adolesc Health, 19*(2), 124-131.

U.S. Department of Education, Office of Special Education Programs. (2002). Annual report to Congress. Data analysis system (DANS): Web site: http://www.ideadata.org/tables24th/ar_ad3htm.

Vessey, J. & Miola, E.S. (1997). Teaching adolescents self-advocacy skills. *Pediatr Nurs, 23*(1), 53-56.

Viner, R. (1999). Transition from paediatric to adult care: Bridging the gaps or passing the buck. *Arch Dis Child, 81,* 271-275.

Wagner, M.M. & Blackorby, J. (1996). Transition from high school to work or college: how special education students fare. *Special Education for Students with Disabilities, 6*(1), 103-119.

Wehman, P., Targett, P., Eltzeroth, H., Green, H., Brooke, V., et al. (1999). Development of business supports for persons with mental retardation in the workplace. *Journal of Vocational Rehabilitation, 13*(3), 175-181.

Wehmeyer, J. (1996). Self-determination for youth with significant cognitive disabilities, from theory to practice. In L. Powers, G. Singer, & J. Sowers (Eds.). *On the road to autonomy, promoting self-competence in children and youth with disabilities.* Baltimore: Paul H. Brookes.

White, P.H. (2002). Access to health care: Health insurance considerations for young adults with special health care needs/disabilities. *Pediatrics, 110*(Suppl 6), 1328-1335.

Wirt, J., Choy, S., Gerald, D., Provasnik, S., Rooney, P., et al. (2002). *The condition of education.* Washington, DC: National Center for Education Statistics.

Wolkstein, D. (2002). *Second annual conference on substance abuse and co-existing disabilities. Baltimore RTTC in drugs and disability.* Dayton, OH: Wright State University.

Younger, J.B. (1991). A theory of mastery. *ANS Adv Nurs Sci, 14*(1), 76-89.

PART TWO

Chronic Conditions

10 Allergies

Elizabeth Sloand and Jennifer Thate

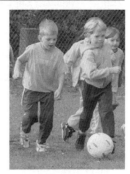

Etiology

Allergy is an unwanted response of the body to what is perceived as a "foreign" substance, or allergen. Allergens or foreign substances are not always harmful and can also trigger a positive response. A positive or beneficial response results in the development of immunity, whereas a negative or unwanted response results in the development of atopy or immunoglobulin E (IgE) mediated disease. The term "atopy" is often interchanged with allergy and contributes to the confusion surrounding the disease. Atopy indicates a hypersensitivity reaction that results in allergy symptoms (Kay, 2000) and often causes inflammation of the body tissues. Allergens are usually proteins, and numerous ones have been identified, including dust mites, animal dander, cockroaches, molds and spores, and pollen. Foods can also cause allergic symptoms and include cow's milk, eggs, peanut, soy, and others (Box 10-1). Although allergy is a broad topic, this chapter will specifically cover the common chronic conditions of allergic rhinoconjunctivitis and food allergies. Medication allergies, allergic reactions to insect bites and venom, and allergic dermatitis will not be comprehensively covered in this chapter.

Allergy is the result of an immunologically based acquired change in the body of an individual child. In most cases, the response to a foreign substance can be classified as either a TH1 or a TH2 response. This refers to the type of cytokine that is activated. A TH1 response is linked to the development of immunity, and a TH2 response contributes to atopy and allergy symptoms (Kay, 2000; Turvey, 2001). Allergic reactions all involve the production of antigen-specific mediators and a complex cascade of reactions. Histamines or other mediators are released from a mast cell or basophil, which causes inflammation. The resulting respiratory, dermatologic, and eye symptoms vary with the individual's sensitivities and may include sneezing; itching of the nose, ears, and eyes; rhinitis; wheezing; conjunctivitis; and rash. When the offending agent is a particular food, the child may experience abdominal pain, diarrhea, vomiting, and skin rashes, alone or in addition to respiratory symptoms.

Food allergies that are specifically IgE-mediated reactions occur in infants and children. However, this term is also commonly used for less specific food reactions and intolerances that are a result of nonallergic causes, such as pharmacologic, toxic, or metabolic mechanisms, as well as gastrointestinal intolerances, such as lactose. This chapter will specifically cover food allergies that are immunologically based. The most common food allergy is cow's milk, followed by eggs, peanut, soy, wheat,

tree nuts, fish, and shellfish (Chan et al, 2002; Spergel & Pawlowski, 2002).

In the past, many people have seen allergy, particularly allergic rhinitis and conjunctivitis, as an insignificant health issue. It has become increasingly clear, however, that it is a significant disease in many ways. As clinicians and researchers look deeper into this issue they are recognizing the tremendous impact allergy has, based on the number of persons affected, the economic burden, and the effect of the disease on quality of life and productivity. In children ages 12 years and under, allergy accounts for well over 2 billion dollars in direct health care costs (Ray et al, 1999). Total economic burden is much greater when the impact on school performance, family function, and parents' work productivity is considered.

Beyond the disease, with its cost, symptoms, and adverse effects of sedating medications, allergic rhinitis has a significant role in the development of life-threatening co-morbidities, such as asthma (Bousquet et al, 2001). Managing allergy more consistently and aggressively will lessen the burden associated with the disease and may also prevent the development of asthma or minimize its severity.

Known Genetic Etiology

A positive family history for allergy, especially maternal allergy, is a risk factor for the development of allergic disease (Sicherer, 2002). Although some genes have been recognized as possible contributors to the development of allergy, no definitive candidates have been identified (Bousquet et al, 2001; Turvey, 2001). There are two reasons for this. First, multiple genes in various combinations are responsible for a variety of allergy phenotypes. Second, it is difficult to interpret and compare studies that use different definitions and phenotypes of allergy (Bousquet et al, 2001; Haagerup et al, 2001; Turvey, 2001).

Although there is no specific gene identified for atopic disease and allergies, there is clear indication of a hereditary factor leading to increased susceptibility to asthma, eczema, and allergies in affected families. There are two methods for identifying the genes responsible for allergy. One is a search for candidate genes, genes that are in regions known to be involved in the immunologic response to allergens. The second is a genome-wide search for potentially involved genes (Bousquet et al, 2001).

Atopy has been linked to some human leukocyte antigen (HLA) histocompatibility types and various chromosome locations (Behrman et al, 2000). Researchers have recently been turning their attention to the multiple factors that either impact

---
BOX 10-1
Common Allergens

ENVIRONMENTAL ALLERGENS
Dust mites
Animal dander
Cockroaches
Molds and spores
Pollen

FOOD ALLERGENS
Cow's milk
Eggs
Peanuts, tree nuts
Soy
Wheat
Fish and shellfish

---

the expression of particular genes or trigger their expression. Scientists are targeting various chromosomes and genes as potential contributors to atopy. Work by Haagerup (Haagerup et al, 2001) has suggested that chromosome 16 is not associated with the development of atopy despite the previous work suggesting that it is. Many other genes are still under investigation. It is likely that multiple genes are responsible for various parts of the inflammatory pathway (including inhibitors, modifiers, and enhancers) and that different combinations of such genes are responsible within a particular individual or family.

Understanding allergy and the rising prevalence will depend not only on continued research in the field of genetics, but also on a greater understanding of the contributing environmental factors. Clearly, the dramatic rise in disease prevalence cannot be attributed to an equally significant change in the existing gene pool (Alm et al, 1999; Doull, 2001; Troye-Blomberg, 2002; Turvey, 2001).

Incidence and Prevalence

Allergy is the most common chronic illness in children (Aria Workshop Report, 2001). More than 40 million people in the United States have allergies, and most of those had an onset in infancy or childhood (Berger, 2001a; Schoenwetter, 2000). The incidence and prevalence of allergy are very low until the age of 2 years. From the age of 2 years and extending throughout childhood, there is a steady increase in the prevalence of allergy (Berger, 2001b; Kulig et al, 2000).

Rhinoconjunctivitis affects up to an estimated 40% of all children (Aria Workshop Report, 2001; Berger, 2001a; Bernstein & Shelov, 1996). Exact numbers are elusive because of varying definitions of the disorder, underdiagnosis, and the existence of co-morbid conditions (Schoenwetter, 2000; Wang et al, 2002). Clinicians and epidemiologists report that the prevalence of allergic rhinitis has increased worldwide over the past few decades (Fineman, 2002; Schoenwetter, 2000; Skoner, 2001).

Food allergy affects approximately 6% of all children (Chan et al, 2002; Yale & La Valle, 2002). Prevalence in infancy is higher, with approximately 2% to 8% affected by cow's milk or soy allergy. Food allergy decreases to less than 2% by

adulthood (Spergel et al, 2002). These numbers reflect those allergies confirmed by history and challenges, and contrast with the number of people who believe they have a food allergy but are not formally diagnosed, which includes approximately 25% to 30% of Americans (Spergel & Pawlowski, 2002). Peanut allergy, which is most often responsible for serious and fatal reactions, has a prevalence of 0.4% to 0.7% (Primeau et al, 2000).

The rising numbers of children affected by allergic rhinitis parallels the increase in atopic diseases in general (Berger, 2001b). Although the reasons for these increases are not fully known, they are most likely multifactorial. Some theories include the increased insulation of homes, the rising popularity of carpeting and upholstered furniture, and a change in lifestyle that results in children spending more time indoors (Schoenwetter, 2000). These factors put children in increasing contact with rising levels of common indoor allergens, such as house dust mites and animal dander.

One of the leading proposals to explain the increasing prevalence of atopy is the hygiene hypothesis. Encompassed in this hypothesis are several theories. One theory proposes a relationship among the increased use of antibiotics, the subsequent decrease in infection, and the increased prevalence of atopy. Many writers have suggested that decreased exposure to infection discourages the development of TH1-type cytokine response and in turn increases the TH2 response, leading to atopy (Turvey, 2001; Doull, 2001; Holt et al, 1999; Illi et al, 2001; Kay, 2000; Martinez & Holt, 1999).

A second theory involves family size and its inverse relationship to allergy. Several studies have suggested that an increased number of siblings results in a decrease in atopy, particularly for the younger siblings (Bodner et al, 1998; Jarvis et al, 1997; Svanes et al, 1999). Scientists theorize that an increased number of siblings directly correlates with increased exposure to infection and therefore a switch from a TH2 default response to a TH1 immunity response. Similarly, exposure to pets at birth or early in life has been related to a decrease in atopic diseases later in childhood, including allergic rhinitis, asthma, and eczema (Nafstad et al, 2001; Ownby et al, 2002; Platts-Mills, 2002; Weiss, 2002). Such early pet exposure may have a protective effect against the development of allergy.

Third, researchers found that there is a lower prevalence of atopy and allergic rhinitis in children who have lived on farms (Doull, 2001; Leynaert et al, 2001). Other reports also suggest that an anthroposophic lifestyle is protective against atopy into adulthood (Alm et al, 1999). An anthroposophic lifestyle restricts the use of antibiotics, limits immunizations, and includes a diet that contains live lactobacilli because of the production and preservation of foods (Alm et al, 1999). Although it is yet to be determined which aspects of this lifestyle affect the decreased development of atopy, the possibilities include diet, decreased antibiotic use, having had measles, increased allergen exposure at a young age, and increased exposure to infection via a greater number of siblings (Alm et al, 1999; Leynaert et al, 2001).

Other hypotheses to explain the rising prevalence of allergy and atopy include increased exposure to pollution (Hajat et al, 2001), increased early vitamin D exposure (Wjst & Dold,

1999), and prenatal influences on immune system development (Troye-Blomberg, 2002).

Clinical Manifestations at Time of Diagnosis (Box 10-2)

Allergic Rhinitis (Hay Fever)

Symptoms of allergic rhinitis include nasal itching, nasal congestion, rhinorrhea with clear nasal discharge, and bouts of sneezing. Clinical signs include pale, bluish, boggy nasal mucosa and turbinates; clear nasal discharge; and nasal obstruction. Specific signs of allergic rhinitis include a crease across the nose (referred to as an "allergic salute"), allergic shiners (dark circles under the eyes, Figure 10-1), Dennie sign (lines under the lower lid margin), throat clicking or clucking, and nose twitching and facial grimacing. Experts have made recent attempts to standardize the definition of allergic rhinitis in order to ultimately enhance the quality of life for those affected. The International Consensus Report defines allergic rhinitis as presenting with one or more of the classic symptoms (e.g., nasal itching, rhinorrhea, nasal obstruction, sneezing), with the affected person exhibiting at least two of the symptoms on most days (Wang et al, 2002). Symptoms can be seasonal or year-round. The World Health Organization (WHO) recommends using the terms "intermittent allergic rhinitis" and "persistent allergic rhinitis" instead of the older terms of "seasonal" and "perennial" (Box 10-3) (Aria Workshop Report, 2001).

Occasionally, a child may present with epistaxis, especially in the winter, because of excessive dryness in the home. Some children exhibit a characteristic facial development. This adenoid-type facies (Figure 10-2) is a result of chronic nasal

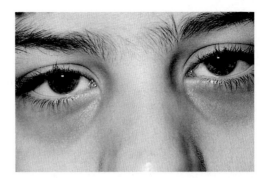

FIGURE 10-1 Allergic shiners, or dark circles beneath the eyes, in patient with allergic rhinitis. (From Zitelli, B.J. & Davis, H.W. [2002]. *Atlas of pediatric physical diagnosis* [4th ed.]. St. Louis: Mosby. Reprinted with permission.)

BOX 10-2

Clinical Manifestations at Time of Diagnosis

ALLERGIC RHINITIS
Symptoms
  Nasal itching
  Nasal congestion
  Clear nasal discharge
  Sneezing
Clinical signs
  Blue or pale boggy nasal mucosa and turbinates
  Clear nasal discharge
  Nasal obstruction
  Allergic salute
  Allergic shiners and Dennie sign
  Throat clicking and facial grimacing

ALLERGIC CONJUNCTIVITIS
Symptoms
  Itching of eyes
  Tearing
Clinical signs
  Bilateral redness of conjunctiva
  Profuse watery discharge
  Cobblestone appearance of palpebral conjunctiva
General symptoms
  Dry sore throat
  Itchy throat or ears
  Dry cough
  Ear popping and fullness
  Headache

FOOD ALLERGY
Symptoms
  Stomachache
  Nausea or diarrhea

  Sneezing
  Nasal congestion
  Feeding difficulties
Clinical signs
  Rash
  Impaired growth in infants

SKIN MANIFESTATIONS
Symptoms
  Pruritus (varies in severity)
  Rash may be very transient, with each lesion lasting less than 24 hours
Clinical signs
  Edematous plaques or wheals with pale centers
  Erythematous borders
  Rash may be confluent

BEHAVIORAL MANIFESTATIONS
Symptoms
  Irritability, sleep disorders
  Fearfulness, anxiety, fatigue
Clinical sign
  Decreased ability to concentrate

ANAPHYLAXIS
Symptoms
  Rash, pruritus
  Cough
  Difficulty breathing
Clinical signs
  Facial edema
  Lip, throat, and tongue swelling
  Urticaria
  Wheezing

BOX 10-3
Classification of Allergic Rhinitis

"Intermittent" means that symptoms are present:
   <4 days/wk,
   or
   <4 wk
"Persistent" means that symptoms are present:
   >4 days/wk
   and
   >4 wk
"Mild" means that none of the following items are present:
   Sleep disturbance
   Impairment of daily activities, leisure, and/or sport
   Impairment of work or school
   Troublesome symptoms
"Moderate-severe" means that one or more of the following items are present:
   Sleep disturbance
   Impairment of daily activities, leisure, and/or sport
   Impairment of work or school
   Troublesome symptoms

From Aria Workshop Report. (2001). Allergic rhinitis and its impact on asthma. *Journal of Allergy and Clinical Immunology, 108*(5), 1-205. Reprinted with permission.

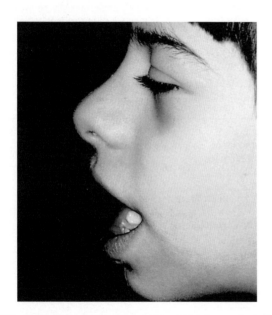

FIGURE 10-2 Characteristic adenoid-type facies in a patient with long-standing allergic rhinitis. Note the open mouth and gaping habitus. (From Zitelli, B.J. & Davis, H.W. [2002]. *Atlas of pediatric physical diagnosis* [4th ed.]. St. Louis: Mosby. Reprinted with permission.)

obstruction and subsequent mouth breathing, which forces currents of breathed air through the mouth and changes the growth pattern of the soft bones of the face. The result typically includes an open gaping mouth, dental malocclusion, and a high arched hard palate.

Allergic Conjunctivitis

Allergic conjunctivitis may present in combination with allergic rhinitis, or it may occur alone. The hallmark symptom is significant itching of the eyes. In addition, there is usually bilateral redness with profuse clear discharge. Stringy white mucus can sometimes be seen in the conjunctival sac, and the conjunctiva often has a "cobblestone" appearance (McManaway & Frankel, 2001).

General Symptoms

In addition to rhinitis and/or conjunctivitis, other more general symptoms may be present. These include dry sore throat, itching of throat and ears, dry cough, ear popping and fullness, and headache (Nash, 1998). Any of these symptoms may be intermittent or persistent. Symptoms may be present for weeks or months and may look like "a cold that never quite goes away." There is typically no fever or adenopathy to accompany these symptoms.

Food Allergy

Food allergy may manifest with a wide variety of mild symptoms, such as skin rash, stomachache, nausea, diarrhea, nasal congestion, and sneezing. Some children have much more severe symptoms, such as respiratory distress and anaphylaxis. Usually severe symptoms appear immediately after ingestion of the causative food. Infants who are allergic to cow's milk or soy may have colic, feeding difficulties, vomiting, and impaired growth.

Skin Manifestations

Urticaria (or hives) that is IgE mediated is sometimes caused by foods, although medications are the most frequent causative agents (Hooper, 1999). The clinician should carefully elicit a complete history; however, the exact cause of the lesions is often not discovered. Urticarial lesions appear as edematous plaques or wheals with pale centers and erythematous borders. The rash may be confluent, and lesions are transient. An individual lesion lasts for less than 24 hours, and new lesions may be continually appearing, giving the rash a sort of migratory nature. Pruritus may be present and varies in severity.

Behavioral Manifestations

Some children with allergy show behavioral manifestations, such as irritability, sleep disorders, and decreased ability to concentrate. Children may be so uncomfortable during allergy season that they act out at school or home. Shyness, depression, fearfulness, anxiety, and fatigue have also been associated with allergy (Fireman, 2000). Clinicians must take care not to confuse these symptoms with those of attention deficit hyperactivity disorder or other behavioral disorders (see Chapter 12). Many believe that these behavioral signs may be due to a lack of sleep or to the use of over-the-counter medicines, many of which have sedating side effects.

Anaphylactic Reactions

Anaphylaxis is a systemic reaction to an allergen, rather than an organ- or system-limited response. Although rare, occurring in approximately 0.6% of children and up to 2% of the general population, it can be life threatening (Gold & Sainsbury, 2000). In children, studies indicate that at least one half of anaphylactic events occur at home, with the most common offending agent being food (Dibs & Baker, 1997; Novembre et al, 1998). Peanuts and tree nuts are by far the most common causative foods, followed by seafood and milk (Bock et al, 2001; Novembre et al, 1998; Sampson, 2002). Initial symptoms of anaphylaxis are predominantly dermatologic, which are then followed by respiratory symptoms (Dibs & Baker, 1997; Novembre et al, 1998). Most frequently seen are facial edema, urticaria, pruritus, lip swelling, tongue swelling, difficulty breathing, wheezing, cough, and throat swelling (Dibs & Baker, 1997). Reactions are more likely to be fatal in children and adolescents with a history of asthma (Bock et al, 2001; Dibs & Baker, 1997). Therefore those children with asthma who concurrently experience food allergy should be identified as high risk for an anaphylactic reaction. Parents and caregivers should be educated on the potential signs and symptoms of anaphylaxis in order to ensure rapid recognition and treatment.

Treatment

The first line of defense against allergies is avoidance (Box 10-4). In some cases, such as the child with a dust mite allergy, that may be nearly impossible. Other potential components of the treatment plan include medications, education of child and parents, referral to an allergist, and immunotherapy ("allergy shots"). The treatment plan must be individualized for each child and developed in partnership with the family and affected child (Box 10-5).

Avoidance

Rhinitis and Conjunctivitis. The health care provider can assist the family in identifying the allergens for a particular child and then endeavoring to avoid, minimize, or control them. Families can try to avoid aerosol products as much as possible. Tobacco smoke is a great offender for many children with respiratory allergy, and smoking should not be allowed in the family's home or car. Molds can be controlled using dehumidifiers, especially in the basement of the home.

Furry pets, unfortunately, are common allergens. The best clinical option is to keep all such pets out of the home. When this is not acceptable to the child or family, the pet should at least be confined to areas of the house where the child is least present. At the very minimum, the animal must be kept out of

---

BOX 10-4
Avoidance of Allergens at Home

Do not use aerosol products.
Utilize humidifiers in damp places, such as basements.
Do not allow smoking in the family's home or car.
Control dust with vacuuming, air filtration systems, wet mopping, and keeping dust catchers, such as stuffed toys and open shelving, out of bedrooms.
Keep windows closed or use air conditioning.
Enclose pillows and mattresses in hypoallergenic covers.

BOX 10-5
Allergy Treatment Strategies

Avoidance
Medication
Parent and child education
Immunotherapy

---

the bedroom. Frequent washing of a cat has been proposed and studied as a possible strategy; however, clinical studies have not shown this to be effective even when done weekly (Klucka et al, 1995).

Dust mite is the most common indoor allergen, and frequent cleaning to control house dust can be helpful in decreasing symptoms. Vacuuming, air filtration systems, and wet mopping of wood floors are worthwhile strategies. Bedrooms, in particular, should be kept free of as many "dust catchers" as possible, including stuffed toys, carpets, big pillows, and open shelving filled with books and toys. In addition, mattresses and pillows can be encased in hypoallergenic covers, and only hypoallergenic pillows and bedding ought to be used. Some studies investigating measures to decrease dust mite exposure indicate that such efforts are not effective in improving asthma (see Chapter 11) (2001). Very few studies have been conducted to investigate the same in allergic rhinitis. Limited clinical trials show that measures to avoid dust mites as described above may be somewhat effective in the reduction of symptoms, but more work needs to be done in this area to provide clear recommendations regarding the role of dust mite control in the management of disease (Sheikh et al, 2002) (Box 10-4).

When a child has allergies to specific seasonal allergens, such as various pollens, it is wise to limit time outdoors during days with high pollen counts. Keeping windows closed and using an air conditioner will also help control symptoms.

Food Allergy. Most children with food allergy must completely avoid all offending foods. Careful reading of food labels is essential (see Resources), and children must be taught to avoid particular foods as they grow more independent and spend more time away from home and parents. They must learn to avoid any sharing of foods in daycare, in school, or at the homes of friends. Clinicians must educate parents, schools, daycare providers, and any other caretakers of the affected child, so that they are fully informed of significant food allergies (Jackson, 2002). Special care must be taken when eating in restaurants, because restaurant food is an increasingly important source of allergens, particularly peanuts and tree nuts, and these agents are frequently "hidden" in foods and difficult to visually identify (Bock et al, 2001; Furlong et al, 2001). Parents and caretakers must routinely ask about food components in restaurants in order to avoid serious or fatal food reactions. For highly allergic children, ingestion may not even be required for all allergic reactions, since reactions have been reported following superficial contact or merely being in the vicinity of the offending food (Furlong et al, 2001).

Infancy presents special challenges. Breast feeding is best in almost all cases. Babies may have allergic reactions to infant formulas, and changes to soy-based formula are sometimes necessary. The infant who is soy allergic must be switched to protein hydrolysate formulas. When babies who are at a high risk for allergic disease because of a positive atopic family history are fed exclusively with breast milk or partial whey hydrolysate formula, there is some evidence that they will have a lower incidence of atopic disease and food allergy. However, it seems that this effect may not persist throughout childhood (Chandra, 1997). Although all the lifelong consequences of infant feeding are not perfectly clear, a conservative approach of advocating breast milk or partial whey hydrolysate formula seems reasonable for the high-risk infant (De Jong et al, 2002; Zeiger & Heller, 1995).

Food allergies may manifest as reactions to the foods the breast-feeding mother eats. The mother may need to eliminate certain offending foods from her diet. In extreme cases, the health care provider may recommend a hypoallergenic infant formula, such as Alimentum, Nutramigen, or Pregestimil (Dibs & Baker, 1997; Zeiger, 1999; Zeiger et al, 1999).

Cow's milk allergy is particularly significant in infancy, when a child's nutritional need for milk is great. It must be carefully diagnosed, since elimination of it from the diet may have serious implications for growth and development.

Medications

Rhinitis and Conjunctivitis. Many over-the-counter and prescription medications can be employed in controlling allergy symptoms (Table 10-1). Antihistamine preparations are the mainstay of treatment, and there are numerous ones to choose from. They are used to target clinical symptoms such as sneezing, rhinorrhea, and pruritus (Nash, 1998) that are a result of histamine release in the allergic response (Figure 10-3).

Most over-the-counter antihistamines are readily available, effective, and reasonable in price. They are prepared in both tablet and liquid form and include diphenhydramine hydrochloride (Benadryl), brompheniramine maleate (Dimetapp), clemastine fumarate (Tavist), and chlorpheniramine maleate (Chlor-Trimeton). These first-generation antihistamines may be reasonable choices for intermittent, mild symptoms or acute flares that do not require daily medications. The most common troublesome side effect of these medications is drowsiness (Van Cauwenberge et al, 2000). Because of their sedative effect, bedtime dosing is often recommended to avoid daytime drowsiness and allow children to be awake and alert for school and activities. The practice of using first-generation antihistamines is not well supported in the literature, and use of the second-generation antihistamines is encouraged when possible (Nash, 1998).

There are many second-generation antihistamines available. They are not necessarily more effective, but most have minimal sedating side effects and a longer duration of action and so are better choices for the child with more severe or persistent symptoms. Those that have been approved for use in young children include fexofenadine hydrochloride (Allegra), loratadine (Claritin), and cetirizine hydrochloride (Zyrtec). Cetirizine appears to be more sedating than the other two (Philpot, 2000).

Rhinitis. Topical nasal steroid sprays are the first-line treatment for persistent nasal symptoms, especially nasal discharge, obstruction, and sneezing (Holm & Fokkens, 2001). They include budesonide (Rhinocort Nasal, Rhinocort Aqua), fluticasone propionate (Flonase), mometasone furoate monohydrate (Nasonex), and triamcinolone acetonide (Nasocort AQ). Several are now available in long-acting preparations. As with all steroids, the lowest possible dose should be employed to minimize side effects. The health community remains cautious about the use of steroids in children, and there are no topical steroids recommended for allergy use in children less than 6 years of age (Nash, 1998; Childhood Asthma Management Program Research Group, 2000). Studies continue to be conducted to investigate the impact of steroid use on children's growth and on the suppression of the hypothalamic-pituitary-adrenal axis (Agertoft & Pedersen, 2000; Skoner et al, 2000). Since there is still uncertainty on this issue, the use of nasal steroids should be time limited and only be employed when symptoms are persistent and have a significant impact on daily functioning such that the benefits outweigh the potential risks.

There are a variety of topical nonsteroidal nasal sprays to choose from to manage the symptoms of rhinitis. Cromolyn sodium (Nasalcrom) spray, a nonsteroidal, antiinflammatory agent, is a mast cell stabilizer. It is a very safe medication; however, its usefulness is limited by the need for frequent dosing (Berger, 2001b). For full effect it must be used four to six times per day during the allergy season or continually for perennial symptoms. Adherence to such a rigorous medication schedule is nearly impossible for children who spend most full days in daycare, school, or camp. Another option in the form of a nasal spray is azelastine hydrochloride (Astelin), a topical antihistamine that can be used in children 5 years of age and older.

Decongestants, both oral and topical, may be helpful for a child with significant nasal congestion. Oral decongestants can be used alone or in a combination preparation with antihistamines. Caretakers must be alert for irritability, a frequent side effect of decongestants (Staff of Physicians, 2001). Decongestant nasal sprays are readily available over the counter in pharmacies and are very effective for fast relief of nasal symptoms. They can cause severe rebound congestion (rhinitis medicamentosa) when used for more than 3 days. Their use must be restricted to 1 or 2 days when optimum nasal clearing is absolutely essential. For example, the child who has a championship soccer game and another who is to perform in a vocal concert may be reasonable candidates for a few doses of a decongestant nasal spray. Providers must emphasize the significance of the rebound effect in these preparations to the child and parent, and their long-term or repeated use must be strongly discouraged.

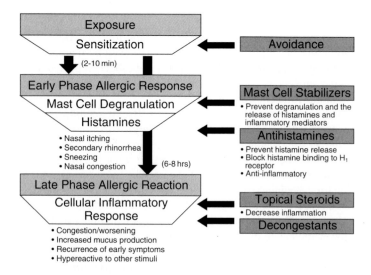

FIGURE 10-3 Etiology of allergic response and the corresponding treatment.

TABLE 10-1
Medications Used in the Treatment of Allergic Rhinoconjunctivitis

	Route	Age	Dosing	Adverse Effects
Systemic Antihistamines				
Allegra (fexofenadine HCl)	Oral	≥12 yr	180 mg once daily or 60 mg twice daily	Headache
		6-11 yr	30 mg twice daily	
Claritin *OTC* (loratadine)	Oral	≥6 yr	10 mg once daily	≥12 yr: headache, somnolence, fatigue, dry mouth
				<12 yr: nervousness, wheezing, fatigue
		2-5 yr	5 mg (1 tsp) once daily	≥12 yr: somnolence, fatigue, dry mouth
Zyrtec (cetirizine HCl)	Oral	≥12 yr	5-10 mg once daily	<12 yr: headache, somnolence
		6-11 yr	5-10 mg (1-2 tsp) once daily	
		2-5 yr	2.5 mg ({1/2} tsp) once daily; max 5 mg/day	
Benadryl *OTC* (diphenhydramine HCl)	Oral	≥12 yr	25-50 mg every 4-6 hr; max 300 mg/day	Drowsiness, excitability
		6-11 yr	12.5-25 mg every 4-6 hr; max 150 mg/day	
Chlor-Trimeton *OTC* (chlorpheniramine maleate)	Oral	6-12 yr	1/2 tablet (2 mg) every 4-6 hr	Drowsiness, excitability
		>12 yr	4 mg every 4-6 hr	
Dimetapp *OTC*	Oral	6 mo+	Liquid by weight	CNS stimulation, dizziness, blurred vision, palpitations, GI upset, anxiety, weakness, insomnia, excitability, drowsiness, anticholinergic effects
		6-12 yr	1 capsule every 4 hr, maximum 4 doses/day	
Tavist *OTC* (clemastine fumarate)	Oral	≥12 yr	1 tablet (1.34 mg) twice daily	Drowsiness, excitability
Topical Antihistamines				
Astelin (azelastine HCl)	Nose	≥12 yr	2 sprays per nostril twice daily	Bitter taste, headache, somnolence
		5-11 yr	1 spray per nostril twice daily	
Emadine (emedastine)	Eyes	≥3 yr	1 drop up to 4× daily	Transient burning, stinging, discomfort
Livostin (levocabastine HCl)	Eyes	>12 yr	1 drop per affected eye twice daily	Local irritation immediately after instillation
Topical Mast Cell Stabilizers				
Nasalcrom (cromolyn sodium)	Nose	≥2 yr	1 spray each nostril every 4-6 hr; prevention: begin 1 wk before exposure to known allergen	Transient stinging, sneezing
Opticrom (cromolyn sodium)	Eyes	≥4 yr	1-2 drops per affected eye 4× to 6× daily	Transient stinging or burning on instillation
Alomide (lodoxamide tromethamine)	Eyes	≥2 yr	1-2 drops 4× daily for up to 4 mo	Burning, stinging, or discomfort
Zaditor (ketotifen fumarate)	Eyes	>3 yr	1 drop per affected eye every 8-12 hr	Conjunctival infection, headache, rhinitis
Alocril	Eyes	≥3 yr	1-2 drops in affected eyes 4× daily	Headache, burning, irritation, stinging, unpleasant taste, nasal congestion
Topical Steroids				
Flonase (fluticasone propionate)	Nose	≥12 yr	2 sprays per nostril once daily	Epistaxis, headache, pharyngitis
		4-11 yr	1 spray per nostril once daily	
Nasocort AQ (triamcinolone acetonide)	Nose	≥12 yr	2 sprays per nostril once daily	Epistaxis, pharyngitis, increase in cough
		6-12 yr	1 spray per nostril once daily	
Nasonex (mometasone furoate monohydrate)	Nose	≥12 yr	2 sprays per nostril once daily	Epistaxis, headache, viral infection, pharyngitis
Rhinocort (budesonide)	Nose	3-11 yr	1 spray per nostril once daily	
Nasal inhaler		≥6 yr	2 sprays per nostril twice daily (morning, evening) or 4 sprays per nostril once daily (morning)	Epistaxis, nasal irritation, pharyngitis, cough
Aqua Nasal Spray		≥6 yr	1 spray per nostril once daily	Epistaxis, pharyngitis, bronchospasm, cough, nasal irritation
Mast Cell Antihistamine				
Patanol (olopatadine HCl)	Eyes	≥3 yr	1 drop per affected eye 2× daily	Headache, asthenia, blurred vision
NSAID				
Acular (ketorolac tromethamine)	Eyes	Adults	1 drop per affected eye 4× daily	Transient stinging and burning on instillation
Anaphylaxis				
Epinephrine Auto-injector	IM, thigh only	>30 kg	EpiPen, 0.3 mg	Palpitations, tachycardia, sweating, nausea and vomiting, respiratory difficulty, pallor, dizziness, weakness, tremor, headache, apprehension, nervousness, anxiety
		<30 kg	EpiPen Jr, 0.15 mg	

From Crisalida, T., Kaline, M.A., & Turkeltaub, M. (2002). *Allergy and asthma pocket guide.* New York: Adelphi Inc. Modified with permission.
OTC, Over the counter; *CNS,* central nervous system; *GI,* gastrointestinal; *NSAID,* nonsteroidal antiinflammatory drug; *IM,* intramuscular.

Conjunctivitis. A wide variety of eye drops are available to relieve symptoms of allergic conjunctivitis. The mast cell stabilizers are very effective and include cromolyn sodium (Opticrom), lodoxamide tromethamine (Alomide), nedocromil sodium (Alocril), and ketotifen fumarate (Zaditor). They vary in frequency of administration, which can be particularly important with a younger child who is fearful or combative with eye drops. Some of the mast cell stabilizers are approved for children as young as 2 years old. Olopatadine HCl (Patanol) is a mast cell stabilizer that also has antihistamine properties. Nonsteroidal antiinflammatory eye drops can also be employed and include ketorolac tromethamine (Acular). Another classification of eye drops is the antihistamines, such as emedastine difumarate (Emadine) and levocabastine (Livostin). Eye drops containing steroids are not usually recommended for children. In addition to pharmacologic treatment, the child may gain some relief from ocular itching with the application of cool compresses, especially during a period of acute discomfort.

Food Allergies. Medications are used in two specific circumstances related to food allergies: to treat food-induced urticaria and to give immediate treatment for anaphylaxis. In the case of food-induced urticaria, a course of oral antihistamines, usually diphenhydramine, is useful to decrease itching and inflammation.

Anaphylaxis. The key to treating anaphylaxis is early recognition and rapid treatment with self-administered epinephrine (EpiPen, EpiPen Jr). (Lee & Greenes, 2000). Unfortunately studies show that in many cases epinephrine is not readily available or used because of lack of prescribing by providers, poor instruction and lack of understanding on how to use the device, or not having the device on hand when an episode occurs. In addition, there is confusion on the part of the provider regarding whether to use the EpiPen or EpiPen Jr (Sicherer et al, 2000).

Injectable epinephrine for the treatment of anaphylaxis should be dosed at 0.01 mg/kg. The EpiPen Jr is 0.15 mg, and the EpiPen is 0.3 mg. There is a lack of definitive guidelines from the academic, clinical, or pharmaceutical literature regarding what dose to use when a child's weight does not fit in either dose category. For example, a 23-kg child would be underdosed using the EpiPen Jr and overdosed using the standard EpiPen. In this case, determining which to prescribe is guided by the provider's clinical judgment. Factors to consider are weight of the child, severity of previous reactions (although this can be misleading), and proximity to an emergency facility (Simons et al, 2002). Epinephrine should never be withheld in an emergency because of concerns regarding possible overdosing. Whereas the potential side effects of an overdose of epinephrine are minimal, the potential consequence of withholding treatment is death.

In order to facilitate proper administration, use of the EpiPen device should be clearly taught and reinforced during routine visits (Figure 10-4). The most critical steps for proper use of the device include removing the gray cap, placing the black end flush against the thigh, applying pressure to the end opposite the black end until a click is heard, and holding the autoinjector in place for 10 seconds (Gold & Sainsbury, 2000). After administration of epinephrine the child should be immediately transported to an emergency facility.

1. Pull off gray safety cap.

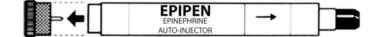

2. Place black tip on outer thigh (always apply to thigh).

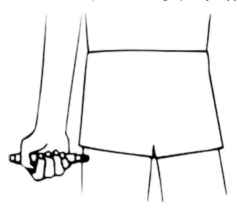

3. Using a quick motion, press hard into thigh until Auto-Injector mechanism functions. Hold in place and count to 10. The EpiPen® unit should then be removed and discarded. Massage the injection area for 10 seconds.

How to Dispose of an EpiPen®
After using an EpiPen®, throw away the gray cap. Place a penny in the bottom of the plastic tube, slip the EpiPen® into the tube, and close it. Return the used EpiPen® to your doctor for disposal.

FIGURE 10-4 How to treat anaphylaxis with self-administered epinephrine. (From The Food Allergy & Anaphylaxis Network, www.foodallergy.org/anaphylaxis.html. Reprinted with permission.)

Education of Child and Parent

As with almost all chronic conditions, the education and involvement of the family are essential parts of the treatment plan and will promote the optimum health of affected children (Scadding et al, 2000). All family members must have some understanding of the condition, its chronic nature, the offending agents (allergens), and the goals of treatment. When working on environmental measures, the family may benefit from additional home-based intervention. For instance, clinicians can seek out the local chapter of an allergy support organization, local health department, university program, or home health agency with an appropriate supportive or intervention program.

A clear understanding of any medications to be used and their proper administration is critical. For instance, some of the nasal sprays and eye drops are preventive in nature, such as steroid nasal sprays and mast cell stabilizer ophthalmic preparations. The family and child must understand that for optimum effectiveness, the medications should not be used only when symptoms are present but must be used regularly throughout the allergy season.

Young children can be very fearful of eye drops, kicking and fighting to prevent administration. Clinicians can help teach caretakers the least traumatic ways to administer eye drops. First, the parent must hold the lower lid down and then dispense the drop into the pocket created by the palpebral and bulbar

Education Points Regarding Allergy and Use of Medications

DISEASE

Parent and child should have an age-appropriate understanding of the chronic nature of allergy and role of allergens

Identification of allergens for individual child and best strategies for avoidance

MEDICATIONS

Action of each medication, and whether it is preventive or prn

Proper timing, frequency, and indications for each medication

No sharing of prescription medicines with family members or friends

---

conjunctiva. Parents must be cautioned not to splash the eye drop into the center of the eye. Another effective method, useful in the younger child who has his or her eyes squeezed shut, is to simply dispense the eye drop on the closed eye, holding the child's head back. Eventually, the child will open his or her eyes, and the drop will roll into the eye.

Children and parents must be proficient in reading food labels when the child has food allergies. This is particularly important with prepared foods, which often have a long list of ingredients. Parents must also be able to identify hidden sources of foods in unfamiliar ingredients (see Resources). In addition, they must be assertive in talking with restaurant managers and food handlers at daycare, school, camp, and other such arenas. Clinicians can educate the children and parents about these matters and demonstrate needed skills.

A vast array of family education and support groups are available in many regions of the United States, and there is a growing list of reliable Web sites (see Resources). Box 10-6 highlights the most important teaching points that should be covered by providers when caring for children with allergy.

Immunotherapy

Immunotherapy is an effective treatment in carefully selected situations. Children who have severe disease, and for whom avoidance and medications are not effective in relieving nasal symptoms, or children who experience recurrent related infections such as otitis media, sinusitis, or pharyngitis, may benefit from immunotherapy (Kay, 2000; Van Cauwenberge, 1998; Nash, 1998). In these cases, a pediatric allergist is consulted and will usually test the child for specific allergies, and an individualized serum will be prepared. The serum is administered in a series of frequent injections, which desensitizes the child to the specific allergens. Immunotherapy is most effective for pollen allergies, at approximately 80% effectiveness, but may also be used for dust mite allergies, with approximately 50% effectiveness (Turvey, 2001; Van Cauwenberge, 1998). Allergy shots must be administered frequently and for several years, so they must be employed judiciously. Parents and providers can work together to help children and adolescents through the difficulties of immunotherapy. A developmental approach will help the child to understand the basic facts on immunotherapy and the reasons that parents and providers believe it is a good idea for them. Such information will help the child accept and cooperate with the plan of frequent injections, in hoping that the resultant decrease in allergy symptoms will be worth the

initial investment and pain. Examples of developmentally based client education include allowing a young child to inject a doll or teddy bear with a play syringe, use of a star chart that marks successful injection visits and is linked to a reward system, and recommending one of the child- or teen-focused allergy Web sites (see Web sites in Resources). There is also a risk of serious reactions with immunotherapy, including anaphylaxis, especially in the early induction stage of therapy. Although allergists make attempts to minimize those risks, they are quite real and must be kept in mind. Immunotherapy is not used for the treatment of ocular symptoms alone or food allergy.

Complementary and Alternative Therapies

The use of complementary or alternative therapies for allergy treatment has been on the rise (Eisenberg et al, 1998). This can be correlated with the rising prevalence of allergy but is also a result of parental and child frustration in not finding adequate relief for allergy symptoms with conventional therapies. The limited understanding of the etiology of allergy, the pervasive nature of offending allergens, nonadherence with prescribed therapies, the lack of a standardized classification system for the diagnosis and management of allergy, and the impact of symptoms on the daily lives of those affected all contribute to treatment failure.

Treatments that have been used by families seeking complementary and alternative therapies include herbal remedies, relaxation, supplementation, elimination diets, and rotation diets (Eisenberg et al, 1998). The literature delineating the use of these therapies in children is lacking. Much work remains to be done by researchers regarding the clinical effectiveness and usefulness of these modalities.

Probiotics, the use of live microbial food ingredients to treat many different kinds of allergy, is a therapy garnering some recent attention. The theory regarding the use of probiotics suggests that atopic individuals are lacking specific microbes in the commensal gut microflora, making them susceptible to the development of allergy (Kalliomaki et al, 2001; Zeiger et al, 1999). Some studies report that *Lactobacillus rhamnosus GG*, a probiotic strain, is effective in the treatment of allergic inflammation (Isolauri et al, 2000; Majamaa & Isolauri, 1997; Pessi et al, 2000). One study has even suggested its usefulness in the prevention of atopic eczema when given to mothers during pregnancy and breast feeding (Kalliomaki et al, 2001). Other researchers have shown no benefit from *Lactobacillus rhamnosus GG* (Helin et al, 2002). The positive findings regarding *Lactobacillus* and its availability have contributed to its use outside conventional therapies, particularly for food allergy where little other treatment is available.

Anticipated Advances in Diagnosis and Management

The most notable advance in the diagnosis and management of allergic disorders is the recommendation to classify allergies similar to that of asthma. It is evident when reviewing current literature that discrepancies exist in the definition of allergic disease, particularly allergic rhinitis and conjunctivitis. This poses problems in making an accurate diagnosis, adequately managing the disease, and comparing studies done in this area.

Because of the variable nature of allergy and its clinical manifestations, a diagnostic structure that considers these differences would be helpful to classify the severity of disease and guide management.

A panel associated with WHO in a report from the workshop Allergic Rhinitis and its Impact on Asthma (Bousquet et al, 2001) has suggested a new classification system for allergy. Use of this classification system (Box 10-3) could be instrumental in guiding practitioners in the development of a management plan to improve symptom control. In addition, the panel has introduced the terms "intermittent," "persistent," "mild," and "moderate-severe" to describe and classify allergic rhinitis.

Advances in the treatment of allergy consist of improvements in existing medications as well as the discovery of new treatments to prevent disease and manage disease-related symptoms. A new medication category in the treatment of allergic rhinitis is the antileukotrienes or leukotriene receptor antagonists. This medication has been devised to target yet another pathway in the process of IgE-mediated allergic responses. Several studies with adults show the effectiveness of montelukast both alone and in combination with antihistamines (Meltzer et al, 2000; Storms, 2002; Wilson et al, 2002). Studies using antileukotrienes in children have yet to be done. A less well-studied advance is the use of intranasal heparin to protect against the development of allergy symptoms in asthma and allergic rhinitis. A recent report indicates that heparin used intranasally reduces eosinophil activity, thereby preventing nasal symptoms (Vancheri et al, 2001). Future work regarding intranasal heparin may offer another option in the management of allergy.

Advances in genetic therapy for allergy include deoxyribonucleic acid (DNA) vaccines aimed at inducing TH1 responses to allergens and the use of naturally occurring isoforms for immunotherapy that may decrease anaphylactic reactions (Kay, 2000; Turvey, 2001). Future advances regarding allergy and atopy will depend on identifying not only the genes responsible but also the complex interaction between genes and the environment.

Associated Problems

Children with allergy often present to the clinician with one or more clinical manifestations and associated conditions (Rachelefsky, 1999). Associated problems include asthma, atopic dermatitis (eczema), sinusitis, pharyngitis, middle ear effusion, otitis media, and sleep apnea (Box 10-7).

Asthma

One of the most prominent associated conditions is asthma (see Chapter 11). It has become clear that asthma and allergic rhinitis are interrelated in several ways (Lack, 2001). These two conditions often co-exist, and because of some shared symptomatology, the diagnosis of asthma often is confounded by the presence of allergic rhinitis. When a child is affected by both these conditions, both must be aggressively treated. Fortunately, there is some evidence to suggest that treatment of children with allergic rhinitis partly improves co-existing asthma, which emphasizes the importance of vigilant allergic rhinitis treatment (Aria Workshop Report, 2001; Lack, 2001). In addition,

---

> **BOX 10-7**
>
> ## Allergy-Associated Problems
>
> Asthma
> Atopic dermatitis (eczema)
> Eustachian tube obstruction
> Respiratory infections
> Sleep apnea
> Dental malocclusion

when aggressive allergen avoidance is successful, both conditions may improve since they both have the common underlying cause of allergic sensitization.

Atopic Dermatitis (Eczema)

Atopic dermatitis (AD) is a chronic inflammatory rash characterized by severe pruritus, overall dryness of the skin, and a pattern of exacerbation and remission (Thestrup-Pedersen, 2000). Like asthma, the incidence and prevalence of AD are rising and the environmental risk factors are similar to those of allergic rhinitis and asthma (Fennessy et al, 2000). Food allergies are also implicated in AD, and elimination diets hold some promise of symptom relief (Yale & La Valle, 2002).

Eustachian Tube Obstruction

Allergies often involve inflammation of the ears, which may lead to eustachian tube obstruction, accumulation of fluid in the inner ear, and infection. Hearing can then be affected, potentially followed by speech problems. This is especially worrisome at the ages of 6 months and 3 years, which are critical times for speech development.

Upper Respiratory Infections

Sinusitis, pharyngitis, or acute otitis media sometimes complicates allergic rhinitis. Clinicians should be careful to follow the current treatment guidelines and thereby avoid overuse of antibiotics. Some children have recurrent bouts of these related infections. In such cases, a pediatric otolaryngologist may be consulted. In cases of persistent cough or recurrent respiratory tract infections, a pediatric pulmonologist may be consulted.

Sleep Apnea

Because of upper airway edema and lymphoid hypertrophy, children with allergic rhinitis may be more prone to obstructive sleep apnea. One study reports an increased prevalence of snoring and the occurrence of obstructive sleep apnea in children with allergy (McColley et al, 1997). Guidelines developed by the American Academy of Pediatrics regarding childhood obstructive sleep apnea syndrome (OSAS) recommend that *all* children be screened for snoring as a part of routine health maintenance visits (American Academy of Pediatrics, 2002). Children with allergy who present with habitual snoring or evidence of disturbed sleep should receive a further work-up for OSAS.

Once snoring is recognized in a child, a more focused history and examination are necessary to identify the child's potential for OSAS. Detailed information regarding the quality of the snoring and the subsequent pauses, snorts, or gasps is important in distinguishing OSAS from primary snoring. History and physical alone are not diagnostic but are useful in determining which children need further testing and treatment as well as in avoiding unnecessary and expensive interventions (American Academy of Pediatrics, 2002). Parents can audiotape their child sleeping to help in the diagnosis and treatment plan. The timely diagnosis and management of this disorder are important to avoid the complications associated with OSAS.

Dental Malocclusion

Allergic rhinitis causes mouth breathing for many children. The result may be dental malocclusion, causing an overbite that could benefit from an orthodontic referral.

Prognosis

Allergic rhinitis and conjunctivitis are chronic conditions that may come and go over time. Approximately 10% to 20% of affected children with allergic rhinitis have a lessening or disappearance of symptoms within 7 years (Schoenwetter, 2000; Sly, 1999). Of those with symptoms that persist into adulthood, improvement generally occurs in the majority of people over the years, although skin test reactivity may not change. Exacerbations and remissions often occur throughout the person's lifetime as a result of environmental changes.

Milder food allergies often resolve over time, although some more severe allergies, such as allergies to peanuts, persist throughout life (Sampson, 2002).

PRIMARY CARE MANAGEMENT

Health Care Maintenance

Growth and Development

Allergy may affect inadequate intake of food and therefore growth in several ways. Chronic congestion may cause a child to have a poor appetite, or allergy to any common foods may severely limit a child's intake. Research has also shown a relationship between steroid use and stunted growth (Skoner et al, 2000). In most cases the effect on growth is insignificant but should be considered when growth is a concern for the child with allergy.

Decreased ability to concentrate, disordered sleep, or sedative effects from allergy medications can compromise a child's success in school (Lack, 2001). There is some evidence that allergic rhinitis can even affect memory and decision making (Fineman, 2002). Providers must be sure to consider allergy when developmental delay or poor school performance is the presenting problem.

The child with severe seasonal allergies may need to avoid being outdoors, even when fully medicated. When this is the case, providers, parents, and child can work together to identify other age-appropriate activities that would be enjoyable for the child and enhance development.

Diet

The child with allergy as noted above may have a poor appetite (Lack, 2001). Sore throats from persistent postnasal drip may also deter a child from eating. Ensuring adequate intake of a well-balanced variety of foods may take extra effort for the child with allergy.

Clinicians should caution parents with a family history of food allergies to wait until the age of 6 months before offering any solid foods, because allergy is more likely to develop when solid foods are introduced sooner (Zeiger, 1999b). At 6 months, parents are encouraged to proceed slowly with the introduction of each new food. Parents may carefully introduce a small amount, approximately 1 teaspoon, of one food, at a time. After 3 to 5 days, another food can then be introduced. This allows parents to more easily identify an offending food if any reactions occur. Avoid giving high-risk children certain foods that are more likely to cause symptoms. These include citrus fruits and juices, peanuts and peanut butter, eggs, and wheat. After 1 year of strict avoidance, some foods can be introduced successfully. Particular care should be taken with peanut allergy because of the greater risk of anaphylaxis. Peanut challenges in very controlled settings may be offered to parents, since it would be a clear advantage for the family to know that the child is no longer allergic (Skolnick et al, 2001).

Managing the diet of a child with food allergies can be particularly challenging. Because avoidance is the mainstay of treatment, parents must become experts in deciphering food labels and be continually vigilant for hidden sources of the offending food. Several Web sites provide useful tips for identifying hidden foods on product labels (see Resources). Equally challenging is making sure the child with food allergy is getting all nutrients in adequate amounts. For instance, a child who has an allergy to milk and milk products must consume other sources of calcium or take a supplement. Helping parents to find alternatives is an important aspect of the primary care provider's role in promoting good health. In situations of multiple food allergies, providers may refer the family to a dietitian.

Safety

Children with allergy to foods must be assessed regarding the need for injectable epinephrine. Factors that contribute to a greater risk of anaphylactic reactions to foods include a past medical history for asthma, young age, and eczema (Bock et al, 2001; Dibs & Baker, 1997; Furlong et al, 2001; Sampson, 2002). The foods most commonly implicated in anaphylaxis include peanuts, tree nuts, seafood, and milk, with peanuts being the most common in the United States (Dibs & Baker, 1997; Furlong et al, 2001; Sampson, 2002). Peanut and tree nut allergy reactions are worse with each subsequent exposure in most children, which makes these children at an even greater risk for anaphylaxis (Bock et al, 2001; Sicherer et al, 2001a, 2001b; Vander Leek et al, 2000). It is critical that health care providers be knowledgeable in prescribing and instructing families in using self-injectable epinephrine (EpiPen). An EpiPen can be a lifesaving medication if available and used promptly and properly. Unfortunately, in many cases of anaphylaxis, either an EpiPen is not available or it is improperly used (Bock et al, 2001; Dibs & Baker, 1997; Gold & Sainsbury, 2000; Novembre et al, 1998; Sicherer et al, 2001b). Parents and providers all need to be better educated about the use of EpiPens, and in turn, need to educate all others who may be caring for their children. This includes teachers, day-care providers, and whoever else may be the first person to recognize early allergic reaction symptoms (Sicherer et al, 2001a). The child should be instructed in self-injection techniques when developmentally appropriate. Emergency plans should be developed and on file in schools and daycare centers to detail the plan of action in the case of anaphylaxis. Including a picture of the child with the plan is helpful when multiple caregivers or teachers are involved.

Immunizations

Routine immunizations are recommended for most children with allergies. In addition, providers may recommend administration of the influenza vaccine in children who are at high risk of developing respiratory complications, such as those with asthma and allergy. Providers must be alert for the small number of children with allergy who have serious contraindications to immunizations. Those who are receiving long-term, high-dose steroid therapy should have live virus vaccines (MMR, varicella) postponed until after steroid treatment is completed (Committee on Infectious Diseases, 2000). It is also imperative for providers to carefully screen all children who have a history of anaphylaxis. Those with anaphylaxis to eggs should not receive influenza vaccine; those with anaphylaxis to gelatin should not receive MMR or varicella (Committee on Infectious Diseases, 2000). If there is known anaphylaxis to gelatin before the first dose of MMR, the vaccine should be given in a facility prepared to handle an anaphylactic reaction. If anaphylaxis is discovered after the first dose, titers should be checked to confirm immunity and the second dose should be deferred (Committee on Infectious Diseases, 2000).

Screening

Vision. Routine screening is recommended for all children. In addition, ocular symptoms or use of ocular medications may require increased evaluation of a child's eyes on physical examination.

Hearing. The child with allergy may require more frequent hearing screens to check for hearing deficit that may be secondary to recurrent otitis media or transient and caused by congestion.

Dental. Routine screening is recommended.

Blood Pressure. Routine screening is recommended.

Hematocrit. Routine screening is recommended.

Urinalysis. Routine screening is recommended.

Tuberculosis. Routine screening is recommended.

Condition-Specific Screening

In primary care practices, allergy is most often diagnosed based on the clinical presentation and response to antihistamine therapy. Diagnostic tests are typically reserved to confirm suspected diagnoses or to identify specific allergens.

Skin Testing. Skin testing, specifically IgE antibody testing, is usually done in the allergist's office. This process involves pricking the skin in order to expose the individual to a small amount of allergen. A positive test results in a reaction caused by IgE antibodies to the allergen. Before skin testing, children must be reminded to discontinue their antihistamines for at least 36 to 48 hours to avoid masking a reaction (Bock et al, 2001; Skoner, 2001). Conversely, false-positive results may also occur and must be fully evaluated.

In the case of food allergy, negative skin tests rather that positive skin tests are more useful in identifying or ruling out a possible allergen. Positive results should be confirmed with double-blind placebo-controlled food challenges before a food is implicated (Hay et al, 2001). This should not be done if anaphylaxis to a food is suspected. Often, food allergens are identified by the relief from symptoms following elimination of a food from the diet; this is a useful method if a particular food is strongly suspected.

RAST. IgE antibody testing can also be accomplished by in vitro serum testing, also known as radioallergosorbent tests (RASTs). This method is more expensive and less specific than skin testing but can be useful if particular issues make skin testing impossible, such as overwhelming atopic dermatitis, failure to discontinue antihistamines, possible anaphylaxis, or client refusal (Skoner, 2001).

Elevated total serum IgE is consistent with atopy but is not a specific indicator for allergy. Blood eosinophilia may also be used as a screening test, but it too has a low sensitivity. A nasal smear with eosinophils clearly indicates allergy but does not implicate a specific allergen.

In summary, no single screening test is recommended for identifying persons with allergy. When needed, skin testing is the standard diagnostic tool. The entire clinical picture, including a thorough family history, is the most valuable and practical diagnostic tool, used either in conjunction with diagnostic testing or alone.

Common Illness Management
Differential Diagnosis (Box 10-8)

Asthma. Asthma can be mistakenly diagnosed as allergy and vice versa. The most frequent reason for this is the existence of the shared symptom of cough, which constitutes an area of clinical overlap between rhinitis and asthma. In young children, cough is often the result of postnasal drip but is sometimes diagnosed as asthma or cough-variant asthma. When this happens, the child may appear to have more severe asthma and therefore may be overtreated with asthma medications. This is particularly problematic when the medications include steroids.

Acute Viral Rhinitis. Acute viral rhinitis, or upper respiratory infection (URI), is the most frequent infection in all children and is easily confused with allergic rhinitis. Both may present with cough, nasal congestion, and discharge. Usually, the nasal discharge in URI is time limited, lasting less than 2 weeks. However, this situation is more difficult to evaluate when the

---

BOX 10-8
Differential Diagnosis of Allergy

Asthma
Acute viral rhinitis
Vasomotor rhinitis
Acute infectious sinusitis, pharyngitis, and conjunctivitis
Rhinitis medicamentosa
Substance abuse
Dermatitis
Gastroenteritis and other gastrointestinal problems

child has the more complicated history of recurrent bouts of URI, a common case in the school-aged child or child in daycare.

The diagnosis of seasonal allergic rhinitis is usually straightforward. The clinician who is knowledgeable about local environmental pollens can simply correlate the clinical signs and symptoms with the time frame and personal and family health history and make the diagnosis. The clinician can also differentiate URI from allergy by evaluating for erythematous nasal mucosa, fever, and purulent nasal discharge, all of which are commonly seen in URI.

Vasomotor Rhinitis. Vasomotor rhinitis is a poorly defined nasal disease that is manifested by some degree of nasal obstruction, profuse rhinorrhea, and mucoid or clear nasal discharge (Fox, 1997; Hoekelman et al, 2001). Symptoms often occur with exposure to nonspecific factors, such as exercise, temperature changes, or air pollution, and generally appear and depart quite suddenly. There is usually a negative family history. The etiology is unclear, and the symptoms rarely improve with environmental controls or medications.

Acute Infectious Sinusitis, Pharyngitis, and Conjunctivitis. Acute sinusitis, pharyngitis, and conjunctivitis can be mistaken for allergy. The affected child may present with nasal obstruction, sore throat, headache, red eyes, and fatigue. In these cases, the clinician must be alert for signs of infection, such as lymphadenopathy, fever, erythema, and purulent discharge. There is often a history of contagious contacts in the family, school, or daycare setting. Some of the hallmark signs of allergy, such as pruritus and clear discharge, are not present with infections. An atopic history may be absent. A rapid strep test or throat culture can help provide a prompt answer in the child with pharyngitis when the clinical picture is unclear.

Often, the child with allergies can develop one of these infectious conditions in addition to the allergic disease. The clinician must be alert for this episodic situation and treat it with antimicrobial agents as appropriate. Allergy medications should be continued. For the child who has recurrent pharyngitis, recurrent otitis media, or snoring, a referral to a pediatric otolaryngologist should be considered.

Rhinitis Medicamentosa. Rhinitis medicamentosa is severe rebound nasal congestion that occurs as a result of frequent prolonged use of proprietary nasal decongestant sprays. When the child stops using the spray, the rebound congestion is acute and intensely uncomfortable. When eliciting the health history, the provider must directly question the child and parent on the use of over-the-counter medications, specifically nasal sprays.

Substance Abuse. Adolescents who are snorting cocaine or abusing other medications may show symptoms that are very suggestive of allergic disease, including rhinorrhea, rhinitis, nasal polyps, conjunctivitis, and nasal congestion (Barker et al, 1995; Bock et al, 2001; Chrostowski & Pongracic, 2002). Chronic use can also cause perforation of the nasal septum (Chrostowski & Pongracic, 2002). Clinicians should watch for these symptoms, especially when other components of the history or physical suggest substance abuse. Behavioral and developmental indicators, such as school failure, increased chaotic relationships with family or peers, mood alterations, or changes in sleep and eating patterns, may reinforce such diagnostic exploration. Another key to diagnosis is when adolescents do not improve with standard allergic rhinitis medical treatment, which may point to underlying substance abuse, not allergic disease. Physical examination may assist in the diagnosis, since the nasal mucosa in substance abuse may bleed easily and is often erythematous, instead of the pale and boggy mucosa that is typical of allergy.

Dermatitis and Other Skin Manifestations. Urticaria (hives) that are related to food allergy often present a confusing dilemma to the clinician. When an offending food cannot be identified, other diagnoses are entertained. Urticarial wheals may mimic many conditions, including insect bites, adverse medication reactions, contact dermatitis, and urticarial vasculitis. If a medication is suspected, future avoidance is paramount. Treatment of most urticaria with antihistamines is the same, regardless of cause. Although the exact cause of many cases of urticaria remains a mystery, the history, distribution, and progression of the rash often provide the clinician with important diagnostic clues.

Gastroenteritis and other Gastrointestinal Problems. Stomach upset, diarrhea, and vomiting are common symptoms in children, with a myriad of causes besides food allergy. These include lactose intolerance, acute gastroenteritis, parasitic infestations, and colic.

Intolerance to a food is not an allergy in that it is not an IgE-mediated response. Differentiating between actual allergy and intolerance can be difficult based on clinical presentation alone. Typically, the child with allergy to a food will have skin and respiratory symptoms in addition to gastrointestinal symptoms.

Acute gastroenteritis has an onset of less than 1 week, may or may not be accompanied by a fever, and is always time limited. With a bacterial cause, critical aspects of the history include presence of bloody diarrhea, fever, chills, and cramps. When caused by a virus, the diarrhea is typically watery. A wait and see approach is reasonable in the case of mild gastroenteritis, focusing more on adequate intake of fluids and maintaining hydration. Other helpful clues for discriminating between food allergy and gastroenteritis include the season at time of presentation (viral more likely in winter and summer) and contact with other sick individuals. Differentiating this from a parasitic infestation depends ultimately on stool cultures; other history points include blood or mucus in the stool and travel history.

Colic is most commonly seen beginning in the second week of life, with a peak at 1 to 2 months and a decline by 3 to 4 months. Although some authors suggest that colic is secondary to gastrointestinal upset, there is no clear evidence for this theory (Dixon & Stein, 2000). A trial of a lactose-free formula for a short time (1 to 2 weeks) may be helpful in teasing this out. Lactose intolerance can be either primary or secondary. In primary intolerance, the infant has diarrhea following feedings, the infant may vomit, and the stool is typically frothy. More common is secondary or acquired intolerance. This is seen usually at about 3 to 5 years of age and more often in children of black or Asian descent (Hay et al, 2001). The primary symptom is stomachache after drinking or eating milk or milk products.

Diagnosing food allergy is a long and arduous process. A definitive diagnosis is only made with a double-blind, placebo-controlled food challenge.

Other Less Common Conditions. When the clinical picture is unclear or when treatment is unsuccessful, the clinician must explore other less common conditions. These include adenoidal hypertrophy, nasal foreign body, nasal polyps as a result of the aspirin triad or cystic fibrosis, congenital syphilis, rhinorrhea of cerebrospinal fluid, or nasopharyngeal tumors (Bernstein & Shelov, 1996; Hoekelman et al, 2001).

Developmental Issues

Sleep

Nasal obstruction and itching can disrupt the sleep of children with allergy. They can result in restlessness, shortened naps, and waking during the night. In addition, the child with allergy may also be experiencing obstructive sleep apnea (see section on associated problems). The resulting sleep deprivation can cause irritability and an inability to concentrate, disturbing home and school activities. When this happens, providers should be careful not to mislabel a child with attention deficit hyperactivity disorder or a learning disability. In turn, daytime sleepiness may be attributed to the sedative effects of some antihistamines rather than a lack of sleep. The clinician must be alert for these more subtle signs of allergy, be certain that the child's treatment plan is appropriately aggressive, and be sure the plan is well understood by the child and family in order to promote adherence. In addition, clinicians must encourage a reasonable bedtime and consistent bedtime ritual.

Toileting

Food allergy with accompanying symptoms of diarrhea can cause additional hurdles in the toddler who is toilet training. When this occurs, it is best to caution the parent to wait until the diarrhea subsides before proceeding with toilet training.

Discipline

Caretakers must be reminded that behavioral manifestations may be due to inadequately treated allergies (Fireman, 2000). Itching of the eyes, nose, and ears can be extremely uncomfortable. Children can feel totally miserable but be unable to fully verbalize the symptoms. This is especially true with young children but can also apply to the older child or adolescent. Sometimes, children just feel bad, get irritable, and cry or act out in some other way. The whole family can be disrupted, and parents may feel compelled to employ stronger disciplining methods. However, if the true underlying cause of the misbehavior is allergy, caretakers should be encouraged to seek help in reevaluating the treatment plan with the provider and adapt it as necessary to get allergy symptoms under better control.

Child Care

Child care providers are usually very vigilant about contagious diseases, and it is not unusual for a child with red teary eyes or a runny nose to be sent home for fear that other children will be exposed to the illness. Parents of children with allergy can be quite frustrated when this happens repeatedly. If the red eyes or runny nose are exclusively allergy related, the clinician can work with the parents to reassure the daycare center that the child poses no threat to the other children. Usually, a statement from the clinician verifying that this is not a contagious disease is sufficient. It may also be helpful to send additional written information to reinforce the facts. There are excellent resources for parents and caretakers that can be used, or the clinician can adapt a patient information sheet, such as one from Schmitt's patient education book (Schmitt et al, 1999).

One important issue in daycare concerns the child who has a severe food allergy. Daycare providers must be informed of the allergy and given whatever additional information they need to fully understand the problem and how it should be handled. In cases of severe food allergy, an EpiPen Jr and diphenhydramine hydrochloride (Benadryl) should be kept at the daycare center with explicit instructions. When there are multiple food allergies, a list of offending foods can be posted in both the daycare kitchen and classroom areas, especially if the daycare center employs multiple caretakers. Clear distinctions should be made among food intolerances, mild food allergy, and severe food allergy. Information should be distributed to other parents who may also bring food into the daycare setting in order to avoid accidental exposure to an offending food. Peanut butter craft projects in daycare and school account for many accidental ingestions, so teachers ought to keep peanut butter completely out of the kitchen as well as out of the arts and crafts area (Sicherer et al, 2001a).

Schooling

Up to 25% of individuals with allergic rhinitis miss time from school or work. Those who do manage to go to school or work are significantly less productive and less able to learn. These problems are due to the symptoms of the disease but also to the sedating effects of some of the medications used to treat allergic rhinitis (Fineman, 2002).

The school setting can be a source of many allergens. Common sources of allergic triggers in school include chalk dust, classroom pets, plants, upholstered furniture or pillows, and carpeting. School-aged children should be seated as far away from the blackboard as possible if it is used. This will minimize exposure to chalk dust. Other less obvious sources of allergens include mold and industrial cleaning agents. If a child's allergies are much worse during school days, with improvement during the weekends or vacations, vigilant parents and clinicians will suspect that the school is the primary site of allergen exposure. For children with specific environmental allergies, school personnel can be instructed to close the windows when grass is being cut or leaves are being raked. Depending on particular school regulations, the school nurse or designated person may be able to administer as-needed medications, such as antihistamines, to a child with acute symptoms.

Physical education, recess period activities, and after-school sports programs do not usually cause additional problems for the child with allergy, unless such activities take place outside during the high pollen season. School personnel may have to alter the child's schedule to avoid being outside on such high pollen days. The family and the school nurse can collaborate to be aware of those days and make appropriate adjustments.

School nurses and teachers must be informed about a school child with allergic rhinitis or allergic conjunctivitis. Even with appropriate treatment, the child may sometimes have inflamed eyes or a runny nose. Similar to daycare providers, school personnel will usually take any potential exposure to infectious disease very seriously, so they must be reassured that the child is not contagious and is getting proper treatment. As in the daycare situation, clinicians and parents must provide the same needed documentation to allay any fears of school personnel.

The school-aged child who is treated with first-generation antihistamines may be drowsy during school, decreasing school performance. Researchers report a statistically significant difference in the learning capacity of school children with allergic rhinitis. Children with allergic rhinitis did better if treated with a second-generation antihistamine vs. no treatment but performed worse if given diphenhydramine (a first-generation antihistamine) vs. no treatment. Conversely, the school-aged child who is taking a decongestant may be overactive and therefore have trouble focusing on school work. For both these reasons, providers must be careful to recommend the minimum medication with the least adverse side effects, while achieving optimum symptom control.

Anaphylactic reactions that occur outside the hospital are most commonly related to food allergy (Sicherer et al, 2001a). Discussion with school administrators and thorough education of the school nurse, teachers, cafeteria workers, and other school personnel are imperative, because school policies are frequently inadequate (Rhim & McMorris, 2001). An emergency health care plan should be devised in conjunction with the clinician, parent, and school nurse. This plan should include specifics regarding the child's allergies, typical reactions, symptoms of anaphylaxis, and a plan to administer epinephrine. In addition, the plan should include notifying an emergency medical team (EMT) and the parent. Last, the plan should explain typical effects of epinephrine and other care the child requires until the EMT arrives. It is essential that parents and guardians of affected children keep school emergency information up to date, with all phone numbers and other contact information kept current. The complete school emergency plan should be updated at least yearly. All school personnel who may be in a setting to respond to an anaphylactic emergency should have a copy of the plan. Attaching a photo of the child is useful for rapid identification.

Sexuality

Age-appropriate anticipatory guidance regarding sexuality should be provided for preadolescents and adolescents with allergy, similar to that given to their peers. If there is a known allergy to latex, information about avoidance of latex condoms and diaphragms should be discussed. In this case the child must also be aware of their risk for anaphylaxis, along with a plan of action including epinephrine (see section on associated problems).

Transition into Adulthood

The majority of children with allergy will progress to adulthood with some allergy symptoms. For this reason, children and adolescents must be encouraged to move gradually toward independence in their allergy care. As with most chronic conditions, such a transition must start early, with young children learning the basics of their disease and care. By adolescence, the parents can assume a supportive role while the teenager predominantly practices self-care. Parents, however, must remain actively aware of their adolescent's moods, behaviors, and subtle allergy symptoms. With the often-chaotic haze of adolescence, this can be challenging for parents. It is well worth the effort, however, because a miserable and itchy adolescent can quickly get his or her whole life out of perspective. Attention to alleviating allergy symptoms will often go a long way in improving adolescent mood and function.

Family Concerns and Resources

When managing the child with allergy it is important to recognize the strong familial link and the likelihood that several other family members may also be experiencing an allergy. The provider should inquire about allergies in other family members to ascertain how they are managing their disease and discourage the sharing of medications. Patient handouts such as Schmitt's (Schmitt et al, 1999) or others that are readily available on the Internet are helpful additions to the teaching done in the office (see Web sites in Resources).

Food allergies require the vigilance of the whole family. Avoiding foods often necessitates change on the part of the entire family. Utilizing nutritionists specializing in food allergy can help the family to maintain a balanced diet while avoiding offending foods. Linking families to resources and support groups is a critical aspect of management. Peanut allergies, when severe, can be particularly disruptive for the child and family because of fear of the child's risk of death (Primeau et al, 2000). For this reason, a careful and accurate diagnosis must be made, followed by vigilant education and emotional support.

In the case of allergic rhinitis and conjunctivitis, total avoidance is a challenging goal. Television and newspaper weather reports are good sources of daily information regarding the pollen count. In addition, Web sites routinely report the pollen count for a given region on a daily basis (see Resources). This may be an integral part of the family's regular routine in high-pollen seasons. Altering the home environment by installing air conditioning, removing carpeting, or even getting rid of the family pet may be essential to controlling allergen exposure. Treating allergy, whether or not others in the family share the disease, will always include treating the family as a unit.

WEB RESOURCES

Allergic-child
Good materials on how to read a food label; also provides links to many other useful sites
www.allergicchild.com

Allergy & Asthma Network, Mothers of Asthmatics
Excellent site with a wide variety of information from avoidance tips to developing anaphylaxis action plan; includes information on both asthma and allergy, including food allergy
www.aanma.org

Allergy, Asthma and Sinus Relief, National Supply, Inc
Provides a resource for ordering supplies used to decrease allergens in the home
(800) 522-1444
www.Nationalallergy.com

American Academy of Allergy Asthma & Immunology
Resources for patients and providers, includes a special "Just for Kids" section;

provides local pollen count and maps with pollen seasons identified
www.aaaai.org

The American Academy of Environmental Medicine
A resource for referrals to local providers specializing in environmentally
affected diseases
(316) 684-5500
www.AAEM.com

Anaphylaxis.com
Excellent resource for providers and patients about anaphylaxis and EpiPens
from the company that manufactures them; even includes an animated movie
on how to use an EpiPen
www.anaphylaxis.com

Asthma and Allergy Foundation of America
Site primarily focused on asthma; however, it also discusses allergy; provides
a link to connect with a local support group; also provides information devised
for different age-groups
www.aafa.org

The Food Allergy and Anaphylaxis Network
Provides good information about food allergy and anaphylaxis; provides
information about unlabeled sources of common allergic foods; downloadable
tools for school action plan and excellent information on anaphylaxis;
supported with references and reviewed by Medical Advisory Board
www.foodallergy.org

Food Allergy Initiative
Nonprofit organization providing information on eating in restaurants with food
allergies and food labeling
www.foodallergyinitiative.com

OTHER RESOURCE

The Allergy Self Help Cookbook by Marjorie Hurt Jones, RN
Provides excellent information on allergy, nutrition, and methods for preparing
foods with atypical ingredients or substitutions

Summary of Primary Care Needs for the Child with Allergy

HEALTH CARE MAINTENANCE
Growth and Development

Chronic congestion and restrictions secondary to food allergy
may adversely affect intake; offer a wide variety of healthful foods,
and monitor for impact on growth.

Prolonged intranasal steroid use may affect growth; consider
when growth is a concern for the child with allergy.

Allergy medications and disordered sleep secondary to allergy
can impede a child's ability to learn and concentrate. The goal for
treatment should be adequate control of symptoms with minimal
side effects to enhance school performance.

Age-appropriate alternatives for outdoor activities may be necessary to promote development during high-pollen days.

Diet

In infancy, solid foods should not be introduced before 6 months
of age to prevent the development of food allergy. When solids are
introduced it should be one food every 3 to 5 days in order to monitor
for adverse reactions to new foods.

Avoid giving high-risk children citrus fruits and juices, peanuts
and peanut butter, eggs, and wheat. After 1 year of strict avoidance
some foods are often successfully tolerated.

Parents of children with food allergies may need guidance in
selecting appropriate substitutions or supplementations to ensure a
balanced diet. A referral to a dietitian may be necessary.

Poor appetite secondary to congestion and sore throat secondary
to postnasal drip may inhibit adequate intake of foods.

Safety

Children with food allergy that are at high risk for anaphylaxis
(past medical history for asthma, young age, eczema) may need a prescription for injectable epinephrine.

Most common foods implicated in anaphylaxis include tree nuts,
peanuts, seafood, and milk; peanut allergy is the most common in the
United States.

Providers, parents, and children need regular instruction regarding the use of epinephrine.

Emergency plans are an important aspect for the care of children
with food allergy attending daycare or school.

Immunizations

Routine immunizations are recommended.

Live virus vaccines should be used cautiously in children receiving long-term, high-dose steroid therapy and may need to be delayed
until treatment has ended.

Children with a history of anaphylaxis to eggs or gelatin should
be identified before administration of influenza, MMR, or varicella
vaccines.

Influenza vaccine is recommended for children with asthma or
allergy.

Screening

Vision. Routine screening is recommended. Ocular symptoms or
use of ocular medications may require increased evaluation of a
child's eyes on physical examination.

Hearing. The child with allergy may require more frequent
hearing screens to evaluate for hearing deficit that may be secondary
to recurrent otitis media or transient and caused by congestion.

Dental. Routine screening is recommended.

Blood pressure. Routine screening is recommended.

Hematocrit. Routine screening is recommended.

Urinalysis. Routine screening is recommended.

Tuberculosis. Routine screening is recommended.

Condition-Specific Screening

Skin testing for IgE antibodies is usually done in the allergist's
office; families must be reminded to discontinue antihistamines 36
to 48 hours before testing.

Double-blind, placebo-controlled food challenges are the best
method for confirming suspected food allergy; use caution if anaphylaxis is suspected.

Radioallergosorbent tests (RASTs) can be used when atopic dermatitis, failure to discontinue antihistamines, possible anaphylaxis,
or client refusal makes skin testing impossible.

Summary of Primary Care Needs for the Child with Allergy—cont'd

COMMON ILLNESS MANAGEMENT

Differential Diagnosis

Asthma. Cough is a common presenting symptom in both asthma and allergy. Distinguish between cough-variant asthma and cough secondary to postnasal drip to avoid inappropriately medicating.

Acute viral rhinitis. Nasal discharge is purulent and time limited, lasting less than 2 weeks; fever and erythematous nasal mucosa are present.

Vasomotor rhinitis. Nasal obstruction, profuse rhinorrhea, and mucoid or clear nasal discharge are secondary to exposure to nonspecific factors such as exercise, temperature changes, or air pollution and generally appear and depart suddenly.

Acute infections, sinusitis, pharyngitis, and conjunctivitis. Signs of an infectious process include lymphadenopathy, fever, erythema, and purulent discharge in conjunction with a history of a sick contact.

Rhinitis medicamentosa. Severe rebound nasal congestion occurs secondary to overuse of decongestant nasal sprays. Their use should be strongly discouraged.

Substance abuse. When allergy symptoms in an adolescent fail to improve with standard treatment, consider underlying substance abuse. Keys to diagnosis may be perforated nasal septum, erythematous nasal mucosa with a tendency to bleed, and behavioral changes.

Dermatitis and other skin manifestations. Urticaria or hives may manifest secondary to food exposure; although is it often difficult to determine the offending agent, treatment is with antihistamines.

Gastrointestinal problems. Clues to distinguishing among acute gastroenteritis, parasitic infections, and food allergy are characteristics of diarrhea (bloody, mucous, frothy, watery), fever, length of symptoms, associated cramping and vomiting, age of child, past history of signs and symptoms, sick exposure, time of year, and travel history.

Other less common conditions. Nasal foreign body, adenoidal hypertrophy, drug interactions, nasal polyps, nasopharyngeal tumors, congenital syphilis, and rhinorrhea of cerebrospinal fluid can all mimic the symptoms of allergy.

DEVELOPMENTAL ISSUES

Sleep Patterns

Nasal obstruction, itching, and obstructive sleep apnea can all disrupt the sleep of the child with allergy. Aggressive allergy symptom control may help.

A regular and reasonable bedtime routine is advisable.

Daytime use of first-generation antihistamines may cause drowsiness.

Toileting

Diarrhea secondary to food allergy may interfere with toilet training; training should be postponed until diarrhea subsides.

Discipline

Behavioral manifestations of allergy may provoke unwarranted discipline; good control of allergy symptoms is necessary to avoid this.

Child Care

Child care providers may need documentation from the primary care provider of a child's diagnosis of allergy and that it is not contagious to avoid being excluded from daycare programs.

Care providers of children with food allergy must be informed in writing of the child's allergy, typical reaction, signs of anaphylaxis, and plans for emergency action (including administration of epinephrine). Other children's parents must also be aware of a child's allergy to avoid accidental exposure from foods.

Schooling

Schools are often the source of many allergic triggers, including chalk dust, classroom pets, plants, upholstered furniture or pillows, and carpeting. Measures should be taken to decrease the presence of these allergens for the child with allergy.

Alternatives to physical education and school sports may be necessary on days where the pollen count is extremely high.

School personnel should be informed of typical allergic symptoms so as not to confuse them with infectious disease symptoms. Medications for symptom relief may need to be given in school. Some medications may make the child drowsy.

Schools must be prepared with an emergency plan for the child with food allergy at risk for anaphylaxis.

Sexuality

Age-appropriate anticipatory guidance is indicated for the child with allergy as with any other child.

Allergy to latex may be a concern for the sexually active adolescent; risk should be assessed and information provided.

Transition into Adulthood

For some children, allergy symptoms diminish or completely subside as they enter their adult years.

Children and adolescents should be encouraged to gradually assume responsibility in managing their allergy care as appropriate.

Family Concerns

It is important to recognize that several family members may also be experiencing allergy; medication sharing should be discouraged.

Avoidance of food allergens requires vigilance of the entire family and may require a change in diet for the entire family; a referral to a dietitian may be useful.

Avoidance of triggers for allergic rhinitis and conjunctivitis may also require changes that will impact the entire family, including installing air conditioning, removing carpeting, and getting rid of the family pet.

REFERENCES

Agertoft, L. & Pedersen, S. (2000). Effect of long-term treatment with inhaled budesonide on adult height in children with asthma. *N Engl J Med, 343*, 1064-1069.

Alm, J.S., Swartz, J., Lilja, G., Scheynius, A., & Pershagen, G. (1999). Atopy in children of families with an anthroposophic lifestyle. *Lancet, 353*, 1485-1488.

American Academy of Pediatrics. (2002). Clinical practice guidelines: Diagnosis and management of childhood obstructive sleep apnea syndrome. *Pediatrics, 109*(4), 704-712.

Aria Workshop Report. (2001). Allergic rhinitis and its impact on asthma. *J Allergy Clin Immunol, 108*, 1-205.

Barker, L.R., Burton, J.R., & Zieve, P.D. (1995). *Principles of ambulatory care*. (4th ed.). Baltimore: Williams & Wilkins.

Behrman, R.E., Kleigman, R.M., & Jenson, H.B. (2000). *Nelson textbook of pediatrics* (16th ed.). Philadelphia: W.B. Saunders Company.

Berger, W.E. (2001a). Allergic rhinitis in children. *Curr Allergy Asthma Rep, 1*, 498-505.

Berger, W.E. (2001b). Treatment update: Allergic rhinitis. *Allergy Asthma Proc, 22*, 191-198.

Bernstein, D. & Shelov, S.P. (1996). *Pediatrics*. Baltimore: Williams & Wilkins.

Bock, S.A., Munoz-Furlong, A., & Sampson, H.A. (2001). Food and drug reactions and anaphylaxis. *J Allergy Clin Immunol, 107*(1).

Bodner, C., Godden, D., & Seaton, A. (1998). Family size, childhood infections and atopic diseases. The Aberdeen WHEASE Group. *Thorax, 53*, 28-32.

Bousquet, J., Van Cauwenberge, P., & Khaltaev, N. (2001). Allergic rhinitis and its impact on asthma. *J Allergy Clin Immunol, 108*, S147-S334.

Chan, Y.H., Shek, L.P., Aw, M., Quak, S.H., & Lee, B.W. (2002). Use of hypoallergenic formula in the prevention of atopic disease among Asian children. *J Pediatr Child Health, 38*, 84-88.

Chandra, R.K. (1997). Five-year follow-up of high-risk infants with family history of allergy who were exclusively breast-fed or fed partial whey hydrolysate, soy, and conventional cow's milk formulas. *J Pediatr Gastroenterol Nutr, 24*, 380-388.

Childhood Asthma Management Program Research Group. (2000). Long-term effects of budesonide or nedocromil in children with asthma. *N Engl J Med, 343*, 1054-1063.

Chrostowski, D. & Pongracic, J. (2002). Control of chronic nasal symptoms: Directing treatment at the underlying cause. *Postgrad Med, 111*, 77-84, 87.

Committee on Infectious Diseases. (2000). *2000 Red book: Report of the Committee on Infectious Diseases* (25th ed.). Elk Grove, IL: American Academy of Pediatrics.

De Jong, M.H., Scharp-Van Der Linden, V.T. Aalberse, R., Heymans, H.S., & Brunekreef, B. (2002). The effect of brief neonatal exposure to cows' milk on atopic symptoms up to age 5. *Arch Dis Child, 86*, 365-369.

Dibs, S.D. & Baker, M.D. (1997). Anaphylaxis in children: A 5-year experience. *Pediatrics, 99*, E7.

Dixon, S.D. & Stein, M.T. (2000). *Encounters with children: Pediatric behavior and development* (3rd ed.). St. Louis: Mosby.

Doull, I.J. (2001). Does pregnancy prevent atopy? *Clin Exp Allergy, 31*, 1335-1337.

Eisenberg, D.M., Davis, R.B., Ettner, S.L., Appel, S., Wilkey, S., et al. (1998). Trends in alternative medicine use in the United States, 1990-1997: Results of a follow-up national survey. *JAMA, 280*, 1569-1575.

Fennessy, M., Coupland, S., Popay, J., & Naysmith, K. (2000). The epidemiology and experience of atopic eczema during childhood: A discussion paper on the implications of current knowledge for health care, public health policy and research. *J Epidemiol Community Health, 54*, 581-589.

Fineman, S.M. (2002). The burden of allergic rhinitis: Beyond dollars and cents. *Ann Allergy Asthma Immunol, 88*, 2-7.

Fireman, P. (2000). Therapeutic approaches to allergic rhinitis: Treating the child. *J Allergy Clin Immunol, 105*, S616-S621.

Fox, J.A. (Ed.). (1997). *Primary health care of children*. St. Louis: Mosby.

Furlong, T.J., DeSimone, J., & Sicherer, S.H. (2001). Peanut and tree nut allergic reactions in restaurants and other food establishments. *J Allergy Clin Immunol, 108*, 867-870.

Gold, M.S. & Sainsbury, R. (2000). First aid anaphylaxis management in children who were prescribed an epinephrine autoinjector device (EpiPen). *J Allergy Clin Immunol, 106*, 171-176.

Haagerup, A., Bjerke, T., Schoitz, P.O., Binderup, H.G., Dahl, R., et al. (2001). Allergic rhinitis—a total genome-scan for susceptibility genes suggests a locus on chromosome 4q24-q27. *Eur J Hum Genet, 9*, 945-952.

Hajat, S., Haines, A., Atkinson, R.W., Bremner, S.A., Anderson, H.R., et al. (2001). Association between air pollution and daily consultations with general practitioners for allergic rhinitis in London, United Kingdom. *Am J Epidemiol, 153*, 704-714.

Hay, W.W., Hayward, A.R., Levin, M.J., & Sondheimer, J.M. (2001). *Current pediatric diagnosis and treatment, 72*. (15th ed.). New York: Lange Medical Books/McGraw-Hill.

Helin, T., Haahtela, S., & Haahtela, T. (2002). No effect of oral treatment with an intestinal bacterial strain, Lactobacillus rhamnosus (ATCC 53103), on birch-pollen allergy: A placebo-controlled double-blind study. *Allergy, 57*, 243-246.

Hoekelman, R.A., Adam, H.M., Nelson, N.M., Weitzman, M.L., & Hoover Wilson, M. (2001). *Primary pediatric care* (4th ed.). St. Louis: Mosby.

Holm, A.F. & Fokkens, W.J. (2001). Topical corticosteroids in allergic rhinitis; effects on nasal inflammatory cells and nasal mucosa. *Clin Exp Allergy, 31*, 529-535.

Holt, P.G., Macaubas, C., Prescott, S.L., & Sly, P.D. (1999). Microbial stimulation as an aetiologic factor in atopic disease. *Allergy, 5*(suppl. 49), 12-16.

Hooper, B.J. (1999). *Primary dermatologic care*. St. Louis: Mosby.

Illi, S., von Mutius, E., Lau, S., Bergmann, R., Niggemann, B., et al. (2001). Early childhood infectious diseases and the development of asthma up to school age: A birth cohort study. *BMJ, 322*, 390-395.

Isolauri, E., Arvola, T., Sutas, Y., Moilanen, E., & Salminen, S. (2000). Probiotics in the management of atopic eczema. *Clin Exp Allergy, 30*, 1604-1610.

Jackson, P.L. (2002). Peanut allergy: An increasing health risk for children. *Pediatr Nurs, 28*, 496-498.

Jarvis, D., Chinn, S., Luczynska, C., & Burney, P. (1997). The association of family size with atopy and atopic disease. *Clin Exp Allergy, 27*, 240-245.

Kalliomaki, M., Salminen, S., Arvilommi, H., Kero, P., Koskinen, P., et al. (2001). Probiotics in primary prevention of atopic disease: A randomised placebo-controlled trial. *Lancet, 357*, 1076-1079.

Kay, A.B. (2000). Overview of 'allergy and allergic diseases: with a view to the future.' *Br Med Bull, 56*, 843-864.

Klucka, C.V., Ownby, D.R., Green, J., & Zoratti, E. (1995). Cat shedding of Fel d I is not reduced by washings, Allerpet-C spray, or acepromazine. *J Allergy Clin Immunol, 95*, 1164-1171.

Kulig, M., Klettke, U., Wahn, V., Forster, J., Bauer, C.P., et al. (2000). Development of seasonal allergic rhinitis during the first 7 years of life. *J Allergy Clin Immunol, 106*, 832-839.

Lack, G. (2001). Pediatric allergic rhinitis and comorbid disorders. *J Allergy Clin Immunol, 108*, S9-S15.

Lee, J.M., & Greenes, D.S. (2000). Biphasic anaphylactic reactions in pediatrics. *Pediatrics, 106*, 762-766.

Leynaert, B., Neukirch, C., Jarvis, D., Chinn, S., Burney, P., et al. (2001). Does living on a farm during childhood protect against asthma, allergic rhinitis, and atopy in adulthood? *Am J Respir Crit Care Med, 164*, 1829-1834.

Majamaa, H. & Isolauri, E. (1997). Probiotics: A novel approach in the management of food allergy. *J Allergy Clin Immunol, 99*, 179-185.

Martinez, F.D. & Holt, P.G. (1999). Role of microbial burden in aetiology of allergy and asthma. *Lancet, 354*(suppl.), SII12-SII15.

McColley, S.A., Carroll, J.L., Curtis, S., Loughlin, G.M., & Sampson, H.A. (1997). High prevalence of allergic sensitization in children with habitual snoring and obstructive sleep apnea. *Chest, 111*, 170-173.

McManaway, J.W., III, & Frankel, C.A. (2001). Red eye. In R.A. Hoekelman, H.M. Adam, N.M. Nelson, M.L. Weitzman, & M.H. Wilson (Eds.). *Primary pediatric care* (4th ed., pp. 1240-1245). St. Louis: Mosby.

Meltzer, E.O., Malmstrom, K., Lu, S., Prenner, B.M., Wei, L.X., et al. (2000). Concomitant montelukast and loratadine as treatment for seasonal allergic rhinitis: A randomized, placebo-controlled clinical trial. *J Allergy Clin Immunol, 105*, 917-922.

Nafstad, P., Magnus, P., Gaarder, P.I., & Jaakkola, J.J. (2001). Exposure to pets and atopy-related diseases in the first 4 years of life. *Allergy, 56*, 307-312.

Nash, D.R. (1998). Allergic rhinitis. *Pediatr Ann, 27*, 799-808.

Novembre, E., Cianferoni, A., Bernardini, R., Mugnaini, L., Caffarelli, C., et al. (1998). Anaphylaxis in children: Clinical and allergologic features. *Pediatrics, 101*, E8.

Ownby, D.R., Johnson, C.C., & Peterson, E.L. (2002). Exposure to dogs and cats in the first year of life and risk of allergic sensitization at 6 to 7 years of age. *JAMA, 286*, 963-972.

Pessi, T., Sutas, Y., Hurme, M., & Isolauri, E. (2000). Interleukin-10 generation in atopic children following oral Lactobacillus rhamnosus GG. *Clin Exp Allergy, 30*, 1804-1808.

Philpot, E.E. (2000). Safety of second generation antihistamines. *Allergy Asthma Proc, 21*, 15-20.

Platts-Mills, T.A. (2002). Paradoxical effect of domestic animals on asthma and allergic sensitization. *JAMA, 288*, 1012-1014.

Primeau, M.N., Kagan, R., Joseph, L., Lim, H., Dufresne, C., et al. (2000). The psychological burden of peanut allergy as perceived by adults with peanut allergy and the parents of peanut-allergic children. *Clin Exp Allergy, 30*, 1135-1143.

Rachelefsky, G.S. (1999). National guidelines needed to manage rhinitis and prevent complications. *Ann Allergy Asthma Immunol, 82*, 296-305.

Ray, N.F., Baraniuk, J.N., Thamer, M., Rinehart, C.S., Gergen, P.J., et al. (1999). Direct expenditures for the treatment of allergic rhinoconjunctivitis in 1996, including the contributions of related airway illnesses. *J Allergy Clin Immunol, 103*, 401-407.

Rhim, G.S., & McMorris, M.S. (2001). School readiness for children with food allergies. *Ann Allergy Asthma Immunol, 86*, 172-176.

Sampson, H.A. (2002). Clinical practice. Peanut allergy. *N Engl J Med, 346*, 1294-1299.

Scadding, G.K., Richards, D.H., & Price, M.J. (2000). Patient and physician perspectives on the impact and management of perennial and seasonal allergic rhinitis. *Clin Otolaryngol, 25*, 551-557.

Schmitt, B.D., Jacobs, J.T., & Fletcher, J. (1999). *Instructions for pediatric patients* (2nd ed.). Philadelphia: W.B. Saunders Company.

Schoenwetter, W.F. (2000). Allergic rhinitis: Epidemiology and natural history. *Allergy Asthma Proc, 21*, 1-6.

Sheikh, A., & Hurwitz, B. (2002). House dust mite avoidance measures for perennial allergic rhinitis. *Cochrane Database of Systematic Reviews, 2*.

Sicherer, S.H. (2002). The impact of maternal diets during breastfeeding on the prevention of food allergy. *Curr Opin Allergy Clin Immunol, 2*, 207-210.

Sicherer, S.H., Forman, J.A., & Noone, S.A. (2000). Use assessment of self-administered epinephrine among food-allergic children and pediatricians. *Pediatrics, 105*, 359-362.

Sicherer, S.H., Furlong, T.J., DeSimone, J., & Sampson, H.A. (2001a). The US Peanut and Tree Nut Allergy Registry: Characteristics of reactions in schools and day care. *J Pediatr, 138*, 560-565.

Sicherer, S.H., Furlong, T.J., Munoz-Furlong, A., Burks, A.W., & Sampson, H.A. (2001b). A voluntary registry for peanut and tree nut allergy: Characteristics of the first 5149 registrants. *J Allergy Clin Immunol, 108*, 128-132.

Simons, F.E., Gu, X., Silver, N.A., & Simons, K.J. (2002). EpiPen Jr versus EpiPen in young children weighing 15 to 30 kg at risk for anaphylaxis. *J Allergy Clin Immunol, 109*, 171-175.

Skolnick, H.S., Conover-Walker, M.K., Koerner, C.B., Sampson, H.A., Burks, W., et al. (2001). The natural history of peanut allergy. *J Allergy Clin Immunol, 107*, 367-374.

Skoner, D.P. (2001). Allergic rhinitis: Definition, epidemiology, pathophysiology, detection, and diagnosis. *J Allergy Clin Immunol, 108*, S2-S8.

Skoner, D.P., Rachelefsky, G.S., Meltzer, E.O., Chervinsky, P., Morris, R.M., et al. (2000). Detection of growth suppression in children during treatment with intranasal beclomethasone dipropionate. *Pediatrics, 105*, E23.

Sly, R.M. (1999). Changing prevalence of allergic rhinitis and asthma. *Ann Allergy Asthma Immunol, 82*, 233-248.

Spergel, J.M. & Pawlowski, N.A. (2002). Food allergy: Mechanisms, diagnosis, and management in children. *Pediatr Clin North Am, 49*, 73-96, vi.

Staff of Physicians. (2001). *Physicians' desk reference 2002* (56th ed.). Montvale, NJ: Medical Economics Company.

Storms, W.W. (2002). Rethinking our approach to allergic rhinitis management. *Ann Allergy Asthma Immunol, 88*, 30-35.

Svanes, C., Jarvis, D., Chinn, S., & Burney, P. (1999). Childhood environment and adult atopy: Results from the European Community Respiratory Health Survey. *J Allergy Clin Immunol, 103*, 415-420.

Thestrup-Pedersen, K. (2000). Clinical aspects of atopic dermatitis. *Clin Exp Dermatol, 25*, 535-543.

Troye-Blomberg, M. (2002). T-cell reactivity in neonates: Influence of environmental and genetic factors. *Allergy, 57*, 69-72.

Turvey, S.E. (2001). Atopic diseases of childhood. *Curr Opin Pediatr, 13*, 487-495.

Van Cauwenberge, P. (1998). Management of rhinitis—the specialist's opinion. *Clin Exp Allergy, 28*(suppl 6), 29-33.

van Cauwenberge, P., Bachert, C., Passalacqua, G., Bousquet, J., Canonica, G.W., et al. (2000). Consensus statement on the treatment of allergic rhinitis. European Academy of Allergology and Clinical Immunology. *Allergy, 55*, 116-134.

Vancheri, C., Mastruzzo, C., Armato, F., Tomaselli, V., Magri, S., Pistorio, M.P., et al. (2001). Intranasal heparin reduces eosinophil recruitment after nasal allergen challenge in patients with allergic rhinitis. *J Allergy Clin Immunol, 108*, 703-708.

Vander Leek, T.K., Liu, A.H., Stefanski, K., Blacker, B., & Bock, S.A. (2000). The natural history of peanut allergy in young children and its association with serum peanut-specific IgE. *J Pediatr, 137*, 749-755.

Wang, D.Y., Niti, M., Smith, J.D., Yeoh, K.H., & Ng, T.P. (2002). Rhinitis: Do diagnostic criteria affect the prevalence and treatment? *Allergy, 57*, 150-154.

Weiss, S.T. (2002). Eat dirt—the hygiene hypothesis and allergic diseases. *N Engl J Med, 347*, 930-931.

Wilson, A.M., Orr, L.C., Coutie, W.J., Sims, E.J., & Lipworth, B.J. (2002). A comparison of once daily fexofenadine versus the combination of montelukast plus loratadine on domiciliary nasal peak flow and symptoms in seasonal allergic rhinitis. *Clin Exp Allergy, 32*, 126-132.

Wjst, M. & Dold, S. (1999). Genes, factor X, and allergens: What causes allergic diseases? *Allergy, 54*, 757-759.

Yale, S., & La Valle J.B. (2002). Food allergies and atopic dermatitis. *Alternative & Complementary Therapies, 8*, 76-80.

Zeiger, R.S. (1999). Food allergy: Current knowledge and future directions. Prevention of food allergy in infants and children. *Immunol Allergy Clin North Am, 19*(3).

Zeiger, R.S. & Heller, S. (1995). The development and prediction of atopy in high-risk children: Follow-up at age seven years in a prospective randomized study of combined maternal and infant food allergen avoidance. *J Allergy Clin Immunol, 95*, 1179-1190.

Zeiger, R.S., Sampson, H.A., Bock, S.A., Burks, A.W. Jr., Harden, K., Noone, S., Martin, D., Leung, S., & Wilson, G. (1999). Soy allergy in infants and children with IgE-associated cow's milk allergy. *J Pediatr, 134*, 614-622.

11 Asthma

Gail Kieckhefer and Marijo Ratcliffe

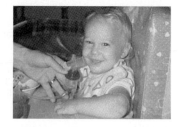

Etiology

Although asthma is still difficult to define, the *Global Strategy for Asthma Management and Prevention Report* (Global Initiative for Asthma Executive Committee, 2002, p. 2) states the following:

Asthma is a chronic inflammatory disease of the airways in which many cell types play a role, in particular mast cells, eosinophils, and T lymphocytes. In susceptible individuals the inflammation causes recurrent episodes of wheezing, breathlessness, chest tightness and cough particularly at night and/or early morning. These symptoms are usually associated with widespread but variable airflow obstruction that is at least partly reversible either spontaneously or with treatment. The inflammation also causes an associated increase in airway responsiveness to a variety of stimuli.

Our current understanding of asthma includes the knowledge, based on research over the past 20 years, that asthma is a heterogeneous disorder with variable expression in different individuals (Lemanske, 2002; Payne et al, 2001). Exposure to an agent, often called a trigger, leads to a cascade of further physiologic changes creating the acute inflammatory episode that occurs on an often already chronically inflamed airway and leads to the usual symptoms of asthma exacerbation: cough, wheeze, and shortness of breath.

Although much current research is aimed toward finding a strategy or treatment to prevent or cure asthma, at this time there is no specific prevention or cure. There is much, however, that can be done by the health care provider, child, and family to reduce the number or minimize the severity of acute exacerbations of the asthma.

An acute asthma episode is initiated by at least one of two types of offending triggers: (1) inflammatory triggers (e.g., allergens, chemical sensitizers, viral infections) and (2) noninflammatory triggers (e.g., dust, cold air, other irritants). Inflammatory triggers are considered asthmogenic insofar as they cause symptoms by increasing the frequency and severity of airway smooth muscle contraction and enhance airway responsiveness through inflammatory mechanisms. Noninflammatory triggers cause a bronchospastic response that may become more severe depending on the existing level of responsiveness in the airway. This initial bronchospastic response can lead to subsequent inflammatory changes in the airway.

Early, late, and mixed responses can occur as a result of an asthma trigger (Busse & Busse, 2002). An early-phase response will occur within the first 10 to 20 minutes of an airway's exposure to a trigger. The allergen/antigen binds to the allergen-specific immunoglobulin E (IgE) surface, causing activation of resident airway mast cells and macrophages. Proinflammatory mediators, such as histamine and leukotrienes, are released. These provoke contraction of the airway's smooth muscles,

increased mucous secretion, and vasodilation. Consequently, microvascular leakage and exudation of plasma into the airway walls cause them to become thickened and edematous with subsequent airway lumen constriction. In addition, the plasma may pass through the epithelial layer to collect in the airway lumen itself, causing further problems in mucous removal and increasing airflow obstruction. The early-phase response is therapeutically addressed through short-acting beta-agonist medications.

During the late-phase response, occurring up to 6 to 9 hours later, the initial bronchospastic reaction may have moderated. However, recruitment and activation of CD+4 T cells, eosinophils, neutrophils, basophils, prostaglandins, and other macrophages by the initial early-phase stimulation and mediator release cause further airway wall inflammation and bronchospasm (Bousquet et al, 2000). An ongoing cycle of proinflammatory mediator release leads to further cell activation, recruitment, and ultimately, persistently inflamed airways. The treatment for this process not only involves smooth muscle relaxation through short- or long-acting beta-agonists but also may require routine antiinflammatory medication.

Children can experience both early- and late-phase responses. If the ongoing inflammatory cycle is not interrupted, it may be the start of a more chronic phase with the creation of nonspecific bronchial hyperresponsiveness, which may initiate the process of airway wall remodeling. Remodeling of the airway causes submucosal damage with airway smooth muscle hypertrophy, mucous gland enlargement, and collagen deposition in the connective tissue (Bousquet et al, 2000; Lemanske, 2000). Although the bronchial epithelial layer may heal well, the submucosal layer regenerates abnormally. At our current stage of understanding, the greatest concern with chronic airway inflammation is that unless treated early and aggressively in children, the process of airway remodeling may ultimately cause irreversible reduced pulmonary function and an accelerated decline in forced expiratory volume in 1 second (FEV_1) beyond that of normal aging (Bousquet et al, 2000; Lemanske, 2000). Current research is directed toward further elucidation of this serious problem and identification of more specific and efficacious prevention and treatment.

Known Genetic Etiology

Specific multiple genetic etiologies of asthma are now being actively investigated (Lemanske, 2002). Evidence to date indicates the involvement of multiple genes and multiple expressions of any one gene (Busse & Busse, 2002; Gern et al, 1999; Palmer et al, 2001). It is this multifaceted genetic predisposition coupled with complex environmental influences that makes asthma a truly multifactorial condition.

Although genetic factors predispose the individual to the possibility of developing asthma, environmental factors contribute to the presence of clinically recognized asthma (Busse & Busse, 2002; Gern et al, 1999). Historically asthma has been characterized as an obstructive airway disease caused primarily by bronchoconstriction (i.e., smooth muscle contraction). Over the last decade the roles and mechanisms of inflammation and mucous secretion have become increasingly recognized and inflammation is now believed to be the most important component of asthma (National Heart, Lung and Blood Institute [NHLBI], 1997, 2002). The prenatal environment (maternal smoking) and infant environment (exposure or lack thereof to various immunologic stimuli, such as viruses and animal dander) are currently being investigated for their role in contributing to the rise in prevalence of asthma in Western cultures during the 1980s and 1990s (Jaakkola & Jaakkola, 2002; Montalbano & Lemanske, 2002). It is now thought that the overall microbial burden experienced vs. any one isolated illness during infancy primes the immunologic system for the child's later phenotypic expression of a genetic asthma predisposition (Martinez, 2001a, 2002).

Incidence and Prevalence

The National Center for Health Statistic's annual National Health Interview Survey (NHIS) from 1997 to 1999 determined the prevalence of asthma over 12 months of age as well as the 12-month asthma attack prevalence in children. Both prevalence parameters were increased in children from 5 to 14 years and in blacks compared with whites. The most recent rates indicate that 1995 had the highest prevalence rate of 7.5% with current stabilization at 5.4% reported in 1997 (Akinbami & Schoendorf, 2002).

In the United States, the poor, especially of black or Hispanic background, experience disproportionally high rates of both asthma prevalence and morbidity (Castro et al, 2001; Mannino et al, 2002a). Stapleton (2002) noted the following attack rates per 1000 for differing ethnic groups in 2000: white, 53.4; black, 76.8; and Hispanic, 42.2. There is great worldwide variability in prevalence, with industrialized areas having consistently high rates (International Study of Asthma and Allergies in Children, 1998). Although public health officials have recently reported decreases in some aspects of childhood asthma morbidity in the United States others remain unimproved (Mannino et al, 2002a), and much work remains to be done in implementing effective identification and treatment systems of care for children with asthma.

Surveys such as the NHIS are always subject to error because of the required assumption that the diagnosis of asthma and the parent's recall of the diagnosis are correct. Diagnosing asthma still remains difficult. In children under the age of 3 years, it is often difficult to differentiate asthma from other obstructive lung disorders, such as bronchiolitis. In these very young children who wheeze, especially with upper respiratory infections, treatment may be empiric and/or the diagnosis singularly clinically based. Parents too may either overreport or underreport a diagnosis of childhood asthma, depending on the

wording of a survey question. Regardless, it appears there had been a real increase in the prevalence rates of childhood asthma overall between 1980 and 1996 concomitant with the increase in office, hospital-based clinic, and emergency room visits. The current decline of mortality and morbidity may be linked to not only earlier diagnosis and aggressive treatment but also comprehensive, focused asthma education and intervention programs having a positive impact on family management of this significant public health problem (Clark & Partridge, 2002; Mannino et al, 2002a).

Clinical Manifestations at Time of Diagnosis (Box 11-1)

Acute Symptoms

Many children with asthma initially present with an acute episode of wheezing and shortness of breath associated with or following an upper respiratory infection (URI). URI symptoms typically include a 2- to 3-day history of rhinitis and slight fever. As these common symptoms persist, a cough, increased wheeze, or both emerge. The children may have tachypnea and use of accessory muscles (e.g., intercostals) and nasal flaring. Children with sternocleidomastoid retraction and supraclavicular in-drawing most often have severe airway obstruction and need rapid assessment of their cardiorespiratory status—including pulse oximetry (if available in the office setting) and interventions immediately initiated. Observations of body position, use of abdominal muscles to expel air, and alterations in mental status should also be noted. Auscultation for adventitious sounds can elicit the following manifestations of increasing airway obstruction: prolongation of the expiratory phase, expiratory wheeze, inspiratory and expiratory wheeze, and absence or distancing of breath sounds. This last is an ominous sign indicative of little air exchange and possible impending respiratory arrest. The child's chest wall may appear to have an increased anteroposterior (AP) diameter, which can indicate long-standing pulmonary obstruction. If an AP and lateral chest

---

BOX 11-1

Clinical Manifestations at Time of Diagnosis

ACUTE SYMPTOMS
Prolongation of expiratory phase
Wheezing and/or chest tightness/pain and cough
Tachypnea, accessory muscle use, retractions, nasal flaring
Agitation or altered mental status
X-ray evidence of hyperinflation

CHRONIC SYMPTOMS
Chronic cough, especially at night
Allergic signs and symptoms
Enlarged anteroposterior diameter of chest wall
Wheeze, although it may only be evident during acute episodes or with activity
Atopic dermatitis
Recurrent pneumonia and/or sinusitis
Shortness of breath on exercise (EIB)
Seasonal pattern
Response to beta-agonist therapy

film is indicated, hyperinflation may be present, as noted by flattened diaphragms and increased AP diameter. In severe obstructive disease, the liver may be palpated below the costal margin. Even with severe asthma, however, clubbing of extremities in a child is rare.

Chronic Symptoms

When examining a child with asthma who is not acutely ill, a different set of chronic findings may be present on history and physical examination. Chronic cough in the absence of wheezing and persistent nocturnal cough or wheeze are the most frequently noted symptoms. Also common are the presence of allergic symptoms (see Chapter 10). An increase in the AP diameter of the chest wall occurs in children with chronic symptoms of increased pulmonary effort. Breath sounds are often clear except during an acute exacerbation; a soft wheeze might be heard on expiration or elicited from the child during a forced expiration. It is important to discern if dry skin patches, keratosis pilaris, or evidence of eczema is present or if there is a family history of asthma or atopy since these conditions should heighten the suspicion of asthma in children of all ages. Other conditions that may prompt consideration of an asthma diagnosis include recurrent pneumonia or sinusitis.

In older children and teenagers, decreased ability to exercise with complaints of shortness of breath, chest pain or pressure, and a history of cough or wheeze *after* exercise are all indicative of exercise-induced bronchospasm (EIB). Although 6% to 13% of children without asthma will have EIB, 60% to 80% of children with asthma have EIB (Anderson & Daviskas, 2000; Fowler, 2001; O'Hallaren, 2002).

A seasonal pattern to asthma symptoms is likely when airborne allergens trigger the child's exacerbations.

Other Conditions Causing Cough and Wheeze

Because children display a variety of symptoms with asthma, other diseases must be considered and ruled out.

Children who have recurrent pneumonia or sinusitis—even with no evidence of malabsorption—should have a quantitative pilocarpine ionophoresis (i.e., sweat chloride test) for cystic fibrosis (see Chapter 22). In young children, monophonic expiratory wheezing or expiratory stridor (sometimes difficult to distinguish from one another) may indicate foreign body aspiration, tracheal compression, stenosis, tracheomalacia, or bronchomalacia. Referral to a pulmonologist or otolaryngologist for bronchoscopy may be necessary for diagnosis when response to asthma treatment is atypical.

Treatment

The current approach to asthma treatment reflects the understanding that airway inflammation is predominant in most phases of the condition. Although therapy must be individualized to the particular child, it is now recognized that it is critical in children with persistent asthma to prevent symptoms caused by underlying inflammation with long-term controllers in addition to treating the acute symptoms caused by bronchoconstriction with quick-acting rescue medication.

BOX 11-2
Treatment

NHLBI GUIDELINES FOR THE DIAGNOSIS AND MANAGEMENT OF ASTHMA
Education for shared management (Box 11-3)
Treatment appropriate to level of severity (Tables 11-1 and 11-2)
   Mild intermittent
   Mild persistent
   Moderate persistent
   Severe persistent
Written action plan
Medications
   Quick relievers (i.e., rescue medications)
   Nonsteroidal antiinflammatory agents
   Inhaled corticosteroids
   Long-acting beta$_2$-agonists
   Systemic corticosteroids
   Leukotriene modifiers
   Methylxanthines
Treatment of exercise-induced bronchospasms
Environmental manipulation

NHLBI, National Heart, Lung, and Blood Institute.

Prevention of airway remodeling through appropriate and timely antiinflammatory treatment may help to preserve the child's pulmonary function and activity tolerance as an adult (Lemanske, 2001).

It is also recognized that asthma is a chronic condition that requires lifelong learning and family participation in shared management with the health care provider. Medications and environmental manipulations will all be necessary to control asthma for most children. For treatment to be effective it will need to be comprehensive and multipronged (Box 11-2).

National Heart, Lung and Blood Institute (NHLBI) Guidelines for the Diagnosis and Management of Asthma

The primary goal of treatment is to allow the child to live as normal a life as possible with as close to normal lung function as possible. The child should be able to participate in normal childhood activities, experience exercise tolerance similar to peers, and attend school to grow intellectually and develop socially. The 1997 NIH *Expert Panel Report II (EPR-II)* and the 2002 *Update on Childhood Asthma Management* articulate current best practices on the diagnosis and comprehensive management of asthma (NHLBI, 1997, 2002). These documents provide a framework to guide clinical decision making by the primary care provider. They serve as the basis for recommendations advocated in this chapter. Because knowledge is rapidly expanding in regard to asthma, providers must regularly review updated on-line reports on best practice, evidence-based management strategies from NHLBI (www.nhlbi.nih.gov), and relevant professional organizations (www.aap.org; www.napnap.org).

Education for Shared Management. Educating the family and maturing child to become effective partners with the primary care provider in the day-to-day management of asthma remains a primary treatment goal (Kieckhefer & Trahms, 2000; NHLBI, 1997). Instruction in shared management is a necessary cornerstone in regular health care and requires age-appropriate sharing of responsibilities among family members and the primary care provider. The purposes of shared management education are to help prevent episodes of asthma exacerbation, minimize the severity of episodes that cannot be prevented, enhance the family's ability to understand and implement treatment strategies, and provide healthy responses to life changes that may be necessitated by asthma.

Family education in shared management should promote a sense of teamwork (Bonner et al, 2002). The foundations should be laid early at diagnosis, with primary care providers drawing families into treatment decisions as their basic knowledge and skills increase. Community organizations recruiting families from a variety of providers have offered formal education programs and developed and extensively tested curricular guides for several programs that are useful, relatively inexpensive, and easy to implement. Other approaches have successfully used games, camp experiences, books, on-line materials, and community activism (most commonly coupled with a formal education program) to educate the child and family. But consistent with the *EPR-II*, the primary care provider should play a central role with the family in ensuring a comprehensive mix of ongoing educational experiences for the family and child. This requires knowledge of community programs and other available age-appropriate resources, ongoing documentation of what has been taught or learned, and the family's and child's response to the information (Pinkerton & Kieckhefer, 2002). On-line and comprehensive printed compilations of resources are available (Friedman, 2002).

Most asthma education programs contain information on the basic pathophysiology of asthma and control of triggers; knowledge of early warning signs that signal the onset of a problem; how to manage an exacerbation, including when to contact the primary care provider; knowledge of strategies for relaxation, controlled breathing, and problem solving; medication names, actions, and when to alter their use according to set guidelines; and proper use of equipment. Programs have shown effectiveness in reducing child and family anxiety, increasing asthma management behavior, improving school attendance, and reducing costly emergency room and hospital use (Homer et al, 2000; Jones et al, 2001). Before a program is implemented or a child is referred to a program, the primary care provider must review the program to ensure it is consistent with the provider's treatment philosophy; know whether it is an individualized or group approach; and identify the age, child, and type of family for whom the program has previously worked best. When the provider is knowledgeable about the shared management program and can reinforce learning during routine health care visits with the family, a true child-parent-provider partnership is enhanced to ultimately improve the child's overall health status.

Education must be viewed in the context of lifelong learning. Changes in the child's and family's capabilities and in treatment modalities necessitate ongoing evaluation and provision of education. This ongoing education helps ensure that the family gains experience in managing the child's asthma and the

---

BOX 11-3
NHLBI Asthma Education Program

EDUCATIONAL COMPONENTS
Basic facts about asthma
Roles of medications
Skills: inhaler/spacer/holding chamber/peak flowmeter use
Self-monitoring
Environmental control measures
When and how to take rescue actions
When to call health care provider
Lifelong learning

NHLBI, National Heart, Lung, and Blood Institute.

---

depth of their knowledge and skills is enhanced and keeps pace with current treatment guidelines.

When the diagnosis of asthma is made during an acute exacerbation, the family first needs education on immediate care, signs of deterioration that require immediate contact with the provider, immediate and relatively inexpensive environmental changes they can implement, such as dust mite covers for pillows and mattresses (Rijssenbeek-Nouwens et al, 2002), and actions and side effects of medications being taken. Once the crisis has passed, the provider will want to plan with the family for ongoing, comprehensive asthma education. Families have noted that it takes them up to 1 year to gain any sense of ease with the full perspective of asthma management. The components of an asthma education program suggested by the *EPR-II* are listed in Box 11-3.

Treatment Appropriate to Level of Severity. Because asthma is a chronic disease with episodic symptoms, asthma management entails treatment based on the needs or severity of the child's underlying airway pathologic condition. The following four categories of asthma severity are currently used: mild intermittent, mild persistent, moderate persistent, and severe persistent. These categories, based on the frequency of cough, wheeze, and other asthma symptoms together with the child's age, are depicted in Tables 11-1 and 11-2. These tables come directly from the *EPR-II* 2002 update for severity categorization and treatment consideration (NHLBI, 2002). The philosophy underlying this approach is that asthma treatment is not static but based on the current symptom presentation. It requires the provider to "step up" treatment if asthma symptoms emerge and remain uncontrolled or "step down" treatment after control has been achieved (NHLBI, 1997, 2002). The approach advocates using the least amount of medication needed to control symptoms with a systematic plan for ongoing evaluation of results.

Timely treatment of an asthma exacerbation requires recognition of early warning signs of an acute exacerbation in a child and rescue treatment appropriate to the level of severity. Early warning signs may be unique to a particular child (e.g., tickle in the throat, frequent yawning or sighing, fatigue) or fairly common (e.g., a cough, especially at night; tightness in the throat with URI symptoms of a runny nose and congestion; a decreased peak expiratory flow rate [PEFR]).

Written Action Plans. All children with asthma need a written action plan they and their family can implement in times of exacerbation. Children with any severity of *persistent asthma*

TABLE 11-1

Stepwise Approach for Managing Infants and Young Children (≤5 Yr) with Acute or Chronic Asthma

Classify Severity: Clinical Features before Treatment or Adequate Control		Medications Required to Maintain Long-Term Control
	SYMPTOMS/DAY SYMPTOMS/NIGHT	DAILY MEDICATIONS
Step 4: Severe Persistent	Continual Frequent	**Preferred treatment** **High-dose inhaled corticosteroids** *and* **Long-acting inhaled beta$_2$-agonists** *and; if needed,* Corticosteroid tablets or syrup long term (2 mg/kg/day, generally do not exceed 60 mg/day) (Make repeat attempts to reduce systemic corticosteroids and maintain control with high-dose inhaled corticosteroids.)
Step 3: Moderate Persistent	Daily >1 night/wk	**Preferred treatments** **Low-dose inhaled corticosteroids and long-acting inhaled beta$_2$-agonists** *or* **Medium-dose inhaled corticosteroids** Alternative treatment Low-dose inhaled corticosteroids and either leukotriene receptor antagonist or theophylline *If needed (particularly in patients with recurring severe exacerbations):* **Preferred treatment** **Medium-dose inhaled corticosteroids and long-acting beta$_2$-agonists** Alternative treatment Medium-dose inhaled corticosteroids and either leukotriene receptor antagonist or theophylline
Step 2: Mild Persistent	>2/wk but <1×/day >2 nights/mo	**Preferred treatment** **Low-dose inhaled corticosteroid (with nebulizer or MDI with holding chamber with or without face mask or DPI)** Alternative treatment (listed alphabetically) Cromolyn (nebulizer is preferred or MDI with holding chamber) *or* leukotriene receptor antagonist
Step 1: Mild Intermittent	≤2 days/wk ≤2 nights/mo	No daily medication needed
Quick Relief: All Patients		Bronchodilator as needed for symptoms. Intensity of treatment will depend on severity of exacerbation. **Preferred treatment: Short-acting inhaled beta$_2$-agonists** by nebulizer or face mask and space/holding chamber Alternative treatment: Oral beta$_2$-agonist With viral respiratory infection Bronchodilator every 4–6 hrs up to 24 hrs (longer with physician consult); in general, repeat no more than once every 6 wk Consider systemic corticosteroid if exacerbation is severe or patient has history of previous severe exacerbations Use of short-acting beta$_2$-agonists >2 times per wk in intermittent asthma (daily or increasing use in persistent asthma) may indicate the need to initiate (increase) long-term control therapy.

↓ **Step down**
Review treatment every 1 to 6 mo; a gradual stepwise reduction in treatment may be possible.

↑ **Step up**
If control is not maintained, consider step up. First, review patient medication technique, adherence, and environmental control.

Note
The stepwise approach is intended to assist, not replace, the clinical decision making required to meet individual patient needs.
Classify severity: assign patient to most severe step in which any feature occurs.
There are very few studies on asthma therapy for infants.
Gain control as quickly as possible (a course of short systemic corticosteroids may be required); then step down to the least medication necessary to maintain control.
Provide parent education on asthma management and controlling environmental factors that make asthma worse (e.g., allergies, irritants).
Consultation with an asthma specialist is recommended for patients with moderate or severe persistent asthma. Consider consultation for patients with mild persistent asthma.

Goals of Therapy: Asthma Control

Minimal or no chronic symptoms day or night	Minimal use of short-acting inhaled beta$_2$-agonist (<1×/day, <1 canister/mo)
Minimal or no exacerbations	
No limitations on activities; no school/parent's work missed	Minimal or no adverse effects from medications

From NHLBI. (2002). *NAEPP expert panel report guidelines for diagnosis and management of asthma—update on selected topics 2002.* U.S. DHHS.
MDI, Metered dose inhaler; *DPI,* dry powder inhaler.

TABLE 11-2

Stepwise Approach for Managing Asthma in Adults and Children >5 Yr: Treatment

Classify Severity: Clinical Features before Treatment or Adequate Control			Medications Required to Maintain Long-Term Control
	SYMPTOMS/DAY SYMPTOMS/NIGHT	PEF OR FEV$_1$ PEF VARIABILITY	DAILY MEDICATIONS
Step 4: Severe Persistent	Continual Frequent	≤60% >30%	**Preferred treatment** **High-dose inhaled corticosteroids** *and* **Long-acting inhaled beta$_2$-agonists** *and, if needed,* Corticosteroid tablets or syrup long term (2 mg/kg/day, generally do not exceed 60 mg/day) (Make repeat attempts to reduce systemic corticosteroids and maintain control with high-dose inhaled corticosteroids.)
Step 3: Moderate Persistent	Daily >1 night/wk	>60% to <80% >30%	**Preferred treatment** **Low to medium dose inhaled corticosteroids and long-acting inhaled beta$_2$-agonists** Alternative treatment (listed alphabetically) Increase inhaled corticosteroids within medium-dose range or Low to medium dose inhaled corticosteroids and either leukotriene modifier or theophylline *If needed (particularly in patients with recurring severe exacerbations):* **Preferred treatment** **Increase inhaled corticosteroids within medium-dose range and add long-acting inhaled beta$_2$-agonists** Alternative treatment Increase inhaled corticosteroids within medium-dose range and add either leukotriene modifier or theophylline
Step 2: Mild Persistent	>2/wk but <1×/day >2 nights/mo	≥80% 20% to 30%	**Preferred treatment** **Low-dose inhaled corticosteroids** Alternative treatment (listed alphabetically): cromolyn, leukotriene modifier, nedocromil, *or* sustained-release theophylline to serum concentration of 5–15 µg/ml
Step 1: Mild Intermittent	≤2 days/wk ≤2 nights/mo	≥80% <20%	**Preferred treatment** **No daily medication needed** Severe exacerbations may occur, separated by long periods of normal lung function and no symptoms. A course of systemic corticosteroids is recommended.
Quick Relief: All Patients			Short-acting bronchodilator: 2–4 puffs **short-acting inhaled beta$_2$-agonists** as needed for symptoms. Intensity of treatment will depend on severity of exacerbation; up to 3 treatments at 20-min intervals or a single nebulizer treatment as needed. Course of systemic corticosteroids may be needed. Use of short-acting beta$_2$-agonists >2 times per week in intermittent asthma (daily or increasing use in persistent asthma) may indicate the need to initiate (increase) long-term control therapy.

↓ Step down
Review treatment every 1–6 mo; a gradual stepwise reduction in treatment may be possible.

↑ Step up
If control is not maintained, consider step up. First, review patient medication technique, adherence, and environmental control.

Note
The stepwise approach is meant to assist, not replace, the clinical decision making required to meet individual patient needs.
Classify severity: assign patient to most severe step in which any feature occurs (PEF is percent of personal best; FEV$_1$ is percent predicted).
Gain control as quickly as possible (consider a short course of systemic corticosteroids); then step down to the least medication necessary to maintain control.
Provide education on self-management and controlling environmental factors that make asthma worse (e.g., allergens, irritants).
Refer to an asthma specialist if there are difficulties controlling asthma or if step 4 care is required. Referral may be considered if step 3 care is required.

Goals of Therapy: Asthma Control

Minimal or no chronic symptoms day or night
Minimal or no exacerbations
No limitations on activities; no school/parent's work missed

Maintain (near) normal pulmonary function
Minimal use of short-acting inhaled beta$_2$-agonist (<1×/day, <1 canister/mo)
Minimal or no adverse effects from medications

From NHLBI. (2002). *NAEPP expert panel report guidelines for diagnosis and man agement of asthma—update on selected topics 2002.* U.S. DHHS. Reprinted with permission.
PEF, Peak expiratory flow; *FEV,* forced expiratory volume.

TABLE 11-3
Usual Dosages for Long-Term Control Medications

Medication	Dosage Form	Adult Dose	Child Dose*
INHALED CORTICOSTEROIDS (SEE TABLE 11-4)			
SYSTEMIC CORTICOSTEROIDS (Applies to all three corticosteroids.)			
Methylprednisolone	2-, 4-, 8-, 16-, 32-mg tablets	7.5-60 mg daily in a single dose in AM or qod as needed for control	0.25-2 mg/kg/day in single dose in AM or qod as needed for control
Prednisolone	5-mg tablets: 5 mg/5 cc; 15 mg/5 cc	Short-course "burst" to achieve control: 40-60 mg/day as single or 2 divided doses for 3-10 days	Short-course "burst": 1-2 mg/kg/day, maximum 60 mg/day for 3-10 days
Prednisone	1-, 2.5-, 5-, 10-, 20-, 50-mg tablets: 5 mg/cc; 5 mg/5 cc		
LONG-ACTING INHALED BETA$_2$-AGONISTS (Should not be used for symptom relief or for exacerbations. Use with inhaled corticosteroids.)			
Salmeterol	MDI, 21 μg/puff	2 puffs every 12 hr	1-2 puffs every 12 hr (>4 yr)
	DPI, 50 μg/blister	1 blister every 12 hr	1 blister every 12 hr (>4 yr)
Formoterol	DPI, 12 μg/single-use capsule	1 capsule every 12 hr	1 capsule every 12 hr
COMBINED MEDICATION			
Fluticasone/salmeterol	DPI, 100, 250, or 500 μg/50 μg	1 inhalation bid; dose depends on severity of asthma	1 inhalation bid; dose depends on severity of asthma (>4 yr)
CROMOLYN AND NEDOCROMIL			
Cromolyn	MDI, 1 mg/puff	2-4 puffs tid-qid	1-2 puffs tid-qid
	Nebulizer, 20 mg/ampule	1 ampule tid-qid	1 ampule tid-qid
Nedocromil	MDI, 1.75 mg/puff	2-4 puffs bid-qid	1-2 puffs bid-qid
LEUKOTRIENE MODIFIERS			
Montelukast	4- or 5-mg chewable tablet	10 mg qhs	4 mg qhs (2-5 yr)
	10-mg tablet		5 mg qhs (6-14 yr)
			10 mg qhs (>14 yr)
Zafirlukast	10- or 20-mg tablet	40 mg daily (20-mg tablet bid)	20 mg daily (7-11 yr) (10-mg tablet bid)
Zileuton	300- or 600-mg tablet	2400 mg daily (give tablets qid)	
METHYLXANTHINE (Serum monitoring is important [serum concentration of 5-15 μg/ml at steady state].)			
Theophylline	Liquids, sustained-release tablets, capsules	Starting dose, 10 mg/kg/day up to 300 mg max; usual max, 800 mg/day	Starting dose 10 mg/kg/day; usual max: <1 yr of age: 0.2 (age in wk) +5 = mg/kg/day ≥1 yr of age: 16 mg/kg/day

From NHLBI. (2002). *NAEPP expert panel report guidelines for diagnosis and management of asthma—update on selected topics 2002.* U.S. DHHS.
MDI, Metered dose inhaler; *DPI,* dry powder inhaler.
*Children ≤12 yr of age.

require this emergency action plan *and* a written daily management plan. For example, a written plan for every day may include twice daily inhaled steroids per metered dose inhaler (MDI) with spacer. An action plan to implement during exacerbation might also include the following: (1) begin or increase rescue medication up to every 4 hours at home, (2) start oral steroid "burst" at prescribed dose if symptoms are not improved after first step of action plan, and (3) notify primary care provider of progress within 24 hours. This type of action plan is meant to reduce the severity and the length of the exacerbation so that emergent medical care is not needed (NHLBI, 1997, 2002). The daily management plan is to control underlying inflammation and daily symptoms and prevent exacerbations.

If symptoms do not respond to home management, the child needs further evaluation and treatment in a primary care provider's office, if appropriate monitoring and treatment equipment is available, or in an emergency room or hospital setting. These settings offer the added ability to monitor the child's air movement, oxygenation, and blood gases; administer oxygen as needed; perform spirometry; continuously monitor cardiac and respiratory status; and give medications frequently in a controlled environment.

Medications
Asthma therapy has changed to reflect the need to focus on reducing the chronic inflammatory processes and combine bronchodilatory medications with antiinflammatory medications during acute exacerbations. Delineated treatment modalities for management of all four severity categories of asthma are available to facilitate decision making in any setting (Tables 11-1 and 11-2; NHLBI, 2002). Several types of medications are currently used in treatment. For quick relief, "rescue" medications of short-acting, inhaled beta-agonists are used. During severe exacerbations, anticholinergics and/or systemic corticosteroids may be added (Table 11-3). A wider array of long-term controller medications includes inhaled or systemic corticosteroids, long-acting beta$_2$-agonists, cromolyn sodium and nedocromil, leukotriene modifiers, and methylxanthines. Specific long-term controller medications, drug forms, and child dosages are summarized in Table 11-4, which provides a comparative listing of strengths of inhaled corticosteroids.

TABLE 11-4
Estimated Comparative Daily Dosages for Inhaled Corticosteroids

Drug	Low Daily Dose		Medium Daily Dose		High Daily Dose	
	Adult	Child*	Adult	Child*	Adult	Child*
Beclomethasone CFC 42 or 84 µg/puff	168–504 µg	84–336 µg	504–840 µg	336–672 µg	>840 µg	>672 µg
Beclomethasone HFA 40 or 80 µg/puff	80–240 µg	80–160 µg	240–480 µg	160–320 µg	>480 µg	>320 µg
Budesonide DPI 200 µg/inhalation	200–600 µg	200–400 µg	600–1200 µg	400–800 µg	>1200 µg	>800 µg
Inhalation suspension for nebulization (child dose)		0.5 mg		1.0 mg		2.0 mg
Flunisolide 250 µg/puff	500–1000 µg	500–750 µg	1000–2000 µg	1000–1250 µg	>2000 µg	>1250 µg
Fluticasone						
MDI: 44, 110, or 220 µg/puff	88–264 µg	88–176 µg	264–660 µg	176–440 µg	>660 µg	>440 µg
DPI: 50, 100, or 250 µg/inhalation	100–300 µg	100–200 µg	300–600 µg	200–400 µg	>600 µg	>400 µg
Triamcinolone acetonide 100 µg/puff	400–1000 µg	400–800 µg	1000–2000 µg	800–1200 µg	>2000 µg	>1200 µg

From NHLBI. (2002). *NAEPP expert panel report guidelines for diagnosis and management of asthma—update on selected topics 2002.* U.S. DHHS. Reprinted with permission.
*Children ≤12 yrs of age.

BOX 11-4
Quick-Relief Medications

Short-acting beta-agonists: Therapy of choice for relief of acute symptoms and prevention of EIB.

Anticholinergics: Ipratropium bromide may provide some additive benefit to inhaled beta₂-agonists in severe exacerbations. May be an alternative bronchodilator for children who do not achieve optimal benefit from inhaled beta₂-agonists alone.

IV systemic corticosteroids: Used for moderate to severe exacerbations to speed recovery and prevent hospitalization.

IV, Intravenous.

Quick-Relief or "Rescue" Medications. For most children the first medication chosen for symptomatic treatment of an acute exacerbation (Box 11-4) is a quick-acting beta-adrenergic agent, such as albuterol (Proventil, Ventolin), that inhibits the early-phase bronchospastic response. All beta-adrenergic agents can cause increased heart rate and may cause tremor of the fingers or hands. Some parents of young children also note hyperactivity, irritability, and sleeplessness.

Using an air compressor with an updraft nebulizer to deliver a beta-adrenergic medication is common; but children as young as 4 years of age may be able to use a metered dose inhaler (MDI [puffer]) if a spacer is used. Even infants and toddlers can use this modality successfully if a face mask is used with the spacer (Anhoj et al, 2002; Ploin et al, 2000). A spacer is a chamber that attaches to the MDI, allowing the medicine to be puffed into the chamber. The child can then inhale from the spacer to receive the medication, which avoids having to coordinate compressing the MDI while slowly inhaling. Dry powder inhalers (DPIs), which involve inhaling a powdered form of the medication but do not require a coordinated effort like an MDI, are now being used to deliver a variety of medications. Delivery devices are also now being altered to reduce environmental chlorofluorocarbons (CFCs). Because of the wide variety of delivery devices available, each with unique steps to activate, maneuvers to inhale, and cleaning requirements, the provider must know and diligently review the directions for proper use and have office staff consistently teach and review proper techniques with the child and family.

Nebulized treatments with a face mask offer several advantages, including (1) direct deposition of aerosolized medication in the respiratory tract, (2) decreased side effects as opposed to oral medication, (3) better delivery than an MDI when the tidal volume is reduced during an acute episode, and (4) the ability to mix beta-adrenergic medications with other medications (e.g., cromolyn sodium or ipratropium sulfate).

Oral syrups containing beta-adrenergic agents are also available, but onset of action comes only after 30 minutes, they may cause greater hyperactivity in many children, and they are not currently recommended as preferred treatment (NHLBI, 2002). For convenience, some older children favor a pill rather than an MDI, and therapeutic adherence may be improved if given this choice (Maspero et al, 2001). However, any oral preparation will have a longer onset compared with an inhaled medication, which is less than ideal in a "rescue" medication.

Nonsteroidal Antiinflammatory Agents. Antiinflammatory agents are used as the first-choice daily preventive medication for children with persistent asthma because they affect both the early- and the late-phase response. These agents are best known as mast cell stabilizers but may have other inhibitory effects on inflammatory cells.

Although low-dose inhaled corticosteroids are now considered the preferred treatment for persistent symptoms, cromolyn (Intal, Nasalcrom) delivered by nebulizer or MDI given three or four times daily remains an alternative for mild persistent asthma (NHLBI, 2002). One treatment per day is not sufficient for maintenance therapy, however, and the frequency of needed administration can affect adherence to the schedule. Cromolyn is compatible for delivery by a hand-held nebulizer when mixed with beta-adrenergic or anticholinergic agents. Nedocromil (Tilade) is another nonsteroidal, antiinflammatory medication that is unique in chemical structure and appears to have a synergistic effect with inhaled steroids (McEvoy, 2002). Nedocromil inhibits the release of inflammatory chemotactic and smooth muscle–contracting mediators from eosinophils, neutrophils, and mast cells. It has been more effective than cromolyn with regard to antigen and exercise-induced symptoms in some individuals and might be considered as part of a preventive therapeutic plan. Although usually well tolerated, the most significant disadvantage to nedocromil has been its undesirable taste, so it is best administered with a spacer to minimize this effect. Recommended dosage is two puffs three or four times per day initially, which, based on the response, may then be reduced to twice daily.

Inhaled Corticosteroids. Corticosteroids inhibit the late-phase asthmatic response and are used to treat inflammation and edema associated with asthma. Thus preferred treatment of children with more than mild intermittent asthma now includes the long-term use of inhaled corticosteroids. The lowest effective dose should be used. Even young children may be able to use inhaled corticosteroids via MDI with a spacer or other device and reduce their need for systemic treatment (Williams et al, 2001). Spacers with masks are also an option for children under 4 years of age who require inhaled steroids. Children using a spacer with inhaled steroids should always rinse their mouth and spit and wipe the facial area that was covered by the mask after use to prevent development of thrush. Pulmicort Respules (a budesonide suspension) are now available for nebulized corticosteroid treatment to children older than 1 year of age. The nebulized medication should be administered via mask to prevent the theoretic potential complication of cataract formation.

Triamcinolone acetate (Azmacort) and beclomethasone (Beclovent, Vanceril) have long been used as inhaled corticosteroids. Budesonide (Pulmocort) and fluticasone (Flovent) are two other inhaled corticosteroids that appear to reduce airway obstruction, as well as reduce the number of inflammatory cells in the airways and the number of asthma exacerbations. Both are highly potent corticosteroids that have low systemic bioavailability as measured by plasma cortisol. Fluticasone is available in three different concentrations and for both MDI and DPI devices.

Long-Acting Beta$_2$-Agonists. For the child with moderate or severe persistent asthma whose symptoms remain uncontrolled with medium- to high-dose inhaled corticosteroids, a long-acting inhaled beta-agonist, such as salmeterol (Serevent) or formoterol (Foradil), should be added to the regimen and effects evaluated. Current recommendations include considering a trial of the addition of a long-acting beta$_2$-agonist to any child with persistent asthma using an inhaled corticosteroid before increasing the steroid dose (NHLBI, 2002).

Systemic Corticosteroids. Children who continue to have frequent symptoms even with this combined therapy or high-dose inhaled corticosteroid treatment may require systemic corticosteroid treatment in either a short burst (3 to 10 days) or for a longer period (NHLBI, 2002). In children requiring prolonged treatment or repeated short treatments with oral steroids, reevaluation is needed every 2 to 3 months so the effects of treatment can be reviewed and documented and a "step up" or "step down" regimen considered. At each visit a thorough interval history is necessary to determine any adverse effects from corticosteroid therapy. Growth and blood pressure should be monitored at each well-child visit and plotted so con-

cerning trends can be appreciated if they occur. Referral to the pulmonary-allergy specialist is warranted for all children with moderate or severe persistent asthma and when adverse side effects of corticosteroid therapy are detected (NHLBI, 2002).

To prevent problems with growth suppression, impaired bone mineralization, or an effect on the hypothalamus-pituitary-adrenal (HPA) axis, the total dose of oral, inhaled, and topical corticosteroids should be adjusted to the cumulative lowest level necessary to maintain symptom control whenever possible. An awareness of cumulative corticosteroid effects must be maintained even with children receiving medium- to high-dose inhaled corticosteroids (Price et al, 2002a; Wong et al, 2002). Table 11-4 provides comparative daily dosages for inhaled corticosteroids so careful selection can occur (NHLBI, 2002).

Growth and steroid use are a frequent concern for parents and providers alike (Purucker & Malozowski, 2001). Several studies appear to concur on the short- and long-term implications. In general, children with both mild and moderate persistent asthma who use daily inhaled corticosteroids have been found to have reduction in growth velocity during the first year of up to 20%, but final predicted adult height has been attained (Agertoft & Pedersen, 2000). In all studies, growth slowing was most evident during the first year of treatment. Concerns regarding the use of inhaled corticosteroids are not confined to growth. The rate of bone loss has been examined in 109 premenopausal women 18 to 45 years of age with asthma. Some took inhaled corticosteroids, whereas others did not require them. A dose-dependent loss of bone in the hip and trochanter was noted but not in the femoral neck or spine. Whether these results can be extrapolated to children has yet to be determined. Although no normative data are available for children less than 12 years of age, the researchers suggested routine assessment of bone density over time for children receiving moderate-to high-dose therapy and attention to utilizing the minimum inhaled corticosteroid dose possible to control symptoms (Harris et al, 2001; Israel et al, 2001).

Anticholinergic agents (e.g., ipratropium bromide [Atrovent]) block cholinergic reflex bronchoconstriction and may be most useful in children with bronchitic symptoms of increased mucous secretion when used with beta-agonists and/or anti-inflammatory agents. These agents, however, are not particularly helpful against allergic challenges and do not block late-phase response nor do they inhibit mediators from mast cells. Ipratropium bromide is the only anticholinergic drug currently approved for treatment of airway disease. Delivery of ipratropium is by MDI or nebulizer. It can be mixed with albuterol and cromolyn sodium for the convenience of providing three medications with one aerosol treatment. Side effects include dry mucous membranes, cutaneous flush, and fever. Behavioral and neurologic symptoms can occur with central nervous system (CNS) toxicity (McEvoy, 2002).

Leukotriene Modifiers. Leukotriene modifiers are a relatively new class of medications that intervene to stop the inflammatory cascade. Montelukast (Singulair), a leukotriene antagonist, is approved for children 2 years of age and older as opposed to zafirlukast (Accolate) and zileuton (Zyflo), which are approved for 12 years of age and older. Montelukast decreases arachidonic acid metabolites that lead to potent inflammatory mediator release of cysteinyl leukotrienes, which activate neutrophils and eosinophils, cause microvascular leakage, produce mucus, and constrict airways. Antileukotrienes have been investigated as a possible first-line treatment in place of inhaled corticosteroids in individuals with mild and moderate persistent asthma. However, when compared with low-dose inhaled corticosteroids in 14 different randomized controlled trials, children and adults receiving antileukotrienes were 60% more likely to experience an exacerbation requiring systemic steroids (Ducharme & Hicks, 2002). Secondary outcomes, including nocturnal awakenings, rescue medication use, quality of life, and improvement of FEV_1 and PEFR, were also more favorable for those taking inhaled corticosteroids compared with leukotrienes alone. Antileukotriene agents were noted to be more efficacious in mild persistent as opposed to moderate persistent asthma. Further investigation into the use of leukotriene modifiers as a steroid-sparing medication for children with atopy and children with EIB is under way (Ducharme & Hicks, 2002; NHLBI, 2002).

Methylxanthines (Long-Acting Bronchodilators). Some children may benefit from the addition of theophylline if antiinflammatory and beta-adrenergic agents do not control their asthma symptoms. Methylxanthines in combination with beta-adrenergic agents work synergistically to produce bronchodilation and may improve control of nocturnal asthma symptoms in particular. A high level of provider and family monitoring is necessary, however. Metabolism of theophylline varies among individuals and age-groups, as does serious toxicity with possible permanent CNS side effects; therefore the dose must be individually adjusted by monitoring theophylline levels in the blood. For children in the ambulatory setting, a level of 15 mg/ml should be the upper limit because theophylline metabolism is affected by many factors, and this level provides a safe buffer if the theophylline level rises. Some children have a therapeutic response with a level as low as 5 mg/ml, and the lowest therapeutic level should be used.

Theophylline levels should be initially obtained after 2 to 4 days because a steady state is reached in an average of 40 hours in adults. Levels also must be rechecked at least every 6 to 12 months. The theophylline dose may need to be significantly adjusted and levels rechecked when there are signs of toxicity or viral illness or when the child experiences persistent or recurring asthma episodes while receiving maintenance medications. Side effects of theophylline include nausea, hyperactivity, and restlessness. Signs of toxicity that indicate an immediate need to determine the theophylline level include severe headaches, abdominal pain, vomiting, or any combination of these. Seizures are also a sign of severe toxicity and require immediate intervention and hospital admission.

Treatment of Exercise-Induced Bronchospasm. When a child experiences EIB, either a beta$_2$-agonist or a specific antiinflammatory agent (e.g., cromolyn) can be used to block the symptoms that inhibit the child's continued exercise. When used to prevent EIB, these agents should be taken approximately 15 minutes before participation in scheduled exercise. Complete protection lasts 1 to 2 hours with some coverage lasting 3 to 6 hours (Fowler, 2001; Milgrom & Taussig, 1999; O'Hallaren, 2002). Salmeterol or formoterol, both long-acting beta-agonists, can be administered via an MDI, for those who need long-lasting protection against exercise-induced symptoms (Milgrom & Taussig, 1999) can use a DPI. Neither, however, is to be used for rescue treatment of acute symptoms. Prescription of a short-acting beta-agonist medication, such as albuterol, is still required for rescue from any emergent acute symptoms (NHLBI, 2002). Although leukotriene modifiers may reduce symptoms of EIB in those taking the medication as part of a daily regimen, they are not currently advised as monotherapy for EIB (NHLBI, 2002).

Environmental Manipulations

It is well known that avoidance of common environmental triggers to asthma exacerbation can lead to improved asthma control in children. Environmental smoke is a trigger in most children. Tobacco smoke is best avoided, along with smoke from wood-burning stoves or campfires. Using motivational interviewing with parents and guiding them to smoking cessation support services when they are ready to quit can be helpful. Health care providers should discuss the damage smoking will do as the child moves into later childhood and throughout adolescence. Helping youth to develop risk avoidance behaviors to smoking or to position themselves to avoid the smoke of peers is critical.

Dust mites and cockroaches are also common triggers for asthma problems, especially when these are found in the child's sleeping room. Biweekly damp mopping, pillow and mattress covers, and elimination of mold may all reduce the number of asthma exacerbations. Outside air pollution, especially high levels of particulate matter, can exacerbate asthma. Some families have found it useful to monitor these levels along with pollen levels through the Asthma and Allergy Foundation of America Web page (www.aafa.org) and adapt the child's outdoor activity when levels are high.

Cats, dogs, rodents, and other furry pets can also trigger exacerbations in some children with allergies. These pets should never be allowed into the child's sleeping room or on furniture where the child will recline. If the pets are suspected to be triggers they can be removed from the home; however, it may take months for the allergens to be removed. This means any evaluation of the effects of such removal needs to be for an extended time. If proven to exacerbate the asthma, removal from the home is advised.

Complementary and Alternative Therapies

Fifty-one percent of families in one survey reported use of complementary therapy either alone or in concert with allopathic medicine for treatment of childhood asthma (Kemper & Lester, 1999). Those with persistent asthma, receiving high-dose corticosteroids, with poorly controlled symptoms, with frequent health care visits, and with adverse reactions to bronchodilators are most likely to use complementary therapies.

The most common therapies used are breathing techniques, yoga, herbal remedies, acupuncture, diet, homeopathy, and over-the-counter medications (Andrews et al, 1998; Malthouse, 1997). Buteyko breathing, advocated to restore normal breathing patterns and reduce hyperventilation, has shown a reduction in rescue medication use but no changes in corticosteroid use, hospitalization rates, or quality of life in one randomized clinical trial (Opat et al, 2000). Yoga, with its stress management results, may prove useful. Although some herbal remedies may be harmless, others, such as ephedra or ma huang, have been found dangerous (Kemper & Lester, 1999). If herbal supplements are taken they should be listed in the medication history so consideration of interaction or adverse effects can be made. The cost and the variability of content in herbal supplements should be discussed with the family.

Dietary addition of onion, quercetin, garlic, coffee, tea, or licorice has been advocated by some authors; however, scientific evidence of positive effect is lacking at this time (White, 2000). Reliance on over-the-counter medications, if used as a substitute for medically supervised management, can be harmful although some (antihistamines) may be helpful in managing allergic reactions. A provider's willingness to understand a family's rationale for using complementary therapies as well as an openness to explore evidence of help or harm is critical to successfully integrating complementary and allopathic treatments.

Anticipated Advances in Diagnosis and Management

There is increasing thought that delayed diagnosis and undertreatment of childhood asthma may contribute to increased pulmonary dysfunction in adults (Busse & Busse, 2002; Cokugras et al, 2001). Since irreversible remodeling of the airways may take place in the early years of a child's life, more aggressive identification and treatment methodologies are being proposed (Lemanske, 2002; NHLBI, 2002). Earlier treatment of even mild persistent asthma with inhaled corticosteroids is fueling much research into beneficial and potential negative long-term impacts of inhaled steroids, and these studies will serve as the evidence base for future early treatment approaches (Reddington, 2001; Spahn & Szefler, 2002). Provider resistance to use of inhaled corticosteroids with young children is also receiving attention (Adams et al, 2002). The resistance is often linked to past practice patterns, but at times lack of knowledge regarding established vs. feared side effects is central. In addition, school-based aggressive screening processes have been suggested to identify children with undiagnosed or undertreated asthma in hopes of reducing morbidity. However, few such programs are in place other than for research purposes.

There is a growing need for noninvasive measures of pulmonary inflammation. Exhaled nitric oxide (eNO) and breath condensate of inflammatory markers are currently being examined in research and may have potential for clinical tracking in the future since they can be used with young and old alike (American Thoracic Society, 1999; Barreto et al, 2001; Kharitonov & Barnes, 2001; Shahis et al, 2002).

Similarly, the link between asthma and respiratory syncytial virus (RSV) continues to be investigated. Whether infection with RSV early in life has a causative role in asthma or merely heralds asthma in a genetically predisposed child is under investigation (Wenzel et al, 2002). Improved prevention and treatment could follow once the link is better understood.

Since immune responses mediated by IgE are thought to be critical to asthma progression in those with an allergic component, the effect of providing recombinant humanized monoclonal antibody, referred to as anti-IgE, to persons with moderate to severe asthma has been tested (Milgrom & Taussig,

1999). Symptom scores in a high-dose anti-IgE group were lowered after 12 and 20 weeks, and more persons in the high vs. placebo group were able to decrease or discontinue their corticosteroids. The treatment was not effective in improving FEV_1, however. Although high-dose anti-IgEs were well tolerated, these mixed results indicate the treatment is still inconclusive in its potential for future use.

New medications are being developed and approved for use in children. Formoterol (Foradil) is a new long-acting beta-agonist, dry powder bronchodilator similar to salmeterol (Serevent) but with a faster onset of action. As a result, formoterol is useful for preventing exercise-induced asthma when used 15 minutes before activity. It is currently approved for prevention of EIB for children 12 years of age and older. As a long-acting beta-agonist it is approved for children 5 years of age or older when used in conjunction with an inhaled corticosteroid.

Advair is a relatively new dry powder formulation that combines Serevent at the standard dose of 50 μg with one of three different strengths of fluticasone (Flovent): 100 μg, 250 μg, or 500 μg. These convenient combinations allow variation in the inhaled corticosteroid dose but require only one puff of the ordered dose to administer the two medications, simplifying the child's regimen when persistent asthma is diagnosed and the two types of long-term control medications are needed. Current US Food and Drug Administration (FDA) approval is for children older than 12 years (Palacioz, 2001).

Advances in Knowledge of Genetic Etiology or Treatment

Investigation of the relationship between the development of asthma and the immune system is actively being explored. It appears that both genetic susceptibility and environmental influences will determine the expression of asthma in a child (Busse & Busse, 2002). Genetic factors indicate that asthma is a multifactorial, polygenic disease with not one or two but rather multiple specific gene sites responsible for the pathology of asthma. T-lymphocytes are known to be one of the many cell types involved in the inflammation of the airways characteristic of asthma. Genetic factors may determine the direction of T-lymphocytic cytokine production tendency toward one of two different subtypes, Th-1 cytokine response or Th-2 cytokine response, both present and known to be circulating in an infant's body. Allergic sensitization results from a Th-2 cell response to produce proinflammatory cytokines to stimulate IgE production and tissue eosinophilia with airway hyperreactivity. If the infant's response can be directed toward a stronger balance of Th-1 vs. Th-2 response, the hope is that ultimately atopic asthma will be repressed (Gern et al, 1999).

In utero and infancy, more Th-2 lymphocytes are produced than Th-1. Environmental factors occurring early, perhaps even in utero or the first year of life, may lead to further expression or an up-regulation of the Th-2 cytokine response. These factors include respiratory infections, allergen exposure, and pollutants. Viral bronchiolitis, use of antibiotics, living in a clean vs. dirty environment, having few if any siblings, and receiving immunizations also seem to promote a more Th-2–like response. As a result, the child experiences the characteristic response of bronchospasm, inflammation, and mucous production.

Conversely, attempting to repress the Th-2 response or increase the Th-1 response during the sensitive time of life is another approach being explored. It appears to be protective against the development of asthma if a child has older siblings; attends daycare; develops a bacterial infection, measles, or hepatitis A; or acquires an acute gastrointestinal infection (Ball et al, 2000; Sabina et al, 2001). Ongoing research continues to explore attempts to promote Th-1 expression in utero as well as through the use of medications, probiotics, and vaccinations to modify the neonatal tendency toward the Th-2 immune response (Gern et al, 1999).

Associated Problems (Box 11-5)

Allergies

All children who have allergies do not have asthma, but the majority of children with asthma have allergies. These allergies can also be expressed in the form of atopic dermatitis or allergic rhinitis (see Chapter 10). If there is a strong history of allergic reactions associated with respiratory symptoms, skin testing to determine specific problematic allergens may be beneficial. Antihistamines for treatment of allergic rhinitis may also help relieve the postnasal drip that can accompany sinusitis symptoms, which can trigger an asthma episode (Larsen, 2001).

Sensitivity to Aspirin and Nonsteroidal Antiinflammatory Drugs

Aspirin and nonsteroidal antiinflammatory drugs (NSAIDs) may precipitate an asthma episode in adults and possibly in children. Although aspirin is rarely indicated in children, these substances should be avoided and parents taught about reading over-the-counter drug labels because aspirin can be combined with other substances in certain drugs—especially cold remedies. If NSAID sensitivity is suspected referral to a specialist for confirmatory testing can be done.

Gastroesophageal Reflux

Gastroesophageal reflux (GER) is found in many children with chronic lung disease. Reflux of gastric secretions into the esophagus can initiate a reflex vagal response with an increased production of airway secretions and cough. Theophylline is known to increase gastric secretions and decrease esophageal pressure and thus may aggravate GER in some children. Management of GER includes upright positioning following thickened feedings for infants, smaller feedings, and use of medications that reduce acidity or increase gastric motility.

Swallowing Disorders

Some young children have other swallowing disorders that may cause episodes of microaspiration, with or without obvious

---

symptoms of cough. The aspiration of food or formula into the lungs will trigger a chronic inflammatory response that will exacerbate a child's asthma requiring escalating therapy. If a swallowing disorder is suspected, a videofluoroscopic swallowing study may be necessary to document aspiration with resulting feeding adaptations required until, and if, the swallow is normally developed. Adaptations may include thickened feedings, positioning, and occupational therapy feeding evaluation.

Vocal Cord Dysfunction

Vocal cord dysfunction, defined as adduction instead of abduction of the vocal cords during the respiratory cycle, may mimic sounds much like an asthmatic wheeze. The "wheeze" does not respond to asthma medications, and the child has near normal spirometry findings and oxygen saturations. A reduced voice quality may be noted and/or the inspiratory loop on the flow volume curve during spirometry may be flattened during times of breathlessness. This disorder may be clinically recognized but is definitively diagnosed via flexible laryngoscopy during an acute episode of symptoms (Zelcer et al, 2002). Speech therapy and relaxation techniques may be recommended for treatment.

Allergic rhinitis may predispose the child to chronic or recurrent sinusitis. Chronic infections of the sinuses with fever, pain, and thick postnasal secretions can irritate lower airways and trigger an asthma exacerbation. Treatment of the infection is necessary to reduce this trigger and may involve routine nasal washes with saline and intermittent nasal or oral steroids and antibiotics over a prolonged period, since chronic sinusitis is a notoriously difficult infection to eradicate.

Obesity

The link between asthma and childhood obesity is being explored. Although obesity has been known to result from inactivity that may be associated with asthma, more recent explorations are examining the role obesity may play in the emergence of asthma (Castro-Rodriguez et al, 2001; Rodriguez et al, 2002; von Kries et al, 2001).

Prognosis

The development of asthma or wheezing disorders as well as the natural history of asthma is currently an area of great discussion and research (Martinez, 1995, 2001b). The consensus of studies indicates that young children who have mild wheezy bronchitis fewer than five times before age 7 years are unlikely to be diagnosed with asthma or to have reduced pulmonary function when they reach adulthood unless they increase their risk by smoking or being exposed to secondhand smoke (Martinez, 2001b). Oswald et al (1994) found children who had recurrent wheezy bronchitis or wheezed even in the absence of URIs were likely to have frequent or persistent asthma symptoms by age 35 years. The more severe the child's asthma at an early age, the more likely it was that the child would continue to exhibit persistent asthma symptoms in adulthood (Oswald et al, 1994). Several long-term longitudinal studies (Grohl et al, 1999; Jenkins et al, 1994; Oswald et al, 1994, 1997; Strachan et al, 1996) noted few significant changes in lung function after 7 to 10 years of age, indicating that most of the loss in

BOX 11-5
Associated Problems

Additional allergies
Medication (aspirin/NSAIDs) and other sensitivities
Gastroesophageal reflux
Swallowing disorders
Vocal cord dysfunction
Chronic sinusitis

pulmonary function occurred during the early years. In addition, children who start to wheeze in the second decade of life may also have their symptoms remit unless they have atopy as well. The main predictors of persistent wheezing into adulthood are childhood reduced level of lung function and significant bronchial hyperresponsiveness to histamine in the childhood years (Martinez, 2001b).

The mild to moderate asthma of many children can be well controlled with effort from the child, family, and health provider. Some children, however, will have refractory asthma, which may be caused by poor implementation of the treatment plan, continued exposure to offending environmental triggers, severe labile asthma, or corticosteroid resistance or relative insensitivity (Busse & Busse, 2002). Psychosocial difficulties in families also can complicate asthma and its management. Chronic uncontrolled asthma may lead to persistent airway inflammation and airway remodeling and possibly irreversible pulmonary changes (Rasmussen et al, 2002).

Mortality from asthma remains a threat, especially at the age extremes. The highest mortality is currently occurring in blacks, leading some to believe this population may carry an underlying propensity for more severe disease (Mannino et al, 2002b). Many factors may contribute to these mortality data, including increased severity of the disease, under or inappropriate pharmacologic treatment, and failure to recognize severity of asthma symptoms with subsequent delay in initiating treatment. Psychosocial disruption in the family is consistently linked to morbidity. Regardless of cause, it remains clear that asthma can and does cause death in some children and thus needs to be addressed with families.

PRIMARY CARE MANAGEMENT

Health Care Maintenance

Growth and Development

Investigators continue to explore whether asthma has a direct influence on growth. It is essential that the practitioner measure height and weight, calculate body mass index (BMI), and record these measurements on the child's growth charts. Any major deviation from the population norms (i.e., less than the 10th or above the 90th percentile) or departure (i.e., two or more zones) from the child's individualized curve should be noted and assessed in further detail. Genetic, social, and nutritional factors that are potentially unassociated with asthma must be considered when evaluating patterns in growth. Alterations may need to be monitored over time for their significance to be appreciated. During a series of acute exacerbations of asthma, the primary care provider may note a plateau or small drop in weight; but with improved health status, catch-up growth should occur. If it does not occur, the cause of the weight loss should be further explored.

The first year of inhaled corticosteroid use may lead to a temporary decrease in growth velocity, but this should disappear in subsequent years (Price et al, 2002b). Primary care providers should always be concerned with growth when a prepubescent or pubescent child uses inhaled corticosteroids at medium to high doses. They need to carefully monitor growth at least every 6 months to evaluate cost/benefit ratios of the treatment protocol (NHLBI, 2002). Concern might necessitate reevaluation of the comprehensive management regimen with knowledge that the fewer the symptoms or acute exacerbations, the more likely full height will be obtained at the age-appropriate time.

Asthma has been associated with delay in the onset of puberty even when growth is adequate. Although the adolescent growth spurt may be slightly delayed, with optimal management of the disease, maximal height attainment is thought possible (Agertoft & Pedersen, 2000; Childhood Asthma Management Research Group, 2000).

Standard infant, child, and adolescent assessment tools are appropriate for use in assessing development. Research has rarely documented delayed development in children with asthma, and when found, the delayed development is not necessarily related to the physiologic severity of the asthma but to the imposed limitations placed on a child's experiences. Limitations typically involve reductions in physical activity and social experiences, including daycare and school attendance. Therefore practitioners should encourage normalization of experiences whenever possible and provide treatment adequate to allow normative activities to reduce the unnecessary negative effect on development (Kieckhefer & Trahms, 2000).

If there are instances when age-typical experiences must be discouraged to avoid specific asthma triggers, primary care providers should assist parents and children to identify alternative experiences that could provide similar developmental stimulation. For example, if the child cannot play competitive soccer because of grass allergy, poor response to medication or immunotherapy, or refusal to take preventive medication, the child and family should be helped to identify an alternate sport. Sports such as basketball or swimming allow the child to exercise and participate in a competitive team and provide the opportunity to engage in an age-appropriate social and skill-building activity but without outdoor allergen exposure. Helping a child find an enjoyable sport or physical activity should be a significant goal for primary care providers. Without these normal experiences a child's self-image, self-esteem, perception of body control, and overall level of health are likely to be reduced and anxiety, fear, and dependent behavior increased (Ortega et al, 2002). If these feelings and/or behaviors develop, consultation with or referral to a mental health practitioner should be considered.

Parents and children may limit strenuous activity because of repeated cough or fear of exacerbations. If this happens the primary care provider should assist family members in building an exercise habit into their daily routine and devising a treatment plan that supports such activity. This will help avoid a sedentary life pattern that may lower the child's sense of physical accomplishment and result in unwanted weight gain.

There are reports of impaired academic achievement in children with repeated brief school absences. Similar concerns have been linked to some medications used to manage asthma or allergies that trigger a child's asthma, but the demonstrated negative effect of medications on cognitive capabilities is not universal. Prevention and swift adequate management of exacerbations will reduce the number and length of school absences, thus limiting the factor thought to contribute most to problems with academic achievement.

Diet

If the BMI rises, especially if it approaches greater than the 85th percentile, the provider should discuss opportunities to increase the child's exercise (with appropriate pharmacologic support) and reduce intake of high-calorie and high-fat foods with the child and family. Advocating changes by the entire family rather than focusing just on the child's habits has been found to be more effective in stabilizing the child's weight.

Today's children and families eat many meals away from home, so dietary restrictions could affect family habits. Sulfites, which were previously used to enhance the appearance of many fresh foods, have been implicated in severe asthma exacerbations in some children and once such sensitivity is identified, sulfites need to be avoided. Although sulfite levels and uses have decreased, the FDA has ruled that foods containing sulfites must be clearly labeled. Sulfites can still be found in processed potatoes, shrimp, dried fruits, molasses, nonfrozen lemon and lime juice, wine, and labeled bulk preparations of fruits and vegetables. See Chapter 10 for additional discussion on food allergies.

Safety

Electrical burns are possible when equipment (e.g., nebulizers) is run in the child's presence. Infants and young children should never be left alone where they can reach the equipment, cord, or open socket. School-aged children and adolescents should be properly instructed in the safe use of electrical equipment and should demonstrate its use to parents or the primary care provider before being encouraged to use the equipment independently.

Medications kept in the home must be safely stored in their original containers in a locked location that is inaccessible to infants and young children. Because children will ultimately need to develop age-appropriate responsibility for medication administration, families may benefit from help to evaluate how to do this safely.

Practitioners can help parents identify their child's developmental capabilities and limits for safely assisting in the medication regimen by providing age-normative suggestions. For example, when a child is an infant or toddler, the parents must speak about the medications as such—not as candy. With maturation, toddlers can be taught how to hold the nebulizer mask or take slow breaths from a spacer with face mask to assist in therapy. Preschool-age children typically have the manual dexterity to take part in the medicinal therapy by helping parents assemble inhalers or count doses in the parent's presence. Young, school-aged children may be asked to get the medication and take it in the presence of a parent. When older school-aged children can tell time, they can assume greater responsibility to prompt the parent when the medication is needed, get the medication, take the medication in the parent's presence, and return it to its proper storage place. School-aged children should also become increasingly responsible for taking needed medication while at school. Parents can monitor and encourage safe and knowledgeable use by discussing or having a child count and record on a calendar the number of times medication was taken as required. As a child grows to adolescence, more autonomy should be given for independently purchasing, taking, and replenishing both controller and rescue medication and ensuring the medication is in all necessary locations. Parents need to be reminded, however, that one consistent finding in successful adolescent adherence to prescribed regimens is the continued support and age-appropriate assistance of their parents. This support is not shown by "doing for" or "nagging" adolescents but by demonstrating faith in their capabilities and offering assistance with problems that arise. Thus parents can maintain an interested, interdependent attitude to best assist an adolescent in growing in the shared management of asthma (Kieckhefer & Trahms, 2000).

Parents and children may need help in monitoring the number of doses remaining in the child's rescue medication. Although several new powder dose inhalers show the number of remaining puffs or require a capsule for each dose, other MDIs do not have these advantages. The typical MDI contains 200 actuations; therefore, with a two-puff dose, it should take 100 doses to empty the MDI. Although historically families were told they could estimate how much medication remained in the MDI by observing its sinking or floating in a water container, this is less often advised since this process would destroy DPI medication. Most pharmacies now recommend families count the actual doses the child takes or keep an extra albuterol MDI on hand to ensure they do not run out of medication the child may need for rescue.

The child's skill in using the inhaler should be observed at each visit with the practitioner. Up to 50% of children who do not receive such monitoring and corrective prompting for proper technique do not use the inhaler effectively. Use of spacers with MDIs for all age-groups lessens these problems and enhances widespread medication deposition. New breath-activated devices may also help in children old enough to inhale with adequate inspiratory effort. Usually children able to perform spirometry are able to appropriately inhale medication from these dry powder inhalers.

With age and increasing time spent away from parents, children must independently recognize when their treatment is not as effective as expected and seek the assistance of their parent or another adult. An episode that does not respond to treatment as expected may herald a particularly severe exacerbation requiring medical assistance. Simple mnemonic devices are helpful in this regard. A rhyme of "twice is nice but three needs more than me" could be a mnemonic device used to teach children their individual asthma plan (i.e., they can try their quick-relief inhaler twice, but if symptoms persist and they feel the need to use it a third time, they need to talk with a parent or health care provider as soon as possible). In addition to mnemonics, however, a written action plan for daily long-term control is needed, as well as a plan to be implemented if an acute exacerbation begins. Although the specific benefits of such written plans remain to be documented, they serve as an ideal way to communicate the treatment plan to the child, the parent, teachers, and other persons who provide care to the child (NHLBI, 2002).

Immunizations

The most recent recommendations of the Committee on Infectious Diseases (2000) should guide immunization decisions. Although the committee notes that vaccination with live-virus vaccines may lead to airway inflammation and therefore increased hyperresponsivity in children with asthma, the standard schedule of childhood immunizations is still recommended with some considerations for the corticosteroid load. Accordingly, guidelines for live-virus vaccination of children receiving corticosteroids are as follows:

- Topical therapy: Administration of topical corticosteroids, either on the skin or in the respiratory system by aerosol, usually does not result in immunosuppression that would contraindicate administration of live-virus vaccines. If clinical or laboratory evidence of systemic immunosuppression results from their prolonged application, however, live-virus vaccines should not be given until corticosteroid therapy has been discontinued for at least 1 month.
- Low or moderate doses of systemic corticosteroids given daily or on alternate days: Children receiving prednisone or its equivalent, less than 2 mg/kg/day or less than 20 mg or more daily if they weigh more than 10 kg, can receive live-virus vaccines while on treatment.
- High doses of systemic corticosteroids given daily or on alternative days for less than 14 days: Children receiving prednisone or its equivalent, 2 mg/kg/day or more or 20 mg or more daily if they weigh more than 10 kg, can receive live-virus vaccines immediately after discontinuation of treatment. Some experts, however, would delay immunization until 2 weeks after corticosteroid therapy has been discontinued if possible.
- High doses of systemic corticosteroids given daily or on alternate days for 14 days or more: Children receiving prednisone or its equivalent, 2 mg/kg/day or more or 20 mg or more daily if they weigh more than 10 kg, should not receive live-virus vaccines until steroid therapy has been discontinued for at least 1 month.

Although infants and children with asthma may have signs of respiratory infection more often, these signs alone—in the absence of specific published contraindications—should not be the basis for deferring immunizations (Committee on Infectious Diseases, 2000). Inadequate immunization with subsequent risk of infection is of great concern. Individualized assessment of the child with respiratory symptoms, including progressive signs of pulmonary dysfunction, should guide decisions about immunization. Delayed immunizations should be rescheduled as soon as possible. Special brief appointments may be needed to ensure adequate immunization during early childhood.

Oral acyclovir should be considered for unvaccinated children exposed to varicella who have been receiving short intermittent aerosolized corticosteroids. If a child has egg sensitivity, treatment equipment for anaphylactic reactions should be readily available in the office and the child should be observed for up to 90 minutes after immunization.

Children with asthma may experience complications with influenza (e.g., increased wheezing, fluctuating theophylline levels, bronchitis, pneumonia, increased school absences, increased medical care visits). Therefore, despite recent or current prednisone bursts, children with asthma should annually receive an influenza vaccine after the age of 6 months (Committee on Infectious Diseases, 2000). The subviron (split) vaccine is given to children under 13 years of age in the fall before influenza season. Children less than 9 years of age

without prior influenza vaccination may require two doses to develop a satisfactory antibody response. If a child has previously had a related strain of influenza (by infection or immunization), one dose is thought to be adequate to confer protection. Children with severe anaphylactic reactions to chicken or eggs generally should not receive influenza immunization given the risk, the need for yearly vaccination, and the availability of chemo prophylaxis (Committee on Infectious Diseases, 2000). Before 6 months of age and in the presence of contraindications to influenza vaccination, alternative treatment methods should be considered. These methods include immunization of contacts or treatment of influenza with amantadine or rimantadine if the child is older than 1 year (Committee on Infectious Diseases, 2000). The influenza vaccine may be given at the same time as measles-mumps-rubella (MMR), DTP or DTaP, Varivax hepatitis A and B, and polio vaccines.

Screening (Box 11-6)

Vision. Routine screening is recommended unless the child is taking daily high-dose corticosteroids because these drugs are known to cause inflammatory changes, cataracts, and glaucoma in adults. If abnormal findings are identified during an eye examination the child should be referred to an ophthalmologist.

Hearing. Routine screening is recommended.

Dental. Routine screening is recommended.

Blood Pressure. Blood pressure should be evaluated at each visit because of possible elevation with sympathetic medications or corticosteroids.

Hematocrit. Routine screening is recommended.

Urinalysis. Routine screening is recommended unless the child is taking high-dose corticosteroids daily, which may cause glycosuria. If glycosuria is present the child should be referred to a pulmonary specialist for evaluation.

Tuberculosis. Routine screening is recommended.

Condition-Specific Screening

Lung Function. Monitoring of lung function is essential to assess current function, as well as to identify long-term trends. Pulmonary function testing should be done at diagnosis and when the child is well to establish baseline lung function.

BOX 11-6
Screening

ROUTINE CHILDHOOD SCREENING
Vision—see text
Hearing—routine
Dental—routine
Blood pressure—see text
Urinalysis—see text
Tuberculosis—routine

CONDITION-SPECIFIC SCREENING
Lung function
Spirometry
Peak expiratory flow rate
Theophylline levels
Allergic triggers

Referral to a specialist for spirometry may be warranted in children with persistent disease to best monitor lung function and direct treatment. Spirometry tests are also recommended when significant treatment changes have been made and minimally every year thereafter (NHLBI, 1997). Spirometry can assess severity of both small and larger airway obstruction. Table 11-5 lists pulmonary function norms.

Peak flowmeters are commonly used in the primary care office to measure the greatest rate of airflow during a forced exhalation. This measurement is labeled the peak expiratory flow rate (PEFR). PEFR, however, is effort dependent and predominantly reflects large airway function. Thus if a child is obviously in respiratory distress or unwilling to cooperate, a PEFR may not be obtainable or easily interpreted. Measurements of PEFR over time will establish an individual's baseline personal best effort. These may or may not reflect average expected PEFR values listed in Table 11-5. PEFRs should not be expected to replace spirometry measurements, but they have a role in home management by the family since they can allow for ongoing daily assessment.

Children who cannot or will not recognize airway obstruction or those with very labile asthma can use a home peak flowmeter to monitor their asthma. Indeed, many primary care providers advocate the systematic use of peak flowmeters for all children with moderate to severe asthma (NHLBI, 2000). These meters are inexpensive, are easy to use, and can provide a record of airway reactivity if used in the morning and evening. These objective data can be used to individualize the child's treatment plan—often in the form of a three-zone action plan (Table 11-6). These meters can help the child, family, and

TABLE 11-5
Pulmonary Function Norms

Height		FVC (L)		FEV₁ (L)	PEFR (L/min)	FEF 25-75 (L/sec)
cm	in	Boys	Girls			
100	39.4	1.00	1.00	0.70	100	0.90
102	40.2	1.03	1.00	0.75	110	0.99
104	40.9	1.08	1.07	0.82	120	1.08
106	41.7	1.14	1.10	0.89	130	1.16
108	42.5	1.19	1.19	0.97	140	1.25
110	43.3	1.27	1.24	1.01	150	1.34
112	44.1	1.32	1.30	1.10	160	1.43
114	44.9	1.40	1.36	1.17	174	1.51
116	45.7	1.47	1.41	1.23	185	1.60
118	46.5	1.52	1.49	1.30	195	1.69
120	47.2	1.60	1.55	1.39	204	1.78
122	48.0	1.69	1.62	1.45	215	1.86
124	48.8	1.75	1.70	1.53	226	1.95
126	49.6	1.82	1.77	1.59	236	2.04
128	50.4	1.90	1.84	1.67	247	2.12
130	51.2	1.99	1.90	1.72	256	2.21
132	52.0	2.07	2.00	1.80	267	2.30
134	52.8	2.15	2.06	1.89	278	2.39
136	53.5	2.24	2.15	1.98	289	2.47
138	54.3	2.35	2.24	2.06	299	2.56
140	55.1	2.40	2.32	2.11	310	2.65
142	55.9	2.50	2.40	2.20	320	2.74
144	56.7	2.60	2.50	2.30	330	2.82
146	57.5	2.70	2.59	2.39	340	2.91
148	58.3	2.79	2.68	2.48	351	3.00
150	59.1	2.88	2.78	2.57	362	3.09
152	59.8	2.97	2.88	2.66	373	3.17
154	60.6	3.09	2.98	2.75	384	3.26
156	61.4	3.20	3.09	2.88	394	3.35
158	62.2	3.30	3.18	2.98	404	3.44
160	63.0	3.40	3.27	3.06	415	3.52
162	63.8	3.52	3.40	3.18	425	3.61
164	64.6	3.64	3.50	3.29	436	3.70
166	65.4	3.78	3.60	3.40	446	3.78
168	66.1	3.90	3.72	3.50	457	3.87
170	66.9	4.00	3.83	3.65	467	3.96
172	67.7	4.20	3.83	3.80	477	4.05
174	68.5	4.20	3.83	3.80	488	4.13
176	69.3	4.20	3.83	3.80	498	4.22

From Polgar, G. & Promadhar, V. (1971). *Pulmonary function testing in children: techniques and standards.* Philadelphia: W.B. Saunders. Modified with permission.
FVC, Forced vital capacity; *FEV,* forced expiratory volume; *PEFR,* peak expiratory flow rate; *FEF,* forced expiratory flow.

TABLE 11-6
Zone Action Plan

Zone	PEFR (Best or Predicted for Age)	Action
Green	80% to 100%	All clear, continue regular management plan
Yellow	50% to 80%	Caution, implement action plan predetermined with primary care provider
Red	50% or less	Medical alert, implement action plan predetermined with primary care provider; if PEFR does not return to yellow or green zone, call provider

PEFR, Peak expiratory flow rate.

TABLE 11-7
Factors Affecting Serum Theophylline Levels

	Factors Increasing Serum Levels Because of Decreased Clearance	Factors decreasing Serum Levels Because of Increased Clearance
Age	Infants	12 mo to 12 yr
Medications	Erythromycin—alone or in combination	Phenobarbital
	Azithromycin (Zithromax)	Phenytoin (Dilantin)
	Clarithromycin (Biaxin)	Rifampin (Rifadin)
	Cimetidine (Tagamet)	
	Oral contraceptives	
	Propanolol (Inderal)	
	Carbamazepine (Tegretol)	
	Zileuton (Zyflo)	
Illnesses	Liver or heart dysfunction	
	Acute viral illnesses	
Other	Obesity	Cigarette or marijuana smoking
	Fever for over 24 hr	

provider decide when to initiate early treatment and to evaluate response to treatment.

Theophylline Levels. Theophylline remains an alternative treatment adjunct in persistent asthma (NHLBI, 2002). Because theophylline preparations come in quick-release (i.e., every 6 to 8 hours), sustained-release (i.e., every 8 to 12 hours), or ultra–sustained-release (i.e., every 24 hours) forms, monitoring theophylline levels is determined by the preparation. In general, it is best to follow the manufacturer's guidelines for measuring theophylline levels. The level should be drawn at the same time (e.g., always 4 hours after the dose of a sustained-release preparation) to ensure consistency in level monitoring. In the case of suspected theophylline toxicity, levels should be obtained immediately (Table 11-7).

Allergic History. A biannual review of possible environmental allergens and irritants is helpful. If it appears that allergies are implicated in asthma exacerbations it can be done more frequently and consideration given for initial or repeat skin testing. In addition to identification of asthma triggers, this review provides a time to discuss other health issues (e.g., parent or adolescent smoking, avoidance of triggers, dust control, desirability of allergy skin testing). Asthma shared-management education can be updated at this time to ensure an

BOX 11-7
Differential Diagnosis

Wheezing—may not be asthma only
Respiratory infections—trigger asthma exacerbation
Vomiting and diarrhea—may indicate theophylline toxicity, GER
Headache—may indicate sinusitis or theophylline toxicity
Fever—not associated with asthma unless underlying infection present

GER, Gastroesophageal reflux.

increasingly mature understanding of the condition and its management.

Bone Density. Currently bone scans are encouraged for children older than 12 years receiving systemic corticosteroids, and some believe children receiving high-dose inhaled corticosteroids should also have bone scans. As data emerge from this recommendation, evidence-based policies may emerge regarding future routine screening.

Common Illness Management
Differential Diagnosis (Box 11-7)

Wheezing. It is well known that all wheezing is not asthma, so when a child presents with recurrent or persistent cough or wheeze, other diagnoses should be considered. Such diagnoses include foreign body aspiration (particularly in the toddler), vocal cord dysfunction, infections (e.g., bronchitis, bronchiolitis, pneumonia), other underlying airway diseases (e.g., cystic fibrosis, bronchiectasis), structural abnormalities (e.g., a vascular ring), or aspiration as a result of a primary swallowing disorder or GER or secondary to underlying neuromuscular disease.

Respiratory Infections. Viral respiratory infections are the most common cause of exacerbations of asthma in children. Treatment is usually supportive. Parents can give antipyretics for fever if indicated and should provide rest and extra fluids. A step up in asthma therapy medications may be necessary. For example, the child who only receives prn albuterol may need to temporarily take albuterol up to every 4 hours for 24 hours (longer with provider consultation or continuation of asthma symptoms) or even add systemic corticosteroids under the direction of the provider if the exacerbation is severe (NHLBI, 2002).

Vomiting and Diarrhea. Children with asthma who present with vomiting should be evaluated for theophylline toxicity if they are taking theophylline preparations, especially if the vomiting is associated with headache. When gastroenteritis occurs in a child with asthma, the usual supportive care is advised. The child should continue receiving his or her usual asthma therapy but may be at increased risk for mucous plugging if dehydration occurs. Controlling the respiratory symptoms with nebulized medications and providing extra fluids should be considered. Hospitalization may be necessary if the child's asthma worsens, medications cannot be tolerated, or fluid intake is extremely reduced.

Headache. Sinusitis can present as a headache, especially if associated with complaints of purulent nasal drainage, foul breath odor, or nighttime cough. Because sinusitis can trigger an asthma episode, there may also be increased wheezing. When diagnosed, sinusitis must be treated early and aggressively to minimize the occurrence of asthma exacerbations. The common cold and symptoms of allergic rhinitis do not, however, require antibiotic treatment.

Fever. Asthma exacerbations are not associated with fever unless there is an underlying infection (e.g., viral infections, sinusitis, pneumonia, otitis media). The cause of the fever must be evaluated by the usual methods. Increased fluids should be given to keep the child hydrated and to avoid mucous plugging, which can occur with asthma. In a child taking a theophylline preparation, a febrile viral illness may alter metabolism, necessitating a theophylline level to evaluate for toxicity.

Drug Interactions

Several factors cause theophylline levels to rise or fall and should be considered when a child's overall health care plan is assessed (Table 11-7). Medications that affect theophylline clearance should be avoided, or the theophylline dose should be appropriately adjusted and levels monitored. These drugs include erythromycin, cimetidine, zileuton (Zyflo), and oral contraceptives. Zafirlukast (Accolate) inhibits the cytochrome P-450 isoenzyme system, which interacts with other drugs metabolized by this system. Warfarin, phenytoin, carbamazepine, and erythromycin interactions are known, but those of cyclosporin, calcium channel blockers, and astemizole are yet unknown, although monitoring is advised. Because zileuton is metabolized by the cytochrome P-450 isoenzyme system, similar monitoring is advised. It is known that zileuton coadministration with theophylline approximately doubles the serum theophylline levels, necessitating a reduction in the dose (Levien & Bailer, 1999).

Cough suppressants should generally be avoided because they will be largely ineffective and may delay diagnosis and appropriate treatment. Cough suppressants are occasionally helpful to control nighttime or continuous postviral cough in which coughing itself is a trigger for increased cough because of irritation of the trachea and bronchi. Antihistamines are now available without medical prescription and may be helpful in relieving allergic rhinitis, but they are not useful in treating the asthma per se.

Children with asthma are often atopic and receive topical steroids in addition to inhaled steroids. The provider must be aware of the potential cumulative effects since it is the total body load of steroid that is related to side effects (Allen, 2002).

Developmental Issues

Sleep Patterns

The sleep of young children is often disrupted during asthma exacerbations. Even when an exacerbation is not evident, a child may routinely awaken and cough during the night or early morning hours (Lentz et al, 2002; Sadeh et al, 1998). Perception of these nocturnal symptoms by parents as indicators of poor asthma control may be as low as 40% (Cabral et al, 2002). This tendency for early morning problems probably represents the normal circadian rhythm in airway caliber and steroid production (Kraft et al, 2001). Because the symptom pattern represents an exaggeration of existing bronchial hyperresponsivity, optimizing daytime control and reducing environmental irritants in the sleeping room minimize the symptoms. Persistent difficulty may necessitate an evening dosage of a short-acting theophylline preparation, long-acting time-release theophylline preparation, long-acting beta-agonist, or leukotriene modifier. Treatment choice is based on the child's response. In general, review of the child's controller medication needs is warranted, as is a complete review of the bedroom environment.

Carpets, stuffed toys, curtains, or anything that retains dust should be removed from the sleeping room and the change in symptoms noted. Dust mite covers for the pillow and mattress can be tried with cost as little as $100. Pets should remain out of the sleeping room, and windows should remain closed, reducing pollen and grass allergens. Mold-producing agents, such as houseplants, should be removed.

Parents have reported that some medications disrupt their children's sleep, but systematic documentation is scarce. Most providers attempt an alternative medication regimen if the sleep disturbance does not resolve within 1 or 2 weeks of beginning any medication.

Most young children find a nighttime ritual soothing. Primary care providers should help parents establish a bedtime ritual that is relaxing and can be easily implemented by the family. A consistent bedtime is helpful because frequent deviation of more than 30 minutes may cause difficulty in settling a child and delay sleep onset.

Toileting

Toileting needs are typically not altered by a child's asthma. Bowel and bladder training is achieved at the expected ages. Clinicians have noted that a small proportion of children experience problems with enuresis when taking theophylline preparations, possibly because of its diuretic action. The exact incidence, however, is undocumented. If standard behavioral interventions are not effective in eliminating enuresis, most primary care providers recommend an alternative medication regimen. Constipation could occur if the child becomes dehydrated during exacerbations.

Discipline

Parents may report that it is difficult to deal with discipline for fear of upsetting the child and initiating an asthma exacerbation. Because children with asthma may experience some degree of bronchospasm with intense crying, parental concern is understandable. Crying cannot be entirely avoided, but parents should be reassured that most discipline can be implemented by rewarding desirable behaviors, if this is done routinely and begun early in a child's life. Inconsistent limit setting for undesirable behavior only confuses children and makes it more difficult for them to learn and internalize the limits chosen by the parents.

Another parental concern is that the child's irritability, refusals, or acting-out behavior is caused by illness or medications. Medications and illness may influence the child's behavior, but consistency of expectations is of greater importance. Blaming the illness or medication does not remove the necessity to help a child develop behaviors desired by the family and social networks. A child will ultimately need to develop a strong sense of internal control to effectively participate in asthma shared management. Early consistent positive expectations set by the parents will form the foundation for a child's later self-discipline and sense of mastery and control. Avoiding discipline early in a child's life will not make the ensuing years more pleasant for parents or help the child in learning socially expected behaviors. Thus primary care providers should initiate discussion about positive discipline early during an infant's first year of life, assuring parents that with time this issue should become less burdensome as the child is able to verbally express emotion without excessive crying leading to bronchospasm.

Child Care

Most families find it necessary to use child care services on either a regular or sporadic basis. Having a child with asthma should not prohibit the use of child care. Because URIs trigger exacerbations of asthma in many children under 5 years of age, a smaller daycare with less chance of exposure to these infections may reduce the number of asthma exacerbations. Parents should evaluate the child care environment for any known triggers. Licensed daycare centers prohibit exposure to secondhand smoke and are evaluated for cleanliness, molds or mildew, and animals. If unlicensed, private or in-home daycare arrangements do not need to meet state requirements so parents must take the initiative to evaluate for these known or common triggers. The local chapter of the American Lung Association or Asthma and Allergy Foundation of America may be of assistance in this regard along with the local health department. With proper communication and explanation, child care can be safely accomplished with a responsible, interested caretaker. Whether child care is at a center or is home based, provided by a relative, neighbor, or professional, information must be shared by parents to ensure success.

Parents must be responsible for providing all relevant information to the caretaker; that is, what triggers the child's asthma, early warning signs of an impending asthma episode, what the caretaker should do first, what should be done next if the action is not fully effective, how the parent and other responsible parties (i.e., including health care provider) can be reached, and what information must be passed on to emergency personnel if they are called. The best way to provide this information is in written format, such as an asthma management plan. Examples of these written plans can be found on-line (www.nhlbi.nih.gov; www.aafa.org; www.aanma.org).

If the child care provider is to give any treatments, the parent must demonstrate the procedures and observe the provider's repeat performance. In addition, center-based programs may require written prescriptions from the primary health care provider and written permission of the parent for the child care provider to perform the treatment. Parents must maintain close contact with the child care provider to learn about changing triggers, medications, or early warning signs. Anyone in repeated contact with the child who observes responses to treatments should also relay that information to the parent. This information can then be integrated into the overall routine reevaluation of the treatment plan. Any treatment changes should be immediately related to the child care provider so that a consistent approach is provided to the child regardless of setting. Frequent and open communication is the key to successful child care arrangements.

Schooling

Surveys of children with asthma report increasing numbers of school days missed because of asthma. National data show there were 6.6 million and 14 million absence days in 1980 to 1982 and 1994 to 1996, respectively (Mannino et al, 2002a). School absence days are often scattered throughout the year. This pattern of frequent, brief absences has been thought more harmful to academic progress than infrequent long absences; thus efforts should be made to avoid this tendency.

Parents report that communicating with school personnel is essential but often difficult. Many fears and misconceptions about children with asthma still exist in the general public. Many teachers do not recognize a cough as a symptom of asthma. They may believe the child has an infectious disease that should restrict school attendance. Teachers and administrators may attempt to limit the child more than the parents or primary care provider believes necessary—especially in regard to sports participation. With proper therapy and education, only those children with severe persistent asthma should require regular limitations (NHLBI, 2002). With appropriate warm-up, pacing, hydration, and preventive pharmacologic therapy, almost all children with asthma will be able to participate in active school activities on a regular basis.

Scheduling an annual parent-teacher conference to discuss the child's current treatment regimen is essential. Teachers and sports coaches should have the same written information plan earlier suggested for child care providers. In addition, the teacher should be informed of the child's skills for shared management. The school nurse may provide support to the parent during annual conferences and should have a copy of the child's written routine and emergency action plans. Provider-prescribed emergency medications that may be needed should be given to the nurse or designated individual. If school personnel hesitate to assume this responsibility, the parents or primary care provider should discuss with them their legal responsibility to allow all children access to medications they need to enable school attendance. After proper instruction and with the permission of the parent, health care provider, and school, the child may be allowed to carry the rescue medication on his or her person for quick access in times of need. Mutual problem solving is essential to finding workable solutions to problems as they emerge. Many on-line resources are available for the health care provider to support the parent in working with school personnel (www.cdc.gov/healthyyouth/healthtopics/asthma).

Fitting in with school peers and maintaining positive peer relationships are essential to the child's full development. Parents can actively arrange peer gatherings, encourage the child to join clubs or organizations, and allow the child age-appropriate independence in visiting friends to ensure social experiences. Friends may question why the child is taking medications or has special equipment in the home. Simple explanations about the child's asthma should be given with the assurance that asthma is not contagious. This might also be done in school as a class presentation with the teacher's assistance. Parents are encouraged to discuss their child's asthma with parents of their child's peers so that all may have an honest understanding of the child's condition and abilities, as well as of any temporary limitations or needs for treatment. The American Lung Association's program "Open Airways" for school-aged children is available from local chapters as is the "Asthma Care Training" program from the Asthma and Allergy Foundation of America.

Sexuality

As noted earlier, sexual development may be delayed if asthma has not been adequately controlled to allow regular growth. Systemic corticosteroids historically have been associated with delay in sexual development because of their effect on the adrenal glands and corticosteroid production. Current treatment regimens that rely heavily on inhaled corticosteroids or more rarely oral corticosteroids every other day with morning dosage schedules appear to have reduced the adverse effect on general and sexual growth patterns.

If an adolescent becomes sexually active and wishes to use contraceptives, drug interactions must be considered. It is known that oral contraceptives may interfere with the breakdown of theophylline, thus increasing the likelihood of toxicity. As new asthma management drugs are developed, their effect on the efficacy of any pharmacologic means of birth control must be explored.

Transition into Adulthood

As youths with asthma enter adulthood, it is important that they continue to increase and periodically update their understanding of asthma and its management with the goal of achieving complete control. Reviewing and updating the education might take place before a move to college or a switch in primary care providers. Persons with a history of moderate to severe asthma who are currently without symptoms should be reminded to inform their new provider of this history because symptoms may return later in life. If the history is complex, a formal request for transfer of records to the adult health care provider should be made. Maintaining a smoke-free work environment is essential. Some vocations that involve inhaled irritants or allergens and overexposure to known triggers (e.g., work with laboratory animals, cleaning fluids, painting products) may be best avoided.

Family Concerns and Resources

Because of the genetic nature of asthma, some family members express guilt during the child's exacerbations. Parents should be reminded that there is nothing they could have done to prevent asthma and that in regard to acute exacerbations; hindsight is always better than foresight. Eliminating all exacerbations may be an ideal but impossible goal to achieve. A more realistic goal is to limit the number and extent of problems and to learn something about prevention or management from each episode.

If many family members have a history of asthma, the family may retain outdated beliefs and habits regarding treatment. The primary care provider must respect the family history but also stress new knowledge and discuss the development of new therapies to encourage the family to take advantage of current information.

Given the familial nature of asthma, cultural and ethnic considerations are important. In the United States, minority ethnicity and poverty continue to be linked to increased prevalence, potentially reduced access to care, lower quality of care, and reduced implementation of recommended care with subsequent higher risks of morbidity and mortality (Castro et al, 2001). Primary care providers need to consider their role in changing this reality. Providers must be child advocates for reducing environmental exposures of children to causes of asthma and its exacerbation (e.g., prenatal tobacco smoke, preterm birth, housing with poor ventilation, mold and mildew, early URI). Providers can continue to support policies and legislation that ensure universal access to health care and the care system's ability to meet the needs of all children with asthma. Exploring values, beliefs, and health practices of the families should enable the creative primary care provider to individualize critical elements of practice guidelines with the individual family. This individualization may help to ensure the greatest acceptance and implementation of the recommended care by tailoring the management program to the cultural realities of the child and family and foster adaptation (Brazil & Krueger, 2002). It is within the ongoing trusting relationship of the family and caregiver that further information regarding cultural beliefs and practices can be discussed.

Although prenatal exposure to tobacco is linked to developing asthma (Busse & Busse, 2002), smoking by a family member is also associated with increased asthma flare-ups (Mannino et al, 2002b). Changing the smoking habits of family members is difficult for health care providers and family members alike. When advising families to eliminate smoke from their child's environment, the practitioner should convey resources for smoking cessation or, at minimum, risk avoidance. Parents must be reminded to only smoke outside (i.e., not in another room, near an open window, or in a car) and wear a "smoking jacket" (i.e., an outer layer to prevent smoke retention on clothes). In some cases, in-home smoking can be viewed as child endangerment and possibly child neglect.

Many parents express ambivalence about long-term medication regimens, especially when the child has been taking medications for many years (Kieckhefer & Ratcliffe, 2000). Although most parents acknowledge the effectiveness of these regimens, most also hold the belief that long-term medication—especially steroids—can be harmful to their child. Helpful approaches for supporting parents include acknowledging and discussing these common feelings while presenting the fact that the most detrimental effects of asthma seem to come from poor control. It is also useful to reinforce that the long-term treatment program will continue to be tailored to their child while trying to decrease medication to the minimum amount needed for symptom control. In addition, providing the family with resources to ensure their ability to stay informed regarding new asthma treatments and research may help the family to become better partners in determining the best care for their child.

Asthma, like all chronic illnesses, can disrupt the life of the child's family (Gustafsson et al, 2000). This disruption is marked when the child is young but can be minimized by actively involving all family members in concrete, daily management tasks. Disruption comes not only from the disease but also from management activities. It is important to recognize the effort families exert and point out successes for them to reflect on as well as continuing to implement the simplest, most effective treatment regimen.

Resources

Primary care providers should become familiar with the local offices of national organizations (see the list that follows) to identify community-based services in local areas that can complement their health care services. Many of these community-based services have programs that are useful to children and parents in managing day-to-day effects of asthma. These programs typically offer education about asthma and training in shared management skills for the child and parents.

If the primary care provider's practice is large enough, educational programs for similar-aged children with asthma may be effectively implemented. A well-stocked lending library of reading materials and videotapes on asthma helps parents and children learn how to manage asthma effectively. Practitioners must provide families with information on how to obtain these materials for their own use. Many Internet resources of high-quality, up-to-date information are now easily accessed from public libraries or home computers (Pinkerton & Kieckhefer, 2002). Printed listings are also available (Friedman, 2002) as well as information on the evaluation of the current asthma Web sites that are available to patients and families (Croft & Peterson, 2002).

Self-Management Curricular Guides

American Lung Association
Super Stuff: Open Airways for Schools

Asthma and Allergy Foundation of America
Asthma Care Training for Kids (ACT)

Media

American Lung Association
A is for Asthma (VHS), 1998
Also available in Spanish

KidSafety America
Asthma, Asthma: You Can't Stop Me and *At Ease with Asthma* (VHS),1998
KidSafety America
4750 Chino Ave, Suite D
Chino, CA
(909) 902-1340

Organizations

Allergy and Asthma Network/Mothers of Asthmatics, Inc
(800) 878-4403
http://www.aanma.com/

American Academy of Allergy, Asthma, and Immunology
(800) 822-ASTHMA
http://www.aaaai.org

American Association for Respiratory Care
(972) 243-2272
http://www.aarc.org

American College of Allergy, Asthma, and Immunology
(800) 842-777
http://allergy.mcg.edu

American Lung Association
(800) LUNG-USA
http://www.lungusa.org

American Pharmaceutical Association
(202) 628-4410
http://www.aphanet.org

American Thoracic Society
(212) 315-8700
http://thoracic.org

Asthma and Allergy Foundation of America
(800) 7-ASTHMA
http://www.aafa.org

National Asthma Education and Prevention Program
(301) 251-1222
http://www.nhlbi.nih.gov/nhlbi/lung/lung.htm

US Environmental Protection Agency
(800) 296-1996
http://www.epa.gov/ozone

Internet

NHLBI: Expert Panel Report II: Guidelines for the Diagnosis and Management of Asthma http://www.nhlbi.nih.gov/nhlbi/lung/asthma/prof/asthgdln.htp

On-line comparison shopping for dust mite bedding covers http://www.dealtime.com/dt-app/SE/FN-Bedding/KW-dust_cover/FD-565/CR-5/compare-prices.html

Summary of Primary Care Needs for the Child with Asthma

HEALTH CARE MAINTENANCE

Growth and Development

It is important to measure and record height, weight, and body mass index. Variations from the expected norms must be investigated.

Prolonged or systemic use of steroids, including inhaled steroids, may affect growth; must be monitored carefully.

Delayed adolescent growth is associated with poor control, with exacerbations or chronic oral corticosteroids.

Delayed development is only noted when unnecessary limitations are imposed on the child.

Impaired cognitive development is most clearly linked to repeated school absences.

Diet

The role of obesity in asthma is unclear. Children who are overweight or obese should be encouraged to increase exercise and decrease excess calorie intake. A family approach to weight management is important.

Children may have allergies to sulfites or foods.

Safety

Electrical burns are possible from nebulizers or steamers.
Medication safety varies with developmental age.
Caution is needed on repeated use of quick-relief medications if improvement is not achieved.
Adherence is an issue with adolescents.

Immunizations

Routine immunizations are recommended.
Caution is necessary with use of live-virus vaccines in children receiving systemic or long-term steroids.
If a child has a documented egg sensitivity, vaccines using other media must be considered.

Summary of Primary Care Needs for the Child with Asthma—cont'd

Influenza vaccine is recommended for children older than 6 months. Pneumococcal immunization (Prevnar) is currently recommended in the schedule advocated for all children at 2, 4, 6, and 12 to 15 months of age. Pneumococcal polysaccharide vaccine, the 23-valent pneumococcal vaccine, is still recommended to expand serotype coverage to children 24 months of age and older deemed at high risk for invasive pneumococcal disease, including those children with significant chronic pulmonary disease (Committee on Infectious Diseases, 2000).

Screening

Vision. Routine screening is recommended unless daily high-dose corticosteroids are taken, which may result in cataracts or glaucoma; then referral to an ophthalmologist is required for complete eye examination.

Hearing. Routine screening is recommended.

Dental. Routine screening is recommended.

Blood pressure. Blood pressure should be evaluated at each visit because of possible sympathetic stimulation from medications or corticosteroids.

Hematocrit. Routine screening is recommended.

Urinalysis. Routine screening is recommended unless daily doses of corticosteroids are taken, which may result in glycosuria. If glycosuria is present, refer to specialist for reevaluation of asthma management.

Tuberculosis. Routine screening is recommended.

Condition-Specific Screening

Lung function tests. Testing of PEFR should be done at each primary care office visit and on a routine schedule in the home based on individualized management plan. Spirometry should be done at diagnosis, when major changes in treatment are contemplated, and routinely every year in age-appropriate children.

Theophylline levels. Theophylline levels should be monitored with change in therapy, growth, and illness.

Allergy testing. Skin testing may be indicated depending on history and therapy response.

Bone density scans. Children receiving high-dose inhaled corticosteroids or systemic corticosteroids should be screened for bone density after 12 years of age.

COMMON ILLNESS MANAGEMENT

Differential Diagnosis

Recurrent or persistent cough or wheeze. Rule out infection, GER, aspiration, and structural anomalies, and consider cystic fibrosis.

Viral respiratory infections. URI may require change in asthma therapy to prevent or modify exacerbation of asthma.

Gastrointestinal symptoms. Rule out theophylline toxicity and GER.

Headache. Rule out theophylline toxicity and sinusitis.

Fever. Fever is not associated with asthma alone. When fever is present, prevention of dehydration is important to prevent mucous plugs.

Drug Interactions

Antihistamines are not contraindicated but will only mediate allergic responses.

Leukotriene modifiers of some types affect or are affected by the cytochrome P-450 isoenzyme system; thus several drug interactions are documented and others suspected.

Medications such as erythromycin, cimetidine, zileuton, or oral contraceptives will raise theophylline levels.

Phenobarbital will decrease theophylline levels.

Codeine cough suppressants may mask symptoms of asthma.

DEVELOPMENTAL ISSUES

Sleep Patterns

Exacerbation may interfere with sleep.

It is important to reduce environmental allergens in sleep area.

If medications disturb sleep, an alternative regimen should be tried.

Toileting

Toileting is routine.

Few children experience enuresis while taking theophylline.

Discipline

There may be concern over discipline initiating asthma attack.

Rewarding desirable behavior should be encouraged.

The influence of medication and illness on behavior is often a concern of parents and needs discussion.

Consistency of expectations is important.

Child Care

Evaluate child care environment for known or common triggers.

Child care workers must be provided with information on asthma triggers, early warning signs of asthma, a written action plan for treatment, emergency contacts, and medications used in daycare.

Schooling

Repeated school absences may interfere with academic performance.

School personnel must be educated to evaluate child's symptoms and use of medications.

School personnel need a written copy of the asthma action plan.

Encourage participation in asthma education programs if available.

Enhancing the child's strengths in all areas will support peer acceptance.

Participation in sports and activities should be encouraged.

Sexuality

Sexual development may be delayed in severe cases or with prolonged corticosteroid use.

Oral contraceptives may interfere with breakdown of theophylline.

Transition into Adulthood

Begin plan for transitioning responsibilities of care throughout the child's life.

Continued

Summary of Primary Care Needs for the Child with Asthma—cont'd

Update knowledge and develop shared management roles as child matures.

Inform new primary care provider.

Discuss vocational issues.

FAMILY CONCERNS

Familial nature of asthma may contribute to outdated beliefs of treatment.

Parents may be ambivalent regarding long-term medication regimens.

Smoking in home is detrimental to children with asthma. Parents who smoke need support and assistance in quitting.

Ethnic minority and poverty have been linked with increased prevalence, morbidity, and mortality.

System changes to improve access to care are necessary, especially for uninsured children.

PEFR, Peak expiratory flow rate; *GER,* gastroesophageal reflux; *URI,* upper respiratory infection.

REFERENCES

Adams, R.J., Fuhlbrigge, A., Guilbert, T., Lozano, P., & Martinez, F. (2002). Inadequate use of asthma medication in the United States: Results of the Asthma in America national population survey. *J Allergy Clin Immunol, 110*(1), 58-64.

Agertoft, L. & Pedersen, S. (2000). Effects of long-term treatment with inhaled budesonide on adult height in children with asthma. *N Engl J Med, 343*(15), 1064-1069.

Akinbami, L. & Schoendorf, K. (2002). Trends in childhood asthma: Prevalence, health care utilization and mortality. *Pediatrics, 111*(2), 315-322.

Allen, D. (2002). Safety of inhaled corticosteroids in children. *Pediatr Pulmonol, 33*(3), 208-220.

American Thoracic Society. (1999). Recommendations for standardized procedures for the online and offline measurement of exhaled lower respiratory nitric oxide and the nasal oxide in adults and children. *Am J Respir Crit Care Med, 160,* 2104-2117.

Anderson, S. & Daviskas, E. (2000). The mechanism of exercise-induced asthma is . . . *J Allergy Clin Immunol, 106*(3), 453-459.

Andrews, L. et al. (1998). The use of alternative therapies by children with asthma: A brief report. *J Paediatr Child Health, 34,* 131-134.

Anhoj, J., Bisgaard, A.M., & Bisgaard, H. (2002). Systematic activity of inhaled steroids in 1-to 3-year-old children with asthma. *Pediatrics, 109*(3), NIL_8-NIL_11.

Ball, T.M., Castro-Rodriguez, J.A., Griffith, K.A., Holberg, C.J., Martinez, F.D., et al. (2000). Sibling daycare attendance and the risk of asthma and wheezing during childhood. *N Engl J Med, 343,* 538-543.

Barreto, M., Villa, M.P., Martell, A.S., Ronchetti, F., Darder, M.T., et al. (2001). Exhaled nitric oxide in asthmatic and non-asthmatic children: Influence of type of allergen sensitization and exposure to tobacco smoke. *Pediatr Allergy Immunol, 5,* 247-256.

Bonner, S., Zimmerman, B.J., Evans, D., Irogoyen, M., Resnick, D., et al. (2002). An individual intervention to improve asthma management among urban Latino and African-American families. *J Asthma, 39*(2), 167-179.

Bousquet, J., Jeffrey, P.K., Busse, W.W., Johnson, M., & Vignola, A.M. (2000). Asthma from bronchoconstriction to airway inflammation and remodeling. *Am J Respir Crit Care Med, 161,* 1720-1745.

Brazil, K. & Krueger, P. (2002). Patterns of family adaptation to childhood asthma. *J Pediatr Nurs, 17*(3), 167.

Busse, P. & Busse, W. (2002). Pathogenesis of asthma. In R. Slavin & R. Reisman (Eds.). *Asthma.* Philadelphia: American College of Physicians.

Cabral, A.L., Conceicao, G.M., Saldiva, P.H., & Martins, M.A. (2002). Effect of asthma severity on symptom perception in childhood asthma. *Braz J Med Biol Res, 35,* 319-327.

Castro, M., Schechtman, K., Halstead, J., & Bloomberg, G. (2001). Risk factors for asthma morbidity and mortality in large metropolitan city. *J Asthma, 38*(8), 625-635.

Castro-Rodriguez, L.A., Holberg, C.J., Morgan, W.J., Wright, A.L., & Martinez, F.D. (2001). Increased incidence of asthma-like symptoms in girls who become overweight or obese during the school years. *Am J Respir Crit Care Med, 163*(6), 1344-1349.

Childhood Asthma Management Program Research Group. (2000). Long-term effects of budesonide or nedocromil in children with asthma. *N Engl J Med, 343,* 1054-1063.

Clark, N.M. & Partridge, M.R. (2002). Strengthening asthma education to enhance disease control. *Chest, 121*(5), 1661-1669.

Cokugras, H., Akcakaya, N., Camciogla, Y., Sarimurat, N., & Aksoy, F. (2001). Ultrastructural examination of bronchial biopsy specimens for children with moderate asthma. *Thorax, 56,* 25-29.

Committee on Infectious Diseases. (2000). *Redbook 2000* (25th ed.). Chicago: American Academy of Pediatrics.

Croft, D.R. & Peterson, M.W. (2002). An evaluation of the quality and content of asthma education on the world wide web. *Chest, 4,* 1301-1307.

Ducharme, F.M. & Hicks, H. (2002). Anti-leukotrienes as add-on therapy to inhaled glucocorticoids in patients with asthma: Systematic review of current evidence. *BMJ, 324*(7353), 1545A-1548A.

Fowler, C. (2001). Preventing and managing exercise-induced asthma. *Nurse Pract, 26*(3), 25.

Friedman, A. (2002). *The complete directory for pediatric disorders.* Millerton, NY: Grey House Publishing, Inc.

Gern, J.E., Lemanske R.F., & Busse, W.W. (1999). Early life origins of asthma. *J Clin Invest, 7,* 837-843.

Global Initiative for Asthma Executive Committee. (2002). *Global strategy for asthma management and prevention.* NIH publication no. 02-3659.

Grohl, M.H., Gerritsen, J., Vonk, J.M., Schouten, J.P., Loeter, G.H., et al. (1999). Risk factors for growth and decline of lung function in asthmatic individuals up to age 42 years: A 30 year follow-up study. *Am J Respir Crit Care Med, 160,* 1830-1837.

Gustafsson, D., Olofsson, N., Andersson, F., Lindberg, B., & Schollin, J. (2000). Intervention models on psycho-social health in families with an asthmatic child. *Pediatr Allergy Immunol, 11,* 241-245.

Harris, M., Hauser, S., Nguyen, T., Kelly, P., Rodda, C., et al. (2001). Bone mineral density in prepubertal asthmatics receiving corticosteroid treatment. *J Paediatr Child Health, 37*(1), 67-71.

Homer, C., Susskind, O., Alpert, H. R., Owusu, M., Schneider, L., et al. (2000). An evaluation of an innovative multimedia educational software program for asthma management: Report of a randomized, controlled trial. *Pediatrics, 106*(1), S210-S215.

International Study of Asthma and Allergies in Childhood (ISAAC) Steering Committee. (1998). Worldwide variation in prevalence of symptoms of asthma, allergic rhinoconjunctivitis, and atopic eczema: ISAAC. *Lancet, 351,* 1225-1232.

Israel, E., Banerjee T.R., Fitzmaurice, G.M., Kotlov, T.V., LaHive, K., et al. (2001). Effects of inhaled glucocorticoids on bone density in premenopausal women. *N Engl J Med, 345,* 941-947.

Jaakkola, J.J. & Jaakkola, M.S. (2002). Effects of environmental tobacco smoke on the respiratory health of children. *Scand J Work Environ Health, 28*(suppl. 2), 71-83.

Jenkins, M.A., Hopper J.L., Bowes, G., Carlin, J.B., Flander, L.B., et al. (1994). Factors in childhood as predictors of asthma in adult life. *BMJ, 309,* 90-93.

Jones, J., Wahlgren, D., Meltzer, S., Meltzer, E., Clark, N., et al. (2001). Increasing asthma knowledge and changing home environments for Latino families with asthmatic children. *Patient Educ Couns, 42*(1), 67-79.

Kemper, K. & Lester, M. (1999). Alternative asthma therapies: An evidence-based review. *Contemp Pediatr, 16*(3), 162-195.

Kharitonov, S. & Barnes, P. (2001). Exhaled markers of pulmonary disease. *Am J Respir Crit Care Med, 163,* 1693-1722.

Kieckhefer, G. & Ratcliffe, M. (2000). What parents of children with asthma can tell us. *J Pediatr Health Care, 14,* 122-126.

Kieckhefer, G. & Trahms, C. (2000). Supporting development of children with chronic conditions: From compliance toward shared management. *Pediatr Nurs, 26*(4), 354-363.

Kraft, M. Gamid, Q., Chrousos, G.P., Martin, R.J., & Leung, D.Y. (2001). Decreased steroid responsiveness at night in nocturnal asthma. *Am J Respir Crit Care Med, 5,* 1219-1225.

Larsen, J.S. (2001). Do antihistamines have a role in asthma therapy? *Pharmacotherapy, 21*(3), S28-S33.

Lemanske, R.F. (2001). Choosing therapy for childhood asthma. *Paediatr Drugs, 3*(12), 915-925.

Lemanske, R.F. (2000). Inflammatory events in asthma: An expanding equation. *J Allergy Clin Immunol, 105,* S633-S636.

Lemanske, R.F. (2002). Issues in understanding pediatric asthma: Epidemiology and genetics. *J Allergy Clin Immunol, 109*(6), S521-S524.

Lentz, M., Kieckhefer, G., Gau, B., & McMillion, J.C. (2002). Influence of sleep on respiratory function in children with asthma: A pilot study. *Commun Nurs Res.*

Levien, T.L. & Bailer D.E. (1999). Selected interaction caused by cytochrome P450 enzymes. *Prescriber's Letter, 4,* 150401.

Malthouse, S. (1997) Homeopathic remedies for asthma. *Can Fam Physician, 43,* 1917.

Mannino, D.M., Homa, D.M., Akinbami, L.J., Mooorman, J.E., Gwynn, C., et al. (2002a). Surveillance for asthma—United States, 1980-1999. *MMWR Morb Mortal Wkly Rep, 51*(SS01), 1-13.

Mannino, D.M., Homa, D.M., & Redd, S.C. (2002b). Involuntary smoking and asthma severity in children—Data from the Third National Health and Nutrition Examination Survey. *Chest, 122*(2), 409-415.

Martinez, F.D. (1995). Asthma and wheezing in the first six years of life. *N Engl J Med, 3,* 133-138.

Martinez, F.D. (2001a). The coming-of-age of the hygiene hypothesis. *Respir Res, 2*(3), 129-132.

Martinez, F.D. (2001b). Links between pediatric and adult asthma. *J Allergy Clin Immunol, 107,* S449-S455.

Martinez, F.D. (2002). Development of wheezing disorders and asthma in preschool children. *Pediatrics, 2,* 362-367.

Maspero, J.F., Duenas-Meza, E., Volovitz, B., Pinacho Daza, C., Kosa, L., et al. (2001). Oral montelukast versus inhaled beclomethasone in 6- to 11-year-old children with asthma: Results of an open-label extension study evaluating long-term safety, satisfaction, and adherence with therapy. *Curr Med Res Opin, 17*(2), 96-104.

McEvoy, G.K. (2002). *American hospital formulary service drug information.* Bethesda, MD: American of Health-Systems Pharmacists, pp. 1234-1240, 3608-3693.

Milgrom, H. & Taussig, L.M. (1999). Keeping children with exercise induced asthma active. *Pediatrics, 3*(e38), 1-5.

Montalbano, M.M. & Lemanske, R.F. (2002). Infection and asthma in children. *Curr Opin Pediatr, 14*(3), 334-337.

National Heart, Lung, and Blood Institute. (1997). *National Asthma Education and Prevention Program Expert Panel report guide II guidelines for the diagnosis and management of asthma. National asthma education program expert panel report II.* Publication no. 97-4051A. U.S. Department of Health and Human Services.

National Heart, Lung, and Blood Institute. (2002). *National Asthma Education and Prevention Program Expert Panel report guide II guidelines for the diagnosis and management of asthma. Update on selected topics 2002. National asthma education program expert panel report II.* U.S. Department of Health and Human Services. *J Allergy Clin Immunol* (online serial), *2*(110), 5; Web site: http://www.nhlbi.nih.gov/guidelines/asthma/index.htm.

O'Hallaren, M. (2002). Exercise induced asthma. In Slavin & Reisman (Eds.). *Asthma.* Philadelphia: American College of Physicians.

Opat, A.J., Cohen, M.M., Bailey, M.J., & Abramson, M.J. (2000). A clinical trial of the Buteyko breathing technique in Asthma as taught by a video. *J Asthma, 37*(7), 557-564.

Ortega, A.N., Huertas, S.E., Canino, G., Ramirez, R., & Rubio-Stipec, M. (2002). Childhood asthma, chronic illness, and psychiatric disorders. *J Nerv Ment Dis, 190*(5), 275-281.

Oswald, H., Phelan, P.D., Lanigan, A., Gibbert, M., Bowes, G., et al. (1994). Outcome of childhood asthma in mid-adult life. *BM J, 309,* 95-96.

Oswald, H., Phelan, P.D., Lanigan, A., Hibbert, M., Carlin, J.B., et al. (1997). Childhood asthma and lung function in mid-adult life. *Pediatr Pulmonol, 1,* 14-20.

Palacioz, K (2001). Advair Diskus. *Prescriber's Letter, 4,* 170406.

Palmer, L., Cookson, W., James, A., Musk, W., & Burton, P. (2001). Gibbs sampling-based segregation analysis of asthma-associated quantitative traits in a population-based sample of nuclear families. *Genet Epidemiol, 20*(3), 356-372.

Payne, D., Wilson, N., Hablas, J., Agrafiioti, C., & Bush, A. (2001). Evidence of different subgroups of difficult asthma in children. *Thorax, 56,* 345-350.

Pinkerton, C. & Kieckhefer, G. (2002). Educating children with asthma. *Nurse Pract, 27*(3), 12-13, 81.

Ploin, D., Chapuis, F.R., Stamm, D., Robert, J., David, L., et al. (2000). High-dose albuterol by metered-dose inhaler plus a spacer device versus nebulization in preschool children with recurrent wheezing: A double-blind, randomized equivalence trial. *Pediatrics, 106*(2), 311-317.

Price, J., Hindmarsh, P., Hughes, S., & Efthimiou, J. (2002a). Evaluating the effects of asthma therapy on childhood growth: What can be learned from the published literature? *Eur Respir J, 19*(6), 1179-1193.

Price, J., Lenney, W., Duncan, C., Green, L., Flood, Y., et al. (2002b). HPA-axis effects of nebulised fluticasone propionate compared with oral prednisolone in childhood asthma. *Respir Med, 96*(8), 625-631.

Purucker, M.. & Malozowski, S. (2001). Asthma, corticosteroids, and growth. *N Engl J Med, 344*(8), 607.

Rasmussen, F., Taylor, D., Flannery, E., Cowan, J., Greene, J., et al. (2002). Risk factors for airway remodeling in asthma manifested by a low postbronchodilator FEV_1/vital capacity ratio: A longitudinal population study from childhood to adulthood. *Am J Respir Crit Care Med, 165*(11), 1480-1488.

Reddington, A. (2001). Step one for asthma treatment: Beta (2)-agonists of inhaled corticosteroids? *Drugs, 61*(9), 1231-1238.

Rijssenbeek Nouwens, L., Oosting, A.J., De Monchy, J., Bregman, I., Postma, D.S., et al. (2002). The effect of antiallergic mattress encasings on house dust mite-induced early and late airway reactions in asthmatic patients: A double-blind, placebo-controlled study. *Clin Exp Allergy, 32*(1), 117-125.

Rodriguez, M.A., Winkleby, M.A., Ahn, D., Sundquist, J., & Kraemer, H.C. (2002). Identification of population subgroups of children and adolescents with high asthma prevalence: Findings from the Third National Health and Nutrition Examination Survey. *Arch Pediatr Adolesc Med, 156*(3), 269-275.

Sabina, I., Von Mutius, E., Lau, S., Bergmann, R., Niggerman B., et al. (2001). Early childhood infectious diseases and the development of asthma up to school age: A birth cohort study. *BMJ, 322,* 390-395.

Sadeh, A., Horowitz, I., Wolach-Benodis, L., & Wolach, B. (1998). Sleep and pulmonary function in children with well-controlled, stable asthma. *Sleep, 21*(4), 379-383.

Shahis, S.K., Kharitonov, S.A., Wilson, N.M., Bush, A., & Barnes, P.J. (2002). Increased interleukin-4 and decreased interferon-gamma in exhaled breath condensate of children with asthma. *Am J Respir Crit Care Med, 165*(9), 1290-1293.

Spahn, J.D. & Szefler, S.J. (2002). Childhood asthma: New insight into management. *J Allergy Clin Immunol, 10*(1, pt. 1), 3-13.

Stapelton, S. (2002). Childhood asthma rates are leveling off, but disparities remain; Web site: http:www.ama-asssn.org/sci-pubs/amnews/pick_02/hlsa0826.htm.

Strachan, D.P., Butland, B.K., & Anderson, H.R. (1996). Incidence and prognosis of asthma and wheezing illness from early childhood to age 33 in national British cohort. *BMJ, 312,* 1195-1199.

von Kries, R., Hermann, M., Grunert, V.P., & von Mutius, E. (2001). Is obesity a risk factor for childhood asthma? *Allergy, 56*(4), 318-322.

Wenzel, S., Gibbs, R., Lehr, M., & Simoes, E. (2002).Respiratory outcomes in high-risk children 7 to 10 years after prophylaxis with respiratory syncytial virus immune globulin. *Am J Med, 112*(8), 627-633.

White, L. (2000). *The herbal drugstore.* London: Signet Publications.

Williams, R.O., Patel, A.M., Barron, M.K., & Rogers, T.L. (2001). Investigation of some commercially available spacer devices for the delivery of glucocorticoid steroids from a MDI. *Drug Dev Ind Pharm, 27*(5), 401-412.

Wong, J., Zacharin, M.R., Hocking, N., & Robinson, P.J. (2002). Growth and adrenal suppression in asthmatic children on moderate to high doses of fluticasone propionate. *J Paediatr Child Health, 38*(1), 59-62.

Zelcer, S., Henri, C., Tewfik, T., & Mazer, B. (2002). Multidimensional voice program analysis (MDVP) and the diagnosis of pediatric vocal cord dysfunction. *Ann Allergy Asthma Immunol, 88*(6), 601-608.

12 Attention Deficit Hyperactivity Disorder

Janice Selekman and Carol Kerrigan Moore

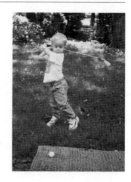

Etiology

Attention deficit hyperactivity disorder (ADHD) was identified as a condition in 1902, although it was described in a German nursery rhyme, "Fidgety Phil," in 1863 (Wender, 2000). The current diagnosis of ADHD has been preceded by many other labels, including brain damaged, minimal brain dysfunction, hyperactive child syndrome, hyperkinetic disorder of childhood, and attention deficit disorder with and without hyperactivity (Stubbe, 2000).

The definition of ADHD also continues to evolve; it is currently defined by the *Diagnostic and Statistical Manual of Mental Disorders IV (DSM-IV)* as a "persistent pattern of inattention and/or hyperactivity-impulsivity that is more frequent and severe than is typically observed in individuals at a comparable level of development" (American Psychiatric Association [APA], 2000, p. 85).

This disorder is intrinsic to an individual and presumed to be the result of central nervous system (CNS) dysfunction. Even though ADHD can occur with other handicapping conditions (e.g., sensory impairment, mental retardation, serious psychosocial and emotional disturbances) or extrinsic influences (e.g., insufficient or inappropriate instruction or parenting), it is not the direct result of those conditions or influences (Wender, 2000). ADHD is a nonprogressive neurologic condition.

Barkley (2000) has proposed that ADHD is not a disorder of attention but rather a defect or delay in response inhibition that results in difficulty "self-regulating" one's impulsive motor behavior. Consequently, one becomes hyperresponsive to stimuli, and hyperactivity results. This neurologic defect in inhibition and self-control leads to alterations in an individual's ability to carry out executive functions (e.g., deflecting distractions, recalling goals by using hindsight and taking steps to reach them by using forethought). It also includes changes in the ability to follow rules, control emotions and behaviors, and exhibit flexibility. This lack of self-regulation interferes with one's ability to inhibit a response that has not yet started, stop one in progress, and prevent interference by extraneous stimuli (Solanto, 2001).

It is recognized that there are conditions that can result in symptoms of ADHD. Brain damage can occur as a result of brain infections, hypoxic and/or anoxic episodes, or trauma; and approximately 20% of this population, especially those with damage to the prefrontal cortex, develop impulsivity and inattention (Jensen, 2000). In the history of ADHD, the first cases were described following cases of encephalitis. Prema-

ture birth is another risk factor for the symptoms of ADHD, especially for infants weighing less than 2.2 lb (1 kg) at birth, who are at a greater risk of developing impulsivity and have trouble with concentration and with social interactions (Hille et al, 2001). Maternal alcohol and tobacco use during pregnancy as well as fetal exposure to other substances of abuse, especially crack cocaine, has also been correlated with the development of alterations in behavior and attention (Barkley, 2000; Jensen, 2000; Silver, 1999). Exposure to high levels of lead in young children can also result in the development of hyperactivity and inattention (Anastopoulos & Shelton, 2001). Questions have been raised as to whether the above conditions actually *cause* ADHD or are merely associated with it.

The causes and the exact mechanisms involved remain unknown, although multiple areas are under investigation. The primary contributors to ADHD appear to be neurologic and genetic. The proposed neurologic causes being explored are neurobiologic and neuroanatomic. The neurobiologic hypothesis focuses on the dysregulation of neurotransmitters—especially catecholamines (dopamine, norepinephrine, and possibly serotonin) (Anastopoulos & Shelton, 2001). It is believed that there is a deficit in catecholaminergic neurotransmission resulting in not enough catecholamine being available to hold onto a task, such as attention (Solanto, 2001). Because most of the medications with proven efficacy for ADHD stimulate receptors to increase dopamine release and inhibit reuptake of neurotransmitters, deficits in this system seem to be supported as one of the primary causes of ADHD (Barkley, 2000).

The neuroanatomic research attempts to identify structural anomalies of, or damage to, the brains of children with ADHD. The prefrontal cortex is rich in dopamine receptors and is therefore the subject of much exploration. In some studies using neurologic scanning techniques, it appears that the right prefrontal cortex and parts of the cerebellum may be smaller in children with ADHD, with decreased blood flow to the area and decreased electrical activity in the area compared with those without the disorder (Barkley, 2000; Castellanos, 2001). The blood flow deficits appear to be reversed following administration of stimulant medication (Anastopoulos & Shelton, 2001). The right prefrontal cortex is involved in inhibiting behavior and sustaining attention; the identified areas of the cerebellum are responsible for allowing the cortex time to process stimuli and coordinate input among the regions of the cortex. The research findings, although potentially helpful from an etiologic aspect, are not useful tools for diagnosis in individuals at this time.

Known Genetic Etiology

ADHD is considered to be a complex genetic disorder; "genetic factors are principal in the etiology of ADHD" (Solanto, 2001, p. 11). The idea of genetic predisposition is supported for ADHD in a significant number of cases. Genetic studies with both twins and adopted children have suggested that the condition is polygenic. There is an 82.7% concordance rate for monozygotic twins and a 37.9% concordance rate for dizygotic twins (Solanto, 2001). "Siblings of children with ADHD are between five and seven times more likely to develop the syndrome than children from unaffected families . . . and the children of a parent who has ADHD have up to a 50 percent chance of experiencing some difficulties" (Barkley, 1998). "If a child has ADHD, then, there is a 500% increase in the risk to other members in that family" (Barkley, 2000, p. 73). In the twin studies, the effect of a "shared environment" was not significant. It was also found that deficient parenting and family adversity did not cause ADHD and accounted for only 10% of the variance in the occurrence of ADHD (Solanto, 2001).

Because of the belief that the symptoms of ADHD are due to pathophysiology of the neurotransmitters and their receptors, investigators are studying the genes that encode for these transmitters and their receptors as well as the neurocircuitry of the frontal lobe (Jensen, 2000). Research is now being done to examine the dopamine transporter gene (*DAT1*), which has a number of sections that repeat themselves. It is hypothesized that the increased number of repeats may result in a rapid turnover of dopamine at the synapse, leading to a greater increase in the hyperactive/impulsive type of ADHD (Solanto, 2001). Another gene being investigated is the dopamine receptor gene (*DRD4*), as well as the genes that regulate the dopamine pathways that direct neural activity in the frontal basal ganglia (Jensen, 2000; Solanto, 2001).

Incidence and Prevalence

ADHD is the most common neurobehavioral disorder of childhood and is considered to be "among the most prevalent chronic health conditions affecting school age children" (AAP, 2000, p. 1158). As the diagnostic criteria have changed over time, so have the prevalence rates. Estimates of the number of children with ADHD range from 3% to 14.4% (Scahill & Schwab-Stone, 2000), depending on the population tested and the methods used. Earlier literature frequently combined ADHD with learning disabilities. The two have been better differentiated in the literature over the past decade.

Early estimates suggested that 3% to 5% of the school-aged population had ADHD; that number is now thought to be between 5% and 10% of those between 5 and 18 years of age and 4% to 5% of adults (Anastopoulos & Shelton, 2001; Wender, 2000). This converts into 4 million children and 4 to 5 million adults in the United States. Children with ADHD account for 4% of all primary care office visits but make up 50% of children seen in child psychiatric clinics (Stubbe, 2000). This range may be because those who display aggressive behavior are more likely to be identified early and referred to a clinic.

The prevalence of ADHD appears to decrease somewhat with age after elementary school (National Institutes of Health [NIH] Consensus Statement, 1998, 2000), perhaps because of

symptomatology that is less well defined for the teenager. The rate of ADHD does appear to decline in adulthood "by 50% approximately every 5 years, leading to the estimates of adult ADHD as 0.8% at age 20 and 0.005% at age 40" (Greenhill, 1998). The American Academy of Child and Adolescent Psychiatry (AACAP, 1997), however, indicates that the frequency in adults is similar to that of children (2% to 7%).

More boys than girls have been diagnosed with ADHD. This is thought to be due to the fact that more males have noticeable signs of hyperactivity and more females exhibit symptoms consistent with the inattentive type of ADHD, leading to a delayed or missed diagnosis. Although the ratios differ by the setting, the general ratio of males to females with this condition is approximately 3:1, with ratios ranging from 9:1 in clinical settings for elementary-aged children to 2:1 for the predominantly inattentive type of ADHD (Carlson & Mann, 2000; Scahill & Schwab-Stone, 2000; Solanto, 2001).

ADHD is found throughout the world in individuals from all cultures and ethnic backgrounds (Anastopoulos & Shelton, 2001). In other countries, the number of cases of ADHD depends on the definition, diagnostic criteria, and diagnostic tools used. During the past decade, studies report the prevalence ranging from 29.2% in India to 10.9% in Germany, 9% in Canada, 7.7% in Japan, 5.8% in Brazil, 2% to 6% in New Zealand, and 3% to 4% in Norway (Weyandt, 2001).

Clinical Manifestations at Time of Diagnosis

The past emphasis on hyperactivity as the primary component of ADHD has changed; impulsivity, inattention, and hyperactivity are now recognized as equally important. These manifestations occur in all facets of a child's life and often become worse in situations requiring sustained attention. Therefore the school setting is frequently where these features result in a referral for evaluation. The current subtypes of ADHD are the predominantly inattentive type (ADHD-I), the predominantly hyperactive-impulsive type (ADHD-H/I), and the combined type (inattentive, hyperactive, and impulsive) (ADHD-C) (APA, 2000).

According to the *DSM-IV*, for an individual to be labeled ADHD predominantly inattentive, at least six of the nine symptoms must have persisted for at least 6 months (Box 12-1). For ADHD predominantly hyperactive-impulsive, at least six of the nine characteristics in that category must have persisted for at least 6 months. A diagnosis of the combined type requires at least six symptoms from each of the sets of categories. Regardless of the type of ADHD, some symptoms must have been present before the age of 7 years (APA, 2000). The criteria have been found to be valid for children as young as 4 years (Lahey et al, 1998). In a practical sense, any child who is experiencing significant dysfunction across settings should be evaluated further.

Although symptoms are often identified in early childhood, they may not be identified until after a child enters a structured school environment. Even then, children (most often girls) with the inattentive type are less likely than other children with ADHD to be referred for evaluation. Children with the inattentive form of ADHD are less likely to exhibit the level of behavior difficulty observed in those with the combined or

---

BOX 12-1

Diagnostic Criteria for Attention Deficit Hyperactivity Disorder

A. Either (1) OR (2):

(1) Six (or more) of the following symptoms of inattention have persisted for at least 6 mo to a degree that is maladaptive and inconsistent with developmental level:

Inattention:

a. Often fails to give close attention to details or makes careless mistakes in school work, work, or other activities

b. Often has difficulty sustaining attention in tasks or play activities

c. Often does not seem to listen when spoken to directly

d. Often does not follow through on instructions and fails to finish school work, chores, or duties in the workplace (not because of oppositional behavior or failure to understand instructions)

e. Often has difficulty organizing tasks and activities

f. Often avoids, dislikes, or is reluctant to engage in tasks that require sustained mental effort (e.g., school work or homework)

g. Often loses things necessary for tasks or activities (e.g., toys, school assignments, pencils, books, tools)

h. Is often easily distracted by extraneous stimuli

i. Is often forgetful in daily activities

(2) Six (or more) of the following symptoms of hyperactivity-impulsivity have persisted for at least 6 mo to a degree that is maladaptive and inconsistent with developmental level

Hyperactivity:

a. Often fidgets with hands or feet or squirms in seat

b. Often leaves seat in classroom or in other situations in which remaining seated is expected

c. Often runs about or climbs excessively in situations in which it is inappropriate (in adolescents or adults, may be limited to subjective feelings of restlessness)

d. Often has difficulty playing or engaging in leisure activities quietly

e. Is often "on the go" or often acts "as if driven by a motor"

f. Often talks excessively

Impulsivity:

g. Often blurts out answers before questions have been completed

h. Often has difficulty awaiting turn

i. Often interrupts or intrudes on others (e.g., butts into conversations or games)

B. Some hyperactive-impulsive or inattentive symptoms that caused impairment present before age 7 yr

C. Some impairment from the symptoms present in two or more settings (e.g., at school or work and at home)

D. Clear evidence of clinically significant impairment in social, academic, or occupational functioning

E. Symptoms do not occur exclusively during the course of a pervasive developmental disorder, schizophrenia, or other psychotic disorder and are not better accounted for by another mental disorder (e.g., mood disorder, anxiety disorder, dissociative disorder, personality disorder)

From American Psychiatric Association. (2000). *Diagnostic and statistical manual of mental disorders* (4th ed.). Washington; DC: Author. Reprinted with permission.

---

hyperactive-impulsive types (APA, 2000). The average age for diagnosis of ADHD-I is 9.8 years compared with 8.5 years for the combined type (Carlson & Mann, 2000), although symptoms were obvious to most parents and teachers 3 to 5 years earlier (Anastopoulos & Shelton, 2001). Increased motor activity—including alterations in sleeping and eating routines, however, has been identified by parents in children as young as 10 to 18 months (Greenhill, 1998).

The *DSM-IV* (APA, 2000) changed the wording of the symptomatology to better address symptoms experienced or observed in preschoolers as well as in adolescents or adults with ADHD. Some controversy has been raised regarding the *DSM-IV* age-of-onset criterion of 7 years for ADHD, particularly in light of the increasing interest in diagnosis of adolescents and adults with ADHD. Diagnostic issues include the following: (1) the validity of historical recollection and self-report of symptoms; (2) the later awareness of impairment, especially with the predominantly inattentive subtype of ADHD; (3) the problem of separating out symptoms of frequent co-morbid disorders in adolescents and adults with ADHD; (4) the coupling of a diagnosis of ADHD with eligibility for federally mandated disability services; and (5) the fact that an onset before the age of 7 years was selected without empiric field trials (Greenhill, 1998; Spencer et al, 1998). The individual who cannot document symptoms of ADHD before the age of 7 years but who does meet the criteria at the time of diagnosis is usually labeled, ADHD—Not Otherwise Specified (APA, 2000). It is important to note that all children under the age of 7 years are likely to manifest some of the behaviors associated with ADHD at times as part of the normal developmental process.

ADHD in Older Adolescents and Adults

Although most researchers have acknowledged that many children with ADHD have the disorder into adulthood, it has been implied that there are many older adolescents and adults with ADHD who were never identified as having the disorder as children. Older adolescents and adults suspected of having ADHD exhibit symptoms slightly different from those in the *DSM-IV.* These symptoms include poor social interaction with possible antisocial behavior, substance and/or alcohol use disorders, high levels of school failure, anxiety disorders, poor work histories, and low self-esteem. Other symptoms include heightened motor activity, such as fingers tapping and knees going up and down fairly continuously, restlessness, distractibility, failure to stay on task, disorganization with schedules, and executive function difficulties. These symptoms may reflect sequelae of undiagnosed and consequently unmanaged ADHD. These adults are often undereducated and assume lower occupational levels (Silver, 2000; Wender, 2000).

Diagnostic Measures

Because no gold standard exists, no one test or tool can diagnose a child as having ADHD. Therefore a diagnosis of ADHD must be viewed with caution. The primary care provider (PCP) needs to know which criteria were used to make the diagnosis and which differential diagnoses were ruled out. Multiple data sources collected over time should have been used to make the diagnosis. These sources include the following: (1) family history, (2) perinatal history, (3) developmental history with current developmental assessment, (4) assessment of past and current temperament of the child, (5) health history, (6) assessment of academic performance, (7) comprehensive age-

TABLE 12-1

Selected Behavior Rating Scales for Screening and Assessing Treatment Efficacy in ADHD

Scales	Source	Age	Method	Comments
Achenbach's Child Behavior Check List (CBCL)	Center for Children, Youth, and Families University of Vermont 1 S Prospect St Burlington, VT 05401	4-18 yr	Observation Interview	Screening provides overview of child's behavior
Conners Parent and Teacher Rating Scale	A.D.D. Warehouse 1-800-233-9273 www.addwarehause.com	3-14 yr (long version) 3-17 yr (short version)	Observation	Screening
ACTeRS	Meritech, Inc 111 N. Market St Champaign, IL 61820	5-13 yr	Teacher observation	Screening
Attenfon Deficit Disorders Evaluation Scale (ADDES)	Catalog: Hawthorne Educational Services (800) 542-1673	5-18 yr	—	—
AD/HD Rating Scale Behavioral Assessment System for Children—Parent Rating Scale (BASC-PRS)	Catalog: American Guidance Systems (800) 328-2560	4-18 yr	—	—

Data from American Academy of Pediatrics (2000). Clinical practice guideline: Diagnosis and evaluation of the child with attention-deficit/hyperactivity disorder. *Pediatrics, 105*(5), 1158-1170; Guyer, B. (2000); *ADHD: Achieving success in school and in life.* Boston: Allyn & Bacon; Hechtman, L. (2000a). Assessment and diagnosis of attention-deficit/hyperactivity disorder. *Child and Adolescent Psychiatric Clinics of North America; 9*(3), 481-498; Weyandt, L. (2001). *An ADHD primer.* Boston: Allyn & Bacon.

appropriate psychologic and intelligence testing, and (8) comprehensive physical assessment with an emphasis on neurologic and motor abilities.

According to the American Academy of Pediatrics [AAP] guidelines, evidence must be directly obtained from parents or caregivers regarding the symptoms displayed in various settings, the age of onset, the duration of the symptoms, and the degree of functional impairment (AAP, 2000). Evidence should also be provided by the classroom teacher or other school personnel. Although it is helpful for a clinician to observe a child's performance and behavior in structured and unstructured activities, it is usually not realistic. Whereas these criteria are used for diagnostic purposes, the same criteria are also used to monitor the child's response to treatment regimens. Therefore it is important for the PCP to be familiar with them.

A variety of behavior rating scales (Table 12-1) can be used by parents and teachers for providing supplemental, standardized data when screening for ADHD and assessing treatment efficacy (AAP, 2000). Comparing a teacher's objective evaluation of a child's behavior with that of his or her same-age peers or using a symptom frequency count with the parent's assessment can be especially valuable. Although hyperactivity can be rated as a physical measurement, inattention cannot be measured directly; it must be "inferred" by the rater (Greenhill, 1998).

Many conditions may mimic symptoms seen in ADHD; a complete assessment will rule out these conditions. Box 12-2 contains a list of common conditions that should be considered as possible alternative causes for the symptomatology. Allergy-based signs and symptoms can result in a child being tired, irritable, or restless (Wender, 2000) (see Chapter 10). Symptoms, such as difficulty breathing or pruritus, can interrupt a child's attention. Obstructive sleep disorders, such as apnea or upper airway resistance syndrome, can result in fatigue and inattention (Chervin et al, 2002). Even hypoglycemia from

BOX 12-2

Differential Diagnosis*

Allergies
Asthma
Hearing and vision problems
Seizure disorders—especially absence seizures, which may be misinterpreted as Inattentive ADHD
Brain injury or brain infection
Brain tumor
Neurologic trauma
Thyroid abnormalities
Congenital adrenal hyperplasia (rare)
High blood lead levels
Hypoglycemia
Obstructive sleep problems
Nutritional deficiency, especially iron deficiency anemia
Use of over-the-counter or prescribed medications where the side effects may be overactivity or sluggishness
Learning disabilities
Other psychiatric conditions, such as anxiety disorders, Asperger syndrome, autism, depression, conduct disorder (CD), oppositional defiant disorder (ODD), or Tourette's syndrome
Family disruptions or dysfunctional family
Child abuse

Data from Chervin, R. et al. (2002). Inattention, hyperactivity and symptoms of sleep-disordered breathing. *Pediatrics, 109*(3), 449-456; Magyary, D., Brandt, P., & Kovalesky, A. (1999). *Children and ADHD: A manual with decision tree—clinical path.* Seattle: University of Washington; Weyandt, L. (2001). *An ADHD primer.* Boston: Allyn & Bacon.
*For conditions with ADHD-like behaviors.

skipped breakfasts can result in irritability and inattention. These conditions can easily be identified and treated. In addition, many psychiatric conditions, especially bipolar and oppositional defiant disorder, may mimic the signs and symptoms of ADHD.

Trials of stimulant medications to determine their effect on the child without a complete assessment are both inappropriate and unethical; this practice has no place in the diagnostic process. As with any chronic condition, the diagnostic period may be especially difficult for the parents, and guidance and support by the knowledgeable PCP are especially helpful.

Treatment

ADHD is a chronic condition that generally causes significant functional impairment across several domains at home, at school, and in the community. Because of this, effective treatment must necessarily address behavioral, educational, and health care needs. This multimodal approach typically requires involvement of the family and primary care clinician and a number of other professionals, such as teachers, administrators, school psychologists, social workers, psychiatrists, psychologists, and the school nurse.

Many primary care clinicians are likely to see individuals who have already been diagnosed and are currently under treatment. In such cases, the effectiveness of the current management needs to be evaluated and maintained or adjusted as necessary, based on parent, teacher, and child feedback and/or consultation with the treating clinician.

Multimodal Treatment

Multimodal treatment addresses the core symptoms of ADHD. The premiere study that systematically evaluated the efficacy of various approaches to treatment was the Multimodal Treatment Study of Children with ADHD (Jensen et al, 1999). The results of this landmark study suggested that pharmacologic management involving close follow-up and feedback from school personnel or a combination of pharmacologic management and behavioral intervention were more effective than intensive behavioral treatment alone. In addition, those children with combined treatment could be effectively treated with lower doses of medications.

In response to primary care clinicians' need for an evidence-based approach to treatment for 6- to 12-year-old children with ADHD without major co-existing conditions, the American Academy of Pediatrics released its first clinical practice guideline for management of ADHD (AAP, 2001). This guideline reiterated some of the approaches enumerated in the previously released "Parameters for Assessment and Treatment of Children, Adolescents, and Adults with Attention Deficit Hyperactivity Disorder" (AACAP, 1997) but from a primary care perspective. The key components of the AAP guideline are (1) that a collaborative approach with the clinician, parents, child, and school personnel is both necessary and desirable in targeting outcomes, (2) that stimulant medication and/or behavioral therapy may be used as appropriate to achieve desired outcomes, and (3) that lack of improvement in symptom management needs to be thoroughly evaluated in terms of adherence and potential co-morbidities. Careful follow-up underlies all these interventions.

Behavioral Intervention

Behavioral interventions comprise a wide array of strategies that may be recommended by specialists in mental health (psychiatrists, psychologists, counselors, social workers) or primary care clinicians (Box 12-3). Recommended interventions and strategies are likely to be most effective if they are implemented relatively consistently across settings by parents, caregivers, and teachers. This is one of the aspects of ADHD management that makes it a very complex undertaking.

Behavior management skills are generally based on behavioral principles, such as positive reinforcement, withdrawal of privileges (cost-response intervention), and token economies, or a combination of these. Response to these interventions can be highly variable, even in the same individual. Examples of functional disparities in the child with ADHD may include difficulties engaging in and completing schoolwork, homework, and chores; consistently negative interactions with siblings; lack of compliance with directions from parents, teachers, or other authority figures; disorganization and forgetting; and impaired social skills. In general, most activities that require sustained mental effort (except those that are highly stimulating and of the child's choosing, such as video or computer games) will present problems to the child with ADHD. "Tangible reinforcers are more effective at improving . . . behavior and academic performance than are teacher attention or other social reinforcers" (Anastopoulos & Shelton, 2001, p.174).

Because ADHD manifests itself primarily through excessive activity, inattention, and academic or behavioral problems, parents (particularly mothers) are frequently targeted as ineffective and responsible for their child's difficulties. Parents frequently do feel as though they must be doing something wrong, particularly if the affected child is their first. Clinicians can help to dispel the myth of poor parenting as a cause of ADHD. These children may not respond to conventional parenting wisdom and discipline strategies, leaving parents with few effective options for managing misbehavior. The core symptoms of ADHD frequently preclude the child from responding to cues,

---

BOX 12-3

Behavior Management Strategies

STRATEGY: POSITIVE REINFORCEMENT
Description: Immediate reward given for desired behavior; tangible reinforcers, such as small treats, stickers, or inexpensive toys, are the most effective. Other reinforcers include special privileges or activities.
Example: Child performs targeted behavior and receives previously agreed on reinforcer. Child completes task, receives praise and small treat.

STRATEGY: WITHDRAWAL OF PRIVILEGES (COST-RESPONSE INTERVENTION)
Description: Undesirable behavior results in loss of desired privilege.
Example: Access to computer time or favorite TV show is withdrawn if targeted misbehavior occurs. Alternatively, time-out removes child temporarily from setting where misbehavior occurred.

STRATEGY: TOKEN ECONOMIES
Description: Tokens are awarded for each appropriate behavior, which can be accumulated and used to acquire a desired activity or object. Alternatively, the child starts with a given number of tokens, and each incidence of targeted misbehavior results in loss of a token. A certain number of tokens must be acquired or retained by child to access special privileges or items.
Example: Desired behavior occurs; token is awarded. Alternatively, undesirable behavior occurs; token is withdrawn. Different numbers of tokens can be traded for small toys, games, or special privileges at the end of a specified time period.

learning from past disciplinary actions, or generalizing a set of rules to a different setting.

Clinicians can be most helpful by recognizing and validating the inherent difficulties of parenting a child with ADHD and facilitating healthy coping through information and knowledge of community resources. Referral for instruction in behavioral management techniques specific to the child with ADHD may be beneficial.

Behavior rating scales, such as the Connors Parent and Teacher Rating Scales, are useful in assessing baseline status and as an evaluation tool for selected interventions and for periodic assessments of the effectiveness of intervention modalities. In general, the more structured and predictable the environment (both home and school), the better the child with ADHD is likely to function. Daily routines should be as consistent as possible, allowing extra time for the child to overcome his or her frequently limited organizational skills. For the younger child, picture charts or written reminder lists can be helpful in getting mornings off to a productive start. If medications are administered, it may be helpful to give the morning dose before the child gets out of bed so that some absorption and effect have occurred at the beginning of the day, facilitating a smoother morning routine.

In addition to pharmacologic and behavioral interventions, children affected by ADHD may benefit from involvement in recreational or competitive sports activities. Summer camps or experiential education activities can offer opportunities for social and emotional growth and enhanced self-esteem. Some children can manage in regular camp situations; others may benefit from camps or programs specific to the child affected with ADHD. It is helpful for the clinician to support and encourage these opportunities where available and to be familiar with community resources.

Although pharmacotherapy can significantly improve the behavior of the child with ADHD, education of the child, parents, and teachers is a key component of treatment (AACAP, 1997). Academic and social adjustments are most difficult for these children because of deficient behavioral and executive function skills. Behavioral interventions are helpful adjuncts to pharmacotherapy, and this combination can offer synergistic and cost-effective benefits. Health care professionals, educators, and parents must help these children set appropriate goals and then guide them to organize and prioritize strategies to obtain them. The support of professionals for child-parent training is important in helping a family and child effectively cope with a chronic, difficult situation.

Pharmacologic Intervention

Strong evidence supports the use of stimulant medications in the treatment of the core symptoms of ADHD; 80% to 90% of children with ADHD respond favorably to stimulants (AAP, 2001; Anastopoulos & Shelton, 2001; Greenhill, 2001). Stimulant medications are among the most studied of all the pharmacologic interventions for ADHD, with over 200 controlled studies in school-aged children. They have excellent effectiveness and safety profiles and are the mainstay of therapeutic medications for ADHD symptoms. It should be noted, however, that few studies on long-term use have been done and that improvement in ADHD symptoms usually only occurs while the medication is being used. There are only a few studies of stimulant medication use in preschool populations.

The goal is to maximize desired effect and minimize adverse effect. The widely held belief that stimulants have a paradoxic calming effect on children with ADHD is erroneous; they are thought to work by affecting certain neurotransmitters, such as serotonin, dopamine, and norepinephrine, which have to do with selectivity, focus, and attention. Indeed, ADHD itself can be conceptualized as paying attention to every stimulus at once, instead of selectively focusing on the most important one. In addition to being effective for the core symptoms of ADHD, stimulant medications may help with oppositional behavior and aggression (Pelham et al, 2001).

The increased use of stimulant medications, although hotly debated in the popular press, probably reflects increased recognition and diagnosis in children, adolescents, and adults (Solanto, 2001; Wilens & Spencer, 2000). Although there are some documented regional differences in use of stimulant medications in the pediatric population, the estimated prevalence rate of ADHD in the United States still exceeds the percentage of children being treated with stimulant medication (Solanto, 2001).

The National Institutes of Health, responding to controversies over the rising use of stimulants in the treatment of ADHD, convened a consensus development conference in 1998. The conclusion was that although stimulant medications are indeed effective in the short term, there are areas that demand attention, such as a lack of long-term use studies, widely variable prescribing practices, and risks/benefits of use (NIH, 2000).

Stimulant Medication–Prescribing Principles. Stimulant dosing is not weight dependent, with recommended acceptable ranges for each medication used instead (Table 12-2). When prescribing medications for the pediatric population, providers should be aware of the following factors: (1) as children grow, changes in the ratio of body fat to muscle affect the bioavailability of lipid-soluble drugs; (2) as a child's age increases, the metabolism of medications decreases; and (3) gender differences in body fat percentage are generally seen in puberty, with females having more fat than males (Tosyali & Greenhill, 1998).

The stimulant dose-response curve is highly variable in its effect among individuals and with respect to specific behaviors and learning. Recommended strategy for initiating stimulant medication is to begin with a low dose and slowly titrate upward at intervals of approximately 1 week, with feedback from parents, teachers, and the child himself or herself to assess for effectiveness and any adverse effects. The effectiveness of stimulants is measured by behavioral changes (e.g., decreased motor activity, increased attention span and concentration). Behavioral changes can be identified within 30 to 90 minutes of ingestion. If a child does not respond to one stimulant, others should be tried before moving on to second-line agents, since efficacy may occur with one stimulant but not another (AACAP, 1997). It is recommended that new doses or medications be started on Saturday mornings so that parents can observe the child for the first 2 days and so that teachers would have 1 week to evaluate if any changes in the child are noted (Anastopoulos & Shelton, 2001).

The most commonly used stimulant medications include methylphenidate products (Ritalin, Methylin, Concerta, Metadate, Focalin) and amphetamines and their derivatives

TABLE 12-2
Psychostimulants Used for ADHD

Drug	Dosage (Individualized)	Range	Approximate Duration	Notes
METHYLPHENIDATE				
Ritalin, Methylin	5-, 10-, 20-mg tablets	5-60 mg/day in divided doses	4 hr	
Focalin	2.5-, 5-, 10-mg tablets	2.5-30 mg/day in divided doses	4 hr	
Ritalin SR, Methylin ER	10-, 20-mg tablets		Up to 8 hr	May be used in place of Ritalin when Ritalin SR dose = titrating 8 hr dosing of Ritalin
Concerta	18-, 36-, 54-mg tablets		10-12 hr	Slow constant release; initial total dose should equal total daily dose
Metadate CD	20-mg capsules	20-60 mg/day	Up to 12 hr	6 mg released immediately; 14 mg over the next 12 hr
Metadate ER	10-, 20-mg tablets	10-60 mg/day	Up to 8 hr	½ released immediately and ½ 4 hr later
Ritalin LA	20-, 30-, 40-mg caps	20-60 mg/day	Up to 8 hr	Bimodal plasma concentration produces 2 distinct peaks 4 hr apart
DEXTROAMPHETAMINE				
Dexedrine	5-mg tablet; 5-, 10-, 15-mg Spansules	10-40 mg in divided doses	4-6 hr	
Dextrostat	5-, 10-mg tablets	5-60 mg/day	4-6 hr	
MIXED SALTS OF DEXTRO AND LEVO AMPHETAMINE				
Adderall	5, 7.5, 10, 12.5, 15, 20, 30 mg	10-40 mg/day in divided doses	4-6 hr	
Adderall XR	5-, 10-, 15-, 20-, 25-, 30-mg capsules	10-60 mg/day	12 hr	½ immediately and ½ over time

Data from *Nurse practitioners' prescribing reference.* (2001-2002). New York: Prescribing Reference, Inc.; Solanto, M., Amsten, A., & Castellanos, F.X. (2001). *Stimulant drugs and ADHD: Basic and clinical neuroscience.* New York: Oxford University Press; Wilens, T. & Spencer, T. (2000). Stimulants and attention-deficit/hyperactivity disorder. *Child and Adolescent Psychiatric Clinics of North America, 9*(3).

(Dexedrine, Dextrostat, Adderall, Adderall-XR). Contraindications to the use of stimulant medications include symptomatic cardiovascular disease, moderate to severe hypertension, marked anxiety or agitation, glaucoma, or a history of drug abuse. The use of stimulants in children with tic disorders is controversial because some children experience worsening of tic problems with stimulant use (Popper, 2000). Short-acting medications typically require several daily doses, whereas the sustained-release preparations may require only a morning dose, with the advantage of avoiding the potential problems of in-school administration.

Of the medications listed in Table 12-2, only Adderall and Dexedrine are labeled for children under the age of 6 years. Although Ritalin SR and Methylin ER have been labeled as longer acting than the original formulations, recent advances in delivery systems have resulted in once-daily dosing recommendations for Adderall XR, Metadate-CD, and Concerta, with similar long-acting agents expected from other manufacturers. Medications in capsule form can usually be opened and sprinkled to aid in administration for children who are unable to swallow tablets whole; however, the granules cannot be chewed. The long-acting methylphenidate medications may sometimes need to be augmented with a short-acting one if symptoms are not well controlled during evening homework time.

Treatment with pemoline (Cylert), another long-acting stimulant, has declined significantly following reported problems with liver toxicity, including liver failure. Pemoline should not be considered a first-line medication, nor is it being considered an appropriate treatment for children newly diagnosed with ADHD (Wender, 2000). For children who are being successfully treated with this drug, concurrent monitoring of liver enzymes should occur every 2 weeks indefinitely (Greenhill, 2001).

One of the greatest concerns of parents is that stimulant use will lead to an addiction. This is not the case. The stimulants are not addictive when taken in the doses prescribed and for the conditions for which they are needed and children with ADHD do not get high from the stimulants they take (Wender, 2000). The stimulants are also not a cure; their use is frequently compared with the use of insulin for the diabetic child or glasses for the child who has visual difficulties.

Management of Adverse Effects: The most common side effects of the stimulant classes of medications are appetite suppression and sleep disturbances. These effects are variable for any given preparation, even if the medication (e.g., methylphenidate) is the same. Other common side effects are rebound behavioral difficulties when the drug is wearing off, irritability, stomachache, headache, dizziness, and growth problems. Suggested solutions to some of these effects include taking medication just before or with meals for appetite suppression, use of supplements such as Ensure as needed to add necessary calories, dosing earlier in the day or using short-acting stimulants to avoid sleep problems, using long-acting stimulants to avoid rebound and irritability, and evaluating the child for mood disorders or medication side effects (Wilens & Spencer, 2000).

Consideration of a "drug holiday" for children taking stimulants for ADHD needs to be evaluated on the basis of the child's academic performance and behavior without medication and the impact these have on the child and family. School vacations and weekends are the best times for trials off medication, when there is generally less pressure on the child. However, if there is an expectation that homework or projects are to be

TABLE 12-3

Nonstimulant Medications for Treating ADHD

Drug	Dosage	Maximum	Side Effects
SELECTIVE SEROTONIN REUPTAKE INHIBITORS (SSRIs)			
Fluoxetine (Prozac)	Start 2.5 mg to 10-20 mg	80 mg	Few significant side effects; occasional GI distress, anxiety, insomnia, agitation
Paroxetine (Paxil)	Start 2.5 mg to 10-20 mg	60 mg	
Citalopram (Celexa)	Start 2.5 mg to 10-20 mg	50 mg	
Sertraline (Zoloft)	Start 12.5 mg to 50-100 mg	200 mg	
Fluvoxamine (Luvox)	Start 25 mg to 50-300 mg	300 mg	
SEROTONIN NOREPINEPHRINE REUPTAKE INHIBITORS (SNRIs)			
Venlaxafine (Effexor-XR)	Start 37.5 mg to 75-112.5 mg	375 mg	Nausea, constipation, nervousness, dry mouth, dizziness, headache, sedation, weight gain
Nefazodone (Serzone)	Start 37.5 mg to 75-112.5 mg	500 mg	
Mirtazapine (Remeron)	Start 37.5 mg to 75-112.5 mg	60 mg	
TRICYCLIC ANTIDEPRESSANTS			
Imipramine (Tofranil)	Start 10-25 mg/day (child) (1.5-5.0 mg/kg/day) 30-40 mg/day (adolescent) (Increase 1-1.5 mg/kg/day at 3- to 5-day intervals.)	2.0-5.0 mg/kg/day (child) 100 mg/day (adolescent)	*Common:* cardiac conduction slowing, mild tachycardia, anticholinergic effects
Desipramine (Norpramin)	Start 10-15 mg/day (2.5-5.0 mg/kg/day) 25-100 mg/day (adolescent)	2.0-5.0 mg/kg/day 150 mg/day (adolescent)	*Uncommon but serious:* heart block or arrhythmias, induction of psychosis, confusion, seizures, hypertension
Amitriptyline (Elavil)	Start 10-25 mg/day (Average: 20-150 mg/day) 40-100 mg/day (adolescent)	2.0-5.0 mg/kg/day 100 mg/day (adolescent)	*Occasional:* rash, tics, gynecomastia
Nortriptyline (Pamelor)	10-25 mg/day 30-50 mg/day (adolescent)	1.0-3.0 mg/kg/day	May worsen tics and lower seizure threshold
Clomipramine (Anafranil)	Starts 25 mg/day (Average: 85 mg/day)	200 mg or 3.0 mg/kg/day, whichever is less	
ATYPICAL ANTIDEPRESSANT			
Bupropion (Wellbutrin)	3 mg/kg in divided doses	6 mg/kg/day or 450 mg/day	Lowers seizure threshold
ALPHA-ADRENERGIC AGONISTS			
Clonidine (Catapres)	8-12 yr: 0.25-0.3 mg/day 0.3-0.4 mg/day, give tid with meals and at HS	Rarely 0.5 mg/day	*Common:* sedation, hypotension (usually not clinically significant), headache and dizziness, stomachache, nausea, vomiting
Clonidine transdermal patches	5-day application		*Uncommon but serious:* rebound hypertension, depression
Guanfacine (Tenex)	Start 0.5 mg/day	3 mg	*Occasional:* enhances sedation and hypotension (but less than appetite, Raynaud syndrome with clonidine)

From Guitierrez, K. (1999). *Pharmacotherapeutics: Decision-making in nursing.* Philadelphia: Saunders; Popper, C. (2000). Pharmacologic alternatives to psychostimulants for the treatment of attention-deficit/hyperactivity disorder. *Child and Adolescent Psychiatric Clinics of North America, 9*(3), 605-646; Rushton, J., Clark, S., & Freed, G. (2000). Pediatrician and family physician, prescription of selective serotonin reuptake inhibitors. *Pediatrics, 105*(6).

accomplished on weekends or over holidays, it is likely to put the school-aged child at a serious disadvantage if medication is withdrawn during these times.

Nonstimulant Medications. Nonstimulant medications (Table 12-3), such as selective serotonin reuptake inhibitors (SSRIs), selective norepinephrine reuptake inhibitors (SNRIs), alpha-adrenergic agonists, and tricyclic antidepressants (TCAs), are sometimes used as adjunct treatment or in place of stimulant medications, particularly if there are co-morbid mood disorders or if the child is not a candidate for or cannot tolerate stimulant medications. Use of these agents seems to be increasing, but limited data are available regarding relative safety and efficacy (Guevara et al, 2002; Rushton et al, 2000). Although most studies of nonstimulant medications for ADHD have involved administration of TCAs or other atypical antidepressants, such

as bupropion, SSRIs have a better safety profile with little risk of cardiotoxicity and have largely replaced TCAs in the management of ADHD and comorlid mood disorders. In any case, full therapeutic effects may not be achieved until 3 to 6 weeks after therapy has been initiated (Wender, 2000).

A baseline electrocardiogram (ECG) needs to be obtained before treatment is initiated and then is rechecked at regular intervals while the child is taking TCAs, because they may prolong the conduction of electrical activity of the heart (Wender, 2000). After the maintenance dose is reached, ECGs can be twice yearly. Nortriptyline (Pamelor) or imipramine (Tofranil) is favored over desipramine (Norpramin) (AACAP, 1997). Bupropion (Wellbutrin), a heterocyclic antidepressant, has been suggested as a second-line drug for treating ADHD. Several well-conducted studies have found bupropion to be similar in efficacy to methylphenidate (AACAP, 1997). Adverse effects with this agent may include agitation.

Antidepressants can be used in children with both ADHD and Tourette syndrome without risk of tic exacerbation (Popper, 2000; see Chapter 40). Recommendations for starting doses are presented in Table 12-3. Dosing should begin at a low, subtherapeutic dose and be titrated up until the maximum dose is reached or untoward effects are observed. "Low doses [of antidepressants] can increase vigilance and decrease impulsivity, as well as reduce disruptive and aggressive behavior" but these treatment effects lessen over time (Anastopoulos & Shelton, 2001, p. 173). Drugs should be tapered over 2 to 3 weeks when they are being discontinued to prevent withdrawal effects (e.g., nausea, vomiting, fatigue, abdominal pain; AACAP, 1997).

Clonidine (Catapres), an alpha-adrenergic agonist, has been widely used in the treatment of ADHD, especially in individuals with a co-morbid tic disorder. The availability of transdermal patches (applied every 5 days) is an advantage, and clonidine can be useful in improving a child's ability to fall asleep. Although not approved by the US Food and Drug Administration (FDA) for these indications, clonidine has been prescribed both alone and in combination with stimulants, reportedly increasing frustration tolerance and cooperation while decreasing distractibility in children with ADHD (AACAP, 1997).

There are no published studies of the efficacy or safety of the use of a stimulant in combination with clonidine (AACAP, 1997). Practice parameters established by the AACAP caution combining clonidine with other medications because four children who had reportedly been taking both clonidine and methylphenidate died. Although the evidence was sparse in linking the medication with the fatalities, a careful cardiovascular history and an ECG should precede onset of clonidine treatment until the details are clarified. Guanfacine (Tenex), a longer-acting, less-sedating, more receptor–specific alphaadrenergic agonist than clonidine, has also been reported to be effective in ADHD treatment (AACAP, 1997). In general, a child with ADHD whose condition seems to require more than one medication should be referred for specialty consultation with a mental health professional after a comprehensive physical examination by the PCP.

Anticipated Advances in Diagnosis and Management

New Advances: Investigational Drugs

At least two investigational drugs show some initial promise in treating the core symptoms of ADHD: Atomoxetine and a compound known as GW 320659. GW 320659 is an active metabolite of bupropion (Wellbutrin) that thus far appears to be safe and effective in a small sample of school-aged children with ADHD, with less risk of seizure than bupropion. Identified adverse effects include headache, gastrointestinal discomfort, and mood and sleep disorders that resolved without sequelae in early trials (Glaxo SmithKline). These new agents promise to enhance the available options for children who do not respond to or cannot tolerate traditional therapies. Atomoxetine is a selective noradrenergic enhancer with a different mechanism of action but an effect similar to methylphenidate. Atomoxetine (Strattera) was FDA approved and became available for pre-

scription use in January 2003. Its main side effect is appetite suppression; no cardiac adverse effects have been noted thus far in clinical trials. It is also being evaluated for use in individuals with ADHD who have tics or have developed them while taking traditional stimulant agents (Heiligenstein, 2001).

Complementary and Alternative Therapies

There is no empiric support for dietary chemicals, such as sucrose or aspartame, as causes for ADHD (Wender, 2000). Although it is proposed that a very small percentage of children with ADHD may demonstrate a high degree of sensitivity to certain food additives, withdrawal of the suspected substances should eliminate the symptoms and no further treatment would be needed. These children do not exhibit hyperactivity but may demonstrate decreased attention and behavior problems and are not considered to have ADHD (Wender, 2000). Other myths related to the causes of ADHD that have no validity include fluorescent lighting, tar and pitch, soaps and detergents, disinfectants, yeast, insect repellants, vitamin deficiencies, stress, and social adversity in the family. Although poor child-rearing and teaching styles have been ruled out as causes of ADHD, certain styles can exacerbate or lessen symptomatology (Barkley, 2000).

Many parents elect to explore alternative therapies for their children with ADHD because of concerns regarding initiating psychopharmacologic agents. Alternatives to traditional therapies include dietary regimens, vitamin and mineral supplements, herbal preparations, supplements, and homeopathic remedies (Chan et al, 2000). Dietary supplements and herbal preparations are not regulated for safety, efficacy, or standardized contents (Wender, 2000). One diet that has now lost favor is the Feingold diet, or elimination of sorbitol, caffeine, and refined sugars (Barkley, 2000). Even though caffeine is a stimulant, "coffee does not have a useful place in the treatment of the ADHD child" (Wender, 2000, p. 93). There is no evidence that megavitamin therapy is beneficial in any way to children with ADHD; in fact, work is beginning to appear that indicates that it may be harmful and that the behaviors exhibited with ADHD may actually get worse (Barkley, 2000). However, if dietary changes have been initiated by the family, it is essential that the health care provider ensure that it is nutritionally balanced for carbohydrates, proteins, fats, and vitamins and minerals.

Use of herbals in the treatment of ADHD has not been systematically evaluated, in part because such studies are not required before marketing herbals or supplements. Labeling is not regulated and may not reflect actual ingredients, and parents should be so advised. Nonetheless, herbals and supplements remain popular and are likely to continue to be sought by parents who prefer a "natural" approach to symptom management. Thus it is helpful for the clinician to be aware of those substances.

Sedative herbs commonly used to promote sleep and decrease restlessness that are recognized by the FDA include lemon balm, chamomile, and valerian. The use of these, while generally recognized as safe, does not imply effectiveness for ADHD treatment. Melatonin, a hormone produced in the pineal gland, has proved to be beneficial as a treatment for sleep problems in children with ADHD, although there is some concern that there may be potential suppression of puberty because of inhibition of gonadotropin (Chan et al, 2000).

Other popular agents that have yet to undergo scientific scrutiny for the treatment of ADHD symptoms include gingko biloba and blue-green algae. Gastrointestinal effects and headache are the most common adverse effects. Gingko's use in enhancing memory and cognitive function in the older adult seems to hold some promise for children affected by ADHD as well (Chan et al, 2000). The NIH is actively engaged in funding and reviewing research on complementary and alternative medicine, but no federally funded studies on the use of herbals or supplements in the management of ADHD have been done at the time of this publication.

Other controversial therapies include cognitive therapy, biofeedback, sensory integration training, and visual training. Although optometric training, sensory integration therapy, and applied kinesiology are often listed in the treatment sections for ADHD, they were primarily earmarked for those with learning disabilities and were not separated out as the conditions were later differentiated. While some children with ADHD also have coordination difficulties, "there is no evidence whatsoever that coordination training will help the ADHD child's learning difficulties. The same statement applies to specific treatment programs of eye exercises" (Wender, 2000, p. 132). Biofeedback is based on programs that change the electrical activity of the brain, yet no deficit in the electroencephalogram (EEG) has been identified for ADHD. This lengthy, time-consuming, costly program does not have scientific evidence supporting its efficacy (Barkley, 2000).

Because scientific evidence is lacking, the American Academy of Pediatrics does not support or recommend any of these programs for children with either learning disabilities or ADHD (Silver, 1999). The NIH, however, maintains an on-line database of published scientific findings on supplements, as does the FDA's Center for Food Safety and Applied Nutrition http://vm.cfsan.fda.gov. Primary care clinicians need to actively inquire about usage of alternative regimens and be knowledgeable about potential interactions, toxicology, and relative effectiveness of the various intervention strategies.

Associated Problems

It is estimated that 12% to 50% of children with ADHD also have another psychiatric condition (Hechtman, 2000a; Pliszka, 2000) (Box 12-4). The increased recognition of significant co-morbidities with ADHD has complicated the diagnosis of ADHD and both the pharmacologic and nonpharmacologic

---

BOX 12-4
Associated Problems

Learning disabilities
Oppositional defiant disorder (ODD)
Conduct disorder (CD)
Psychologic sequelae: low self-esteem, inadequate social skills, anxiety, depression, academic difficulties, multiple failures, family conflict, exercising of poor judgment, altered peer relationships, antisocial behavior (especially with ADHD and CD), psychosomatic complaints, failure to reach potential, labeling

---

management strategies. The presence of co-morbid conditions may decrease the individual's response to stimulant medication and may result in more or different side effects than those seen in children with ADHD alone (Greenhill, 2001). Most guidelines are designed for the child who presents with ADHD without co-morbidity. The most common conditions seen with ADHD include learning disabilities (LDs), oppositional defiant disorder (ODD), and conduct disorder (CD).

Learning Disabilities

In earlier literature, learning disabilities and ADHD were frequently merged together. Estimates of the prevalence of LDs are between 5% and 10%, although some estimate it could be as high as 20% of the population as a whole (MacMillan et al, 1998). Approximately 25% of children with ADHD have an LD, although some argue it is as high as 40%, and approximately 25% of those with LDs have ADHD (Pliszka, 2000; Silver, 1999). LDs are very different from ADHD; LDs affect the brain's *ability* to learn in a particular way, whereas ADHD interferes with the individual's *availability* for learning (Silver, 1999). Neurotransmitters are not implicated in the cause of LDs. Although many of the environmental and behavioral interventions are similar for the two conditions, no medications are appropriate in the treatment of LDs.

The diagnosis of LD requires that one must have at least a normal intelligence quotient (IQ), whereas "ADHD can be found across all levels of intelligence" (Anastopoulos & Shelton, 2001, p. 50). ADHD does not affect one's intelligence (Wender, 2000). LDs can be diagnosed by psychologic testing on multiple parameters, with the evaluators looking for discrepancies among and between the components (Fletcher et al, 1999). Whereas symptoms of ADHD should be present before the age of 7 years, there is no age requirement for learning disabilities.

Oppositional Defiant Disorder and Conduct Disorder

According to Pliszka, "almost all children younger than 12 years of age who meet criteria for ODD or CD will almost always meet criteria for ADHD" (2000, p. 526); however, others believe that only 20% of children with CD also have ADHD (Ward & Guyer, 2000). Between 10% and 42.7% of children with ADHD also have CD whereas ODD ranges from 19% to 44% (Scahill & Schwab-Stone, 2000). The combination of ADHD with CD or ODD significantly increases the risk of later delinquency, substance abuse, and antisocial behaviors. Individuals with these co-morbidities have high levels of aggression, increased anxiety, decreased self-esteem, and increased rates of psychopathology among family members (Pliszka et al, 1999; Wilens et al, 2000).

Those with combined ADHD and CD have higher rates of morbidity, with many of them going on to develop antisocial personality disorder and alcohol and substance abuse problems in adulthood (Wender, 2000). Positive or negative outcomes appear to be mediated by factors such as age at diagnosis, individualized treatment measures instituted, coping mechanisms, mental health of family members, intelligence, cultural expectations, co-morbidity of other conditions, and persistence of symptoms. ADHD with co-morbid conditions, especially CD or ODD, "seems to result in more negative outcomes, particularly adult antisocial behavior and antisocial personality disorder" (Hechtman, 2000b, p. 446).

Co-morbidity rates are much higher in clinic populations than in community samples. Other conditions that are often found in conjunction with ADHD include mood disorders and depression, anxiety disorders, obsessive-compulsive disorder, and Tourette syndrome (Brown, 2000; see Chapter 40). "A diagnosis of Pervasive Developmental Disorder or Early Infantile Autism 'preempts' the ADHD diagnosis, even if the patient meets all criteria for the ADHD disorder" (Greenhill, 2001, p. 43; see Chapter 13). The PCP needs to ensure that referrals are made for children who have co-morbid psychiatric conditions.

One of the greatest concerns regarding the prognosis for individuals with ADHD is the potential for future illicit drug use. Taking stimulants does not predispose the child with ADHD to substance abuse of other drugs later in life; in actuality, those teens who continued to use stimulant medication during adolescence "had a significantly lower likelihood of substance use or abuse than did children with ADHD who were not taking medications during adolescence" (Barkley, 2000, p. 273).

Psychosocial Sequelae

Children who are misdiagnosed or not diagnosed in grade school may experience many years of academic difficulties that may lead to frustration and failure. The psychologic sequelae of multiple failures can result in poor self-esteem. Chronic school pressures and failure can result in frustration, anxiety, depression, an inner sense of restlessness, psychosomatic complaints, and school absenteeism or resignation (Greenhill, 1998). Teachers may misinterpret their behaviors and label these children as lazy or insensitive or dismiss them from the classroom. On average, children with ADHD are rated by their teachers as less popular, less assertive, and less cooperative than their classmates (Lahey et al, 1998). Teachers and parents may unintentionally label the children as "bad," "terrible," or "troublemakers," further aggravating the psychologic sequelae. One important point for health care providers is to remember that increased emotional lability or "spacey" behavior may be a result of the side effects of the psychotropic medication being taken (Silver, 1999).

A number of children with ADHD have difficulty with peer relationships. This difficulty is especially true for those who have significant psychomotor dysfunction or a restricted use of language, or those who are in special education classes or singled out and labeled as "different" in a regular classroom. Some of the social behavior problems may be the result of the child's low frustration tolerance, temper tantrums, impulsivity, and difficulty in reading nonverbal social cues. These may result in misjudgment of acceptance or rejection by or increased aggression to peers (Weyandt, 2001). Family relationships are also affected.

One problem in identifying children as having ADHD is the effect of labeling. The label allows the child to receive necessary services to compensate for deficits and adjust to the consequences but may also result in a self-fulfilling prophecy.

Prognosis

Although many individuals with ADHD grow up to become successful adults, up to 80% of children with ADHD manifest symptoms as adolescents, and 50% to 65% still meet all or part of the criteria into adulthood (Barkley, 2000). Of those with ADHD 18% to 53% "will be academic underachievers, performing significantly below their level of intelligence" (Anastopoulos & Shelton, 2001, p. 49). Studies of long-term outcomes in ADHD demonstrate considerable variation in results. Adults report increased interpersonal problems resulting in having fewer friends, increased job terminations (especially in jobs requiring adult problem solving, prioritizing, task completion, and self-control), and restlessness. Other symptoms seen more frequently in adults who had ADHD as a child include impaired academic functioning with significantly less formal schooling, an increased risk of antisocial problems, and an increased risk of nonalcohol substance use, especially cocaine and marijuana in young people with ADHD who had not received stimulant medication as treatment (Anastopoulos & Shelton, 2001; Mannuzza & Klein, 2000; Wilens & Spencer, 2000).

PRIMARY CARE MANAGEMENT

Health Care Maintenance

Growth and Development

Careful attention must be given to routinely (i.e., about every 6 months) measuring weight and physical growth parameters if a child is taking stimulant medication for symptom management. The effect of stimulant medication on growth appears to be temporary and minimal, with no significant differences seen by adolescence (Wender, 2000). The growth rate may be slowed for 1 to 2 years, but then it approaches normal with no long-term effects on health (Greenhill, 2001). "The concern about growth is no longer an issue" for children with ADHD who are taking stimulants (Silver, 1999, p. 190).

Children with ADHD should demonstrate the normal progression of attaining developmental milestones, especially in the early years. As the child reaches the preschool years, some delay in the development of a longer attention span as well as the increased activity level of the child may signal a need for a referral for psychoeducational evaluation.

ADHD is not routinely diagnosed until a child begins school. The Individuals with Disabilities Education Act requires that children at risk for developing ADHD be assessed in the first 3 years of life if signs and symptoms are evident (see Chapter 5). This places more responsibility on health care providers to develop and use tools that can identify the components of ADHD at an earlier age. Because children learn to compensate for their disability, and in some cases the nature of their disability changes as they grow and develop, it is important to reevaluate a child's cognitive, motor, and psychosocial level of development at each well-child visit. Whichever screening tools were used in the initial assessment of ADHD can be used periodically to monitor the child's progress with the treatment interventions.

Diet

There are no dietary restrictions, and no empiric evidence suggests that diets that restrict sugars, refined carbohydrates, food additives, or colors result in any improvement in the symptomatology, nor do they cause ADHD (Barkley, 2000; Weyandt, 2001).

Children taking stimulant medication may have a decreased appetite, and their increased activity level may warrant an increased caloric intake. These children may be easily distracted from the meal and leave the table before they are finished eating. They may also experience a stomachache as a side effect of the medications; if this is the case, medication should be taken on a full stomach. Meals and snacks that are high in protein and calories and easy to eat should be encouraged to enhance nutritional status; because of the timing of medications, it may be easier to promote a healthy intake for breakfast and at bedtime, before and after the action of the stimulants has peaked. Establishing a mealtime routine may also be beneficial. Parents and caregivers should look for windows of opportunities to provide nutritious foods, such as after school and at bedtime.

The side effect of anorexia, resulting in weight loss of 0.5 to 2.25 kg, may be controlled by the timing of the administration of stimulant medications. In many children, this side effect abates after 6 months. The weight loss does not occur to a "medically serious degree" (Wender, 2000, p. 82).

Safety

There are a number of safety issues for children and adolescents with ADHD. Children with ADHD "have more than their share of accidents and are much more likely than non-ADHD children to be seen in Emergency Rooms" (Wender, 2000, p. 13). They have a decreased ability to tolerate delays or to think before acting; they often act without considering potential outcomes. Because of this impulsive behavior and altered judgment, they are at higher risk for engaging in unsafe activities. These children are more likely to sustain injuries, especially closed head injuries, because of behavioral inattentiveness and impulsivity (Gerring et al, 1998). Children with ADHD were reported to have more injuries and more severe injuries related to means of transportation (i.e., motor vehicle, pedestrian, bicycle, motorcycle, all-terrain vehicles, recreational vehicles) than children with no preexisting condition, and pedestrian injuries were noted as the major cause of hospital admission for trauma in the ADHD population (DiScala et al, 1998).

A significant number of adolescents with ADHD have decreased judgment of speed, space, and distance. These deficits, plus a decreased ability to pay attention to things such as conditions of the road and driving speed, result in an increase in motor vehicle accidents in this population (Barkley, 2000). Driving is an activity that requires multiple tasks and decision making simultaneously. Adolescents who have difficulty in these areas are advised to delay driving for a few years.

Although no data support abuse of stimulant medications, medication safety should always be a consideration in teaching. Using containers that mark the pills for each day of the week may be helpful for children who are self-administering their medications. Standard precautions for keeping medications safely secured should be followed not only for the child with ADHD but also for siblings and classmates because many of the medications can be easily sold on the street.

Immunizations

No changes in the routine schedule of immunizations are needed.

Screening

Vision. Comprehensive vision testing should be performed during the diagnostic period; poor vision could also be a reason why a child might appear inattentive in the classroom. Routine screening at recommended intervals should then occur.

Vision therapy that includes ocular exercises and the use of colored lenses or prisms was initially recommended for children with visual perceptual learning disabilities. There is no research to demonstrate their efficacy for either LDs or ADHD, and this type of therapy is not recommended (Baumgaertel, 1999).

Hearing. Comprehensive audiometric testing should also be performed during the diagnostic period; poor hearing might be a reason a child appears to be inattentive and in his or her own world. Routine screening at recommended intervals should then occur.

Dental. Routine screening is recommended.

Blood Pressure. Blood pressure alterations may occur as a result of receiving stimulants, tricyclics, clonidine, or guanfacine; thus blood pressure should be monitored every few months (Barkley, 2000). Mild elevations from the stimulants usually disappear within 1 month (Greenhill, 2001). Children not taking medication for ADHD should have routine blood pressure screening.

Hematocrit. Routine screening is recommended.

Urinalysis. Routine screening is recommended.

Tuberculosis. Routine screening is recommended.

Condition-Specific Screening

Speech and Language. Speech and language assessments should be initiated for children demonstrating receptive or expressive language disorders.

Liver Function. Children taking pemoline need liver function tests every few months because of the reported incidence of occasional liver failure.

Thyroid Function. A rare genetic resistance to thyroid hormone has been linked to the symptoms of ADHD. Thyroid function should be checked if a child has any symptoms or a family history of hypothyroid or hyperthyroid function (AACAP, 1997).

Cardiac Function. Children taking TCAs and clonidine will need baseline ECGs repeated with dose increments (AACAP, 1997). Mild increases in pulse rate as a result of stimulant medication usually disappear within 1 month (Greenhill, 2001).

Common Illness Management

The diagnostic and recovery phases of illness may sometimes be compromised by the symptoms or treatments for ADHD. It is important to differentiate the clinical manifestations of ADHD, such as irritability and inability to attend to a task, with those same symptoms seen when a child is ill or experiencing emotional trauma. Absence seizures can be mistaken as inattentive ADHD.

Side effects of stimulant medications or the characteristics of the conditions themselves (e.g., anorexia, weight loss, stomachache, headache, insomnia) may mask the symptoms of other physical and psychologic illness. The lack of appetite, insomnia, and difficulty resting the body may interfere with the healing process as well as with taking in the fluids and nutrients needed in recovery.

Psychologic conditions such as chronic anxiety, fear of failure, and those that develop from family stress (i.e., divorce, illness, and death in the family; teen pregnancy; poverty; malnutrition) may result in difficulty attending to academic tasks but should not be confused with a worsening of the disability. Adolescents who are found to have LDs or depression may have their diagnosis of ADHD delayed because the learning and behavior problems displayed may be classified as secondary to the depression.

Drug Interactions

Medications used to treat ADHD have a number of interactive effects when given with other drugs (Table 12-4). Psychostimulants, the most common medications used to treat ADHD, fortunately have few clinically significant drug-to-drug interactions (Ten Eick et al, 1998). When administered simultaneously with sympathomimetic medications used for cold and allergy symptoms (ephedrine, pseudoephedrine) or other stimulants, a dangerously heightened stimulant effect can result (Deglin & Vallerand, 2001). In addition, monoamine oxidase inhibitors (MAOIs) retard the metabolism of psychostimulants, which can lead to toxic effects; and the co-administration of MAOIs and stimulants is contraindicated, since it can lead to a potentially lethal hypertensive crisis.

Dextroamphetamines can impair the hypotensive effects of guanethidine (Ismelin), possibly resulting in arrhythmias. Clearance of amphetamines is enhanced by urinary acidifiers, resulting in lower levels of the amphetamine; alkalinizers result in impaired renal tubular clearance.

Some psychostimulants have specific precautions that need to be addressed. Methylphenidate may elevate levels of tricyclic antidepressants (TCAs) and warfarin. Dextroamphetamine may increase the risk of cardiovascular effects with beta-blockers, and phenothiazines may decrease the effect of dextroamphetamine (Dexedrine) (Deglin & Vallerand, 2001).

TCAs can cause increased effects with stimulants, CNS depressants (e.g., MAOIs, sympathomimetics, alcohol or other substance-abuse medications), anticholinergics, thyroid preparations, and seizure-potentiating medications. TCAs can decrease the effects of clonidine. The effects of the tricyclics are increased by phenothiazine, cimetidine, and oral contraceptives. The effects of the tricyclics are decreased by barbiturates and smoking.

Increased CNS depression is noted with concurrent use of clonidine or guanfacine with TCAs, and the antihypertensive effect of clonidine may be antagonized with TCA use. Clonidine increases the effects of CNS depressants and anticholinergic preparations, although usually less in children than adults. Clonidine decreases the effects of beta-adrenergic blockers, which heightens the rebound hypertension that can occur when it is discontinued (Deglin & Vallerand, 2001).

Developmental Issues
Sleep

Sleep problems (especially the amount of time it takes to fall asleep) are identified by parents as a chronic problem in children with ADHD. Some parents may present to the primary health care provider with complaints of the child's sleep problems; they may describe their child's difficulty falling asleep, waking frequently, or rising early in the morning (Wender, 2000). These problems may not always be related to use of stimulant medications but do result in fewer total sleep hours (Greenhill, 2001).

In children with ADHD, medication timing or inability to settle down may affect falling asleep. The drug administration schedule should be assessed. Insomnia is a common side effect of stimulant medication and often resolves after a few weeks of stimulant use as a child develops a tolerance to the medication (Silver, 1999). If insomnia does not resolve, however, decreasing the doses, scheduling administration earlier in the day, and changing between long- and short-acting preparations may help. Some clinicians recommend a second medication to assist with the onset of sleep; however, as a general rule, it is best not to treat one medication's side effect with another medication. Practitioners should be alerted to the fact that extreme sleepiness may be a sign of overmedication.

Toileting

Enuresis and encopresis may occur in the child with ADHD because of inattention to body cues. This may result in a lengthened time for toilet training. Routine toilet breaks should be a part of the daily schedule. Elementary schools should also be sensitive to this need and incorporate toileting into daily activities.

Discipline

All children act out and misbehave at various intervals in the developmental process. As with other children, discipline should fit the seriousness of the misbehavior. Children with ADHD, however, do not learn well from past experiences and may not be able to control their behavior. Even after these children have done something wrong, they may not relate their activity to the discipline and will need frequent clarification from adults. Frequent feedback related to progress is important.

Behavior modification techniques over a prolonged period may help a child develop self-control. If time-outs are used, children must be told when the period of restriction has ended. They need to be reminded of the reasons for the punishment and consistently helped to differentiate between "the act being wrong or bad" and "the child being bad." Although behavior modification helps to improve targeted behaviors and skills, it does not reduce inattention, hyperactivity, or impulsivity (AACAP, 1997). Rewards for good behavior are effective, especially if given immediately after the behavior is identified or the short-term task completed.

For hyperactive children, parents need help determining to what degree their child's normal behavior requires discipline. Parenting classes may help them to make this differentiation

TABLE 12-4

Drug Interactions Relevant in Treating ADHD

Drug A	Combined with Drug B	Interaction
Stimulants	Sympathomimetics, other stimulants	Significantly increased stimulant effect
	monoamine oxidase inhibitors (MAOIs)	Toxic stimulant effect; hypertensive crisis; may be lethal
	Beta-blockers	Hypertension; bradycardia
	Hypoglycemic agents	Increased glucose lability
	Neuroleptics	Decreased seizure threshold
	TCAs	Increased TCA effect; risk of cardiotoxicity
	SSRIs	Increased SSRI effect
	Insulin	Decreased requirements of insulin if eating less
Amphetamines	Phenytoin	Increased level of phenytoin
	Urinary acidifiers	Decreased amphetamine effect
	Urinary alkalinizer	Decreased amphetamine effect
	Guanethidine	Guanethidine effect (arrhythmias); hypotension
Methylphenidate	Warfarin	Anticoagulant level
	TCA	Increased TCA levels
Dextroamphetamine	Beta-blockers	Beta-blocker action
	Phenothiazine	Action of both drugs
Pemoline	Antiepileptic medications	Seizure threshold
Tricyclic antidepressants	Stimulants	Effects of stimulants; increased plasma levels of TCA; increased risk of cardiotoxicity
	CNS depressants (MAOI, alcohol sympathomimetics)	CNS depressant effect; hyperpyretic crisis
	Anticholinergics	Effect of anticholinergics
	Thyroid preparations	Thyroid activity
	Seizure potentiating medications	Seizure potentiation
	Carbamazepine	Decreased TCA action; increased plasma level of anticonvulsant
	Valproic acid	Increased TCA effect
	Clonidine or guanfacine	Effect of clonidine, guanfacine
	Phenothiazines	TCA effect
	Oral contraceptives	TCA effect; increased plasma levels of TCA
	Barbiturates	TCA effect; increased plasma levels of TCA; increased CNS depression
	Smoking	Decreased TCA effect
	CNS depressants	Additive sedation
Clonidine	Anticholinergic preparations	Drug B
	Beta-adrenergic blockers	Drug B effect; attenuation or reversal of antihypertensive effect
	Fenfluramine	Clonidine effect
	Thiazide diuretics	Clonidine effect
	Antihypertensive agents	Clonidine effect
	TCAs	Hypotensive effect of clonidine; decreased hypertensive effect
	Nonsteroidal antiinflammatory drugs (NSAIDs)	Hypotensive effect of clonidine
	Sympathomimetic drugs	Hypotensive effects of clonidine
Bupropion	MAOIs, levodopa	Increased adverse effects
All selective serotonin reuptake inhibitors (SSRIs)	MAOIs	Hypertensive crisis
	Valproate, carbamezapine	Increased anticonvulsant levels
	TCAs	Increased TCA level; increased risk of cardiotoxicity
	Beta-blockers	Bradycardia; syncope
	Insulin	Increased insulin sensitivity

Data from Guitierrez, K. (1999). *Pharmacotherapeutics: Decision-making in nursing.* Philadelphia: Saunders; *Nurse practitioners' prescribing reference.* (Winter 2001-2002). New York: Prescribing Reference, Inc.; Wynne, A., Woo, T., & Millard, M. (2002). *Pharmacotherapeutics for nurse practitioner prescribers.* Philadelphia: F.A. Davis.

and provide clear instructions with positive reinforcement. Parent support groups are also helpful, such as those provided through ChADD (Children and Adults with Attention Deficit Disorder). Attention should also be paid to siblings of children with ADHD. Parents must be sensitive to the child with ADHD's inability to self-regulate behavior and make necessary modifications in their own discipline techniques while balancing sibling needs and discipline issues as well.

Discipline should be part of the daily routine and must be consistent. Limit setting is an important component of the day. Structuring the daily routine of the home environment helps these children establish acceptable patterns of behavior. Parents should be reminded to also teach the recommended behavioral approaches to a child's significant others (e.g., grandparents, caregivers). It is also important for the teachers and other school personnel to differentiate the behaviors caused by the ADHD from defiant behavior that is counter to the rules of the school when discipline is being determined.

PCPs may need to help families and older children develop plans to structure their environment and their activities. Breaking down activities into component parts and using checklists may help children be more aware of their behavior. Parents should be advised that normal activities may take more time, and they should keep the child's schedule simple to prevent it from becoming overloaded.

Child Care

Child care that has a small class or group size, a structured and safe environment, constant adult supervision, and an opportunity to engage in gross motor play outdoors should be selected. Predictability of schedule and personnel is reassuring to children with ADHD because they often do not handle surprises or changes well. It is important to talk with personnel about ADHD and to listen to them when they express concern about the child in their care.

Schooling

ADHD has a major effect on the education of children and adolescents. Children should be evaluated for school readiness before kindergarten. Children who are not yet diagnosed when they enter school may experience a series of barriers. Teachers are not permitted to identify a child as hyperactive, lest they be making a diagnosis. Neither teachers nor principals may mandate that children be placed on medication before being able to return to school; those are medical decisions.

Some districts discourage staff from recommending testing to parents because it is then the district's responsibility to pay for the testing. Practitioners should be familiar with the internal policies of the school districts in which they practice and support parents in their requests for testing and evaluation through special education if a child's history and physical findings are consistent with ADHD. There is no benefit in waiting to see if a child "outgrows" the condition if school failure is already occurring.

Federal and state laws requiring schools to provide accommodations for children with ADHD do not ensure that this help is readily available in any given school system or that there are quality services. Obtaining these services requires a working knowledge of the process; clinicians have a responsibility to either be familiar with or have a referral source to help parents negotiate the complexities of the special education system. It is helpful for the clinician to question parents about which strategies they have used and what has been useful thus far in managing behavioral difficulties, if present.

Children with ADHD may be covered under Section 504 of the Rehabilitation Act, making them eligible for reasonable accommodations and the development of an accommodation plan. Children who are severely affected with ADHD or have an identified learning disability may qualify for an individualized education plan (IEP) instead (see Chapter 5).

Any child experiencing school difficulties should be evaluated for learning and behavioral disorders, and this evaluation can be provided through the public school district at no expense to the parents. It is on the basis of this evaluation (if diagnosed with ADHD) that the school is required by law to implement an accommodation plan, if one is appropriate. These accommodations apply to both the classroom and disciplinary policies. If the symptoms are significant enough to interfere with learning, then the child may qualify under the Individuals with Disabilities Education Act (IDEA) for the development of an IEP. The parent who disagrees with the evaluation findings may request an independent evaluation. Educators must be careful not to use the label to separate or identify children in a mainstreamed classroom.

Children with ADHD benefit from small, structured classes. They may be educated in regular classrooms, use the resource room, attend special education classes, be tutored, or use a combination thereof. The goal is inclusion into normal classrooms, but special education classrooms and resource rooms are also very acceptable therapies. In resource rooms (supplementary help) and special education (self-contained) classrooms, teachers can limit the number of students in the classroom, decrease the amount of distraction, and provide specific interventions based on a child's needs (Box 12-5). Parents, with support from the PCP, can work with school personnel to help plan the child's school day. Information on when would be the best times of the day for the child to learn, where the child should sit, how to break content into short segments, and how frequently breaks are needed would be important and helpful for the teachers.

Children who continue to have academic difficulty resulting in failure need counseling support and assistance in dealing with related stress. By high school, the inattention of ADHD may be manifested as chronic academic underachievement and motivation problems. Children with ADHD need to understand that even though they failed a course (or examination), they are not failures. It is not appropriate to tell children to "try harder." A child's decreased performance is not often because of a lack of effort or anyone's fault. These children need to be reassured that they are not stupid and that requests for repetition of directions and clarification of content are not a nuisance.

A significant part of the educational plan is to help children learn to compensate for their particular disability. Children need to understand which accommodations work best for them. It may be more helpful to present material in writing, pictorially, or with hands-on demonstration. Short lists of directions, calendars, or check-off sheets also help with organization.

Constant feedback to ensure their understanding of subject matter is essential. These children should be given extra time to answer questions; timed or competitive testing may be extremely stressful. It may be helpful to highlight texts to help them find the important information. A second set of textbooks that can be kept at home can minimize the effect of forgetting to bring them home.

Administration of medication during school hours has presented some problems for children. Some children forget to get their lunchtime dose because they often have to leave their friends to go to the school nurse or office, are involved in group activities, or may feel guilty or self-conscious about having to take pills—especially if "drug-free schools" information is being promoted. In addition, state and local policies on administration of medication in schools must be considered when prescribing medicines (see Chapter 5).

BOX 12-5

Behavioral, Educational, and Environmental Strategies for the Child with ADHD

Identify the child's strengths, and build on them.
Provide immediate and specific positive reinforcement for effort and achievement; only reinforce the positive.
Make a hierarchy of rules; implement rules and consequences consistently.
Provide parent coaching and child coaching.
Provide learning activities when medication is at its peak.
Get child's attention first; put child's head or shoulders gently in your hands; ask child what he or she was just told (speak in a neutral tone).
Give verbal *and* written instructions.
Remind the child of critical behavior before an activity.
Help child distinguish between feelings and actions.
Help child understand labels and teasing.
Use physical activities (e.g., role playing) for instruction.
Use a notebook for daily homework assignments.
Institute classroom rule that no laughing is allowed when someone makes a mistake.
Help the child to develop a relationship with an adult (e.g., college student, Big Brother) to promote social interaction and supervised learning experiences.
Decrease the length of tasks, plan frequent breaks, divide large projects into smaller parts.
Keep a second set of books at home.
Post a daily schedule, and make to-do lists (use pictures if necessary).
Pace the child; do not let the child get overloaded.
Allow extra time for child to overcome limited organizational skills.
Use a kitchen timer to keep child on task.
Anticipate change, and frequently tell child what is going to happen.
Build the child's self-esteem and self-confidence at every opportunity.

LEARNING ENVIRONMENT

Use muted wall colors.
Decrease clutter (desks, worksheets, classroom).
Seat child in front of room, away from doors, windows, and distractions.
Seat child near on-task peer.
Structured environment is preferred over open, unstructured environment.
Have a place for everything with a picture on it.
Provide consistency; keep daily routines.
Use calendars, assignment books, structured schedule, untimed and oral testing and/or testing in separate quiet room.
Give extra time to answer questions.
Use technologic assistive devices (e.g., tape recorders, word processors).

Sexuality

Providing sex education for children and adolescents is an important role for the PCP. Sex education must be individualized to the child and be repetitive and developmentally appropriate. Role playing can be helpful because problem solving may be difficult. Using a calendar for girls to predict oncoming menses may be helpful. Because of impulsivity and the lack of attention to planning ahead, parents need to constantly reinforce to adolescents with ADHD that they do not have to engage in high-risk activities for peer approval. Opportunities for open dialogue regarding puberty and sexuality must be made available by parents, counselors, or clinicians. Adolescents need to be made aware of community resources that offer information and services related to their developing sexuality.

Transition into Adulthood

The transition of older adolescents into adulthood is a critical point for families of children with ADHD. The underlying condition and its associated risks do not go away, so adolescents working on the developmental tasks of separation from parents and family, establishing a sense of identity, and formulating personal and occupational goals often require professional help. Youth with ADHD often have unresolved issues from earlier developmental phases, less developed executive functioning skills and problem-solving skills, and less confidence and may have limited awareness of the ramifications of their disability.

As the children enter adolescence, they should begin to be responsible for taking their medication. However, parents must maintain control of the medications, since many are controlled substances. Keeping records of how many pills are in the vial, getting confirmation that the school nurse has received the number of pills sent to the school, and keeping the medications stored in a secure site away from other children in the family are essential for assisting the adolescent in transitioning to full responsibility for his or her own health.

Family Concerns and Resources

Unlike many children's chronic health problems, ADHD is not likely to generate a sympathetic response from school administrators, teachers, other family members, and the health care system itself. Parents must frequently be tireless advocates to accomplish any type of effective intervention. Rewards are few, and the barriers to success are many.

Many parents benefit from the step-by-step information available through support groups, such as Children and Adults with Attention Deficit Disorder (ChADD), local parent information centers, and books about the special education process. These may especially be helpful for those parents who themselves have ADHD but who never received assistance during their formative years. An advocate of the parent's choosing (frequently a mental health professional) may accompany the parents to school accommodation or IEP planning meetings.

The continuous contact with health care providers recommended in the multimodal approach can rapidly become cost prohibitive if families are underinsured or uninsured. Mental health insurance coverage typically has its own set of restrictions and may not allow sufficient coverage for the long-term treatment of ADHD and its associated behavioral problems.

Parents and siblings of a child with ADHD must learn strategies to facilitate their abilities. Children with ADHD and their families will need to readjust to the child's condition at every new developmental stage. The psychologic effect of ADHD results in specific psychosocial needs. Building a child's self-esteem and self-confidence, as well as an accurate self-perception, becomes even more important when the child is experiencing chronic academic difficulty.

Environmental control in the home is similar to that discussed for the classroom. Decreasing clutter, developing routines, scheduling ample time for activities, and providing clear directions in the format that best meets the child's needs may be beneficial. Parents typically give more commands, directions, and supervision to these children than to a "normal" child. Parents are concerned about the child's potential for schooling and vocational choices, as well as the child's ability to assume an independent lifestyle. This concern may result in increased parental stress, depression, and marital discord. Parents, as well as their children, need coping strategies and consistent support.

RESOURCES

Books on ADHD for Parents and Teachers

Barkley, R.A. (2000). Taking charge of ADHD: The complete authoritative guide for parents. New York: Guilford Press.

Bender, W. (1997). Understanding ADHD: A practical guide for teachers and parents. Upper Saddle River, NJ: Prentice-Hall.

The ChADD information and resource guide to attention deficit/hyperactivity disorder. (2001). Landover, Md: Author.

Cooper, P. & Ideus, K. (1996). Attention deficit/hyperactivity disorder: A practical guide for teachers. London: David Fulton Publishers.

Greene, R. (1998). The explosive child. New York: Harper Collins.

Levine, M. (2002). *A mind at a time.* New York: Simon and Schuster.

McEwan, E. (1998). *The principal's guide to attention deficit hyperactivity disorder.* Thousand Oaks, Calif: Corwin Press.

Osman, B. (1997). *Learning disabilities and ADHD: A family guide to living and learning together.* New York: John Wiley & Sons, Inc.

Strip, C. (2000). *Helping gifted children soar: A practical guide for parents and teachers.* Scottsdale, Ariz: Gifted Psychology Press, Inc.

Web Sites

American Association of Child and Adolescent Psychiatry
www.aacap.org

National Institute of Mental Health, ADHD
http://www.nimh.nih.gov/publicat/adhd.cfm

Books on ADHD for Children

Gantos, J. (2000). *Joey Pigza loses control.* New York: Farrar, Strauss, & Giroux.

Gordon, M. (1991). *Jumpin' Johnny: Get back to work: A child's guide to ADHD/hyperactivity.* DeWitt, NY: GSI Publications.

Levine, M. (1992). *All kinds of minds: A young student's book about learning abilities and learning disorders.* Cambridge, Mass: Educators Publishing Service, Inc.

Mosa, D. (1989). *Shelly, the hyperactive turtle.* Bethesda, Md: Woodbine House.

Quinn, P. & Stern, J. (1991). *Putting on the brakes: Young people's guide to understanding attention deficit hyperactivity disorder.* New York: Magination Press.

Organizations and Sources of Information

ADD Warehouse
300 Northwest 70th Ave, Suite 102
Plantation, FL 33317
(800) 233-9273
sales@addwarehouse.com

Attention Deficit Disorder Association (ADDA)
1788 Second St, Suite 200
Highland Park, Il 60035
(847) 432-ADDA
http://www.add.org

Children and Adults with Attention Deficit Disorders (ChADD)
8181 Professional Pl, Suite 201
Landover, MD 20785
(800) 233-4050
http://www.chadd.org

Health Resource Center (National Clearinghouse for Postsecondary Education for People with Disabilities)
1 DuPont Circle NW, Suite 800
Washington, DC 20036-1193
http://www.acenet.edu/Programs/heath/home.html

Learning Disabilities Association of America
4156 Library Rd
Pittsburgh, PA 15234
(412) 341-1515
http://www.ldanatl.org

National Center for Learning Disabilities (NCLD)
381 Park Ave S, Suite 1401
New York, NY 10016
(212) 545-7510
http://www.ncld.org

National Information Center for Children and Youth with Disabilities (NICHCY)
PO Box 1492
Washington, DC 20013-1492
(800) 695-0285
http://www.nichcy.org

Summary of Primary Care Needs for the Child with Attention Deficit Hyperactivity Disorder

HEALTH CARE MAINTENANCE

Growth and Development

Medications for hyperactivity cause appetite suppression; assess height and weight every 6 months.

Manifestations of ADHD vary with development.

Early identification is beneficial and supported under the Individuals with Disabilities Education Act (IDEA).

Diet

Children may be poor eaters. Decreased appetite may occur if they are taking stimulant medication. A nutritious diet with adequate protein and calories for growth is important.

Stomachache may be a side effect of stimulant medication.

Safety

There is a risk of injury because of impulsive behaviors and altered judgment.

Children with ADHD have increased incidence of injuries related to means of transportation.

Medication should be safely kept out of reach of young children. No data support abuse of stimulant medications.

Immunizations

Routine schedule is recommended.

Screening

Vision. Comprehensive visual testing is done initially as part of differential diagnosis.

Summary of Primary Care Needs for the Child with Attention Deficit Hyperactivity Disorder—cont'd

Hearing. Comprehensive audiometric testing is done initially as part of differential diagnosis. Children may have difficulty with audiometric testing because of attention needed.

Dental. Routine screening is recommended.

Blood Pressure. Routine screening is recommended. If a child is taking medication for ADHD, screening must be done more often because of possible hypotension or hypertension.

Hematocrit. Routine screening is recommended.

Urinalysis. Routine screening is recommended.

Tuberculosis. Routine screening is recommended.

Condition-Specific Screening

Speech and Language. Specialized testing is done if a problem is observed.

Liver Function Tests. These tests are necessary for children taking pemoline.

Thyroid Function. Thyroid function may need to be tested.

Electrocardiogram (ECG) Monitoring. ECG is necessary for children taking tricyclic antidepressants and clonidine.

COMMON ILLNESS MANAGEMENT

Differential Diagnosis

Irritability, anorexia, weight loss, and insomnia are side effects of stimulants.

Illness or need for a change in dose or dosing schedule for medications must be ruled out.

Co-morbidity is common in developmental and/or behavioral deviations and must be evaluated.

Change in inattention pattern may require ruling out seizure disorder.

Change in mood may suggest referral for anxiety, depression, and decreased self-esteem.

Injury pattern may be associated with possible abuse or need for greater supervision and/or safety practices.

Drug Interactions.

See Table 12-4.

Developmental Issues

Sleep Patterns. Children with ADHD taking stimulant medication may have insomnia if it is given late in the day or in large doses.

Toileting. Enuresis or encopresis may be present as a result of inattention to body cues.

Discipline. Children may have difficulty responding to directions and may not understand discipline or learn from past experiences. Consistency in expectations is important.

Behavior modification may be effective. A bad deed must be differentiated from a bad child.

Child Care. Children perform better in a small, structured safe environment with constant adult supervision.

Schooling. Education strategies to decrease distraction in a regular classroom, in addition to creative teaching modalities appropriate to the specific learning needs of the child, should be implemented. Building a child's self-esteem and confidence is essential. Children should be helped to learn to compensate for their disability. Development of the individualized education plan (IEP) or accommodation plan is a team effort.

Sexuality. Learning techniques individualized for particular adolescents must be used when teaching sexuality and birth control material.

Transition into Adulthood

Professional help may be necessary to facilitate the transition to more autonomous living and work situations; peer coaching may be helpful.

Career development counseling may be helpful in identifying an appropriate vocation based on a child's strengths and weaknesses.

Family Concerns

The child and the family need to readjust to this disability at every new developmental stage. Family counseling can provide information and emotional support.

REFERENCES

American Academy of Child and Adolescent Psychiatry. (1997). Practice parameters for the assessment and treatment of children, adolescents, and adults with attention-deficit/hyperactivity disorder, *J Am Acad Child Adolesc Psychiatry, 36*(10), 85S-112S, 1997.

American Academy of Pediatrics. (2000). Clinical practice guideline: Diagnosis and evaluation of the child with attention-deficit/ hyperactivity disorder. *Pediatrics, 105*(5), 1158-1170.

American Academy of Pediatrics. (2001). Clinical practice guideline: Treatment of the school-aged child with attention-deficit/hyperactivity disorder, *Pediatrics, 108*(4), 1033-1044.

American Psychiatric Association. (2000). *Diagnostic and statistical manual of mental disorders: Text revision* (4th ed.). Washington, DC: Author.

Anastopoulos, A. & Shelton, T. (2001). *Assessing attention-deficit/hyperactivity disorder.* New York: Kluwer Academic/Plenum Publishers.

Barkley, R. (1998, September). Attention-deficit hyperactivity disorder. *Scientific American;* Web site: http://www.sciam.com/1998/0998issuebarkley.html.

Barkley, R. (2000). *Taking charge of ADHD.* New York: The Guildford Press.

Baumgaertel, A. (1999). Alternative and controversial treatments for attention-deficit/hyperactivity disorder. *Pediatr Clin North Am, 46*(5), 977-992.

Brown, T. (2000). *Attention-deficit disorders and comorbidities in children, adolescents, and adults.* Washington, DC: American Psychiatric Press, Inc.

Carlson, C. & Mann, M. (2000). Attention-deficit/hyperactivity disorder, predominantly inattentive subtype. *Child Adolesc Psychiatr Clin North Am, 9*(3), 499-510.

Castellanos, F.X. (2001). Neuroimaging studies of ADHD. In M. Solanto, A. Arnstein, & F.X. Castellanos (Eds.). *Stimulant drugs and ADHD: Basic and clinical neuroscience.* New York: Oxford University Press (pp. 243-258).

Chan, E., Gardiner, P., & Kemper, K. (2000). "At least it's natural": Herbs and dietary supplements in ADHD. *Contemp Pediatr, 17*(9), 116-126.

Chervin, R., Archbold, K., Dillon, J., Panahi, P., Pituch, K., et al. (2002). Inattention, hyperactivity and symptoms of sleep-disordered breathing. *Pediatrics, 109*(3), 449-456.

Deglin, J. & Vallerand, A. (2001). *Davis's drug guide for nurses.* Philadelphia: FA Davis Co.

DiScala, C., Lescohier, I., Barthel, M., & Li, G. (1998). Injuries to children with attention deficit hyperactivity disorder. *Pediatrics, 102*(6), 1415-1421.

Fletcher, J., Shaywitz, S., & Shaywitz, B. (1999). Comorbidity of learning and attention disorders: Separate but equal. *Pediatr Clin North Am, 46*(5), 885-597.

Gerring, J.P., Brady, K.D., Chen, A., Vasa, R., Grados, M., et al. (1998). Premorbid prevalence of ADHD and development of secondary ADHD after closed head injury. *J Am Acad Child Adolesc Psychiatry, 37*(6), 647-654.

Glaxo SmithKline; Web site: http://science.gsk.com.

Greenhill, L. (2001). Clinical effects of stimulant medication in ADHD. In M. Solanto, A. Arnsten, & F.X. Castellanos (Eds.). *Stimulant drugs and ADHD: Basic and clinical neuroscience.* New York: Oxford University Press (pp. 31-72).

Greenhill, L. (1998). Diagnosing attention-deficit hyperactivity disorder in children. *J Clin Psychiatry, 59*(suppl. 7), 31-41.

Guevara, J., Lozano, P., Wickizer, T., Mell, L., & Gephart, H. (2002). Psychotropic medication use in a population of children who have attention-deficit/hyperactivity disorder. *Pediatrics, 109*(5), 733-739.

Guitierrez, K. (1999). *Pharmacotherapeutics: Decision-making in nursing.* Philadelphia: Saunders.

Hechtman, L. (2000a). Assessment and diagnosis of attention-deficit/hyperactivity disorder. *Child Adolesc Psychiatr Clin North Am, 9*(3), 481-498.

Hechtman, L. (2000b). Subgroups of adult outcome of attention-deficit/hyperactivity disorder. In T. Brown (Ed.). *Attention-deficit disorders and comorbidities in children, adolescents, and adults.* Washington, DC: American Psychiatric Press, Inc. (pp. 437-453).

Heiligenstein, J. (2001, October). *Atomoxetine efficacy vs. placebo in school-age girls with ADHD.* Poster Presented at 49th Annual Meeting of the American Academy of Child and Adolescent Psychiatry, Honolulu.

Hille, E.T., den Ouden, A.L., Saigal, S., Wolke, D., Lambert, M., et al. (2001). Behavioural problems in children who weigh 1000 g or less at birth in four countries. *Lancet, 357,* 1641-1643.

Jensen, P. (2000). ADHD: Current concepts on etiology, pathophysiology and neurobiology. *J Am Acad Child Adolesc Psychiatry, 9*(3), 557-572.

Jensen, P., Arnold, L., Richters, J., et al. (1999). 14 month randomized clinical trial of treatment strategies for attention deficit hyperactivity disorder. *Arch Gen Psychiatry, 56,* 1073-1086.

Lahey, B.B., Pelham, W.E., Stein, M.A., Loney, J., Trapani, C., et al. (1998). Validity of DSM-IV attention-deficit/hyperactivity disorder for younger children. *J Am Acad Child Adolesc Psychiatry, 37*(7), 695-702.

MacMillan, D., Gresham, F., & Bocian, K. (1998). Discrepancy between definitions of learning disabilities and school practices: An empirical investigation. *J Learn Disabil, 31*(4), 314-326.

Magyary, D., Brandt, P., & Kovalesky, A. (1999). *Children and ADHD: A manual with decision tree—clinical path.* Seattle: University of Washington.

Mannuzza, S. & Klein, R. (2000). Long-term prognosis in attention-deficit/hyperactivity disorder. *Child Adolesc Psychiatr Clin North Am, 9*(3), 711-726.

National Institute of Health Consensus Statement. (1998, November). *Diagnosis and treatment of attention deficit hyperactivity disorder (ADHD)*; Web site: http://odp.od.nih.gov/consensus/cons/110/110_statement.htm.

National Institute of Health Consensus Statement. November 16-18, 1998. (2000). Diagnosis and treatment of attention deficit hyperactivity disorder (ADHD). *J Am Acad Child Adolesc Psychiatry, 39,* 182-193.

Nurse Practitioners' Prescribing Reference. (2001-2002, Winter). New York: Prescribing Reference, Inc.

Pelham, W.E., Gnagy, E.M., Burrows-Maclean, L., Williams, A., Fabiano, G.A., et al. (2001). Once a day Concerta methylphenidate versus three-times-daily methylphenidate—in laboratory and natural settings. *Pediatrics, 107*(6).

Pliszka, S. (2000). Patterns of psychiatric co-morbidity of attention-deficit/hyperactivity disorder. *Child Adolesc Psychiatr Clin North Am, 9*(3), 525-540.

Pliszka S., Carlson, C., & Swanson, J. (1999). *ADHD with comorbid disorders.* New York: The Guildford Press.

Popper, C. (2000). Pharmacologic alternatives to psychostimulants for the treatment of attention-deficit/hyperactivity disorder. *Child Adolesc Psychiatr Clin North Am, 9*(3), 605-646.

Rushton, J., Clark, S., & Freed, G. (2000). Pediatrician and family physician prescription of selective serotonin reuptake inhibitors. *Pediatrics, 105*(6), 2000.

Scahill, L. & Schwab-Stone, M. (2000). Epidemiology of ADHD in school-age children. *Child Adolesc Psychiatr Clin North Am, 9*(3), 541-555.

Silver, L. (1999). *ADHD: A clinical guide to diagnosis and treatment for health and mental health professionals.* Washington, DC: Psychiatric Press, Inc.

Silver, L. (2000). Attention-deficit/hyperactivity disorder in adult life. *Child Adolesc Psychiatr Clin North Am, 9*(3), 511-523.

Solanto, M. (2001). Attention-deficit/hyperactivity disorder: Clinical features. In M. Solanto, A. Arnsten, & F.X. Castellanos (Eds.). *Stimulant drugs and ADHD: Basic and clinical neuroscience.* New York: Oxford University Press (pp. 3-30).

Spencer, T., Biederman, J., Wilens, T.E., & Faraone, S.V. (1998). Adults with attention-deficit/hyperactivity disorder: A controversial diagnosis. *J Clin Psychiatry, 59*(suppl. 7), 59-68.

Stubbe, D. (2000). Attention-deficit/ hyperactivity disorder overview: Historical perspective, current controversies, and future directions. *Child Adolesc Psychiatr Clin North Am, 9*(3), 469-479.

Ten Eick, A.P., Nakamura, H., & Reed, M.D. (1998). Drug-drug interactions in pediatric pharmacology. *Psychiatr Clin North Am, 45*(5), 1233-1264.

Tosyali, M. & Greenhill, L. (1998). Child and adolescent psychopharmacology: Important developmental issues. *Psychiatr Clin North Am, 45*(5), 1021-1035.

Ward, J. & Guyer, K. (2000). Medical management of ADHD. In B. Guyer (Ed.). *ADHD: Achieving success in school and in life.* Boston: Allyn & Bacon (pp. 38-54).

Wender, P. (2000). *ADHD: Attention-deficit hyperactivity disorder in children and adults.* New York: Oxford University Press.

Weyandt, L. (2001). *An ADHD primer.* Boston: Allyn & Bacon.

Wilens, T. & Spencer, T. (2000). Stimulants and attention-deficit/hyperactivity disorder. *Child Adolesc Psychiatr Clin North Am, 9*(3), 573-604.

Wilens, T., Spencer, T., & Biederman, J. (2000). Attention-deficit/hyperactivity disorder with substance use disorders. In T. Brown (Ed.). *Attention-deficit disorders and comorbidities in children, adolescents, and adults.* Washington, DC: American Psychiatric Press (pp. 319-339).

Wynne, A., Woo, T., & Millard, M. (2002). *Pharmacotherapeu.tics for nurse practitioner prescribers.* Philadelphia: F.A. Davis Co.

13 Autism

Maureen Sheehan

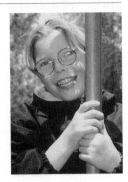

Etiology

Autism was initially described by Leo Kanner in 1943, who thought that children with autism were of normal intelligence and the product of cold and distant parenting. His description of the 11 children he studied focused on their social impairment and, to a lesser extent, their insistence on "sameness" (Kanner, 1943). Autism is now known to be a neurodevelopmental disorder recognized as one of a spectrum of pervasive developmental disorders (PDDs) (American Psychiatric Association, 1994). Children with autism have impaired communication skills and social interactions and one or more repetitive and stereotyped behaviors. Autism becomes apparent in a child by the age of 3 years, although delays in diagnosis can occur. Many children with autism are also mentally retarded. To be diagnosed with autism, a child must meet the criteria for autistic disorder of the American Psychiatric Association in the fourth edition of the *Diagnostic and Statistical Manual of Mental Disorders (DSM-IV)* (Box 13-1).

The variation in the clinical manifestations of autism among all children with autism, monozygotic twins and siblings with autism, and other family members with autistic spectrum disorders has led to research into environmental factors that might interact with genetic susceptibility for autism or cause autism. In addition, while most children with autism do not experience a period of normal social and language development, there is a group who do and have developmental regression of unknown origin (Davidovitch et al, 2000). Many potential environmental causes of this regression have been proposed and are being studied.

In 1998, Wakefield et al proposed a link among the measles-mumps-rubella (MMR) vaccine, colitis, and the development of PDD in 12 children. Since then numerous epidemiologic studies have been unable to find any evidence to support the idea that the MMR vaccine induces autism. In their sample of 262 children with autism, 98 of whom had not received the MMR, Fombonne & Chakrabarti (2001) found that developmental regression did not differ between the two groups in the study, indicating introduction of the MMR had not resulted in a higher rate of developmental regression among children with autism. A study of 498 children with autism in the United Kingdom found they were diagnosed at the same age whether they received the MMR before or after the age of 18 months or not at all (Taylor et al, 2002). Kaye et al (2001) found that although the number of cases of autism in boys 2 to 5 years old in the United Kingdom increased fourfold from 1988 to 1993, the rate of MMR vaccination remained constant at 95%. In children born in California between 1980 and 1994 and enrolled in California kindergartens, there was a 373% increase in the

diagnosis of autism whereas MMR vaccine coverage increased only 14% (Dales et al, 2001).

Numerous studies have identified prenatal, perinatal, and neonatal factors that have occurred in children with autism. The problems observed (e.g., hypertension, use of prescription medication, nonvertex presentation, hyperbilirubinemia) have not been consistently seen, are not specific to autism, and cannot be used to either predict or prevent autism (Bolton et al, 1997; Juul-Dam et al, 2001). There does seem to be a consistent association between complications during pregnancy, labor and delivery, and the neonatal period and the later development of autism (Juul-Dam et al, 2001). Mothers of children with autism were found to have a significantly higher incidence of uterine bleeding than the general population (Juul-Dam et al, 2001). Children with autistic spectrum disorders are more likely than their siblings to have had mothers with minor obstetric complications (Zwaigenbaum et al, 2002). Among unaffected siblings of children with autism, those with the largest proportion of relatives with manifestations of the autism phenotype also had a higher rate of complications (Zwaigenbaum et al, 2002). These studies provide evidence that the minor obstetric complications observed were more likely to be the result of genetically determined preexisting fetal developmental anomalies than the cause of them (Bolton et al, 1997; Juul-Dam et al, 2001; Zwaigenbaum et al, 2002).

Neuropathologic studies of brain tissue from people with autism have found abnormalities in the hippocampus, amygdala, limbic system, Purkinje cells, and cerebellum—structures important to processing social and environmental information (Fatemi et al, 2001; Kemper & Bauman, 1998; Sparks et al, 2002). More recently, a reduction in some proteins found in brain tissue and thought to be involved in several neuropsychiatric disorders has been discovered in the brains of people with autism (Blatt et al, 2001; Fatemi et al, 2001). The differences found in these areas of the brain indicate a developmental disorder early in gestation that leads to dysregulation of cell growth and death (Blatt et al, 2001; Fatemi et al, 2001). This pathologic process is thought to continue into adulthood, as evidenced by the larger than expected brains of children and adults with autism (Hardan et al, 2001).

Magnetic resonance imaging (MRI), positron emission tomography (PET), and single-photon emission computed tomography (SPECT) studies have all found abnormalities in children with autism, but most studies have been done with very few subjects and often without controls. The largest MRI study showed excessive brain growth early in life that then slowed to below normal growth during the school-age years (Courchesne et al, 2001). This pattern was observed in both the

Diagnostic Criteria for Autistic Disorder

A total of six (or more) items from (1), (2), and (3), with at least two from (1) and one each from (2) and (3):

(1) Qualitative impairment in social interaction, as manifested by at least two of the following:

Marked impairment in the use of multiple nonverbal behaviors, such as eye-to-eye gaze, facial expression, body postures, and gestures to regulate social interaction

Failure to develop peer relationships appropriate to developmental level

Lack of spontaneous seeking to share enjoyment, interests, or achievements with other people (e.g., by a lack of showing, bringing, or pointing out objects of interest)

Lack of social or emotional reciprocity

(2) Qualitative impairments in communication as manifested by at least one of the following:

Delay in, or total lack of, the development of spoken language (not accompanied by an attempt to compensate through alternative modes of communication, such as gesture or mime)

In individuals with adequate speech, marked impairment in the ability to initiate or sustain a conversation with others

Stereotyped and repetitive use of language or idiosyncratic language

Lack of varied, spontaneous make-believe play or social imitative play appropriate to developmental level

(3) Restricted repetitive and stereotyped patterns of behavior, interests, and activities, as manifested by at least one of the following:

Encompassing preoccupation with one or more stereotyped and restricted patterns of interest that is abnormal either in intensity or focus

Apparently inflexible adherence to specific, nonfunctional routines or rituals

Stereotyped and repetitive motor mannerisms (e.g., hand or finger flapping or twisting, complex whole-body movements)

Persistent preoccupation with parts of objects

Delays or abnormal function in at least one of the following areas, with onset before age 3 yr: (a) social interaction, (b) language as used in social communication, or (c) symbolic or imaginative play

The disturbance is not better accounted for by Rett disorder or childhood disintegrative disorder

From American Psychiatric Association (APA). (1990). *Diagnostic and statistical manual of mental disorders* (4th ed.). Washington, DC: Author, pp. 70-71. Reprinted with permission.

gray and white matter, a finding that may help explain why the deficits of autism are pervasive and lifelong (Courchesne et al, 2001). Electroencephalographic (EEG) studies in a number of individuals with autism provide further evidence of abnormal brain development, but there is no singular EEG pattern exclusive and universal to autism (Tanguay, 2000).

The most consistent neurochemical finding in autism is hyperserotoninemia (Rapin & Katzman, 1998; Tanguay, 2000). Because of the frequency of sleep disorders in children with autism, melatonin abnormalities have been hypothesized (Rapin & Katzman, 1998). Levels of oxytocin, dopamine, norepinephrine, endogenous opioids, and cortisol have all been found to be abnormal in some children with autism (Korvatska et al, 2002; Rapin & Katzman, 1998). The relationship of these findings to the pathology of autism is unclear.

Fetal exposures to thalidomide, valproic acid, ethanol, and misoprostol appear to account for a tiny percentage of children with autism (Rodier, 2002). A number of prenatal viral infections have also been associated with autism in some individuals (Hornig & Lipkin, 2001).

The evidence that a wide variety of factors are implicated in the etiology of autism suggests that it is a neurodevelopmental disorder with a broad continuum of behavioral symptoms that has a strong genetic component. The genes may interact with prenatal infectious, environmental, or autoimmune factors to produce abnormal brain development and function.

Known Genetic Etiology

Over the past decade, the evidence has mounted that genetic factors play a primary role in the etiology of autism (Korvatska et al, 2002). Three epidemiologically based twin studies report an average concordance rate of 70% among monozygotic (identical) twins and a 0% concordance rate among dizygotic (fraternal) twins (Folstein & Rosen-Sheidley, 2001). The difference between the concordance rates for monozygotic and dizygotic twins suggests that the inheritance pattern is nonmendelian (Szatmari et al, 1998). The mode of genetic transmission for autism must be heterogeneous (Szatmari et al, 1998).

Siblings of children with autism have autism at a rate of about 3% (Folstein & Rosen-Sheidley, 2001). This may be an artificially low estimate of the rate of recurrence of familial autism because "stoppage rules" indicate that many parents with one child with autism will decide not to have more children (Slager et al, 2001). By only considering the rate of recurrence of autism in siblings born after the child with autism, the risk of autism in subsequent children increases to 8.6%, which represents a 50-fold to 100-fold increase in the expected prevalence of autism in siblings (Szatmari et al, 1998). Studies of family members of children with autism found that twins without autism and a significant minority of first-degree relatives were more likely to have social difficulties, language delays, and affective and anxiety disorders (Bailey et al, 1998). These problems range from one of the milder PDDs, such as Asperger syndrome, to isolated social, communication, or personality traits, such as shyness, rigidity, and sensitivity to experience, that bear some resemblance to the core deficits of autism (Bailey et al, 1998; Murphy et al, 2000).

Although there is a strong genetic component to autism, no specific genes for autism have yet been found (Monaco & Bailey, 2001). Across the globe genetic researchers have identified a number of chromosome regions that may be involved. These include chromosome 15q and, to a lesser extent, 7q and 16p (Monaco & Bailey, 2001; Tanguay, 2000). Chromosomes 2, 4, 10, 19, and 22 have also been implicated, but many of these findings have not been replicable (Monaco & Bailey, 2001; Tanguay, 2000). Clearly, there is a great deal of genetic heterogeneity in autism, and the search for specific genes will be long and arduous.

Incidence and Prevalence

Studies over the past 15 years have shown an increase in the rate of autism. Prevalence of autism is now estimated to be 15 to 17 children in 10,000 (Chakrabarti & Fombonne, 2001; Croen et al, 2002a). Higher rates of as many as 60 per 10,000 have been reported, but these studies involved small and regionally defined populations (Bertrand et al, 2001; Hyman et al, 2001; Kadesjo et al, 1999). The rate for all PDDs combined is now thought to be 45 to 60 children in 10,000 (Bertrand et al,

2001; Chakrabarti & Fombonne, 2001; Hyman et al, 2001). Autism is now recognized as a common disorder of childhood.

Several factors might explain this increase in the rate of autism. As specific behavioral criteria for a diagnosis of autism have been delineated by the American Psychiatric Association *(DSM-IV)* (1994) and the World Health Organization's *International Classification of Diseases* *(ICD*-10; 1994) a wider spectrum of children and adults with autism has been identified. A population-based study of eight successive California birth cohorts from 1987 to 1994 found that the incidence of autism increased by 9.1 cases per 10,000 (Croen et al, 2002a). At the same time the incidence of mental retardation of unknown etiology decreased by 9.3 cases per 10,000 (Croen et al, 2002a). This suggests that changes and improvements in the diagnosis of autism and reclassification of diagnosis for some children from mental retardation to autism account for the increase in the prevalence of autism.

Public awareness of autism has increased, as has the availability of information regarding autism through the Internet. For example, the age when children with autism entered the service delivery system in California in the Croen study (2002a) decreased every year and went from a mean age of 6.9 years in 1987 to 3.3 years in 1994, indicating that children with autism are now being identified through primary care before they reach school age. It is also possible that as intensive treatments for children with autism became the standard of care in many areas, children previously diagnosed as having one of the autistic spectrum disorders were reclassified as having autism so that they might qualify for services not generally available to children without the diagnosis of autism (Croen et al, 2002a).

Autism is found in all ethnic and socioeconomic groups. It is generally more common in boys than in girls, by a ratio of 2.1 to 5:1, although the ratio between boys and girls approaches 1:1 as severity of co-existing mental retardation increases (Bertrand et al, 2001; Croen et al, 2002a; Fombonne, 1999; Magnusson & Saemundsen, 2001). In the California population of Croen et al (2002b), increasing maternal age, being born to a black mother or a mother with a postgraduate degree, and being part of a multiple birth all increased the risk of autism. The finding that simply being a twin increases a child's risk for autism has also been demonstrated in two other studies (Betancur et al, 2002; Greenberg et al, 2001).

Finally, it is possible that that the actual incidence of autism has increased over the past 2 decades. Studies with consistent and rigorously defined diagnostic criteria conducted with defined populations over a period of years could more precisely define the actual incidence of autism. Changes in diagnostic criteria over time, however, preclude a definitive answer to the question of whether the incidence and prevalence of autism have actually increased. What is important is the knowledge that autism is a common condition, more common in the pediatric population than cancer, diabetes, spina bifida, and Down syndrome (Filipek et al, 1999).

Clinical Manifestations at Time of Diagnosis

The fourth edition of the *Diagnostic and Statistical Manual of Mental Disorders* has established a set of diagnostic criteria with which to make the diagnosis of autism (American

---

BOX 13-2

Clinical Manifestations at Time of Diagnosis

DELAYED OR ABSENT COMMUNICATION
Expressive language delay
Receptive language delay

IMPAIRMENT OF SOCIAL INTERACTION
Avoidance of eye contact
Fascination with objects rather than people
Interactions revolve around obtaining desired objects rather than emotional responses

RESTRICTIVE AND REPETITIVE BEHAVIOR, INTERESTS, AND ACTIVITIES
Organizes toys, rather than manipulates them
Throws tantrums when repetitive behaviors are interrupted
Hand flapping, twirling, toe walking

RESISTANCE TO CHANGES IN SCHEDULE OR ENVIRONMENT
Narrow food preferences
Auditory hypersensitivity

Psychiatric Association [APA], 1994) (Box 13-1). The principal symptoms of autism fall into three categories: impaired communication skills (both verbal and nonverbal); impaired social interactions; and restricted and rigid play, activities, and interests (Wing, 2001) (Box 13-2). Although all children with autism will exhibit the triad of symptoms above, the severity of these symptoms varies widely among children, which can lead to a delay in diagnosis. The majority of children with autism have cognitive deficits, but there are individuals with normal or even superior intelligence quotients (IQs; Filipek et al, 1999). Although autism may present in infancy as a lack of attention to faces, people, or the environment; interest in objects instead of faces; and inability to point or wave bye-bye; most children with autism are diagnosed as toddlers (i.e., between their first and third birthdays) when their delayed language is quite apparent.

Delayed Communication and Impaired Social and Play Skills

Parents of young children with autism typically raise one or more of three concerns with their child's primary care provider (Filipek et al, 1999). These concerns are a delay in the development of language or social skills of their child or delayed development in the younger sibling of a child with known or suspected autism (Filipek et al, 1999). Further questioning by the provider may uncover impairment in play including the absence or impoverishment of imaginative play, preoccupation with certain toys or objects, and an inflexible adherence to routine (National Institute of Neurological Disorders and Stroke, 2002). Although language delay is not an uncommon complaint among parents, paired with concerns about social skills and behavior it needs prompt investigation (Filipek et al, 1999; Box 13-3).

Parental concerns regarding delays in the language, motor, and cognitive development of children 4 years and older have been shown to be highly sensitive predictors of developmental problems, whereas the absence of concerns in these areas had

BOX 13-3

Parental Concerns that are Red Flags for Autism

COMMUNICATION CONCERNS
Does not respond to his or her name
Cannot tell me what he or she wants
Language delayed
Does not follow directions
Appears deaf at times
Seems to hear sometimes but not others
Does not point or wave bye-bye
Used to say a few words but does not now

SOCIAL CONCERNS
Does not smile socially
Seems to prefer to play alone
Gets things for himself or herself
Is very independent
Does things "early"
Has poor eye contact
In his or her own world
Tunes us out
Is not interested in other children

BEHAVIORAL CONCERNS
Tantrums
Is hyperactive uncooperative or oppositional
Does not know how to play with toys
Gets stuck on things over and over
Toe walks
Has unusual attachments to toys (e.g., always is holding a certain object)
Lines things up
Is oversensitive to certain textures or sounds
Has odd movement patterns

ABSOLUTE INDICATIONS FOR IMMEDIATE FURTHER EVALUATION
No babbling by 12 mo
No gesturing (pointing, waving bye-bye, etc.) by 12 mo
No single words by 16 mo
No two-word spontaneous (not just echolalic) phrases by 24 mo
Any loss of *any* language or social skills at *any* age

From Filipek P.A. et al. (1999). The screening and diagnosis of autistic spectrum disorders. *J Autism Dev Disorders, 29*(6). Reprinted with permission.

high specificity in identifying typically developing children (Glascoe, 1997). Parents were accurate in their concerns regardless of education, income, or parenting experience (Glascoe, 1997). In a study of 1300 families with children with autism, the average age of diagnosis was 6 years, although most parents felt something was wrong by the age of 18 months and had expressed their concerns to a health care professional by their child's second birthday (Howlin & Moore, 1997). A small retrospective video study found subtle symptoms of autism present at 9 to 12 months of age in children later diagnosed with autism and that parents attempted to engage their children in play and social interactions to compensate for these symptoms (Baranek, 1999).

The mean age for diagnosis is now 30 months (Chakrabarti & Fombonne, 2001). While most toddlers and preschoolers with autism have consistent delays in communication, social interactions, and play skills, there is a minority of approximately 30% who appear to have a period of normal development followed by either a plateauing or regression of skills

(Bertrand et al, 2001; Tuchman & Rapin, 1997). This regression is a common event in the natural course of autism for many children, yet one that appears to lead to feelings of guilt in mothers of children with autism (Davidovitch et al, 2000). Parents of children with regression found the first symptoms of autism at virtually the same age as those with children who did not regress (Fombonne & Chakrabarti, 2001).

Screening and Diagnosis

In 2000 the Quality Standards Subcommittee of the American Academy of Neurology and the Child Neurology Society published a practice parameter for the screening and diagnosis of autism (Filipek et al, 2000). This parameter was based on consensus decisions reached by representatives from 11 professional organizations, four parent organizations, and the National Institutes of Health who gathered their information from a biography of over 2750 sources (Filipek et al, 1999). It recommends a dual process for the identification of children with autism: routine developmental screening for autism for all children and then comprehensive evaluation and diagnosis of children identified to be at risk for autism. This process has been put into an algorithm (Filipek et al, 2000; Figure 13-1).

Evaluation of a child for autism includes an audiology exam to rule out hearing impairment as the primary reason for the child's speech delay. The audiology exam often requires brainstem auditory evoked response (BAER) testing because of the challenging behavior of children with autism. If the audiology exam and a lead screen do not indicate any abnormalities, then the primary care provider should use a screening tool specifically for autism such as the Checklist for Autism in Toddlers (CHAT) of the Autism Screening Questionnaire to objectively elicit the clinical manifestations of autism (Filipek et al, 2000; Scambler et al, 2001). A modified CHAT (M-CHAT) is now being tested. The M-CHAT is a simple questionnaire that can be completed by parents of 24-month-old children while they are at their child's well-child visit (Robins et al, 2001). There are six items on the M-CHAT that have the strongest predictive value for autism. They are as follows: a lack of pointing, not following a parent's pointing, not bringing things to show parents, little or no interest in other children or in imitation, and the child's inability to respond to his or her name (Robins et al, 2001). If the results of these procedures indicate the child has autism, the child and family should then be referred for formal diagnostic testing by clinicians experienced with autism and to the local school district or early intervention program (Filipek et al, 2000).

After a child has been diagnosed with autism, the primary care provider can help the child and parents by coordinating additional work-up aimed at identifying possible causes. This work-up includes a skin examination with a Wood's lamp looking for the hypopigmented macules of tuberous sclerosis, high-resolution chromosomes, and deoxyribonucleic acid (DNA) analysis for fragile X syndrome (Filipek et al, 2000; Shevell et al, 2001). Routine metabolic testing and electroencephalogram (EEG) studies are necessary only if the child has symptoms of metabolic disease, epilepsy, or a clinically significant loss of language skills (Filipek et al, 2000). There is inadequate evidence to recommend routine hair or stool analysis; allergy, immunology, micronutrient, or urinary peptide testing;

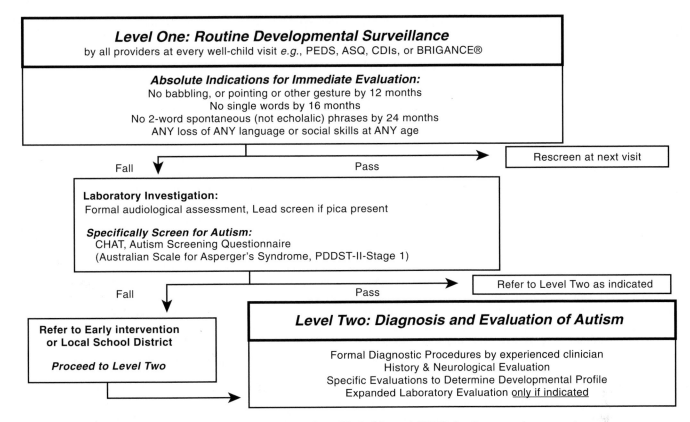

Level One: Routine Developmental Surveillance
by all providers at every well-child visit *e.g.*, PEDS, ASQ, CDIs, or BRIGANCE®

Absolute Indications for Immediate Evaluation:
No babbling, or pointing or other gesture by 12 months
No single words by 16 months
No 2-word spontaneous (not echolalic) phrases by 24 months
ANY loss of ANY language or social skills at ANY age

Fall   Pass   Rescreen at next visit

Laboratory Investigation:
Formal audiological assessment, Lead screen if pica present

Specifically Screen for Autism:
CHAT, Autism Screening Questionnaire
(Australian Scale for Asperger's Syndrome, PDDST-II-Stage 1)

Fall   Pass   Refer to Level Two as indicated

Refer to Early Intervention or Local School District

Proceed to Level Two

Level Two: Diagnosis and Evaluation of Autism

Formal Diagnostic Procedures by experienced clinician
History & Neurological Evaluation
Specific Evaluations to Determine Developmental Profile
Expanded Laboratory Evaluation only if indicated

FIGURE 13-1 Practice parameter algorithm. (From Filipek, P.A. et al. [2002]. Practice parameters: screening and diagnosis of autism. *Neurology, 55*, 469. Reprinted with permission.)

or mitochondrial disorder and thyroid function tests (Filipek et al, 1999). Because of the low yield of diagnostic testing, a thorough history and physical should be the guide for all further evaluation of a child with autism (Hyman et al, 2001).

Treatment

Just as there is no cure for autism, there is no one treatment that works for every child (Box 13-4). Improved long-term outcomes are associated with early, intensive, and sustained behavioral and educational interventions (American Academy of Child and Adolescent Psychiatry [AACAP], 1999). As the genetic and neurobiologic basis for the deficits of autism has become more apparent, approaches to treatment have focused on the specific symptoms of autism. A comprehensive treatment plan for a child with autism must include both education and behavior management and often pharmacologic treatment. The plan should define language, social, and educational goals, define and prioritize target behavioral symptoms for intervention, and provide for periodic assessment of the child's functioning at home and school (AACAP, 1999). For some children, medication management will also be necessary (AACAP, 1999). This comprehensive treatment must be planned, coordinated, and delivered by a multidisciplinary team that includes the child's parents; primary care provider; school personnel; psychiatrist; and behavioral, speech, physical, and occupational therapists as needed (AACAP, 1999).

BOX 13-4
Treatment

Early intervention and education
   One-on-one discrete trial learning
   Therapeutic preschools
   Social communication and interaction skills
Behavioral management
Pharmacologic intervention
   Stimulants
   Selective serotonin reuptake inhibitors (SSRIs)
   Neuroleptics
   Other pharmacologic treatments
Complementary and alternative therapies

Early Intervention and Education

The most significant treatment for autism is early and consistent education, which has been shown to improve the child's long-term outcome (AAP, 2001). There is a lack of research, however, to indicate which educational methods are the most effective (AAP, 2001). Since early intervention has been shown to improve outcomes, parents should be referred to the local early intervention program and school district as soon as the diagnosis of autism is suspected, without waiting for definitive diagnosis (AAP, 2001). Eligibility for these programs is based on the presence of delays, not on a categoric diagnosis (AAP, 2001).

Early intervention (i.e., between birth and 4 years old) has been shown to improve children's level of functioning and decrease the frequency of aberrant behaviors (Howlin, 1998). Therapeutic education during the preschool years takes advantage of the child's most rapid period of development and greatest degree of brain plasticity. This type of early treatment can result in some children with autism, who are cognitively intact, no longer meeting the criteria for autism by the school-age years (Rapin & Katzman, 1998). What form this intervention should take is a matter of some debate.

Many clinicians in the field of autism recommend that preschoolers with autism receive 40 hours per week of one-to-one discrete trial learning based on the methods used by Lovaas (1987) in the Early Intervention Project (Siegel, 1996). Children whose parents, under the direction of a behavior therapist, implemented intensive behavioral treatment as developed by Lovaas (1987) had significant improvements in IQ and decreases in symptom severity as compared with children in conventional school-based settings (Sheinkopf & Siegel, 1998). This type of treatment is expensive (as much as $50,000 per year) and very time and energy consuming. Clearly not all families have the financial resources and community support necessary to carry out 30 to 40 hours per week of one-to-one teaching. Parents are increasingly turning to their school districts for help with one-to-one early intervention and often meeting with resistance, resulting in litigation (Gresham & MacMillan, 1998).

Other early educational approaches include therapeutic preschools employing Greenspan's developmental approach, which is based on learning through floor play and behavioral one-to-one interventions in an academic setting rather than at home (Elder, 2002). Children between the ages of 31 and 65 months who were younger (M = 42 months) when they began intensive behavioral treatment in a therapeutic preschool were more likely to be in a regular classroom 4 to 6 years later (Harris, 2000). Preschools that use the Treatment and Education of Autistic and Related Communication-Handicapped Children (TEACCH) approach rely primarily on group instruction and extensive teaching through visual means to compensate for the verbal deficits of children with autism (Cohen, 1998). The Autism Society of America (2002) has criticized this approach as not intense enough and without enough emphasis on language skills.

A growing number of studies suggest that young children with autism, particularly nonverbal and preverbal children, require early training in social communication and interaction skills (Hwang & Hughes, 2000; Rogers, 2000). Although most of this training occurs in controlled settings, evidence suggests that training that occurs in a child's natural home, school, and play settings promotes generalization of the skills learned (Hwang & Hughes, 2000).

Speech therapy is an essential part of any early intervention program for children with autism. Functional spoken language by the age of 5 years is an important predictor of future outcome (AACAP, 1999). Sign language and the Picture Exchange Communication System (PECS) are important alternatives to spoken language that some children with autism can master,

thus allowing them to communicate with family members and at school and reducing the frustration of unmet needs that can lead to behavioral outbursts (Elder, 2002).

Behavioral Management

Behavioral management is an essential part of the treatment plan for a child with autism and should begin as soon after diagnosis as possible, before problematic behaviors are deeply entrenched. Parents may be reluctant to set the firm limits that even a very young child with autism requires to prevent the establishment of inappropriate behaviors. As Howlin (1998) describes, parents can be reminded that removing a screaming 3-year-old from a store is embarrassing, but removing a screaming 13-year-old may be impossible.

Behavioral interventions are generally based on the principles of behavior modification and can help a child with autism acquire language, social, and self-care skills and reduce aberrant behavior. The most commonly used approaches are based on the work of Oscar Lovaas and variously referred to as discrete trial learning, intensive behavior intervention, or applied behavior analysis (Elder, 2002). In this approach, the child is rewarded with something highly desirous to him or her (e.g., candy) every time the child responds correctly to a command, for example, to make eye contact. If the child is unable or unwilling to respond to the command "Look at me," the teacher may gently turn the child's head and reward the child for the most fleeting of glances. Once this behavior is established, the teacher will expand on it by requiring eye contact of 1 or 2 seconds before rewarding the child. This approach is often implemented with 1:1 teaching for 30 to 40 hours per week, beginning with children as young as 2 or 3 years.

Functional analysis with antecedent-based interventions is gaining popularity (Elder, 2002). With this technique, the child's behavior is first observed and then analyzed for events that may prompt the child to behave in certain ways. Interventions are then tailored to change the events provoking inappropriate behavior.

Pharmacologic Intervention

Medication is not a substitute for appropriate education and behavioral management but may be a useful adjunct and enable a child to make full use of other therapies. Medications are generally used to treat targeted, specific symptoms of autism. Medication is most often used to reduce self-injurious and aggressive behaviors, attention deficits, hyperactivity, compulsive behavior, psychotic symptoms, and affective lability (Tsai, 1999). A trial of any medication should include concrete, objective behavioral goals that are measurable and a predetermined time period for the use of the medication, during which its performance will be evaluated. At the end of this period, the parents and provider should have enough information to feel comfortable about a decision to either continue or stop the medication.

The primary care provider may want to consult a child psychiatrist, pediatric neurologist, or personnel from developmental disorders clinics for their expertise about antiepileptic and psychoactive medications that may be useful in treating specific behaviors. No medication has been approved by the US Food and Drug Administration (FDA) for use specifically in autism,

TABLE 13-1

Medications with Demonstrated Efficacy in Autism by Double-Blind, Placebo-Controlled Studies

Drug Name	Symptom Improvement	Comments
Haloperidol	Aggression, hyperactivity, irritability, stereotypes, withdrawal	No controlled data in adults
Pimozide	Aggression	No controlled data in adults
Risperidone	Aggression, irritability, repetitive behavior	No controlled data in children
Clomipramine	Aggression, irritability, repetitive behavior	
Fluvoxamine	Aggression, repetitive behavior	Controlled data in children not promising
Clonidine	Aggression, hyperactivity, irritability	Small studies
Methylphenidate	Hyperactivity	Small studies
Naltrexone	Hyperactivity	Modest effect, no effect on core symptoms of autism

From Posey, D.J. & McDougle, C.J. (2001, April). Pharmacotherapeutic management of autism. *Expert Opin Pharmacother, 2*(2), 587-600. Reprinted with permission.

and many of the medications used for children with autism are not approved for use in children, facts that should be disclosed to parents as part of the informed consent process. A growing number of studies have demonstrated the safety and efficacy of psychoactive medications in children but with small numbers of children and with some untoward effects and reactions reported (Tables 13-1 and 13-2).

Stimulants. Stimulants may decrease hyperactivity and impulsiveness and increase attention (Posey & McDougle, 2001; Tsai, 1999). Several very small studies of the use of methyphenidate (Ritalin) demonstrated an increase in attention but also insomnia and continued aggression in some children (Posey & McDougle, 2000). These side effects can be managed in some children with dosage reduction and the addition of an antipsychotic medication (Posey & McDougle, 2000). In children with autism and epilepsy, stimulants can lower the child's seizure threshold and precipitate an increase in seizures. This may necessitate an adjustment in the child's antiepileptic regimen or discontinuation of the stimulant. Longer-term controlled trials with larger numbers of children are needed to determine whether the psychostimulants are both safe and efficacious (Posey & McDougle, 2000). As with the use of any medication, a risk-benefit analysis can be useful.

Selective Serotonin Reuptake Inhibitors (SSRIs). Fluoxetine (Prozac) has been shown to improve behavior, cognition, language, affect, and social skills in some children with autism (DeLong et al, 1998; Fatemi et al, 1998; Posey & McDougle, 2000). Not all children treated responded, however, and some had increases in hyperactivity. DeLong and colleagues (1998) reported that a response to fluoxetine (Prozac) in their subjects correlated with a family history of a major affective disorder (i.e., bipolar disorder or major depression). Some studies with adults with autism suggest that fluvoxamine (Luvox) may reduce anxiety and obsessive-compulsive–like behaviors (AACAP, 1999; Elder, 2002). As a group, a number of the SSRIs seem to be somewhat useful for decreasing agitation, preoccupations, and restlessness (Tanguay, 2000). No SSRI has been shown to be more effective than any other (Tanguay, 2000). Fenfluramine (Pondimin) was originally thought to have a number of positive effects on behavior and learning in children with autism. Placebo-controlled studies have not confirmed these initial reports, and safety concerns about fenfluramine (Pondimin) have been raised. It is now specifically contraindicated in autism (Malone et al, 2002; Tsai, 1999).

TABLE 13-2

Medications with Possible Efficacy in Select Target Symptoms of Autism

Symptom	Medication
Inattention/hyperactivity	Alpha$_2$-adrenergic agonists
	Methylphenidate
	Antipsychotics
	Clomipramine
Aggression/self-injury	Alpha$_2$-adrenergic agonists
	Antipsychotics
	Anticonvulsants
	SSRIs
	Clomipramine
Sleep disturbance	Alpha$_2$-adrenergic agonists
	Antipsychotics
	Mirtazapine
	Clomipramine
Anxiety/agitation	Alpha$_2$-adrenergic agonists
	Antipsychotics
	SSRIs
	Mirtazapine
	Buspirone
	Clomipramine

From Posey, D.J. & McDougle, C.J. (2001, April). Pharmacotherapeutic management of autism. *Expert Opin Pharmacother, 2*(2), 587-600. Reprinted with permission.
SSRIs, Selective serotonin reuptake inhibitors.

Neuroleptics. Only haloperidol (Haldol) has demonstrated in more than one study that it is better than placebo at treating aggressive and self-injurious behavior in children with autism (Research Units on Pediatric Psychopharmacology Autism Network [RUPPAN], 2002). The risks of dyskinesias and extrapyramidal symptoms cause many clinicians to avoid prescribing haloperidol (Haldol) (Barnard et al, 2002). The new-generation neuroleptics, which include risperidone (Risperdal), olanzapine (Zyprexa), quetiapine (Seroquel), and ziprasidone (Geodon), are characterized by a lower incidence of tardive dyskinesia. They are now being tested and used in children with autism (Barnard et al, 2002; Posey & McDougle, 2001). As with all other medications used with children with autism, the response is variable, but some children achieve a marked reduction in the targeted symptoms of aggression, irritability, and repetitive behavior (Malone et al, 2002; Posey & McDougle, 2001).

In a multisite, randomized, double-blind trial with school-aged children with autism, risperidone (Risperdal) was found safe and effective for short-term treatment of tantrums, aggression, and self-injurious behavior (RUPPAN, 2002). There was no significant improvement in social skills or communication, however. The withdrawal rate from this study was 35% for children in the placebo group and only 6% in the risperidone (Risperdal) group, attesting to parent satisfaction with the treatment. Side effects included sedation, tremor, and constipation, all of which were time limited (RUPPAN, 2002).

The most significant side effect widely reported in studies of the new neuroleptics is weight gain, as much as 1 lb/wk. Although the risk of neuroleptic malignant syndrome, a potentially life-threatening side effect marked by hyperthermia and muscle rigidity, appears to be lower than with traditional neuroleptics, it can occur.

Other Pharmacologic Treatments. Carbamezapine (Tegretol, Carbatrol), divalproex sodium (Depakote), and lamotrigine (Lamictal) are anticonvulsants that may also be useful for decreasing irritability and aggression. There are case reports and small clinical trials regarding a variety of other medications frequently used in children with neuropsychiatric disorders. Clonidine (Catapres), naltrexone (Trexan), imipramine (Tofranil), trazodone (Desyrel), steroids, and buspirone (BuSpar) have all been reported to ameliorate the behavioral and social problems of some children with autism (AACAP, 1999; Elder, 2002; Tanguay, 2000). All these claims have been refuted by other studies. None of the studies, either in support of these medications or suggesting caution in their use, have been conducted with large enough populations or with appropriate randomization and control groups to definitively rule them in or out in the pharmacotherapy of autism.

Children with autism often require sedation for medical and dental procedures. Many medications used for sedation, however, produce paradoxic effects in children with autism (Sigman & Capps, 1997). Primary care providers may want to work with parents to give test doses of agents such as chloral hydrate and diphenhydramine (Benadryl) at home before attempting to use them for sedation for a medical or dental procedure.

Complementary and Alternative Therapies

Autism is a clinical, not laboratory-based, diagnosis. The deficits of autism are profound and to many parents seem to appear out of nowhere after their child has been developing typically. It comes as no surprise that parents have sought out and tried every possible type of treatment, and a number of alternative treatments for autism are available. They fall into three broad categories: those that are unproven but relatively benign (e.g., low-dose vitamin supplements), those that pose a risk to the child and family in terms of time and money that are redirected from treatments with some proven efficacy to those that may disrupt ongoing education and management (e.g., patterning and holding therapy), and those that present an actual danger to the child (e.g., injection of sheep brain extract) (AACAP, 1999).

Megadose vitamin B_6 and magnesium have been tried to improve speech and behavior (Rimland & Baker, 1996) but can cause diarrhea and peripheral neuropathy so their use should be monitored by a care provider. Dietary treatments include colostrum and gluten-free and/or dairy-free diets; the latter is currently the subject of a randomized, double-blind study (Elder, 2002). Intravenous immunoglobulin administration to 10 children with autism only led to significant improvement in one child, who reverted to his previous autistic behavior when treatment was stopped (Plioplys, 1998). Dimethylglycine (DMG), a dietary supplement, was found to be no different in improving behavior from placebo in a double-blind, placebo-controlled study (Kern et al, 2002).

Secretin, a gastrointestinal hormone, was proposed as a treatment for the social and communication deficits of autism after a report of a single child given a single injection of porcine secretin who appeared to show dramatic improvement in these areas (Carey et al, 2002). A number of studies, including a randomized, double-blind, placebo-controlled multisite study with 56 subjects, found no evidence that secretin improved the development of the children treated with either a single dose of porcine or synthetic secretin (Carey et al, 2002; Owley et al, 2001). It seems clear that placebo effect was involved in the early reports of the efficacy of secretin (Sandler et al, 1999).

In 1998 the Committee on Children with Disabilities of the American Academy of Pediatrics published a statement on the use of auditory integration training and facilitated communication for autism that concluded that these treatments are only warranted as part of research protocols.

Regardless of the alternative therapy the parents choose to use, the primary care provider should endeavor to become familiar with it and approach its use as objectively and compassionately as possible (Committee on Children with Disabilities, 2001a). Primary care providers can help the family set objective, measurable goals regarding the symptoms to be treated and assist in defining a length of time the treatment will be used before its efficacy is evaluated. Parents should be cautioned to try only one new treatment at a time so that any changes observed can be ascribed to the alternative therapy. The primary care provider must balance his or her role as an advocate and guardian for the child's well-being with a commitment to family-centered care (Committee on Children with Disabilities, 2001b).

Anticipated Advances in Diagnosis and Management

Numerous questions about autism are still in need of investigation. In 2001 the National Institutes of Health (NIH) announced a research grant program aimed at some of the key questions regarding autism (National Institutes of Health [NIH], 2001). Areas that the government identified as needing further research include epidemiology, early diagnosis, genetics, brain mechanisms, communication skills, cognition, and behavioral and biologic interventions (NIH, 2001). These studies must be scientifically rigorous and multidisciplinary and must enroll sufficient numbers of children and adults with autism to arrive at significant conclusions.

The quest for autism susceptibility genes is complicated by the complex and extremely variable behavioral phenotype of autism and the now-established genetic heterogeneity of autism (Monaco & Bailey, 2001). At times this appears to be an overwhelming task, but only 25 years ago it was believed that genes played no role in autism (Szatmari et al, 1998). Because of the wide continuum of behavioral phenotypes observed in autism, future research will need to include assessment of family members in order to delineate the boundaries of the milder phenotypes (Bailey et al, 1998). Primary care providers can assist with this search by referring families to genetics clinics for education regarding their recurrence risk and for direction to studies in which they might participate.

Neuroimaging and neuropathologic studies have discovered abnormalities in the brains of both children and adults with autism. Courchesne & colleagues (2001) believe that the unusual brain growth pattern they found with MRI may have important consequences for the consideration of infectious, immunologic, and environmental causes in the etiology of autism. Abnormal regulation of immunity by autistic genes may interact with environmental factors to produce central nervous system (CNS) pathologic findings that result in autism (Korvatska et al, 2002). The NIEHS (2002) has established two centers, one at the University of California at Davis and the other at the University of Medicine and Dentistry in New Jersey, to study environmental factors that may be related to autism. Neuropathologic studies may be advanced if families of children with autism who die for any reason are encouraged by primary care providers to consent to tissue donation by calling 1-800-BRAIN-BANK.

Psychopharmacology may be the answer to some of the most troubling behavioral manifestations of autism, although medications have not been shown to be effective in improving social and communication skills. There is a dearth of rigorously conducted, placebo-controlled, large, long-term studies of both the efficacy and safety of the many neuropsychiatric medications being tried empirically in children. Future research in psychopharmacology using systematic, double-blind, placebo-controlled studies of medications that will benefit individuals with autism is needed (Rapin, 2002).

Associated Problems

Approximately 90% of children with autism do not have autism that is caused by or associated with a specific medical disorder (Tanguay, 2000). Associated medical conditions (Box 13-5) increase in proportion with degree of mental retardation (Barton & Volkmar, 1998).

Mental Retardation

Children with autism may have IQs ranging from profound retardation to superior intelligence. Epidemiologic surveys

---

BOX 13-5
Associated Problems

Mental retardation
Epilepsy
Tuberous sclerosis
Fragile X syndrome
Tourette's syndrome
Psychiatric disorders

---

indicate approximately 80% of children with autism have mental retardation, with more severe retardation seen in children with associated medical conditions and more severely impaired social and language skills (Fombonne, 1999). The largest epidemiologic studies have shown that about 50% of children with autism are severely to profoundly retarded, 30% have mild to moderate retardation, and 20% have normal IQs (Fombonne, 1999). The rate of mental retardation may be trending downward as testing of children with challenging behaviors improves. Some small studies indicate that the rate may be closer to 50% than 80% (Bertrand et al, 2001). Children with autism usually have higher nonverbal than verbal IQ scores, and testing must be done by an experienced psychologist who can work with the child's potential negativity, distractibility, and comprehension difficulties (Geiger et al, 2002). Because a child's cognitive ability can help predict the child's future course and outcome, accurate assessment of a child's IQ provides the child's family with important information for treatment planning (Korkmaz, 2000).

Epilepsy

Twenty to twenty-five percent of people with autism have been reported to develop epilepsy (see Chapter 25), with a bimodal peak onset of seizures during early childhood and again in adolescence (Filipek et al, 1999). The risk of developing epilepsy is slightly higher in individuals with autism who are also profoundly retarded, which is consistent with the incidence of epilepsy in people who are profoundly retarded, and in children with tuberous sclerosis and autism (Filipek et al, 1999). One epilepsy syndrome, infantile spasms, may precede the onset of autism. In other cases of epilepsy in autism, the epilepsy is most likely a symptom of the same brain dysfunction that is responsible for the child's autism (Barton & Volkmar, 1998). As many as 8% of children with autism and without epilepsy have abnormal EEGs with epileptiform discharges (Tuchman & Rapin, 1997). Some children with abnormal EEGs may have behavioral improvement after treatment with a mood-stabilizing antiepileptic medication, such as divalproex sodium. Before an empiric trial of an antiepileptic drug, parents and the primary care provider or neurologist should determine measurable behavioral goals in order to assess the efficacy of the medication. Because of the high incidence of epilepsy in children with autism, primary care providers should not hesitate to obtain an EEG if parents report any behavior that could be seizures. Primary generalized, complex partial, atypical absence, and other types of seizures—alone or in combination—have all been reported (Rapin, 1997).

Tuberous Sclerosis

Tuberous sclerosis, a neurocutaneous syndrome, is found in 1% to 4% of individuals with autism and in as many as 8% to 14% of individuals with autism and epilepsy (Smalley, 2002), which is the most significant association between autism and a known, genetically determined medical condition (Lainhart & Piven, 1995). Epilepsy, particularly infantile spasms, and mental retardation are significant risk factors in the development of autism in tuberous sclerosis (Smalley, 2002). The mechanism for this association is unclear. The genes for tuberous sclerosis probably directly influence the development of autism, although it is possible autism susceptibility genes lie in close proximity to the tuberous sclerosis genes (Smalley, 2002). The primary care provider should thoroughly examine the skin of any child with autistic symptoms to look for the hypopigmented macules (i.e., ash-leaf spots) characteristic of tuberous sclerosis (Coleman & Gillberg, 1985).

Fragile X Syndrome

In a large review of 17 studies, the prevalence of autism in individuals with fragile X syndrome (see Chapter 26) was found to be 0% to 16%, with a mean of 4% (Dykens & Volkmar, 1997). Although many individuals with fragile X syndrome may exhibit some autistic traits (e.g., poor eye contact, vocal perseveration), relatively few meet the *DSM-IV* criteria for a diagnosis of autism (Feinstein & Reiss, 1998). Fragile X syndrome is an uncommon cause of autism, but the rate of this syndrome in individuals with autism is higher than in the general population (Feinstein & Reiss, 1998).

Tourette Syndrome

A large-scale prospective study found the prevalence of Tourette syndrome (see Chapter 40) to be 6.5% in children previously diagnosed only with autism, significantly greater than the general population rate of 0.5 per 1000 (Baron-Cohen et al, 1999). The Tourette syndrome found in these children had previously been overlooked in 100% of the cases (Baron-Cohen et al, 1999). In addition, one quarter of the children observed had either vocal or motor tics but not both; therefore they did not qualify for the diagnosis of Tourette syndrome (Baron-Cohen et al, 1999). Tics can be distinguished from the usual stereotypies of autism in a number of ways. Tics are typically short lived, interrupt the flow of behavior, are contextually inappropriate, and are seen more often in the face, shoulders, and arms than hands and fingers (Baron-Cohen et al, 1999). Alleviation of tics through medication can improve quality of life. Tourette syndrome also has an extensive family history. There may be some common etiologic factors at work in autism and Tourette syndrome (Baron-Cohen et al, 1999; see Chapter 40).

Psychiatric Disorders

A number of psychiatric conditions, including attention deficit hyperactivity disorder (see Chapter 12), obsessive-compulsive disorder, and mood disorders (e.g., depression; see Chapter 32) may co-exist with autism (Tsai, 1999). Clinical symptoms may vary with age, e.g., in early childhood hyperactivity, irritability, and stereotypies may be more common while aggressiveness and self-injury appear later in childhood (Tsai, 1999). Adolescents and adults, particularly higher functioning individuals, may develop depression and obsessive-compulsive disorder, which can cause further deterioration in their functioning (Tsai, 1999). It has been estimated that 24% to 43% of individuals with autism will have self-injurious behavior at some point in their lives (Tsai, 1999).

Landau-Kleffner Syndrome

Landau-Kleffner syndrome is not an associated condition of autism but is discussed here because of the interest in the autism community in this syndrome and the belief by many parents of children with autism that Landau-Kleffner syndrome might be responsible for their child's developmental problems.

Landau-Kleffner syndrome (i.e., a syndrome of acquired aphasia with convulsive disorder in children) was originally described in 1957 by Drs. Landau and Kleffner. It was based on six children they studied who had had normal language and development and then, after the age of 3 years, had rapid onset of aphasia accompanied by seizures. All the children subsequently recovered, most completely, over a period of weeks to several years. Recovery occurred spontaneously in some children and after treatment with antiepileptic medications and speech therapy in others (Landau & Kleffner, 1998).

Landau-Kleffner syndrome has two necessary symptoms, acquired aphasia and a sleep-activated epileptiform EEG maximal over the temporal regions (Tatum et al, 2001). The epilepsy of Landau-Kleffner syndrome, which occurs in about 70% of diagnosed individuals, is usually easily and well controlled (Tatum et al, 2001). Intelligence and social skills are preserved, and behavioral stereotypes are not seen. There may be behavioral problems, such as hyperactivity and personality changes, although it is not clear if these are a result of the Landau-Kleffner syndrome itself, the child's reaction to the sudden loss of well-established language skills, or both. The onset of the aphasia is rapid, occurring over days, and with receptive aphasia usually preceding expressive (Tatum et al, 2001). Evaluation and diagnosis require EEG monitoring of deep sleep that can only be accomplished with an overnight EEG, either in the home or as an inpatient in an epilepsy monitoring unit. Treatment usually involves antiepileptic medication, speech therapy, and often steroids. Surgery may be an option for children who do not respond to medication.

Other Conditions

Several epidemiologic studies over the past decade have concluded that there is no statistically significant relationship between autism and any other conditions other than those described previously. Specifically, phenylketonuria; congenital rubella and cytomegalovirus infection; lactic acidosis; purine disorders; autosomal and sex chromosome anomalies; and Williams, Möbius, Sotos and other syndromes have all been found with autism but at rates not exceeding their prevalence in the general population (Fombonne et al, 1997; Lauritsen et al, 2002; Tanguay, 2000). Autism can co-exist with Down syndrome (see Chapter 24), as it can with any of the disorders listed above, but without a causal relationship (Rasmussen et al, 2001). Children with Down syndrome and autism may have a delay of years until the diagnosis of autism is made, preventing them from receiving appropriate education and intervention (Rasmussen et al, 2001). Primary care providers must recognize that children with any medical condition might also have autism and that children with autism can also have another unrelated condition.

When possible, treatment of the co-morbid condition often results in an improvement in the child's autistic symptoms. In addition, information about associated problems—even when a problem cannot be treated—can be important for genetic counseling and educating the family about their child's diagnosis and prognosis (Gillberg & Coleman, 1996).

Prognosis

There is no cure for autism. It is a lifelong condition that cannot be outgrown, although all children with autism have the potential to learn and develop new skills. Children may learn self-care skills, how to play with toys rather than just ritualistically manipulate them, and how to tolerate small changes in their routines. The development of useful language and some social skills by the age of 5 years is the best predictor of future outcome, hence the emphasis on early diagnosis and early intensive treatment (Harvard, 2001).

The outcome for children with autism, similar to the expression of the syndrome itself, varies. At one end of the spectrum are individuals with average or above average cognitive abilities who have attended college, have careers, and can live independently. This group is a small minority, about 2% (Harvard, 2001). Fifteen to thirty percent are able to live semiindependently through the support of sheltered workshops and job and residence coaches funded by private and governmental agencies. About two thirds of adults with autism are totally dependent and must live either with their parents or in group homes or institutions (Harvard, 2001). Rarely is any adult with autism able to work at a job that requires social interaction or flexibility or be involved in intimate relationships. Even adults with average intelligence and academic achievement may have such serious social and judgment deficits that living completely independently is impossible (Rapin & Katzman, 1998). The one caveat to this rather grim picture is that these results are from adults not generally exposed to early, intensive, and continual therapeutic education and treatment. As research on autism continues and findings are put into clinical practice, more children may be able to function independently or semiindependently when they reach adulthood.

The development of useful language by the age of 5 years is an important prognostic factor (Korkmaz, 2000). Approximately one half of children with autism will not develop usable language (Mauk, 1993). Young children who demonstrate joint attention behaviors (i.e., communication signals such as pointing to direct someone's attention to an experience they want to share) are more likely to have better language skills. Children without language—either verbal or sign—by the age of 5 years are not likely to attain socially usable language skills. They function poorly socially and remain dependent as adults. A nonverbal IQ less than 50 in combination with the absence of meaningful speech by 5 years old is currently predictive of serious deficits that will be lifelong (Korkmaz, 2000).

The natural course of autism varies over time. It is unclear if children with autism present with symptoms during the first year of life. Most parents first report differences in a child's communication, social, and play skills during the second year of life. Children with milder autism, however, may not be diagnosed until school age. Many parents report that the behavior of children with autism is particularly problematic during the preschool years (Tonge et al, 1994). With intensive interventions, these children may experience an improvement in their symptoms as they enter the school-age years. The duration and intensity of the treatment required to produce positive changes have not been determined, nor have the characteristics of children most likely to respond to intensive treatment (AACAP, 1999). With the onset of puberty, many of a child's disturbed behaviors may reappear and then fade somewhat in adulthood (Wing, 2001).

Increases in behavioral disturbances (e.g., self-injurious, aggressive, obsessive, and anxious behaviors) have been reported in adolescents, as well as improvement in these symptoms (Korkmaz, 2000). A decline in functioning may be due to hormonal influences, the onset of other co-existing conditions, a response to increased demands, or their own increased awareness of their limitations (Tonge et al, 1994).

Individuals with autism have reduced life expectancy, with a greater reduction for girls compared with boys and with a mortality rate that increases with degree of mental retardation (Shavelle et al, 2001). Hyperthermia associated with neuroleptic malignant syndrome has caused the death of a few individuals with autism (Shavelle et al, 2001).

PRIMARY CARE MANAGEMENT

Health Care Maintenance

Growth and Development

Perhaps the most challenging aspect of monitoring the growth and development of a child with autism is enlisting the child's cooperation. Before a child's visit to the provider, consultation with the parents regarding the child's behavioral symptoms, fears, and likes can give the provider information to make the child's visit a success (Seid et al, 1997). With the parents' permission, the provider may also find it useful to talk with the child's teacher or behavioral therapist about the best ways to approach the child (Seid et al, 1997). Together, the provider and the parents can devise a plan for the examination that will help the provider and child begin to form a working relationship and lead the provider from the child's most to least favorite parts of the exam. A flexible unhurried approach is best. A reward at the completion of the exam can be planned, available, and referred to during the examination as necessary. Because many children with autism are highly distractible, time spent in the waiting room with other children and parents can leave them overstimulated and unable to fully cooperate. Therefore many providers find it best to schedule a child with autism as the first morning or afternoon appointment.

Children with autism may have their growth affected by disease symptomatology or pharmacologic therapies. Weight gain and height increases may falter as the result of decreased caloric intake secondary to restricted food preferences. The use of stimulant medication can decrease a child's appetite. Conversely, valproic acid and, especially, the atypical neuroleptics can result in unwanted weight gain because of their appetite-stimulating effects. Parents should be educated about the possible effects of medication on the child's growth and encouraged to monitor the child's growth and consult a provider if there are concerns. Parents of children taking the atypical neuroleptics need nutritional guidance as their child begins taking them, including advice to limit portion sizes and restrict snacks to water and low-fat foods. Children with risk factors for altered growth should be measured every 6 months.

Neonatal head circumferences are generally normal for children with autism (Courchesne et al, 2001). Large head circumferences occur in early and mid-childhood in about 25% of children with autism (AAP, 2001; Filipek et al, 2000). These large head circumferences are nonpathologic and do not require further investigation with neuroimaging unless the child's neurologic exam reveals focal or cranial nerve abnormalities (Filipek et al, 2000). Head circumferences should be measured until the age of 5 years and annually if a child also has tuberous sclerosis.

Routine screening for autism should occur at every well-child visit with one of the recommended screening tools: the Ages and Stages Questionnaire, the BRIGANCE Screens, the Child Development Inventories, or the Parents' Evaluation of Developmental Status (see Chapter 2; Filipek et al, 2000). The Denver-II is specifically not recommended because of its lack of sensitivity and specificity (Filipek et al, 2000). In addition to failure of any of these screening tools, further evaluation should begin immediately if a child has no babbling or gesturing by their first birthday, no single words by 16 months, or no two-word spontaneous (not echolalic) phrases by the second birthday (Filipek et al, 2000).

Children with autism generally develop normally or with differences too subtle to detect until 12 to 18 months of age (Mauk, 1993). Between 18 and 30 months of age, the child's parents and primary care provider often note abnormal or delayed social skill development, a red flag for autism (AAP, 2001). When combined with a language delay or reported developmental regression, referral for further evaluation is indicated (AAP, 2001; Filipek et al, 2000). As soon as the diagnosis of autism is considered, the child should be referred for a multidisciplinary developmental evaluation that includes thorough neuropsychologic, speech and language, and motor skill testing (AAP, 2001; Filipek et al, 2000). Primary care providers should not delay this referral in the hope that the child will "outgrow" a language delay.

The success of a child's treatment for autism is measured empirically. Therefore the child will need to be annually reevaluated by the multidisciplinary team during the first few years of treatment and thereafter every few years. These evaluations will serve as the basis for treatment planning.

Primary care providers should continue to monitor motor, cognitive, language, and social-emotional development at all well-child care visits, using a standardized developmental questionnaire completed by the primary caregiver and/or an objective screening tool of the primary care provider's choice (AAP, 2001).

Diet

Throughout the lifetime of a child with autism, parents, teachers, therapists, and providers are faced with decisions about when and when not to accommodate the child's insistence on sameness (Cohen, 1998). There is no one right answer for every child and family. Each family, with the help of their child's provider, should assess their own values, needs, and level of tolerance and make decisions accordingly.

Many children with autism have feeding and eating difficulties. Adequacy of dietary intake should be evaluated at each well-child visit. A small study comparing the intake of children with autism on a regular diet with those on a gluten- and casein-free diet found a substantial proportion of children

in both groups were not receiving recommended minimum nutrient intake (Cornish, 2002). An excessive adherence to routine and an abhorrence of changes in the environment may lead children with autism to reject their parents' efforts to provide them with a balanced diet. These children may have periods when they eat only one or a few foods (Wing, 2001). The hypersensitivity of some children with autism to smell, taste, and touch seems to result in the rejection of certain foods and food textures (Rapin, 1997; Sigman & Capps, 1997).

The feeding patterns of typically developing children have not been well studied, leaving uncertainty about just how abnormal the food rejection behaviors of some children with autism are (Ahearn et al, 2001). Some of these difficulties may be ameliorated through the interventions of the child's behavioral therapist. If the child insists on using certain dishes and cups for eating, the provider may advise the parents to have multiple sets of the preferred items. A daily multivitamin supplement is recommended to ensure adequate vitamin and mineral intake. Parents of children taking valproic acid and atypical neuroleptics should be encouraged to provide them with plenty of low-calorie, low-fat snacks and water instead of juice or soda, to prevent excessive weight gain.

Safety

The parents of children with autism are faced with a number of safety issues that arise from the cognitive and behavioral deficits of autism. Because of their poor judgment and lack of impulse control, children with autism must be supervised at all times. Their ability to recognize a potentially dangerous activity (e.g., tree climbing) is usually far behind their chronologic age and gross motor capabilities (Sigman & Capps, 1997). Children with autism have been known to swallow an entire bottle of medication in the time it takes a parent to turn away and answer the telephone.

Morbidity and mortality can be the result of momentary lapses in supervision. Deaths in children with autism during seizures, drowning, and suffocation were more than three times higher compared with the general population (Shavelle et al, 2001). Children between 5 and 10 years old were particularly at risk for premature death, perhaps because teenagers with autism engage in fewer high-risk behaviors such as driving and recreational drug use than their typically developing peers (Shavelle et al, 2001). Children with autism, especially those with autism and epilepsy, must never be left alone in a bathtub or near a spa or any body of water. Providers will often find that parents need education regarding this precaution. They often do not realize that "never" includes those few seconds it may take to answer the phone or doorbell. Supervision during swimming means a specific adult being assigned to watch the child with autism while in the water. Drowning has occurred when a group of children is swimming with a group of adults nearby but no single adult is responsible for observing the child with autism.

Childproofing the home of a child with autism is essential. Medications must be out of reach and securely locked. Other dangerous objects (e.g., knives, matches) must be kept out of reach. Hot stoves and liquids present a constant danger to children with autism.

Children with autism may develop self-injurious behaviors such as head banging, hand biting, and scratching or picking at their skin (Siegel, 1996). Some of these behaviors may be gentle and are probably self-stimulatory (Siegel, 1996). Other self-injurious behavior, however, can cause significant body harm, and parents must stop this behavior even if the child becomes aggressive. Parents of children with self-injurious behavior must work with the child's primary care provider and autism treatment team to devise a plan for responding to this behavior. This plan may include pharmacotherapy and behavior modification techniques such as immediate removal from the situation and a firm "no." Self-injurious behaviors are extremely upsetting to parents, so they will need a great deal of support and assistance as they attempt to manage and prevent these behaviors.

The presence of self-injurious behaviors is complicated by an apparent decreased sensitivity to pain in many children with autism (Rapin, 1997). That is, they may fail to respond with tears or a painful outcry to painful stimuli (e.g., a hot stove, a laceration). They often fail to approach their parents for comfort when they have been injured or are ill. Because of their lack of communication and social skills, the only sign that a child with autism is in pain may be an exacerbation of their autistic symptomatology. Children with autism have died from gastrointestinal bleeding and bowel rupture that may not have been diagnosed rapidly enough because of the child's inability to communicate. The provider must pay attention to parental reports that their child's behavior is different for no apparent reason because this may be the only clue that the child has suffered an injury or is in pain.

Immunizations

Children with autism should be vaccinated following the schedule recommended by the American Academy of Pediatrics, including receiving the MMR. Both *The Lancet* (2002) and the Centers for Disease Control (2002) have concluded that the evidence is in favor of the MMR being given to all children consistent with published guidelines.

Because of their insensitivity to pain and inability to report discomfort, children with autism may be given acetaminophen or ibuprofen prophylactically 1 hour before and periodically for 24 hours following the administration of vaccinations.

Children with autism who also have epilepsy should be vaccinated following the guidelines of the American Academy of Pediatrics for children with neurologic disorders (see Chapter 25).

Screening

Vision. A child with autism needs a thorough ophthalmologic examination at the time of diagnosis to look for the ocular signs of tuberous sclerosis: hypopigmented spots in the iris and choroid hamartomas. Following this initial screening, routine screening is recommended.

Hearing. Following an initial evaluation by an audiologist (which often requires BAER) to rule out hearing loss as a cause of communication delay, routine screening is recommended.

Dental. Routine screening is recommended. Children with autism who are also taking phenytoin for epilepsy are prone to development of gum hyperplasia and need to have their gums checked at least semiannually. Referral to a dentist familiar with treating children with developmental disabilities is essential. Some children with autism will not be able to tolerate routine dental screening and dental work without sedation.

Blood Pressure. Routine screening is recommended. Children with autism may take clonidine either to treat a concomitant tic disorder or to decrease hyperactivity and improve attention. Clonidine can cause both hypotension and hypertension. Blood pressure should be monitored before initiation of therapy. Lowering the dose of clonidine or stopping it completely must be done very slowly with blood pressure monitoring after each dose change. A rapid decrease in the clonidine dose can precipitate potentially dangerous rebound hypertension (Posey & McDougle, 2001).

Hematocrit. Routine screening is recommended. Children with autism who are taking carbamezapine or valproic acid should have complete blood counts (CBCs) with platelets before initiation of therapy and several weeks after establishment of the maintenance dose. These tests should be repeated annually and should also be done if the child develops symptoms of thrombocytopenia or liver dysfunction, such as unusual bruising or petechiae, unusual bleeding, jaundice, vomiting, or hepatomegaly.

Urinalysis. Routine screening is recommended.

Tuberculosis. Routine screening is recommended.

Condition-Specific Screening

Liver function tests (AST, ALT) should be performed before a child begins taking either carbamezapine or valproic acid. Several weeks after the maintenance dose is reached and annually after that, liver function tests and serum drug levels should be obtained. Slight elevations in liver functions are usually nonpathologic if asymptomatic and should be checked semiannually.

Common Illness Management
Differential Diagnosis (Box 13-6)

Because of their social, communication, and cognitive deficits, most children with autism cannot accurately report symptoms of illness to their parents or providers. Parents or caretakers of children with autism are the experts on their child's baseline behavior and level of functioning (Seid et al, 1997). Regression in a child's skills, a negative change in behavior, or self-injurious behavior is often the first indication that a child with

---

BOX 13-6
Differential Diagnosis

Communication and cognitive deficits make assessment difficult
Change in behavior may indicate underlying medical problem
Injury vs. sequelae from self-injurious behavior vs. nonaccidental injury
Seizures vs. repetitive or stereotypical behaviors of autism
Medication side effects (e.g., gastrointestinal symptoms, ataxia, lethargy, tremulousness)

autism is ill (Oliver & Petty, 2002). Therefore it is important for primary care providers to listen carefully to parental reports of children who are not behaving in their customary ways. Head banging or other self-injurious or aggressive behaviors may suddenly begin as a response to a painful illness, such as otitis media (Cohen, 1998).

Injury. Children with autism are at high risk for injury. The frequency of accidental injury may obscure the occurrence of nonaccidental injury that can result from caretaker fatigue and the extremely trying and sometimes dangerous behavior of a child with autism. Self-injurious behaviors (e.g., hand biting, head banging) can also cause injuries that may require both treatment of the injury and behavioral and pharmacologic intervention to prevent further injury.

Seizures. Children with autism may have any one of the various types of seizures: simple or complex partial seizures, absence seizures, or generalized tonic and/or clonic seizures. Many of the self-stimulatory behaviors seen in children with autism can appear to be seizure activity. Nonepileptic events, such as self-stimulatory behaviors, tics, and staring and inattention, can be differentiated from epileptic events in several ways. Nonepileptic events are usually asymmetric and arrhythmic, they can be interrupted by physical stimulation from the caregiver, and children remain responsive during them. Children who manifest signs of seizure activity (e.g., rhythmic jerking, stiffening, staring with unresponsiveness to physical stimulation, eye fluttering or deviation) should have an EEG at a diagnostic laboratory experienced in obtaining EEGs in children. An abnormal EEG indicates the need for referral to a pediatric neurologist (see Chapter 25). When there is suspicion that the child has experienced language regression that may be Landau-Kleffner syndrome, an overnight EEG to obtain deep sleep is necessary for diagnosis. This can be obtained as a 24-hour ambulatory EEG in the child's home or with a overnight inpatient stay in an epilepsy monitoring unit.

Medication Side Effects

Although there are no routinely prescribed medications for children with autism, many affected children take medications for controlling seizures or behavioral disturbances. Primary care providers should know what medications a child is taking and the common and adverse side effects and signs of toxicity of each. Although these medications will have been prescribed by the child's neurologist or psychiatrist, parents will call the primary care provider first if the child develops nausea and vomiting, ataxia, lethargy, tremor, or other potential symptoms of toxic drug levels. It is up to primary care providers to be aware of what medications, if any, a child is taking and their possible adverse side effects (Table 13-3).

Priapism is a potential adverse side effect of trazodone (Desyrel), so it should be used cautiously in postpubertal males (Kem et al, 2002).

Drug Interactions

The use of erythromycin in children taking carbamazepine should be avoided. Erythromycin increases carbamazepine blood levels, which can result in toxicity (see Chapter 25 for other antiepileptic drug interactions).

TABLE 13-3

Important Adverse Effects of Medications Commonly Used in Treatment of Autism

Medication	Important Potential Adverse Effects
Typical antipsychotics	Sedation, EPS, hyperprolactinemia, TD
Atypical antipsychotics	Weight gain, sedation, hyperprolactinemia, EPS (at high doses), TD (rare)
Clomipramine	Seizures, ECG changes, anticholinergic side effects
SSRIs	Activating effects, especially in children
Alpha$_2$-adrenergic agonists	Sedation, hypotension
Psychostimulants	Agitation and irritability in significant minority of patients, insomnia, weight gain
Anticonvulsants	Blood cell abnormalities, liver toxicity (often requires regular blood monitoring)

From Posey, D.J. & McDougle, C.J. (2001, April). Pharmacotherapeutic management of autism. *Expert Opin Pharmacother, 2*(2), 587-600. Reprinted with permission.
EPS, Extrapyramidal symptoms; *TD*, tardive dyskinesia; *ECG*, electrocardiogram; *SSRIs*, selective serotonin reuptake inhibitors.

Developmental Issues
Sleep

Sleep diaries kept by parents of children with autism show that their children sleep less and wake more frequently than typically developing children (Patzold et al, 1998). Many children with autism seem to need less sleep than other children their age and refuse naps, fall asleep late, awaken during the night, and stay awake for long periods (Siegel, 1996). As they get older, children with autism may repeatedly attempt to leave their room at night, causing parents to take them into their bed (Siegel, 1996). This disturbing sleep pattern may be related to circadian rhythm dysfunction and abnormally low levels of melatonin (Patzold et al, 1998). Comparing parental reports of their child's sleeping behaviors with actual monitoring of the children during sleep has shown, however, that children with autism differ from their typically developing peers only in awakening earlier (Hering et al, 1999). This discrepancy might be explained by parental hypervigilance regarding the sleep of their children with autism. In addition, it is now known that children with typical development or chronic conditions are much more likely to have sleep disorders than previously thought (Stores, 2001). Before embarking on medication management of reported sleep disturbances, the primary care provider should seek evaluation of the child at a sleep disorders clinic experienced in working with children.

Sleep disturbances may respond to behavioral intervention. Children with autism need highly structured bedtime rituals (Siegel, 1996; Wing, 2001) and may need a parent at their bedside until they fall asleep. Parents can gradually move themselves farther and farther from their child's bed until their presence is no longer needed. This is a process that may take weeks or even months (Wing, 2001). Because they may awaken and get out of bed during the night, their rooms must be safe and free of objects with which the children could harm themselves. Some children with autism learn to play alone in their room, even in the dark (Siegel, 1996). The door of the room must be secured, however, so that a child cannot wander about the house and engage in potentially dangerous behavior. A Dutch door is a useful alternative for some families. Parents will need reassurance that this aberrant sleep pattern is not unusual for some children, both with and without autism, and that it is alright for the child to be awake and playing at night.

Melatonin is the first-choice medication for sleep disturbances (Tsai, 1999). It is a naturally occurring hormone with few side effects. Doses of 1 to 10 mg have been found effective in some children with autism (Tsai, 1999). Antihistamines, such as diphenhydramine and hydroxyzine, can be tried next (Tsai, 1999). Parents have reported paradoxic effects in children with autism, however. When given as part of the bedtime ritual, trazodone may help the child both fall asleep and stay asleep (Siegel, 1996; Tsai, 1999). A child receiving a neuroleptic or tricyclic antidepressant for behavioral symptoms may derive some sedative effect from it if given in the evening. Trazodone (Desyrel) is a better alternative than neuroleptics or tricyclic antidepressants when they are only used to promote sleep because trazodone has fewer side effects. Trazodone should be taken with food to promote absorption. There is no evidence, however, that any medication helps without highly structured and consistent bedtime routines used simultaneously (Lord, 1998).

Toileting

Children with autism are often very difficult to toilet train and may not respond to toilet training before age 7 years (Tsai, 1999). Children with performance IQs below the equivalent of 30 months of age are generally not ready for toilet training, and parents should be advised not to initiate toilet training until this performance level is obtained (Siegel, 1996). Children with autism do not respond to many of the standard toilet training strategies parents use (e.g., being encouraged to imitate the parent or wear "big kid underwear") but can often be toilet trained by using a behavioral approach with food as a reward (Siegel, 1996).

Toilet training should be initiated by taking the child to the bathroom at set times when the child is most likely to urinate. These times include soon after getting up in the morning, after meals and snacks, before and after going to school, and before going to bed. It is helpful if all the child's caretakers work on toilet training together, using a very structured and consistent approach and including the same language and rewards. Parents should be advised that toilet training can take months or even longer if a child has both autism and mental retardation.

Discipline

Discipline is an all-day, every-day affair with children with autism. As questions arise about appropriate behavior management, providers will want to consult the child's treatment team. Parents will need guidance about establishing and prioritizing behavioral goals and target symptoms for intervention (AACAP, 1999). A highly structured and consistent environment is necessary for a child to learn socially appropriate behavior and refrain from dangerous behavior. Behavior modification techniques that can be taught to parents and other caregivers may be the most successful interventions for challenging behaviors such as tantrums, aggression, and self-injury (Tanguay, 2000). The use of positive reinforcers (e.g., play with favorite objects, food) is essential. Time-out for negative behaviors can also be employed if positive reinforcement is not totally successful. Negative reinforcement, such as a firm "no" and restraint or removal from the situation, may be necessary for potentially dangerous or self-injurious behaviors, but parents should be warned that children with autism do not readily generalize from one situation to another and often only attend to one very specific component of a situation (Cohen, 1998).

In certain situations, parents may feel the need to discipline their child with autism even when they are not sure that the child will understand the discipline. For example, Harris (1994) relates the story of a mother who sent her daughter with autism for a time-out after she broke her brother's favorite toy. Although she knew her daughter might not learn from the time-out, she thought it was important for her son to see his sister receive appropriate consequences for her actions.

Child Care

There are two types of child care that may be essential for children with autism: traditional child care during the hours the child's parents are working and respite care (i.e., care provided so that the child's parents may have time away from the constant responsibility of caring for their child with autism). In addition, families of children with chronic conditions have identified a third type of child care they need: care for their unaffected children during the time the parents are taking the child with the chronic condition to clinic appointments and therapy sessions (Garwick et al, 1998).

Children with autism are often easily overstimulated and can respond by withdrawing into self-stimulatory behaviors. They generally cannot interact with peers without teaching and supervision from adults. For these reasons, large-group child care is inadvisable unless a child has an accompanying aide to ensure that the child is appropriately occupied or the daycare provider has been taught specifically to care for children with autism. When both parents and daycare providers are educated and supported through lectures and on-site consultation, children with autism who attended child care with trained providers made significant gains in language as compared with children with autism whose parents and providers were not trained and supported (Jocelyn et al, 1998). Parents also expressed greater satisfaction with their child's care. Small family daycare arrangements can work well (Siegel, 1996). The daycare provider must be educated about the special behavior training and safety needs of the child with autism and willing to take on the challenge of integrating the child into activities with other children.

Therapeutic after-school programs are increasingly becoming available for school-aged children with autism and may be covered under the related services clause of the Individuals with Disabilities Education Act (IDEA; see Chapter 5). These programs feature a low staff/child ratio and activities designed to teach social skills and appropriate public behavior. Although some children with autism can be fully included in regular after-school programs, many find these programs too unstructured and unpredictable.

Respite care is sometimes provided in the home by a trained respite care worker. Out-of-home respite care is provided by a licensed worker in the worker's home or in a group home designed to provide short-term respite care (Howlin, 1998). The primary care provider can be instrumental in referring the family to local respite services. Parents may be reluctant to use these services because they are fearful that their child will not be adequately cared for and that their need for respite services is a reflection on their parenting. The provider can reassure the parents that by taking care of themselves and the other children in the family, they will have more energy with which to meet the needs of their child with autism. Respite care is also excellent practice for the transition to living away from home that many children with autism make in young adulthood.

Schooling

Public Law 101-426 has made free and appropriate education the right of every child in America. For children with autism, however, what is "appropriate" is often debated by educators, clinicians, and parents. School services that are available to children with autism vary widely but should always provide consistent structure and focus on developing functional communication and social skills and decreasing problematic behaviors (AAP, 2001).

Preschool and school-aged children with autism may be offered educational programs ranging from full inclusion in a standard classroom with an aide to time divided between a regular classroom and special resources (e.g., speech therapy) to placement in a special day class solely for children who qualify for special education. Children who are "fully included" are placed in regular classrooms, usually with the assistance of an aide (Elder, 2002). Regular classrooms may be overstimulating and make it impossible for the child with autism to attend and learn (AACAP, 1999). Although increased opportunities for socialization seem to exist in a class with typically developing children, research has shown that children with autism find it impossible to interact with their peers without specific guidance from adults and peers who have been taught how to play and work with children with autism (Laushey & Heflin, 2000). Children as young as kindergarten age can be trained to use a "stay, play, and talk" approach with their peers with autism in order to improve their social skills (Laushey & Heflin, 2000). Regardless of the setting, education for children with autism needs to take place year-round in a structured and predictable environment that limits the opportunities for repetitive and ritualistic behaviors and consistently rewards appropriate behaviors (AACAP, 1999; National Institute of Mental Health [NIMH], 1997).

Throughout a child's school years, parents need to participate in individualized education plan (IEP) meetings. During these meetings the child's school placement is determined. Parents must carefully evaluate all alternatives for their child, choose the one that they and the treatment team feel is most appropriate, and be prepared to present the reasons for their choice at the planning meeting because federal law neither guarantees the best education for the child nor adequately funds programs to provide the highest standard of care (Siegel, 1996). Many parents find it helpful to attend IEP training classes or bring a friend or advocate with them to IEP meetings.

Parents should work closely with their child's speech therapist and consider adding augmentative communication methods (e.g., pictures, sign language, computers) to their child's program if the child does not begin to develop functional language spontaneously. There is no evidence that introducing augmentative communication methods delays or prevents the development of spoken language; in fact, the evidence is to the contrary (Autism Society of America, 2002).

Primary care providers should work with parents and the child's educational team to ensure that regular evaluation of the various domains of the child's functioning occurs (AACAP, 1999). This includes addressing the child's behavioral adjustment, adaptive daily living skills, academic skills when appropriate, communication skills, and social interaction with family members and peers (AACAP, 1999).

Sexuality

Children with autism must be taught appropriate behaviors regarding their sexuality that are tailored to their developmental level and educated to refrain from the inappropriate behaviors they may exhibit. Because of their cognitive, communication, and social deficits, children with autism will not necessarily independently learn behaviors such as refraining from masturbating or undressing in public and shutting the door when using the bathroom. Two small studies found that a majority of adolescent and adult males and a significant minority of females with autism masturbated (Konstantareas & Lunsky, 1997; Van Bourgondien et al, 1997). Many of these individuals engaged in this and other sexual behaviors in community settings, although most were able to state that these activities should take place in their bedrooms. Specific rules about private behavior can be taught using repetition, redirection, positive reinforcement, and modeling. The parents of the individuals in this study reported that almost two thirds of their children had touched their private parts in public, and approximately one quarter had removed clothing in public or masturbated in public. There was no significant difference in the frequency of these behaviors between individuals with autism who were verbal and high functioning and those without language who were low functioning.

Primary care providers can work with parents to identify problematic sexual behaviors and solicit help from the child's treatment team in developing a plan to ameliorate them. No research indicates that teaching children with autism about their sexuality encourages the development of aberrant behaviors, although many parents fear this (Konstanareas & Lunsky, 1997). The provider can reassure parents that many children with autism display inappropriate sexual behaviors but that these behaviors can be dealt with using the behavior management techniques for nonsexual behaviors. To prevent the development of inappropriate behaviors, parents should be guided to teach their children very specific and concrete rules about acceptable and unacceptable sexual behavior throughout the child's life, not waiting until adolescence when such behavior may increase.

Transition into Adulthood

There is a paucity of research regarding adults with autism, especially compared with what is available regarding children with autism (Brereton & Tonge, 2002). Research has primarily focused on adults without cognitive deficits, although this is a minority of individuals with autism (Brereton & Tonge, 2002). What is known is that children with autism grow up to be adults with autism. For the majority of those with autism, it is a severely disabling condition into adulthood (Brereton & Tonge,

2002). Adults who have cognitive deficits in addition to autism will require lifelong care, support, and supervision (Lainhart & Piven, 1995; Wing, 2001). These services may include residential placement, sheltered workshop employment, continued education, and behavioral management (Ballaban-Gil et al, 1996; Wing, 2001). In their follow-up study of 102 children with autism, Ballaban-Gil and associates found that 69% continued to experience behavior problems in adolescence and adulthood. Over 90% of these individuals with autism still had social deficits. Despite one third of the children having near-normal to normal intelligence, only 11% of the adults had jobs—and all were menial. Previous follow-up studies done in the United States and Europe found even smaller proportions of the adults employed.

As treatment of autism has improved, so have these statistics. The National Institute of Mental Health (NIMH) (2002) states that about one third of all adults with autism can live and work in the community with some degree of independence. The persistent social deficits of autism (e.g., poor judgment in social situations, limited conversation skills, impaired problem-solving) preclude most adults with autism from completely independent employment and marriage. Work skills based on an individual's abilities, communication skills, and interests and that incorporates the adult's propensity for structure and repetition can be taught (NIMH, 2002). Most individuals with autism will qualify for SSI. Parents may be directed to their local Social Security office by either their child's school counselor or the primary care provider.

The parents of children with autism must be encouraged and counseled by their child's primary care provider to plan for the child's future. Education is mandated for children with significant disabilities until they are 22 years of age. At age 14 years, the parents and treatment team will need to begin planning the child's transition from school to sheltered or supervised work through a public or private community agency. Those few individuals able to attend college will still need a great deal of support and assistance with organization and planning. The end of mandated education may also be an appropriate time for a young adult to enter residential or community placement. Planning for this and locating a suitable home with an opening can take years. In early adolescence, the child's primary care provider should guide parents to begin exploring their options.

Finally, the pediatric primary care provider must help the parents find adult primary care for their child. As increasing numbers of children with developmental disabilities grow to adulthood and live and work in the community, family and adult providers will need to learn how to care for individuals who are often nonverbal and have continuing behavioral disturbances.

Family Concerns and Resources

Receiving a diagnosis of autism is intensely painful for most families. It may be months or even years from the time a toddler's delayed speech development is first recognized until the final diagnosis of autism is made. During this time, parents may have heard from several different providers in various specialties, including the child's primary care provider, that something is wrong with their child and it might be autism. The wait for the final diagnosis can be agonizing and delays implementation of appropriate interventions. The presentation of the diagnosis should be given in a setting that provides adequate time for discussion of test results and needs of the child and family (AACAP, 1999). Because there is no biologic marker for autism, the diagnosis is made based on neuropsychologic testing, careful history taking, and observation of the child's behavior. This relatively subjective way of diagnosing such a serious and lifelong condition is often difficult for parents to understand. This method of diagnosis, the apparently typical period of development of children with autism during the first year of life, and the lack of a cure have contributed to a plethora of alternative diagnostic procedures and treatments that parents consider pursuing. Primary care providers can play a crucial role in educating parents about the diagnosis, how it is determined, and the evidence-based treatments that are available.

Many health insurance plans exclude autism and mental retardation as conditions for which they will pay for behavioral health services (Peele et al, 2002). A number of states, which is growing, have enacted legislation requiring these conditions to be covered (Peele et al, 2002). Even when autism is a covered condition, many plans are reluctant to pay for the neuropsychologic testing necessary for the diagnosis and follow-up of a child with autism. Primary care providers must advocate for the child and family in pursuing appropriate referrals and payment for them.

All parents of children with autism should receive counseling to inform them of the fiftyfold risk of having another child with autism (Filipek et al, 1999). Referral to a genetics clinic is appropriate since knowledge about the genetics of autism increases constantly and there are a number of research studies involving families of children with autism of which family members should be made aware.

As families raise their child with autism, they will often meet professionals and lay people who view autism as a psychiatric disorder engendered by deficient mothering. Families will hear unkind remarks about their child's behavior and poor social skills and be given conflicting advice about how their child should be parented, treated, and educated. They will often have to struggle with school systems and after-school programs that are not designed to meet the special needs of a child with autism. Parents will need to educate all those who interact with their child about autism, their child's individual case, and the latest advances in the field of autism. In addition to educating parents, primary care providers will need to be open to receiving information from the parents about their child and the subject of autism in general.

Parenting a child with autism can be a tremendous physical, emotional, and financial challenge. A great deal of time and energy may be directed toward the child with autism and away from other relationships and family members—especially siblings (Harris, 1994; Tonge et al, 1994). Siblings may be embarrassed or afraid of the behavior of their sibling with autism and thus reluctant to bring friends home (Harris, 1994). Parents may be at increased risk for depression and stress-related illness, secondary both to possible genetic predisposition related to their child's autism and the strain of caring for a child with such deficient communication and social skills (AACAP, 1999). Siblings are at increased risk for developmental problems, also adding to the parents' burden (AACAP, 1999). Primary care providers can direct families to support groups, social services, and organizations that can address these issues.

ORGANIZATIONS

Autism Society of America
7910 Woodmont Ave, Suite 650
Bethesda, MD 20814-3015
(800) 3-AUTISM
http://www.autism-society.org

CAN (Cure Autism Now)
5225 Wilshire Blvd, Suite 503
Los Angeles, CA 90036
(213) 549-0500
http://www.canfoundation.org

NAAR (National Alliance for Autism Research)
414 Wall St, Research Park
Princeton, NJ 08540
(609) 430-9160 or (888) 777-NAAR
http://www.naar.org

INFORMATION

For information on research programs contact the following:
BRAIN
PO Box 5801
Bethesda, MD 20824
www.ninds.nih.gov

Clinic for the Behavioral Treatment of Children
(O. Ivar Lovaas, Director)
Department of Psychology
128A Franz Hall, PO Box 951563
University of California
Los Angeles, CA 90095-1563
(310) 815-2319

Division TEACCH
The Division for Treatment and Education of Autistic and Related Communication Handicapped Children
University of North Carolina, Chapel Hill
School of Medicine
310 Medical School, Wing E, CB 7180
Chapel Hill, NC 27599-7180
(919) 966-2174
http://www.unc.edu/depts/teacch/teacch.htm

The Family Connection
Beach Center on Families and Disability
31111 Haworth Hall
University of Kansas
Lawrence, KS 66045
(800) 854-4938
http://www.lsi.ukans.edu/beach/beachp.htm

National Institute of Mental Health
6001 Executive Blvd
Bethesda, MD 20892-9663
(301) 443-4513
www.nimh.nih.gov

Summary of Primary Care Needs for the Child with Autism

HEALTH CARE MAINTENANCE

Growth and Development

Height and weight are usually within normal range but maybe altered by medication side effects or restricted food preferences.

Measure head circumference annually until age 5 yr. If child also has tuberous sclerosis, annual measurement of head circumference should continue after age 5 yr.

Delayed language development is usually noticed between 18 and 30 mo of age.

Do not delay referral for diagnostic evaluation.

Diet

Child's insistence on sameness may affect food intake.
Well-balanced diet is encouraged.
Multiple vitamin supplements may be indicated.
Valproic acid may cause increased hunger and excessive weight gain.

Safety

Risk of injury is increased because of lack of impulse control, inability to generalize safety rules from one situation to another, and motor abilities more advanced than judgment. Constant supervision is required.

Childproofing the environment is required.

Self-injurious behavior can result in injury because of increased pain tolerance and inability to communicate injury.

There is an increased risk of drowning. Children with autism and epilepsy must follow safety guidelines for children with epilepsy, including no unsupervised baths or swimming.

Diagnosis of acute and chronic medical conditions can be delayed by child's inability to report symptoms.

Immunizations

Routine schedule is recommended, including MMR.

Children with autism and epilepsy should follow the guidelines for children with epilepsy.

Screening

Vision. Routine screening is recommended after initial ophthalmologic examination to look for signs of tuberous sclerosis.

Hearing. Routine screening is recommended after initial audiology evaluation, which may include brainstem auditory evoked response testing to rule out hearing loss as a cause of communication delay.

Dental. Routine dental care is recommended.

Children receiving phenytoin therapy require more frequent dental care for gum hyperplasia.

Sedation for dental care of the child with autism may be necessary.

Blood Pressure. Routine screening is recommended.

Children receiving clonidine therapy require blood pressure monitoring before initiation of therapy and with all dosage changes.

Hematocrit. Routine screening is recommended.

Children receiving carbamezapine or valproate therapy should have a complete blood count (CBC) with platelets done before

Summary of Primary Care Needs for the Child with Autism—cont'd

initiation of therapy, after establishment of maintenance dose, and annually thereafter.

Urinalysis. Routine screening is recommended.

Tuberculosis. Routine screening is recommended.

COMMON ILLNESS MANAGEMENT
Differential Diagnosis

Communication and cognitive deficits make assessment difficult.

Change in behavior can indicate injury or illness.

Injury. Cause of injury, accidental injury, self-injury, and nonaccidental injury must be determined and appropriate intervention identified.

Seizures. Seizure activity must be differentiated from repetitive or stereotypical behaviors.

Medication side effects must be considered.

Drug Interactions

Erythromycin can increase plasma levels of carbamazepine.

Developmental Issues

Sleep Patterns. Difficulty falling asleep and staying asleep is commonly reported by parents.

Highly structured, consistent bedtime rituals are a necessity.

Bedrooms must be thoroughly childproofed and secured so children cannot wander out alone or harm themselves at night.

Pharmacologic management using melatonin or antihistamines or scheduling trazodone, neuroleptics, or antidepressants for evening dosing may help with sleep.

Toileting. Training is often delayed.

Child must have performance IQ of 30 before training should be attempted.

Structured, behavioral approach with reward system is usually needed.

Mimicking parental behavior is usually not effective.

Discipline. Highly structured and consistent approach is necessary.

Continuous discipline is necessary because children with autism do not readily generalize from one situation to another.

Concrete positive reinforcement (e.g., food) is essential.

Negative reinforcement may be needed for dangerous behavior.

Child Care. Family daycare or therapeutic child care setting is recommended.

After-school care may be covered under the related services clause of the Individuals with Disabilities Education Act (IDEA).

Respite care can be important for primary caretaker and other family members.

Schooling. Early, intense intervention, which may include 1:1 teaching, is often needed and most effective.

Families will need support during the individualized education plan (IEP) process to advocate for their child.

Year-round structured schooling is important.

Augmentative communication methods are often helpful.

Parents must choose from a range of options from full inclusion to self-contained schools for children with autism.

Sexuality. Appropriate sexual behavior must be taught using behavior management techniques.

Specific and concrete rules about sexuality are necessary.

Transition into Adulthood

Most adults with autism require lifelong care, support, and supervision.

Work that involves concrete and repetitive tasks and little social interaction may be most suitable.

Most individuals will qualify for SSI.

Parents need to plan for child's future, including finding appropriate adult primary care.

Family Concerns

Diagnosis is based on neuropsychological testing and observation and appears relatively subjective; families may find it hard to comprehend.

Heath insurance plans often exclude behavioral health services for autism.

Lack of understanding of autism in the community contributes to lack of supportive services.

Siblings and others may be afraid of or embarrassed by behavior of the child with autism.

REFERENCES

Ahearn, W.H., Castine, T., Nault, K., & Green, G. (2001). An assessment of food acceptance in children with a pervasive developmental disorder—not otherwise specified. *J Autism Dev Disord, 31*(5), 505-511.

American Academy of Child and Adolescent Psychiatry. (1999). Practice parameters for the assessment and treatment of children, adolescents, and adults with autism and other pervasive developmental disorders. *J Am Acad Child Adolesc Psychiatry, 38,* 32S-54S.

American Academy of Pediatrics. (2001). The pediatrician's role in the diagnosis and management of autistic spectrum disorder in children. *Pediatrics, 107*(5), 1221-1226.

American Psychiatric Association. (1994). *Diagnostic and statistical manual of mental disorders* (4th ed.). Washington, DC: Author.

Autism Society of America. (2002). *Autism treatments;* Available: www.autism-society.org.

Bailey, A., Palferman, S., Heavey, L., & Le Couteur, A. (1998). Autism: The phenotype in relatives. *J Autism Dev Disord, 28*(5), 369-392.

Ballaban-Gil, K., Rapin, I., Tuchman, R., & Shinnar, S. (1996). Longitudinal examination of the behavioral, language, and social changes in a population of adolescents and young adults with autistic disorder. *Pediatr Neurol, 15*(3), 217-223.

Baranek, G.T. (1999). Autism during infancy: A retrospective video analysis of sensory-motor and social behaviors at 9-12 months of age. *J Autism Dev Disord, 29*(3), 213-224.

Barnard, L., Young, A.H., Pearson, J., Geddes, J., & O'Brien, G. (2002). A systematic review of the use of atypical antipsychotics in autism. *J Psychopharmacol, 16*(1), 93-101.

Baron-Cohen, S., Mortimore, C., Moriarty, J., Izaguirre, J., & Robertson, M. (1999). The prevalence of Gilles de Tourette syndrome in children and adolescents with autism: A large scale study. *Psychol Med, 29*(5), 1151-1159.

Barton, M. & Volkmar, F. (1998). How commonly are known medical conditions associated with autism? *J Autism Dev Disord, 28*(4), 273-278.

Bertrand, J., Mars, A., Boyle, C., Bove, F., Yeargin-Allsopp, M., et al. (2001). Prevalence of autism in a United States population: The Brick Township, New Jersey, investigation. *Pediatrics, 108*(5), 1155-1161.

Betancur, C., Leboyer, M., & Gillberg, C. (2002). Increased rate of twins among affected sibling pairs with autism. *Am J Hum Genet, 70,* 1381-1383.

Blatt, G.J., Fitzgerald, C.M., Guptill, J.T., Booker, A.B., Kemper, T.L., et al. (2001). Density and distribution of hippocampal neurotransmitter receptors in autism: An autoradiographic study. *J Autism Dev Disord, 31*(6), 537-544.

Bolton, P.F., Murphy, M., & MacDonald, H. (1997). Obstetric complications in autism: Consequences or causes of the condition? *J Am Acad Child Adolesc Psychiatry, 36,* 272-281.

Brereton, A. & Tonge, B.J. (2002). Autism and related disorders in adults. *Curr Opin Psychiatry, 15*(5), 483-487.

Carey, T., Ratliff-Schaub, K., Funk, J., Weinle, C., Myers, M., et al. (2002). Double-blind placebo-controlled trial of secretin: Effects on aberrant behavior in children with autism. *J Autism Dev Disord, 32*(3), 161-167.

Centers for Disease Control. (2002). *MMR vaccine and autism;* Available: www.cdc.gov/nip/vacsafe/concerns/autism/autism-mmr-facts.htm.

Chakrabarti, S. & Fombonne, E. (2001). Pervasive developmental disorders in preschool children. *JAMA, 285*(24), 3093-3099.

Charman, T., Baron-Cohen, S., Baird, G., Cox, A., Swettenham, J., et al. (2002).

Cohen, S. (1998). *Targeting autism.* Berkeley, CA: University of California Press.

Coleman, M. & Gillberg, C. (1985). *The biology of the autistic syndromes.* New York: Praeger Publishers.

Committee on Children with Disabilities. (1998). Auditory integration training and facilitated communication for autism. *Pediatrics, 102*(2, pt 1), 431-433.

Committee on Children with Disabilities. (2001a). Counseling families who choose complementary and alternative medicine for their child with chronic illness or disability. *Pediatrics, 107*(3), 598-601.

Committee on Children with Disabilities. (2001b). The pediatrician's role in the diagnosis and management of autistic spectrum disorders in children. *Pediatrics, 107*(5), 1221-1226.

Cornish, E. (2002). Gluten and casein free diets in autism: A study of the effects of food choice and nutrition. *J Hum Nutr Diet, 15*(4), 261-269.

Courchesne, E., Karns, C.M., Davis, H.R., Ziccardi, R., Carper, R.A., et al. (2001). Unusual brain growth patterns in early life in patients with autistic disorder. *Neurology, 57,* 245-254.

Croen, L.A., Grether, J.K., Hoogstrate, J., & Selvin, S. (2002a). The changing prevalence of autism in California. *J Autism Dev Disord, 32*(3), 207-215.

Croen, L.A., Grether, J.K., & Selvin, S. (2002b). Descriptive epidemiology of autism in a California population: Who is at risk? *J Autism Dev Disord, 32*(3), 217-224.

Dales, L., Hammer, S.J., & Smith, N.J. (2001). Time trends in autism and in MMR immunization coverage in California. *JAMA, 285*(22), 2852-2853.

Davidovitch, M., Glick, L., Holtzman, G., Tirosh, E., & Safir, M.P. (2000). Developmental regression in autism: Maternal perception. *J Autism Dev Disord, 30*(2), 113-119.

DeLong, G.R., Teague, L.A., & Kamran, M.M. (1998). Effects of fluoxetine treatment in young children with idiopathic autism. *Dev Med Child Neurol, 40,* 551-562.

Dykens, E.M. & Volkmar, F.R. (1997). Medical conditions associated with autism. In D.J. Cohen & F.R. Volkmar (Eds.). *Handbook of autism and pervasive developmental disorders* (2nd ed). New York: Wiley.

Elder, J.H. (2002). Current treatments in autism: Examining scientific evidence and clinical implications. *J Neurol Nurs, 34*(2), 67-73.

Fatemi, S.H., Stary, J.M., Halt, A.R., & Realmuto, G.R. (2001). Dysregulation of reelin and Bcl-2 proteins in autistic cerebellum. *J Autism Dev Disord, 31*(6), 529-536.

Fatemi, S.H., Realmuto, G.M., Khan, L., & Thuras, P. (1998). Fluoxetine in treatment of adolescent patients with autism: A longitudinal open trial. *J Autism Dev Disord, 28*(4), 303-307.

Feinstein, C. & Reiss, A.L. (1998). Autism: The point of view from fragile X studies. *J Autism Dev Disord, 28*(5), 393-405.

Filipek, P.A., Accardo, P.J., Ashwal, S., Baranek, G.T., Cook, E.H., Jr., et al. (2000). Practice parameter: Screening and diagnosis of autism. *Neurology, 55,* 468-479.

Filipek, P.A., Accardo, P.J., Baranek, G.T., Cook, E.H., Jr., Dawson, G., et al. (1999). The screening and diagnosis of autistic spectrum disorders. *J Autism Dev Disord, 29*(6), 439-484.

Folstein, S.E. & Rosen-Sheidley, B. (2001). Genetics of autism: Complex aetiology for a heterogeneous disorder. *Nat Rev Genet, 2*(12), 943-955.

Fombonne, E. (1999). The epidemiology of autism: A review. *Psychol Med, 29*(4), 769-786.

Fombonne, E. & Chakrabarti, S. (2001). No evidence for a new variant of measles-mumps-rubella-induced autism. *Pediatrics, 108*(4), e58.

Fombonne, E., Du Mazaubrun, C., Cans, C., & Grandjean, H. (1997). Autism and associated medical disorders in a French epidemiological survery. *J Am Acad Child Adolesc Psychiatry, 36,* 1561-1569.

Garwick, A.W., Kohrman, C., Wolman, C., & Blum, R.W. (1998). Families' recommendations for improving services for children with chronic conditions. *Arch Pediatr Adolesc Med, 152*(5), 440-448.

Geiger, D.M., Smith, D.T., & Creaghead, N.A. (2002). Parent and professional agreement on cognitive level of children with autism. *J Autism Dev Disord, 32*(4), 307-312.

Gillberg, C. & Coleman, M. (1996). Autism and medical disorders: A review of the literature. *Dev Med Child Neurol, 38,* 191-202.

Glascoe, F.P. (1997). Parents' concerns about children's development: Prescreening technique or screening test? *Pediatrics, 99*(4), 522-528.

Greenberg, D.A., Hodge, S.E., Sowinski, J., & Nicoll, D. (2001). Excess of twins among affected sibling pairs with autism: Implications for the etiology of autism. *Am J Hum Genet, 69*(5), 1062-1067.

Gresham, F.M. & MacMillan, D.L. (1998). Early intervention project: Can its claims be substantiated and its effects replicated? *J Autism Dev Disord, 28*(1), 5-13.

Hardan, A.Y., Minshew, N.J., Mallikarjuhn, M., & Keshavan, M.S. (2001). Brain volume in autism. *J Child Neurol, 16*(6), 421-424.

Harris, J.C. (1995). *Developmental neuropsychiatry: assessment, diagnosis, and treatment of developmental disorders* (Vol 2). Oxford: Oxford University Press.

Harris, S.L. (2000). Age and IQ at intake as predictors of placement for young children with autism: A four-to six-year follow-up. *J Autism Dev Disord, 30*(2), 137-142.

Harris, S.L. (1994). *Siblings of children with autism.* Bethesda, Md: Woodbine House.

Harvard Mental Health Letter. (2001). Autism–Part II, Harvard Health Online. Available: www.health.harvard.edu/medline/Mental/M701a.html.

Hering, E., Epstein, R., Elroy, S., Iancu, D.R., & Zelnik, N. (1999). Sleep patterns in autistic children. *J Autism Dev Disord, 29*(2), 143-147.

Hornig, M. & Lipkin, W.I. (2001). Infectious and immune factors in the pathogenesis of neurodevelopmental disorders: Epidemiology, hypotheses, and animal models. *MRDD Research Reviews, 7,* 200-210.

Howlin, P. (1998). Practitioner review: Psychological and educational treatments for autism. *J Child Psychol Psychiatry, 39*(3), 307-322.

Howlin, P. & Moore, A. (1997). Diagnosis in autism: A survey of over 1200 patients in the UK. *Autism, 1,* 135-162.

Hwang, B. & Hughes, C. (2000). The effects of social interactive training on early social communicative skills of children with autism. *J Autism Dev Disord, 39*(4), 331-343.

Hyman, S.L., Rodier, P.M., & Davidson, P. (2001). Pervasive developmental disorders in young children. *JAMA, 285*(24).

Jocelyn, L.J., Casiro, O.G., Beattie, D., Bow, J., & Kneisz, J. (1998). Treatment of children with autism: A randomized controlled trial to evaluate a caregiver-based intervention program in community day-care centers. *J Dev Behav Pediatr, 19*(5), 326-334.

Juul-Dam, N., Townsend, J., & Courchesne, E. (2001). Prenatal, perinatal, and neonatal factors in autism, pervasive developmental disorder—not otherwise specified, and the general population. *Pediatrics, 107*(4), e63.

Kadesjo, B., Gillberg, C., & Hagberg, B. (1999). Brief report: Autism and Asperger syndrome in seven-year-old children: A total population study. *J Autism Dev Disord, 29*(4), 327-331.

Kanner, L. (1943). Autistic disturbances of affective contact. *The Nervous Child, 2,* 217-250.

Kaye, J.A., del Mar Melero-Montes, M., & Jick, H. (2001). Mumps, measles, and rubella vaccine and the incidence of autism recorded by general practitioners: A time trend analysis. *BMJ, 322*(7284), 460-463.

Kem, D.L., Posey, D.J., & McDougle, J. (2002). Priapism associated with trazodone in an adolescent with autism. *J Am Acad Child Adol Psychiatry, 41,* 758.

Kemper, T.L. & Bauman, M. (1998). Neuropathology of infantile autism. *J Neuropathol Exp Neurol, 57*(7), 645-652.

Kern, J.K., Van Miller, S., Evans, P.A., & Trivedi, M.H. (2002). Efficacy of porcine secretin in children with autism and pervasive developmental disorder. *J Autism Dev Disord, 32*(3), 153-160.

Konstantareas, M.M. & Lunsky, Y.J. (1997). Sociosexual knowledge, experience, attitudes, and interests of individuals with autistic disorder and developmental delay. *J Autism Dev Disord, 27*(4), 397-413.

Korkmaz, B. (2000). Infantile autism: Adult outcome. *Semin Clin Neuropsychiatry, 5*(3), 164-170.

Korvatska, E., Van de Water, J., Anders, T.F., & Gershwin, M.E. (2002). Genetic and immunologic considerations in autism. *Neurobiol Dis, 9*, 107-125.

Lainhart, J.E. & Piven, J. (1995). Diagnosis, treatment, and neurobiology of autism in children. *Curr Opin Pediatr, 7*, 392-400.

Lancet. (2002). Time to look beyond MMR in autism research. *Lancet, 359*, 637.

Landau, W.M. & Kleffner, F.R. (1998). Syndrome of acquired aphasia with convulsive disorder in children. *Neurology, 51*(5), 1241-1249.

Lauritsen, M.B., Mors, O., Mortensen, P.B., & Ewald, H. (2002). Medical disorders among inpatients with autism in Denmark according to ICD-8: A nationwide register-based study. *J Autism Dev Disord, 32*(2), 115-119.

Laushey, K.M. & Heflin, L.J. (2000). Enhancing social skills of kindergarten children with autism through the training of multiple peers as tutors. *J Autism Dev Disord, 30*(3), 183-193.

Lord, C. (1998). What is melatonin? Is it a useful treatment for sleep problems in autism? *J Autism Dev Disord, 28*(4), 345-346.

Lovaas, O. (1987). Behavioral treatment and normal educational and intellectual functioning in young autistic children. *J Consult Clin Psychol, 55*(1), 162-164.

Magnusson, P. & Saemundsen, E. (2001). Prevalence of autism in Iceland. *J Autism Dev Disord, 31*(2), 152-163.

Malone, R.P., Maislin, G., Choudhury, M.S., Gifford, C., & Delaney, M.A. (2002). Risperidone treatment in children and adolescents with autism: Short- and long-term safety and effectiveness. *J Am Acad Child Adolesc Psychiatry, 41*, 140-147.

Mauk, J.E. (1993). Autism and pervasive developmental disorders. *Child Dev Disabil, 40*(3), 567-587.

Monaco, A.P. & Bailey, A.J. (2001). The search for susceptibility genes. *Lancet, 358*(1), 3.

Murphy, M., Bolton, P.F., Pickles, A., Fombonne, E., Piven, J., et al. (2000). Personality traits of the relatives of autistic probands. *Psychol Med, 30*(6), 1411-1425.

National Institutes of Health. (2001). *Program announcement number PA-01-051.* Available: http://grants.nih.gov/grants/guide/pa-files/PA-01-051.html.

National Institutes of Health. (2002). *Research on autism and autism spectrum disorders;* Available: http://grants.nih.gov/grants/guide/pa-files/PA-01-051.html.

National Institute of Mental Health. (2002). *Autism.* Available: http://www.nim.nih.gov/publicat/autism.cfm.

National Institute of Neurological Disorders and Stroke. (2002). *Autism fact sheet.* Available: http://www.ninds.nih.gov/health_and_medical/pubs/autism.htm.

NIEHS News. (2002). New centers to focus on autism and other developmental disorders. *Environ Health Perspect, 110*(1). Available: ehpnet1.niehs.nih.gov/docs/2002/110-1/niehsnews.html.

Oliver, C. & Petty, J. (2002). Self-injurious behavior in people with intellectual disability. *Curr Opin Psychiatry, 15*(5), 477-481.

Owley, T., McMahon, W., Cook, E.H., Laulhere, T., South, M., et al. (2001). Multisite, double-blind, placebo-controlled trial of porcine secretin in autism. *J Am Acad Child Adolesc Psychiatry, 40*, 1293-1299.

Patzold, L.M., Richdale, A.L., & Tonge, B.J. (1998). An investigation into sleep characteristics of children with autism and Asperger's disorder. *J Paediatr Child Health, 34*(6), 528-533.

Peele, P.B., Lave, J.R., & Kelleher, K.J. (2002). Exclusions and limitations in children's behavioral health care coverage. *Psychiatr Serv, 53*(5), 591-594.

Plioplys, A.V. (1998). Intravenous immunoglobulin treatment of children with autism. *J Child Neurol, 13*, 79-82.

Posey, D.J. & McDougle, C.J. (2001). Pharmacotherapeutic management of autism. *Expert Opin Pharmacother, 2*(4), 587-600.

Posey, D.J. & McDougle, C.J. (2000). The pharmacotherapy of target symptoms associated with autistic disorders and other pervasive developmental disorders. *Harv Rev Psychiatry, 8*(2), 45-63.

Rapin, I. (2002). The autistic-spectrum disorders. *N Engl J Med, 347*(5), 302-303.

Rapin, I. (1997). Autism. *N Engl J Med, 337*(2), 97-104.

Rapin, I. & Katzman, R. (1998). Neurobiology of autism. *Ann Neurol, 43*, 7-14.

Rasmussen, P., Borjesson, O., Wentz, E., & Gillberg, C. (2001). Autistic disorders in Down syndrome: Background factors and clinical correlates. *Dev Med Child Neurol, 43*(11), 750-754.

Research Units on Pediatric Psychopharmacology Autism Network (RUPPAN). (2002). Risperidone in children with autism and serious behavioral problems. *N Engl J Med, 347*(5), 314-321.

Rimland, B. & Baker, S.M. (1996). Brief report: Alternative approaches to the development of effective treatments for autism. *J Autism Dev Disord, 26*(2), 237-241.

Robins, D.L., Fein, D., Barton, M.L., & Green, J.A. (2001). The Modified Checklist for Autism in Toddlers: An initial study investigating the early detection of autism and pervasive developmental disorders. *J Autism Dev Disord, 31*(2), 131-144.

Rodier, P.M. (2000). The early origins of autism. *Sci Am, 282*(2), 56-63.

Rodier, P.M. (2002). Environmental influences as etiologic factors in autism. National Institute of Child Health and Human Development NIH/ACC 2001 Conference. Available: http://www.nichd.nih.gov/autism/abstracts/rodier.htm.

Rogers, S.J. (2000). Interventions that facilitate socialization in children with autism. *J Autism Dev Disord, 30*(5), 399-409.

Sandler, A.D., Sutton, K.A., DeWeese, J., Girardi, M.A., Shepard, V., et al. (1999). Lack of benefit of a single dose of synthetic human secretin in the treatment of autism and pervasive developmental disorder. *N Engl J Med, 341*, 1801-1806.

Scambler, D., Rogers, S.J., & Wehner, E.A. (2001). Can the Checklist for Autism in Todldlers differentiate young children with autism from those with developmental disabilities? *J Am Acad Child Adolesc Psychiatry, 40*, 1457-1463.

Seid, M., Sherman, M., & Seid, A.B. (1997). Perioperative psychosocial interventions for autistic children undergoing ENT surgery. *Int J Pediatr Otorhinolaryngol, 40*, 107-113.

Shavell, R.M., Strauss, D.J., & Pickett, J. (2001). Causes of death in autism. *J Autism Dev Disord, 31*(6), 560-576.

Sheinkopf, S.J. & Siegel, B. (1998). Home-based behavioral treatment of young children with autism. *J Autism Dev Disord, 28*(1), 15-23.

Shevell, M.I., Majnemer, A., Rosenbaum, P., & Abrahamowicz, M. (2001). Etiologic yield of autistic spectrum disorders: A prospective study. *J Child Neurol, 16*(7), 509-512.

Siegel, B. (1996). *The world of the autistic child.* Oxford, England: Oxford University Press.

Sigman, M. & Capps, L. (1997). *Children with autism.* Cambridge, Mass: Harvard University Press.

Slager, S.L., Foroud, T., Haghighi, F., Spence, M.A., & Hodge, S.E. (2001). Stoppage: An issue for segregation analysis. *Genet Epidemiol, 20*(3), 328-339.

Smalley, S.L. (2002). Autism and tuberous sclerosis. *J Autism Dev Disord, 28*(5), 407-414.

Sparks, B.F., Friedman, S.D., Shaw, D.W., Aylward, E.H., Echelard, D., et al. (2002). Brain structural abnormalities in young children with autism spectrum disorder. *Neurology, 59*(2), 184-192.

Stores, G. (2001). *A clinical guide to sleep disorders in children and adolescents.* New York: Cambridge University Press.

Szatmari, P., Jones, M.B., Zwaigenbaum, L., & MacLean, J.E. (1998). Genetics of autism: Overview and new directions. *J Autism Dev Disord, 28*(5), 351-368.

Tanguay, P. (2000). Pervasive developmental disorders: A 10-year review. *J Am Acad Child Adolesc Psychiatry, 39*, 1079-1095.

Tatum, W., Genton, P., Bureau, M., Dravet, C., & Roger, J. (2001). Less common epilepsy syndromes. In E. Wylie (Ed.). *The treatment of epilepsy: Principles and practice* (3rd ed.). Philadelphia: Lippincott Willliams & Wilkins.

Taylor, B., Miller, E., Lingam, R., Andrews, N., Simmons, A., et al. (2002). Measles, mumps, and rubella vaccination and bowel problems or developmental regression in children with autism: Population study. *BMJ, 324*, 393-396.

Tonge, B.J., Dissanayake, C., & Brereton, A.V. (1994). Autism: Fifty years on from Kanner. *J Paediatr Child Health, 30*, 102-107.

Tsai, L.Y. (1999). Psychopharmacology in autism. *Psychosom Med, 61*(5), 651.

Tuchman, R.T. & Rapin, I. (1997). Regression in pervasive developmental disorders: Seizures and epileptiform electroencephalogram correlates. *Pediatrics, 99*(4), 56-66.

Van Bourgondien, M.E., Reichle, N.C., & Palmer, A. (1997). Sexual behavior in adults with autism. *J Autism Dev Disord, 27*(2), 113-125.

Wakefield, A.J., Murch, S.H., Anthony, A., Linnell, J., Casson, et al. (1998). Ileal-lymphoid-nodular hyperplasia, non-specific colitis, and pervasive developmental disorder in children. *Lancet, 351,* 637-641.

Wing, L. (2001). *The autistic spectrum.* Berkeley, Calif: Ulysses Press.

World Health Organization. (1994). *International classification of diseases* (10th rev). Geneva: Author.

Zwaigenbaum, L., Szatmari, P., Jones, M.B., Bryson, S.E., MacLean, J.E., et al. (2002). Pregnancy and birth complications in autism and liability to the broader autism phenotype. *J Am Acad Child Adolesc Pschyiatry, 41,* 572-579.

14 Bleeding Disorders

Susan Karp

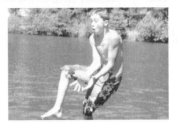

Etiology

Hemophilia and von Willebrand disease are the most common inherited bleeding disorders resulting from deficiencies or abnormalities of specific coagulation proteins. The von Willebrand protein is activated when the endothelium is damaged. This protein promotes formation of an initial platelet plug by enabling platelet adhesion. Multiple coagulation proteins, including those that are deficient in individuals with hemophilia, are critical components of the secondary or intrinsic hemostatic mechanism that is activated when collagen fibers are exposed in a damaged blood vessel. These proteins are required for the formation of the final fibrin clot (Jones, 2002; Mannucci et al, 2002).

Hemophilia

Hemophilia involves a defect in the intrinsic hemostatic mechanism (Figure 14-1; Jones, 2002). Factor VIII deficiency (e.g., classic hemophilia, hemophilia A) accounts for approximately 80% to 85% of hemophilia cases, whereas factor IX deficiency (e.g., Christmas disease, hemophilia B) accounts for 15% to 20% of such cases (Kulkarni & Lusher, 2001). Less common factor deficiencies exist but are not specifically discussed in this chapter. Severity of hemophilia is defined by the percentage of activity of the deficient coagulation protein (Table 14-1).

von Willebrand Disease

Generally a mild bleeding disorder, von Willebrand disease is closely related to hemophilia. The von Willebrand factor, a high–molecular weight glycoprotein, plays an essential role in the initiation of hemostasis by promoting platelet adhesion (Figure 14-1). Von Willebrand factor carries factor VIII in plasma; and when von Willebrand protein is deficient, the amount of circulating factor VIII may also be reduced. Thus individuals with von Willebrand disease usually have a dual hemostatic defect characterized by a prolonged bleeding time (secondary to poor platelet adhesion) and low plasma factor VIII levels (Jones, 2002; Rodeghiero, 2002).

Three main variants of the disorder exist (Rodeghiero, 2002). In the most common and generally the mildest variant, type 1, there is a partial quantitative deficiency of von Willebrand factor. In type 2 (which includes subtypes 2A, 2B, 2M, and 2N), there is a qualitative deficiency of the von Willebrand factor. It is important to note that individuals with subtype 2B should not be treated with desmopressin (DDAVP). The potential for thrombocytopenia with desmopressin use in subtype 2B, in which the large multimers are absent in the plasma, should be noted (Batlle et al, 2002).

Known Genetic Etiology

Hemophilia is inherited in an X-linked pattern (Figure 14-2). Most frequently, female carriers pass the disorder to their sons. The severity of hemophilia remains constant within families, although clinical symptoms may vary based on lifestyle and treatment regimens. Approximately one third of all hemophilia cases are sporadic (e.g., negative prior family history; Kulkarni & Lusher, 2001). A woman is considered to be an obligate carrier if hemophilia has been diagnosed in her father, two of her sons, or one son and one other relative. Carriers of hemophilia A or B are expected to have, on average, factor VIII or IX levels that are approximately 50% of normal. Because of lyonization, however, some carriers have very low factor levels with resultant symptoms of excessive or unusual bleeding—particularly menorrhagia, which validates the need for determination of factor VIII/IX coagulant levels—even in obligate carriers (Lee, 1999; Miller, 1999).

A single performance of carrier testing for hemophilia using a factor VIII coagulant/antigen ratio has an accuracy rate of approximately 90% (Shetty et al, 1999). The use of deoxyribonucleic acid (DNA) testing to detect carriers has an estimated accuracy of 95% to 99%, depending on the number of probes used. However, it is expensive and requires blood samples from an affected male (Ljung, 1999; Lozier & Kessler, 2000). The factor VIII inversion is a genetic defect found in approximately 50% of people with severe hemophilia A and occurs when the distal end of the X chromosome containing part of the factor VIII gene flips over so that the factor VIII message is interrupted by irrelevant genetic material. If an affected male has this inversion, all female relatives who are carriers will also have it. This inversion test has an accuracy rate of 100% (Ljung, 1999). Carrier testing for factor IX hemophilia using DNA analysis is also available (Ljung, 1999).

Prenatal diagnosis may be performed by amniocentesis as early as 13 to 16 weeks' gestation, by chorionic villus sampling at 10 to 13 weeks' gestation, or by fetal blood sampling (i.e., using percutaneous umbilical blood sampling) at 18 to 20 weeks' gestation. Male fetuses can be diagnosed as having hemophilia in utero by the use of DNA testing or the inversion test. If percutaneous umbilical blood sampling is performed, the hemophilia diagnosis is made by either DNA testing or a factor VIII or IX level (Kulkarni & Lusher, 2001).

In von Willebrand disease inheritance of types 1 and 2 is autosomal dominant. Type 3 is a severe autosomal recessive form of the disorder marked by the absence of detectable von Willebrand factor (Almeida et al, 2002). Decreased penetrance and variable expressivity are peculiar to type 1 disease (Jones, 2002; Rodeghiero, 2002).

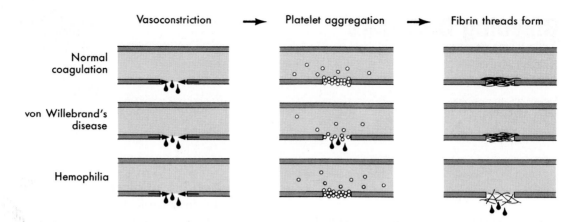

FIGURE 14-1 Comparison of the defect in hemophilia and von Willebrand disease with normal coagulation after a break in a vessel wall. Defect in von Willebrand disease is in platelet aggregation. Defect in hemophilia is in fibrin thread formation.

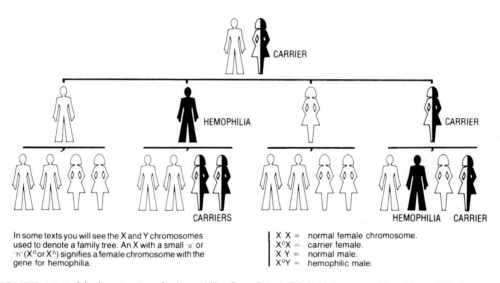

In some texts you will see the X and Y chromosomes used to denote a family tree. An X with a small "o" or "h" (X°or Xʰ) signifies a female chromosome with the gene for hemophilia.

X X =	normal female chromosome.
X°X =	carrier female.
X Y =	normal male.
X°Y =	hemophilic male.

FIGURE 14-2 Inheritance pattern for hemophilia. (From Eckert, E.F. [1990]. *Your child and hemophilia*. New York: The National Hemophilia Foundation. Reprinted with permission.)

TABLE 14-1
Severity of Hemophilia

Severity	Factor VIII and IX Coagulant Activity (%)	Frequency and Type of Bleeding
Severe	<1	By school age, several bleeding episodes that require treatment often occur each month. Bleeding may be spontaneous or the result of injury.
Moderate	1-5	Frequency of bleeding is variable. Spontaneous bleeding is less common.
Mild	>5	Bleeding is generally only a result of trauma or surgery.

Note that normal factor VIII and IX coagulant levels are generally 50%-150% (0.50-1.5 U/dl) but vary slightly between laboratories.

Incidence and Prevalence

Hemophilia occurs in all ethnic groups, with an incidence of 1 in 5000 live male births (Kulkarni & Lusher, 2001; Lozier & Kessler, 2000). The Centers for Disease Control and Prevention estimate there are approximately 17,000 people with hemophilia in the United States (U.S. Department of Health and Human Services [U.S. DHHS], 2002). Although the true incidence of von Willebrand disease is not known, it is thought to be the most common inherited bleeding disorder. Many scientists estimate that von Willebrand disease is present in more than 1% of the general population (Dilley et al, 2001). Many cases are not diagnosed because of the mild nature of the symptoms.

Clinical Manifestations at Time of Diagnosis

Diagnosis in infancy most commonly occurs because of a positive family history. It is confirmed by cord blood coagulation assays, intracranial hemorrhage, excessive bruising and hematomas, cephalohematoma, or bleeding following circumcision and venipuncture (Kulkarni & Lusher, 2001). Bleeding from the umbilical cord stump may be indicative of factor XIII deficiency (Almeida et al, 2002). Intracranial hemorrhage may be life threatening and occurs in approximately 1% to 5% of newborns with moderate to severe hemophilia; one half of these newborns develop neurologic deficits (Kulkarni & Lusher, 1999).

It is recommended that male newborns of known carriers not diagnosed prenatally be tested for hemophilia by cord or peripheral blood sampling (Kulkarni & Lusher, 2001). In addition, neonates with no family history of hemophilia and unexplained subgaleal or intracranial hemorrhage, and who present with an intracranial hemorrhage, should be screened for a hereditary bleeding disorder (Kulkarni & Lusher, 2001). Cesarean delivery is not routinely recommended in nontraumatic situations (Kulkarni & Lusher, 2001).

Although factor VIII levels generally rise above 50% during pregnancy, carriers whose baseline levels are below 50% may be at particular risk for postpartum hemorrhage. Factor VIII and IX levels should be checked several weeks before anticipated delivery to assess the possible need for hematologic intervention at delivery. Factor IX levels do not rise in pregnancy, and carriers with low levels of factor IX are more likely to need hematologic support with delivery (Kadir & Aledort, 2000; Kulkarni & Lusher, 1999, 2001). When a newborn has a family history of hemophilia, circumcision, heel sticks, and intramuscular immunizations and injections should ideally be delayed until a definitive diagnosis is made. Vitamin K may be given subcutaneously instead of intramuscularly to reduce the risk of hematoma development. Diagnosis is performed prenatally or by using cord or peripheral blood to test factor levels.

By 12 to 18 months of age, most children with severe hemophilia are diagnosed because of positive family history or unusual bleeding (Box 14-1; Jones, 2002). Before diagnosis, parents may be questioned about child abuse because of excessive bruising. Children who first show signs of bleeding later in childhood or in adolescence more often have mild to moderate hemophilia. A frequent misconception is that children with hemophilia can bleed to death from a typical childhood cut or scratch. They may, however, demonstrate joint bleeding (i.e., hemarthrosis); muscle hematomas; excessive postoperative bleeding; or excessive or prolonged oral bleeding following frenulum tears, lost deciduous teeth, tooth eruption, and dental extractions (Jones, 2002).

Von Willebrand disease is commonly manifested by bleeding from the mucous membranes. Although epistaxis is most frequently noted, excessive oral, gastrointestinal (GI), and menstrual bleeding also occurs (Batlle et al, 2002). Diagnostic testing is often requested when there is a positive family history of the disorder or when an increased partial thromboplastin time is obtained during routine preoperative screening. Because the levels of the von Willebrand protein and factor VIII may vary over time, coagulation testing may need to be repeated to establish a diagnosis (Rodeghiero, 2002). Despite the relatively high incidence of this disorder, it is often not diagnosed because the common symptoms of epistaxis and heavy menstrual bleeding are often not brought to medical attention.

Treatment (Box 14-2)

Comprehensive Care in Hemophilia Treatment Centers

The standard of care in hemophilia is a collaborative interdisciplinary approach facilitated by local hemophilia treatment centers (HTCs). These centers, which are funded in part by the US government, provide comprehensive management of inherited coagulation disorders. The core team consists of a pediatric hematologist, nurse coordinator, and social worker. A genetic counselor and physical therapist are other integral team members. A pediatric dentist and orthopedic surgeon provide consultative services. With the advent of human immunodeficiency virus (HIV), HTCs have also been mandated by the government to either provide or procure comprehensive management for clients exposed to HIV. Individuals exposed to hepatitis C are often seen by a liver specialist. Services of the

---

BOX 14-1

Clinical Manifestations at Time of Diagnosis

HEMOPHILIA
Bleeding following circumcision and/or heel stick
Excessive bruising
Hematomas after venipuncture or minimal injury
Bleeding from the umbilical cord stump
Intracranial bleeding
Cephalohematoma
Prolonged oral bleeding (i.e., after frenulum tear, dental extraction, tooth loss)
Hemarthrosis (i.e., generally not the first symptom)

VON WILLEBRAND DISEASE
Prolonged or repeated epistaxis
Prolonged or excessive menstrual bleeding
Gastrointestinal bleeding

BOX 14-2

Treatment

Comprehensive treatment in hemophilia centers
General treatment guidelines to control bleeding
Pharmacologic treatment for hemophilia (Table 14-2)
   Clotting factor concentrates
   Recombinant factor VIII and factor IX
   Plasma-derived factor IX complex concentrates and coagulation factor IX products
   Desmopressin acetate (DDAVP)
   Allergic and inhibitor response to infused factor VIII
   Dosing and cost of pharmacologic treatment
Pharmacologic treatment for von Willebrand disease
   Use of synthetic and plasma-derived products (Table 14-2)
   Desmopressin acetate treatment choice for types 1 and 2A: intravenous or intranasal spray administration
Estrogen therapy (von Willebrand disease) for women
Oral antifibrinolytic agents
Topical hemostatic agents
Pain management
Physical therapy
Surgery (e.g., synovectomy, joint replacement)

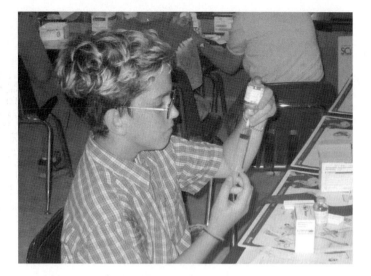

FIGURE 14-3 Adolescent learns the steps for self-injection. (Photo by Ken Hatfield.)

HTC include interdisciplinary comprehensive evaluations, counseling and support services, patient and family education, carrier detection, access to new technology treatment products through clinical trials, and instruction on home infusion (Soucie et al, 2000).

All children and adolescents (Figure 14-3) with hemophilia and von Willebrand disease should receive regular comprehensive evaluations at the nearest HTC. The frequency of these evaluations should be every 3 to 12 months, depending on the severity of the child's bleeding disorder, use of prophylaxis, and other problems the child or family may be having. At these visits, children and their families are seen by the members of the interdisciplinary team. The family and primary care provider receive updated information on the status of a child's health and development, treatment options, new treatment products, and readiness for home therapy is evaluated. HTCs work closely with primary care practitioners to provide comprehensive, coordinated, and accessible care for day-to-day management of pediatric health care. A federally funded study found that individuals receiving care at a hemophilia comprehensive care treatment center were 30% less likely to die than were those who did not receive hemophilia comprehensive care (Soucie et al, 2000).

General Guidelines to Control Bleeding

The goals of treatment are to rapidly initiate clotting when bleeding occurs, to prevent bleeding during high-risk procedures, and in many persons with moderate or severe hemophilia, to prevent joint bleeding through prophylactic infusions of factor concentrate (Box 14-2). The treatment product of choice should be determined by consulting with the child's hematologist. This information should be updated at least yearly to incorporate changes in manufacturing technologies. The current recommended treatment products are the recombinant factor VIII and factor IX products (Medical and Scientific Advisory Council of the National Hemophilia Foundation [MASAC NHF], 2002). Some families whose children

are not receiving home therapy keep a supply of factor concentrate in their home refrigerators to expedite treatment of their child in local emergency rooms. Factor concentrate does not need to be kept at school unless infusions are performed there.

Significant head trauma or bleeding into the iliopsoas muscle (retroperitoneal), hip, GI tract, neck, or posterior pharynx constitutes bleeding episodes that frequently require hospital admission and hematologic consultation. Such consultation is also recommended for bleeding that requires more than two treatments (i.e., concern that an inhibitor may be developing, the dosage is incorrect, or that the injury is severe) and when there is any doubt about the need to treat an injury or bleeding episode. When there is doubt, it is safest to provide treatment if a bleeding episode is suspected (Jones, 2002).

School personnel and families often ask providers to recommend first-aid measures to be instituted while a child is waiting for evaluation and possible infusion. For soft tissue, joint, and muscle bleeding, elevating the affected area and applying an elastic bandage and ice may help to reduce swelling. The child should be allowed to fully rest the affected joint (Jones, 2002). Firm pressure applied over a clean dressing is often sufficient to stop bleeding from surface lacerations in children with both hemophilia and von Willebrand disease. Firm pressure applied to the nares is recommended for nose bleeding. Universal precautions must be used whenever blood or body secretions are encountered. Although ice may help to reduce the superficial swelling from a head hematoma, it should never replace a medical evaluation because intracranial bleeding is unaffected by its application.

Pharmacologic Treatment for Hemophilia (Table 14-2)

Compared with fresh frozen plasma and cryoprecipitate, clotting factor concentrates revolutionized the treatment of hemophilia in the early 1970s because of their ease of administration, fewer allergic side effects, and the ease of home storage. Each vial of these factor concentrates contains the plasma of thousands of donors. Before 1986, production methods did not inactivate HIV. It is important to note that there have been no seroconversions to HIV, hepatitis B, or hepatitis C using products that are currently available (Kasper 2002a, 2002b).

The newest technologic advance in factor replacement is the use of recombinant DNA to manufacture recombinant factor VIII and factor IX concentrates. Some of these factor products are not entirely plasma free because they are stabilized using albumin. However, one factor VIII product and one factor IX product contain no added albumin in the final products (Lozier & Kessler, 2000; MASAC NHF, 2002; Table 14-2).

In addition, two types of plasma-derived factor IX products are available for use: prothrombin-complex concentrates, which are also known as factor IX–complex concentrates, and coagulation factor IX products. The prothrombin-complex concentrates contain clotting factors II, VII, IX, and X and are thrombogenic when given often and in large doses. The coagulation factor IX products contain only factor IX and do not induce thrombosis. Therefore children who are having surgery, have experienced trauma, or are having a severe bleeding

TABLE 14-2
Products Available to Treat Patients with Bleeding Disorders

FACTOR VIII PRODUCTS LICENSED IN THE UNITED STATES
Recombinant Factor VIII Products

Product Name	Manufacturer	Method of Viral Depletion or Inactivation	Stabilizer	Human or Animal Protein Used in Culture Medium	Specific Activity of Final Product (IU Factor VIII/mg Total Protein)	Hepatitis Safety Studies in Humans with This Product
Helixate FS	Bayer (distributed by Aventis Behring)	Immunoaffinity chromatography	Sucrose	Human plasma protein fraction	4,000*	Yes
Kogenate FS	Bayer	Immunoaffinity chromatography	Sucrose	Human plasma protein fraction	4,000*	Yes
Recombinate	Baxter	Immunoaffinity chromatography	Human albumin	Bovine calf serum	1.65-19	Yes
ReFacto	Wyeth	Immunoaffinity chromatography Solvent/detergent (TNBP and Triton X-100)	Sucrose	Human serum albumin	11,200-15,500	Yes

Immunoaffinity Purified Factor VIII Products Derived from Human Plasma

Product Name	Manufacturer	Method of Viral Inactivation	Specific Activity of Final Product (IU Factor VIII/mg Total Protein)	Hepatitis Safety Studies in Humans with This Product	Hepatitis Safety Studies in Humans with Another Product but Similar Viral Inactivation Method
Hemofil M	Baxter	Immunoaffinity chromatography Solvent/detergent (TNBP and Octoxynol 9)	2-15	Yes	No
Monarc-M	Manufactured by Baxter for American Red Cross (ARC) from ARC-collected plasma (distributed by ARC)	Immunoaffinity chromatography Solvent/detergent (TNBP and Octoxynol 9)	2-15	No	Yes
Monoclate-P	Aventis Behring	Immunoaffinity chromatography Pasteurization (60° C, 10 hr)	5-10	Yes	Yes

Factor VIII Products Derived from Human Plasma That Contain von Willebrand Factor

Product Name	Manufacturer	Method of Viral Inactivation	Specific Activity of Final Product (IU Factor VIII/mg Total Protein)	Hepatitis Safety Studies in Humans with This Product	Hepatitis Safety Studies in Humans with Another Product but Similar Method	FDA Approved for von Willebrand Disease
Alphanate	Alpha	Affinity chromatography Solvent/detergent (TNBP and polysorbate 80) Dry heat (80° C, 72 hr)	8-30	No	Yes	No
Humate-P	Aventis Behring GmbH (Marberg, Germany)	Pasteurization (60° C, 10 hr)	1-2	Yes	No	Yes
Koate-DVI	Bayer	Solvent/detergent (TNBP and polysorbate 80) Dry heat (80° C, 72 hr)	9-22	No	Yes	No

TNBP; Tri(n-butyl)phosphate; *FDA*, U.S. Food and Drug Administration; *IV*, intravenous; *SQ*, subcutaneous.
*Valid as long as product is kept under refrigeration as recommended by the manufacturer.

Continued

TABLE 14-2

Products Available to Treat Patients with Bleeding Disorders—cont'd

FACTOR VIII PRODUCTS LICENSED IN THE UNITED STATES—cont'd
Porcine Factor VIII Products (for Use in Patients with Inhibitors to Human Factor VIII)

Product Name	Manufacturer	Method of Viral Inactivation	Specific Activity of Final Product (IU Factor VIII/mg Total Protein)	Hepatitis Safety Studies in Humans with This Product	Hepatitis Safety Studies in Humans with Another Product but Similar Method
Hyate: C	Ipsen, Inc (Wales)	None (but no report of transmission of any viruses to humans)	>50	No	No

FACTOR IX PRODUCTS LICENSED IN THE UNITED STATES
Recombinant Factor IX Products

Product Name	Manufacturer	Method of Viral Depletion or Inactivation	Stabilizer	Human or Animal Protein Used in Culture Medium	Specific Activity (IU Factor IX/mg Total Protein)	Hepatitis Safety Studies in Humans with This Product
Benefix	Wyeth	Affinity chromatography Ultrafiltration	Sucrose	None	≥200	Yes

Coagulation Factor IX Products Derived from Human Plasma

Product Name	Manufacturer	Method of Viral Depletion or Inactivation	Specific Activity of Final Product (IU Factor IX/mg Total Protein)	Hepatitis Safety Studies in Humans with This Product	Hepatitis Safety Studies in Humans with Another Product but Similar Viral Inactivation Method
Alpha-Nine SD	Alpha	Dual affinity chromatography Solvent/detergent (TNBP and polysorbate 80) Nanofiltration (viral filter)	229 ± 23	Yes	Yes
Mononine	Aventis Behring	Immunoaffinity chromatography Sodium thiocyanate Ultrafiltration	>160	Yes	No

Prothrombin Complex Concentrates Derived from Human Plasma That Contains Factors II, VII, IX, X (for Use in Patients with Deficiencies of Factors II, VII, X; Content Varies by Lot and Product)

Product Name	Manufacturer	Method of Viral Inactivation	Specific Activity of Final Product (IU Factor IX/mg Total Protein)	Hepatitis Safety Studies in Humans with This Product	Hepatitis Safety Studies in Humans with Another Product but Similar Viral Inactivation Method
Bebulin VH	Baxter (Vienna)	Vapor heat (10 hr 60° C, 1190 mbar pressure plus 1 hr, 80° C, 1375 mbar)	2	Yes	No
Profilnine SD	Alpha	Solvent/detergent (TNBP and polysorbate 80)	4.5	No	Yes
Proplex T	Baxter	Dry heat (60° C, 144 hr)	3.9	No	No

Antiinhibitor Coagulation Complex (Activated Prothrombin Complex Concentrates) Derived from Human Plasma (for Use in Patients with Inhibitors to factor VIII or IX)

Product Name	Manufacturer	Method of Viral Depletion or Inactivation	Specific Activity of Final Product (IU Factor/mg Total Protein)	Hepatitis Safety Studies in Humans with This Product	Hepatitis Safety Studies in Humans with Another Product but Similar Viral Inactivation Method
Autoplex T	Baxter (distributed by Nabi)	Dry heat (60° C, 144 hr)	5	No	No
FEIBA VH	Baxter (Vienna)	Vapor heat (10 hr, 60° C, 1190 mbar plus 1 hr, 80° C, 1375 mbar)	0.8	Yes	Yes

TNBP; Tri(n-butyl)phosphate; *FDA*, U.S. Food and Drug Administration; *IV*, intravenous; *SQ*, subcutaneous.

TABLE 14-2
Products Available to Treat Patients with Bleeding Disorders—cont'd

FACTOR VII PRODUCTS LICENSED IN THE UNITED STATES
Recombinant Factor VIIa

Product Name	Manufacturer	Method of Viral Depletion or Inactivation	Stabilizer	Human or Animal Protein Used in Culture Medium	Hepatitis Safety Studies in Humans with This Product
NovoSeven	Novo Nordisk (Bagsvaerd, Denmark)	Affinity chromatography	Mannitol	Bovine calf serum	Yes

DESMOPRESSIN FORMULATIONS USEFUL IN DISORDERS OF HEMOSTASIS

Product Name	Manufacturer	US Distributor	Formulation	Recommended Dosage and Administration
DDAVP injection	Ferring AB (Malmo, Sweden)	Aventis Pharma	For parenteral use (IV or SQ), 4 μg/ml in a 10-ml vial	0.3 μg/kg, mixed in 30 ml normal saline solution, infused slowly over 30 min IV 0.4 μg/kg subcutaneously; maximum dose 24 μg once every 24 hr; may repeat after 24 hr
Stimate nasal spray for bleeding	Ferring AB (Malmo, Sweden)	Aventis Behring	Nasal spray, 1.5 mg/ml; metered dose pump delivers 0.1 ml (150 μg) per actuation; bottle contains 2.5 ml with spray pump capable of delivering 25, 150-μg doses or 12, 300-μg doses	In patients weighing <50 kg, one spray in one nostril delivers 150 μg; >50 kg, give one spray in *each nostril* (total dose 300 μg); may repeat after 24 hr

FRESH FROZEN PLASMA PRODUCTS

Product Name	Manufacturer	Distributor	Method of Viral Depletion or Inactivation	Pool Size, Number of Donor Units
Donor retested fresh frozen plasma	Some community blood centers	Some community blood centers	Donors must test negative on second donation for first donation to be released	1

TNBP, Tri(n-butyl)phosphate; *FDA*, U.S. Food and Drug Administration; *IV*, intravenous; *SQ*, subcutaneous.

episode and require factor IX therapy more than once daily for several days in a row should be treated with one of the coagulation factor IX products or recombinant factor IX. There have been no reported cases of thrombosis with the coagulation factor IX products or the recombinant factor IX product (Lozier & Kessler, 2000).

Unfortunately, a number of children were reported to have developed severe allergic reactions along with the development of a factor IX inhibitor within the first 10 to 20 treatment episodes with factor IX. The median age of these children was 16 months (Jadhav & Warrier, 2000). These reactions did not occur with any specific brand of factor IX, but all of the children had either a complete deletion or major derangements of the factor IX gene. The study investigators suggest that the first 10 to 20 infusions of factor IX be given in a medical setting where the child can be monitored (Jadhav & Warrier, 2000).

Desmopressin acetate (DDAVP) is also effective in raising the levels of factor VIII in many children with mild factor VIII deficiency and von Willebrand disease (MASAC NHF, 2001b). The benefits of DDAVP include relatively few major side effects and the lack of viral contaminants because it is not derived from human blood. DDAVP is discussed in greater detail in reference to von Willebrand treatment options.

A number of studies have documented that prophylactic factor treatment can reduce the incidence of chronic hemophilic synovitis and joint damage when begun as early as 1 to 2 years of age. When prophylaxis is begun at a later age, such treatment may prevent further deterioration even when arthropathy is present (Fischer et al, 2002). Typical dosing schedules are 20 to 40 units/kg/dose administered three times each week for children with hemophilia A and 25 to 40 units/kg/dose administered two or three times each week for children with hemophilia B (MASAC NHF, 2001a).

The use of implanted venous access devices (IVADs) has been helpful when prophylactic or frequent treatment is needed in children with poor venous access. IVADs have been used successfully in many children with hemophilia, but the incidence of line sepsis and clotting has reportedly been relatively high in children with hemophilia (MASAC NHF, 2001a).

Studies have shown that as many as 20% of persons with factor VIII deficiency will develop an inhibitor (i.e., antibody) to infused factor VIII (Feinstein, 2000). The level of inhibitor severity is measured in Bethesda units. Most individuals who will develop an inhibitor do so at an early age, after an average of 9 treatment days. A much smaller percentage (i.e., less than 5%) of persons with factor IX deficiency will develop an inhibitor (Feinstein, 2000). Many inhibitors are transient, or levels may be so low as to be clinically insignificant; however, one half of persons with inhibitors develop significant inhibitors and cannot be treated with conventional factor VIII or IX therapy. Treatment options in this situation include immune tolerance regimens, high doses of certain factor concentrates that can bypass part of the standard clotting cascade, porcine factor VIII, and recombinant factor VIIa (Feinstein, 2000; Kulkarni et al, 2001). The use of immune tolerance regimens is a commonly accepted and desirable option. These treatment regimens call for large doses of factor VIII or IX to be given daily in an effort to suppress or eradicate the inhibitor. When laboratory measurements indicate that suppression has been achieved, the frequency of administration and dose of factor concentrate can be tapered. Success rates have averaged 70%. Immune tolerance therapy is extremely costly, often requires use of an IVAD, and necessitates a great deal of compliance from the family.

The unit of measurement for products that replace the deficient factor protein is calculated in international units of factor VIII or IX activity. Choice of a particular dose is based on the type of hemophilia, the child's weight, the severity of the bleeding episode, the half-life of the chosen product, and the occurrence of bleeding in a chronically affected joint (Table 14-3). Repeat doses may be given if significant improvement has not occurred (Jones, 2002). Treatment is initiated as soon as a bleeding episode is identified. For bleeding into a joint, treatment may begin when a child notes tingling in the joint. Many children have come to know this as the first indicator of oozing blood into the joint. For some children, mild swelling, mild pain, or loss of range of motion of a joint may be the first recognizable indicators. In other children with high pain tolerances or little self-awareness of body changes, the bleeding episode may not be recognized until there is severe swelling, major limitation of joint motion, and severe pain. Joint and bone radiographic examinations are generally not needed unless the child has a history of trauma and a broken bone is suspected. Treatment is usually given on demand as soon as bleeding is identified but may be given prophylactically to facilitate healing when bleeding is recurrent or severe or before high-risk or invasive procedures (e.g., surgery, dental extractions, physical therapy of a chronically affected joint).

Vials of factor concentrate come in various sizes with varying numbers of factor units per vial. When a child is prescribed a specific dose of factor (i.e., expressed in factor VIII or IX units), this is considered a minimum dose and the child should be given the full number of vials that provide the desired dose without discarding any of the factor from an individual vial. This minimum dosing rule is due to the high cost of the medication and the lack of adverse sequelae from a dose slightly higher than that originally prescribed. Factor concentrates are given by slow intravenous (IV) push over 5 to 10 minutes. Because most of these concentrates are blood products, those who reconstitute the lyophilized factor should always wear gloves and dispose of supplies that contact the factor in approved infectious waste containers.

High-purity products, such as the recombinant VIII and IX concentrates, are extremely costly. A school-aged child with severe hemophilia who is receiving prophylactic therapy may use close to 180,000 units of factor VIII or IX per year; a 1-year supply of recombinant factor costs approximately $200,000.

Pharmacologic Treatment for von Willebrand Disease

The standard treatment for von Willebrand disease encompasses both synthetic and plasma-derived products. Primary care providers are urged to consult the child's hematologist, local HTC, or the National Hemophilia Foundation for the most current treatment recommendations (MASAC NHF, 2001b).

Desmopressin acetate (Table 14-2), which is a synthetic analogue of vasopressin, is the treatment of choice for persons with types 1 and 2A von Willebrand disease but not subtype 2B (Batlle et al, 2002; MASAC NHF, 2001b). Although the mechanism of action is not completely understood, it is thought that desmopressin releases stores of factor VIII and the von Willebrand protein from the endothelial lining of the blood vessels. Stores may be depleted, however, if treatment is repeated more often than every 24 hours. The IV dosage is 0.3 μg/kg diluted in 30 to 50 ml of normal saline and infused over 30 minutes (Batlle, 2002; Revel-Vilk et al, 2002).

Effectiveness of this medication for various bleeding episodes depends on the rise in coagulation protein activity. Peak response is generally obtained 30 minutes after IV infusion is complete. Individuals should have a test dose of this product to determine response before using it therapeutically. The response varies among individuals, and it should be determined if an individual is a candidate for this therapy before it is used for a bleeding episode or before an invasive procedure. Individuals tend to show consistency in the degree of response over time. Desmopressin has also been given subcutaneously at a slightly higher dose with good results in some children (Batlle, 2002; Revel-Vilk et al, 2002).

A concentrated intranasal form of desmopressin is now available as Stimate Nasal Spray (Ferring AB; 1.5 mg/ml). The peak effect of this form is obtained 1 to 2 hours after administration. Studies have shown significant clinical response with the use of this intranasal form in children with mild hemophilia A and von Willebrand disease who responded well to the IV form. If a child has had prior desmopressin testing with the IV form, repeat laboratory testing with the intranasal form is still indicated before clinical use because results may not be consistent for the two forms of administration (Revel-Vilk et al, 2002). It should be noted that the less-concentrated DDAVP Nasal Spray (Ferring AB; 0.1 mg/ml) is ineffective in treating children with bleeding disorders.

Desmopressin has an antidiuretic effect, so children and parents must be cautioned to limit fluid intake for the remainder of the day that the drug is administered (Lozier & Kessler, 2000).

If a blood product is needed to control bleeding in children with von Willebrand disease, virally inactivated intermediate-purity factor VIII concentrates containing von Willebrand factor are preferable to cryoprecipitate, which cannot be virally inactivated (MASAC NHF, 2001b).

TABLE 14-3

Assessment and Treatment of Common Bleeding Episodes

Site of Bleeding	Signs and Symptoms	Treatment
Subcutaneous and/or soft tissue	Mild: not interfering with ROM, not enlarging	Ice, Ace wrap
	Moderate: occurring in wrist, volar surface of forearm, plantar surface of foot; interferes with ROM or is enlarging	Ice, splint/Ace wrap
		FVIII, 20-30 U/kg, or desmopressin*
	Severe: pharyngeal; areas listed in "moderate" category accompanied by change in neurologic signs	FIX, 30-50 U/kg
		Admit to hospital
		FVIII, 50 U/kg and follow-up doses
		FIX, 80-100 U/kg and follow-up doses
Joint	Earlier: moderate swelling, mild to moderate pain, warmth, stiffness, limited motion	Rest, splint/crutches
		FVIII, 20-25 U/kg, or desmopressin†
		FIX, 30-50 U/kg
	Later: tense swelling, moderate to severe pain, marked decrease in ROM; hip bleeding; limited abduction or adduction	Rest, splint/crutches
		PT plan
		May need repeat doses
		FVIII, 30-40 U/kg
		FIX, 40-50 U/kg
		Ultrasound follow-up for hip bleed
Muscle	Mild: swelling does not greatly affect ROM, mild discomfort	Rest, crutches, PT plan
		Ice, splint/Ace wrap
		FVIII, 20-30 U/kg, or desmopressin*
		FIX, 30-40 U/kg
	Severe: swelling with neurologic changes, decreased ROM	Rest, splint/Ace wrap
		PT plan
		FVIII, 50 U/kg and follow-up doses
		FIX, 80-100 U/kg and follow-up doses
	Iliopsoas: abdominal, inguinal, or hip area pain, limited hip extension, numbness from nerve compression	Strict bedrest/hospitalization
		Will need repeat doses
		FVIII, 50 U/kg
		FIX, 80-100 U/kg
Nose	Mild: 10 min	Pressure to nares
	Severe: prolonged or recurrent	Collagen hemostat fibers and nasal pack
		vWd: desmopressin, EACA
		FVIII, 20 U/kg, or desmopressin*
		FIX, 40 U/kg
Oral areas	Dental extractions; frenulum, tongue, or lip bleeding	Topical hemostatic agent
		Epsilon amino caproic acid (caution with prothrombin complex concentrates)
		May need follow-up doses
		May need hospitalization if hard to control or severe anemia
		vWd: desmopressin*
		FVIII, 30-40 U/kg, or desmopressin*
		FIX, 50-100 U/kg
Gastrointestinal system	Abdominal pain, hypotension, blood in emesis, tarry or bloody stools, weakness	Hospitalization likely
		vWd: desmopression*/FVIII product with high level vWd
		FVIII, 50 U/kg and follow-up doses
		FIX, 100 U/kg and follow-up doses
Central nervous system	Head, neck, or spinal injury; presence of blurred vision, headaches, vomiting, unequal pupils, change in speech or behavior, drowsiness; if no symptoms yet significant injury, treat and observe	Hospitalization and immediate consult with hematologist depending on injury
		CT scan
		vWd: desmopressin*/FVIII product with high level vWd factor
		FVIII, 50 U/kg 2-3 times/day
		FIX, 80-100 U/kg 2 times a day
		May require f/u prophylaxis if positive
		MRI or CT
Urinary tract	Gross hematuria (bright red to brown); if clots present, more likely to infuse with factor concentrate	Push oral fluids, rest
		Prednisone (2 mg/kg/day, maximum 60 mg/day) for 5 days
		Factor concentrate/DDAVP
		EACA contraindicated

Follow-up: By daily telephone contact or office visits through resolution of bleeding episode. If family is receiving home therapy, they should have telephone or office consultation if head, neck, or throat injury occurs; if more than 2 treatments are needed; or if bleeding occurs in hip, iliopsoas muscle, or urinary tract.

Data from Jones P. (2002). *Living with haemophilia* (5th ed.). Oxford England: Oxford University Press; Hemophilia of Georgia, Inc. (2002). *The hemophilia handbook* (4th ed.). Atlanta: Author; C. R. Kessler, & J. N. Lozier, (2000). Clinical aspects and therapy of hemophilia. In R. Hoffman et al. (Eds.). *Hematology: Basic principles and practice* (3rd ed.). New York: Churchill Livingstone.
Note: Specific dosages may vary for individual patients; consult with the child's hematologist.
ROM, Range of motion; FVIII, factor VIII hemophilia; FIX, factor IX hemophilia; U/kg, units of factor VIII or IX per kilogram (factor concentrate vial contains a given number of FVIII or FIX activity units); PT, physical therapy; vWd, von Willebrand disease; EACA, antifibrinolytic: epsilon-aminocaproic acid; CT, computed tomography; MRI, magnetic resonance imaging.
*Desmopressin may be used if, after a test dose, the child with mild hemophilia has achieved a factor VIII coagutant level equal to the level that would be achieved after the recommended dose of factor VIII concentrate. Example: For a moderate soft tissue bleeding in the calf, a dose of 20-30 U/kg should raise a child's factor VIII level to 40% to 60%. If after desmopressin the child reached a peak of only 25%, it is likely desmopressin would not be beneficial.

Estrogen may be useful in the management of excessive menstrual and other types of bleeding in women because it may increase levels of factor VIII and the von Willebrand protein (Lee, 1999).

Oral Antifibrinolytic Agents

Children with hemophilia and von Willebrand disease often have oral bleeding that requires additional medication to keep the clot stable once it has formed. Because of digestive enzymes in the saliva that lyse fibrin clots, an antifibrinolytic agent should be given orally for 7 to 10 days or until the site of oral bleeding has completely healed (Harrington, 2000; Stubbs & Lloyd, 2001). The only such agent currently licensed is epsilon-aminocaproic acid (Amicar).

Topical Hemostatic Agents

Collagen hemostat (Avitene) fibers can be applied to nasal packing or salt pork pledgets to control epistaxis or at the site of frenulum tears or tooth extraction. When nasal packing is used, it is generally left in place for 24 to 36 hours to promote stable clot formation. Nosebleeds can often be prevented or diminished by using petroleum jelly or antibiotic ointment in the nares as well as humidification of room air. Less conventional topical agents have been used successfully in the treatment of oral bleeding. Moistened tea bags containing tannic acid may provide local hemostasis. Fibrin glue has been used to promote local hemostasis in some circumcisions; cryoprecipitate is the source of fibrinogen in this treatment (Lozier & Kessler, 2000).

Pain Management

Uncontrolled bleeding into a joint or muscle can produce significant pain. Prompt replacement of the deficient coagulation protein, to stop the bleeding, is the most effective way to prevent severe pain. Mild pain may be treated with acetaminophen (*not* aspirin), ice, and elevation of the affected extremity. If pain is moderate or severe, acetaminophen with codeine every 4 to 6 hours is recommended. Pain medication is generally not necessary after the first day of factor replacement. Continued pain may suggest ineffective control of bleeding because of inadequate dosing of the factor concentrate, development of an inhibitor, or a more severe bleeding episode than previously thought. Swelling caused by irritation of the synovial lining may be more effectively treated with a nonsteroidal antiinflammatory agent. These agents should be used with caution, however, because they can cause GI bleeding secondary to interference with platelet aggregation (Lozier & Kessler, 2000).

Physical Therapy

Splinting and immobilization for 1 to 2 days after acute bleeding often aid in resolution of the episode. A resting splint that places the extremity in a comfortable position is recommended for night use for several days following a significant hemarthrosis to prevent further bleeding secondary to twisting during sleep and to quiet the joint. Following severe bleeding or prolonged immobilization, a physical therapy program should be prescribed to enable children to achieve their baseline range of motion and regain muscle mass. Factor replacement is often needed with vigorous physical therapy (Anderson et al, 2000).

Surgical Intervention

Destruction of joint cartilage secondary to repeated bleeding episodes can result in significant pain, decreased strength and range of motion, and an impaired ability to use the affected extremity. Several orthopedic procedures have been successful in individuals with hemophilia and can provide them with significantly reduced joint pain, decrease in number of bleeding episodes, and greater range of motion and endurance. Open synovectomy is successful in reducing pain and bleeding episodes, but mobility is often lost and progression of the arthropathy continues. Arthroscopic synovectomy reduces the pain and frequency of bleeding episodes without loss of mobility (Wiedel, 2002). Injection of a radioactive isotope into the affected joint to eradicate overgrown and inflamed synovium, which is a less invasive procedure, has been successful in improving range of motion and decreasing bleeding episodes in individuals who are not surgical candidates (Hilgartner, 2002). Once a child is fully grown and the epiphyseal plates are closed, total joint replacements—particularly of the knee—have been quite successful in individuals with hemophilia, as measured by increased function and decreased pain and frequency of bleeding episodes (Lozier & Kessler, 2000; Rodriguez-Merchan, 2002).

Complementary and Alternative Treatments

No complementary or alternative therapies were identified in the literature for the treatment of hemophilia or von Willebrand disease.

Anticipated Advances in Diagnosis and Management

Attainment of a cure for hemophilia has been explored through liver transplantation and gene-insertion therapy. Liver transplantation has been found to cure both hemophilia A and B because both factor VIII and factor IX are synthesized in the liver (Wilde et al, 2002). Liver transplantation, however, is both an extremely costly and a high-risk procedure and requires immunosuppressive therapy for life. At this time, liver transplantation is only performed in individuals with end-stage liver disease. In the future, successful gene-insertion therapy may provide a cure for hemophilia or at least convert persons with severe hemophilia to a milder form of the disorder. Research is under way to find the best vector for gene expression (Walsh, 2002).

Associated Problems (Box 14-3)

Anemia

Anemia can occur as a result of slow, persistent oozing from the mouth or nose or bleeding or pooling of blood in muscle hemorrhages. In persons with von Willebrand disease, excessive or prolonged menstrual bleeding or persistent or recurrent epistaxis can result in anemia.

Neurologic Problems

Intracranial hemorrhage is the most frequent cause of death in children with hemophilia (Lozier & Kessler, 2000). Intracranial hemorrhage also can result in spastic quadriplegia and devel-

BOX 14-3
Associated Problems

Anemia
Neurologic deficits from intracranial hemorrhage, bleeding around spinal
   column, compartment syndrome compression of nerves
Airway obstruction as a result of bleeding
Hepatitis
Gastrointestinal bleeding
Human immunodeficiency virus (HIV)
Musculoskeletal problems
Genitourinary bleeding

---

opmental delay. In some cases of intracranial bleeding, no known prior injury is identified. Therefore any injury or neurologically related symptom should be treated aggressively. There may be significant intracranial bleeding without the presence of a "goose egg" because the most significant bleeding occurs from internal shearing of the brain and cranium. The presence of a hematoma, however, indicates that the cranium may have met with significant force. Because of the high risk of rebleeding after intracranial hemorrhage, prophylactic factor treatment is continued for an extended period. Individuals with von Willebrand disease also are at increased risk for this type of bleeding. Bleeding within or around the spinal column can also produce enough pressure to cause neurologic damage. Compartment syndrome resulting from nerve compression may occur after untreated bleeding into the forearm or calf (Anderson et al, 2000).

Airway Obstruction as a Result of Bleeding

Posterior pharyngeal bleeding, which increases the potential for asphyxia, can result from a traumatic throat culture, bronchoscopy, or dental extractions or deep injection of anesthetic without pretreatment with factor concentrates or desmopressin. Intubation should only be attempted after pretreatment with factor concentrate.

Hepatitis

In the past, exposure to blood products resulted in a high incidence of infection with hepatitis B and C in the population with hemophilia. Approximately 75% of those with hemophilia have been exposed to hepatitis B; the majority have developed immunity, but a small percentage are chronic carriers. Of individuals with hemophilia, approximately 80% to 90% have been exposed to hepatitis C (Goedert et al, 2002; US DHHS, 2002; Yee et al, 2000). With the use of the hepatitis B vaccine series, the incidence of hepatitis B has been greatly reduced. In addition, the factor products currently on the market are considered to have a negligible risk of hepatitis transmission as a result of current screening and processing methods (Kasper, 2002a).

A new combination therapy that uses subcutaneous pegylated alfa-interferon 2b in combination with oral ribavirin has been successful in treating chronic hepatitis C. This treatment has resulted in undetectable serum hepatitis C virus (HCV) ribonucleic acid (RNA) levels after completion of treatment and in improving liver histology as detected by liver biopsy in over 50% of individuals treated for as long as 48 weeks. Success of

the therapy depends to a large extent on the individual's HCV genotype. The success rate of 80% in individuals with genotypes 2 and 3 is much higher than the 45% success rate in individuals with genotype 1 (Lee & Dusheiko, 2002; Manns et al, 2001). Unfortunately, the side effects of this therapy often include severe anemia, flulike symptoms, and severe psychiatric symptoms, so some individuals need to discontinue treatment before completing the full course (Lee & Dusheiko, 2002; Manns et al, 2001). It is recommended that individuals with hepatitis C infection be immunized with hepatitis A vaccine because these individuals have a substantial risk of fulminant hepatitis and death if infected with hepatitis A (MASAC NHF, 2002; Vento et al, 1998).

Gastrointestinal Bleeding

Bleeding into the GI tract may occur in children with von Willebrand disease and in those with hemophilia. The fragile mucous membrane–lined digestive system is prone to bleeding that can result from ulcers, gastritis, hemorrhoids, rectal fissures, and endoscopic procedures. This type of bleeding should be considered when there is an unexplained drop in hemoglobin levels or abdominal pain.

HIV Infection

Approximately 50% of those exposed to untreated factor concentrates between 1978 and 1985 (i.e., approximately 9200 persons) have developed HIV infection (Lozier & Kessler, 2000). However, currently less than 20% of persons with hemophilia are HIV positive (US DHHS, 2002). The incidence of HIV infection in persons with von Willebrand disease who were exposed to cryoprecipitate is much lower, however, because of the decreased risk with exposure to single-donor units of cryoprecipitate.

Musculoskeletal Problems

The normally smooth synovial lining of a joint produces synovial fluid that with the cartilage serves as a shock absorber for the joint (Figure 14-4). The synovium is also supplied with many blood vessels. When bleeding into a joint ceases with the administration of the deficient coagulation protein, enzymes clear away the blood from the synovial fluid. These enzymes, however, do not seem to focus their destruction solely on the unwanted blood cells; they begin to eat away at the smooth synovial lining, producing breaks in the surface that can make it easier for bleeding to recur in that joint. Eventually they may destroy the cartilaginous surface of the bones. The nonintact synovial lining can cause the synovium to produce abnormal amounts of fluid in an inflammatory response known as synovitis. Even when actual bleeding into the joint does not occur, the joint may become swollen and stiff. Synovitis is differentiated from a hemarthrosis by its gradual onset, mild or absent pain, and fuller range of motion. The more blood that accumulates in the joint capsule, the more enzymes that are released. This destructive process can ultimately lead to severe osteoarthritic-like conditions and joint contractures. A single hip hemarthrosis can produce aseptic necrosis of the femoral head if bleeding is not fully resolved. When bleeding recurs in a specific joint, it may be referred to as a "target joint" (Anderson et al, 2000). Thus a strong case is made for early

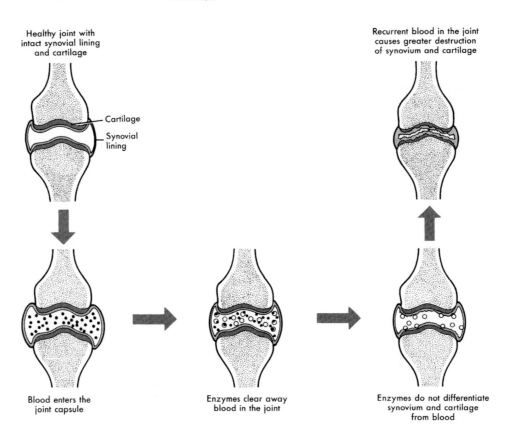

FIGURE 14-4 Progression of joint destruction in hemophilia.

detection and treatment of bleeding episodes and ultimately for the use of prophylactic treatment for children with severe hemophilia (Fischer et al, 2002).

Genitourinary Problems

If a boy has bleeding into the testicle that is not treated promptly, future fertility and maintenance of a patent urinary tract may be compromised. This type of bleeding can result from performing bicycle stunts or taking part in vigorous play on a rocking horse or playground toy.

Hematuria occurs most commonly in adolescents with hemophilia, is usually of short duration, is not a result of trauma, and often stops spontaneously. Clots can sometimes cause renal or ureteral obstruction with temporary renal colic and, at times, hydronephrosis. Treatment with epsilon-aminocaproic acid (Amicar) should be avoided during periods of hematuria because of the risk of developing clots in the genitourinary system (Jones, 2002).

Prognosis

The major factors contributing to morbidity in hemophilia are neurologic sequelae of intracranial bleeding, disability from chronic joint disease (arthropathy), liver disease secondary to hepatitis, and HIV infection. Intracranial bleeding that occurs at or soon after birth may result in spastic quadriplegia and brain damage, whereas intracranial bleeding that occurs later in life may affect the achievement of developmental milestones. Because of the availability of clotting factor concentrates, disabling arthropathy in childhood is now much less common.

The rate of HIV infection among adolescents with hemophilia in the United States is currently less than 3% (US DHHS, 2002). The lower incidence reflects the fact that there have been very few HIV seroconversions since 1986, so many individuals with HIV have now reached adulthood. In addition, many individuals with hemophilia and HIV have died.

For the child with hemophilia born today, life expectancy approaches that of the general population (Ljung, 2002). HIV-related disease is the leading cause of death in persons with hemophilia (Chorba, 2001; Soucie et al, 2000). In those not infected with HIV, however, the leading cause of death is bleeding, especially from intracranial hemorrhage (Diamondstone et al, 2002).

Data regarding morbidity and mortality of persons with von Willebrand disease are not readily available. Because of the generally mild nature of the disorder, life expectancy is thought to be normal. The relatively small number of individuals infected with HIV or hepatitis B or C through infusions of cryoprecipitate have a decreased life expectancy.

PRIMARY CARE MANAGEMENT

Health Care Maintenance

Growth and Development

Monitoring a child's weight is especially important because obesity places added stress on joints and muscles. Limb length may be increased by bony overgrowth of the epiphysis from chronic arthropathy.

Repeated bleeding into a joint may result in a permanent contracture of that joint, with leg length discrepancy. Gait disturbances caused by scoliosis may predispose individuals with hemophilia to joint or muscle bleeding.

A thorough baseline and ongoing assessment of developmental parameters and neurologic status are useful in follow-up for head trauma and screening of potentially undiagnosed or unreported intracranial bleeding. Normal development is anticipated unless there is a history of intracranial bleeding.

Diet

It is especially important for children with bleeding disorders to meet the recommended requirements for protein and calcium intake because of their role in bone and muscle formation. A nonconstipating diet may prevent the rectal bleeding that can occur when hard stools are passed. When a child has mouth bleeding, a soft diet and avoidance of foods that are hot or have sharp edges (e.g., chips) and straws (i.e., because the sucking action can disturb the clot) are recommended. As mentioned previously, weight management to prevent obesity is important to decrease stress on weight-bearing joints.

Safety

Protection against head injury is of primary importance. Some hemophilia providers feel that a protective helmet for children with hemophilia who are learning to walk may reduce the risk of head injury. Other providers feel that it may make the child more unbalanced and lead to an increased incidence of falls. Knee pads may be used for toddlers prone to knee hematomas. From the time they start to walk, children at risk for hemarthroses should wear high-top leather sneakers and shoes. Walkers are never recommended for young children but may be particularly hazardous for children with bleeding disorders. Care must also be taken that the child is safely strapped in when using portable swings and high chairs.

Contact sports (e.g., football, soccer, hockey, wrestling, boxing, competitive basketball) are strongly discouraged because of the increased chance of head trauma. Appropriate physical activity is encouraged, however, to maintain strong muscles that promote joint stability and normal social adjustment. Swimming is an ideal aerobic activity. Although recommended for all children, helmets are particularly important for those with bleeding disorders when riding bikes or scooters or using roller skates or blades. Knee and elbow pads are also recommended for roller skating or blading and skateboarding. Activities that increase the chances for testicular trauma (dirt-bike riding, horseback riding, gymnastics) should be discouraged in boys with moderate to severe hemophilia.

Use of a medical identification emblem that includes diagnosis and treatment recommendations is required for safety. Infants can have the emblem pinned to their car seats or jackets when traveling. A wallet identification card may be used if a child or adolescent refuses to wear the emblem. Medical information should be checked yearly and updated as necessary.

Families participating in a home infusion program should follow accepted guidelines for infection control, including the use of gloves to mix and administer factor concentrates and the disposal of infectious wastes in approved containers that are disposed of appropriately.

Arterial blood samples should only be drawn after pretreatment with factor concentrate.

Immunizations

Routine injectable vaccines should be given subcutaneously when possible because intramuscular injections may cause muscle bleeding (Centers for Disease Control and Prevention [CDC], 2002). When any injectable vaccine is given, the following interventions can help to prevent hematoma development: using a 25-gauge needle, applying firm pressure to the site for 5 minutes after injection, and using a factor concentrate before intramuscular injection.

The hepatitis A and B vaccine series are recommended for all children likely to be exposed to blood products (Jones, 2002). If an at-risk child did not receive the vaccine as an infant, the hepatitis B vaccine should be administered immediately and again at 1 month and 6 months after the first dose. Hepatitis A vaccine has been recommended for use in individuals with bleeding disorders who are at least 2 years of age and seronegative for the hepatitis A virus. The recommendations are currently a two-dose series for adults (i.e., the vaccine is again administered 6 to 12 months later) and a two- or three-dose series for children at least 2 years of age (i.e., again administered 1 and 6 months later [for the three-dose series]). The number of dosages for children depends on the vaccine brand and dose per vial.

Screening

Vision. Following an eye injury, referral to an ophthalmologist is recommended, with follow-up until resolution is obtained. Otherwise, routine office screening and attention to the fundal examination are sufficient. Individuals with HIV should have yearly eye exams to screen for cytomegalovirus (CMV).

Hearing. Routine screening is recommended.

Dental. Invasive dental procedures can often be prevented through careful oral hygiene (including flossing under parental supervision), fluoride treatments, and regular dental evaluations. An initial dental evaluation is recommended at 2 to 3 years of age, in part to help the child establish a positive relationship with the dentist, as well as to impress on parents the importance of preventive care. Pediatric dentists with expertise in the management of persons with bleeding disorders are often associated with the local HTC. If necessary, local dentists can manage most procedures with consultation from the HTC. The HTC should be consulted about whether prophylactic treatment with factor concentrate or desmopressin is necessary for routine dental cleaning or anesthetic infiltrates close to the gum line for a particular child. For dental extractions, desmopressin or factor concentrate plus an antifibrinolytic agent is recommended (Harrington, 2000). If a child has an implantable port, external venous catheter, or joint replacement, some treatment centers advocate the use of subacute bacterial endocarditis (SBE) antibiotic prophylaxis (see Chapter 21).

Blood Pressure. Routine screening is recommended.

Hematocrit. Annual screening for anemia is recommended. Nosebleeds that are short in duration but occur frequently may not be regularly reported by families and may lead to significant anemia. If venipuncture is required, a 23-gauge butterfly needle should be used and firm pressure applied to the site for at least 5 minutes afterward to prevent hematoma formation. Trauma may be reduced if a skilled pediatric phlebotomist performs venipuncture. Females with von Willebrand disease and females who are carriers of hemophilia and have low factor levels may have menorrhagia. This may result in a lower than normal hematocrit. Menorrhagia may be controlled by the use of birth control pills or other estrogen-containing medications or the high concentration intranasal DDAVP product, Stimate.

Urinalysis. An annual urinalysis is recommended to screen for microscopic hematuria.

Tuberculosis. Routine screening is recommended. No factor pretreatment is needed for tine or purified protein derivative (PPD) skin testing.

Condition-Specific Screening

Children who have received any blood bank products (excluding factor concentrates) in the past year should have liver function studies performed. A factor VIII or IX inhibitor screen should also be performed for those with hemophilia and is usually performed during comprehensive evaluations at the HTC. HIV antibody testing with pretest and posttest counseling is recommended for adolescents exposed to blood products before 1986 who have not previously been tested.

Common Illness Management

Differential Diagnosis

Headaches and Head Injury. Intracranial bleeding must be ruled out whenever there is a history of injury within the past several days, focal headaches, or vomiting without GI distress. A computed tomographic (CT) scan is often helpful in ruling out intracranial bleeding. If either significant history or physical symptoms are present, however, providers often treat a child with factor concentrate prophylactically to achieve a 100% factor VIII or IX level. This conservative approach is often adopted because of the serious implications of a delay in diagnosis. Therapy may cease after the resolution of symptoms if scans remain normal. If bleeding is documented, the child would need hospitalization and factor replacement regularly for several weeks or longer.

Visual Disturbance. In the presence of acute changes in visual acuity, it is necessary to rule out intraocular bleeding by performing a thorough funduscopic examination. Documented bleeding, ocular injury, or persistent visual changes, however, warrant referral to an ophthalmologist.

Fever. When children with IVADs develop a fever, blood cultures should be drawn and IV antibiotics started until the cultures are shown to be negative. These indwelling devices present a significant risk for infection even in children whose immune systems are not suppressed.

If pretreated with factor concentrates or desmopressin, children with hemophilia may safely have lumbar punctures if required for a sepsis work-up.

Sore Throat. If a throat culture is indicated, extreme caution must be exercised because of the potential for posterior pharyngeal bleeding. A throat culture should not be attempted in an uncooperative child. If streptococcal pharyngitis is suspected, a course of penicillin should be initiated based on history and physical findings.

Mouth Bleeding. Although oral bleeding may not appear profuse in children with hemophilia, persistent slow oozing can cause a significant drop in hemoglobin levels. Topical measures and antifibrinolytics alone are often not sufficient to control bleeding well. In most cases, factor replacement or the use of desmopressin is also required. Rebleeding can be prevented with a soft diet and avoidance of placing straws, hot foods, chips, and toys in the mouth.

Abdominal Pain. Primary care practitioners should have a high suspicion of GI bleeding with acute abdominal pain or a significant drop in hemoglobin levels in the absence of other bleeding in children with hemophilia or von Willebrand disease. Testing stool or emesis for blood can easily be done in the office as a screening tool. In hemophilia, iliopsoas bleeding (i.e., a combination of the iliacus muscle [origin, iliac fossa; insertion, greater trochanter] and psoas muscle [origin, thoracic and lumbar vertebrae; insertion, lesser trochanter]) can cause pain in the abdomen or in the inguinal area. Children with iliopsoas bleeding are unable to straighten their leg at the knee joint and hold their hip in a flexed position. Psoas bleeding can result in a large amount of blood loss and nerve damage that necessitates hip joint replacement in some men later in life. Hospital admission for strict bedrest and aggressive treatment with factor is generally required for iliopsoas and GI bleeding. Strict bedrest is recommended with iliopsoas bleeding.

Gait Disturbance. Gait disturbance may be the result of bleeding in or around the ankle, knee, hip, or iliopsoas muscle. Inability to fully extend the hip and, later, leg paresthesias are characteristics of iliopsoas bleeding. Ultrasonography is useful for confirmation. Bleeding into the hip socket, which is rare in children, is characterized by limitation of hip abduction and adduction.

Dysuria and Hematuria. Pressure within the urinary tract can cause dysuria. Testicular bleeding, however, must be ruled out. Bleeding into the testicular area is often quite pronounced with obvious bruising and swelling. Hospitalization may be required for aggressive therapy and bedrest. Hematuria may be spontaneous and directly related to the bleeding disorder. Whenever bleeding occurs, however, its origin within the urinary tract and any potential infection should be considered. Increased fluid intake, bedrest, and avoidance of antifibrinolytic agents, which may cause obstructive clots, are routinely recommended as part of a treatment plan. The benefits of treatment with factor concentrate or corticosteroids, however, are debated among clinicians.

Heavy Menstrual Bleeding. Females who are carriers of hemophilia or have von Willebrand disease may have heavy menstrual flow, resulting in anemia. Once other causes have been ruled out, these females may benefit from treatment with estrogen therapy in the form of oral contraceptives or the high-dose form of intranasal DDAVP, Stimate.

Numbness, Tingling, and Pain. Compression of nerves caused by deep or superficial hematomas should be suspected in individuals with changes in sensation or focal pain. Bleeding in or near the calf, spine, buttock, iliopsoas muscle, and volar surface of the forearm can lead to neurologic changes.

Drug Interactions

All products that contain aspirin are contraindicated. Caution should also be exercised with prolonged use of other medications that can affect platelet aggregation (e.g., non-steroidal antiinflammatory agents). It is important to educate parents on how to read medication labels (e.g., choosing those with acetaminophen over those with acetylsalicylic acid) and enlist the help of the pharmacist when they are in doubt about the use of a particular product.

Developmental Issues

Sleep Patterns

Standard developmental counseling is advised. Parents are often advised to pad their child's crib rails to prevent bruising. Crib side rails should be lowered and pillows placed on the floor below as soon as the child begins to crawl out of his or her crib.

Toileting

Standard developmental counseling is advised.

Discipline

Some families tend to overprotect children with a bleeding disorder and may be more strict with unaffected siblings. Positive disciplinary techniques that are age appropriate and developmentally appropriate and do not include physical punishment should be recommended for all children. Pulling a child with a bleeding disorder by the arm is a specific action that may result in serious shoulder bleeding and radial head subluxation. Primary care providers should evaluate the disciplinary style of the parents and offer counseling on alternative discipline measures if potentially injurious methods are used. Families should be counseled about the use of noncontact limit-setting measures (e.g., time-outs, distraction, activity limitations).

Child Care

Contact with the proposed source of child care can help allay fears and clarify the caretaker's responsibilities with regard to the prevention and management of bleeding episodes. HTC personnel or the primary care provider may provide this service. It is helpful to emphasize that early recognition of bleeding (e.g., mild swelling or slight change in range of motion) and rapid access to medical evaluation and treatment are of primary importance for children with hemophilia. Spontaneous bleeding may occur, however, despite diligent safety efforts. Child care providers should be discouraged from trying to make treatment decisions without the input of the parents, which is especially important when seemingly mild head "bumps" occur. To find the safest environment possible, parents may be encouraged to seek out sources of child care that have smaller numbers of children per provider, protective ground cover under outside activity spaces, and a staff willing to learn about the special needs and activity requirements of a child with a bleeding disorder. Some facilities may be fearful of admitting children with bleeding disorders because of their fear of liability. Health care providers can provide education and help allay concerns.

Schooling

Teachers, school nurses, and athletic coaches should be informed of a child's bleeding disorder. Families and children may be reticent to disclose the diagnosis to others for fear of discrimination because of the connection between hemophilia and HIV. School personnel are more often concerned with prevention of bleeding (which may not be possible), emergency management, and HIV infection. Many HTCs offer school visits by the program's nurse coordinator and social worker. These educational visits are most helpful on entrance to a new school and should be done with the permission and—ideally—participation of the child and parents. It is not uncommon for children and adolescents with hemophilia to encounter peer disbelief that the disability and the need for crutches or a sling created by an acute bleeding episode can resolve in 1 to 2 days.

Alterations in body image and self-esteem may be precipitated by chronic joint arthropathy or limitations on physical activity caused by the bleeding disorder. From the time of diagnosis, parents may be assisted in guiding their child toward skills, careers, and sports that place less stress on joints and are not associated with high rates of injury. It is critical that children have activities and skills at which they can excel. The advent of prophylaxis has enabled more "normal" active play without the fear of increased injury and bleeding.

Children with learning problems resulting from intracranial bleeding must be fully evaluated and provided with appropriate support.

Sexuality

Safe-sex counseling (i.e., including decision-making skills; values clarification; and instruction in the use of condoms to prevent transmission of HIV, hepatitis B and C, and other sexually transmitted diseases) should be offered to all adolescents. Some adolescents who test HIV-antibody positive may avoid sexual relationships because of fear of rejection once their status is known to a potential partner.

The genetic counselor at the HTC may first interact with children concerning basic education on the inheritance of the bleeding disorder and eventually include a discussion of reproductive options.

Transition into Adulthood

The transition from adolescence to adulthood can be particularly stressful for some individuals with bleeding disorders. When they approach adulthood, such individuals have their comprehensive HTC medical care transferred from the pediatric hematology service to the adult hematology service. Some young men experience feelings of anger and rejection because of the need to develop relationships with new providers and sever nurturing relationships they have had with the pediatric team since infancy. This is usually the time when the responsibility for medical care is transferred from the parents to the young adult. It is helpful if this expected transition is discussed with the child and family when the child is still young. Open and ongoing discussion about this expected transition of care may help allay some of the stress, sadness, and anger the child and family feel when they must transfer care to new providers.

Choice of college may also be influenced by the availability of specialized medical care in the area, and choice of career may be influenced by physical limitations.

As adolescents make the transition to adulthood, they may no longer be eligible for medical coverage under their parent's policy and may have difficulty finding coverage that will accommodate their disorder. In many states, there are special programs that cover individuals with hemophilia, or individuals may be eligible for a federal government program (e.g.,

Medicare, Medicaid, Supplemental Security Income [SSI]) as a result of disability.

Family Concerns and Resources

If a child with a bleeding disorder has excessive bruising before and after diagnosis, parents often encounter questions about suspected child abuse from health care providers or stares from friends, relatives, teachers, and strangers. Compounding the parents' distress may be guilt regarding the inheritance of the bleeding disorder.

It is difficult for parents to cope with their inability to prevent bleeding episodes despite diligent efforts to prevent injury. Fear of injury to the infant may even interfere with parent-infant bonding. When a child requires an infusion of blood products to stop bleeding, parents often continue to question the viral safety of the product despite current data on product safety.

Reimbursement for high-priced factor replacement has become an area of real concern as families reach the maximum lifetime amount of insurance reimbursement. Families who may face this problem need early intervention and counseling about insurance options. This is generally provided by the social worker at the HTC.

Different racial and ethnic groups may have varying feelings about and experiences of disability and chronic illness. As a result, individuals with hemophilia may receive little under-standing from their own ethnic community and may even encounter racial bias in the delayed diagnosis of a hemarthrosis (e.g., a black man presenting with a swollen joint may be assumed to be having a sickle cell episode instead of being treated with a prompt infusion of factor concentrate). In many Asian cultures, it is a sign of weakness to tell others about an illness or disease. Many Hispanics are hesitant to join organized support networks for their disorder because they fear stigmatization. Women are another minority group in whom the effect of bleeding disorders or carrier status has been overlooked.

RESOURCES

The National Hemophilia Foundation (116 West 32nd St, 11th floor, New York, NY 10001; [212] 328-3700 and [800] 424-2634; www.hemophilia.org) and its local chapters disseminate information on recent advances in therapy not only for hemophilia and von Willebrand disease but also for HIV and hepatitis C infection. Active members of the foundation include consumers, families, and health care providers at HTCs. The local chapters provide educational programs and support services to meet the members' needs.

Hemophilia treatment centers (HTCs) also provide educational programs and support groups for individuals with bleeding disorders and their families. A list of HTCs is available from the National Hemophilia Foundation in New York or from local National Hemophilia Foundation chapters.

Summary of Primary Care Needs for the Child with Bleeding Disorders: Hemophilia and von Willebrand Disease

If a child or adolescent with a bleeding disorder also has an HIV infection, please see additional guidelines given in Chapter 28.

HEALTH CARE MAINTENANCE

Growth and Development

Monitoring and preventing obesity is important due to added stress on joints. Leg length discrepancy may occur due to chronic arthropathy.

Developmental screening should be done as a follow-up for head trauma or screening for undiagnosed or unreported intracranial bleeding.

Diet

Adequate protein and calcium intake is of particular importance because of the role of both in bone and muscle formation. Non constipating diet will help prevent rectal bleeding. A soft diet and avoiding foods with sharp edges is necessary when a child has mouth bleeding.

Obesity should be avoided because it places extra stress on joints.

Safety

A protective helmet may be recommended for children who are learning to walk to reduce the risk of head injury. Use of a helmet is controversial because it restricts peripheral vision.

Knee pads in the pants of toddlers may decrease knee hematomas.

High-top sneakers and shoes (i.e., not canvas type of shoes) are recommended for children at risk for hemarthroses from the time they start to walk.

Participation in noncontact sports should be encouraged. Helmets and joint pads are recommended.

The child should wear a medical identification emblem that includes information regarding diagnosis, treatment product, and blood type. The information should be updated annually.

Activities that increase the chance of testicular bleeding, particularly in boys, should be discouraged.

Families participating in a home infusion program should follow accepted guidelines for universal precautions and disposal of infectious wastes.

Arterial blood samples should only be drawn after treatment with factor concentrate.

Immunizations

Some sources recommend that the hepatitis A and B, DTaP, and HIB vaccines be given intramuscularly, despite risk of bleeding, whereas other sources recommend giving all immunizations subcutaneously.

Summary of Primary Care Needs for the Child with Bleeding Disorders: Hemophilia and von Willebrand Disease—cont'd

Some children may require factor replacements before immunization injections if given intramuscularly.

Injectable vaccines should be given with a 25-gauge needle.

Firm pressure should be applied over the immunization site for 5 minutes. Ice may be applied after pressure.

Screening

Vision. Examination for eye injury should be done by an ophthalmologist. Routine office screening with attention to funduscopic examination is recommended.

Hearing. Routine screening is recommended.
Do not curette wax aggressively.

Dental. Teeth should initially be evaluated at 2 to 3 yr of age, followed by regular routine examinations. Hygiene should include flossing under supervision. Factor replacement or desmopressin is recommended for regional blocks; an antifibrinolytic should be added for dental extractions. If child has an imported port, indwelling venous catheter, or joint replacement, bacterial endocarditis prophylaxis may be recommended.

Blood Pressure. Annual screening is recommended.

Hematocrit. Annual screening is recommended.
Use a 23-gauge butterfly needle for venipuncture in persons of any age.

Urinalysis. Annual screening for microscopic hematuria is recommended.

Tuberculosis. Routine screening is recommended.

Condition-Specific Screening

If blood product has been received in the past year, a factor VIII or IX inhibitor screen (i.e., specifically for persons with hemophilia) and liver function studies are indicated. HIV antibody testing with precounseling and postcounseling is recommended for those exposed to blood products before 1986 if not previously performed.

COMMON ILLNESS MANAGEMENT

Differential Diagnosis

Headaches and Head Injury. Rule out intracranial bleeding, especially with concurrent vomiting and absence of GI symptoms.

Visual Disturbance. Rule out intraocular bleeding.

Fever. If indwelling venous access device is present, blood cultures must be drawn and IV antibiotics started.

Sore Throat. Throat cultures present a risk for posterior pharyngeal bleeding. Cultures should not be taken from an uncooperative child.

Mouth Bleeding. Mouth bleeding often requires factor replacement in addition to topical measures and antifibrinolytic agents.

Abdominal Pain. Rule out GI bleeding. Rule out iliopsoas muscle bleeding with groin pain and decreased hip extension.

Gait Disturbance. Rule out bleeding. in and around the ankle, knee, hip, and iliopsoas muscle. Rule out scoliosis.

Dysuria and Hematura. Rule out testicular bleeding, renal or ureteral bleeding and infection.

Heavy menstrual Bleeding. May occur in hemophilia carriers or women with von Willebrand disease. DDAVP or estrogen therapy may be helpful.

Numbness, Tingling, and Pain. Rule out nerve compression caused by bleeding.

Drug Interactions. Products that contain aspirin are contraindicated.

Prolonged use of other substances that can affect platelet aggregation (e.g., nonsteroidal antiinflammatory agents) should be avoided.

DEVELOPMENTAL ISSUES

Sleep Patterns

Standard developmental counseling is advised. Safety of sleeping environment must be assessed.

Toileting

Standard developmental counseling is advised.

Discipline

Recognize the potential for overprotection of the affected child and the use of deferential disciplinary methods when compared with unaffected siblings.

Pulling a child by the arm may result in shoulder joint bleeding.

Physical punishment may result in internal bleeding.

Parents should be counseled about use of time-outs and other nonphysical methods of limit setting.

Child Care

Contact with the proposed source of care by the primary health care provider or hemophilia treatment center staff is often useful to allay fears and clarify responsibilities with regard to prevention and management of bleeding episodes and trauma. The importance of early recognition and treatment of bleeding should be stressed. Child care centers with smaller numbers of children, protective ground cover, and low child-provider ratio are suggested.

Recognize that the child care provider may have fears regarding liability for injuries.

Schooling

School visits are most helpful on enrollment in a new school and ideally include the child and parent or parents.

Because of the difficulty in understanding acute onset and resolution of bleeding episodes, peer acceptance may initially be poor.

Acknowledge potential fear of HIV infection among school personnel, and educate regarding transmission and current safety of treatment.

Recognize potential alterations in body image and self-esteem because of chronic joint arthropathy or limitations on physical activity.

Intracranial bleeding may result in learning problems.

Continued

Summary of Primary Care Needs for the Child with Bleeding Disorders: Hemophilia and von Willebrand Disease—cont'd

Sexuality

Delay circumcision until the child with a positive family history is screened for a bleeding disorder.

Safe-sex counseling is recommended to prevent sexually transmitted diseases.

Transition into Adulthood

The transfer of medical care from a pediatric center to an adult hemophilia center may be difficult.

Educational and career opportunities may be restricted because of physical limitations and the need to be near a treatment center.

Obtaining health care coverage for a bleeding disorder may be difficult and may limit employment opportunities. Individuals may be eligible for SSI if disabilities are significant.

FAMILY CONCERNS

Child abuse may be suspected.

Parents may experience guilt regarding hereditary nature of a bleeding disorder.

The fear of injury to an infant may decrease parent-infant bonding.

Parents may fear the inability to prevent bleeding episodes despite attempts to prevent injury.

The potential for undiscovered HIV and hepatitis C infection may be a concern.

The family may experience uncertainty regarding the viral safety of blood products.

Insurance problems may occur as children and adults reach lifetime maximum amounts of reimbursement.

REFERENCES

Almeida, A., Khair, K., Hann, I., & Liesner, R. (2002). Unusual presentation of factor XIII deficiency. *Haemophilia, 8*(5), 703-705.

Anderson, A., Holtzman, T.S., & Masley, J. (2000). *Physical therapy in bleeding disorders.* New York: National Hemophilia Foundation.

Batlle, J., Noya, M.S., Giangrande, P., & Lopez-Fernandez, M.F. (2002). Advances in the therapy of von Willebrand disease. *Haemophilia, 8*(3), 301-307.

Centers for Disease Control and Prevention. (2002). *General Recommendation on Immunizations, 51,* RR-2.

Chorba, T.L. (2001). Effects of HIV infection on age and cause of death for persons with hemophilia A in the United States. *Am J Hematol, 66,* 229-240.

Diamondstone, L.S., Aledort, L.M., & Goedert, J.J. (2002). Factors predictive of death among HIV-uninfected persons with haemophilia and other congenital coagulation disorders. *Haemophilia, 8*(5), 660-667.

Dilley, A., Drews, C., Miller, C., Lally, C., Austin, H., et al. (2001). Von Willebrand disease and other inherited bleeding disorders in women with diagnosed menorrhagia. *Obstet Gynecol, 97*(4), 630-636.

Feinstein, D.I. (2000). Inhibitors in hemophilia. In R. Hoffman et al. (Eds.). *Hematology: Basic principles and practice* (3rd ed.). New York: Churchill Livingstone.

Fischer, K., van der Bom, J.G., Mauser-Bunschoten, E.P., Roosendaal, G., Prejs, R., et al. (2002). The effects of postponing prophylactic treatment on long-term outcome in patients with severe hemophilia. *Blood, 99*(7), 2337-2341.

Goedert, J.J., Eyster, M.E., Lederman, M.M., Mandalaki, T., De Moerloose, P., et al. (2002). End-stage liver disease in persons with hemophilia and transfusion-associated infections. *Blood, 100*(5), 1584-1589.

Harrington, B. (2000). Primary dental care of patients with haemophilia. *Haemophilia, 6*(suppl. 1), 7-12.

Hilgartner, M.W. (2002). Current treatment of hemophilic arthropathy. *Curr Opin Pediatr, 14*(1), 46-49.

Jadhav, M. & Warrier, I. (2000). Anaphylaxis in patients with hemophilia. *Semin Thromb Hemost, 26*(2), 205-208.

Jones, P. (2002). *Living with haemophilia* (5th ed.). Oxford, England: Oxford University Press.

Kadir, R.A. & Aledort, L.M. (2000). Obstetrical and gynaecological bleeding: A common presenting symptom. *Clin Lab Haematol, 22*(suppl. 1), 12-16.

Kasper, C.K. (2002a). Concentrate safety and efficacy. *Haemophilia, 8*(3), 161-165.

Kasper, C.K. (2002b). *Principles of clotting factor therapy in hemophilia.* Los Angeles: Orthopedic Hospital.

Kulkarni, R. & Lusher, J.M. (1999). Intracranial and extracranial hemorrhages in newborns with hemophilia: A review of the literature. *J Pediatr Hematol Oncol, 21*(4), 289-295.

Kulkarni, R. & Lusher, J. (2001). Review: Perinatal management of newborns with haemophilia. *Br J Haematol, 112,* 264-274.

Kulkarni, R., Aledort, L.M., Berntorp, E., Brackman, H.H., Brown, D., et al. (2001). Therapeutic choices for patients with hemophilia and high-titer inhibitors. *Am J Hematol, 67*(4), 240-246.

Lee, C.A. (1999). Women and inherited bleeding disorders: Menstrual issues. *Semin Hematol, 36*(3, suppl. 4), 21-27.

Lee, C. & Dusheiko, G. (2002). The natural history and antiviral treatment of hepatitis C in haemophilia. *Haemophilia, 8*(3), 322-329.

Ljung, R.C. (1999). Prenatal diagnosis of haemophilia. *Haemophilia, 5*(2), 84-87.

Ljung, R. (2002). Paediatric care of the child with haemophilia. *Haemophilia, 8*(3), 178-182.

Lozier, J.N. & Kessler, C.R. (2000). Clinical aspects and therapy of hemophilia. In R. Hoffman et al. (Eds.). *Hematology: Basic principles and practice* (3rd ed.). New York: Churchill Livingstone.

Manns, M.P., McHutchison, J.G., Gordon, S.C., Rustgi, V.K., Shiffman, M., et al. (2001). Peginterferon alfa-2b plus ribavirin compared with interferon alfa-2b plus ribavirin for initial treatment of chronic hepatitis C: A randomised trial. *Lancet, 358,* 958-965.

Mannucci, P.M., Chediak, J., Hanna, W., Byrnes, J., Ledford, M., et al. (Alphanate Study Group). (2002). Treatment of von Willebrand disease with a high-purity factor VIII/von Willebrand factor concentrate: A prospective, multicenter study. *Blood, 99*(2), 450-456.

Medical and Scientific Advisory Council of the National Hemophilia Foundation. (2001a). *MASAC recommendations concerning prophylaxis (prophylactic administration of clotting factor concentrate to prevent bleeding). MASAC Recommendation #117.* New York: National Hemophilia Foundation.

Medical and Scientific Advisory Council of the National Hemophilia Foundation. (2002). *MASAC recommendations concerning the treatment of hemophilia and other bleeding disorders. MASAC Document #135.* New York: National Hemophilia Foundation.

Medical and Scientific Advisory Council of the National Hemophilia Foundation. (2001b). *MASAC recommendations regarding the treatment of von Willebrand disease. MASAC Recommendation #112.* New York: National Hemophilia Foundation.

Miller, R. (1999). Counseling about diagnosis and inheritance of genetic bleeding disorders: Haemophilia A and B. *Haemophilia, 5,* 77-83.

Revel-Vilk, S., Blanchette, V.S., Sparling, C., Stain, A.M., & Carcao, M.D. (2002). DDAVP challenge tests in boys with mild/moderate haemophilia A. *Br J Haematol, 117*(4), 947-951.

Rodeghiero, F. (2002). Von Willebrand disease: Still an intriguing disorder in the era of molecular medicine. *Haemophilia, 8*(3), 292-300.

Rodriguez-Merchan, E.C. (2002). Orthopaedic surgery of haemophilia in the 21st century: An overview. *Haemophilia, 8*(3), 360-368.

Shetty, S., Ghosh, K., Pathare, A., & Mohanty, D. (1999). Carrier detection in haemophilia A families: Comparison of conventional coagulation parameters with DNA polymorphism analysis—first report from India. *Haemophilia, 5*(4), 243-246.

Soucie, J.M., Nuss, R., Evatt, B., Abdelhak, A., Cowan, L., et al. (2000). Mortality among males with hemophilia: Relations with source of medical care. *Blood, 96*(2), 437-442.

Stubbs, M. & Lloyd, J. (2001). A protocol for the dental management of von Willebrand's disease, haemophilia A and haemophilia B. *Aust Dent J, 46*(1), 37-40.

U.S. Department of Health and Human Services. (2002). *Report on the Universal Data Collection Program (UDC). 4*(1). Atlanta: Centers for Disease Control and Prevention.

Vento, S., Garofano, T., Renzini, C., Cainelli, F., Casali, F., et al. (1998). Fulminant hepatitis associated with hepatitis A virus superinfection in patients with chronic hepatitis C. *N Engl J Med, 338*(5), 286-290.

Walsh, E.C. (2002). Gene therapy for the hemophilias. *Curr Opin Pediatr, 14*(1), 12-16.

Wiedel, J.D. (2002). Arthroscopic synovectomy: State of the art. *Haemophilia, 8*(3), 372-374.

Wilde, J., Teixeira, P., Bramhall, S.R., Gunson, B., Mutimer, D., et al. (2002). Liver transplantation in haemophilia. *Br J Haematol, 117*(4), 952-956.

Yee, T.T., Griffioen, A., Sabin, C.A., Dusheiko, G., & Lee, C.A. (2000). The natural history of hepatitis C in a cohort of patients with hemophilia. *Gut, 47,* 845-851.

15 Bone Marrow Transplantation

Karen Marie Kristovich

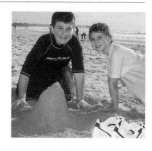

Etiology

Bone marrow transplantation, or hematopoietic stem cell transplantation (HSCT), as it is more recently referred to, is a treatment option for children with cancer, conditions that affect the hematopoietic and immune systems, and some metabolic conditions. Significant advances in HSCT in the past 2 decades have led to increased sources of stem cells and donors as well as improved outcomes (Trigg, 2002). Diseases and disorders that can be treated or cured by HSCT have also increased and now include a variety of leukemias, solid tumors, immune deficiencies, other deficiencies from marrow-derived cells, and some genetic disorders (Box 15-1). Sources of stem cells have expanded, going beyond bone marrow as the original source, to include peripheral blood and umbilical cord blood. Improved understanding of human leukocyte antigens (HLAs) has improved the accuracy of donor typing for matched-related, as well as mismatched and haplo-identical family donors and volunteer unrelated adult donors.

As a treatment option HSCT is used to (1) maximize treatment of malignancies by intensifying cytotoxic chemotherapy such that hematopoietic toxicity becomes dose limiting, combining this high-dose chemotherapy with stem cell infusion to restore hematopoiesis; and (2) correct acquired or congenital defects in marrow production and/or immune function. There are three basic types of HSCT: *autologous,* when the individual acts as his or her own donor, having stem cells collected and stored before the myeloablative therapy; *syngeneic,* when a genetically identical twin is used as the donor; and *allogeneic,* when the child receives stem cells from a related or unrelated donor. The type of transplant and source of stem cells used in transplantation are primarily determined by the diagnosis and clinical condition of the child and donor availability. Autologous HSCT is most commonly used for children with high-risk neuroblastoma, recurrent lymphomas, recurrent Wilm tumor, and some brain tumors and sarcomas. Autologous HSCT has a lower mortality rate from acute toxicities but a higher incidence of recurrent disease (Molina et al, 2000; Weisdorf et al, 2002).

Hematopoietic conditions, both malignant and nonmalignant, and genetic disorders are usually treated with allogeneic transplantation. The preferred donor source for allogeneic transplantation is an HLA-identical family member, which most often is a sibling. Alternative donor sources are frequently sought since only 30% of children have an HLA-identical family member. Although the overall incidence of disease recurrence is lower in allogeneic transplants, there is a higher posttransplant morbidity and mortality rate because of the host immunosuppression required to achieve donor engraftment and prevent graft-vs.-host disease (GVHD) (Molina et al, 2000; Weisdorf et al, 2002). These risks are greater when an unrelated or mismatched family member donor is utilized (Gross et al, 2001). Allogeneic transplants owe their antitumor effect not only to the cytotoxic treatment but also to the potential immune effect mediated by the donor lymphocytes, which has been termed the graft-vs.-tumor or leukemia (GVL) effect (Gustafsson et al, 2003).

Indications for HSCT have changed over the years. In the 1980s the most common indication was salvage therapy for children with acute lymphoid leukemia (ALL) who failed to maintain or achieve remission from conventional therapy. With the improvements in treatment for childhood cancer, combined with the significant advances in HSCT and supportive care, this treatment option is used now more often as primary therapy for children with certain high-risk leukemias, including acute myelogenous leukemia (AML), chronic myelogenous leukemia (CML), juvenile myelomonocytic leukemia (JMML), and infant ALL. The majority of children with ALL are now cured using conventional chemotherapy, and therefore HSCT is used to treat children with high-risk leukemias and recurrent disease. Other indications for HSCT include salvage therapy for children with recurrent solid tumors and recurrent lymphomas that demonstrated responsiveness to chemotherapy, as well as first-line therapy for some children with aplastic anemia and other nonmalignant conditions outlined in Box 15-1.

There are important fundamental differences between allogeneic HSCT and solid organ transplantation (see Chapter 34) which should be mentioned. In solid organ transplantation there are a limited number of donor cells with immunologic activity being transferred into the host through the transplanted organ. The immune system of the recipient will recognize the organ as foreign without adequate immune suppression. The primary concern after transplant is with preventing the rejection of the organ by the recipient's immune system. This usually requires lifelong administration of immunosuppressive medications. In HSCT the preparative regimen the recipient receives before transplantation, typically high-dose chemotherapy with or without total body irradiation, eliminates most elements of the immune system. The transplant of donor stem cells contains all the necessary cellular elements for complete reconstitution of the hematopoietic and immune system in the recipient. The immune system following transplantation therefore is generated by the graft and comes from the donor.

The primary concerns after HSCT are threefold: (1) preventing graft rejection mediated by recipient T-lymphocytes that survived the preparative regimen, (2) preventing donor cells from activating an immunologic response against the

Conditions for Use of Autologous and/or Allogeneic Hematopoietic Stem Cell Transplants

MALIGNANCIES
Leukemia/preleukemia
  Chronic myeloid leukemia
  Acute myeloid leukemia
  Acute lymphoblastic leukemia
  Juvenile chronic myeloid leukemia
  Myelodysplastic syndromes (MDSs)
  Therapy-related MDS/leukemia
  Chronic lymphocytic leukemia
Non-Hodgkin and Hodgkin lymphoma
Multiple myeloma
Solid tumors
  Breast cancer
  Testicular cancer
  Ovarian cancer
  Small cell lung cancer
  Neuroblastoma
  Wilms tumor
  Other pediatric solid tumors

NONMALIGNANT CONDITIONS
Severe aplastic anemia
Paroxysmal nocturnal hemoglobinuria
Hemoglobinopathies
  Thalassemia
  Sickle cell anemia
Congenital disorders of hematopoiesis
  Fanconi anemia
  Diamond-Blackfan syndrome
  Kostmann agranulocytosis
  Familial erythrophagositic histiocytosis
  Dyskeratosis congenita
  Shwachman-Diamond syndrome
Severe combined immunodeficiencies
  Wiskott-Aldrich syndrome
  Inborn errors of metabolism

From Horowitz, M.M. (1999). Uses and growth of hematopoietic cell transplantation. In E.D. Thomas, K.G. Blume, & S.J. Forman (Eds.). *Hematopoietic cell transplantation* (2nd ed.). Boston: Blackwell, pp. 12-17. Reprinted with permission.

recipient causing tissue injury and GVHD, and (3) allowing for immunologic reconstitution so that the donor-derived cells recognize and control pathogens in the host body. Immunosuppressive medications are used to prevent and treat GVHD. Immune tolerance can be achieved between the donor and recipient usually in 6 to 12 months. This allows for discontinuation of immunosuppressive medications following allogeneic HSCT in the majority of children.

Known Genetic Etiology

The majority of HSCTs occur in children with a malignant disease. Chapter 17 reviews known genetic etiologies for childhood cancers. HSCT is also used as a potentially curative treatment option for some children with genetic disorders characterized by deficits involving hematopoiesis or metabolic disorders caused by specific enzyme deficiencies. For example, hemoglobinopathies, such as severe beta-thalassemia and sickle cell disease, could potentially be corrected by allogeneic HSCT, which would correct the underlying genetic disease by provid-

ing a new donor-derived hematopoietic system. The use of HSCT for these conditions is actively being studied (Mentzer, 2000). Other genetic disorders treated by transplant include some mucopolysaccharidoses (MPSs), such as MPS I (Hurler syndrome), and some leukodystrophies (Kaye, 2001; Krivit, 2002). For these metabolic disorders the donor hematopoietic stem cells provide a source of macrophages and other marrow-derived cells that produce the deficient enzymes or proteins. Correction of the underlying enzyme deficiency prevents future deposition of abnormal storage products that are the cause of organ dysfunction in most metabolic diseases. However, any preexisting damage caused by the disorder up to the time of transplant may not be reversible.

Incidence and Prevalence

According to the International Bone Marrow Transplant Registry/Autologous Blood & Marrow Transplant Registry (IBMTR/ABMTR) there were an estimated 40,000 HSCTs carried out worldwide in 2000: an estimated 15,000 allogeneic and over 25,000 autologous transplants (IBMTR/ABMTR, 2002). The IBMTR/ABMTR collects and analyzes data from blood and marrow transplant centers nationally and internationally. More than 450 centers now participate in the IBMTR, and over 200 autologous transplant centers participate in the ABMTR. Data from the IBMTR/ABMTR between 1998 and 2000 reveal that approximately 30% of the autologous and allogeneic transplants were in individuals 20 years of age or younger. Hematopoietic stem cell sources for allogeneic transplants in this group report 70% from bone marrow, 18% from peripheral blood, and 12% from umbilical cord blood. Of the almost 8000 children with allogeneic transplants, 6000 utilized related donors, and the remaining 2000 required unrelated donors. The stem cell sources for autologous transplants in children during the same period were 80% from peripheral blood and the remaining 20% from bone marrow or a combination of peripheral blood and bone marrow.

Clinical Manifestations at Time of Diagnosis

The majority of children with malignant conditions are in remission or have minimal residual disease when they are referred for HSCT. They may, however, exhibit treatment-related side effects, such as alopecia, anorexia, weight loss, or organ dysfunction (see Chapter 17). Children with severe aplastic anemia will be pancytopenic and may have petechiae and bruising from thrombocytopenia.

Treatment (Box 15-2)

Referral and Consultation

Children being considered for transplantation are referred to an HSCT team by their pediatric hematologist/oncologist, immunologist, or geneticist. Consultation is particularly important in identifying suitable candidates at an early stage of their disorder. Box 15-3 reviews the responsibilities of the HSCT team during this process. Children and their families require a comprehensive evaluation and counseling by an experienced multidisciplinary team. The timing and type of transplant depend on

Treatment

REFERRAL AND CONSULTATION
Pretransplant work-up
   Human leukocyte antigen (HLA) typing
   Peripheral blood stem cell (PBSC) collection

PERITRANSPLANT PHASE
Preparative regimens
   Chemotherapy
   Total body irradiation
   Total lymphoid irradiation
Transplant day

POSTTRANSPLANT PHASE
Immunosuppressive management
   Nonspecific immunosuppressive drugs
   Specific T-lymphocyte immunosuppressive drugs
   Antibodies
Infection prevention
   High-efficiency particulate air (HEPA) filter system in hospital rooms
   Antiinfective agent prophylaxis
   Passive antibody prophylaxis
   Infection reduction techniques
Consolidative radiation therapy/chemotherapy for malignancies

Responsibilities of the Hematopoietic Stem Cell Transplant Center for Referral and Consultation Process

Referral is obtained. The following data are gathered:
   Basic demographic information
   Review of medical history and summary
   Reason for referral

Transplant and referral teams discuss disease and remission status, performance status, role of transplantation within the disease trajectory, and logistical variables.

Transplant team discusses child's eligibility, appropriateness for transplantation, potential stem cell sources, and best curative intent. Child is placed on an upcoming/new patient list.

In the case of allogeneic transplantation: HLA typing is ordered or obtained and a search for a donor begins. If an unrelated donor search is expected, an international search is initiated based on the best available, highest resolution typing. Family, umbilical cord, and marrow options are discussed, and all results are compared to determine the best source for the individual child's circumstances.

In the case of autologous peripheral/marrow transplantation: Dates for marrow/peripheral harvest(s) are scheduled, in conjunction with the planned date of the transplant. If PBSC is planned, the appropriate catheter is also discussed and may be placed at this time.

A thorough psychosocial assessment of the child and family is undertaken to evaluate financial resources; social supports; religious, cultural, and ethnic variables; and family dynamics. In addition, issues surrounding compliance, follow-up, and aftercare demands are explored with the family.

Multiple visits and counseling sessions are scheduled in the weeks following referral to consolidate the preparation and evaluation of the child and family. Extensive verbal and written information and education are provided to the family and referring physician or institution. In out-of-state referrals, these can be conducted via teleconferencing.

Search results and/or total stem cell doses (cord nucleated cell counts, yields from peripheral stem cell collections) are reviewed, and the best stem cell source and total targeted nucleated cell dose are obtained.

Financial coverage for the transplant is secured. Insurance benefits are reviewed, and authorization for transplantation is obtained before the scheduled transplant. A letter of medical necessity is formulated, and information is communicated to the payer, referring physician, and family. When relevant, a global case rate or individual payment contract is negotiated at this time.

From Gonzales-Ryan, L. et al. (2002). Hematopoietic stem cell transplantation. In C.R. Baggot, K.P. Kelly, D. Foctman, & G.V. Foley (Eds.). *Nursing care of children and adolescents with cancer* (3rd ed.). Philadelphia: W.B. Saunders, pp. 212-255. Reprinted with permission.

the child's diagnosis and stage of disease. Excellent communication among the transplant team, referring physician, and primary care practitioner is essential.

Pretransplant Work-up

A thorough clinical evaluation of the child and donor (if applicable) takes place within 4 weeks of the proposed admission (Box 15-4). Special attention is given to the evaluation of organ function in the child receiving transplantation to determine if he or she can withstand high-dose cytotoxic therapy. The majority of the testing takes place at the referring or transplant centers, but some tests may be obtained locally. This is usually a time of anxiety and uncertainty for the child and family, and these feelings are intensified by any delays or unexpected problems, such as infection or relapse of the disease.

HLA Typing. Tissue typing, or HLA typing, is used to identify genetically compatible hematopoietic stem cell donors. Human leukocyte antigens are proteins found on the surface of almost all nucleated cells in the body. These antigens regulate the immune response in specific ways and are responsible for the body's ability to recognize "self" from "nonself" on a cellular level.

There are two main classes of HLA antigens: class I antigens (HLA-A, -B, -C) and class II antigens (HLA-DR, -DQ, -DP), both of which are key in determining histocompatibity in transplantation. There are many different specific HLA proteins within each class of antigens. The genes that encode these antigens are on the short arm of chromosome 6. These genes are closely linked and inherited within families as clustered groups, or *haplotypes*. Each person has two haplotypes, one set being inherited from each parent. The best donor for an allogeneic HSCT is an HLA-identical sibling, that is, an individual who shares two sets of identical haplotypes with the recipient. Family HLA typing is obtained for children requir-

ing an allogeneic transplant. Children receiving the same HLA haplotype from each parent would be HLA identical and express the same HLA antigens on the surface of their cells. There is a 25% chance that a child's sibling will be HLA identical. Parents should always be HLA typed whenever possible. Parents may have one or more alleles in common, a recombination of alleles or sharing of haplotypes, which may increase the chance of identifying an HLA-identical family donor by an additional 5%.

If an allogeneic transplant is required and an appropriate sibling or family donor is not identified or available, an unrelated donor search is initiated. National and international donor registries are accessed by the search coordinator at the transplanting institution. The National Marrow Donor Program (NMDP) is the largest volunteer donor registry and was estab-

Comprehensive Pre-HSCT Evaluation

STAGING AND DISEASE-RELATED TESTS (AS APPROPRIATE)
Bone marrow aspirate and biopsy
Spinal tap/cerebrospinal fluid assessment
Radiologic tests (computed tomography, magnetic resonance imaging, bone
scans, x-rays, gallium scans)
Tissue biopsy (liver, reevaluation or staging surgery)
Tumor markers

COMPREHENSIVE ASSESSMENT AND ORGAN PERFORMANCE STATUS
Catheter/venous access issues
Psychosocial assessment
Nutritional evaluation
Occupational and physical therapy evaluation
Ancillary support evaluation (education/academic support, child life, clergy)
Transfusion history and support planning
Blood product donor screening and preparation
Significant drug intolerance or allergies
Genetic disease status evaluation (if applicable)
Dental evaluation
Hearing evaluation
Multiple gated acquisition (MUGA), echocardiogram, electrocardiogram (ECG)
Chest x-rays
Pulmonary function tests
Sinus films
Sperm or ova banking

LABORATORY TESTS
Complete blood count
Renal, hepatic, electrolyte, endocrine serum tests
Hepatitis screen (A, B, C)
Human immunodeficiency virus (HIV)
Cytomegalovirus (CMV)
Herpes simplex virus
Human T-cell leukemia/lymphoma virus (HTLV)
Rapid plasma regain (RPR; syphilis screen)
Prothrombin time (PT), partial thromboplastin time (PTT)

From Gonzales-Rya, L. et al. (2002). Hematopoietic stem cell transplantation. In C.R. Baggot, K.P. Kelly, D. Foctman, & G.V. Foley (Eds.). *Nursing care of children and adolescents with cancer* (3rd ed.). Philadelphia: W.B. Saunders, pp. 212-255. Reprinted with permission.

lished in 1986. There are more than 4.8 million potential donors registered with the NMDP and approximately 3000 searches taking place at any time (NMDP, 2003). If an unrelated donor is being used, the transplant center closest to the donor is responsible for the donor evaluation and cell collection.

Peripheral Blood Stem Cell Collection. Children who will receive an autologous HSCT will require peripheral blood stem cell (PBSC) collection. This process, *apheresis,* involves the use of a commercially available automated blood cell separator, with the collection occurring weeks or months before the planned transplant. Hematopoietic stem cells normally reside in the bone marrow and are rarely detected in peripheral blood. Mobilization of the stem cells into the peripheral blood can be accomplished during the recovery phase of myelosuppressive chemotherapy and is enhanced by the administration of recombinant hematopoietic growth factors. Granulocyte colony-stimulating factor (G-CSF, filgrastim) is the most commonly used recombinant human growth factor and is administered by subcutaneous injection daily until collection is complete.

Complete blood cell counts (CBCs) are obtained daily and followed closely by both the transplant and pheresis teams. PBSC collection starts as the white blood cell (WBC) count begins to rise. Careful consideration is given to the vascular access device of the child, and temporary pheresis catheters can be placed if the child's indwelling central venous catheter (CVC) is too small to accommodate the pheresis procedure. In older children or teenagers, large peripheral intravenous (IV) lines can be used in place of indwelling central catheters. Multiple daily collections are commonly required to obtain an adequate stem cell dose.

Side effects of G-CSF include bone pain, headache, myalgia, and fatigue (*Physicians' Desk Reference [PDR], 2003*). A small percentage of children will have poor mobilization of PBSCs resulting in inadequate collection of stem cells. This most frequently occurs in children who have been heavily pretreated with chemotherapy or radiation. In this circumstance, a bone marrow harvest may be used to attempt to reach the desired stem cell dose.

Stem Cell Manipulation. Stem cells for autologous and allogeneic transplantation may be manipulated before infusion to reduce the risk of some complications or disease recurrence. A blood cell separator is generally used for this purpose. In autologous PBSC collection, particular stem cells may be selected for inclusion in the infusion, allowing the remainder of the pheresis product to be discarded and facilitating removal of potential tumor cell contamination. A technique used at some transplant centers for allogeneic transplants is the removal of T-lymphocytes from unrelated donor bone marrow in an effort to decrease the risk of GVHD. Although T-lymphocyte depletion of donor marrow is an effective method of GVHD prophylaxis, children who receive T cell—depleted grafts are at increased risk for graft rejection, disease recurrence, and delayed immunologic recovery after HSCT.

Peritransplant Phase

Children begin the conditioning, or preparative regimen, 5 to 10 days before the cell infusion date. Admission to the transplant unit occurs when the preparative regimen begins, or on the day of transplantation, and will vary at institutions. Preparative regimens consist of high-dose chemotherapy with or without total body irradiation (TBI). The most common regimens utilize high-dose cyclophosphamide (CY) given in combination with busulfan (BU) or TBI. Other chemotherapeutic agents used in various combinations include high-dose etoposide (VP-16), carmustine (BCNU), melphalan, and thiotepa. Total lymphoid irradiation (TLI) may be used as an alternate form of radiation therapy (XRT).

Regimen selection is determined by the underlying disease and type of HSCT and serves multiple functions: (1) tumor cytoreduction and ideally disease eradication in the case of malignancy, (2) marrow ablation to allow for space in the bone marrow for new stem cells and to remove any dysfunctional stem cells, and (3) sufficient immunosuppression to overcome host-mediated rejection of the donor cells. The child usually becomes neutropenic shortly after beginning the preparative regimen. Treatment side effects include severe mucositis, pancytopenia, venoocclusive disease, nausea, vomiting, and renal insufficiency.

On transplant day, or day zero, the stem cells are infused into the child, a process that is similar to a blood product infusion. If the stem cells are from marrow of a related donor, the bone marrow harvest takes place the same day in an operating room suite. In an autologous transplant, the cryopreserved stem cell product is thawed and infused into the child. When an unrelated donor is used, the freshly harvested marrow or stem cell product is escorted from the donor center, usually requiring air transportation, to the transplant center. The marrow is processed by a specialized lab at the transplanting institution and must be infused within 24 hours from the time it is harvested. The child begins strict isolation per institutional policy when the stem cells are infused or when the child becomes neutropenic. Once the cells are infused intravenously they migrate to the bone marrow, and within 10 to 21 days production of normal blood cells usually occurs. This is called hematopoietic *engraftment*. The child is usually confined to the transplant unit or a specific transplant room until engraftment has occurred. This too may differ at institutions, since some are performing outpatient autologous HSCT and may only require admission for fever or other complications.

Posttransplant Phase

Immunosuppressive Management. Immunosuppressive regimens may vary according to the child's underlying diagnosis, stem cell source, or treatment or institutional protocol. Almost all allogeneic transplant recipients receive immunosuppressive medications to prevent GVHD. Exceptions to this include syngeneic transplants and those for severe combined immunodeficiencies (SCIDS), when little to no immunosuppression is required. Cyclosporine (CSA, Neoral) has been the core of prophylactic therapy since the 1980s and is typically combined with a short course of methotrexate (MTX) or corticosteroids. Tacrolimus (Prograf, FK-506) has recently replaced CSA as the prophylactic immunosuppressive drug for unrelated donor transplants at many centers after showing a lower incidence of moderate to severe GVHD (Jacobson et al, 1998). Other common immunosuppressive agents include antithymocyte globulin (ATG) and mycophenolate mofetil (CellCept, MMF). Table 15-1 outlines toxicities of these agents.

Specific T-lymphocyte immunosuppressive drugs. Cyclosporine (CSA) interferes with the activation of T-lymphocytes,

or T cells, the cells responsible for stimulating GVHD. It is initially given intravenously in the early phase of transplantation and then switched to liquid or capsules for oral use after resolution of mucositis and adequate gastrointestinal absorption resumes. Dosage is usually protocol driven; however, the goal is to achieve a therapeutic blood level with higher loading doses and eventual tapering of the medication. Only steady state trough levels are useful in determining if a therapeutic level has been achieved. Values of CSA levels drawn at other times are usually uninterpretable for drug dosing management. Tacrolimus (Prograf, FK-506), although structurally different from CSA, has the same cellular function, interrupting T-cell activation. Similar to CSA, it is first administered intravenously and later given orally. Mycophenolate mofetil (MMF) has multiple properties, including antibacterial, antifungal, antiviral, and immunosuppressive.

Nonspecific immunosuppressive drugs. Corticosteroids can be used alone or in combination with other agents for the prevention of GVHD or treatment of acute or chronic GVHD. The mechanism of action of corticosteroids is not fully understood, but they may suppress proinflammatory cytokines as well as interfere with T-lymphocyte function. Corticosteroids are given intravenously or orally when children are able to eat sufficiently and have adequate absorption. Methotrexate (MTX) is a highly efficient and toxic antimetabolite. The exact mechanism of action in prevention of GVHD is not known, but it has been shown to induce tolerance when administered before stem cell engraftment. MTX is usually administered intravenously in three or four doses within the first 2 weeks after transplant and may be used in combination with CSA or tacrolimus. However, in some protocols it is used as a single agent with weekly infusions up to day +100 after HSCT.

Antibodies. Antithymocyte globulin (ATG) is a product of serum immunoglobulins produced by injecting horses or rabbits with human thymocytes. The horse or rabbit antibodies produced are capable of reacting with and eliminating human T-lymphocytes. Regimens that include this therapy infuse ATG before the donor cell infusion to decrease the incidence of graft rejection or afterward to prevent GVHD. Serum sickness can occur since ATG is a foreign xenogeneic protein, and premedication and treatment with acetaminophen, corticosteroids, and H1 and H2 blockers are usually required.

TABLE 15-1

Toxicities of Immunosuppressive Agents

Cyclosporine	Tacrolimus	Methotrexate	Corticosteroids	ATG	Mycophenolate Mofetil
Nephrotoxicity	Nephrotoxicity	Mucositis	Hyperglycemia	Infection risk	Leukopenia
Hypertension	Hypertension	Delayed engraftment	Muscle wasting	Fever, chills	Anemia
Decreased magnesium	Decreased magnesium	Hepatotoxicity	Infection risk	Skin reactions	Thrombocytopenia
Tremors (hand)	Tremor		GI hemorrhage	Hypersensitivity	GI effects
Neurotoxicity	Neurotoxicity		Hypertension	Serum sickness	Headaches
Hyperkalemia	Hyperkalemia				
Hirsutism	HUS				
HUS					

From Gonzales-Ryan, L. et al. (2002). Hematopoietic stem cell transplantation. In C.R. Baggot, K.P. Kelly, D. Foctman, & G.V. Foley (Eds.). *Nursing care of children and adolescents with cancer* (3rd ed.). Philadelphia: W.B. Saunders, pp. 212-255. Reprinted with permission.
ATG, Antithymocyte globulin; *GI,* gastrointestinal; *HUS,* hemolytic-uremic syndrome.

Infection Prevention. Special precautions are taken to reduce the risk of infections in children who have undergone HSCT. Transplanting institutions utilize either high-efficiency particulate air (HEPA) filter systems or laminar airflow rooms to decrease potential environmental pathogens during the acute phase of transplantation. With no functioning immune system and alterations in mucosal integrity from treatment-related mucositis, these children are susceptible to bacterial, fungal, and viral infections. Several antiinfective agents are prescribed prophylactically for the prevention of *Pneumocystis carinii* pneumonia (PCP), reactivation of herpes simplex virus (HSV), cytomegalovirus (CMV), and fungal disease. Most allogeneic and some autologous recipients receive passive antibody prophylaxis with intravenous immunoglobulin (IVIG) after transplantation (Sokos et al, 2002). The dose and frequency vary by protocol or institutional policy and may be administered weekly, every other week, or every 4 weeks.

To further reduce the risk of infection, children and their families receive extensive counseling on prevention of infections by hand washing, appropriate foods and food preparation, as well as protective isolation guidelines, the details of which may vary among institutions. These guidelines typically include the use of a respirator or filter mask by the child when in the medical center or associated buildings and the need to avoid crowds, public buildings, and ill persons. Children are not allowed to return to school and will therefore attend hospital-based schools or home tutoring for the duration of isolation, which is commonly 6 to 12 months.

Tolerance and Chimerism. Tolerance of the donor cells to the host is primarily achieved by thymic education of the donor precursor T-lymphocytes that derive from donor stem cells in the marrow. Donor-derived precursor T-lymphocytes migrate to the host's thymus, where they are programmed to distinguish "self" from "nonself." These new donor-derived T-lymphocytes are educated to recognize the host as "self." The T-lymphocytes primarily involved in activating GVHD are the mature lymphocytes infused at transplantation that were previously coded in the donor's thymus and therefore would recognize the new recipient as "nonself."

Routine surveillance of donor- and recipient-derived hematopoiesis is obtained in children after allogeneic transplantation utilizing a variety of molecular methods to distinguish between and quantify the percentage of donor-derived vs. residual recipient-derived hematopoiesis. Serial testing allows the transplant team to assess for graft rejection and relapse. Molecular techniques are applied at most centers utilizing marrow and/or blood samples at specific time periods after HSCT. The transplanting institutional policy or patient protocol determines the frequency and timing of the testing.

Consolidative Radiation Therapy and Chemotherapy. Some children require further antineoplastic treatment after HSCT. In children with high-risk neuroblastoma, improvement in remission rates after HSCT were noted with the addition of consolidative radiation therapy (XRT) to their tumor bed region (Matthay et al, 1999). Following XRT they receive a 6-month treatment course of 13–cis–retinoic acid (isotretinoin, cis-RA, Accutane), an oral retinoid that is a differentiating agent for neuroblastoma and is believed to help control minimal residual disease (Kohler et al, 2000; Reynolds & Lemons,

2001). Children with Hodgkin disease usually receive post-HSCT XRT to the areas of previous disease after hematopoietic recovery. Children receiving consolidative XRT are monitored closely by the transplant team for treatment-related side effects and symptom management of XRT (see Chapter 17). Children with ALL may receive intrathecal MTX for central nervous system (CNS) prophylaxis after transplant at some institutions.

Complementary and Alternative Treatments

Children may use a variety of complementary and alternative treatments during the conditioning phase and in recovery after HSCT to control or alleviate symptoms of their disease or treatment (i.e., pain, nausea, fatigue, depression, anxiety). Acupuncture, acupressure, imagery/relaxation, therapeutic touch, massage, and aroma therapies are the most common. These therapies are employed as adjuncts to conventional medical therapy, as opposed to those that replace standard care, and are often encouraged by the HSCT team or oncology team managing the subspecialty interventions.

Biologically based natural therapies that are ingested or injected are contraindicated in children who have received HSCT because of multiple concerns: (1) products made from plant matter can be contaminated with fungal spores, (2) many natural products have definite biologic activity that can cause harmful side effects or interactions with other medications, and (3) the lack of product standardization and formal oversight of the herbal and dietary supplement industry fails to ensure product consistency and purity (Barnes, 2003).

Anticipated Advances in Diagnosis and Management

Research is improving survival in children receiving HSCT. The shortcomings of this treatment option include toxicities from the conditioning regimen, GVHD in allogeneic transplant recipients, and disease recurrence. Medical and scientific improvements in the past 3 decades have led to increased understanding of the hematopoietic and immune systems, directly affecting the outcomes in HSCT. Improvements in supportive care have further enhanced the chance of survival for children undergoing HSCT. Improved characterization of HLA antigens to identify optimal donors and novel stem cell selection technologies are examples of ongoing scientific investigations that continue to move the HSCT field forward. Treatment approaches to improve tumor kill and manipulate the immune system to decrease the risk of relapse show promise (Noga, 2000; Schouten, 2002; Waldmann, 2001).

Peripheral Blood Stem Cells

In the past 10 years there has been a shift from the use of bone marrow as the preferred source of hematopoietic stem cells to peripheral blood in autologous transplantation for both adults and children. Now, more than 80% of children undergoing autologous HSCTs receive PBSCs as the source of stem cells. Benefits of PBSCs include elimination of hospital admission, general anesthesia, and multiple bone marrow aspirates required for harvesting bone marrow as a source of hematopoietic stem cells. Hematopoietic recovery (engraftment) is also more rapid following the infusion of the PBSCs compared with bone marrow. The successful use of PBSCs in autologous recipients led to the investigation of PBSCs as a possible stem cell source in the allogeneic recipients using related and unrelated donors. Healthy allogeneic donors require G-CSF to mobilize stem cells to the peripheral blood, where they can be harvested by apheresis. Besides the multiple injections of G-CSF, temporary placement of a pheresis catheter may be required in donors with small veins.

During the last few years, mobilized PBSCs have been used more frequently for adults receiving allogeneic HSCT. Initial studies from adult transplants appeared promising; however, recent published reports show an increased frequency of chronic GVHD (Uharek et al, 2000). This finding has also been documented in small pediatric studies (Levine et al, 2000; Nagatoshi et al, 2002). Pediatric transplant centers utilize PBSCs in allogeneic transplantation in certain circumstances, but this remains limited because of several areas of concern. Further study is needed to evaluate the risk of chronic GVHD and risks to the healthy donor. The sibling donor for the child who is a transplant candidate is usually a minor. Since the long-term impact of G-CSF administration on healthy children is uncertain, ethical issues must be considered.

Nonmyeloablative (NMA) Transplants

This newer form of transplantation is also known as subablative transplants or minitransplants. It shows promise in the treatment of both nonmalignant and some malignant hematologic disorders. Traditionally, conditioning regimens for allogeneic transplantation rely on maximally tolerated doses of cytotoxic chemotherapy to eradicate malignancy and the allograft serves to rescue the child from treatment-related marrow aplasia. This conventional form of HSCT results in significant morbidity and mortality.

In an attempt to avoid this problem, immunosuppressive therapy combined with myelosuppressive but not myeloablative therapy has been used to try to achieve engraftment with less morbidity. Children receive submyeloablative doses of chemotherapy with or without TBI to create a partial but stable graft. In children with sickle cell anemia or thalassemia, only a small portion of hematopoietic stem cells is needed to fully engraft and function to correct the underlying genetic defect. In children with malignancy, especially leukemia, the goal of this approach is to achieve donor chimerism with a nontoxic conditioning regimen. Sufficient immunosuppression is used to achieve engraftment and allow graft-vs.-leukemia/tumor (GVL) effect to reduce minimal residual disease or prevent relapse. The use of nonmyeloablative transplant for hematologic malignancies is currently used primarily for older adults and some children who do not qualify for a standard ablative conditioning regimen because of preexisting organ toxicity (Djulbegavic et al, 2003; Georges & Storb, 2003; McSweeney et al, 2001).

Donor Lymphocyte Infusion (DLI)

DLI has been used for several years in treating both recurrent disease after HSCT and significant post- HSCT viral infections with some success (Bader et al, 1999; Greinix, 2002; Gross, 2001). DLIs are frequently used following NMA regimens to

increase host suppression and engineer full donor chimerism in the recipient (Massenkeil et al, 2003).

Tandem Transplants

Dose intensification, and the sequential use of chemotherapeutic agents to overcome drug resistance, may benefit some children with aggressive or resistant tumors. This treatment approach attempts to reduce residual disease by repeated, closely timed courses of high-dose chemotherapy, each given with a human to hematopoietic stem cell (HSC) rescue to reduce the risks associated with prolonged pancytopenia. Interest has been growing in this concept, and recent studies in children with high-risk neuroblastoma and other solid tumors show promise (Katzenstein et al, 2002; Kletzel et al, 2002).

In Utero Transplantation

In utero transplantation has only recently moved from animal models to humans and is being studied with mixed results in fetuses diagnosed with severe combined immunodeficiency syndrome (SCIDS), alpha-thalassemia, and other fatal or potentially fatal inborn errors of metabolism (Jones, 2001). The migration of fetal hematopoiesis in the first several weeks of gestation, when stem cells move from the yolk sac to the fetal liver before honing into the bone marrow, combined with a relatively incompetent fetal immune system, can allow for engraftment of donor cells in the bone marrow (Carrier, 2000).

Gene Therapy

Hematopoietic stem cells appear to be ideal candidates as vehicles for gene therapy. They are being studied as the mechanism for transferring genetic information in attempts to treat or cure disease at the gene level (Benedict et al, 2000). Box 15-5 reviews potential disorders for treatment with gene therapy.

Associated Problems (Box 15-6)

Anemia and Thrombocytopenia

All children experience prolonged marrow aplasia following the myeloablative conditioning regimen. Supportive platelet and red blood cell (RBC) transfusions are required until

---

BOX 15-5

Possible Disorders for Gene Therapy Using Hematopoietic Stem Cells

INHERITED DISORDERS
Congenital immune deficiencies: severe combined immunodeficiencies (SCIDs), Wiskott-Aldrich syndrome
Lysosomal storage diseases: Gaucher disease, adrenoleukodystrophy
Leukocyte defects: chronic granulomatous disease, Chédiak-Higashi syndrome
Hemoglobinopathies: sickle cell anemia, thalassemia, hemolytic anemias
Stem cell defects: Fanconi anemia

INFECTIOUS DISEASES
HIV-1 infection, AIDS

From Kohn, D.B., Crooks, G.M., & Nolta, J.A. (2000). Gene therapy using hematopoietic stem cells. In A.D. Ho, R. Haas, & R.E. Champlin (Eds.). *Hematopoietic stem cell transplantation.* New York: Marcel Dekker, Inc., pp. 537-552. Modified with permission.
HIV, Human immunodeficiency virus; *AIDS,* acquired immunodeficiency syndrome.

adequate hematopoietic function is restored by the engrafted megakaryocytes and RBC precursors. The recovery time is affected by the source of stem cells (marrow, umbilical cord blood, peripheral blood), manipulation of stem cells (T-cell depletion, purging), infection, and GVHD. Transfusions of platelets are generally required to prevent or treat bleeding complications in the child with thrombocytopenia. Most transplant centers attempt to keep the child's platelet count above 10 to 20×10^9/L and in some circumstances higher (e.g., history of CNS bleed, uncontrolled hypertension). Delayed platelet engraftment is not uncommon in recipients of autologous transplants since their stem cells may lack full hematopoietic potential because of prior exposure to chemotherapy. RBC support is usually required for at least 2 to 4 months after transplantation. This may be required longer in children receiving transplants from ABO-incompatible donors. The ABO and HLA genes are not inherited together; therefore a child may be HLA-A, -B, -DR identical to the donor but have a minor or major incompatibility to the RBCs of the donor. Recipient isohemagglutinins can be present for several weeks after HSCT and react against donor RBCs. This may result in poor erythroid engraftment, and prolonged RBC support may be required (Sniecinski & O'Donnell, 1999). Most transplant centers recommend maintaining a hemoglobin concentration of ≥10 g/dl in children during the acute HSCT phase and ≥8 g/dl for children in the recovery phase after HSCT.

Blood products should always be irradiated to prevent transfusion-associated GVHD in immunocompromised children. Blood products may contain small numbers of T-lymphocytes, which, if viable, can cause a potentially life-threatening reaction in the transfused child. Irradiation prevents the T-lymphocytes from replicating and attacking host cells without altering the normal function of the transfused RBCs or platelets (McCullough, 1999). Transfusion-acquired CMV infection can also be a major cause of morbidity and mortality in severely immunocompromised children; therefore CMV-negative blood

products should be used when available. Alternatively, the use of filters to deplete WBCs from the transfusion product (leukoreduction) has been shown to be highly effective in eliminating transmission of CMV.

Graft-vs.-Host Disease

GVHD is the major cause of morbidity and mortality in children who have received an allogeneic HSCT, affecting 10% to 50% of matching sibling donor transplant recipients (Zecca & Locatelli, 2000). GVHD can be mild, with no lasting effects, or severe, with debilitating or fatal consequences. Historically, GVHD has been divided into two phases: acute and chronic.

Acute GVHD. GVHD is an immune-mediated response in which donor T-lymphocytes react against the host's tissue after becoming sensitized to the host antigens. The activated T-lymphocytes differentiate into effector cells that produce cytokines and mediate cytotoxic activity targeted at specific tissues in the child, most commonly the skin, gastrointestinal tract, and liver. Acute GVHD occurs within the first 100 days following transplantation and may involve one, two, or all three organs. Staging and overall grading are based on the extent of involvement of each organ (Chao, 1999; Table 15-2). Grade I acute GVHD is considered mild, and grade II is moderate; both are associated with a favorable outcome. Grades III and IV are severe and have a significantly higher mortality rate (Sullivan, 1999; Tabbara et al, 2002). Involvement of target organs in GVHD often follows a characteristic clinical pattern and is ultimately defined pathologically (Box 15-7).

Biopsy is the definitive method of diagnosis for acute GVHD involving the skin, gastrointestinal tract, or liver.

BOX 15-6
Associated Problems

Anemia and thrombocytopenia
Graft-vs.-host disease
  Acute GVHD (<100 days after transplant)
    Target organs: skin, gastrointestinal, liver
  Chronic GVHD (>100 days after transplant; Table 15-4)
    Autoimmune reactions
    Severe immunodeficiency
Graft failure or rejection
  Primary
  Late or secondary
Infection
  Preengraftment phase
  Postengraftment phase
  Late phase
  Viral infections
    Cytomegalovirus (CMV)
    Herpes simplex virus (HSV)
    Varicella zoster virus (VZV)
  Fungus
Late effects
Relapse

TABLE 15-2
GVHD Stage and Grading Systems

Staging of Individual Organ System(s)		
Organ	**Stage**	**Description**
Skin	+1	Maculopapular (MP) eruption over <25% of body area
	+2	MP eruption over 25%-50% of body area
	+3	Generalized erythroderma
	+4	Generalized erythroderma with bullous formation and often with desquamation
Gut	+1	Diarrhea >30 ml/kg or >500 ml/day
	+2	Diarrhea >60 ml/kg or >1000 ml/day
	+3	Diarrhea >90 ml/kg or >1500 ml/day
	+4	Diarrhea >90 ml/kg or >2000 ml/day; or severe abdominal pain and bleeding with or without ileus
Liver	+1	Bilirubin 2.0-3.0 mg/dl; SGOT 150-750 IU
	+2	Bilirubin 3.1-6.0 mg/dl
	+3	Bilirubin 6.1-15.0 mg/dl
	+4	Bilirubin >15.0 mg/dl

Overall Grading of Acute GVHD			
Grade	**Skin Staging**	**Liver Staging**	**Gastrointestinal Staging**
I	+1 to +2	0	0
II	+1 to +3	+1 and/or	+1
III	+2 to +3	+2 to +4 and/or	+2 to +3
IV	+23 to +4	+2 to +4 and/or	+2 to +4

From Chao, N.J. (1999). *Graft-versus-host disease* (2nd ed.). Austin, Tex.: R.G. Landes, pp. 63-122. Modified with permission.
GVHD, Graft-vs.-host disease; *SGOT*, serum glutamic oxaloacetic transaminase.

BOX 15-7

Acute Graft-vs.-Host Target Organs

Skin: Skin is the most common organ affected by acute GVHD, with symptoms varying in intensity from mild erythematous maculopapular rash that can be pruritic to generalized erythroderma with bullous lesions and epidermal necrolysis.

Gastrointestinal: Gastrointestinal symptoms are characterized by diarrhea and abdominal cramping and may include intestinal bleeding. This can be the most difficult to treat in children. Staging of gastrointestinal GVHD is usually made by quantifying daily diarrhea output, which can be quite voluminous. Providing adequate fluid and electrolyte balance can be challenging in these children. Infection must also be considered as a cause of diarrhea, and stool cultures are sent for analysis. *Rotavirus* and *Clostridium difficile* are common in children undergoing HSCT.

Liver: Although a common site for acute GVHD, the liver is rarely the site of single-organ involvement. The earliest and most common sign of liver involvement is a rise in the conjugated bilirubin and alkaline phosphatase; however, there are many other causes of liver abnormalities in these children, including venoocclusive disease (VOD), hepatic infections, and drug toxicity.

BOX 15-8

Clinical Manifestations of Chronic Graft-vs.-Host Disease

Dermal	Oral	Ocular	Pulmonary
Erythema	Erythema	Conjunctivitis	Sinopulmonary infections
Lichenoid lesions	Atrophy	Uveitis	Bronchiolitis obliterans
Hypopigmentation	Lichen planus	Blurring	Obstructive lung disease
Hyperpigmentation	Xerostomia	Dryness	
Poikiloderma	Xerophthalmia	Photophobia	
Violaceous papule	Sjögren syndrome		
Progression?			
Induration			
Sclerosis			
Joint contractures			
Ulcers			
Alopecia			
Anhidrosis			

Hepatic	Musculoskeletal	Gastrointestinal
Liver function abnormalities	Arthralgias	Weight loss
Cholestasis	Synovial effusions	Desquamative esophagitis
	Arthritis	Gastroesophageal reflux
	Tendonitis	Malabsorption
	Fasciitis	
	Muscle cramping	

Data from Kansu, E. & Sullivan, K (2000). Late complications of hematopoietic stem cell transplantation. In A.D. Ho, R. Haas, & R.E. Champlin (Eds). *Hematopoietic stem cell transplantation.* New York: Marcel Dekker, Inc.

However, these children are at significant risk for bleeding with any invasive procedure. Liver biopsies pose the greatest threat and can cause intrahepatic and extrahepatic bleeding; transjugular approaches to these biopsies may reduce the bleeding risk (Chao, 1999; McCormack et al, 2001).

Chronic GVHD. Chronic GVHD (cGVHD) occurs after the first 100 days following an allogeneic HSCT, usually presenting between 3 and 18 months after transplantation. The incidence of cGVHD ranges from 33% with an HLA-identical sibling donor to 50% to 70% when an HLA-identical unrelated donor or mismatched family donor is used (Kansu & Sullivan, 2000). cGVHD involves target tissues that may differ from those sites affected by acute GVHD and is clinically more consistent with an autoimmune phenomenon, demonstrating features resembling lupus erythematosus, scleroderma, and rheumatoid arthritis (Chao, 1999) (Box 15-8). cGVHD may occur as a progression of acute GVHD, after a period of quiescence from acute GVHD, or as de novo disease. cGVHD is the single most determining factor of quality of life and morbidity following allogeneic HSCT.

Another serious consequence of cGVHD is severe immunodeficiency; immunosuppression is worsened by cGVHD itself and is further compounded by the treatment, which invariably involves the administration of immunosuppressive agents. Treatment of both acute and chronic GVHD includes the use of steroids, CSA, FK-506, and/or other immunosuppressive agents. Prompt and aggressive treatment of moderate to severe GVHD is necessary to attempt to bring the immune response under control. Complete or partial response occurs in slightly more than one half of these children (Arai & Vogelsang, 2000; Zecca & Locatelli, 2000). Newer treatments show promise, including extracorporeal photochemotherapy for steroid-resistant GVHD (Salvaneschi et al, 2001).

Graft Failure or Rejection

Failure or rejection of the graft is fortunately an infrequent complication in children following HSCT. There are generally two forms of graft failure: *primary*, when there are no signs of hematopoietic recovery following transplantation, and *late* or *secondary*, when persistent pancytopenia is seen weeks or months following initial engraftment. In children who receive autologous HSCT, graft failure can be caused by poor function of their stem cells, likely caused by the child having been heavily pretreated with chemotherapy before stem cell collection. Some drugs or infections can also damage the newly infused stem cells and result in graft failure. The likely causes for graft failure for a child receiving an allogeneic HSCT include a low stem cell dose, T cell–depleted transplantation, ineffective immunosuppression of the recipient, significant HLA disparity between the donor and recipient, and damage to the microenvironmental network during conditioning treatment or infection. Graft rejection is seen only in allogeneic HSCT recipients and is immune mediated leading to graft failure. It is often fatal unless a second graft can be achieved.

Infection

Bacterial, viral, and fungal infections are significant obstacles to both the immediate and long-term survival in children after HSCT. Although improvements in prophylaxis and treatment strategies have been numerous over the years, infections still contribute significantly to the morbidity and mortality of these children (Lujan-Zilbermann & Patrick, 2000). The risk of infection begins with the cytotoxic conditioning regimen used to treat the underlying disease. High-dose chemotherapy destroys

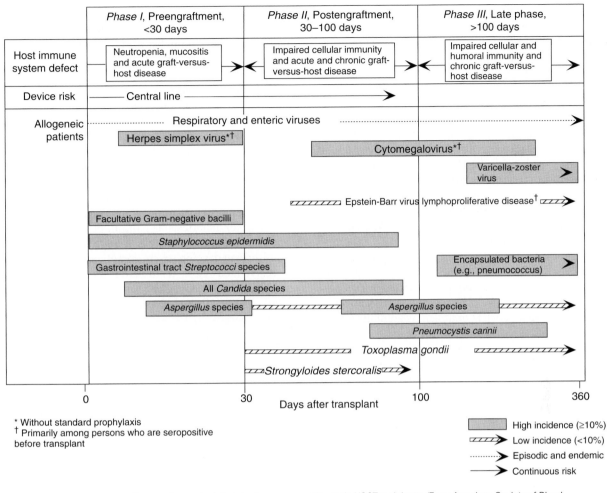

FIGURE 15-1 Phases of opportunistic infections among allogeneic HSCT recipients. (From American Society of Blood and Marrow Transplantation. [2000]. Guidelines for preventing opportunistic infections among hematopoietic stem cell transplant recipients. *Bio Blood Marrow Transplant, 6*(6a), 662. Reprinted with permission.)

the production of WBCs and damages mucosal cells, causing temporary loss of integrity of the mucosal barrier, vascular injury, and decreased ability of the child's body to repair tissue. All children treated with HSCT develop cellular and humoral immunodeficiencies for at least several months after transplantation; this can extend to years if they develop cGVHD. In general, phagocytic function recovers first. Lymphocytic function typically takes much longer to recover and function adequately. The child is at risk for certain types of infections at predictable time periods after HSCT, reflective of the predominant host-defense defect. The time line for the risk of opportunistic infections in these children is outlined in Figure 15-1.

Preengraftment Phase. For a child in the preengraftment phase, prolonged neutropenia and breaks in the mucosal and cutaneous barriers create increased risk of infection. The bacteria and fungi normally present in the gastrointestinal tract may then become a reservoir of potential pathogens. During this time, the risk of infection is the same for children receiving autologous or allogeneic transplantation. Translocated oral and bowel flora, along with indwelling CVCs, are the primary source of gram-positive and enteric gram-negative bacterial infections in children undergoing HSCT. Standard practice may

include the prophylactic or empiric use of antibiotics when bacteremia is suspected. The emergence of drug-resistant bacteria, such as vancomycin-resistant *Enterococcus,* however, has many transplant centers rethinking routine prophylaxis against bacterial infections (Sepkowitz, 2002). Superinfection with fungal organisms continues to be a serious cause of morbidity and mortality in the transplant arena. *Candida* and *Aspergillus* species are the most common causes, the latter resulting in more serious and sometimes fatal infections.

Postengraftment Phase. During the early engraftment (the first 100 days after HSCT), recipients of both autologous and allogeneic grafts have impaired cell-mediated immunity. GVHD and immunosuppressive therapy increase the risk of infection for children who have received an allogeneic transplant. Because these children lack intact T- lymphocyte function, they are at particular risk for viral infections. The most common viral infections in the early posttransplant phase are herpes simplex virus (HSV), cytomegalovirus (CMV) and varicella zoster virus (VZV). Infection can result from primary infection or reactivation of latent virus. These viruses are responsible for significant morbidity and mortality in children undergoing transplantation, and until the past decade there has been little pharmacologic armamentarium to use against them. *Pneumocystis carinii* pneumonia (PCP) is a potential pulmonary pathogen during this time, and although it was historically a frequent cause of serious infection in the immunocompromised child, it is now prevented in almost all cases by the prophylactic administration of trimethoprim-sulfamethoxazole (TMP-SMX, Septra, Bactrim).

Late Phase. During the late recovery phase (more then 100 days after transplantation), autologous recipients are at lower risk of opportunistic infections, with recovery of their immune function and no need for post-HSCT immunosuppressive therapy. Children who undergo an allogeneic transplant are at continued risk for viral and fungal infections until adequate immune function is achieved. Although bacterial infections do not play a large role during this phase, serious infections can still occur in children who have a CVC or cGVHD. Administration of prophylactic penicillin is highly recommended in children with cGVHD for reducing the risk of infection with encapsulated organisms (i.e., *Haemophilus influenzae, Streptococcus pneumoniae, Neisseria meningitides*). Prophylaxis should continue as long as GVHD treatment is administered or there remains clinically active cGVHD.

Viral Infections

Cytomegalovirus. CMV, a common virus from the herpesvirus family, is the most frequent cause of viral-associated morbidity and mortality in children treated with HSCT. Recently, significant improvements in virus detection and treatment have been made; however, CMV infections remain a major infectious complication in children who receive an HSCT. CMV infections most commonly occur between 45 and 60 days after transplantation and can cause multiorgan disease, including pneumonia, gastroenteritis, retinitis, hepatitis, and encephalitis. CMV, similar to other herpesviruses, can establish lifelong, latent infections after primary exposure. In children with a competent immune system the latent infection is asymptomatic; however, reactivation of latent CMV infection in children undergoing HSCT may cause severe and sometimes fatal consequences.

The outcome of therapy for disseminated CMV infection in this population is poor so prevention remains the best treatment. Primary CMV infection may be transmitted by close personal contact, in utero from mother to child, by blood product transfusion, or by infused stem cells. Steps to prevent primary infection include the use of CMV-negative or leukocyte-depleted blood products and choosing a CMV-negative stem cell donor if possible. Prophylaxis and preemptive therapy are possible with the use of ganciclovir. Most transplant centers have adopted one of two plans if the child or the donor is seropositive at the pretransplant evaluation: (1) universal prophylaxis: administer ganciclovir after engraftment until 100 days after HSCT for all children at risk, or (2) monitor children weekly for detection of virus in the blood and initiate preemptive therapy with ganciclovir if reactivation occurs. Prophylaxis with acyclovir during the first 30 days of HSCT may help decrease the risk of CMV reactivation and is incorporated into supportive care guidelines at some centers for CMV-seropositive recipients of unrelated donor HSCT.

Herpes simplex virus. In the early post-HSCT phase, HSV is the most common viral infection seen in children. Reactivation of HSV occurs in 80% of immunocompromised seropositive children. The most common form of infection is gingivostomatitis, but dissemination can occur in the gastrointestinal tract, lungs, and liver. Prophylaxis with acyclovir is administered to children who are seropositive before transplant and continues for at least the first month after HSCT.

Varicella zoster virus. VZV, the cause of both primary varicella (chickenpox) and herpes zoster (shingles), is highly contagious. Similar to herpesviruses, it can be a serious infection in children who are undergoing HSCT. Primary infection with varicella causes fever, malaise, and a vesicular rash. Following the primary infection, the virus resides in ganglia during its latency. Antibodies to VZV can be detected in the blood and provide evidence of past primary infection, immunization, and virus latency. Reactivation of the latent virus causes herpes zoster, which manifests as painful, pruritic vesicular eruptions in a dermatomal distribution. Children who are immunocompromised can develop severe complications from either primary or reactivated VZV if disseminated, including pneumonia, encephalitis, and hepatitis (American Academy of Pediatrics, 2000). The majority of children who are seropositive will develop herpes zoster within the first year after HSCT. If a seronegative child after HSCT has a known exposure to primary varicella and has not received posttransplant IVIG within 3 weeks, varicella zoster immune globulin (VZIG) should be administered (Arvin, 1999). VZIG should be administered within 96 hours, preferably within 48 hours, of exposure and should be repeated if another exposure takes place more than 2 weeks after a VZIG injection.

Localized herpes zoster is the most common viral manifestation in the late post-HSCT phase. Distribution of vesicles in the immunocompromised child is similar to that of the general population with vesicles erupting along dermatomes of the thorax most commonly followed by the cranial dermatomes. Clusters of vesicles may form, and individual vesicles may enlarge to form confluent lesions. Prompt initiation of antiviral treatment with acyclovir is necessary to prevent dissemination.

Fungus. *Candida albicans* has historically been the most common fungal pathogen in children undergoing HSCT. However, prophylaxis with fluconazole has been successfully used for the past decade, decreasing the incidence of *C. albicans* infections in the transplant setting. As a consequence of this practice, however, the emergence of fluconazole-resistant *Candida* species (e.g., *C. tropicalis, C. glabrata*) has been described (Pfaller et al, 1998). Additional fungal problems include an increase in *Aspergillus* infections among HSCT recipients that can be fatal (Marr et al, 2002). Whereas *Candida* infections usually arise from gut contamination via damaged mucosa, *Aspergillus* is exogenous, airborne, and found primarily in soil. Several factors are likely responsible for the rising incidence of *Aspergillus* infections in the immunocompromised population, including the use of more aggressive myeloablative regimens, increased immunosuppression required for mismatched family and unrelated donors, and construction at or around medical centers (Lai, 2001; Marr et al, 2002).

Late Effects

Improvements in the science of transplantation have allowed more children the opportunity for potentially curative therapy. This very aggressive form of therapy has resulted in late effects for the increasing number of children who survive, requiring long-term follow-up and care. The delayed or late sequelae that may develop can be the result of a combination of the following factors: (1) the side effects of the condition for which transplantation was performed, (2) the effects of previous treatment for the underlying disorder, (3) the toxicities associated with the cytotoxic preparative regimen (usually high-dose chemotherapy with or without TBI), and (4) the toxic effects from treatment of posttransplant acute complications, especially prophylaxis and treatment of GVHD with immunosuppressive medications and physical effects of chronic GVHD.

TABLE 15-3

Types of Late Complications: Tissues Affected, Risk Factors, Prevention, and Treatment

Tissue/Organs	Late Complications	Risk Factors	Preventive Measures	Treatment Options
Immunity	Infections	GVHD T-cell depletion Herpesvirus infection Donor source Histocompatibility of donor and recipient	Antibiotic prophylaxis Immunizations Optimization of matching PCP prophylaxis	Targeted antimicrobials for specific infectious pathogens
	Autoimmune syndromes	GVHD	Optimization of matching	IVIG for autoimmune thrombocytopenia Steroids for various autoimmune phenomena
Endocrine glands	Hypothyroidism	Radiotherapy to head, neck, and mantle TBI	Fractionation of TBI Annual thyroid screening	Thyroid replacement
	Hypoadrenalism	Prolonged corticosteroid use	Replacement steroids for surgical procedures or acute medical conditions	
	Gonadal failure	TBI, intensive chemotherapy	Sperm banking	Hormone replacement
Skelelal	Osteopenia	Prolonged corticosteroid usage, TBI, inactivity, ovarian hormonal failure	Screening densitometry, exercise, bisphosphonates, ovarian hormonal replacement	Bisphosphonates
	Avascular necrosis	Corticosteroid usage, male gender, age >16 yr	Minimization of steroids	Joint replacement of affected weight-bearing joints
Liver	GVHD Hepatitis B or C Iron overload		Hepatitis A and B vaccines	Lamivudine or foscarnet for hepatitis B; interferon plus ribavirin for hepatitis C
Ophthalmologic	Cataracts Keratoconjunctivitis	TBI, busulfan, corticosteroids GVHD		Extraction and lens implantation Artificial tear solution and ointment
Musculature	Myopathy Myositis	Corticosteroid therapy Chronic GVHD	Minimization of corticosteroids Exercise	
Nervous system	Leukoencephalopathy	Cranial radiotherapy Intrathecal chemotherapy Fludarabine		
	Peripheral neuropathy	GVHD		Corticosteroid therapy
Respiratory tract	Interstitial fibrosis	Intensive conditioning regimen GVHD		
	Bronchiolitis obliterans	GVHD		Immunosuppressive therapy
Growth	Short stature	CNS irradiation TBI (single dose rather than fractionated) Hypothyroidism Corticosteroid therapy Gonadal insufficiency	Periodic assessment of endocrine status	Hormone replacement
Dentition	Cavities Sicca syndrome	Chronic GVHD	Dental hygiene	Artificial saliva
Bladder	Scarring after hemorrhagic cystitis	Cyclophosphamide, BK virus, adenovirus, CMV	Hyperhydration or mesna Cyclophosphamide administration	Antispasmodics for symptomatic relief
Kidneys	Nephropathy	TBI, prior platinum compounds	Angiotensin-converting enzyme inhibitors	Control of hypertension

GVHD, Graft-vs.-host disease; *PCP*, *Pneumocystis carinii* pneumonia; *IVIG*, intravenous immunoglobulin; *TBI*, total body irradiation; *CNS*, central nervous system; *CMV*, cytomegalovirus.

Most late effects of HSCT are a combination of factors. A review of treatment-related toxicities from childhood cancer can be found in Chapter 17. Table 15-3 (Wingard et al, 2002) outlines the types of late complications, tissues affected, risk factors, prevention, and treatment. Table 15-4 reviews organ involvement in cGVHD, clinical manifestations, evaluation, and interventions. Close attention must be paid to all treatments that can adversely affect the physical and cognitive development of the child.

The most common late effects involve the endocrine system that is particularly vulnerable to damage by radiation and some chemotherapeutic drugs, causing impairment of growth and pubertal development as well as infertility (Cohen et al, 1999; Mayer et al, 1999). Thyroid function can be affected if the child received XRT before transplantation or during the preparative regimen, resulting in overt or compensated hypothyroidism (Sanders, 1999). Bone-related late effects can be the result of both endocrine and nonendocrine causes. Osteochondromas are

TABLE 15-4

Clinical Manifestations of Chronic Graft-vs.-Host Disease (GVHD)

Organ	Clinical Manifestation	Evaluation	Intervention
Skin	Erythematous papular rash (lichenoid) or thickened, tight, fragile skin (sclerodermatous)	Clinical and biopsy to confirm the diagnosis of GVHD	Moisturize (petroleum jelly), treat local infections, protect from further trauma; topical steroid ointment may be used if it gives symptomatic relief to localized areas
Nails	Vertical ridging, fragile	Clinical	Nail polish may help to decrease further damage
Sweat glands	Destruction leading to risk of hyperthermia		Avoid excessive heat
Hair	Scalp and body hair thin and fragile, can be partially or completely lost	Clinical	
Eyes	Dryness, photophobia, and burning Progression to corneal abrasion	Regular ophthalmologic evaluation including Schirmer's test	Preservative-free tears during the day and preservative-free ointment at night
Mouth	Dry; sensitivity to mint, spicy food, tomato; whitish lacelike plaques in the cheeks and tongue identical to lichen planus; erythema and painful ulcerations, mucosal scleroderma with decreased sensitivity to temperature possible	Regular dental evaluation (with appropriate endocarditis prophylaxis; viral and fungal cultures at diagnosis and at any worsening	Avoid foods that are not tolerated; regular dental care preceded by appropriate endocarditis prophylaxis; topical steroid rinses followed by an antifungal agent for symptomatic relief
Respiratory tract	Bronchiolitis obliterans can manifest as dyspnea, wheezing, cough with normal CT scan and marked obstruction at pulmonary function tests; chronic sinopulmonary symptoms and/or infections also common; with abnormal chest CT, must rule out infections; lung biopsy if clinically indicated	Pulmonary function tests including FEV_1, FVC, DLCO, helium lung volumes; CT scan in symptomatic patients	Investigational therapy
Gastrointestinal	Abnormal motility and strictures. Weight loss.	Swallowing studies, endoscopy if clinically indicated; nutritional evaluation	Systemic treatment of GVHD; endoscopic/surgical treatment of strictures; nutritional intervention
Liver	Cholestasis (increased bilirubin, alkaline phosphatase); isolated liver involvement needs histologic confirmation	Liver function tests. Liver biopsy if clinically indicated.	No specific therapy is proven superior; FK-506 may concentrate in liver
Musculoskeletal	Fasclitis. Myositis is rare. Osteoporosis possible secondary to hormonal deficits, use of steroids, decreased activity	Periodical physical therapy evaluation to document range of motion; bone density evaluation especially in patients using steroids	Aggressive physical therapy program
Immune system	Profound immunodeficiency; functional asplenia; high risk of pneumococcal sepsis, PCP, and invasive fungal infections; variable IgG levels	Assume all patients as severely immuno-compromised and asplenic to 6 mo after GVHD has resolved	PCP prophylaxis (until 6 mo after no GVHD) and pneumococcal prophylaxis (lifetime); delay vaccinations
Hematopoietic system	Cytopenias; occasional eosinophilia	Counts. Bone marrow aspirate and biopsy, antineutrophil and antiplatelet antibodies when indicated.	Systemic treatment of GVHD
Others	Virtually all autoimmune disease manifestations have been described in association with chronic GVHD	As clinically indicated	

CT, Computed tomography; *FEV*$_1$, forced expiratory volume in 1 sec; *FVC*, forced vital capacity; *DLCO*, *PCP*, *pneumocystis carinii* pneumonia; *IgG*, immunoglobulin G.

common after HSCT, occurring in approximately 20% of children, and are known to be associated with radiation (Bordigoni et al, 2002; Leiper, 2002b). Avascular necrosis, most commonly in the hip joints, affects fewer than 10% of children and should be considered in children with persistent pain who received therapy with corticosteroids following HSCT (Leiper, 2002b). Osteoporosis and reduced bone mineral density can be a result of growth hormone deficiency, radiation, and corticosteroid use and increases the risk of osteoporotic fractures in these children (Nysom et al, 2000). There are other non–endocrine-related sequelae that may not become evident for months to years after transplantation (Lieper, 2002a, 2002b).

Multidisciplinary evaluations are necessary to fully assess sequelae related to treatment. The schedule for follow-up and surveillance testing is often coordinated by the transplanting and referring institutions and should include the evaluation and recognition of late effects, treatment options for late organ dysfunction, and evaluation for detection of early relapse. To ensure optimum health care for general and specialty issues, communication is critical among the various subspecialties involved and the child's primary care practitioner. The goal of treatment for every child is not only to cure the underlying disorder but also to minimize both the acute and long-term complications.

Prognosis

In children who have received either autologous or allogeneic HSCT, relapse of their primary disorder is the most frequent cause of treatment failure (Box 15-9). The vast majority of relapses occur within the first 2 years after HSCT. Since transplantation is usually the child's best option for cure, additional

treatment holds only a small likelihood of restoring the child to disease-free health. However, in recent years some success has been achieved by adoptive immunotherapy, that is, using the immune system to assist in disease eradication. Most commonly this is attempted by discontinuation of immunosuppressive medications (if the child is still taking them) to create a graft-vs.-leukemia/tumor effect (GVL). Donor lymphocyte infusions (DLIs) may be given, if the stem cell donor is available for pheresis of leukocytes, in an effort to achieve a remission via immunologic mechanisms. Unfortunately, this modality has shown limited utility for the most common hematologic malignancies of childhood. If the child is more than 1 year after HSCT when relapse occurs, a second transplant may be an option if a hematologic remission can be achieved, although the toxicities to the child are significant (Shah et al, 2002). If a child is a candidate for neither DLI nor a second HSCT, he or she will usually return to the care of the referring center for palliative therapy or end-of-life care.

Success of HSCT ranges from 10% to 90% and depends greatly on the child's original diagnosis and response to therapy, the status of organ function before transplant, and the type of transplant and stem cell source. Box 15-9 estimates long-term outcomes after allogeneic HSCT for various conditions. Ten to fifteen percent of children who undergo HSCT will die within the first 1 to 2 months from transplant-related complications that may include organ toxicity, venoocclusive disease, infection, and interstitial pneumonitis. The leading cause of death, however, is from recurrent disease: failure of the transplant to eradicate their underlying condition. Infection is the second leading cause of death. Both these causes of death can occur months to years after transplant.

PRIMARY CARE MANAGEMENT

The primary care provider plays a key role for the child and family in their return home and adjustment toward normalcy following the intensive treatment of HSCT. Most families require some encouragement to reenter the primary health care arena following several months and possibly years of close management by a subspecialist multidisciplinary team often located hundreds of miles away from their home. Good communication between the transplant team and the primary care provider can foster an easy transition and decrease the anxieties of the family.

Health Care Maintenance
Growth and Development

The endocrine system can be affected by chemotherapy and radiation therapy, which may lead to problems with growth and development. Several factors may impair growth in children after HSCT, including hypothyroidism and growth hormone deficiency. The type of HSCT preparative regimen the child receives is the most significant risk factor affecting growth (Sanders, 1999; Shaw, 2000). Children receiving chemotherapy alone have little to no growth disturbance, whereas children receiving a radiation-based regimen are at the greatest risk for growth impairment. This is particularly relevant for children who receive cranial XRT before receiving TBI. Single-dose

---

BOX 15-9

Long-Term Outcomes after Allogeneic Bone Marrow Transplantation

DISEASE STATUS AT THE TIME OF TRANSPLANTATION	DISEASE-FREE SURVIVAL AT 5 YR (%)
Acute myeloid leukemia	
First remission	45-70
First relapse, second or later remission	20-30
Refractory, multiply relapsed	10-15
Acute lymphocytic leukemia	
First or second remission	30-60
Relapse	10
Chronic myelogenous leukemia	
Chronic phase	50-70
Accelerated or blastic phase	10-30
Aplastic anemia	
Untransfused	80-90
Transfused	50-70
Thalassemia major	
Without liver abnormalities	85-95
With liver abnormalities	60-85
Congenital immunodeficiency	50-90
Lymphoma	40-50
Multiple myeloma	20-30

From Tabbara, I.A. et al. (2002, July 22). Allogeneic hematopoietic cell transplantation: Complications and results. *Archives of Internal Medicine, 162.* Reprinted with permission.

TBI has been found to cause more growth dysfunction compared with fractionated TBI. Growth hormone therapy can be effective in children found to be hormonally deficient.

The majority of children who receive transplants before the onset of puberty will experience some delay in onset and progression through puberty, and many will require exogenous hormone replacement to proceed through puberty and achieve maximal growth potential. Children who receive TBI during their preparative regimen are likely to be infertile because of the damaging effects of radiation on follicular development in ovaries and germinal epithelium in testes. Small testicular volume and low to normal testosterone levels are seen in boys after TBI, and some boys will require testosterone therapy for pubertal progression and to maintain normal sexual function as young adults. Production of sex hormones is linked to linear growth; therefore accurate documentation of sexual maturity or Tanner stage is helpful in identifying those children with failure to develop secondary sexual characteristics in an age-appropriate fashion. Referral to a pediatric endocrinologist, if not already coordinated by the transplant team or referring subspecialist, is critical for the management of hormone replacement in survivors of HSCT.

Careful monitoring of both growth by plotting height and weight on standardized growth charts and gonadal function by plotting Tanner stage progression after HSCT is warranted in order to detect disturbances early and ensure normal pubertal development in these children. In addition, significant or continued weight loss may be a sign of chronic GVHD, recurrent disease, secondary malignancy, or thyroid dysfunction.

Relative to other chronic conditions in childhood, survivors of HSCT are few in number. There are few published data addressing the cognitive and behavioral impact of this treatment on children after HSCT. Most information in the literature looks at childhood cancer survivors and infers similar cognitive and psychosocial effects to children having received an HSCT, since the majority of those who received transplants had an underlying malignant condition. These studies, as discussed in Chapter 17, show that children who received cranial irradiation and intrathecal chemotherapy exhibit the most frequent and severe cognitive effects and that age of treatment and dose of radiation are significant predictors of outcome. A recent prospective longitudinal study (Kupst et al, 2002) evaluated children before HSCT, 1 year after HSCT, and 2 years after HSCT for cognitive and psychosocial functioning. The results showed stable cognitive functioning by IQ score over time with the strongest predictor being pretransplant cognitive functioning. Psychosocial functioning showed similar results, with a low incidence of behavioral and social problems, again with pre-HSCT function predictive of later functioning. It is likely that with more children undergoing this aggressive treatment and more children surviving, similar studies will be performed to better understand cognitive and psychosocial sequelae related to HSCT. However, one problematic factor in studying this select population that will not change is the heterogeneity of this group of children.

Assessment of academic performance and behavior should be obtained yearly. Cognitive deficits can be subtle and questioning of the parent and child specifically about school performance may provide early clues.

Diet

Nutrition plays a key role during and after HSCT. Optimal nutrition is required for healing and to maximize long-term growth and development potential. Children usually receive total parenteral nutrition (TPN) for a few weeks during the early transplant phase because of severe mucositis. Once mucositis is healed, children are usually maintained on a modified diet to reduce exposure to environmental food contaminants. These precautions may be institutional specific and often remain in effect until adequate immune reconstitution is documented. A post-HSCT diet is instituted to reduce the child's risk of infection by avoiding unpasteurized products, aged or veined cheeses, undercooked meats or seafood, and other potential sources of infection in food products. Table 15-5 outlines foods that pose a risk for the child and suggestions for safer substitutions (CDC, 1999). Multidisciplinary transplant teams commonly include a nutritionist, who educates parents and children on nutrition and food safety. Parents may be required to keep daily food/fluids records until the child has attained adequate oral nutrition after HSCT. Children receiving steroids for treatment of GVHD often require a low-sodium diet to minimize hypertension. Calcium supplements may be recommended to offset the risk for osteopenia. Changes in taste may be a problem for some children initially, although this usually normalizes by 2 to 4 months after HSCT.

Safety

Child safety should be reviewed with parents at primary care visits. First-time parents whose children become ill during infancy and who are now adjusting to the liberation of protective isolation often need additional anticipatory guidance. Infant and toddler issues that would normally have been reviewed took a back seat to the life-threatening condition and treatment the child required.

Children returning home after transplantation have multiple oral medications, equipment for the care of their CVC, and possibly IV medications as well. All medications should be stored away from children. A "sharps container" should be in the home to properly dispose of any needles and syringes related to the care of the CVC or IV medications. Decreasing the risk of infection at home is important. Hand washing is the single most effective factor in preventing the spread of infection. Parents should supervise the hand washing of small children. No ill contacts should be allowed in the home. Eating utensils, cups, and glasses should not be shared with the immunocompromised child. The child's home should be cleaned frequently and be free of mold. Any construction on the house or surrounding property should be delayed until immune reconstitution is documented. No new pets should be brought into the household for at least 6 to 12 months. Immunocompromised children should have minimal direct contact with their household pets, wash their hands after handling them, avoid contact with animal feces, and avoid contact with reptiles (e.g., snakes, lizards, turtles, iguanas) to reduce the risk of acquiring salmonellosis.

Children are encouraged to resume normal activities that fall within the protective isolation guidelines of the transplanting center. Physical activities may be restricted because of thrombocytopenia. Children with a platelet count below 100,000 are restricted from climbing, contact sports, bike riding, or other physical activities in which the risk of trauma is high. Loss of

TABLE 15-5

Foods That Pose a High Risk for Hematopoietic Stem Cell Transplant (HSCT) Recipients and Safer Substitutions

Foods That Pose a High Risk	Safer Substitutions
Raw and undercooked eggs* and foods containing them (e.g., French toast, omelettes, salad dressings, eggnog, puddings)	Pasteurized or hard-boiled eggs
Unpasteurized dairy products (e.g., milk, cheese, cream, butter, yogurt)	Pasteurized dairy products
Fresh-squeezed, unpasteurized fruit and vegetable juices	Pasteurized juices
Unpasteurized cheeses or cheeses containing molds	Pasteurized cheeses
Undercooked or raw poultry, meats, fish, and seafood	Cooked poultry, well-done meats, cooked fish and seafood
Vegetable sprouts (e.g., alfalfa, bean, other seed sprouts)[+]	Should be avoided
Raw fruits with a rough texture (e.g., raspberries)[‡]	Should be avoided
Smooth raw fruits	Should be washed under running water, peeled, or cooked
Unwashed raw vegetables[§]	Should be washed under running water, peeled, or cooked
Undercooked or raw tofu	Cooked tofu (i.e., cut into $\leq$1-inch cubes and boiled for $\geq$5 min in water or broth before eating or using in recipes)
Raw or unpasteurized honey	Should be avoided
Deli meats, hot dogs, and processed meats[††]	Should be avoided unless further cooked
Raw, uncooked grain products	Cooked grain products including bread, cooked, and ready-to-eat cold cereal, pretzels, popcorn, potato chips, corn chips, tortilla chips, cooked pasta, and rice
Maté tea[¶]	Should be avoided
All moldy and outdated food products	Should be avoided
Unpasteurized beer (e.g., home brewed and certain bottled or canned, or draft beer that has been pasteurized after fermentation	Pasteurized beer (i.e., retail microbrewery beer)
Raw, uncooked brewer's yeast	Should be avoided; HSCT recipients should avoid any contact with raw yeast (e.g., they should not make bread products themselves)
Unroasted raw nuts	Cooked nuts
Roasted nuts in the shell	Canned or bottled roasted nuts or nuts in baked products

*From Centers for Disease Control and Prevention (CDC). (1996). Outbreaks of *Salmonella* serotype enteritidis infection associated with consumption of raw shell eggs—United States, 1994-1995. *MMWR, 45*(34), 737-742.
[+]From Taormino, P.J., Beuchat, L.R., & Slutsker, L. (1999). Infections associated with eating seed sprouts: An international concern. *Emerg Infect Dis, 5*(5), 626-634.
[‡]From Herwaldt, B.L. & Ackers, M.L. (1997). Outbreak in 1996 of cyclosporiasis associated with imported raspberries. *New England Journal of Medicine, 336*(22), 1548-1556.
[§]From CDC. (1998). Foodborne outbrerak of cryptosporidiosis—Spokane, Washington, 1997. *MMWR, 47*(27), 565-567.
[††]From CDC. (1999). Update: Multistate outbreak of listeriosis—United States, 1998-1999. *MMWR, 47*(51), 1117-1118.
[¶]From Kusminksy, G., Dictar, M., Arduino, S., Zylberman, M., & Sanchez Avalos, J.C. (1996). Do not drink Maté: An additional source of infection in South American neutropenic patients. *Bone Marrow Transplant, 17*(1), 127.

muscle mass and endurance is common after lengthy hospitalizations, and physical and occupational therapy are often necessary in the post-HSCT care of the child. Travel to developing countries is not advised because of the risk of contracting opportunistic or unusual infections. The transplant center should be consulted by the family for any planned travel out of state or internationally for the first 1 to 2 years.

Immunizations

Most children lose their immunity to vaccine-preventable diseases following HSCT. It is generally recommended that HSCT recipients initiate reimmunization 1 year following HSCT if there is no evidence of cGVHD and the child is not receiving corticosteroids. Live-virus immunization (MMR, OPV, Varivax) poses the risk of infection in immunocompromised children, and children who are immunosuppressed may not be able to initiate an immune response to immunizations. Siblings, family contacts, and health professionals should all be fully immunized to decrease the potential exposure of the child undergoing HSCT. The Centers for Disease Control (CDC), Infectious Disease Society of America, and the American Society of Blood and Marrow Transplantation issued recommendations for reimmunization of children following HSCT (Table 15-6) (CDC, 2000). The CDC recommends annual influenza immunizations for all household contacts of children

undergoing transplantation as well as for children more then 1 year after transplant and not affected by cGVHD (CDC, 2000).

Screening

Vision. Routine vision screening is advised as well as an annual ophthalmologic examination. Corticosteroid use and radiation can cause posterior subcapsular cataract formation that usually develops within the first 2 years after HSCT (Holmstrom et al, 2002). Small cataracts may not initially interfere with vision but should be monitored by an ophthalmologist in this circumstance. Chronic GVHD can result in keratoconjunctivitis. The ophthalmologic evaluation should include a Schirmer test to assess for adequate tear production. CMV retinitis is another potential complication. An ophthalmologist who is familiar with sequelae from high-dose chemotherapy and radiation therapy should be closely involved in the care of any child who has had HSCT.

Hearing. Routine screening is advised. Hearing loss, usually high frequency, may occur in children who receive ototoxic treatments, such as platinum-based chemotherapy, aminoglycoside antibiotics, loop diuretics or XRT (Landier, 1998; Nagy et al, 1999). It should be anticipated that many children whose pre-HSCT treatment included multiple ototoxic drugs (e.g., children with neuroblastoma) will require hearing aids after HSCT.

TABLE 15-6

Recommended Vaccinations for Recipients of HSCT

Vaccine	Patient Age	Timing of Administration	Comments
Diphtheria, tetanus, pertussis (DTP)	<7 yr	12, 14, and 24 mo after transplantation	No data regarding safety and immunogenecity of pertussis vaccine in this setting. Patients with a contraindication to pertussis should received the DT vaccine.
Diphtheria toxoid–tetanus toxoid (DT)	<7 yr	12, 14, and 24 mo after transplantation	Patients with a contraindication to pertussis should received the DT vaccine.
Tetanus-diphtheria toxoid (Td)	≥7 yr	12, 14, and 24 mo after transplantation	Patients should be reimmunized every 10 yr.
Haemophilus influenzae type B conjugate	All patients	12, 14, and 24 mo after transplantation	
Hepatitis B vaccination	Age <18 yr: susceptible patients Adults: patients with risk factors for infection	12, 14, and 24 mo after transplantation	High-dose vaccine recommended for immunocompromised adults; no data regarding response to high-dose vaccine in children. Response to be assessed 1-2 mo following completion of series of 3 vaccinations. Those without response may undergo a second cycle of 3 vaccinations.
23-Valent pneumococcal polysaccharide vaccine	≥2 yr	12 and 24 mo after transplantation	Vaccine demonstrates limited efficacy in posttransplantation setting with higher response rates later after transplantation.
7-Valent pneumococcal conjugative	All patients	Use age-dependent guidelines*	Antibiotic prophylaxis encouraged in patients with chronic graft-vs.-host disease.
Influenza (inactivated)	All patients	Lifelong seasonal administration beginning before transplantation and resuming at 6 mo after transplantation	Children <9 yr old should receive 2 doses for first vaccination. Children ≤12 yr should receive split vaccine. Patients >12 yr may receive split or whole vaccine.
Inactivated polio (IPV)	All patients	12, 14, and 24 mo after transplantation	IPV vaccine is immunogenic after transplantation although efficacy data are not available.
Measles, mumps, rubella (live vaccine)	All patients	≥24 mo after transplantation	Vaccination reserved for patients with recovered immunity (not for patients receiving immunosuppressive therapy).
Varicella vaccine	Contraindicated	Contraindicated	Contraindicated

Modified from the joint guidelines issued by the Centers for Disease Control, Infectious Disease Society of America and the American Society of Blood and Marrow Transplantation on October 20, 2000.
*MMWR. (October 6, 2000). No. RR-9, (49)21-27.

Dental. During the pretransplant dental evaluation, existing dental caries should be repaired and other risk factors for potential infection should be identified and eliminated. Routine dental examinations are very important and should resume once the child has adequate immune reconstitution. Chemotherapy and XRT, especially TBI, are known to cause dental and skeletal abnormalities in young children, including delay in tooth development, altered root development, enamel hypoplasia, and craniofacial abnormalities (Duggal, 2003). Children who are treated before the development of secondary dentition are at greatest risk for these complications. In addition, children who develop cGVHD involving the mouth will have oral mucosal changes that may increase their risk of oral infections (Woo et al, 1997).

Blood Pressure. Children are commonly placed on medication for hypertension after HSCT. Hypertension is most commonly secondary to renal insufficiency caused by nephrotoxic drugs. Parents are instructed on blood pressure monitoring and administration of antihypertensive medication.

Management of hypertension is usually coordinated by the transplant team, since the tapering of immunosuppressive agents and discontinuation of some antiinfective agents may reduce the need for antihypertensive agents. Blood pressure measurement and documentation by the primary health provider are important even after the child has stopped all nephrotoxic medications, because a small percentage of children will develop chronic renal insufficiency requiring long-term antihypertensive management (Kist-van Holthe et al, 2002).

Hematocrit. During the first year after HSCT, routine hematocrit by the primary care provider is not required because of the multiple CBCs and close hematologic assessment by the transplanting center. Routine screening may resume once the child is off all immunosuppressive medications.

Urinalysis. Routine urinalysis is recommended. Abnormalities should be communicated to the referring subspecialist or transplant team. Hematuria may be seen in children with cystitis or opportunistic urinary viral infections. Children without a competent immune system are at increased risk for urinary tract infections.

Tuberculosis. Routine screening for tuberculosis is advised for children during their reimmunization but not within the first year after HSCT. It is advisable to place controls (e.g., diphtheria-tetanus [dT]) to assess immunocompetency and a false-negative result.

Condition-Specific Screening

Physical examinations and laboratory studies are usually obtained at the transplant center or medical center of the referring subspecialist during the first year after HSCT. After the first year, annual evaluations for complications and late effects are generally requested by the transplant team and include subspecialty evaluations by the transplant team, endocrinologist, and ophthalmologist and periodic echocardiograms and pulmonary function tests.

Screening for Late Complications. The primary care provider plays a key role in screening for possible complications and late effects of treatment. Once the child returns to the community, it is the primary care practitioner's familiarity with the late complications of HSCT (Table 15-3) and clinical manifestations of cGVHD (Table 15-4) that can aid in early recognition of potential problems and result in prompt consultation with the transplant team or referring subspecialist.

Common Illness Management
Differential Diagnosis (Box 15-10)

Infections. Immunocompromised children may not be able to mount a typical response to infection (e.g., fever, erythema, edema) and therefore may not manifest classic physical exam findings despite true infection. A child who is still immunocompromised following HSCT is susceptible to complications from common community respiratory viruses such as

---

BOX 15-10

Differential Diagnosis

Infections
  Respiratory infections
  Fevers
  Central venous catheter infections
  Viral infections
  Asymptomatic infections
Gastrointestinal symptoms
  Opportunistic infections
  Graft-vs.-host disease (GVHD)
  Bacteremia
  Effect on medication absorption
  Effect on hydration and nutrition
Headache
Pain
  Possibility of infection
  Neuropathy
  Myalgias
  Post-HSCT complications
Symptoms associated with primary condition and sequelae of chemotherapy and radiation therapy

---

respiratory syncytial virus (RSV), adenovirus, influenza, parainfluenza, and even rhinovirus, which can result in severe and life-threatening pneumonitis. It is important to limit potential exposure to ill persons by limiting contact with large groups of people (i.e., at movies, airplane travel, school, church, or waiting rooms of medical offices). No rectal temperatures or medications should be administered because these increase the risk of bacteremia from local trauma.

Guidelines for fever management may differ according to the policy of the transplanting institution. Infection and recurrent malignancy are the key differential diagnoses. Any child who is either within the first year after HSCT or is still taking immunosuppressive medication and develops a fever requires consultation with the transplant team for management guidelines. For children still receiving immunosuppressive therapy and for those who have a CVC, any fever requires immediate evaluation; infection is the most likely cause and must be ruled out. Any child who has chills or rigors following flushing or administration of IV fluids or medications through their catheter should be evaluated immediately for possible bacteremia. After a thorough physical examination is performed, laboratory analysis usually includes aerobic and anaerobic blood cultures peripherally and from each lumen of the CVC, urinalysis, urine culture, chest radiograph, and throat culture and nasal swab for rapid testing of viral pathogens if URI symptoms are present.

The primary care provider may be asked to provide the initial evaluation if the child lives more then 1 hour from the transplanting institution or subspecialty clinic setting. Admission to a hospital or transfer to the transplanting institution is usually required. Broad-spectrum IV antibiotics are initiated for a minimum of 48 hours and later modified based on positive cultures and antimicrobial sensitivities.

Viral infections are common in children after HSCT. The herpesviruses HSV, CMV, and VZV are most common. If the child is within the first year after HSCT or still under the direct care of the transplanting institution, the transplant team should be contacted immediately if infection with one of these viruses is suspected. Uncomplicated HSV infection is usually treated with acyclovir (250 mg/m^2/8 hr) intravenously. VZV, whether primary (chickenpox) or secondary (zoster), is treated with acyclovir (500 mg/m^2/8 hr) intravenously. Administration of IV acyclovir commonly requires oral hydration to be supplemented with IV fluids because of the nephrotoxic effects of the anti-viral medication. Treatment for CMV infection includes the use of ganciclovir and IVIG per transplant institutional policy.

Children who are more then 1 year after HSCT, who have demonstrated adequate immune recovery, who are on no immunosuppressive medication, and who have no evidence of cGVHD may have less stringent fever management guidelines as directed by the child's referring subspecialist.

Gastrointestinal Symptoms. In the immunocompromised child, vomiting or diarrhea could be a result of an opportunistic infection or GVHD, and so the transplant team should be consulted. For a child with diarrhea, stool cultures for rotavirus, *Clostridium difficile, Campylobacter, Salmonella,* and *Shigella* should be obtained. It is helpful to ascertain the volume of diarrhea in a 24-hour period and assess the child for dehydration.

If the child is not able to keep down daily medications because of vomiting, the transplant team should be contacted to discuss alternative forms of administration. Blood cultures, as described previously, should be obtained because vomiting and diarrhea may be the presenting symptoms of bacteremia. IV hydration should be administered for children with large fluid losses, symptoms of dehydration, or inability to tolerate oral fluids.

Headaches. Headaches, although a common symptom in childhood and adolescents, can indicate a serious complication in the immunocompromised child following HSCT. The differential diagnosis is lengthy and includes the following: infection, hypertension, dehydration, spinal fluid leak caused by recent lumbar puncture, strain from impaired visual acuity, and medications. A thorough history to obtain a detailed description of the headaches as well as to note any recent changes in medications is important. Parents have usually been instructed not to administer acetaminophen for any symptoms until the child has been assessed for fever.

Pain. A thorough history of the location, onset, precipitating factors, and qualities of the pain will usually identify the cause of pain in most children after HSCT. Because of the immunocompromised status of these children the differential diagnosis primarily focuses on infection. Phone or visual assessment should include assessing for skin or oral lesions. Herpes zoster can cause neuropathy and pain in a dermatomal distribution before visible vesicle formation and should be considered in children who describe recurring pain under the skin. It is not uncommon for children to have mild myalgias after HSCT because their energy level improves and they increase their physical activity. Other pain may also may be related to specific post-HSCT complications and should be discussed with the transplant team.

Drug Interactions

Children are administered multiple medications following HSCT. The addition of any medication, prescriptive or over the counter, has potential drug interactions. Children who have received an allogeneic transplantation are at greatest risk for drug interactions because they are usually receiving CSA or tacrolimus for immunosuppression. The addition or discontinuation of other medications can greatly affect absorption or clearance of the immunosuppressive medications, causing a change in serum drug levels that can lead to organ toxicity or may trigger GVHD. Primary care providers should consult the transplant team before prescribing or advising additional medications for these children.

These children should not receive nonsteroidal antiinflammatory drugs (NSAIDs, e.g., ibuprofen [Motrin]) because they can interfere with platelet function and increase the risk of bleeding.

Developmental Issues

Sleep

It is not uncommon for children recovering from HSCT to have disturbances in their sleep pattern if they are receiving moderate to high doses of corticosteroids. Most children receive TPN during the first month after HSCT, and many children require nighttime supplemental IV fluids for 2 to 3 additional months. Pump malfunctions and alarms may disturb their sleep. IV hydration overnight may prompt multiple trips to the bathroom. It is not uncommon for these children to report awakening three to five times per night to urinate. Children having difficulty sleeping should avoid caffeine and other stimulants that may contribute to insomnia. Keeping a predictable bedtime routine and planning quiet activities in the evening, as well as avoiding overstimulating video games and movies, may be helpful.

Toileting

Diarrhea can be a consequence of GVHD or infection and may affect normal toileting habits. Regression in toileting skills may be seen in very young children during and after long hospitalizations and generally tends to improve as the child's health improves.

Discipline

HSCT is often the last form of treatment children receive. Families may have been dealing with the child's condition and prognosis for months or years before transplantation. Patterns of behavior and discipline are often well established before the child receives HSCT.

During the first 6 to 12 months following the transplant, parents often continue to be very protective of the child and tend to be indulgent and not as strict as they have been with their other children. This practice can be compounded by the difficulty in differentiating between the child's normal developmental acting-out and medication-induced behavioral changes (e.g., behavior changes associated with corticosteroids). In general, children recovering from HSCT are eager to be active and interact with their family, especially their siblings, following the acute phase of transplant when they are often in the hospital and feeling sick for weeks. The primary care provider can be instrumental in helping to facilitate normalcy in family functioning by reviewing with the parents age-appropriate behavior, development, limit setting, and discipline. Parents should strive to achieve consistency in limit setting and discipline for all the children in the household.

Child Care

Children who have received an HSCT and are immunocompromised must avoid child care settings because of the risk of acquiring common community respiratory viruses. If child care is required, in-home care is strongly recommended.

Schooling

School plays a very important role in the development of a child. The transplant team, referring center, and parents work together to ensure alternative forms of education during the child's protective isolation. This period may last between 6 and 12 months and may be longer in children with cGVHD. Arrangements are made for home study or hospital-based schooling until adequate immune function has been obtained. Once the child is no longer in protective isolation and can resume education with his or her peers, an individualized education plan (IEP) should be obtained through the school (see Chapter 5). There are no general limitations placed on children returning to school. They are encouraged to fully participate, including physical education, to a level physically tolerable. A small percentage of children will be fatigued from a full day of school at reentry and a partial or half day may be more appropriate at the beginning.

Sexuality

Many physical changes occur in the child or young adult during and after transplantation because of surgery, medication side effects, transplant-related complications, and late effects. These changes can have negative effects on self-image. Fortunately, many of these changes are temporary, lasting only months, but others are permanent. Physical changes may include alopecia, cushingoid features, scarring, striae, significant weight gain or loss, skin dyspigmentation, short stature, and hirsutism. The physical signs and symptoms of cGVHD may take years to improve and may never completely resolve (Table 15-4).

Delayed pubertal development may also affect self-esteem and peer acceptance. Adolescents who have received HSCT should have access to counseling. Sexually active young adults should be counseled on methods to reduce the risk of sexually transmitted infections and encouraged to practice cleanliness and safe sex with their partner. Barrier methods, particularly the use of condoms, should be encouraged. Intimate oral contact should be avoided until the mouth is completely healed.

Although the overwhelming majority of children and young adults are infertile after HSCT, successful pregnancies have occurred and the likelihood of infertility should not be considered adequate birth control. Appropriate birth control measures should be taken by sexually active young adults.

Transition into Adulthood

The struggle for independence for the adolescent is in sharp contrast to both the protective isolation before adequate immune recovery and the parents' need for close observation of their medically fragile adolescent. Normal adolescent issues still occur in young adults who have received an HSCT. Practitioners caring for long-term survivors of HSCT should emphasize the importance of the routine use of sunscreen and abstinence from tobacco because of increased vulnerability to ultraviolet rays and carcinogens. Body piercing is not advised while the immune system is incompetent or the risk for developing GVHD still exists. Education on developing habits that form a healthy lifestyle is important for these young adults. Maintaining a healthy weight, active lifestyle with routine exercise, varied diet, and limited alcohol consumption may reduce their risk of further disease and complications as they age.

Family Concerns and Resources

There are very little data on the ability of survivors of HSCT to obtain medical and life insurance, to achieve gainful employment, or to successfully form intimate relationships and live independently. There is information, however, on survivors of childhood cancer (a much larger population), which can be found in Chapter 17 and is largely applicable to HSCT survivors. Chapter 17 also outlines the Americans with Disabilities Act of 1990, which protects any person who has had the diagnosis of cancer from discrimination in employment or housing and therefore has a significant impact on the vast majority of survivors of HSCT.

Owing to the rapid improvements of HSCT and the relatively small number of affected individuals, in comparison with other chronic conditions of childhood, there is a gap in our understanding of the psychologic sequelae associated with this procedure. HSCT is a very intense, complicated form of treatment. Parents and children are often balancing the choice of potential long-term survival with the up-front risk of significant morbidity and mortality. There are a series of intense stressors that face the child and family. These stressors include the decision to accept the treatment, the search for a donor, the workup to determine the child's eligibility, enduring the cytotoxic preparative regimen followed by the anticlimactic infusion of the stem cells, the wait for blood count recovery, the potential for death from complications, and discharge from the hospital and eventually the return home. Anxiety comes with each step forward; as blood counts return, whose cells are they? Is there any evidence of the underlying condition? Once the child can finally leave the hospital, the parent becomes responsible for administering daily medications and deciding what problems necessitate calling the transplant team. When these children finally are allowed to return home, they may be at a significant distance from the security of the transplant team and medical center, and although they are home their physical and social isolation has not ended, and parents must juggle their child's complex care with managing a household and meeting the needs of the other children and family members. From the beginning the threat of relapse or severe complications is ever present and looming.

Research is ongoing to make transplant a safer, more successful treatment option to provide more children with a second chance at long-term survival. Since the number of children successfully treated with HSCT is increasing we can expect, in the very near future, more studies assessing the psychosocial functioning and concerns of the children and young adult survivors. More information is needed on this growing population to better fully understand the physical and psychosocial sequelae of HSCT.

ORGANIZATIONS

American Cancer Society
(800) ACS-2345
www.cancer.org

Candlelighters Childhood Cancer Foundation
(800) 366-2223
www.candlelighters.org

Children's Oncology Group
www.chidrensoncologygroup.org

National Cancer Institute (NCI) Childhood Cancers Home Page
www.cancer.gov/cancerinfo/types/childhoodcancers

National Marrow Donor Program
www.marrow.org

Summary of Primary Care Needs for the Child with Bone Marrow Transplant

HEALTH CARE MAINTENANCE

Growth and Development

Height and weight should be measured at each visit and plotted on standard growth curve forms. Hypothyroidism and hormone deficiencies are common side effects of chemotherapy and radiation therapy.

Children who receive transplants before puberty will often experience delay in onset and progression of puberty. Tanner staging should be done at each visit. Hormone replacement therapy may be needed for both males and females.

Cognitive development has had limited study in children with bone marrow transplants. Risks of cognitive impairment are similar to those of children with cancer receiving similar chemotherapy and radiation, especially cranial radiation and intrathecal chemotherapy.

Diet

Optimal nutrition is required for healing and to maximize growth.

A post-HSCT diet is instituted to reduce the risk of infection by avoiding foods with potential vectors for infection, such as unpasteurized products and undercooked meats.

Nutritional support via total parenteral nutrition (TPN) is often needed for few weeks after discharge.

Children receiving steroids may be placed on a low-sodium diet to reduce hypertension and calcium supplements to reduce the risk of osteopenia.

Safety

Anticipatory guidance is important, especially for parents who have only parented when their child was sick and now must care for a child who is more active and mobile.

Hand washing to prevent the spread of infections is critical. Eating utensils should not be shared.

All medicines should be stored safely away from children and needles and syringes deposited in a sharps container.

The child should have minimal direct contact with animals.

Physical activity may be restricted in children with thrombocytopenia.

Travel to developing countries is not advised. Travel away from the transplant center should be arranged with the knowledge of the transplant team.

Immunizations

Most children lose their immunity to previously administered vaccines following HSCT. Reimmunization should occur 1 year after transplant if there is no evidence of graft-vs.-host disease (GVHD) and the child is not receiving steroids.

Live-virus vaccines pose the risk of active disease.

Influenza vaccine should be given annually to the child and all household or close contacts.

Screening

Vision. An opthalmologist familiar with sequelae of high-dose chemotherapy and radiation should be involved in care.

Corticosteroid use can cause cataracts, cGVHD can result in keratoconjunctivitis, and cytomegalovirus (CMV) can cause retinitis.

Vision should be screened at each primary care visit and referral made for visual changes or abnormalities.

Hearing. Routine screening is advised. Hearing loss may occur as a result of ototoxic drug therapy.

Dental. Dental screening and restorative care should be done before transplant to reduce potential sources of infection. Routine dental care should be resumed once the child's immune system is restored.

Blood Pressure. Blood pressure should be taken and recorded at each visit. Children are commonly placed on medication for hypertension after HSCT because of nephrotoxic medications. Parents may be instructed to record blood pressure at home.

Hematocrit. Routine screening is resumed after the child is off all immunosuppressive therapy. Before this the child has frequent complete blood counts (CBCs) done by the transplant center so additional hematocrit testing is not necessary.

Urinalysis. Routine screening is recommended. Abnormalities should be reported to the transplant team.

Tuberculosis. Routine screening is recommended during reimmunization. Controls may need to be in place to determine immunocompetency.

Condition-Specific Screening

Physical and laboratory analysis during the first year after HSCT is usually obtained by the transplant team.

Screening for late complications needs to be done by the primary care provider (Table 15-3).

COMMON ILLNESS MANAGEMENT

Differential Diagnosis

Infections. When a child is immunocompromised, community respiratory infections can result in serious pneumonia.

Children with central venous catheters (CVCs) or still taking immunosuppressants must have fever immediately evaluated for possible bacteremia. Initial evaluation of fever may be done by the primary care provider in conjunction with the transplant center if the child lives more than 1 hour from the transplant center.

Rectal temperatures are not recommended.

Viral Infections. Herpes simplex virus (HSV), CMV, and varicella zoster virus (VZV) are common in children after HSCT.

Gastrointestinal Symptoms. Gastrointestinal symptoms may be caused by opportunistic infections or GVHD.

Headaches. Headaches may be a symptom of serious complications in the immunocompromised child.

Pain. Pain may be the result of prolonged bedrest and treatment side effects but also must be evaluated as a symptom associated with infection. Herpes zoster can cause neuropathy.

Drug Interactions

Children are taking multiple drugs after HSCT, and additions of other medications have the potential to alter absorption or clearance of these medications, leading to possible organ toxicity

Summary of Primary Care Needs for the Child with Bone Marrow Transplant—cont'd

Drug Interactions—cont'd

or GVHD. New pharmacologic therapy must be evaluated by transplant team.

Nonsteroidal antiinflammatory drugs (NSAIDs) are not recommended because they may interfere with platelet function.

DEVELOPMENTAL ISSUES

Sleep Patterns

Disturbance in sleep patterns is associated with high doses of corticosteroids.

TPN and supplemental intravenous (IV) fluids at night may interfere with sleep and increase nighttime voiding.

Caffeine and other stimulants, including television and videos, should be avoided in the evening.

Bedtime routines are encouraged.

Toileting

Diarrhea can be a symptom of GVHD and affect normal toileting habits.

Regression is common after a stressful hospitalization.

Discipline

Family patterns of behavior and discipline are often well established before the child receives HSCT. Children have often had chronic life-threatening conditions for a long time before transplant intervention.

Parents are encouraged to establish common discipline patterns for all children in the family.

Child Care

In-home child care is recommended because of the risk of infection in other child care settings.

Schooling

In-hospital or in-home schooling is required after HSCT for 6 to 12 months until immune function has been obtained because of concern regarding infection exposure.

An individualized education plan (IEP) should be done yearly to identify learning problems. Fatigue may be an issue.

There are no general limitations, and children are encouraged to participate fully in school activities.

Sexuality

Many physical changes occur with treatment that may interfere with body image.

Sex education is important, especially for infection control.

The overwhelming majority of children are infertile after transplant, but birth control is advised.

Oral sexual contact is discouraged until mucositis is completely healed.

Transition into Adulthood

The development of independence is often difficult after prolonged illness and a life-threatening condition.

Healthy life behaviors (i.e., good nutrition, regular exercise, no smoking) are important.

FAMILY CONCERNS

There is very little information on long-term quality of life after HSCT, employment, relationships, and insurability.

Individuals are protected under the Americans with Disabilities Act.

Families experience a great deal of stress during the transplant process, and there is an ongoing fear of recurrent disease, GVHD, and other late complications.

REFERENCES

American Academy of Pediatrics. (2000). Varicella-zoster infections. In L.K. Pickering (Ed.). 2000 *Red Book: Report of the Committee of Infectious Diseases* (25th ed.). Elk Grove Village, Ill.: Author, pp. 624-638.

Arai, S. & Vogelsang, G.B. (2000). Management of graft-versus-host disease. *Blood Rev, 14*(4), 190-204.

Arvin, A. (1999). Varicella-zoster virus infections. In E.D. Thomas, K.G. Blume, & S.J. Forman (Eds). *Hematopoietic cell transplantation* (2nd ed.). Malden, Mass.: Blackwell Science, pp. 591-606.

Bader, P., Klingebiel, T., Schaudt, A., Theurer-Mainka, U., Handgretinger, R., et al. (1999). Prevention of relapse in pediatric patients with acute leukemias and MDS after allogeneic SCT by early immunotherapy initiated on the basis of increasing mixed chimerism: A single center experience of 12 children. *Leukemia, 13*(12), 2079-2086.

Barnes, J. (2003). Quality, efficacy and safety of complementary medicines: Fashions, facts and the future. I. Regulation and quality. *Br J Clin Pharmacol, 55*(3), 226-233.

Benedict, C.A., Zhao, Y., Kashara, N., Cannon, P.A., & Anderson W.F. (2000). Development of retroviral vectors that target hematopoietic stem cells. In A.D. Ho, R. Hass, & R. Champlin (Eds.). *Hematopoietic stem cell transplantation.* New York: Marcel Dekker, pp. 575-593.

Bordigoni, P., Turello, R., Clement, L., Lascombes, P., Leheup, B., et al. (2002). Osteochondroma after pediatric hematopoietic stem cell transplantation: Report of eight cases. *Bone Marrow Transplant, 29,* 611-614.

Carrier, E. (2000). Murine model of in utero transplantation. In A.D. Ho, R. Haas, & R.E. Champlin (Eds.). *Hematopoietic stem cell transplantation.* New York: Marcel Dekker, pp. 195-222.

Centers for Disease Control and Prevention. (2000). Guidelines for preventing opportunistic infections among hematopoietic stem cell transplant recipients: Recommendations of CDC, the Infectious Disease Society of America, and the American Society of Blood and Marrow Transplantation. *Biol Blood Marrow Transplant, 6*(6a), 659-727.

Chao, N.J. (1999). *Graft versus host disease* (2nd ed.). Austin, Tex.: Landes Co.

Cohen, A., Rovelli, A., Bakker, B., Uderzo, C., van Lint, M.T., et al. (1999). Final height of patients who underwent bone marrow transplantation for hematological disorders during childhood: A study by the working party for late effects—EBMT. *Blood, 93*(12), 4109-4115.

Djulbegavic, B., Seinenfeld, J., Bonnell, C., & Kumar, A. (2003). Nonmyeloablative allogeneic stem-cell transplantation for hematologic malignancies: A systematic review. *Cancer Causes Control, 10*(1), 17-41.

Duggal, M.S. (2003). Root surface areas in long-term survivors of childhood cancer. *Oral Oncol, 39*(2), 178-183.

Georges, G.E. & Storb, R. (2003). Review of "minitransplantation": Nonmyeloablative allogeneic hematopoietic stem cell transplantation. *Int J Hematol, 77*(1), 3-4.

Greinix, H.T. (2002). DLI or second transplant. *Ann Hematol, 81*(suppl. 2), S34-S35.

Gross, T.G. (2001). Treatment of Epstein-Barr virus-associated post transplant lymphoproliferative disorders. *J Pediatr Hematol Oncol, 23*(1), 7-9.

Gross, T.G., Egeler, R.M., & Smith, F.O. (2001). Pediatric hematopoietic stem cell transplantation. *Hematol Oncol Clin North Am, 15*(5), 795-808.

Gustafsson, J.A., Remberger, M., Ringden, O., & Winiarski, J. (2003). Graft-versus-leukemia effect in children: Chronic GVHD has a significant impact on relapse and survival. *Bone Marrow Transplant, 31*(3), 175-181.

Holmstrom, G., Borgstrom, B., & Calissendorff, B. (2002). Cataract in children after bone marrow transplantation: Relation to conditioning regimen. *Acta Ophthalmol Scand, 80*(2), 211-215.

International Bone Marrow Transplant Registry/Autologous Blood & Marrow Transplant Registry (IBMTR/ABMTR). (2002). *IBMTR/ABMTR Newsletter, 9*(1), 4-11.

Jacobson, P., Uberti, J., Davis, W., & Ratanatharathorn, V. (1998). Tacrolimus: A new agent for the prevention of graft-versus-host disease in hematopoietic stem cell transplantation. *Bone Marrow Transplant, 22*(3), 217-225.

Jones, D.R. (2001). In utero stem cell transplantation: Two steps forward but one step back? *Expert Opin Biol Ther, 1*(2), 205-212.

Kansu, E. & Sullivan, K.M. (2000). Late complications of hematopoietic stem cell transplantation. In A.D. Ho, R. Haas, & R.E. Champlin (Eds.). *Hematopoietic stem cell transplantation.* New York: Marcel Dekker, p. 422.

Katzenstein, H.M., Kletzel, M., Reynolds, M., Suprina, R., & Gonzalez-Crussi, F. (2002). Novel therapeutic approaches in the treatment of children with hepatoblastoma. *J Pediatr Hematol Oncol, 24*(9), 751-755.

Kaye, E.M. (2001). Lysosomal storage diseases. *Curr Treat Options Neuro, 3*(3), 249-256.

Kist-van Holthe, J.E., Goedvolk, C.A., Brand, R., van Weel, M.H., Bredius, R.G.M., et al. (2002). Prospective study of renal insufficiency after bone marrow transplantation. *Pediatr Nephrol, 17*(12), 1032-1037.

Kletzel, M., Katzenstein, H.M., Haut, P.R., Yu, A.L., Morgan, E., et al. (2002). Treatment of high-risk neuroblastoma with triple-tandem high-dose therapy and stem-cell rescue: Results of the Chicago Pilot II Study. *J Clin Oncol, 20*(9), 2284-2292.

Kohler, J.A., Imeson, J., Ellershaw, C., & Lie, S.O. (2000). A randomized trial of 13-Cis retinoic acid in children with advanced neuroblastoma after high-dose therapy. *Br J Cancer, 83*(9), 1124-1127.

Krivit, W. (2002). Stem cell bone marrow transplantation in patients with metabolic storage diseases. *Adv Pediatr, 49*, 359-378.

Kupst, M.J., Penati, B., Debban, B., Camitta, B., Pietryga, D., et al. (2002). Cognitive and psychosocial functioning of pediatric hematopoietic stem cell transplant patients: A prospective longitudinal study. *Bone Marrow Transplant, 30*, 609-617.

Lai, K.K. (2001). A cluster of invasive aspergillosis in a bone marrow transplant unit related to construction and the utility of air sampling. *Am J Infect Control, 29*(5), 333-337.

Landier, W. (1998). Hearing loss related to ototoxicity in children with cancer. *J Pediatr Oncol Nurs, 15*(4), 195-206.

Leiper, A.D. (2002a). Non-endocrine late complications of bone marrow transplantation in childhood. I. *Br J Haematol, 118*(1), 3-22.

Leiper, A.D. (2002b). Non-endocrine late complications of bone marrow transplantation in childhood. II. *Br J Haematol, 118*(1), 23-43.

Levine, J.E., Wiley, J., & Kletzel, M. (2000). Cytokine-mobilized allogeneic peripheral blood stem cell transplants in children result in rapid engraftment and a high incidence of chronic GVHD. *Bone Marrow Transplant, 25*, 13-18.

Lujan-Zilbermann, J. & Patrick, C.C. (2000). Infections in the hematopoietic stem-cell transplant patient. *Semin Pediatr Infect Dis, 11*(2), 97-104.

Marr, K.A., Carter, R.A., Boeckh, M., Martin, P., & Corey, L. (2002). Invasive aspergillosis in allogeneic stem cell transplant recipients: Changes in epidemiology and risk factors. *Blood, 100*(13), 4358-4366.

Massenkeil, G., Nagy, M., Lawang, M., Genvresse, I., Geserick, G., et al. (2003). Reduced intensity conditioning and prophylactic DLI can cure patients with high-risk acute leukemias if complete donor chimerism can be achieved. *Bone Marrow Transplant, 31*(5), 339-345.

Matthay, K.K., Villablanca, J.G., Seeger, R.C., Stram, D.O., Harris, R.E., et al. (1999). Treatment of high-risk neuroblastoma with intensive chemotherapy, radiotherapy, autologous bone marrow transplantation, and 13-cis-retinoic acid. Children's Cancer Group. *N Engl J Med, 341*(16), 1165-1173.

Mayer, E.I.E., Dopfer, R.E., Klingebiel, T., Scheel-Walter, H., Ranke, M.B., et al. (1999). Longitudinal gonadal function after bone marrow transplantation for acute lymphoblastic leukemia during childhood. *Pediatr Transplant, 3*(1), 38-44.

McCormack, G., Nolan, N., & McCormick, P.A. (2001). Transjugular liver biopsy: A review. *Ir Med J, 94*(1), 11-12.

McCullough, J. (1999). Principles of transfusion support before and after hematopoietic cell transplantation. In E.D. Thomas, K.G. Blume, & S.J. Forman (Eds.). *Hematopoietic cell transplantation* (2nd ed.). Malden, Mass.: Blackwell Science, pp. 685-703.

McSweeney, P.A., Niederwieser, D., & Shizura, J.A. (2001). Hematopoietic cell transplantation in older patients with hematologic malignancies: Replacing high-dose cytotoxic therapy with graft-versus-tumor effects. *Blood, 97*(11), 390-400.

Mentzer, W.C. (2000). Bone marrow transplantation for hemoglobinopathies. *Curr Opin Hematol, 7*(2), 95-100.

Molina, A., Popplewell, L., Kashyap, A., & Nademanee, A. (2000). Hematopoietic stem cell transplantation in the new millennium: Report from City of Hope National Medical Center. *Clin Transpl,* 317-342.

Nagatoshi, Y., Kawano, Y., Watanabe, T., Abe, T., Okamoto, Y., et al. (2002). Hematopoietic and immune recovery after allogeneic peripheral blood stem cell transplantation and bone marrow transplantation in a pediatric population. *Pediatr Transplant, 6*(4), 319-326.

Nagy, J.L., Adelstein, D.J., Newman, C.W., Rybicki, L.A., Rice, T.W., et al. (1999). Cisplatin ototoxicity: The importance of baseline audiometry. *Am J Clin Oncol, 22*(3), 305-308.

National Marrow Donor Program. (2003). *NMDP registry growth: General facts & figures;* Web site: http://www.marrow.org/.

Noga, S.J. (2000). Using allogeneic graft engineering to improve long-term survival. *Semin Oncol, 27*(suppl. 5), 15-21.

Nysom, K. Holm, K.. Michaelson, K.F., Hertz, H., Jacobsen, N., et al. (2000). Bone mass after allogeneic BMT for childhood leukemia or lymphoma. *Bone Marrow Transplant, 25*, 191-196.

Pfaller, M.A., Jones, R.N., Messner, S.A., Edmond, M.B., & Wenzel, R.P. (1998). National surveillance of nosocomial blood stream infection due to species of *Candida* other than *Candida albicans. Infect Diagn Microbiol Dis, 30*(2), 121-129.

Physicians' Desk Reference. (2003). Filgrastim. In *Thomson PDR* (57th ed.), p. 585.

Reynolds, C.P. & Lemons, R.S. (2001). Retinoid therapy of childhood cancer. *Hematol Oncol Clin North Am, 15*(5), 867-910.

Salvaneschi, L., Perotti, C., Zecca, M., Bernuzzi, S., Viarengo, G., et al. (2001). Extracorporeal photochemotherapy for treatment of acute and chronic GVHD in childhood. *Transfusion, 41*(10), 1299-1305.

Sanders, J.E. (1999). Growth and development after hematopoietic cell transplantation. In E.D. Thomas, K.G. Blume, & S.J. Forman (Eds). *Hematopoietic cell transplantation* (2nd ed.). Malden, Mass.: Blackwell Science, pp. 764-775.

Schouten, H.C. (2002). The role of mini-allotransplants in the treatment of solid tumors. *Ann Oncol, 13*(suppl. 4), 281-286.

Sepkowitz, K.A. (2002). Antibiotic prophylaxis in patients receiving hematopoietic stem cell transplantation. *Bone Marrow Transplant, 29*(5), 367-371.

Shah, A.J., Kapoor, N., Weinberg, K.I., Crooks, G.M., Kohn, D.B., et al. (2002). Second hematopoietic transplantation in pediatric patients: Overall survival and long-term follow-up. *Biol Blood Marrow Transplant, 8*(4), 221-228.

Shaw, P.J. (2000). Growth and development of the pediatric recipient. In K. Atkinson (Ed). *Clinical bone marrow and blood stem cell transplantation* (2nd ed.). Boston: Cambridge University Press, pp. 870-877.

Sniecinski, I.J. & O'Donnell, M.R. (1999). Hemolytic complications of hematopoietic cell transplantation. In E.D. Thomas, K.G. Blume, & S.J. Forman (Eds). *Hematopoietic cell transplantation* (2nd ed.). Malden, Mass.: Blackwell Science, pp. 674-684.

Sokos, D.R., Berger, M., & Lazarus, H.M. (2002). Intravenous immunoglobulin: Appropriate indications and uses in hematopoietic stem cell transplantation. *Biol Blood Marrow Transplant, 8*(3), 117-130.

Sullivan, K.M. (1999). Graft-versus-host disease. In E.D. Thomas, K.G. Blume, & S.J. Forman (Eds.). *Hematopoietic cell transplantation* (2nd ed.). Malden, Mass.: Blackwell Science, pp. 515-536.

Tabbara, I.A., Zimmerman, K., Morgan, C., & Nahleh, Z. (2002). Allogeneic hematopoietic stem cell transplantation: Complications and results. *Arch Intern Med, 162*(14), 1558-1566.

Trigg, M.E. (2002). Milestones in the development of pediatric hematopoietic stem cell transplantation—50 years of progress. *Pediatr Transplant, 6*, 465-474.

Uharek, L., Dreger, P., Glass, B., Zeis, M., & Schmitz N. (2000). Peripheral blood stem cells for allogeneic transplantation. In A.D. Ho, R. Haas, & R.E. Champlin (Eds.). *Hematopoietic stem cell transplantation.* New York: Marcel Dekker, pp. 383-402.

Waldmann, H. (2001). Therapeutic approaches for transplantation. *Curr Opin Immunol, 13*, 606-610.

Weisdorf, D., Bishop, M., Dharan, B., Bowell, B., Cahn, J.Y., et al. (2002). Autologous versus allogeneic unrelated donor transplantation for acute lymphoblastic leukemia: Comparative toxicity and outcomes. *Biol Blood Marrow Transplant, 8*(4), 213-220.

Wingard, J.R., Vogelsang, G.B., & Deeg, H.J. (2002). Stem cell transplantation: Supportive care and long-term complications. *Hematology (Am Soc Hematol Educ Program),* 422-444.

Woo, S.B., Lee, S.J., & Schubert, M.M. (1997). Graft -vs-host disease. *Crit Rev Oral Biol Med, 8*(2), 201-216.

Zecca. M. & Locatelli, F. (2000). Management of graft-versus-host disease in paediatric bone marrow transplant recipients. *Paediatr Drugs, 2*(1), 29-55.

16 Bronchopulmonary Dysplasia

Beverly Capper-Michel

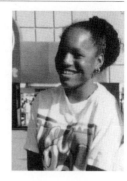

Etiology

Bronchopulmonary dysplasia (BPD) was first described by Northway and colleagues (1967) in a review of chest radiographs of premature infants who were treated with positive pressure ventilation and oxygen for respiratory distress syndrome (RDS). A four-stage radiographic classification was used when the disease was first described.

Philip (1975) broadened the definition to include the following nonradiographic findings and management: (1) institution of positive pressure ventilation within the first week of life for a minimum of 3 days; (2) clinical findings of tachypnea, rales, and retractions persisting beyond 28 days of life; (3) an oxygen requirement to maintain arterial oxygen pressure (PaO_2) above 55 mm Hg for more than 28 days; and (4) chest radiographs showing persistent strands of densities with normal and hyperlucent areas in bilateral lung fields.

With advances in technology, treatment, and research findings the lung injury, inflammation, and lung fibrosis previously described by Rozycki and Kirkpatrick (1993) are seen less frequently today, and these early classification systems are used less often. Today, BPD might be described as "classic" or "late" BPD and is usually classified as mild, moderate, or severe. BPD is often used interchangeably with the term "chronic lung disease (CLD)."

New pathogenetic factors for BPD are being identified (Jobe & Bancalari, 2001). The pathogenesis of BPD describes an interruption in alveolar development, particularly when preterm infants require mechanical ventilation and supplemental oxygen (Eber & Zach, 2001). Inflammation and persistent hypoxia also contribute to the pathogenesis of BPD. Figure 16-1 outlines the pathogenesis of BPD.

The accuracy of defining BPD by an oxygen requirement at 36 weeks' postmenstrual age is challenged as treatment and technology decrease exposure to barotrauma and high oxygen concentrations (Davis et al, 2002; Martin & Walsh-Sukys, 1999). Davis et al (2002) describe the emergence of yet another "new" BPD that extends beyond lung injury and demonstrates a cessation of pulmonary alveolar development. It is this developmental and reparative immaturity of the very preterm infant's lung that increases their susceptibility for BPD (Vaucher, 2002).

Respiratory failure at birth is critical to the etiology of classic or severe BPD because it requires treatment with supplemental oxygen and mechanical ventilation (Hazinski, 1998). Respiratory failure may be a result of several causes but is most often due to RDS (Hazinski, 1998). Other contributing conditions to the development of BPD include neonatal pneumonia, meconium aspiration, patent ductus arteriosus, fluid overload, and lung hypoplasia (Eber & Zach, 2001).

Risk factors that are key indicators of infants prone to develop BPD include lung immaturity, oxygen toxicity, mechanical ventilation, and infection (Vaucher, 2002). Some studies associate a family history of asthma with an increased risk for development of BPD (Ghezzi et al, 1998; Hazinski, 1998).

BPD represents a wide spectrum of clinical entities that are not completely understood and result from a variety of insults and predisposing factors. Current perspectives on CLD suggest that it is a complex disorder resulting from more than just lung injury associated with oxygen toxicity and barotrauma from mechanical ventilation. Specific microbes (e.g., *Ureaplasma histolyticum, Chlamydia trachomatis*) have been implicated along with high levels of inflammatory mediators (e.g., interleukin-8) in the bronchial secretions of premature infants (Ghezzi et al, 1998). Researchers suggest low levels of the antiinflammatory Clara cell–secreted protein (CCSP) place preterm infants at higher risk for developing BPD (Ramsay et al, 1999). Further studies are needed to determine the role of CCSP in BPD. The presence of patent ductus arteriosus (PDA) further contributes to the development of significant CLD. Left-to-right shunting of blood flow through a PDA increases pulmonary blood flow and lung fluid. This process interferes with normal lung mechanics and gas exchange. The combination of neonatal infection and a PDA appears to be a significant risk factor for the development of BPD (Nievas & Chernick, 2002; Groneck et al, 1994).

Known Genetic Etiology

Polymorphisms may increase risks for developing BPD when factors interrupt developmental timing of alveolar and vascular development (Jobe & Bancalari, 2001). Preterm infants are at the greatest risk for developing CLD. Preterm birth is often precipitated by chorioamnionitis and the release of intraamniotic endotoxins (Kramer et al, 2002). These endotoxins interrupt normal alveolar growth and development. Although a family history of asthma may predispose an infant to CLD, there is a lack of evidence to identify it as a causal factor (Eber & Zach, 2001).

Incidence and Prevalence

BPD may be associated with chronic pulmonary dysfunction, recurrent hospitalization, increased incidence of developmental disabilities, growth delay, and even death (Barrington & Finer, 1998; Fillmore & Cartlidge, 1998). As medical

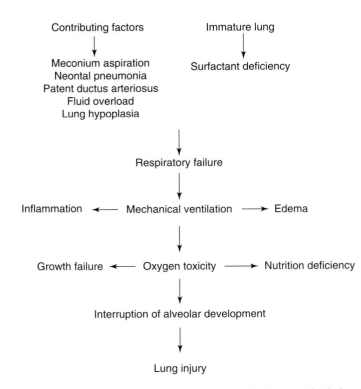

Contributing factors   Immature lung

Meconium aspiration   Surfactant deficiency
Neontal pneumonia
Patent ductus arteriosus
Fluid overload
Lung hypoplasia

Respiratory failure

Inflammation ← Mechanical ventilation → Edema

Growth failure ← Oxygen toxicity → Nutrition deficiency

Interruption of alveolar development

Lung injury

FIGURE 16-1 Outline of pathogenesis of bronchopulmonary dysplasia.

BOX 16-1

Treatment That May Decrease the Incidence of Chronic Lung Disease in High-Risk Infants

Prenatal steroids (maternal)
Early surfactant
Postnatal steroids
Less aggressive ventilator management
Early patent ductus arteriosus (PDA) closure
Conservative fluid management

From Bancalari, E. (1998, May). Bronchopulmonary dysplasia: Then and now. Presented at the American Thoracic Society Conference, Chicago. Reprinted with permission.

BOX 16-2

Clinical Manifestations at Time of Diagnosis

Tachypnea
Wheezing
Rales
Abnormal chest radiograph
Retractions
Cyanotic episodes
Activity/handling intolerance
Poor growth

technology progresses, the survival rates of premature and very low birth weight (e.g., <1500 g) newborns increase (Rimensberger, 2002; Martin & Walsh-Sukys, 1999). These increased survival rates account for the lack of change in the incidence of BPD despite advances in neonatal care. Overall, more than 85% of all perinatal complications are attributed to premature births with BPD reported as the most frequent sequela (Thebaud et al, 2001). Premature infants are at greatest risk for developing CLD, and it is estimated that 75% of infants with BPD are very low birth weight (Hazinski, 1998; see Chapter 36).

Prevention of premature births through improved prenatal care is the key to decreasing the incidence of BPD. Several changes in the early treatment of high-risk premature infants and their mothers have resulted in a shift in BPD severity. The use of antenatal steroids, early use of surfactant, systemic steroids, PDA closure, less aggressive ventilator management, and conservative fluid management may have contributed to the decreased incidence of severe BPD (Box 16-1).

The classic form of BPD or severe CLD is less common with the use of surfactant and prenatal steroids. As a result, a milder form of CLD has emerged as a major entity in the population of high-risk premature infants (Nievas & Chernick, 2002). These infants usually present with a need for ventilatory support for poor respiratory effort but are quickly weaned from the ventilator after a few hours to days. Ventilatory support is at low pressures and low oxygen concentrations; therefore these infants can avoid the initial lung insults of barotrauma and oxygen toxicity. Some of these infants have progressive deterioration, however, despite their early success. Complications such as PDA or infection appear to trigger lung deterioration in the group of infants with mild CLD (Vaucher, 2002).

Clinical Manifestations at Time of Diagnosis

Clinical manifestations of BPD vary depending on the age of the infant at onset and the severity of the disease. The severity can range from an infant having some pulmonary symptoms that require bronchodilator treatment and diuretics to a child requiring a tracheostomy and mechanical ventilatory support for prolonged periods in the hospital and at home.

An infant with BPD displays significant alteration in lung mechanics. Lung compliance is diminished because of (1) the interruption of alveolar vascularization, (2) the increased risk of inflammation as a result of mechanical ventilation, and (3) lung injury (Jobe & Bancalari, 2001). The combination of decreased lung compliance and increased airway resistance produces clinical findings such as tachypnea, wheezing, and increased work of breathing. Fluid leak from cellular damage is manifested as inspiratory and expiratory rales (Box 16-2).

Chest radiographs of infants with BPD reveal interstitial thickening, hyperexpansion, and atelectasis (Eber & Zach, 2001). The abnormality in radiographs may normalize during infancy or may persist into childhood(Carey & Trotter, 2000). Scoring systems for chest radiographs have been developed to correlate films with respiratory support and create a standard for comparison of severity among infants with BPD (Carey & Trotter, 2000).

An abnormal respiratory examination is the key finding in the diagnosis of BPD (Figure 16-2). On visual examination, the respiratory rate may be elevated as much as 20 to 30 breaths/min above the baseline for a child's age. With respiratory distress, the primary care provider will observe a prolonged exhalation with increased use of abdominal and accessory muscles. Umbilical or inguinal hernias may occur as

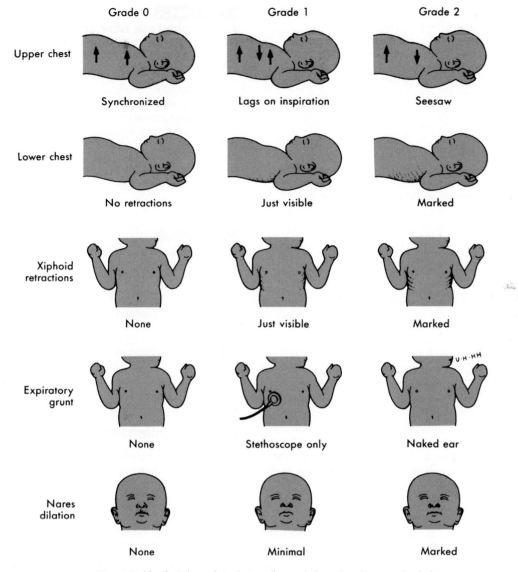

FIGURE 16-2 Manifestations of respiratory distress in bronchopulmonary dysplasia.

a result of increased abdominal pressure from high airway resistance and use of accessory muscles (Hazinski, 1998).

Other clinical manifestations of the preterm infant with BPD include poor gas exchange, bronchospasm, mucous plugging, and poor physical growth. Cyanosis and activity intolerance with feeding and handling are common findings (Hazinski, 1998). Ultimately the task of breathing robs these infants of precious calories needed for physical growth and development.

Treatment (Box 16-3)

Synthetic Surfactant

The BPD process is initiated through cellular injury to the immature lung. Infants born before 28 to 32 weeks' gestation have an insufficient amount of pulmonary surfactant. Surfactant is a lipoprotein that lowers the surface tension of the air-alveolar surface and allows lung expansion, thus maintaining the patency of the alveoli and preventing atelectasis. Synthetic surfactant given in the first 24 hours of life has been shown to

---

BOX 16-3
Treatment

Synthetic surfactant
Systemic steroids
Supplemental oxygen
Diuretics
Bronchodilators
Antiinflammatories
"Tincture of time"

---

decrease neonatal mortality but not significantly reduce the incidence of BPD (Rimensberger, 2002). Some studies have analyzed the outcome of surfactant use in the first 12 hours as prophylaxis in high-risk infants and as treatment for infants with known RDS. Outcomes indicate surfactant use as treatment can reduce medical costs for large infants by decreasing complications and the length of time they need ventilatory

TABLE 16-1

Weaning of an Infant from Supplemental Oxygen: Sample Schedule

Time	Amount of Oxygen (per min)
At hospital discharge	0.5 L at all times
1 mo after discharge*	0.5 L during feedings and sleep; 0.25 L when awake
2 mo*	0.25 L at all times
3 mo*	0.25 L during feedings and sleep; room air when awake

From Hazinski, T.A. (1998). Bronchopulmonary dysplasia. In V. Cerhnick, T.F. Boat, E.L. Kendig, & J. Fletcher. *Kendig's disorders of the respiratory tract in children.* Philadelphia: W.B. Saunders. Reprinted with permission.
*Assumes clinical stability, adequate weight gain, and proof of adequate oxygen saturation (intervals may vary).

BOX 16-4

Diuretics Used to Treat Bronchopulmonary Dysplasia

FUROSEMIDE (LASIX)
1–4-mg/kg/day in 1 or 2 divided doses

CHLOROTHIAZIDE (DIURIL)
30–40-mg/kg/day in 2 divided doses

SPIRONOLACTONE (ALDOCTONE)
2–4-mg/kg/day in 1 or 2 divided doses

Data from Johns Hopkins University. (2000). *The Harriet Lane handbook* (16th ed.). St Louis: Mosby; Benitz, W.E. & Tatro, D. (1996). *The pediatric drug handbook* (3rd ed.). St Louis: Mosby.

support (Nievas & Chernick, 2002). Improved lung compliance induced by surfactant allows for rapid weaning from mechanical ventilation by decreasing the risk of complications associated with mechanical ventilation (Rimensberger, 2002). The early use of surfactant in very small premature infants significantly reduces mortality (Rimensberger, 2002).

Steroids

Use of systemic steroids has become one of the most controversial treatments of BPD (Nievas & Chernick, 2002). Although dexamethasone decreases the need for mechanical ventilation and supplemental oxygen for infants with BPD, it has not improved morbidity or mortality rates (Fernandez & Chernick, 2002; Vermont Oxford Network Steroid Study Group, 2001). Poor neurodevelopmental outcomes have been reported with prolonged use of glucocorticoid therapy (Hack & Fanaroff, 2000). Cole et al (1999) studied the use of inhaled steroids, and although not shown to prevent BPD, inhaled steroids are associated with fewer side effects and a lower use of systemic glucocorticoid therapy.

Treatment also focuses on enhancing the infant's natural healing process, thereby avoiding further complications often associated with BPD. A "tincture of time" is the primary force that leads to stabilization of BPD. In the interim, support is employed until physiologic maturation of lung tissue can support oxygen needs. Such treatment modalities include oxygen therapy, diuretics, bronchodilators, and corticosteroids.

Oxygen

The need for supplemental oxygen varies with the severity of lung dysfunction. Infants who require oxygen after hospital discharge rarely require more than 1 to 2 L/min via nasal cannula. Infants discharged on oxygen must be observed at frequent intervals to assess for hypoxia. Assessments should include a physical examination and noninvasive monitoring of oxygen and carbon dioxide readings. These readings can be obtained via pulse oximeter or transcutaneous oxygen monitoring. Oxygen and carbon dioxide measurements must be done during periods of rest and activity to accurately determine the infant's continuing supplemental oxygen needs (Hazinski, 1998). When the infant appears clinically stable, is gaining weight, and is not anemic, gradual weaning from oxygen is initiated by the neonatal pulmonary team. A typical weaning schedule is presented in Table 16-1. To avoid significant oxygen desaturation during

sleep, a child with BPD should continue nighttime supplemental oxygen until daytime oxygen saturation equals or exceeds 92% in room air (Hazinski, 1998). Oxygen should be restarted if somatic growth slows by more than 20% after discontinuation of supplemental oxygen (Nievas & Chernick, 2002).

Diuretics

Diuretics are often used in the care of infants with BPD. These medications correct fluid retention, prevent fluid overload, decrease pulmonary resistance, and increase pulmonary compliance (Box 16-4; Johns Hopkins University, 2000). Furosemide (Lasix) is a commonly used diuretic effective in eliminating excess fluid in the lungs. In moderate to severe BPD, potassium-sparing spironolactone (Aldactone) and chlorothiazide (Diuril) are often needed for additional diuresis. Because of the potential electrolyte imbalance associated with diuretic therapy, children with BPD must have serum electrolyte values monitored and are often given potassium chloride supplements. Serum electrolytes should be monitored monthly with supplements adjusted to maintain chloride above 92 mEq/L and potassium above 3.5 mEq/L (Johns Hopkins University, 2000). Serious complications may result from prolonged use of diuretics (Fernandez & Chernick, 2002). Nutritional requirements must be balanced with fluid restriction to avoid overloading the already stressed cardiopulmonary system.

Bronchodilators

Infants with BPD may be predisposed to bronchial hyperreactivity and bronchospasm from neonatal lung injury and hyperplasia of smooth muscle (Hazinski, 1998). Bronchodilator therapy is used to reduce the effects of bronchoconstriction by relaxing smooth muscle in the airways. The outcome of this therapy is improved gas exchange through a decrease in airflow resistance and gas trapping (Fok et al, 1998). A positive response from this therapy is clinically shown by a decrease in wheezing, coughing, or supplemental oxygen requirements.

Machines used to administer aerosolized medications can be cumbersome and inconvenient. Spacer devices have become a portable alternative for older children and adults with airway obstruction. Studies on infants indicate that a spacer with a mask is an effective means of administering aerosolized bronchodilators (Fok et al, 1998).

Three categories of bronchodilators are beta-adrenergic agonists (albuterol), anticholinergics (ipratropium [Atrovent]), and methylxanthines (theophylline, caffeine citrate). Albuterol is commonly used via inhalation at a dose of 0.05 to 0.15 mg/kg/dose every 4 to 6 hours depending on response and disease severity (Johns Hopkins University, 2000).

Use of nebulized ipratropium bromide (Atrovent) in combination with albuterol can enhance pulmonary function in infants with BPD. Ipratropium bromide antagonizes muscarinic receptors in the airways, resulting in bronchodilation (Johns Hopkins University, 2000).

Theophylline and caffeine citrate are oral bronchodilators that stimulate respiratory drive. Theophylline is administered two to four times per day, requires monitoring of blood levels, and has reported side effects that include feeding intolerance, tachycardia, irritability, diarrhea, increased gastroesophageal reflux (GER), and lowered seizure threshold (Johns Hopkins University, 2000). As a result, the role of theophylline in bronchodilator therapy is diminished, and the use of caffeine citrate has increased in infants with BPD and apnea of prematurity. Caffeine citrate has a prolonged half-life and is administered once per day with fewer reported side effects (Gannon, 2000). The wide therapeutic range decreases the need for frequent blood samples.

Antiinflammatories

Systemic corticosteroids have been used in the acute and chronic phases of BPD disease. Corticosteroids can reduce pulmonary edema and inflammation in the small airways, as well as potentiate the effects of bronchodilators; however, shorter and less frequent courses are used today to prevent poor neurodevelopmental outcomes associated with prolonged therapy (Hack & Fanaroff, 2000). Prednisone (i.e., 1 to 2 mg/kg/day) given for 3 to 5 days can be effective for acute exacerbations. Watterberg and Scott (1995) speculate that infants with BPD have a decreased ability to secrete cortisol in response to stress, which leaves them more vulnerable to inflammatory lung injury. Infants with severe BPD may benefit from the strong antiinflammatory effect of corticosteroids, which reduces the duration of mechanical ventilation and oxygen therapy (Cherif et al, 2002). Infants using this type of therapy are at risk for adrenal suppression and may require an increase in their usual steroid dose during significant biophysical stressors (e.g., moderate to severe infection or surgical procedures; Hack & Fanaroff, 2000).

The increased use of inhaled corticosteroids (ICSs) for infants with BPD has decreased the use of oral corticosteroid therapy with hope of lowering the incidence and severity of side effects (Cole et al, 1999; Karinski et al, 2000). Studies evaluating the efficacy and safety of nebulized steroids in infants with BPD revealed that those treated had improved extubation rates (Lister et al, 2000). Inhaled steroids are rapidly absorbed from the respiratory tract and can be administered with a metered dose inhaler (MDI). Administration of inhaled steroids such as beclomethasone dipropionate (Beclovent) and budesonide (Pulmicort) demonstrates fewer adverse effects than systemic steroids (Cherif et al, 2002).

Bronchopulmonary disease is often associated with asthma. Research on children with asthma using ICSs (via MDI with spacer) has revealed consistent efficacy in the reduction of airway inflammation (see Chapter 11). Concern about long-term effects on growth, however, has prompted further evaluation of the use of ICSs in prepubertal children. A review of 30 studies revealed that children using relatively high doses of ICSs for 7 to 12 months had documented growth suppression of 1.0 to 1.4 cm/yr (Welch, 1998). It is unclear how to apply this information to infants using ICSs and whether the growth suppression will be permanent or temporary. It is clear, however, that ICSs have systemic bioavailability and should be used cautiously.

Complementary and Alternative Therapies

At this time, there are no known complementary or alternative therapies utilized to increase lung compliance in infants with BPD.

Recent Advances in Diagnosis and Management

The delivery of antenatal steroids has proven successful in reducing the incidence of death and RDS in preterm infants (Battin et al, 1998). Postnatal delivery of high doses of glucocorticoids, however, has adverse effects on the infant's gastrointestinal tract, growth patterns, and neurodevelopment (Jobe & Bancalari, 2001). Recent clinical trials studied the administration of hydrocortisone within the first 12 days of life (Jobe & Bancalari, 2001). Cortisol plays an important role in response to lung injury, and cortisol synthesis is suppressed until the later part of gestation.

Inhaled nitric oxide (iNO) increases pulmonary blood flow and improves oxygenation for infants with severe RDS (Jobe & Bancalari, 2001). Rimensberger (2002) reports randomized clinical trials are under way to determine the efficacy of iNO in the preterm infant and prevention of BPD.

Some clinicians speculate that supplementing deficient nutrients in premature neonates can prevent BPD. Vitamin A promotes healing of epithelial cells, and clinical trials suggest parenteral administration of vitamin A immediately after birth is beneficial in reducing oxygen requirements for infants with BPD (Darlow & Graham, 2000; Vaucher, 2002). Further research is needed to investigate treatment modalities that will reduce the severity of BPD.

Associated Problems (Box 16-5)
Airway Complications

Structural damage to an infant's premature respiratory tree often occurs as a result of endotracheal intubation and positive pressure ventilation. Upper airway anomalies (i.e., including subglottic stenosis, granuloma, tracheal scarring, and polyp formation) can occur immediately after extubation or as a late presentation (Hazinski, 1998). Infants presenting with homophonous wheezing, hypoxia, and bradycardia (i.e., cyanotic "BPD spells") should be evaluated for lower airway anomalies such as tracheomalacia and bronchomalacia (Hazinski, 1998).

Infants who require prolonged ventilatory support and infants who develop respiratory failure from an upper airway obstruction need a tracheostomy. Children with a tracheostomy are now often cared for at home. The most frequent complications are infection of the tracheostomy, obstruction by

Associated Problems

Airway complications
Respiratory infection
Poor growth and nutrition
Gastroesophageal reflux
Cardiac conditions
Neurodevelopmental complications
Seizures
Ophthalmologic sequelae
Renal conditions
Rickets
Stoma care
Otitis media/sinusitis

secretions, or accidental decannulation. Parents and primary care providers must be competent in tracheostomy care. This includes the knowledge and skills necessary for maintaining tracheostomy patency, caring for the stoma, and changing tracheostomy tubes.

Airways of infants with BPD exhibit significant loss of cilia and denudation of their lining, resulting in the absence of the normal cleansing abilities of the lung (Hazinski, 1998). Daily chest physiotherapy (CPT) and postural drainage help mobilize secretions so they can be removed from the airway by coughing or suctioning if an artificial airway is present. During a viral or bacterial illness, secretion production increases and more frequent CPT and drainage may be necessary.

Respiratory Infection

Infants with BPD are at increased risk of lower respiratory tract infections in the first year of life (Piedra, 2002). Infection is the major cause of rehospitalization, late morbidity, and mortality in children with BPD (Piedra, 2002). Therefore early evaluation and close follow-up are recommended for children with BPD with any upper respiratory illness or cold. Community-acquired viruses can exacerbate BPD by making hypoxia, edema, bronchoconstriction, and secondary bacterial infection worse (Hazinski, 1998). Treatment to stabilize such episodes includes an increase in supplemental oxygen, extra doses of diuretics, and administration of aerosolized bronchodilators (Hazinski, 1998). Broad-spectrum antibiotic treatment and a septic work-up may be indicated for a febrile infant with BPD. Nasopharyngeal aspirate for immunofluorescence may be helpful in identifying particularly harmful viruses such as respiratory syncytial virus (RSV), adenovirus, and influenza.

Poor Growth and Nutrition

Growth patterns in children with BPD depend on the nutritional status and the severity of the lung disease. Growth retardation in infants with BPD most commonly occurs as a result of an inability to match caloric intake with energy expenditure (Abrams, 2001). The combination of fluid restrictions, frequent respiratory infections, and an elevated metabolic rate often results in poor weight gain (Hazinski, 1998). Further, infants with BPD who have labored breathing while at rest often have difficulty coordinating their rapid respirations, suck, and swallow.

Early in treatment, total parenteral nutrition is often necessary, followed by supplementation of breast or bottle feedings with gavage feedings. In infants with severe BPD and feeding problems, a gastrostomy tube may be necessary. Caloric requirements are high (i.e., up to 120 to 150 kcal/kg/day). Most infants require formula with a caloric concentration of at least 24 to 30 kcal/30 ml (1 oz) to achieve optimal catch-up growth (Hazinski, 1998). Formula may be fortified with vegetable oil, triglycerides, or glucose polymers to increase the calories per ounce (Hazinski, 1998). In addition, formulas with higher protein, calcium, phosphorus, and zinc may contribute to more linear growth, lean body mass, and bone mass (Mueller, 1998).

As a result of a high risk for growth delay, some infants with BPD benefit from a comprehensive evaluation by a nutritional specialist. In one study, risk factors associated with growth failure included low socioeconomic status, postdischarge days of illness, and "suspect" development (Johnson et al, 1998). Management strategies should be implemented to ensure adequate energy intake, parental support and/or education, and feeding therapy needs.

Gastroesophageal Reflux

Gastroesophageal reflux (GER) is a common gastrointestinal dysfunction seen in children with BPD that is caused by an incompetent lower esophageal sphincter that allows acidic gastric contents to pass back into the esophagus. Symptoms of GER include emesis, apnea, bradycardia, recurrent pneumonia, delayed growth, and esophagitis (Blackburn, 1999). Abnormal lung mechanics leading to abnormal pressure gradients between the chest and abdomen may contribute to the occurrence of GER in infants with BPD (Hazinski, 1998). Infants with BPD are at risk for a more serious pathologic reflux referred to as gastroesophageal reflux disease (GERD) (Blackburn, 1999). Esophageal pH probe monitoring over 18 to 24 hours is used to confirm the diagnosis of GERD (Blackburn, 1999).

Theophylline decreases the tone of the lower esophageal sphincter and should therefore be avoided in infants with both BPD and GERD. Ranitidine (Zantac) and cimetidine (Tagamet) help to buffer the acidity of the stomach after meals and decrease episodes of bronchospasm caused by gastric content irritation. If these medications are not effective in controlling symptoms, metoclopramide (Reglan) should be considered to promote gastric emptying and prevent residual reflux (see the section on drug interactions later in this chapter). Thickening food with rice cereal and using reflux precautions (e.g., keeping head of bed elevated 30 degrees with infant in prone position) may help although the efficacy of such precautions is now being questioned (Blackburn, 1999). A high incidence of swallowing dysfunction is associated with BPD and may need further evaluation to prevent aspiration (Mercado-Deane et al, 2001). If symptoms and the clinical picture do not demonstrate any improvement, Nissen fundoplication surgery is the last option (Blackburn, 1999).

Cardiac Conditions

Chronic cardiac changes persist in children with BPD who have experienced numerous hypoxic insults or have been maintained at a low PaO_2. Pulmonary vasoconstriction occurs in response to alveolar hypoxia, which results in pulmonary hypertension (Hazinski, 1998). Progression of pulmonary hypertension can lead to right ventricular hypertrophy, cor pulmonale, and congestive heart failure. Administration of supplemental oxygen maximizes pulmonary vasodilation when oxygen saturation is maintained between 92% and 95%. Inhaled nitric oxide is a potent vasodilator that decreases pulmonary vascular resistance and improves ventilation and perfusion of impaired lungs (Golombek, 2000). Refractory hypoxemia or sudden fluctuations in PaO_2 may indicate a cardiac defect. PDA, incompetent foramen ovale, or septal defects can cause congestive heart failure or pulmonary hypertension (Hazinski, 1998). Diagnostic tests (i.e., including echocardiogram and cardiac catheterization) are used to confirm cardiac complications.

Neurodevelopmental Complications

Children with BPD are at high risk for developmental delays. All aspects of development can be affected: physical, cognitive, language, and sensorimotor skills. Mild gross motor sequelae (i.e., including hypotonia, hypertonia, and delayed motor development) are often seen in the first year of life (Hack & Fanaroff, 2000; Majnemer et al, 2000). Intraventricular hemorrhage, periventricular leukomalacia, or echodensity in the newborn period is predictive of a poor developmental outcome (Wilson-Costello et al, 1998). Regular assessment with early intervention involving a physical and/or occupational therapist can optimize development. Regular screening exams for vision and hearing are important in a population prone to retinopathy of prematurity (ROP) and recurrent ear infections. A history of CLD seems to add significant risk for poor school performance that is often associated with very low birth weight infants (Hughes et al, 1999).

Seizures

Hypoxic insults and intraventricular hemorrhages occurring in the newborn period predispose an infant to seizures. Even with anticonvulsant therapy the onset of new seizures can be triggered at any time by an infection with a high fever or a hypoxic insult. Children with BPD who have not had a seizure for at least 1 year with electroencephalograms (EEGs) free of epileptiform activity can be considered for weaning of anticonvulsants (see Chapter 25).

Ophthalmologic Sequelae

The incidence of retinopathy of prematurity (ROP) has decreased as the toxic effects of oxygen have become known. Prematurity, however, remains one of the strongest risk factors for ROP (Holmstrom et al, 1998). Central blindness can occur with repeated incidence of severe hypoxia and severe intraventricular hemorrhage. All infants weighing less than 1500 g or under 28 weeks' gestational age should be screened for ROP (Oh & Merenstein, 1997). Infants with BPD who are diagnosed with ROP should be observed closely by an ophthalmologist because of their risk for strabismus and amblyopia (Oh & Merenstein, 1997).

Renal Conditions

One half of infants with BPD who receive long-term furosemide (Lasix) therapy will develop renal calcification (Hazinski, 1998). Infants receiving intravenous (IV) furosemide for over 2 weeks should have a renal ultrasound (Impact-RSV Study Group, 1998). Thiazides (Diuril) decrease calcium excretion and may help prevent nephrocalcinosis. If renal stones are identified, furosemide should be discontinued as soon as possible to allow the calcium to reabsorb.

Rickets

Infants with BPD often develop rickets secondary to prolonged parenteral nutrition and difficulty absorbing calcium and phosphorus. The population most at risk for rickets are infants with a birth weight less than 1000 g. Long-term furosemide administration can also contribute to a negative calcium balance, thus inhibiting normal bone formation.

Stoma Problems

Children with tracheostomy tubes are at risk for irritation around the tracheostomy stoma. Secretions that ooze from tracheostomy stomas may irritate the skin. Meticulous regular care to the tracheostomy stoma generally maintains skin integrity. Fastening tracheostomy ties too tightly can cause skin lacerations on the neck. A small, premeasured protective patch of skin barrier may be placed over the laceration to allow it to heal without continued direct contact with the tracheostomy ties or the flange of the tracheostomy tube.

Some children may develop areas of granulation tissue on and around the tracheostomy stoma. If left unattended, the tissue will continue to grow and can impede or block insertion of the tracheostomy tube into the stoma. The tissue occasionally forms a tight band around the tracheostomy stoma. Applying silver nitrate to the site will promote shrinkage and eliminate tissue. In extreme cases a child must be referred to an otorhinolaryngologist for possible surgical excision with the child under anesthesia. Similar difficulties with granulation tissue occur with gastrostomy stomas, and the same treatment applies. Leakage of feeding around the gastrostomy tube irritates the skin on the abdomen. The cause of such leakage is usually mechanical. Some families are instructed to change gastrostomy tubes on a regular basis because over time the stomach acid alters the integrity of the tube within the stomach.

The primary care provider should examine the tube to determine its type and how it is inserted. Foley catheters, Malecot tubes, and gastrostomy button devices may be used as gastrostomy tubes. Some tubes may be placed securely with a fluid-inflated balloon. The amount of fluid in the balloon should be documented in the discharge plan. If the amount in the balloon is less than the prescribed amount, it can contribute to leakage. It is important to ensure that the internal balloon is pulled up close to the internal abdominal wall to prevent leakage. When leakage is persistent, some practitioners insert a larger tube into the stoma. This technique is controversial because over time the stoma expands and the problem will recur. The less the tube is manipulated, the longer the stoma will remain intact. Secure fastening procedures can minimize movement of the gastrostomy tube.

Otitis Media/Sinusitis

The same bacteria that colonize the lower airways often colonize the upper airways and precipitate upper respiratory infections. Recurrent otitis media is often seen in this population. Hearing loss can occur as a result of chronic infection and chronic IV use of furosemide and aminoglycosides.

The risk of sinusitis is greater in children with CLD and those who have required or continue to require nasogastric tube feedings because the tube is a place for bacteria to seed and interferes with normal defenses in the lining of the epithelium. Postnasal drainage results in coughing and throat clearing, especially after a child awakes. Oral antibiotics taken for at least 3 weeks clear most infections, but prolonged therapy may be needed to treat severe cases.

Prognosis

Survival rates and outcomes are steadily improving for infants with BPD. Improved survival rates are seen in extremely low birth weight infants with advances in steroid therapy, surfactant, and improved mechanical ventilation methods (Martin & Walsh-Sukys, 1999). Expert medical care is now available for these infants through easier access to tertiary care personnel. Although mortality rates continue to decrease, a significant number of infants experience cognitive and neurosensory delays (Hack et al, 2000).

Ventilator parameters, treatment with oxygen for at least 28 days, and persistent clinical features of respiratory distress may provide predictors of sequela from BPD (Jobe & Bancalari, 2001). The duration of oxygen requirement appears to be a controversial predictor of sequela because of the variability in practice (Davis et al, 2002; Martin & Walsh-Sukys, 1999). However, infants who required oxygen beyond 36 weeks' gestational age had more days of readmission for respiratory problems and a lower mean developmental quotient at 18 months of age (Gregoire et al, 1998). In addition, toddlers with a history of BPD were twice as likely to require hospitalization in the first 2 years of life as toddlers without BPD (Gross et al, 1998). Infants with BPD are also more likely to develop asthma (Ng et al, 2000).

For infants with BPD who survive, growth and developmental delays improve over time. When compared with their peers as young children, adolescents, and young adults, however, the effects of BPD appear to linger. After discharge the growth failure rate is between 30% to 67% (Abrams, 2001). Catch-up growth of a child's head circumference in the first year of life may predict neurodevelopmental outcome. Other outcome studies of infants with BPD show that they have poorer motor outcome at age 3 years than unaffected infants.

Overall, school-aged children with a history of BPD demonstrate poorer cognitive performance when compared with their peers (Hughes et al, 1999). Assessments often reveal attention deficit hyperactivity disorder, perceptual-motor integration problems, and language delays (Hack et al, 2000; see Chapter 12). Longitudinal studies reveal that despite increased nursery survival of extremely low birth weight infants over the past 15 years, there has not been an increase in neurodevelopmental morbidity (Hack & Fanaroff, 2000; Schaap et al, 1999).

Although the effects of BPD on the respiratory system diminish in time, 70% of adolescents with BPD demonstrate continued airway obstruction and are at risk for respiratory failure in early adulthood (Pandya & Kotecha, 2001). One study evaluated 7-year-olds with a history of BPD and found that they had more airway obstruction evidenced by reduction of forced vital capacity, forced expiratory flow, and mid flows (Gross et al, 1998). Infants who required supplemental oxygen for at least 1 month after term had a significant degree of gas trapping at 1 year of age (Jacob et al, 1998). There may be a difference, however, in long-term pulmonary function in infants with milder CLD. There are limited follow-up data of pulmonary function in this group, but it appears that the abnormalities are less pronounced and tend to improve during the first 3 years of life (Bancalari, 1998).

PRIMARY CARE MANAGEMENT

Health Care Maintenance
Growth and Development

Length and/or height, weight, and head circumference measurement (i.e., corrected for gestational age) should be obtained and plotted monthly while a child is hospitalized and with each subsequent ambulatory care visit (Trachtenbarg & Golemon, 1998). Growth measurements taken before a child is discharged from the hospital help establish growth trends in the newly discharged infant. Even minor illness in children with BPD may result in weight loss because of their high caloric needs.

The head circumference must be measured and recorded carefully on standardized growth curves for premature infants or corrected for gestational age and plotted on National Center for Health Statistics graphs. The head shape of a premature infant often appears boxy, and the corrected age should be used for 2 years or until the sutures are normally fused. Careful physical examination and documentation of caloric intake should indicate if a cranial ultrasound is needed.

Developmental screening and diagnosis by the primary care provider can be accomplished using the child's corrected age and standard screening tools, such as the Bayley Mental Developmental Index (see Chapter 2). Even with correction for prematurity, these infants often exhibit a developmental lag during the first year of life. Most infants with transient developmental delays test normal after they are 1 year of age. If developmental delays are significant or persist after the first year of life, the child should be referred for further assessment and therapeutic intervention. For optimal long-term prognosis, early intervention referrals should be made before discharge for all children who are high risk (Hussey-Gardner et al, 2002).

Diet

The high caloric requirements caused by prematurity and the increased work of breathing with BPD require creative ways of providing adequate nutrition in an appealing, tasteful manner that does not require a high expenditure of energy for consumption or create fluid overload in a compromised infant. It is important for the primary care provider to regularly assess weight gain and evaluate nutritional needs. It is beneficial to maintain contact with the nutritionist from the discharging hospital and ask for assistance in maintaining adequate caloric intake. As previously mentioned, children with severe BPD or feeding problems may require supplemental feedings via gavage or gastrostomy tube.

The introduction of solid foods is generally initiated between 4 and 6 months of corrected age or when an infant weighs 6 to 7 kg. Oral-tactile hypersensitivity as a result of oral trauma from the passage of nasogastric or orogastric tubes, endotracheal tubes, or repeated suctioning may make it difficult for a child to adequately feed. Early recognition of the problem and intervention by trained health care providers (i.e., nurses, speech pathologist, or occupational therapist) can facilitate feeding and decrease parental frustration and feelings of failure.

Safety

Children with BPD who are tethered by oxygen or ventilator tubing require close supervision. Respiratory equipment should have alarm systems because free-spirited toddlers will wander beyond the length of the tubing. Restricted and supervised areas of play must be set up to create a safe environment for recreation. Children should be supervised at all times to prevent them from manipulating dials on their support equipment. Some devices have safety covers for control dials.

Children with tracheostomy tubes need virtually continuous observation. If they are not directly attended by caregivers, a noninvasive monitoring system with an oxygen saturation or apnea monitor should be in place. An accidental decannulation can cause death or serious physical and developmental sequelae. Security of the tracheostomy tube ties should be assessed every 4 to 8 hours and readjusted if more than one finger can be inserted between the tracheostomy ties and the child's neck. Family members should be taught cardiopulmonary resuscitation (CPR) before the child is discharged from the hospital.

Families with toddlers must be warned against the insertion of small toys into ventilator tubing and artificial airways. When insufficiently supervised or educated, playful siblings can contribute to accidental airway decannulations and equipment disconnections. Older school-aged and adolescent children can be instructed to observe and intervene with specified responsibilities in emergency or routine situations.

Oxygen is a highly flammable gas and must be used with caution in the home. Parents and caretakers must be taught necessary safety precautions. The implementation of these safety measures should be evaluated whenever a home visit is made (Table 16-2).

The primary care provider should review the use of aerosol cans and open flames in the home with the family. Fumes and smoke cause increased irritation to already sensitive airways and present a fire hazard if oxygen is in use. Caregivers and visitors should be warned against smoking in the home and around the child.

Consideration for safety with the use of electrical equipment should be part of the preparation for discharge from the hospital. The primary care provider should also reinforce safety concerns. All medical equipment should be electrically grounded. Extension cords should not be used unless approved by the home care equipment vendor.

Before a child is discharged, contact with emergency services should be established. Contacts include fire, ambulance, police, electric, and telephone services. The contacts should be reviewed with families to reinforce required actions. The inadvertent omission of an essential contact may be identified, thus avoiding needless anxiety or lack of attention in a true emergency.

Immunizations

Infants with BPD should receive all standard immunizations at the appropriate chronologic age (Nievas & Chernick, 2002). Hepatitis B immunization is usually given within the first 12 hours of life to infants whose mother is infected with hepatitis B (Committee on Infectious Disease, 2000). For premature infants whose mother is not infected, hepatitis B immunization is usually given at discharge if they weigh greater than 2 kg or at 2 months' chronologic age (Committee on Infectious Disease, 2000). Because of prolonged hospitalizations and recurrent illnesses, however, the immunization schedules of infants with BPD are often delayed. Before immunizations are initiated in the primary care office, hospital records should be reviewed to determine if any immunizations were administered during hospitalization. If an infant has a history of uncontrolled

---

TABLE 16-2
Safe Use of Oxygen at Home

Safety Guidelines	Rationale
Secure oxygen tank in upright position. Keep oxygen tanks at least 5 ft from heat source and electrical devices (e.g., space heaters, heating vents, fireplaces, radios, vaporizers, humidifiers).	Oxygen tanks are highly explosive; if a horizontally positioned tank explodes, the rapid release of oxygen can catapult it through animate (e.g., human bodies) and inanimate (e.g., walls) objects.
Ensure that no one smokes in the room or in the area of the oxygen tank.	Smoking increases the risk of fire, which could cause the tank to explode; escaped oxygen would feed the fire.
Use lemon-glycerin swabs to relieve dryness around the child's mouth; avoid oil or alcohol-based substances (e.g., petroleum jelly, vitamin A and D ointment, baby oil).	Both alcohol and oil are flammable and increase the risk of fire.
Have the child wear cotton garments.	Silk, wool, and synthetics can generate static electricity and cause fire.
Keep a fire extinguisher readily available.	It is necessary to put out fire immediately.
Turn off both volume regulator and flow regulator whenever oxygen is not in use.	If the volume regulator is on when oxygen is turned on, the child might receive a rapid, forceful flow of oxygen in the face that could be frightening and uncomfortable.
	Oxygen leakage, which might not be detected because oxygen is odorless, can cause fire.

From Hagedorn, M.I. & Gardner, S. (1989). Physiologic sequelae of prematurity: The nurse practitioner's role. Part I. Respiratory issues, *J Pediatr Health Care*, 3, 288-297. Reprinted with permission.

seizures, pertussis may be withheld until the seizures are controlled, or diphtheria and tetanus vaccines may be given without pertussis (see Chapter 25). Infants and children with chronic BPD are at highest risk for serious morbidity with pertussis infection, so pertussis vaccination should not be withheld without cause.

The subviron influenza vaccine should be administered to children over 6 months of age with BPD and their caretakers during the fall or early winter months (Committee on Infectious Disease, 2000). The pneumococcal vaccine (Prevnar) is recommended at 2, 4, 6, and 15 months of age (Committee on Infectious Disease, 2000).

Synagis (palivizumab) should be given as an intramuscular (IM) injection once per month through the RSV season (usually October/November to April/May). This injection is indicated for infants 2 years of age or younger with a diagnosis of BPD who require some form of respiratory therapy in the 6 months before RSV season (Impact-RSV Study Group, 1998). Synagis does not interfere with measles-mumps-rubella (MMR) or the varicella vaccine as previously seen with respiratory syncytial virus immune globulin (RSV-IVIG [RespiGam]) (Committee on Infectious Diseases and Committee of Fetus and Newborn, 1998).

Screening

Vision. Evaluations for ROP should be done by a pediatric ophthalmologist every 2 or 3 months during the child's first year of life. If there is a question of blindness, a visual evoked-response test can be requested. Routine eye examinations with Hirschberg, cover test, tracking, and funduscopic examinations should be done at each primary care visit to check for the common problems of myopia and strabismus. Surgical correction for strabismus is often required.

Hearing. Infants with BPD are at risk for hearing loss as a result of prematurity and the IV administration of furosemide, corticosteroids, and aminoglycosides. A basal auditory evoked response (BAER) test should be completed before discharge from the hospital, and routine screening for hearing should be conducted with each primary care visit. If recurrent otitis media is a problem, regular audiometric examinations should be conducted to identify hearing impairment and speech delays. Speech delays can be anticipated in children with long-term tracheostomies.

Dental. Routine dental care is recommended. Orally ingested ferrous sulfate may stain teeth, but this can be remedied with good dental hygiene. Daily tooth brushing may be a challenge for parents because of a child's oral defensiveness. Primary care providers can recommend using Toothettes or foam-tipped brushes, which are softer, and baking soda instead of toothpaste because of its milder taste.

Blood Pressure. Blood pressure should be measured with every visit and routinely followed to detect early signs of progressive cardiac disease, pulmonary hypertension, or renal dysfunction.

Hematocrit. Premature infants are more susceptible to iron deficiency anemia than full-term infants and must be observed closely during their first year of life. Hematocrit values should be checked monthly for the first 6 months of life and bimonthly for the following 6 months. Anemia of prematurity may be further aggravated by erosive gastroesophageal reflux and frequent blood tests. Children with chronic hypoxia may have elevated hemoglobin and hematocrit values.

Urinalysis. Routine screening is recommended.

Tuberculosis. Routine screening is recommended.

Condition-Specific Screening

Chest Radiographic Films. Chest radiographic studies may need to be obtained if physical symptoms change.

Pulmonary Function Tests. Pulmonary function studies may help the diagnosis of asthma and should be completed if pulmonary factors cause physical impairment.

Common Illness Management
Differential Diagnosis (Box 16-6)

Parents and caretakers must be aware of ongoing health care needs for children with CLD.

BOX 16-6
Differential Diagnosis

DIFFERENTIAL DIAGNOSIS
Respiratory Distress
Pneumonia (viral, bacterial)
Pulmonary edema
Congestive heart failure
Cardiac defect
Bronchospasm

BPD Unresponsive to Therapy
Wilson-Mikity syndrome
Pulmonary interstitial emphysema
Congenital heart disease
Pulmonary hemorrhage
Viral pneumonia
Cystic fibrosis
Pulmonary lymphangiectasia

Cough
Sinusitis
Gastroesophageal reflux (GER)
Reactive airways
Pulmonary edema
Pertussis
Respiratory syncytial virus (RSV)

Fever
Otitis media
Sinusitis
Respiratory tract infection
Urinary tract infection
Septicemia

Gastrointestinal Disturbances (e.g., emesis, feeding intolerance, diarrhea)
Antibiotic therapy
Theophylline toxicity
Gastroesophageal reflux (GER)
Formula density intolerance
Gastroenteritis

Skin and Mucosa Changes
Candida dermatitis
Oral thrush

Respiratory Distress. Respiratory distress is a common cause of urgent visits to the primary care practitioner. A child should be assessed for an elevated respiratory rate, increased work of breathing with substernal and intercostal retractions, nasal flaring, and a change in baseline breath sounds. Oxygenation can be quickly and accurately assessed via pulse oximetry if available in the office. Activity level and appetite may decrease. The child should also be assessed for sources of infection (e.g., a viral illness). Children dependent on respiratory support (e.g., oxygen, aerosolized bronchodilators, or mechanical ventilation) may require an increased level of support to reverse hypoxia and hypercarbia during this period of respiratory workload.

A chest radiograph will determine if a child has atelectasis, aspiration pneumonia, an infectious pulmonary process (e.g., viral or bacterial pneumonia), or increased pulmonary fluid. Respiratory distress with wheezing or prolonged expiratory phase that resolves after bronchodilator treatment indicates bronchospasm.

Significant respiratory distress in the infant with severe BPD may be cardiac in origin. Pallor, diaphoresis, and tachypnea may indicate congestive heart failure. Evaluation with an electrocardiogram (ECG) will reveal right and left ventricular hypertrophy. A heart murmur in an infant with severe BPD necessitates an immediate cardiologic consultation to rule out patent ductus arteriosus, foramen ovale, or septal defects.

An infant with diagnosed BPD will occasionally not respond to treatment as expected. If unresponsiveness occurs, other respiratory disorders related to the neonatal period should be considered. Several conditions may mimic BPD in infants, including the following: (1) Wilson-Mikity syndrome, which presents as increasing respiratory distress in the premature infant at 2 to 6 weeks of life, although cystic changes make it pathologically different from BPD; (2) pulmonary interstitial emphysema, which appears similar to stage III BPD on radiographs; (3) congenital heart disease with left-to-right shunting, which can result in respiratory failure secondary to pulmonary edema; (4) pulmonary hemorrhage that causes complete opacification on chest radiographs, mimicking stage II BPD; (5) viral pneumonia; (6) cystic fibrosis, which may present with respiratory distress and abnormal radiographs similar to BPD; and (7) congenital pulmonary lymphangiectasia, which is an overgrowth of the lung lymphatic vessels that shows mottling and hyperinflation on chest radiographs at birth.

Cough. Cough in an infant with BPD can indicate several possible processes. A productive, persistent, or moist cough without changes in lung sounds or chest radiographs may indicate sinusitis. Intermittent dry cough that is more pronounced after feedings and when the infant is supine may result from undiagnosed or poorly controlled reflux. Cough associated with increased activity may indicate undertreated reactive airway disease. A new cough in combination with tachypnea and crackles without evidence of infection often indicates pulmonary edema. Sudden onset of a staccato cough—with or without apnea—that interferes with feedings may indicate pertussis. If this cough is accompanied by copious, clear rhinorrhea, RSV should be considered.

Fever. If an infant's body temperature persists above 101° F for more than 24 hours despite antipyretic administration, the primary care provider should consider further work-up with a complete blood cell count, secretion culture, and possible chest radiograph. The outcome of the culture and sensitivity test will determine the antibiotic of choice and the route of administration (i.e., either enteral or IV). An infant with BPD who exhibits a toxic or septic appearance should also have a blood culture drawn to rule out septicemia. Otitis media and sinusitis often cause fever in infants with BPD, and their upper respiratory tract processes can lead to lower respiratory tract infection.

Gastrointestinal Disturbances. Disturbances such as diarrhea, nausea, emesis, and feeding intolerances are common in infants with BPD. Gastrointestinal disturbances may be associated with a respiratory infection, antibiotic therapy, theophylline toxicity, feeding intolerance to formulas, or a change in osmotic load as a result of changes in caloric density of the formula. If these reasons have been reviewed and diarrhea persists, a stool specimen should be obtained to rule out bacterial or viral etiology. Frequent emesis may indicate gastroesophageal reflux. Hydration status must be monitored to avoid dehydration. The child may need to be hospitalized for fluid management.

Skin and Mucosa Changes. *Candida* infections are often contracted after a course of antibiotic treatment or prolonged systemic steroid treatment. The warm, moist surfaces of the body, including diaper areas, oral mucosa, and tracheostomy and gastrostomy stomas, are most sensitive. Practicing good skin hygiene and keeping the skin dry prevent the spread of the rash. Topical treatment with antifungal creams such as nystatin is also indicated. Nystatin suspension also is the treatment for oral thrush.

Drug Interactions

Cough suppressants are not recommended for children with BPD; the cause of the cough should be evaluated and treated. Likewise, antihistamines are not recommended for children with artificial airways. The drying effect can thicken airway secretions, presenting the potential for plugging of the smaller peripheral airways and the tracheostomy tube.

Caffeine citrate and theophylline are bronchodilators. Caffeine citrate has become the drug of choice largely because of its efficient administration and management (Gannon, 2000). The maintenance dose of 5 to 10 mg/kg/dose of caffeine citrate can be administered once daily (Johns Hopkins University, 2000). The reduced incidence of side effects and wide therapeutic range of 5 to 25 mg/L serum levels allow for less frequent monitoring of serum levels (Gannon, 2000). Infants receiving theophylline require closer monitoring. If doses are missed, the blood level and resulting effectiveness of the medication may be significantly altered. Theophylline may cause a number of adverse gastrointestinal side effects, including gastric irritability, nausea, and vomiting, but these can be prevented by administering certain preparations with food. If a child is already difficult to feed, this adds an additional challenge. Theophylline levels are altered by some commonly used medications, and serum levels must be checked often when these medications are prescribed. (See Chapter 11 for additional asthma drug interactions.)

Cisapride (Propulsid) is often used in infants with feeding intolerance. It enhances gastric motility by increasing esophageal peristaltic activity and enhancing the tone of the esophageal sphincter (Premji & Paes, 1999). The use of cisapride for promotility effects on the gastrointestinal tract in premature infants, however, is controversial (Johns Hopkins University, 2000; Premji & Paes, 1999). Administration of high doses or in conjunction with other medications causes cardiac arrhythmia with a prolonged QT interval (Premji & Paes, 1999). This adverse effect is enhanced and administration to neonates is contraindicated if the infant is receiving antifungals (fluconazole, itraconazole, ketoconazole); antibiotics (erythromycin, clarithromycin); or protease inhibitors (ritonavir, indinavir) (Johns Hopkins University, 2000; Premji & Paes, 1999).

Developmental Issues

Sleep

Most hospitals preparing to discharge a child with BPD attempt to arrange the child's care to provide for several hours of undisturbed sleep at night. The primary care provider should determine if there has been any change in the child's status as a result of the schedule adjustment. For example, bronchodilator treatments and CPT may be extended from 6 to 8 hours to promote the child's and parents' sleep. If schedules for home life have not been restructured, this is an appropriate time to discuss the schedule with the family and gradually implement changes.

The infant's and parents' sleep patterns may be altered because of the monitors placed in the home for children who require mechanical ventilation, receive oxygen therapy, or have a history of apnea. The primary care provider should inquire about the frequency of alarms and determine what type of alarm is appropriate for the child's condition. Readjustment of alarm limits may be warranted if false alarms are frequent; the limits are set within the physiologic range of the child's heart and respiratory rate. With increasing frequency, the pulse oximeter is the preferred monitor because of its simplicity of use and accuracy of measurement.

It is important to determine how audible the monitor alarm is to the family. If the alarm is so loud that it is very disturbing, the monitor can be placed on a cloth to absorb sound. If the sound is not sufficiently audible, the primary care provider can recommend a commercially available intercom system.

Toileting

Delayed bowel and bladder training may be a result of prolonged hospitalization, prematurity, or neurodevelopmental delay. The use of diuretics may make bladder training more difficult because of increased frequency of urination. Parents must be helped to identify cues that indicate a child's developmental readiness for toilet training.

Discipline

Children with technologic support learn quickly that the sounding of alarms and monitors immediately summons a caregiver. Purposeful disconnections can easily become an attention maneuver. The child and family should be educated with regard to potential risks.

Parents need support and guidance from the primary care provider to recognize that their children need reasonable, consistent discipline. Primary care providers can help families develop consistent responses and discipline approaches that can be used by numerous caregivers (i.e., including parents, siblings, therapists, and nurses). Approaches should be based on the child's cognitive and developmental—not chronologic—age.

Child Care

Children requiring mechanical ventilation often have the support of nursing care during the night that is reimbursed by third-party payers. Children who have an artificial airway may or may not have this coverage, depending on third-party payer guidelines.

Children who do not require technologic support may not qualify for supportive care through insurance. This can present a problem for families who have limited budgets and cannot afford private, in-home baby sitters. Regular daycare services may place the child at high risk for exposure to infections.

Traditional well-child daycare centers may not be equipped or trained to care for a child who is medically fragile. There have been a few medical daycare centers created by individuals or agencies that employ skilled nurses to provide high-quality child care. Primary care providers can help families explore child care options. Hospital discharge programs often incorporate additional family members or neighbors into the teaching plans if requested.

The primary care provider should review the family support systems to determine if the systems are satisfactory to the well-being of the child and family. Nursing care should be used to provide support for families during activity-intensive periods of the day. Time without nursing support can be scheduled to incorporate activities and responsibilities within the context of the family structure and routine.

There is increasingly an awareness of the need for medical daycare facilities that provide services for children requiring supportive treatments. Funding may be supported by insurance. The number of operating facilities is small, but the availability should increase as the need intensifies.

Schooling

All children with BPD should have a thorough developmental evaluation. Plans should be established for outpatient follow-up either at a community-based education center or within the home (i.e., in accordance with Public Laws 99-457 and 101-476). Parents will need ongoing support as the child grows and develops (see Chapter 5).

On entering the school system, a child may note differences in physical build and exercise endurance. Body image and peer acceptance may become an issue. Children with attention deficit hyperactivity disorder or those who are put in special classes for learning disabilities may have difficulty developing social skills (see Chapter 12). Increased absences during the winter season because of respiratory tract infections may further disrupt the school routine. Parents may develop separation anxiety from concern for their loss of control of their "fragile" child.

Primary care providers can assist in the transition from home to school by providing school personnel with specific instructions about the child's medical conditions and medications. Each school has a policy regarding medication administration during school hours. The ultimate goal is to encourage children with special needs to take responsibility for self-care.

Sexuality

There are no specific sexuality problems related to BPD. Children with physical and developmental delays and handicaps will need referrals and follow-up appropriate to their needs. The earliest survivors of BPD are now approximately 30 years of age, and to date no difficulties in the area of sexuality have been documented.

Children with BPD generally become adults with asthma. For women with a history of BPD, pregnancy brings a certain degree of stress on the respiratory system. Airway inflammation and bronchoconstriction should be controlled so both mother and baby receive an adequate oxygen supply (National Institutes of Health [NIH] Executive Summary, 1997). Inhaled bronchodilators and antiinflammatories are considered safe for pregnant women (NIH Executive Summary, 1997).

Transition into Adulthood

Pulmonary dysfunction is common in adolescents and adults with a history of BPD. Airway obstruction and airway hyper-responsiveness persist in a significant percentage of persons with BPD (Eber & Zach, 2001). Anticipatory guidance that includes environmental control and possible future needs for asthma therapy is suggested. Vocational counseling on environmental irritants in the workplace (i.e., secondhand cigarette smoke, construction dust or particles, pollens, factory smoke) and their relationship to asthma should be provided. A yearly influenza vaccine is recommended for individuals with BPD. An educational review of the pathophysiology of airway disease, medication action and indication, use of a peak flowmeter and an MDI or aerochamber, and signs and symptoms of distress that warrant immediate medical attention is essential during adolescence and young adulthood for older individuals to assume self-care.

Family Concerns and Resources

Education and Discharge Planning

Discharge planning ideally starts several weeks before the anticipated discharge date. Family members who will be caregivers must attend teaching sessions and hands-on practice sessions with the hospital nurses and therapists in order to safely care for the infant when at home.

Basic respiratory assessment skills, which include counting a breathing rate during sleep and recognizing fluid overload (puffiness), retractions, flaring, and color changes, are essential for families to monitor their infants at home. Family members should have a basic understanding of the pathophysiology of BPD, its chronic nature, and the need for close follow-up. Caregivers at home should understand the infant's high nutritional needs and appreciate the infant's low respiratory reserve. CPR instruction must be provided before a child is discharged from the hospital. The family must be able to demonstrate use of any medical equipment that will be in the home (i.e., oxygen, apnea monitor, nebulizer and/or compressor).

Family members and friends should practice good hand washing and when ill avoid contact with the infant. Environmental control of airway irritants can be maximized in the home. A smoke-free, pet-free home without mold or mildew and with minimal dust is ideal.

Financial Responsibilities

Most third-party payers—including Medicaid—fund the cost of equipment and rehabilitative and nursing needs. Significant variations exist, however, among plans. The financial strain created by numerous visits from medical and rehabilitative care practitioners can stress family budgets (Miller et al, 1998). Equipment such as mechanical ventilators, compressors, and monitors increases the use of electricity. Calls to physicians, therapists, vendors, and nursing services increase telephone bills. Some utility companies have programs for families with special needs. Other hidden costs (e.g., medications, special formulas, corrective glasses, rehabilitative equipment, higher electricity and heat bills) can create further financial burden (Miller et al, 1998). Loss of parental wages because of a leave of absence from work in order to care for a fragile infant causes families additional financial burden.

Privacy

The increased number of people in the home environment (i.e., nurses, vendors, respiratory therapists, rehabilitative therapists) can seriously limit family privacy. When the family appears capable of assuming care safely and voices concerns about the lack of privacy and the needs of the child are stabilized, the primary care provider, in conjunction with the pediatric respiratory team, can suggest decreasing some of this support.

Once a child has been discharged from the hospital, the reality of the developmental delay may become apparent. Families will need ongoing emotional support to face and adjust to this problem. The primary care provider can assist with investigation of appropriate educational and rehabilitative programs.

RESOURCES

American Association for Premature Infants (AAPI)
http://www.aapi-online.org
National advocacy organization

American Lung Association
(800) 586-4872
www.lungusa.org

Exceptional Parent Magazine
PO Box 3000
Denville, NJ 07834
(877) 372-7368
www.eparent.com

March of Dimes
www.modimes.org/HealthLibrary

Mary Searcy's Resources for Parents of Preemies
http://Members.aol.com/MarAim/preemie.htm
Exhaustive list of resources for parents of preemies

Parent information on kids' health conditions
http://kidshealth.org/parent/medical

Parents of Prematures
PO Box 3046
Kirland, WA 98083-3046
Publishes monthly newsletter

Respiratory Syncytial Virus (RSV)
(877) 568-8171
www.rsvprotection.com

Summary of Primary Care Needs for the Child with Bronchopulmonary Dysplasia

HEALTH CARE MAINTENANCE

Growth and Development

Height and weight are below average in the majority of children—even at 2 years of age.

Plot head circumference, height, and length corrected for gestational age with each visit. Standardized growth curves for premature infants are available.

The head of a premature infant often appears boxy and must be measured carefully until 2 years' corrected age to determine adequate growth.

Review caloric intake for adequacy. Repeated illness can result in insufficient caloric intake to maintain growth.

Developmental delay is often seen during the first year of life.

Early referral to an infant stimulation program is recommended. Continued delays may be seen in children of very low birth weight or with a history of severe BPD.

Learning disabilities are often evident during school years.

Diet

Adequate caloric intake is important for optimal lung repair and growth and development. Increased caloric intake needs to be balanced with concerns regarding fluid load and expenditure of energy with feeding.

Difficulties may arise with oral motor function. Oral feedings may need to be supplemented with enteral feedings via gavage or gastrostomy. Introduction of solids should occur at 4 to 6 months' corrected age, but oral-tactile hypersensitivity may make this difficult.

Early referral to a pediatric nutritionist or occupational therapist can prevent long-term problems.

Safety

Respiratory equipment should have functioning alarms set "on."

Beware of accidental decannulations and disconnections from respiratory support.

Constant supervision and a noninvasive monitoring system are needed.

Security of tracheostomy tube should be assessed frequently. Aspiration of small objects into artificial airway can occur.

Family members should know CPR.

Oxygen should be used with caution in the home. Open flames, smoking, sparks, and aerosol cans all pose increased fire risks.

Electrical safety requires grounded equipment.

Establish emergency service contact with local fire, ambulance, police, electric, and telephone service before a child is discharged from the hospital.

Immunizations

Many children are delayed in receiving immunizations because of prolonged hospitalization. Check hospital records for immunizations given while hospitalized.

Children should be immunized according to a routine schedule based on chronologic—not gestational—age.

Pertussis vaccine should only be withheld with just cause because of the high risk of significant morbidity with active disease in children with BPD. Use a cellular pertussis if appropriate.

Inactivated polio vaccine may be administered in the hospital before discharge.

Influenza vaccine is recommended yearly for children with chronic lung disease (CLD).

Synagis should be given monthly from October/November to April/May for at-risk infants and toddlers 2 years of age and younger.

Screening

Vision. Children should be evaluated by a pediatric ophthalmologist every 2 to 3 months during the first year of life to rule out retinopathy of prematurity (ROP). Cover test should be done and tracking ability screened at each visit.

Myopia and strabismus are common and must be followed in the primary care office and by a pediatric ophthalmologist.

Hearing. A basal auditory evoked response (BAER) test should be done before discharge from the hospital.

There is a risk of hearing loss because of prematurity and medications.

Age-appropriate screening should be done at each office visit.

Audiometry screening should be done with recurrent, serous otitis media.

Speech delays are anticipated in children with tracheostomies.

Dental. Routine screening is recommended.

Hypoplastic and discolored teeth are common.

Oral defensiveness may make dental hygiene difficult. Foam-dipped brushes and baking soda may be recommended.

Blood Pressure. Blood pressure should be taken at each visit. Children with abnormal blood pressure findings should be referred to a pulmonologist.

Hematocrit. Because of prematurity, iron deficiency anemia is common.

Hematocrit screening must be done frequently during the first year of life.

Chronic hypoxia may cause elevated hemoglobin levels.

Urinalysis. Routine screening is recommended.

Tuberculosis. Routine screening is recommended.

Condition-Specific Screening

Chest Radiograph. Radiographic examinations of the lung should be done at discharge and then annually and as needed per clinical indication.

Pulmonary Function Tests. Pulmonary function tests should be done at discharge, annually, and as necessary per clinical indication.

COMMON ILLNESS MANAGEMENT

Differential Diagnosis

Respiratory Distress Rule out bacterial or viral infection, atelectasis, pneumonia, bronchospasm, pulmonary edema, heart

Continued

Summary of Primary Care Needs for the Child with Bronchopulmonary Dysplasia—cont'd

Differential Diagnosis—cont'd

failure, and sinusitis. Consider respiratory syncytial virus (RSV) infections from November to March.

Oxygenation should be checked with pulse oximeter. Chest x-ray is often indicated.

Cough. Rule out sinusitis, gastroesophageal reflux (GER), reactive airway disease, pulmonary edema, pertussis, and RSV.

Fever. Rule out otitis media, sinusitis, upper or lower respiratory tract infection, urinary tract infection, and septicemia.

Gastrointestinal Disturbances. Consider feeding intolerances, bacterial and viral infections, GER, or theophylline toxicity.

Skin. For skin problems around tracheostomy and gastrostomy stomas and diaper areas, consider *Candida* infection and cellulitis.

Drug Interactions

Caffeine citrate administration is preferred over theophylline. Theophylline interacts with other medications (see Chapter 11).

Cough suppressants may mask an underlying condition and are not recommended.

Do not use antihistamines for children with tracheostomy tubes because of the thickening of airway secretions.

Cisapride (Propulsid) use in premature infants is controversial because of possible cardiac arrhythmia.

DEVELOPMENTAL ISSUES

Sleep Patterns

Attempt to evaluate the child's schedule of care to decrease sleep disturbances and provide for the whole family.

Evaluate functioning of monitors. Readjustment of alarm limits may be warranted if false alarms are frequent.

Toileting

Delayed bowel and bladder training may occur as a result of prolonged hospitalization and the use of diuretics and theophylline.

Discipline

Children should receive discipline appropriate to their developmental level of understanding.

A consistent plan should be followed.

Purposeful disconnection from oxygen for attention may occur in toddlers.

Child Care

Recommend that children not supported by oxygen and mechanical ventilation attend home or small daycare centers to reduce exposure to infection.

Children with mechanical support may be eligible for nursing support from third-party payers.

Help family determine availability of medical daycare facilities if child requires technologic support.

Schooling

Help family with developmental evaluations and planning early intervention programs. An individualized family service program (IFSP) should be initiated for children 0 to 2 years, followed by an individualized education program (IEP) for children 3 to 21 years if learning deficit or developmental delay is present.

Sexuality

Care is routine unless associated problems warrant additional care. Pregnancy increases respiratory workload in women who had BPD. Prenatal care is important.

Transition into Adulthood

Abnormal pulmonary function frequently persists into adulthood. Counsel regarding possible environmental irritants in workplace or school. Review and educate concerning disease process and management.

FAMILY CONCERNS

Education on respiratory assessment, CPR, and equipment for home use is needed.

A home free of smoke, pets, mold, mildew, and dust is recommended.

There may be a lack of privacy in the home because of the need for medical caregivers.

Developmental outcome is uncertain. Assist families with adjustment to developmental delays. The potential for developmental delay and persistent medical problems results in great emotional strain on parents. Financial responsibilities are great even with insurance coverage.

REFERENCES

Abrams, S.A. (2001). Chronic pulmonary insufficiency in children and its effects on growth and development. *J Nutr, 131*(3), 938-941.

Bancalari, E. (1998, May). *Bronchopulmonary dysplasia: Then and now.* Presented at the American Thoracic Society conference, Chicago.

Barrington, K.J. & Finer, N.N. (1998). Treatment of bronchopulmonary dysplasia, a review. *Clin Perinatol, 25*(1), 177-202.

Battin, M., Ling, E.W., Whitfield, M.F., Mackinnon, M., & Effer, S.B. (1998). Has the outcome for extremely low gestational age (ELGA) infants improved following recent advances in neonatal intensive care? *Am J Perinatol, 15*(8), 469-477.

Blackburn, S., (1999, July). Understanding gastroesophageal reflux in infants. *Cent Lines, 15*(3), 16-22.

Carey, B.E. & Trotter, C. (2000). Bronchopulmonary dysplasia. *Neonatal Netw, 19*(3), 45-49.

Cherif, A., Marrakchi, Z., Chaouachi, S., Boukef, S., & Sfar, R. (2002). Bronchopulmonary dysplasia and corticosteroid therapy. *Arch Pediatr, 9*(2), 159-168.

Cole, C.H., Colton, T., Shah, B.L., Abbasi, S., MacKinnon, B.L., et al. (1999). Early inhaled glucocorticoid therapy to prevent bronchopulmonary dysplasia. *N Engl J Med, 340*(13), 1005-1010.

Committee on Infectious Disease. (2000). *The Red Book* (25th ed.). Elk Grove Village, Ill.: American Academy of Pediatrics.

Committee on Infectious Diseases and Committee of Fetus and Newborn. (1998). Prevention of respiratory syncytial virus infections: Indications for the use of palivizumab and update on the use of RSV-IVIG. *Pediatrics, 102*(5), 1211-1216.

Darlow, B.A. & Graham, P.J. (2000). Vitamin A supplementation for preventing morbidity and mortality in very low birthweight infants. *Cochrane Database Syst Rev*, no. 2, CD000501.

Davis, P.G., Thorpe, K., Roberts, R., Schmidt, B., Doyle, L.W., et al. (2002). Evaluating "old" definitions for the "new" bronchopulmonary dysplasia. *J Pediatr, 140*(5), 555-560.

Eber, E. & Zach, M.S. (2001, April). Long term sequelae of bronchopulmonary dysplasia (chronic lung disease of infancy). *Thorax, 56,* 317-323.

Nievas, F.F. & Chernick, V. (2002). Bronchopulmonary dysplasia (chronic lung disease of infancy): An update for the pediatrician. *Clin Pediatr, 41*(2), 77-85.

Fillmore, E.J. & Cartlidge, P.H. (1998). Late death of very low birthweight infants. *Acta Paediatr, 87*(7), 809-810.

Fok, T.F., Lam, K., Ng, P.C., So, H.K., Cheung, K.L., et al. (1998). Randomized crossover trial of salbutamol aerosol delivered by metered dose inhaler, jet nebuliser, and ultrasonic nebuliser in CLD. *Arch Dis Child Fetal Neonatal Ed, 79*(2), 100-104.

Gannon, B.A. (2000, December). Theophylline or caffeine: Which is best for apnea of prematurity? *Neonatal Netw, (19)*8, 33-36.

Ghezzi, F., Gomez, R., Romero, R., Yoon, B.H., Edwin, S.S., et al. (1998). Elevated interleukin-8 concentrations in amniotic fluid of mothers whose neonates subsequently develop bronchopulmonary dysplasia. *Eur J Obstet Gynecol Reprod Biol, 78*(1), 5-10.

Golombek, S.G. (2000). The use of inhaled nitric oxide in newborn medicine. *Heart Dis, 2*(5), 342-347.

Gregoire, M.C., Lefebvre, F., & Glorieux, J. (1998). Health and developmental outcomes at 18 months in very preterm infants with bronchopulmonary dysplasia. *Pediatrics, 101*(5), 856-860.

Groneck, P., Gotze-Speer, B., Oppermann, M., Eiffert, H., & Speer, C.P. (1994). Association of pulmonary inflammation and increased microvascular permeability during the development of bronchopulmonary dysplasia: A sequential analysis of inflammatory mediators in respiratory fluids of high-risk preterm neonates. *Pediatrics, 93*(5), 712-718.

Gross, S.J., Iannuzzi, D.M., Kveselis, D.A., & Anbar, R.D. (1998). Effect of preterm birth on pulmonary function at school age: A prospective controlled study. *J Pediatr, 133*(2), 188-192.

Hack, M. & Fanaroff, A.A. (2000). Outcomes of children of extremely low birthweight and gestational age in the 1990s. *Semin Neonatol, 5*(2), 89-106.

Hack, M., Wilson-Costello, D., Friedman, H., Taylor, G.H., Schluchter, M., et al. (2000). Neurodevelopment and predictors of outcomes of children with birth weights of less than 1000 g: 1992-1995. *Arch Pediatr Adolesc Med, 154*(7), 725-731.

Hazinski, T.A. (1998). Bronchopulmonary dysplasia. In Kendig. *Kendig's disorders of the respiratory tract in children.* Philadelphia: W.B. Saunders.

Holmstrom, G., Broberger, U., & Thomassen, P. (1998). Neonatal risk factors for retinopathy of prematurity: A population-based study. *Acta Ophthalmol Scand, 76*(2), 204-207.

Hughes, C.A., O'Gorman, L.A., Shyr, Y., Schork, M.A., Bozynski, M.E., et al. (1999). Cognitive performance at school age of very low birth weight infants with bronchopulmonary dysplasia. *J Dev Behav Pediatr, 20*(1), 1-8.

Hussey-Gardner, B. et al. (2002). Early intervention best practice: Collaboration among an NICU, an early intervention program, and an NICU follow-up program. *Neonatal Netw, 21*(3), 15-22.

Impact-RSV Study Group. (1998). Palivizumab, a humanized respiratory syncytial virus monoclonal antibody, reduces hospitalization from respiratory syncytial virus infection in high-risk infants. *Pediatrics, 102*(3), 531-537.

Jacob, S.V., Coates, A.L., Lands, L.C., MacNeish, C.F., Riley, S.P., et al. (1998). Long-term pulmonary sequelae of severe bronchopulmonary dysplasia. *J Pediatr, 133*(2), 193-200.

Jobe, A.H. & Bancalari, E. (2001). Bronchopulmonary dysplasia. *Am J Respir Crit Care Med, 163*(7), 1723-1729.

Johns Hopkins Hospital. (2000).*The Harriet Lane handbook* (15th ed.). St Louis: Mosby.

Johnson, D.B., Cheney, C., & Monsen, E.R. (1998). Nutrition and feeding in infants with bronchopulmonary dysplasia after initial discharge: Risk factors for growth failure. *J Am Diet Assoc, 98*(6), 649-656.

Karinski, D.A., Balkundi, D., Rubin, L.P., & Padbury, J.F. (2000). The use of inhaled glucocorticosteroids and recovery from adrenal suppression after systemic steroid use in a vlbw premature infant with BPD: Case report and literature discussion. *Neonatal Netw, 19*(8), 27-32.

Kramer, B.W., Kramer, S., Ikegami, M., & Jobe, A.H. (2002). Injury, inflammation, and remodeling in fetal sheep lung after intra-amniotic endotoxin. *Am J Physiol Lung Cell Mol Physiol, 283*(2), 452-459.

Lister, P., Iles, R., Shaw, B., & Ducharme, F. (2000). Inhaled steroids for neonatal chronic lung disease. *Cochrane Database of Systematic Reviews*, no. 3, CD002311.

Majnemer, A., Riley, P., Shevell, M., Birnbaum, R., Greenstone, H., et al. (2000). Severe bronchopulmonary dysplasia increases risk for later neurological and motor sequelae in preterm survivors. *Dev Med Child Neurol, 42*(1), 53-60.

Martin, R.J. & Walsh-Sukys, M.C. (1999). Bronchopulmonary dysplasia—no simple solution. *N Engl J Med, 340*(13), 1036-1038.

Mercado-Deane, M.G., Burton, E.M., Harlow, S.A., Glover, A.S., Deane, D.A., et al. (2001). Swallowing dysfunction in infants less than 1 year of age. *Pediatr Radiol, 31*(6), 423-428.

Miller, V.L., Rice, J.C., DeVoe, M., & Fos, P.J. (1998). An analysis of program and family costs of case managed care for technology-dependent infants with bronchopulmonary dysplasia. *J Pediatr Nurs, 13*(4), 244-251.

Mueller, D.H. (1998). Timeliness of codifying nutrition ABCDE's for BPD. *J Pediatr, 133*(3), 315-316.

National Institutes of Health Executive Summary. (1997). *Management of asthma during pregnancy, National Asthma Education Program, National Heart, Lung and Blood Institute, National Institutes of Health.* Washington, DC: U.S. Government Printing Office.

Ng, D.K., Lau, W.Y., & Lee, S.L. (2000). Pulmonary sequelae in long-term survivors of bronchopulmonary dysplasia. *Pediatr Int, 42*(6), 603-607.

Northway, W.H., Jr., Rosan, R.C., & Porter, D.Y. (1967). Pulmonary disease following respiratory therapy of hyaline membrane disease. *N Engl J Med, 267,* 357-368.

Oh, W. & Merenstein, G. (1997). Fourth edition of the guidelines for perinatal care: Summary of changes. *Pediatrics, 100*(6), 1021-1022.

Pandya, H.C. & Kotecha, S. (2001). Chronic lung disease of prematurity: Clinical and pathophysiological correlates. *Monaldi Arch Chest Dis, 56*(3), 270-275.

Philip, A.G. (1975). Oxygen plus pressure plus time: The etiology of bronchopulmonary dysplasia. *Pediatrics, 55,* 44-50.

Piedra, P.A. (2002). Future direction in vaccine prevention of respiratory syncytial virus. *Pediatr Infect Dis J, 21*(5), 482-487.

Premji, S.S. & Paes, B. (1999). Cisapride: The problem of the heart. *Neonat Netw, 18*(7), 21-25.

Ramsay, P.L. et al. (1999). Attenuation in the postnatal expression of the clara cell secreted protein is associated with the development of bronchopulmonary dysplasia. *Pediatr Res, 45*(4), 316A.

Rimensberger, P.C. (2002). Neonatal respiratory failure. *Pediatrics, 14*(3), 315-321.

Rozycki, H.J. & Kirkpatrick, B.V. (1993). New developments in bronchopulmonary dysplasia. *Pediatr Ann, 22,* 532-538.

Schaap, A.H., Wolf, H., Bruinse, H.W., Smolders-de Haas, H., van Ertbruggen, I., et al. (1999). School performance and behaviour in extremely preterm growth-retarded infants. *Eur J Obstet Gynecol Reprod Biol, 86*(1), 43-49.

Thebaud, B., Lacaze-Masmonteil, T., Watterberg, K. (2001). Postnatal glucocorticoids in very preterm infants: "The good, the bad and the ugly"? *Pediatrics, 107*(2), 413-415.

Trachtenbarg, D.E. & Golemon, T.B. (1998). Office care of the premature infant. Part II. Common medical and surgical problems. *Am Fam Physician, 57*(10), 2383-2390.

Vaucher, Y.E. (2002). Bronchopulmonary dysplasia: An enduring challenge. *Pediatr Rev, 23*(10), 349-358.

Vermont Oxford Network Steroid Study Group. (2001). Early postnatal dexamethasone therapy for the prevention of chronic lung disease. *Pediatrics, 108*(3), 741-748.

Watterberg, K.L. & Scott, S.M. (1995). Evidence of early adrenal insufficiency in babies who develop bronchopulmonary dysplasia. *Pediatrics, 95*(1), 120-125.

Welch, M.J. (1998). Inhaled corticosteroids and growth in children. *Pediatr Ann, 27*(11), 752-758.

Wilson-Costello, D., Borawski, E., Friedman, H., Redline, R., Fanaroff, A.A., et al. (1998). Perinatal correlates of CP and other neurologic impairments among LBW children. *Pediatrics, 102,* 315-322.

17 Cancer

Christina Baggott and Mary Alice Dragone

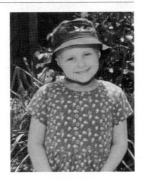

Etiology

An estimated 12,400 children and adolescents under age 20 years are diagnosed with cancer annually in the United States (Ries et al, 1999). Cancer results when the body fails to regulate cell production. A proliferation and spread of abnormal cells then occur, which—if left unchecked—may lead to death of the host. Common sites of malignancy in children include the blood and bone marrow, bone, lymph nodes, brain and central nervous system (CNS), kidneys, and soft tissues (Table 17-1).

Known Genetic Etiology

Although particular genetic factors or environmental exposures are known to place children at risk of developing cancer (as outlined in Table 17-1), the specific etiology of childhood cancer is yet to be identified. The genes associated with many pediatric tumors have been discovered, and scientists are making progress in applying this knowledge to successful therapies (Cripe & Mackall, 2001). Researchers are studying the deoxyribonucleic acid (DNA) point mutations, viral insertions and gene amplifications, deletions, or gene rearrangements to gain an understanding of the process of malignant transformation (Look & Kirsch, 2002; Ruccione, 2002).

Incidence and Prevalence

The overall incidence of malignancy in children under 20 years of age is approximately 15.5:100,000 per year (Ries et al, 2002). Leukemia and CNS tumors account for the majority of pediatric malignancies. A comparison of the incidence of the various childhood malignancies in the United States (Table 17-1 on pp. 300-303) illustrates a wide variation depending on site. Childhood cancer incidence also varies by race. White children have the highest rates of childhood cancer, followed by Hispanic children, Asian/Pacific Islander children, and black children. American Indians have the lowest rate of childhood cancer (Ries et al, 1999).

Clinical Manifestations at Time of Diagnosis

The signs and symptoms of a malignant disease depend on the interval between time of origin and diagnosis, as well as the type and location of the tumor. In general, cancer may manifest in one of the following three ways: (1) as a mass lesion, (2) with symptoms directly related to the tumor, or (3) with nonspecific symptoms. The presence of a mass lesion should alert the primary care provider to the possibility of a malignancy after benign conditions (e.g., constipation, a distended bladder) have been ruled out (Vietti & Steuber, 2002). A biopsy of other lesions should be taken in a timely manner to rule out malignancy. Symptoms related directly to the tumor may include bone pain, limping, unexplained bleeding, bruising or petechiae, morning headache and vomiting, hematuria, pallor, swelling of the face or neck, a white spot in a pupil (leukokoria), airway or urinary tract obstruction, or endocrinologic symptoms from hormone production by the tumor. Nonspecific symptoms include weight loss, diarrhea, low-grade fevers, malaise, or failure to thrive (Box 17-1).

Prompt referral to a pediatric cancer treatment center ensures that specimens for staging are properly obtained and the child is enrolled in multiinstitutional treatment studies. The initial work-up is crucial to the accurate and timely establishment of a diagnosis. One large study of the lag times to diagnosis of pediatric solid tumors found that older children and those with Ewing sarcoma and osteosarcoma had much longer lag times than young children and those with other tumors (Pollock et al, 1991). Children with neuroblastoma had the shortest lag time. After a thorough history and physical examination and laboratory tests, the work-up may include nuclear-radiologic examinations, ultrasound, bone marrow aspirate, bone marrow biopsy, or lumbar puncture, depending on the type of tumor suspected and the most frequent sites for metastases.

Whenever a biopsy is being considered, the primary care provider should consult an oncology treatment center before proceeding. Accurate staging increasingly depends on molecular genetics and the immunocytochemistry of initial diagnostic materials processed in specialty laboratories (American

---

BOX 17-1

Clinical Manifestations at Time of Diagnosis

Mass lesion, particularly in abdomen
Lymph node enlargement that is unresponsive to antibiotic therapy or accompanied by nonspecific symptoms
Unexplained bruising, bleeding, or petechiae
Pallor and fatigue
Unexplained or persistent fevers
Recurrent infection
Bone pain or limping
Morning headache with vomiting
Swelling in the face or neck
White spot in pupil (leukokoria)
Hematuria
Airway or urinary tract obstruction
Nonspecific symptoms: weight loss, diarrhea, failure to thrive, malaise, low-grade fevers

TABLE 17-1

Common Pediatric Cancers

Type	Site	Incidence (ages 0-14 yr)	Etiology	Signs/Symptoms	Treatment
LEUKEMIA		4.7 per 100,000 children per year			

	Bone marrow		*For ALL and AML:*
			Genetic factors
			  Chromosomal abnormalities
			  (trisomy 21, Bloom syndrome,
			  Fanconi anemia, AT)
			Familial predisposition (ALL—
			  infant identical twins)
				For ALL and AML:
				Pallor
				Fatigue, headache
				Fever, infection
				Purpura, bruising
				Organomegaly
				Bone pain	

Acule lymphoblastic leukemia (ALL)			Environmental factors
			  Ionizing radiation
			  Chronic chemical exposure
			  Use of alkylating agents for
			    treatment of malignant
			    disease (AML)
			Possible viral infection
					Combination chemotherapy
					CNS prophylaxis
					  Radiation therapy (for
					    high-risk cases)
					  Intrathecal chemotherapy

Acute myelogenous leukemia (AML)					Combination chemotherapy
					CNS prophylaxis
					  Single-agent intrathecal
					    chemotherapy
					HSCT in first remission

CENTRAL NERVOUS SYSTEM		3.4 per 100,000 children per year	*For all CNS cancers:*		

Infratentorial
  Medulloblastoma
	Cerebellum/brainstem
	Midline cerebellar
			Genetic factors
			  Heritable disease (NF, VHL,
			    LFS)
			  Familial
				Early
				  Decreased
				    academic
				    performance
				    Fatigue
					Anticonvulsants, if symptoms
					  present
					Treatment of hydrocephalus

Ependymoma	Ependymal lining of
	  ventricular system
	  or central canal of
	  spinal cord
			Environmental factors
			  Chronic chemical exposure
				Personality changes
				Intermittent headache
				
				Late
					Corticosteroids
					Shunting
					Surgical resection (if operable)

Brainstem glioma	Brainstem		Ionizing radiation
			Other primary malignancies
			Exogenous immunosuppression
				Morning headache
				  Vomiting
				  Diplopia/visual
				    changes
				Brainstem/cerebellar
				  Deficits of balance/
				    positioning
					Radiation therapy
					Chemotherapy for some tumors
					
					HSCT in rare cases

Supratentorial
  Astrocytomas
	Ventricles, midline
	  diencephalous,
	  cerebrum
				Supratentorial
				Nonspecific
				  headache	

Craniopharyngioma	Sella turcica			Seizures Hemiparesis	
Gliomas	Visual pathway				

Pineoblastoma
  or germ cell
  tumors
	Pineal region				

NON-HODGKIN LYMPHOMA		0.8 per 100,000 children per year	*For all non-Hodgkin lymphomas:*		

Lymphoblastic lymphoma	Usually generalized
	Anterior mediastinum
	Lymph nodes
	Bone marrow
			Immunodeficiency (HIV)
			Exogenous immunosuppression
			Viral—associated with
			  Epstein-Barr virus
				Generally rapid
				  progression
				Lymphoblastic
				  lymphoma
				Dysphagia, dyspnea
				Swelling of neck,
				  face, upper
				  extremities
				Supradiaphragmatic
				  lymphadenopathy
					Treatment of emergent
					  symptoms
					Multiagent chemotherapy
					CNS prophylaxis

Small noncleaved
  lymphoma
  Burkitt lymphoma
	Abdomen
	Bone marrow
	Lymph nodes
				Respiratory distress
				Small noncleaved
				  lymphoma
					Treatment of emergent
					  symptoms and tumor lysis
					  syndrome

AT, Ataxia-telangiectasia; *CNS*, central nervous system; *HSCT*, hematopoietic stem cell transplant; *HIV*, human immunodeficiency virus; *GI*, gastrointestinal; *NF*, neurofibromatosis; *LFS*, Li-Fraumeni syndrome (a germline mutation of the p53 tumor suppressor gene).

TABLE 17-1

Common Pediatric Cancers—cont'd

Type	Site	Incidence (ages 0-14 yr)	Etiology	Signs/Symptoms	Treatment
NON-HODGKIN LYMPHOMA—cont'd					
Small noncleaved—cont'd					
Non-Burkitt lymphoma				Abdominal pain or swelling Change in bowel habits Nausea/vomiting GI bleeding Intestinal perforation (rarely) Inguinal/iliac adenopathy Intussusception	Multiagent chemotherapy CNS prophylaxis Multiagent chemotherapy
Large cell lymphoma	Lymph nodes Cutaneous lesions Mediastinum Abdomen Head, neck			Large cell lymphoma As cited earlier, depending on site	
HODGKIN LYMPHOMA		0.4 per 100,000 children per year			
	Single lymph node or lymphatic chains Mediastinal mass Spleen		Genetic factors Familial predisposition Environmental influence Iatrogenic or acquired immunodeficiency (HIV, AT) Infectious etiology (Epstein-Barr virus)	Lymphadenopathy Organomegaly Fatigue Anorexia/weight loss/ fever	Splenectomy, if surgical staging Multiagent chemotherapy Radiation therapy
NEUROBLASTOMA		0.95 per 100,000 children per year			
	Anywhere along the sympathetic nervous system chain Most commonly Abdomen Adrenal gland Paraspinal ganglion Thorax Neck		Genetic factors Autosomal dominant inherited predisposition in some children Familial predisposition Associated with fetal alcohol syndrome and fetal hydantoin syndrome	Dependent on primary site, site of metastases Metastases present in 70% of cases at diagnosis (especially in bone marrow) Presence of a mass (abdomen, thoracic, cervical, pelvic, liver) Symptoms from compression of mass (Horner syndrome, edema of upper and lower extremities secondary to vascular compression, hypertension caused by compression of renal vasculature, cord compression symptoms [paresis, paralysis, bowel/ bladder dysfunction]) Diarrhea from vasoactive intestinal peptides produced by tumor cells Skin or subcutaneous nodules (infants only) Nonspecific symptoms (fever, weight loss, failure to thrive, generalized pain) Rarely syndrome of opsoclonus-myoclonus	Treatment of emergent symptoms Surgery (staging excision of tumor, evaluation of treatment) Radiation therapy Combination chemotherapy HSCT in some cases

Continued

TABLE 17-1

Common Pediatric Cancers—cont'd

Type	Site	Incidence (ages 0-14 yr)	Etiology	Signs/Symptoms	Treatment
SOFT TISSUE SARCOMAS		0.9 per 100,000 children per year	*For both sarcomas:* Genetic factors Associated with NF, LFS, Beckwith-Wiedemann syndrome Environmental factors Parental use of recreational drugs Possible viral etiology	*For both sarcomas:* Dependent on location and size of tumor	*For both sarcomas:* Surgical removal (if feasible) Radiation therapy for residual tumor Multiagent systemic chemotherapy
Rhabdomyosarcoma	Head and neck (most common)				
Undifferentiated sarcoma	Abdomen Anywhere in body				
KIDNEY		0.8 per 100,000 children per year			
Wilms tumor (nephroblastoma, renal embryoma)	Unilateral, bilateral		Genetic factors Associated with; aniridia, NF, Beckwith-Wiedemann syndrome, hemihypertrophy, Denys-Drash syndrome Familial predisposition Environmental factors Long-term chemical exposure (hydrocarbons/lead)	Asymptomatic mass Malaise, pain Microscopic or gross hematuria Hypertension	Complete surgical excision (if bilateral, nephrectomy of more involved site, excisional biopsy/partial nephrectomy of smaller lesion in remaining kidney) Multiagent chemotherapy Radiation therapy for high-risk tumors
BONE TUMORS		0.6 per 100,000 children per year			
Osteosarcoma	Long bones of extremities		Genetic factors Familial predisposition (hereditary retinoblastoma) Environmental factors Ionizing radiation Use of alkylating agents	Pain over involved area with or without swelling (often 3-6 mo or longer)	Multiagent chemotherapy Surgical excision of tumor with limb salvage or amputation putation if extent of disease or location does not allow complete excision
Ewing sarcoma	Bones of the extremities and central axis		Possible genetic factors No strong or consistent association with constitution of chromosomal abnormalities or congenital diseases	In presence of metastatic disease nonspecific symptoms (fatigue, anorexia, weight loss, intermittent fever, malaise)	Localized radiation therapy or surgical excision Multiagent chemotherapy
RETINOBLASTOMA		0.4 per 100,000 children per year			
	Eye		Genetic factors Gene mutation (nonhereditary) Autosomal dominant (all bilateral retinoblastomas and 15% of unilateral)	Leukokoria (cat's eye reflex) Squint Strabismus Orbital inflammation	Surgery (resection, enucleation with extensive disease; salvage of one eye attempted in bilateral disease) Radiation therapy Chemotherapy (usually palliative) Cryotherapy Laser photocoagulation

Data from Ries, L.A. et al. (Eds.). (2002). *Incidence data from SEER cancer statistics review, 1973-1999.* Bethesda, Md.: National Cancer Institute; Web site: http://seer.cancer.gov/csr/1973_1999/ except incidence for neuroblastoma and retinoblastoma from Ries, L.A. et al. (Eds.). (1999). *Cancer incidence and survival among children and adolescents: United States SEER Program 1975-1995.* NIH Pub. No. 99-4649. Bethesda, Md.: National Cancer Institute, SEER Program. Additional resources: Margolin, J.F., Steuber, C.P., & Poplack, D.G. (2002). Acute lymphoblastic leukemia. In P.A. Pizzo & D.G. Poplack (Eds.). *Principles and practice of pediatric oncology* (4th ed.). Philadelphia: Lippincott Williams & Wilkins, pp. 489-544; Golub, T.R. & Arceci, R.J. (2002). Acute myelogenous leukemia. In P.A. Pizzo & D.G. Poplack (Eds.). *Principles and practice of pediatric oncology* (4th ed.). Philadelphia: Lippincott Williams & Wilkins, pp. 545-589; Strother, D.R. et al. (2002). Tumors of the central nervous system. In P.A. Pizzo & D.G. Poplack (Eds.). *Principles and practice of pediatric oncology* (4th ed.). Philadelphia: Lippincott Williams & Wilkins, pp. 751-824; Magrath, I.T. (2002). Malignant non-Hodgkin's lymphomas in children. In P.A. Pizzo & D.G. Poplack (Eds.). *Principles and practice of pediatric oncology* (4th ed.). Philadelphia: Lippincott Williams & Wilkins, pp. 661-705; Hudson, M.M. & Donaldson, S.S. (2002). Hodgkin's disease. In P.A. Pizzo & D.G. Poplack (Eds.). *Principles and practice of pediatric oncology* (4th ed.). Philadelphia: Lippincott Williams & Wilkins, pp. 637-705; Brodeur, G.M. & Maris, J.M. (2002). Neuroblastoma. In P.A. Pizzo & D.G. Poplack (Eds.). *Principles and practice of pediatric oncology* (4th ed.). Philadelphia: Lippincott Williams & Wilkins, pp. 895-937; Wexler, L.H. Crist, W.M. & Helman, L.J. (2002). Rhabdomyosarcoma and the undifferentiated sarcomas. In P.A. Pizzo & D.G. Poplack (Eds.). *Principles and practice of pediatric oncology* (4th ed.). Philadelphia: Lippincott Williams & Wilkins, pp. 939-971; Grundy, P.E. et al. (2002). Renal tumors. In P.A. Pizzo & D.G. Poplack (Eds.). *Principles and practice of pediatric oncology* (4th ed.). Philadelphia: Lippincott Williams & Wilkins, pp. 865-893; Link, M.P., Gebhardt, M.C., & Meyers, P.A. (2002). Osteosarcoma. In P.A. Pizzo & D.G. Poplack (Eds.). *Principles and practice of pediatric oncology* (4th ed.). Philadelphia: Lippincott Williams & Wilkins, pp. 1051-1089; Ginsberg, J.P. et al. (2002). Ewing's sarcoma family of tumors: Ewing's sarcoma of bone and soft tissue and the peripheral primitive neuroectodermal tumors. In P.A. Pizzo & D.G. Poplack (Eds.). *Principles and practice of pediatric oncology* (4th ed.). Philadelphia: Lippincott Williams & Wilkins, pp. 973-1016; Hurwitz R.L., et al. (2002). Retinoblastoma. In P.A. Pizzo & D.G. Poplack (Eds.). *Principles and practice of pediatric oncology* (4th ed.). Philadelphia: Lippincott Williams & Wilkins, pp. 825-846.

Treatment

Surgery
  Biopsy
  Resection
  Palliation
Chemotherapy
Radiation
Hematopoietic stem cell transplantation
Immunotherapy

Academy of Pediatrics Section on Hematology/Oncology, 1997; Vietti & Steuber, 2002). Prompt referral to a pediatric cancer treatment center will allow a child or adolescent to be enrolled in multiinstitutional treatment studies.

Treatment

Cancer treatment involves the concurrent or sequential use of surgery, chemotherapy, radiation therapy, hematopoietic stem cell transplantation, and immunotherapy (Box 17-2). State-of-the-art treatment is provided by multiinstitutional cooperative study groups and some specialty cancer treatment centers. These centers generally employ a multidisciplinary approach combining the expertise of physicians, advanced practice nurses, social workers, art and child life therapists, and other specialists. More than 90% of children younger than 15 years with cancer in the United States are treated at institutions participating in National Cancer Institute (NCI) sponsored clinical trials (Bleyer, 2002). In the year 2000, the Children's Oncology Group (COG) was formed from a merger of four pediatric clinical trial cooperative groups (the Children's Cancer Group, the Pediatric Oncology Group, the National Wilms Tumor Study Group, and the Intergroup Rhabdomyosarcoma Study Group). Nurses have actively contributed to advancements in pediatric oncology through these cooperative groups (Ruccione & Kelly, 2000). Children under 15 years of age are equally represented in these groups regardless of race (Bleyer, 1997).

Only 20% of adolescents ages 15 to 19 years, however, are treated at institutions offering clinical trials sponsored by the NCI, and only 10% are registered in clinical trials (Bleyer, 2002). Adolescents' lack of equal access to national clinical trials requires further analysis of the effect on survival and quality of life. Although at times adolescents with cancer may be referred to adult oncologists, adolescents treated in pediatric clinical trials showed improved survival over those treated with adult treatment regimens (Stock, 2000).

A child's treatment protocol, determined by the type of cancer and the extent of disease, consists of a schedule and combination of therapies shown to be effective in treating the condition. A particular disease protocol may have several treatment regimens ("arms"), which are based on an accepted standard treatment with slight variations. Because no protocol regimen is known to be more effective than another, ongoing research investigates various therapies that maximize treatment efficacy while minimizing toxicity. Before a child is assigned to a particular protocol, informed consent is obtained from the parents and, if appropriate, the child. If a child is treated on a research protocol, the family may elect to withdraw the child from the study at any time and have the child treated according to standard therapy.

Surgical intervention is used to (1) obtain a biopsy specimen, (2) determine the extent of disease, (3) remove primary or metastatic lesions, (4) evaluate previously unresectable tumors, (5) provide a "second look" to evaluate the effects of chemotherapy and radiation on partially or nonresected tumors, and (6) relieve symptoms. Surgical procedures are also used to place indwelling venous access devices and to displace organs outside the radiation field (e.g., ovaries during pelvic irradiation).

The goal of chemotherapy is to interrupt the cell cycle of proliferating malignant cells while minimizing the damage to normal cells. In combination chemotherapy, different drugs are used to disrupt the cell cycle at different phases, which increases the exposure of the malignant cells to cytotoxic agents. The route of chemotherapy administration includes oral, intramuscular, intravenous, intrathecal, and intraventricular routes. Although most intravenous infusions have traditionally been administered in the hospital setting, certain agents lend themselves to safe administration in the home (NACHRI, 2000). Eligibility for home infusion often depends on stable utilities in the home, parental reliability, and few side effects during an in-hospital trial of the agent.

Chemotherapeutic agents may be either cycle phase specific or nonspecific. Cell cycle–specific drugs kill cells only in a certain stage of the cell's development and are most effective on rapidly growing cells. Along with malignant cells, the cells of the bone marrow, hair follicles, and intestinal epithelium are susceptible to damage from these drugs. Cell cycle–nonspecific drugs kill cells regardless of their stage of development. They act on dormant as well as dividing cells. Chemotherapeutic agents are further classified by their mechanism of action. The major classifications include alkylating agents, antimetabolites, vinca alkaloids, antibiotics, and corticosteroids. Side effects and toxicities vary depending on the specific agent (Table 17-2).

Radiation therapy is often used in conjunction with surgery and chemotherapy. Radiation causes breakage of DNA strands, thus inhibiting cell division. The goal of radiation therapy is to destroy the cancer cells while minimizing complications and long-term sequelae. External beam radiotherapy is the most common delivery method for radiation treatments. Radiation therapy may also be given by brachytherapy (radiation implants placed near the tumor). Generally the surgery is used to place the implants, but they may also be placed in body cavities, such as the vagina. The role of radiation therapy may be definitive, adjunctive, or palliative. Definitive treatment is given with curative intent to a tumor on which a biopsy has been performed or that has been partially resected. In adjunctive radiotherapy, a primary tumor—although totally resected—is at risk for a local recurrence. This area is then treated with a lower dose of radiation than what would be given to control the tumor without surgery. Palliative radiotherapy is used to relieve symptoms of incurable disease after more conservative methods have proved ineffective.

Text continued on p. 308

TABLE 17-2

Summary of Chemotherapeutic Agents Used in the Treatment of Childhood Cancers*

Agent/Administration	Side Effects and Toxicity	Comments and Specific Nursing Considerations
ALKYLATING AGENTS		
	All alkylating agents: Azoospermia, ovarian failure Secondary malignancy (AML)	Sperm banking, egg donation, if feasible
Mechlorethamine (nitrogen mustard, Mustargen) IV	N/V Myelosuppression Alopecia Local phlebitis Mucositis	Vesicant†
Cyclophosphamide (Cytoxan, CTX) PO, IV	N/V Myelosuppression Alopecia Hemorrhagic cystitis Stomatitis (rare) Cardiac toxicity (high dose) Pulmonary fibrosis (high dose) Syndrome of inappropriate secretion of antidiuretic hormone (SIADH)	Give dose early in day to allow adequate fluids afterward Force fluids before administering drug and for 2 days after to prevent chemical cystitis; encourage frequent voiding even during night Warn parents to report signs of burning on urination or hematuria Mesna given with high doses to protect bladder Mesna causes false ketonuria
Ifosfamide (IFEX) IV	N/V Myelosuppression Alopecia Renal tubular damage (Fanconi-like syndrome) Hemorrhagic cystitis Peripheral neuropathy Encephalopathy	See Cyclophosphamide above Mesna given with all doses to protect the bladder
Busulfan (Myleran) PO	N/V Myelosuppersion Excessive dryness of skin and mucous membranes Gynecomastia (rare) Pulmonary fibrosis (long-term therapy) Seizures at high doses	Pulmonary function tests
Melphalan (Alkeran, L-PAM) PO, IV	Myelosuppression N/V Mucositis Diarrhea Alopecia Hypersensitivity reaction Pulmonary fibrosis	Take PO on empty stomach Hydrate well for 24 hr after dose
Procarbazine (Matulane) PO	N/V Myelosuppression Lethargy Dermatitis Myalgia Arthralgia Stomatitis Neuropathy Alopecia Diarrhea Amenorrhea	CNS depressants (phenothiazines, barbiturates) enhance CNS symptoms Monoamine oxidase (MAO) inhibition sometimes occurs; therefore all other drugs are avoided unless medically approved; red wine, fava beans, broad bean pods, tea, coffee, cola, cheese, bananas are to be avoided Give medication in evening to reduce nausea
Dacarbazine (DTIC) IV	N/V Myelosuppression Alopecia Flulike syndrome Burning sensation in vein during infusion (not extravasation)	Vesicant (less sclerosive) Must be given cautiously in individuals with renal dysfunction Decrease IV rate or use cold pack on IV site to decrease burning

Data from Ettinger, A., Bond, A., & Sievers, T.D. (2002). Chemotherapy. In C.R. Baggott, K.P. Kelly, & D. Fochtman. (Eds.). *Nursing care of children and adolescents with cancer* (3rd ed.). Philadelphia: W.B. Saunders, pp. 133-176; Balis, F.M., Holcenberg, J.S., & Blaney, S.M. (2002). General principles of chemotherapy. In P.A. Pizzo & D.G. Poplack (Eds.). *Principles and practice of pediatric oncology* (4th ed.). Philadelphia: Lippincott Williams & Wilkins, pp. 237-308.
AML, Acute myelogenous leukemia; *N/V*, nausea and vomiting; *IV*, intravenously; *PO*, orally; *CNS*, central nervous system; *IM*, intramuscularly; *SC*, subcutaneously; *IT*, intrathecally; *PVC*, polyvinylchloride; *ECG*, electrocardiogram; *BUN*, blood urea nitrogen; *PT*, prothrombin time; *PTT*, partial thromboplastin time.
*Table includes principal drugs used in the treatment of childhood cancers. Other chemotherapeutic agents may be employed in treatment regimens.
†Vesicants (sclerosing agents) can cause severe cellular damage if even minute amounts of the drug infiltrate surrounding tissue. These drugs must be given through a free-flowing IV line. The infusion is stopped *immediately* if any sign of infiltration (pain, stinging, swelling, or redness at needle site) occurs. Additional interventions for extravasation vary.

TABLE 17-2

Summary of Chemotherapeutic Agents Used in the Treatment of Childhood Cancers—cont'd

Agent/Administration	Side Effects and Toxicity	Comments and Specific Nursing Considerations
ALKYLATING AGENTS—cont'd		
Carmustine (BCNU) IV	N/V Myelosuppression Burning pain along IV infusion (usually from alcohol diluent) Flushing and facial burning on pulmonary infiltration and/or fibrosis	Prevent extravasation; contact with skin causes brown spots Reduce IV burning by diluting drug and infusing slowly via IV drip Crosses blood-brain barrier Check pulmonary function tests
Lomustine (CCNU) PO	N/V Myelosuppression Pulmonary infiltrates and/or fibrosis (but more common with carmustine)	Oral form—give on empty stomach Crosses blood-brain barrier Check pulmonary function tests
ANTIMETABOLITES		
Cytarabine (Ara-C, Cytosar, cytosine arabinoside) IV, IM, SC, IT	N/V Myelosuppression Mucosal ulceration Hepatitis (usually subclinical) Conjunctivitis (high dose) Ara-C syndrome: fever, myalgia, malaise, rash 6-12 hr after administration Neurotoxicity with high doses	Crosses blood-brain barrier Use with caution in individuals with hepatic dysfunction Corticosteroid ophthalmic drops to prevent conjunctivitis
Mercaptopurine (6-MP, Purinethol) PO, IV	N/V Stomatitis Myelosuppression Dermatitis Elevated liver enzymes	6-MP is an analog of xanthine; therefore allopurinol (Zyloprim) delays its metabolism and increases its potency, necessitating a lower dose ($\frac{1}{3}$ to $\frac{1}{4}$) of 6-MP
Methotrexate (MTX, amethopterin) PO, IV, IM, SC IT; may be given in conventional doses (mg/m²) or high doses (g/m²)	N/V Diarrhea Mucosal ulceration (2-5 days later) Myelosuppression Dermatitis Photosensitivity Alopecia Hepatitis (fibrosis) Elevated liver enzymes Nephropathy Pneumonitis (fibrosis) Neurologic toxicity with high doses and IT use—arachnoiditis, leukoencephalopathy, seizures	Side effects and toxicity are dose related Potency and toxicity increased by reduced renal function, salicylates, sulfonamides; avoid use of aspirin and ibuprofen High-dose therapy 　Citrovorum factor (folinic acid or leucovorin) decreases cytotoxic action of MTX; used as an antidote for overdose and to enhance normal cell recovery following high-dose therapy; avoid use of vitamins containing folic acid during MTX therapy unless prescribed by physician IT therapy 　Drug *must* be mixed with preservative-free diluent 　Report signs of neurotoxicity immediately
Thioguanine (6-TG) PO	N/V Myelosuppression Stomatitis Dermatitis Liver dysfunction	Side effects unusual
5-Fluorouracil (5-FU, fluorouracil) IV	N/V Myelosuppression Dermatitis Stomatitis	Take at least 2 hr before or after food
PLANT ALKALOIDS		
Vincristine (Oncovin, VCR) IV	Neurotoxicity—paresthesia (numbness), ataxia, weakness, footdrop, hyporeflexia, constipation (adynamic ileus), hoarseness (vocal cord paralysis); abdominal, chest, and jaw pain	Vesicant Report signs of neurotoxicity because this may necessitate cessation of drug Individuals with underlying neurologic problems may be more prone to neurotoxicity

Continued

TABLE 17-2

Summary of Chemotherapeutic Agents Used in the Treatment of Childhood Cancers—cont'd

Agent/Administration	Side Effects and Toxicity	Comments and Specific Nursing Considerations
PLANT ALKALOIDS—cont'd		
Vincristine—cont'd	Fever Myelosuppression Alopecia SIADH	Monitor stool patterns closely; administer stool softener Excreted primarily by liver into biliary system; check bilirubin before administration
Irinotecan IV	Diarrhea Myelosuppression Diaphoresis Abdominal cramping N/V Alopecia Malaise Electrolyte abnormalities	Atropine or loperamide for treatment of diarrhea
Vinblastine (Velban) IV	Neurotoxicity (same as for vincristine but less severe) N/V (rare) Myelosuppression Alopecia	Same as for vincristine
Etoposide, (VP-16, Ve-Pesid) PO, IV	N/V Myelosuppression Alopecia Hypotension with rapid infusion Diarrhea May reactivate erythema of irradiated skin (rare) Allergic reaction with anaphylaxis possible Secondary malignancy (AML)	Give slowly via IV drip over at least 1 hr with child recumbent Have emergency drugs available at bedside[‡] Vital signs with blood pressure every 15 min during infusion
Teniposide (VM-26) IV	Myelosuppression Alopecia N/V Hypotension with rapid infusion Mild neurotoxicity Hypersensitivity reaction with anaphylaxis possible	Irritant Have emergency drugs available at bedside
Paclitaxel (Taxol) IV	Myelosuppression N/V during infusion "Stocking-glove" peripheral neuropathy Mucositis Bradycardia Alopecia	Monitor frequently Premedicate with corticosteroids and antihistamines Avoid PVC bags and tubing
ANTIBIOTICS		
Dactinomycin (actinomycin D, Cosmegen, ACT-D) IV	N/V Myelosuppression Mucosal ulceration Diarrhea Anorexia (may last few weeks) Alopecia Erythema or hyperpigmentation of previously irradiated skin Fever Malaise Hepatic (venooclusive disease)	Vesicant Enhances cytotoxic effects of radiation therapy but increases toxic effects May cause serious desquamation of irradiated tissue

Doxorubicin (Adriamycin, ADR), IV	N/V
	Stomatitis
	Myelosuppression
	Local phlebitis
	Alopecia
	Cumulative-dose toxicity includes:
	  Cardiac abnormalities
	  ECG changes
	  Heart failure
	Secondary malignancy (AML) when used in high doses with cyclophosphamide
		Vesicant (extravasation may *not* cause pain)
		Use only sterile distilled water as diluent
		Observe for any changes in heart rate or rhythm and signs of failure; follow echocardiogram or MUGA (multiple gated uptake) scan
		Recommended cumulative lifetime dose: 450 mg/m^2
		Warn parents that drug causes urine to turn red (for up to 12 days after administration); this is normal, not hematuria

‡Emergency drugs include oxygen and parenteral preparations of epinephrine 1:1000, diphenhydramine or similar antihistamine, aminophylline, corticosteroids, and vasopressors.

TABLE 17-2
Summary of Chemotherapeutic Agents Used in the Treatment of Childhood Cancers—cont'd

Agent/Administration	Side Effects and Toxicity	Comments and Specific Nursing Considerations
ANTIBIOTICS—cont'd		
Daunomycin (Cerubidine, daunorubicin) IV	Similar to doxorubicin	Similar to doxorubicin May tolerate slightly higher cumulative lifetime dose
Bleomycin (Blenoxane) IV, IM, SC	Allergic reaction—fever, chills, hypotension, anaphylaxis Fever (nonallergic) N/V Stomatitis Cumulative dose effects include: Skin—rash, hyperpigmentation, thickening, ulceration, peeling, nail changes, alopecia Lungs—pneumonitis with infiltrate that can progress to fatal fibrosis Raynaud syndrome	Should give test dose (IM) before therapeutic dose administered Have emergency drugs at bedside Hypersensitivity occurs with first one to two doses May give acetaminophen before drug to reduce likelihood of fever Concentration of drug in skin and lungs accounts for toxic effects Cumulative lifetime dose no >400 units Pulmonary function test as baseline and in follow-up
Idarubicin (Ida) IV	Similar to doxorubicin	Similar to doxorubicin
HORMONES		
Corticosteroids (prednisone, prednisolone, dexamethasone) Prednisone—PO Prednisolone—PO, IV Dexamethasone—PO, IV, IM	Moon face, mood changes, increased appetite, insomnia Immunosuppression Aseptic necrosis Pancreatitis Psychiatric disorders Amenorrhea Trunk obesity Muscle wasting and weakness Osteoporosis Poor wound healing Gastric bleeding Hypertension Diabetes mellitus Growth failure Acne	Explain expected effects, especially in terms of body image, increased appetite, and personality changes Monitor weight gain Recommend moderate salt restriction May need to disguise bitter taste (crush tablet and mix with syrup, jam, ice cream, or other high-flavored substance; use ice to numb tongue before administration; place tablet in gelatin capsule if child can swallow it) Observe for potential infection sites; usual inflammatory response and fever are absent Test stools for occult blood Monitor blood pressure Test blood for sugar and urine for acetone Observe for signs of abrupt steroid withdrawal: flulike symptoms, hypotension, hypoglycemia, shock
ENZYMES		
Asparaginase (L-ASP, Elspar) IM, IV	Allergic reactions (including anaphylactic shock) N/V Anorexia Weight loss Low fibrinogen levels Liver dysfunction Hyperglycemia (transient) Renal failure Pancreatitis Somnolence, lethargy	Have emergency drugs at bedside Record signs of allergic reaction (urticaria, facial edema, hypotension, abdominal cramps) Normally, BUN and ammonia levels rise as a result of drug—not evidence of liver damage Check urine for sugar and ketones; treat with insulin as needed Check PT, PTT, fibrinogen—may need fresh frozen plasma Check amylase levels
Pegasparaginase (Oncaspar) IM	See Asparaginase	See Asparaginase Lower incidence of hypersensitivity reaction than use of native asparaginase
OTHER AGENTS		
Cisplatin (Platinol) IV	Renal toxicity (severe) N/V Myelosuppression Ototoxicity Neurotoxicity (similar to that for vincristine) Nephrotoxicity-induced electrolyte disturbances, especially hypomagnesemia Anaphylactic reactions may occur	Renal function (creatinine clearance) must be assessed before giving drug Must maintain hydration before and during therapy (specific gravity of urine is used to assess hydration) Mannitol may be given IV to promote osmotic diuresis and drug clearance Monitor intake and output Monitor for signs of ototoxicity (e.g., ringing in ears) and neurotoxicity; report signs immediately; ensure that routine audiogram is done before treatment for baseline and routinely during treatment

Continued

TABLE 17-2

Summary of Chemotherapeutic Agents Used in the Treatment of Childhood Cancers—cont'd

Agent/Administration	Side Effects and Toxicity	Comments and Specific Nursing Considerations
OTHER AGENTS—cont'd		
Cisplatin—cont'd		Do not use aluminum needle; reaction with aluminum decreases potency of drug
		Monitor for signs of electrolyte loss (i.e., hypomagnesemia—tremors, spasm, muscle weakness, lower extremity cramps, irregular heartbeat, convulsions, delirium)
		Have emergency drugs at bedside
Carboplatin (Paraplatin) IV	N/V	As for cisplatin
	Myelosuppression	
	Ototoxicity (rare)	
	Neurotoxicity	
	Renal toxicity	
	Anaphylaxis	

Some children with CNS tumors have been treated with hyperfractionated radiation delivery. This method uses smaller individual doses of radiation two or more times daily instead of the usual daily dose to affect more of the rapidly dividing tumor cells. The total overall dosage of radiation used is higher. However, this method has failed to provide a treatment advantage compared with daily radiotherapy treatments (Mandell et al, 1999).

The tumor's response to radiation depends on the type of tumor, the type and dose of radiation delivered, and the size of the area irradiated. These factors also influence the type and severity of side effects and long-term sequelae. Many side effects are similar to those of chemotherapy, but, rather than a systemic response, the side effects are generally related to the irradiated area. They include nausea and vomiting, diarrhea, mucositis, cataracts, skin changes, neurocognitive deficits, and growth and endocrine abnormalities (Tarbell & Kooy, 2002).

The use of immunotherapy in the treatment of cancer is one of the newest available treatment modalities. It encompasses both cytokines (interleukins, interferons, tumor necrosis factor) and monoclonal antibodies. This therapy stimulates the body's natural immune system and has the potential to selectively target and destroy malignant cells. Immunotherapy has been more completely studied in adults and is currently being applied to children with cancer (Cheung & Rooney, 2002).

Hematopoietic stem cell transplantation is used in treating some cases of relapsed acute lymphocytic leukemia (ALL), acute myelogenous leukemia (AML), neuroblastoma, and lymphoma and is being investigated for use in recurrent Ewing sarcoma and brain tumors (see Chapter 15). Hematopoietic stem cells for transplantation come from bone marrow, peripheral blood, or umbilical cord blood (Gonzalez et al, 2002; Guinan et al, 2002). Donors of bone marrow or blood stem cells come from three sources: the affected person (autologous), an identical twin (syngeneic), or another histocompatible or incompatible donor (allogeneic). In some institutions, transplantation is the initial therapy of choice for children with high-risk (having clinical and laboratory features at diagnosis that are known to have a poor prognosis) ALL and AML. This procedure allows for potentially lethal doses of chemotherapy and radiation to be given to rid the body of all malignant cells. The donor's marrow or blood stem cells replace the child's destroyed marrow and after engraftment should produce the donor's nonmalignant functioning cells.

An autologous transplantation may be used when there is no available histocompatible donor, the tumor is not in the marrow, or the marrow can be purged of all tumor cells. However, allogeneic transplantation offers the benefit of graft-vs.-leukemia (GVL) effect, in which the immune cells of the donor attack any remaining leukemia cells (Golub & Arceci, 2002). In allogeneic transplantation, the donor is preferably a tissue-identical relative of the child, most often a sibling.

Hematopoietic cell transplantation is a promising treatment modality for certain malignancies in children. It must be realistically viewed, however, in terms of the potentially fatal toxicities, developmental sequelae, and psychosocial and financial effects on the child and family.

Complementary and Alternative Therapies

The category of complementary therapies encompasses a variety of interventions ranging from the use of herbs and dietary supplements in hopes to fight cancer to the use of relaxation techniques, guided imagery, hypnosis, art therapy, and play therapy in the control of symptoms such as pain and nausea (Rhodes & McDaniel, 2001; Sentivany-Collins, 2002).

Parents will often inquire about the use of herbs, special diets, or other dietary interventions to speed the recovery of the blood cell counts or combat the tumor. The majority of children with cancer are using some form of alternative therapy (Neuhouser et al, 2001). Any supplement or major dietary change should be viewed in terms of its potential to interact with chemotherapeutic agents. Recently a commonly used herbal preparation, St. John's wort, was found to interfere with the metabolism of the chemotherapeutic agent irinotecan (Mathijssen et al, 2002). Other drug interactions most likely exist, and further research on herbal preparations is needed. The primary care provider can acknowledge and support the parents' desire to help their child while providing access to information that puts the cost and potential benefits of such treatments in perspective.

Anticipated Advances in Diagnosis and Management

Oncology is a constantly evolving field. Breakthroughs in all types of therapy occur on a daily basis. Although many new therapies are developed, only a small fraction of these treatments become frontline therapy.

Immunotherapy continues to show promise in the treatment of childhood cancer. Types of immunotherapy include monoclonal antibodies (MoAbs), cancer vaccines, and cytokines. MoAbs are hybrid cells made from the fusion of B cells from mice to cancer cells. These MoAbs are most effective in children with minimal residual disease after initial surgery, chemotherapy, and/or radiation therapy. MoAbs are used alone ("naked antibodies") or as conjugates with toxins (immunotoxins), or they may be radiolabeled (often with radioactive iodine as the isotope). Examples of MoAbs include anti-G_{D2} in the treatment of neuroblastoma and rituximab in the treatment of lymphoma (Cheung & Rooney, 2002). Immunotherapy remains investigational rather than frontline therapy.

Most new chemotherapeutic drugs currently arise from the study of molecular biology, often referred to as "targeted therapy." Scientists are examining the molecular defects in cancer cells and how cancer cells differ from normal cells in order to design treatment aimed at these defects (Stephenson, 2002). In particular, scientists are studying pathways that cause malignant transformation or progression of the tumor, such as angiogenesis (blood vessel formation), apoptosis (programmed cell death), cell cycle regulation, receptor signaling, cellular proliferation, and cellular differentiation. Research into methods to block oncogenes (genes that promote tumor progression) and to repair mutations in tumor suppressor genes (genes that inhibit tumor growth) may also lead to effective cancer therapies (Ivy et al, 2002).

Gleevac (STI-571) is a well-publicized new drug in the targeted therapy category. It inhibits tyrosine kinase, a compound found to be important in the malignant transformation of cells, particularly in chronic myelogenous leukemia. The drug may also be effective against high-grade gliomas, neuroblastomas, and types of rhabdomyosarcoma and osteosarcoma because of an alternate pathway (Ivy et al, 2002).

Overexpression of human epidermal growth factor receptor 2 (HER2) is associated with a poor prognosis for individuals with osteosarcoma. Trastuzumab (Herceptin) is an antibody against the HER2 receptor and is being studied in certain people with osteosarcoma (Link et al, 2002).

Many cancer therapies fail because of the development of drug resistance in the cancer cells. The initial agents used to prevent the development of drug resistance, such as verapamil and cyclosporine, have been generally ineffective. However, the study of other methods to block drug resistance is underway (Balis et al, 2002).

A few drugs are being revisited for cancer therapy. Investigations of thalidomide are underway, with use as an antiangiogenic agent (therapy that blocks new blood vessel formation). By blocking the formation of new blood vessels, solid tumor growth could be limited to a maximum of a few millimeters (Thiele & Kastan, 2002). However, careful study is needed when using these agents in growing children with concern about reducing the blood supply to normal tissues (Ivy et al, 2002). There are many other antiangiogenic drugs in development. Arsenic, a well-known poison that was historically used to treat syphilis, is now being used to treat acute promyelocytic leukemia (Higgins & Brown, 2002).

The development of fast and powerful computers along with accurate imaging software supports the delivery of radiotherapy to precise fields. Stereotactic radiosurgery (using a single, highly focused dose of radiation) is an option for some children, particularly to boost a small residual tumor or as treatment for recurrent disease in a person previously irradiated (Tarbell & Kooy, 2002). Treatment with a new stereotactic radiation machine, the Cyberknife, is under investigation (Quinn, 2002). Intensity modulated radiation therapy is a new technique using many fields of radiation treatment, each with varying degrees of intensity. This therapy contrasts with conventional radiation therapy that uses only a few fields each with a fixed intensity (Tarbell & Kooy, 2002).

Advances in hematopoietic stem cell transplantation include the type of conditioning regimen and sources for stem cells. Nonmyeloablative transplants are being performed in select situations in which the recipient's immune system and marrow cells are only partially destroyed. In another type of transplant, haploidentical marrow or peripheral stem cell donors are used (three out of six antigens match). The most common donor in this situation is the child's parent (Gross et al, 2001).

Robotics is an emerging field in surgery. In oncology, robotic techniques can provide greater precision than standard surgical procedures and have been used to obtain biopsy specimens of areas difficult to access in the brain (Cleary & Nguyen, 2001). With modem access, the surgeon can be located many miles away. This treatment may allow children in remote areas, who may be critically ill, to have surgery performed by experts in the field, without the burden of travel.

Advances are also being made in supportive care. Agents are used to mitigate the toxic effects of chemotherapy. These drugs include dexrazoxane, to minimize the cardiotoxic effects of anthracyclines, and amifostine, to minimize the myelotoxicity, nephrotoxicity, and mucositis associated with chemotherapy and radiotherapy (Hensley et al, 1999). A new formulation of granulocyte colony-stimulating factor (G-CSF) is now approved for use. This agent, peg-filgrastim, promotes an increase in the white blood cells following chemotherapy, as does standard G-CSF. However, peg-filgrastim is given as one injection following treatment as opposed to daily injections with standard G-CSF (Holmes et al, 2002).

Advances in Knowledge of Genetic Etiology or Treatment

With microarray technology, scientists are studying the expression of individual genes in relationship to the entire genetic makeup of the cell. This technology aids researchers in further classifying tumors, tailoring therapy to improve the treatment of children with cancer and predicting survival (Raetz et al, 2001). Three types of strategies are being used to counteract cancer based on the genetic changes in the cells. These strategies are genetic manipulation (gene therapy), viral oncolysis (killing cancer cells with certain genetically driven viruses), and immunotherapy (as previously described) (Cripe & Mackall, 2001).

Associated Problems (Box 17-3)
Vascular Access

Children receiving prolonged, intensive treatment are required to endure frequent venipunctures for laboratory tests and the administration of chemotherapy, blood products, antibiotic therapy, and nutritional support. These children are often aided by the placement of a long-term indwelling central venous access device (VAD), which helps minimize the trauma of frequent needle sticks and vein irritation from the chemotherapy. Access devices include tunneled catheters and subcutaneous implanted ports.

Tunneled catheters are single-, double-, or triple-lumen silicone catheters with a Dacron felt cuff that anchors the catheter under the skin and provides a barrier to infection. Tunneled catheters have an internal and external portion, whereas subcutaneous ports are totally implanted below the skin with the catheter tip at the junction of the superior vena cava and the right atrium. Venous access is achieved by puncturing the skin above the reservoir and passing a specially designed needle through the silicone membrane into the port receptacle (Bagnall-Reeb & Perry, 2002). Topical anesthetics may be applied to port sites before accessing to reduce discomfort and fear.

The patency of all long-term VADs is maintained through periodic flushing with heparinized saline. Care of these lines is taught to the child (when appropriate) and parents. Complica-tions of indwelling VADs include infection, occlusion of the catheter from thrombus and fibrin formation, damage to the external portion of the catheter, and rarely, cardiac tamponade (Bagnall-Reeb & Perry, 2002; Shamberger et al, 2002).

Because a child with cancer is at risk for profound neutropenia as a result of therapy, prompt and aggressive treatment of infection at the catheter site is necessary. Most exit site infections can be cleared with oral and topical antibiotics in the nonneutropenic child; but tunnel infections, septicemia, or any catheter-related infection in the neutropenic child requires intravenous antibiotics and possible catheter removal (Bagnall-Reeb & Perry, 2002).

Therapy-Related Complications

Nausea and Vomiting. Nausea and vomiting are common side effects of chemotherapy and radiation. Nausea and vomiting can have profound physiologic and psychologic effects on the child receiving therapy (Panzarella et al, 2002). Problems, including dehydration, chemical and electrolyte imbalances, and decreased nutritional intake, can lead to decreased compliance or termination of treatment.

The mechanisms involved in nausea and vomiting are complex, and no single drug will consistently control these side effects. The situation is further complicated by the wide variation in response of the individual child to both the chemotherapeutic agent and the antiemetic. The antiemetic should be given before nausea and vomiting occur and should be continued until the symptoms have resolved. Nausea and vomiting related to the chemotherapy generally will not last longer than 48 hours after chemotherapy administration.

Serotonin antagonists have a significant role in the management of nausea and vomiting in children. Ondansetron (Zofran) and granisetron (Kytril) inhibit the binding of serotonin to receptors in both the CNS and the gastrointestinal system. These medications do not cause drowsiness and rarely cause extrapyramidal side effects (Culy et al, 2001). Adjunctive methods such as progressive relaxation and guided imagery have had some positive effects when combined with antiemetic medications (Rhodes & McDaniel, 2001).

Anorexia and Weight Loss. During therapy, anorexia and weight loss are common and can be attributed to both the disease and its treatment. The psychologic impact of cancer and the tumor's metabolic influence can contribute to weight loss. Treatment-induced nausea and vomiting, as well as changes in taste acuity, may lead to food aversion. Therefore the child's weight must be closely monitored throughout treatment. Oral supplements and, in some cases, nasogastric or gastrostomy feedings or hyperalimentation may be necessary (DeSwarte-Wallace et al, 2001; Panzarella et al, 2002).

Bone Marrow Suppression. Bone marrow suppression is another side effect of chemotherapy and radiation. Leukopenia, thrombocytopenia, and anemia usually begin within 7 to 10 days after drug administration, with the nadir (i.e., the point at which the blood cell counts are the lowest) occurring at approximately 14 days. The marrow then recovers by 21 to 28 days. The exact time of the nadir varies depending on the specific chemotherapeutic agent. Close monitoring is necessary to determine the extent of marrow suppression.

BOX 17-3
Associated Problems

Vascular access: most children require the use of indwelling central VADs
All lumens must be cultured if any fever
SBE prophylaxis for dental procedures
Nausea and vomiting: use antiemetics before and after chemotherapeutic administration, NOT on an "as needed" (i.e., prn) basis
Anorexia and weight loss: monitor weight regularly, early intervention
Bone marrow suppression:
Hemoglobin <7 to 8 g/dl, consider transfusion
Platelets <10,000 to 20,000 mm³ consider transfusion
ANC <500, high risk for infection. Possible use of erythropoietins for treatment of anemia and G-CSF or GM-CSF for neutropenia
Infection: blood cultures for all fevers
IV antibiotics for fever and neutropenia or for any child with an implanted central venous access device
Alopecia
Late effects: see Table 17-3

VAD, Venous access device; *SBE*, subacute bacterial Endocarditis; *ANC*, absolute neutrophil count; *G-CSF*, granulocyte colony-stimulating factor; *GM-CSF*, granulocyte-macrophage colony-stimulating factor.

Calculation of Absolute Neutrophil Count (ANC)

White blood count (WBC) = 7400 (also expressed as 7.4 K/µl; 7.4 × 10³/mm³)

Neutrophils (poly, segs) = 40%

Nonsegmented neutrophils (bands) = 12%

Step 1: Determine total percent neutrophils (poly. segs + bands)

$$40\% + 12\% = 52\%(0.52)$$

Step 2: Multiply WBC by % neutrophils

ANC = 7400 × 0.52

ANC = 3848 (normal)

WBC = 900 (0.9 k/UL; 0.9 × 10³/mm³)

Neutrophils (poly, segs) = 7%

Nonsegmented neutrophils (bands) = 7%

Step 1: 7% + 7% = 14% (0.14)

Step 2: ANC = 900 × 0.14

ANC = 126/mm³ (severely neutropenic)

Leukopenia refers to the presence of a low number of all white blood cells (WBCs), whereas neutropenia refers specifically to a low neutrophil cell count. Neutrophils are the body's main defense against bacterial infection. It is necessary to determine the absolute neutrophil count (ANC) (Box 17-4) because the incidence and severity of infection are inversely related to the child's ANC. Infections are a major life-threatening complication of cancer and its treatment (Alexander et al, 2002; Groll et al, 2001).

Several precautions can be taken to reduce the risk of infection. Good hand-washing techniques by the child, the parents, and the caregivers are paramount to reducing the spread of pathogens. Good personal hygiene by the child, which includes thorough dental care, is also important. A child with neutropenia should avoid individuals who are ill, crowded situations, and anyone with a communicable disease, especially chickenpox. Rectal temperatures and suppositories should also be avoided because abrading the rectal mucosa increases the risk of introducing bacteria into the bloodstream.

Guidelines for transfusion are based on laboratory parameters and clinical symptoms. The child who is thrombocytopenic may require transfusions of platelets because of the risk of serious hemorrhage. Transfusion is recommended if the platelet count is less than 10,000 to 20,000/mm³ and/or in the presence of bleeding. In a child whose hemoglobin level is less than 7 to 8 g/dl and/or who is symptomatic (e.g., shortness of breath, headache, dizziness), a transfusion is usually indicated (Benjamin & Anderson, 2002; Rossetto & McMahon, 2000).

To reduce the risk of transfusion-acquired infections and graft-vs.-host (GVH) reactions, blood products should be cytomegalovirus (CMV) seronegative, irradiated, and leukocyte depleted for CMV-negative individuals. Granulocyte and granulocyte-macrophage colony-stimulating factors (G-CSFs/GM-CSFs) may be used in high-risk children to reduce the severity and duration of neutropenia (Crawford & Lee, 2000).

Hair Loss. A distinguishing therapy-related complication is alopecia. It is generally a temporary condition that results from damage to the hair follicles by chemotherapy and radiation. Although the hair usually regrows after therapy, the texture and color may be slightly different. Cutting the child's hair into a shorter style may help to reduce some distress when the hair begins to fall out. Younger children and some adolescents prefer to cover their heads with colorful hats, baseball caps, and scarves. Adolescent girls are more likely to consider the use of wigs.

Late Effects

As survival rates continually improve, the long-term effects of therapy are becoming evident. The goal of therapy is not merely improving survival but also reducing physiologic and developmental morbidity. A growing body of knowledge indicates that both chemotherapy and radiation have adverse effects on normal tissues that may not be manifested for months or years after therapy. The development of second malignancies, impaired growth, diminished cognitive functioning, and organ damage are the areas of greatest concern. Factors that appear to influence the development of late effects include the child's age and stage of development at the time of diagnosis, the primary tumor and extent of involvement, and the therapy used (Richardson et al, 1999; Ward, 2000). Although the majority of survivors of childhood cancer in a large study did not demonstrate symptoms of depression or somatic distress, the survivors were more likely than their healthy siblings to demonstrate such symptoms (Zebrack et al, 2002).

Secondary malignant neoplasms (SMNs) are found with greater frequency in children with a genetic predisposition based on the primary tumor or as a result of chemotherapy and radiation therapy. The highest rate of SMNs occurs in children with hereditary retinoblastoma (Moll et al, 2001). There may also be an increased risk of SMN in persons with the genetic forms of Wilms tumor (bilateral), neuroblastoma, and other embryonal tumors. In children with Hodgkin disease treated with radiation and chemotherapy, there is an increased incidence of SMN—especially AML and solid tumors, including breast cancer (Neglia et al, 2001). Treatment with alkylating agents and etoposide increases the risk of AML. Concurrent use of dose-intensive anthracyclines with cyclophosphamide has been associated with an increased risk of SMN (Neglia et al, 2001).

Children receiving treatment directly to the CNS are at risk for negative neurologic and intellectual sequelae. Neurotoxicity is related to the number and sequence of treatment modalities used. The impact of late effects on the various organ systems is described in Table 17-3.

Relapse

Despite the advances in treatment of childhood cancer, some children will experience a relapse of their disease. Relapse, like diagnosis, is a crisis period for the family. It poses a challenge for the oncology team because the best methods of treatment were used at diagnosis. Relapse often requires more

Text Continued on p. 316

TABLE 17-3

Late Effects of Antineoplastic Therapy on Body Systems

Body System	Adverse Effects	Causative Agent	Time Interval	Signs and Symptoms	Predisposing Factors	Preventive/Diagnostic Measures
Cardiovascular system	Cardiomyopathy	Anthracycline chemotherapy	Weeks to years after therapy	Abrupt onset of congestive heart failure; tachycardia; tachypnea; edema; hepatomegaly; cardiomegaly; gallop rhythms; pleural effusions; dyspnea	Increased risk with age <15 yr and females	Careful monitoring with chest radiograph, ECG, echocardiogram, MUGA scan
		Cyclophosphamide (high dose)			Anthracycline therapy; especially lifetime cumulative dose of ≥550 mg/m²	Observation for shortness of breath, exercise intolerance, weight gain, edema
		Irradiation of mediastinum			Stresses such as growth hormone use; cocaine or excessive alcohol use; pregnancy, labor and delivery; anesthesia; isometric exercising such as heavy weight lifting	Partial shielding of mediastinum. Close monitoring of pregnant females, particularly immediately postpartum. Use of cardioprotectant drug, ICRF-187 (dexrazoxane) with anthracyclines under investigation. Referral to cardiologist
	Chronic constrictive pericarditis	Mediastinal irradiation	Few months to years	Chest pain; dyspnea; fever; paradoxic pulse; venous distention; friction rub; Kussmaul sign	Most common with doses of 40-60 Gy	Partial shielding of mediastinum. Referral to cardiologist
	Premature coronary artery disease	Mediastinal or spinal irradiation	Years after therapy	Chest pain with exertion; exercise intolerance; chest pressure; arm pain; heartburn, nausea, or fatigue	Sedentary lifestyle; high-fat diet	Promote healthy lifestyle with moderate aerobic exercise and diet low in fat and salt. Close monitoring with ECG, lipid panel
Pulmonary system	Pneumonitis followed by pulmonary fibrosis	Pulmonary irradiation	Months to years after treatment	Dyspnea; decreased exercise tolerance; pulmonary insufficiency	Increased risk with: • Large lung volume in radiation field • Therapy during periods of pulmonary infection • Use of radiation sensitizing chemotherapy • Doses >40 Gy	Careful monitoring of status with physical examination; chest radiograph; pulmonary function tests
		Bleomycin, carmustine, high-dose cyclophosphamide, busulfan,			Subsequent delivery of high levels of oxygen (as with anesthesia) may exacerbate lung injury	Yearly influenza vaccine. Pneurmovax. Avoid smoking. Encourage frequent rest periods. High-dose steroids for severe cases. Careful use of oxygen therapy after busulfan and bleomycin therapy

Data from Late effects of childhood cancer and its treatment. Dreyer, Z.E., Blatt, J., & Bleyer, A. (2002). In P.A. Pizzo & D.G. Poplack (Eds.). *Principles and practice of pediatric oncology* (4th ed.). Philadelphia: Lippincott Williams & Wilkins, pp. 1431-1461; Hobbie, W. et al. (2002). Care of survivors. In C.R. Baggott, K.P. Kelly, & D. Fochtman (Eds.). *Nursing care of children and adolescents with cancer* (3rd ed.). Philadelphia: W.B. Saunders, pp. 426-464.
ECG, electrocardiogram; *MUGA*, multiple gated acquisition; *WBC*, white blood cell; *IV*, intravenous; *AST*, aspartate transaminase; *ALT*, alanine transaminase; *PCR*, polymerase chain reaction; *RNA*, ribonucleic acid; *CBC*, complete blood count; *BUN*, blood urea nitrogen; T_3, triiodothyronine; T_4, thyroxine; *TSH*, thyroid-stimulating hormone; *LH*, luteinizing hormone; *FSH*, follicle-stimulating hormone; *IT*, intrathecal; *CT*, computed tomography; *MRI*, magnetic resonance imaging; *CNS*, central nervous system; *AML*, acute myelocytic leukemia.

TABLE 17-3

Late Effects of Antineoplastic Therapy on Body Systems

Body System	Adverse Effects	Causative Agent	Time Interval	Signs and Symptoms	Predisposing Factors	Preventive/Diagnostic Measures
Hematopoietic system	Long-term suppression of marrow function	Extensive irradiation of marrow-containing bones Chemotherapy	Months to years following therapy	Fall in WBC and platelet counts; hypoplastic/aplastic bone marrow aspirates; diminished uptake of radioisotopes	Radiation doses; 30-50 Gy in older individuals Concomitant use of chemotherapy	Limitation of areas of marrow irradiated Monitoring of child's status with periodic bone marrow aspirates and peripheral blood cell counts
	Alterations in immune system	Nodal irradiation affects cellular immunity Splenectomy or splenic irradiation affects humoral immunity	Weeks to years following therapy	Predisposition to infection	Adolescents more at risk than younger children	Pneumococcal vaccine and penicillin if splenectomy done Monitoring of child's status with periodic blood counts and tests of immune response
Gastrointestinal system	Hepatic fibrosis-cirrhosis	Chemotherapy	Months to years following therapy	Persistent elevation of liver function tests after cessation of therapy; hepatomegaly; cirrhosis; jaundice; spider nevi	Daily low doses of methotrexate by mouth for long periods Long-term use of mercaptopurine	Monitor child's status with liver function tests Perform liver biopsy if liver function test results remain persistently abnormal
	Chronic enteritis	Radiation therapy	Months to years following therapy	Pain; recurrent vomiting; diarrhea; malabsorption syndrome, weight loss	Radiation doses >50 Gy Children with previous abdominal surgery Chemotherapy as radiation sensitizers (actinomycin, doxorubicin)	Avoid concomitant use of radiation sensitizers Careful monitoring of height and weight Supportive therapy when symptoms develop, including low-residue, low-fat, gluten- and milk-free diet
	Hepatitis C infection	Blood transfusion before 1993	Months to years	Most patients asymptomatic	Other risk factors: IV drug use, sexual promiscuity, tatooing	Screen all recipients of transfusion before 1993 with AST/ALT and hepatitis C antibody; if positive, (or negative with elevated ALT) monitor PCR-based RNA screen for hepatitis C and refer to gastroenterologist
Kidney and urinary tract	Nephritis-glomerular and/or tubular dysfunction	Radiation to renal structures (20-30 Gy)—may be enhanced by chemotherapy	Weeks to years after therapy	Decrease in renal function with elevated BUN and creatinine; proteinuria; anemia; hypertension; may have urinary wasting of magnesium, potassium, and calcium with cisplatin	Other nephrotoxic drugs (aminoglycosides, vancomycin, amphotericin, cyclosporine)	Periodically monitor renal status during and after therapy with blood pressure readings, urinalysis, CBC, BUN, and creatinine
		Ciplatin, ifosfamide, lomustine, carmustine, methotrexate (high doses)			Inadequate alkalinization of urine before methotrexate Urinary tract infections	Once progressive renal failure develops, treatment is supportive Electrotype supplementation as needed

Continued

TABLE 17-3
Late Effects of Antineoplastic Therapy on Body Systems

Body System	Adverse Effects	Causative Agent	Time Interval	Signs and Symptoms	Predisposing Factors	Preventive/Diagnostic Measures
Kidney and urinary tract—cont'd						Child should avoid rough contact sports after nephrectomy to protect remaining kidney
	Renal Fanconi syndrome	Ifosfamide	Weeks to years after therapy	Urinary wasting of phosphorus, glucose, proteins and inability to acidify urine; can lead to renal rickets with inhibition of growth and bone deformity	Age <3 yr at time of treatment, prior renal dysfunction, nephrectomy	Periodically monitor renal status during and after therapy with urinalysis and electrolytes and phosphorus Electrolyte supplementation as needed
	Chronic hemorrhagic cystitis	Cyclophosphamide, ifosfamide Radiation therapy	Months to years after treatment	Sterile, painful hematuria; urinary frequency	Inadequate hydration during cyclophosphamide or ifosfamide therapy	Techniques to reduce bladder exposure during radiation therapy Frequent emptying of bladder during and 24 hr after therapy Adequate hydration before, during, and after therapy Concomitant use of mesna with chemotherapy Treatment of bladder hemorrhage with formalin instillation or cauterization of bleeding sites
Musculoskeletal system	Impaired skeletal growth	Irradiation of skeletal structures and abdomen	Months to years following treatment	Growth retardation, reduction in sitting height, scoliosis, altered growth of facial skeleton	Effect of spinal irradiation to vertebral bodies in doses 10-20 Gy dependent on age of child; known damage >20 Gy Unilateral radiation results in asymmetric deformities Symmetric growth delay during periods of chemotherapy	Careful monitoring of child's status with growth charts, radiographic studies, sitting and standing height Dose radiation reduction during periods of rapid growth
	Delayed or arrested tooth development	Irradiation of maxilla or mandible Chemotherapy	Months to years	Teeth are small with pale enamel; malocclusion	Radiation during period of dental growth and development	Dental examinations every 6 mo Good oral hygiene including flossing Fluoride prophylaxis
	Avascular necrosis (AVN) and osteoporosis	Radiation Steroids (particularly dexamethasone) Methotrexate (usually resolves at end of therapy)	Months to years	AVN—joint pain often accompanied by slipped capital epiphysis of femoral head Osteoporosis—bone fractures	Poor calcium intake Increased body weight	Encourage calcium intake and low impact exercise as preventive measures DEXA scan for osteoporosis Referral to orthopedics

TABLE 17-3

Late Effects of Antineoplastic Therapy on Body Systems—cont'd

Body System	Adverse Effects	Causative Agent	Time Interval	Signs and Symptoms	Predisposing Factors	Preventive/Diagnostic Measures
Endocrine system	Thyroid gland dysfunction	Irradiation of thyroid gland, brain, and total body irradiation	Months to years	Hypothyroidism; may be asymptomatic and have abnormal thyroid function; nodular abnormalities	Reported with varying radiation doses: 25-70 Gy	Monitor thyroid function with T_3, free T_4, and TSH Hormonal replacement therapy for all children with abnormal thyroid tests since elevated TSH is associated with thyroid cancer
	Injuries to gonads	Irradiation of gonads Chemotherapy (alkylating agents)	Months to years	Infertility; sterility, hormonal monal dysfunction, azoospermia, teratogenic during first trimester of pregnancy	Testicular radiation; ovarian radiation Chemotherapy damage dependent on drug used, dose, duration of therapy, child's gender, and age	Tanner staging yearly Protection of testes/ovaries from radiation field Gonadal dysfunction from chemotherapy may be reversible Males (14 yr old): check LH, FSH, testosterone levels Females (12 yr old): check LH, FSH, estradiol levels
	Decreased growth rate	Irradiation of cranium and/or spine Total body irradiation Chemotherapy	Months to years	Reduction in height percentile or growth rate	Radiation therapy at younger age and dose of ≥30 Gy to brain Spinal irradiation at >35 Gy Total body irradiation at >10 Gy	After completion of therapy, check standing and sitting heights 1-2 times each year Thyroid function tests, bone age, and growth hormone testing to be considered if growth rate declines
Nervous system	Peripheral sensory or motor neuropathies	Irradiation of peripheral nerves; chemotherapy (vincristine, etoposide, cisplatin)	Months to years	Deficit in function Pain Decreased tendon reflexes	Radiation doses: 55-120 Gy Chemotherapy with vinca alkaloids	Careful monitoring of child's status during and after therapy Vinca alkaloid damage may be diminished or reversed by reducing or withholding therapy
	Central neuroendocrine dysfunction of hypothalamic pituitary axis	Cranial irradiation; chemotherapy	Months to years	Growth hormone deficiency Panhypopituitarism with short stature; hypothyroidism; Addison disease	Dependent on dose of radiation, age of child, and concomitant use of chemotherapy Younger children who receive >24 Gy at greatest risk	Careful monitoring of child's status with growth charts, Tanner staging, bone age at 9 yr then yearly to puberty Thyroid, hormone, insulin, and cortisol measurement may be necessary Treatment with replacement of deficient hormones
	Encephalopathy	Cranial irradiation; chemotherapy, particularly IV methotrexate (high dose) and IT methotrexate	Months to years	May be asymptomatic but demonstrate abnormalities on head CT scans May have overt symptoms ranging from lethargy to somnolence, dementia, seizures, paralysis, and coma	Cranial radiation alone or with concomitant chemotherapy Frequency increased with chemotherapy Less damage with cranial radiation <18 Gy Younger children more vulnerable	Monitor child's status with careful physical examination, head MRI/CT scans, psychometric testing Reduce chemotherapy dose when preclinical radiographic findings appear

Continued

TABLE 17-3

Late Effects of Antineoplastic Therapy on Body Systems—cont'd

Body System	Adverse Effects	Causative Agent	Time Interval	Signs and Symptoms	Predisposing Factors	Preventive/Diagnostic Measures
Nervous system—cont'd	Intelligence deficits and/or neuropsychologic dysfunctions	Radiation therapy, chemotherapy	Months to years	Abnormal psychologic tests with deficits in perceptual behavior, language development, and learning abilities Personality changes	More common in younger children, those who received cranial irradiation >18 Gy and concomitant chemotherapy Damage may occur in all individuals prophylactic or therapeutic cranial radiation and/or chemotherapy	Careful monitoring with periodic neurocognitive/psychologic evaluations Early intervention with multidisciplinary approach and specialized education programs
Secondary malignancy (multiple systems)	Leukemia, especially AML	Alkylating agents Doxorubicin Etoposide	Years	Leukopenia Anemia Thrombocytopenia Fever Bone pain	Hodgkin disease as primary malignancy	Monitor CBC
	Thyroid cancer	Irradiation of mediastinum, spine, head, or neck		Palpable mass/nodule Anterior cervical adenopathy	Younger age at time of radiation therapy	If thyroid nodule present obtain thyroid scintiscan, tests of thyroid function Biopsy or bone needle aspiration of nodule or node
	Breast cancer	Irradiation of mediastinum, spine, or chest wall		Palpable mass	More common with >20 Gy mantle area Genetic form of Wilms tumor or Hodgkin disease as primary malignancy	Teach adolescents to do breast self-examination Consider baseline mammogram in early 20s May consider chemoprevention for Hodgkin survivors in the future
	Bone and soft tissue tumors	Irradiation of bone or soft tissue		Mass Pain	Retinoblastoma as primary malignancy especially if treated with radiation or bilateral	

experimental modes of treatment. The primary care provider in cooperation with the oncology team can support the family—and especially the child—through this difficult time.

Death

There may come a time when all possible viable treatment options have been exhausted. The care of the child moves from focusing on a cure to providing comfort and as much quality time as possible. The collaboration between the primary care provider and the oncology team can be invaluable during this time. Families often seek guidance and support in making decisions that they can live with long after the child's death. Knowledge of the community- and hospital-based hospice programs in their area can be beneficial in meeting many of the home care and support needs of families. All families need reassurance that they will not be abandoned at this time and that multidisciplinary resources will be made available to them as required.

Prognosis

The prognosis of a malignancy depends on the age of the child, primary site, extent of the disease, and cell type. In the 1960s the overall cure rate for pediatric malignancies was 28% (Landis et al, 1998). Over the past 20 years dramatic advances have been made in the treatment and potential cure of children with cancer (Table 17-4). The current figures estimate an overall 5-year disease-free survival of 72% for pediatric cancers in general (Ries et al, 2002).

PRIMARY CARE MANAGEMENT

Health Care Maintenance

Growth and Development

Although growth retardation secondary to chemotherapy often resolves when therapy is complete, it may persist for some

TABLE 17-4

Relative 5-Yr Survival Rates (%) of Children (0-14 Yr) with Malignant Disease

Site	Year of Diagnosis						
	1974-1976	1977-1979	1980-1982	1983-1985	1986-1988	1989-1991	1992-1998
All sites	55.8	61.5	65.1	67.7	70.2	73.3	77.2*
Bone and joint	54.6†	52.2†	54.6†	56.6	63.4†	61.8	72.5*
Brain and central nervous system (CNS)	54.8	56.1	55.5	61.7	63.0	62.1	69.9*
Hodgkin disease	78.3	83.5	91.0	89.6	89.9	94.0	93.5*
Acute lymphocytic leukemia	53.2	67.1	71.1	69.1	78.1	80.3	85.3*
Acute myelocytic leukemia	14.4	27.4†	24.3†	28.5†	30.2†	35.2†	46.4*
Neuroblastoma	52.6	53.1	52.5	55.0	59.3	67.9	68.6*
Non-Hodgkin lymphoma	44.3	50.2	61.5	70.9	69.7	74.8	81.0*
Soft tissue	60.4	68.3	65.4	76.1	66.5	78.0	72.2*
Wilms tumor	74.4	77.5	87.1	86.5	90.8	92.6	90.3*

From Ries L.A. et al. (Eds.). (2002). *SEER cancer statistics review, 1973-1999*. Bethesda, Md.: National Cancer Institute; Web site: http://seer.cancer.gov/csr/1973_1999/.
Rates are from the SEER 9 areas. They are based on data from population-based registries in Connecticut, New Mexico, Utah, Iowa, Hawaii, Atlanta, Detroit, Seattle–Puget Sound, and San Francisco–Oakland. Rates are based on follow-up of patients into 1999.
*The difference in rates between 1974-1976 and 1992-1998 is statistically significant ($P < .05$).
†The standard error of the survival rate is between 5 and 10 percentage points.

children (Dreyer, Blatt, & Bleyer, 2002). The effect of radiation, however, can be permanent. Radiation affects growth by damaging the epiphyseal plates of the long bones and the glands that are responsible for growth-related hormone production. A child's growth should be observed on a standardized growth curve, with growth patterns examined over time rather than as isolated measurements. Preferably both sitting and standing heights should be obtained. Growth rates should be checked every 1 to 3 months during therapy and for the first year after therapy; then measurements should be taken every 6 months until linear growth is completed. Because of the risk of significant weight loss, weight should also be monitored at each visit.

Primary care providers can play an invaluable role in providing anticipatory guidance for parents about the developmental changes children with cancer will experience. Children with cancer are often limited in their opportunities to develop independence and autonomy. The limitations come from restrictions placed by treatment regimens, therapy-related complications, and protective parents.

Ongoing developmental assessment should be performed during and after therapy. Early identification and intervention are important in assisting the child in maintaining age-appropriate development. Neuropsychologic testing is recommended within the first 2 years after completion of therapy for children receiving cranial radiation. Age-standardized tests should be used to measure intellectual ability, visual perception, visual-motor and motor skills, language, memory and learning, academic achievement, and behavior and social functioning (see Chapter 2). Neuropsychologic testing may need to be repeated to diagnose long-term effects.

Diet

Maintaining adequate nutrition while a child is receiving treatment is challenging because of the child's anorexia. Well-balanced, nutritious meals should be offered. Small, frequent meals may often be more appealing than the standard three meals each day. High-calorie, high-protein snacks may also be helpful.

Children receiving corticosteroids often experience an increased appetite and weight gain, but because corticosteroids usually are administered for limited amounts of time, such symptoms generally are of short duration. Nutritious foods low in sodium should be encouraged.

Constipation and diarrhea are frequent side effects of chemotherapy. Constipation may be relieved by increasing the child's fluid intake and encouraging high-fiber foods and fruits. A stool softener or laxative may be necessary, especially with vincristine therapy. Enemas and suppositories should be avoided, especially if the child is neutropenic. Diarrhea should be monitored closely and the child evaluated for signs and symptoms of dehydration.

Safety

Safety issues for a child with a malignant disease involve balancing normal participation in daily activities with taking appropriate precautions imposed by the treatment of a malignant disease. For the safety of all children, chemotherapeutic agents must be stored securely out of reach. Thorough hand washing should follow the handling of any chemotherapeutic agent. Pregnant women should avoid contact with the chemotherapeutic agents and the urine of children receiving chemotherapy. If circumstances make this impossible, gloves should be worn to avoid direct contact with the medication. Unused portions of chemotherapeutic drugs should be returned to the dispensing pharmacy for disposal with other potent chemicals.

External tunneled VADs must have a clean dressing applied to the exit site and the line secured to the chest to minimize any excessive tension on the catheter. Needles, syringes, and other supplies used to maintain the line should be stored properly out of reach of children. Needles should be disposed of carefully, without recapping, in an approved container.

Children with external tunneled VADs should avoid lake or ocean swimming and hot tubs to reduce the risk of infection. They should also have an extra padded clamp available in case of damage to the catheter lumen.

If the child should have a significant fall or head injury, blood cell counts should be checked to determine the platelet count and the possible need for transfusion. Contact sports may be discouraged if the platelet count is less than 100,000/mm³.

Many chemotherapeutic agents will alter the skin's tolerance for sun exposure. It is important that children receiving chemotherapy take extra caution in using a para-aminobenzoic acid (PABA)-free sun block whenever prolonged sun exposure is anticipated. It is best to avoid sun exposure during midday. If the child has alopecia, a hat and sun block should be worn to protect the scalp.

The primary care provider can play a key role in helping the child and family set realistic expectations and limitations on activities. Limitations are influenced by immunosuppression, hematologic compromise, or extremity dysfunction because of peripheral neuropathy induced by chemotherapy or as a result of amputation or limb salvage procedures.

Immunizations

Live-virus vaccines (e.g., those preventing measles, mumps, and rubella and the oral polio vaccine) are contraindicated for children receiving chemotherapy or radiation therapy (Alexander et al, 2002). The oral polio vaccine must also be avoided in the household contacts of any immunosuppressed individual. Although the Advisory Committee on Immunization Practices (ACIP) of the Centers for Disease Control and Prevention recommends administering inactivated vaccines (e.g., the diphtheria-pertussis-tetanus, hepatitis B, *Haemophilus influenzae* type B, pneumococcal, and inactivated polio vaccines) (Atkinson et al, 2002), many oncology centers hold all routine vaccines during immunosuppressive therapy and for the first 3 to 6 months after cancer treatment because the child's immune system may not be able to mount an appropriate response to the vaccination. However, most pediatric oncology teams recommend the use of the influenza vaccine for children receiving therapy and any household contacts during therapy and for up to 1 year after therapy. Persons at risk for pulmonary fibrosis may also benefit from using the vaccine throughout their lives (Alexander et al, 2002). Normal immunologic response usually returns between 3 and 12 months after discontinuing immunosuppressive therapy (American Academy of Pediatrics [AAP], 2000). Because there is some variation in immunization recommendations among cancer treatment centers, it is best to consult the child's oncology team for specific guidance.

Varicella Exposure Prophylaxis and Vaccination. If a child who is seronegative for antibody to the varicella virus or who has not been vaccinated has a direct exposure to a person with active chickenpox or to a person who develops lesions within 48 hours of the contact, the child must receive varicella-zoster immune globulin (VZIG). This vaccine is available with a physician's order through the regional distribution centers of the American Red Cross Blood Services and should be administered within 48 to 96 hours of exposure. The dose of VZIG is 125 units/ 10 kg, with a maximum dosage of 625 units. Once a child is exposed to chickenpox, the child must be isolated from other children who are immunocompromised from day 10 to day 28 following the exposure.

The live-attenuated varicella vaccine is not currently licensed for children with malignancies. The vaccine is available through a research protocol, however, for children with ALL who have been in remission for at least 1 year and who have an absolute lymphocyte count over 700/mm³ (Gruber, 2001). The vaccine should not be administered within 5 months of the administration of blood products or any form of immune globulin. Transmission of vaccine-induced varicella from healthy children to their immune-compromised siblings has not been documented (Gruber, 2001).

Other Immunizations. Children with Hodgkin disease should receive the pneumococcal and meningococcal vaccines before splenectomy or splenic irradiation. Booster doses of these polysaccharide vaccines should be given in 2 to 3 years and then every 5 to 6 years. In addition, these children should be given twice-daily penicillin, daily amoxicillin, or daily erythromycin to prevent bacterial infection (AAP, 2000).

Screening

Vision. Routine vision screening is advised. A recurring brain tumor may manifest as impaired visual acuity caused by ocular nerve compression or increased intracranial pressure or as blurred vision caused by papilledema. There may be ptosis, visual disturbances, and sixth cranial nerve dysfunction with recurrent orbital rhabdomyosarcoma. Two classic signs of recurrent retinoblastoma are the white eye reflex in place of the normal red reflex and strabismus. Cataracts are also a late effect of radiation therapy. In addition, vincristine and vinblastine may cause ptosis that can interfere with vision.

Hearing. Routine screenings of hearing are advised. Unilateral hearing loss may indicate the presence of a mass. Children receiving radiation or cisplatin or both are at increased risk for hearing loss (Nagy et al, 1999); evaluation by an audiologist every 6 to 12 months is recommended.

Dental. Routine dental care is advised during treatment and after therapy. Both radiation therapy and chemotherapy place a child at risk for stomatitis, dental caries, and periodontal disease. Ideally dental work requiring manipulation of the oral tissues should be performed only if the ANC is greater than 1000/mm³ and the platelet count is greater than 50,000/mm³ (Overholser, 1999). All children with central VADs having dental manipulation should receive antibiotic prophylaxis to prevent subacute bacterial endocarditis (SBE), as recommended by the American Heart Association (Pallasch et al, 1999; see Chapter 21 for SBE guidelines). Daily brushing with a soft-bristled brush and flossing are recommended when the ANC is over 500/mm³, the platelet count is over 100,000/mm³, and stomatitis is not present. Daily fluoride rinses may be indicated in children with a high potential for caries. Good oral hygiene is important in preventing stomatitis and infection. Despite widespread research on numerous agents, no medication clearly shows efficacy in the prophylaxis or treatment of stomatitis (Kostler et al, 2001). Chlorhexidine, a commonly used mouthwash, was no more effective than routine oral rinsing with water in a large randomized clinical trial (Dodd et al, 1996).

Blood Pressure. Blood pressure should be measured at every visit because of possible hypertension from corticosteroids, potential renal toxicity of many chemotherapeutic agents, and cardiac toxicities from anthracyclines.

Hematocrit. Because of frequent hematologic analyses, routine hematocrit screening is not necessary while a child is receiving therapy. After therapy, routine screening is recommended.

Urinalysis. Routine urinalysis is advised because it may reveal red blood cells in children with bladder or kidney tumors. Late effects of radiation therapy may include proteinuria. Children receiving cyclophosphamide may experience hemorrhagic cystitis, although symptoms may occur months to years after the drug has been discontinued. Particular care is required to screen for and treat urinary tract infections in children who have undergone a nephrectomy.

Tuberculosis. Routine screening for tuberculosis of children off therapy is advised. Children receiving therapy may be anergic to skin testing. The placement of controls (e.g., *Candida* and diphtheria-tetanus [dT]) will help assess the individual's responsiveness. A chest radiograph may be necessary if skin testing is unsuccessful.

Children receiving immunosuppressive therapy are at risk for tuberculosis. Children with a significant exposure to tuberculosis should receive 12 months of therapy with isoniazid (AAP, 2000).

Condition-Specific Screening

The primary care provider must keep in mind the possibility of abnormalities because of disease recurrence or the long-term effects of treatment (Table 17-3). Screening for these complications should be done in consultation with either the pediatric oncology team or other subspecialty team.

Common Illness Management

Differential Diagnosis (Box 17-5)

Fever. The presence of fever (i.e., 38.3° C [101° F]) adds a critical dimension to diagnosis and treatment in the face of neutropenia. If adequate therapy is not initiated promptly, the result could be life threatening. The first step in evaluating a fever is obtaining a complete blood count (CBC) with differential to determine if the child is neutropenic, blood cultures from all central VAD lumens, and cultures from other potential sites of infection as indicated by the history and physical exam. Obtain-

ing a chest radiograph is not indicated in the absence of respiratory symptoms (McCullers & Shenep, 2001). The physical exam should focus on the skin, lungs, nose, sinuses, oral cavity, pharynx, catheter site, abdomen, joints, and perineal and perirectal areas. Expected signs of infection such as erythema and edema may be absent or diminished. A history of chills or rigors occurring within 2 hours of flushing a central VAD may indicate the presence of bacteremia (McCullers & Shenep, 2001).

The febrile child with a central VAD should have aerobic and anaerobic blood cultures obtained peripherally and from each lumen of the catheter or port. Parenteral broad-spectrum antibiotics are initiated and later modified based on culture and sensitivity results. If after 48 to 72 hours, the ANC is over 500/mm^3, the cultures are negative, and the child is afebrile, antibiotics may be stopped. If the cultures are positive, a full 10- to 14-day course of antibiotics should be administered (Orudjev & Lange, 2002).

Admission to the hospital for treatment is generally required for the child who is febrile and neutropenic (i.e., ANC < 500/mm^3). In selected cases of moderate neutropenia (i.e., ANC 200 to 500/mm^3), however, the child may be treated as an outpatient with daily examination by the oncologist (Orudjev & Lange, 2002). After cultures are obtained, parenteral broad-spectrum antibiotics should be started immediately under the disection of the oncologic team. Antibiotic choice is based on suspected organism and institutional-regional patterns of antibiotic resistance.

Viral Infections. The human viruses most frequently affecting children with malignant diseases are herpes simplex virus (HSV), varicella-zoster virus (VZV), and cytomegalovirus (CMV). Treatment of HSV infections in children with cancer depends on the site and severity of the infection but is most often with acyclovir (250 mg/m^2 every 8 hours).

In the event that the child contracts a primary (chickenpox) or secondary (shingles) VZV infection, acyclovir (500 mg/m^2 every 8 hours) should be administered intravenously immediately and continued for at least 7 days or until all lesions have crusted. Vigorous hydration and monitoring of blood urea nitrogen (BUN) and creatinine during acyclovir treatment are needed to prevent renal toxicity of the drug.

An acute CMV infection may present with fever, hepatosplenomegaly, retinitis, pneumonia, colitis, CNS manifestations, and a rash. Antiviral therapy for CMV includes the use of gancyclovir and immune globulin intravenously.

Other Infections. Candidiasis and aspergillosis are the two most common fungal infections in children with malignant diseases. Candidiasis is more common and can involve the oral mucosa, gastrointestinal tract, urinary tract, bone, lungs, and, less frequently, the blood. Meticulous oral care and prompt identification of lesions help to reduce morbidity from oral candidiasis. Once an oral infection is documented, systemic oral antifungal agents may be used. Aspergillosis is seen most frequently in the respiratory tract, gastrointestinal tract, and brain. Amphotericin B is the most effective drug for systemic fungal infection; however, it has potent side effects (McCullers & Shenep, 2001).

The child who is immunocompromised and at risk for *Pneumocystis carinii* may take trimethoprim/sulfamethoxazole (Septra, Bactrim) prophylactically. The usual dose is

---

BOX 17-5

Differential Diagnosis

FEVER
Bacterial, viral, fungal, or protozoal infection
Site: blood, VAD, nasopharynx, skin, joints, perineal, perirectal areas

GASTROINTESTINAL SYMPTOMS
Diarrhea: infectious causes or chemotherapy induced
Constipation: vinca alkaloids (paralytic ileus)
Vomiting: chemotherapy induced, anticipatory

HEADACHE
Increased intracranial pressure caused by a mass lesion or shunt malfunction
CSF leak with recent history of lumbar puncture

PAIN
Tumor related: caused by compression of nerves or invasion of bone
Treatment related: mucositis, dermatitis, neurotoxicity, phantom limb pain, infection
Procedure related: bone marrow, lumbar puncture, venipuncture

VAD, Venous access device; *CSF*, cerebrospinal fluid.

150 mg/m^2/day divided and given twice daily for 3 days each week. The prophylaxis is continued for approximately 6 months after the completion of therapy. In children who cannot tolerate Septra or Bactrim, daily oral dapsone or monthly aerosolized or intravenous pentamidine may be used (Alexander et al, 2002). Pneumonitis is the most common clinical manifestation of *Pneumocystis carinii*. Symptoms include a dry cough, fever, tachypnea, cyanosis, and respiratory distress. Onset may be acute (few days) or insidious (months). All significant infections in children who are immunocompromised should be managed by the oncology team.

Gastrointestinal Symptoms. Nausea, vomiting, and diarrhea, which are common side effects of cancer treatment, may be difficult to distinguish from infections caused by bacteria, protozoa, viruses, or *Clostridium difficile* toxin. The primary care provider must establish the relationship of the symptoms to the administration of chemotherapy or radiation. During these periods, it is important to monitor fluid intake and avoid dehydration, especially in children who are currently receiving chemotherapy. In some cases intravenous fluid replacement and antiemetics may be necessary. Stool cultures will help to identify an infectious source of diarrhea. Blood chemistry values, especially BUN, creatinine, aspartate transaminase (AST), and alanine transaminase (ALT), must be monitored closely to avoid damaging vital organs from concentrated levels of the chemotherapeutics and from delayed excretion as a result of dehydration. Many families are taught how to administer antiemetics and intravenous hydration at home.

Vinca alkaloids predispose children to the development of constipation. If dietary intervention is not successful, supplementation with a stool softener or laxative will be needed to prevent paralytic ileus. This is most often needed when frequent repeated doses of vincristine are used. Suppositories and enemas should not be used without consultation with the oncology team because of the potential risk of infection related to reduced WBC counts.

Headaches. Headache pain, which is usually benign late in childhood and adolescence, is indicative of serious underlying difficulties in young children. Morning headaches associated with vomiting and minimal nausea should always arouse suspicion of increased intracranial pressure caused by a mass lesion or shunt malfunction in a child with a brain tumor. Headaches following a lumbar puncture that resolve with lying down may be caused by a slow cerebrospinal fluid leak. This type of headache is best treated by bed rest and adequate hydration. While taking a thorough history, the primary care provider should note onset, any precipitating factors or symptoms, location, severity, and what, if any, medication gives relief. A thorough neurologic examination is imperative. Many headaches may be treated at home with acetaminophen and rest; but if the headache symptoms are unrelieved by medication or there is any change in vision or neurologic function, immediate evaluation is necessary.

Pain. Pain in children is often difficult to assess and requires understanding of normal child development and age-appropriate verbal and behavioral cues. Most important, keep in mind that children rarely fabricate the presence of pain. The child with cancer poses additional challenges because of the multiple etiologies of pain, which may result from the malignancy, treatments, or procedures (e.g., bone marrow and spinal tap).

Tumor-related pain occurs with direct tumor invasion of the bone, impingement of the tumor on nervous tissue, or metastatic lesions. Compression of the spinal cord by a tumor may result in back pain and is accentuated by maneuvers such as coughing, sneezing, and flexion of the spine. Immediate evaluation is imperative because an untreated cord compression can rapidly progress to irreversible neurologic damage (Rheingold & Lange, 2002). Treatment-related pain can occur from mucositis, infection, radiation-induced dermatitis, neurotoxicity from chemotherapy (vincristine), abdominal pain, or phantom limb pain following the amputation of a limb (Berde et al, 2002). Management of disease-related pain relies on pharmacologic and behavioral approaches. Systematic assessment of the child's pain is needed to design an optimal plan.

Pain resulting from procedures is greatly reduced with the use of conscious sedation (e.g., using a combination of a sedative [midazolam, diazepam] and an opioid [fentanyl, morphine]). Some children who experience great psychologic or physical pain during procedures may benefit from the use of short-acting general anesthetics (Anghelescu & Oakes, 2002).

Topical anesthetics are used in combination with sedation to reduce procedural pain. There are three primary methods of achieving topical anesthesia: subcutaneous infiltration with lidocaine, topical lidocaine creams, and use of electric current with anesthetic. Creams are most commonly used. The onset, duration, and depth of analgesia depend on the brand of cream used and the duration of application. Numby Stuff (Iomed) delivers lidocaine into the skin using a low-level electric current from a battery-powered dose control unit. Topical anesthesia for procedures is achieved in 7 to 15 minutes.

Nonpharmacologic therapies to reduce pain and distress include distraction, guided imagery, and hypnosis. Art and play therapy can also assist children and adolescents in coping with the loss of control and pain associated with invasive procedures (Sentivany-Collins, 2002).

Drug Interactions

Children receiving therapy need to avoid aspirin-containing products because they impair platelet function. Acetaminophen is generally recommended; however, its use during periods of neutropenia is discouraged because it may mask a fever. Multivitamins high in folic acid should be avoided because of the interference of folate with methotrexate. Vitamins low in folic acid are acceptable. Because of the number of drugs a child may be taking for therapy and the possibility of interaction, it is advisable that the primary care provider contact the pediatric oncology team before prescribing additional medications.

Developmental Issues
Sleep Patterns

Disturbances in sleep patterns are common. The extent to which the child is affected will depend on the age at diagnosis, medication schedules, the frequency of hospitalizations, and the general coping patterns of the child. Maintaining a consistent bedtime ritual whenever possible provides security during a time when many things are disrupted. Parents should also be encouraged to bring transitional objects (e.g., a teddy bear, favorite blanket) because these may help the child with sleep during periods of hospitalization.

Toileting

Diarrhea and constipation may occur with certain chemotherapy agents. Toilet training may be delayed or regression may occur if treatment occurs during the toddler or preschool period.

Discipline

Discipline for the child with cancer should be the same as for all children. A consistent approach in establishing expectations and setting limits is important to the child's sense of security. The parents should be supported in maintaining normal patterns of discipline, although they may initially be ambivalent about disciplining their child who is ill. Consistency in discipline among siblings is also important (Walker et al, 2002).

Child Care

The intensity of certain phases of therapy may make regular daycare both impractical and potentially harmful to the child with cancer because of the increased risk of acquiring some infectious diseases in these settings. When a child has begun less intensive therapy, a home or small group situation is recommended because it minimizes exposure to the various common pediatric illnesses. The caretaker must be educated about (1) the child's disease and notifying the family immediately of any fever, signs and symptoms of infection, or increased bruising or bleeding; (2) reporting any communicable illness—especially chickenpox—in the other children; and (3) any medication or oral chemotherapeutic agent that must be administered during child care hours. In addition, the importance of good hand washing should be emphasized, especially before and after toileting, food preparation, and meals.

Schooling

With advances in the treatment of children with cancer, more children are surviving into adulthood. The child who is too ill to participate in the regular classroom should be enrolled in a home study program. The role of health care providers, parents, and educators is to work as a team to assist the child in returning to school as soon after diagnosis as is medically possible. The return to school provides a sense of normalcy and contributes to the child's sense of hopefulness (see Chapter 5).

The child's school reentry must be carefully planned. To enhance the child's participation in school activities, anticipatory guidance should include attention to the special precautions that need to be taken for the child's safety and learning needs. Research results support a three-pronged method of school reentry: direct communication with school personnel, education of the child's classmates, and determination of the child's attitude toward school (Walker et al, 2002). This can be achieved by mutual respect between parents and school personnel, a willingness to provide needed resources such as homebound education, and advocacy on the part of parents and the oncology team to educate school personnel to the special needs created by hospitalizations, chemotherapy-induced side effects, and long-term sequelae of surgery, radiation, and chemotherapy on learning abilities.

Establishing an individualized educational plan (IEP) can help define and anticipate the special needs of the child. The teachers and the school staff must be informed of the child's illness and implications that will influence attendance, social interaction, educational capacity, and the restrictions or special needs dictated by medical care. Early recognition of learning disabilities enhances prompt assessment and intervention.

With the family's and child's permission, the child's classmates are taught about the child's illness at an appropriate developmental level. The child also needs to be prepared to answer classmates' questions. The primary care provider can provide the family with support and resources to help ease the transition into school (see Chapter 5).

Sexuality

The child with cancer often struggles with an alteration in body image because of hair loss, weight loss or gain, or disfiguring surgery. A major task of these children is learning to deal with this change, be it temporary or permanent. This is especially true in adolescents, who, in addition to treatment, may be experiencing the normal pubertal changes. Ongoing monitoring of the child's development through the use of Tanner staging is important. Failure to progress through the stages warrants referral to a pediatric endocrinologist.

A young woman receiving chemotherapy may experience delayed development of secondary sexual characteristics and amenorrhea. After the cessation of therapy, development often occurs and the menses will begin. Fertility status of children surviving childhood malignancies varies depending on the type and extent of treatment. Transposition of ovaries from the radiation field has been shown to help preserve ovarian function (Hobbie et al, 2002). It appears that treatment with chemotherapy does not increase the risk of congenital anomalies in the offspring of childhood cancer survivors (Meistrich & Byrne, 2002). Ongoing long-term follow-up is required.

Sperm banking should be offered to pubescent males, if feasible, before therapy because sterility and mutagenicity can occur from cancer treatment. Ongoing assessment of appropriate sexual development and functioning (e.g., libido, impotence) is important. Hormone replacement may be necessary if there is a deficiency. Peer support groups are often useful in helping adolescents to deal with issues of sexuality and body image.

Transition into Adulthood

Because most children diagnosed with cancer are surviving into adulthood, pediatric cancer centers are attempting to create follow-up or "late effects" clinics that meet the needs of young adults or are referring them to adult oncologists who have remained current on issues specific to childhood cancer survivors. Follow-up including the same multidisciplinary approach used during treatment would benefit the young adult (Oeffinger, 2000).

The protections provided by the Americans with Disabilities Act of 1990 apply to persons with cancer—whether it is cured, controlled, or in remission. The Department of Defense generally does not allow cancer survivors to enlist but has provided waivers on a case-by-case basis when the individual has been off therapy with no recurrence for 5 years. To avoid job discrimination, it is advisable for young adults to apply for jobs for which they are clearly qualified, be honest with employers' questions but not volunteer a prior cancer history, and supply a letter from their primary care provider about prognosis and life expectancy if a question arises (Weiner et al, 2002). Health insurance through large employers is much less likely to create a barrier to coverage than individual or small business policies.

Family Concerns and Resources

Advances in medicine that have led to improved survival rates of children with cancer have also brought problems of chronic uncertainty. The uncertainty faced by families centers around the basic issue of the child's survival. Family concerns often reflect the phase of treatment they are experiencing. In the beginning, uncertainty is focused on whether or not remission will be obtained. If remission is achieved, will it be long-term or will relapse occur? If relapse occurs, will the child enter remission again or die? At the end of treatment, families struggle with ambivalent feelings; they are grateful for the end of therapy yet fearful of the loss of their "safety net" of frequent contact with providers and the end of drugs that have maintained remission (Chanock et al, 2002).

In addition to providing illness-related information, the health care team must help families cope with uncertainty (Santacroce, 2002). Learning to cope with uncertainty is important to the health and well-being of all family members. Support for the child and family must be ongoing, not only at diagnosis but also long after completion of therapy or death of the child.

At diagnosis, parents often feel incredible guilt for not having brought the child to medical care sooner or for not being a more vocal advocate if providers did not realize the significance of the symptoms. The pediatric oncology team tries to support families through this difficult time by allowing opportunities for individual and family counseling. Siblings of the child with cancer benefit from an understanding of what happens during clinic and hospital visits and from interventions directly addressing their need for communication and support (Murray, 1999; Sloper, 2000).

Compliance becomes an issue when the child or adolescent's chemotherapy consists primarily of oral medications taken at home. Several factors, including confusion about parental vs. adolescent responsibilities, denial of the illness, and a loss of control, may affect adolescent noncompliance (Spinetta et al, 2002; Walker et al, 2002). Compliance in younger children may encompass a parental inability to get them to take the medication because of its taste or form or because of the timing of doses (Fielding & Duff, 1999). There are many innovative methods that can be shared with parents if they express their difficulties in administering the chemotherapy.

Cultural issues related to how individuals regard and prepare for death are of particular interest in the care of children with cancer. In Korea, for example, dying outside the home is considered very undesirable, which has implications for the importance of home care for these children who are terminally ill (Martinson et al, 1995). With regard to the caretaking of children who are ill, mothers most commonly take on this responsibility in Korea, Japan, and many Hispanic families, whereas in China, fathers often assume this role when the child is ill (Martinson et al, 1995). At an appropriate time, assessing such issues as the family's feelings about disclosure of information to the child, caretaking responsibilities, death rituals, and comfort with asking questions and voicing concerns and disagreement with health care providers is important.

The financial burden of a catastrophic illness is of monumental concern to the family. It not only affects the current financial status of the family but also has far-reaching implications for the child's future insurability. Insurance companies and health maintenance organizations (HMOs) vary in their reimbursement of medications and procedures they deem to be experimental. All these factors place a tremendous amount of stress on an already taxed family unit.

Numerous local, regional, and national organizations provide information and educational resources about childhood malignant diseases. Local hospitals and cancer centers often provide support groups for family members. Informal parent-to-parent interactions based on the sense of having a common understanding of parenting a child with cancer can be a powerful source of support. Identifying local resources will provide a much-welcomed service to these families.

ORGANIZATIONS

American Cancer Society
1599 Clifton Rd, NE
Atlanta, GA 30329
(800) ACS-2345 or (404) 320-3333
www.cancer.org
A volunteer organization offering educational programs, family services, rehabilitation support, and referral to local and regional resources.

Cancer Information Service, National Cancer Institute
Blair Bldg, Rm 414
9000 Rockville Pike
Bethesda, MD 20892
(800) 4CANCER
www.cancernet.nci.nih.gov
A network of regional information centers that provide personalized answers to cancer-related questions from individuals, families, the general public, and health care professionals; also provides referral to local and regional resources.

Candlelighters Childhood Cancer Foundation, Inc
7910 Woodmont Ave, Suite 460
Bethesda, MD 20814
(800) 366-2223 or (301) 657-8401
www.candlelighters.org
An international organization of parents whose children have had cancer; provides guidance and emotional support through local chapters, information, and referral to local and regional resources.

Leukemia and Lymphoma Society
1311 Mamaroneck Ave
White Plains, NY 10605
(800) 955-4572 or (914) 949-5213
www.leukemia.org
A volunteer organization offering educational programs, information, financial assistance, and referral to local and regional resources.

Summary of Primary Care Needs for the Child with Cancer

HEALTH CARE MAINTENANCE

Growth and Development

Growth slows because of chemotherapy and radiation.

Closely monitor weight; child is at risk for significant weight loss because of disease and treatment and is also at risk for weight gain because of steroids.

Periodic developmental screening is done to assess for age-appropriate behaviors.

Neuropsychologic testing is done for children who received cranial radiation.

Diet

Maintain an adequate diet. Offer small frequent meals if the child is experiencing anorexia. Low-sodium foods should be given to children receiving corticosteroid therapy. Increase fluid intake and high-fiber foods for constipation. Monitor diarrhea closely.

Safety

Ensure proper handling of chemotherapeutic agents at home and proper maintenance and protection of indwelling venous access devices.

Check platelet count after significant fall or head injury. The child may need platelet transfusion.

Minimize roughhousing and discourage contact sports if the platelet count is less than 100,000. Because of photosensitivity, protect the child from sun. Use PABA-free sunblock.

Immunizations

No live-virus vaccines are given while the child is receiving therapy or for the first year off therapy.

Some centers recommend administering killed vaccines if the child is scheduled to receive them by age; booster doses, however, may be needed after therapy is complete. Other centers do not give killed vaccines until child has been off treatment for 6 months.

Siblings and household contacts should not receive live polio vaccine because of transmissibility to child who is immunocompromised. Siblings and household contacts may receive measles, mumps, Rabella (MMR) vaccine.

The varicella vaccine, although not routinely recommended for children with malignancies, is available for use in some children with acute lymphocytic leukemia (ALL) who have been in remission for at least 1 year.

Children recovering from hematopoietic stem cell transplantation require special consideration in determining immunization schedule and protocol.

Children with Hodgkin disease should be vaccinated with the pneumococcal and *H. influenzae* type B conjugate vaccines before splenectomy or splenic irradiation.

Screening

Vision. Routine screening is recommended. Thorough assessment is warranted if visual abnormalities are detected.

Hearing. Routine screening is recommended. Children receiving ototoxic drugs should have regular evaluations by an audiologist.

Dental. Routine screening is recommended. A complete blood count (CBC) should be done before an appointment to verify adequate absolute neutrophil count (ANC), platelet count. Meticulous oral hygiene is necessary to prevent infections. Oral subacate bacterial endocarditis (SBE) prophylaxis is needed for children with central venous access devices (VADs).

Blood Pressure. Blood pressures should be taken at each visit to evaluate for hypertension as a result of drug toxicity.

Hematocrit. Hematocrit testing is routine and is done off therapy. It is done as needed while the child is receiving therapy. Critical levels are ANC less than 500, platelets less than 20,000, and hemoglobin less than 7 to 8 g/dl.

Urinalysis. Urinalysis is routine. Protein may be observed after radiation therapy, or hematuria may be seen after cyclophosphamide/ifosfamide therapy. Special caution should be taken when only one kidney is present.

Tuberculosis. Tuberculosis screening is routine and is done off therapy. Possible anergic status requires use of a control if child is tested on therapy.

Condition-Specific Screening

Close assessment is required for signs and symptoms of late effects of therapy or recurrence of malignancy (Table 17-3).

COMMON ILLNESS MANAGEMENT

Differential Diagnosis

Fever. Rule out neutropenia and infection. Do septic work-up as warranted. Prompt intervention is required with neutropenia or the presence of central VAD.

Viral and Other Infections. Varicella-zoster immune globulin (VZIG) is required within 96 hours of exposure if the child does not have antibodies to varicella or has not been immunized. Acyclovir is given intravenously for chickenpox in the immunosuppressed individual. Rule out dissemination of disease.

Give *Pneumocystis carinii* prophylaxis.

Gastrointestinal Symptoms. For chemotherapy-induced constipation, ensure adequate hydration and begin stool softeners or laxatives as needed. Avoid suppositories and enemas.

For nausea and vomiting, determine the relationship to chemotherapy and radiation; rule out viral and bacterial infection. Give hydration fluid and antiemetics as needed.

Headaches. Perform a thorough neurologic examination. Consider possibility of a brain tumor, central nervous system (CNS) involvement, sinusitis, and lumbar puncture cerebrospinal fluid leak.

Pain. Determine the source of pain; rule out cord compression. Premedicate for procedures.

Drug Interactions

No aspirin-containing products should be given. Acetaminophen is recommended except in times of neutropenia to avoid masking a fever.

Low folic acid multivitamins my be taken. Consult with the oncology team before prescribing additional medication because of the risk of drug interaction.

Continued

Summary of Primary Care Needs for the Child with Cancer—cont'd

DEVELOPMENTAL ISSUES

Sleep Patterns

Disturbances are common. Maintain consistent bedtime schedule and routine whenever possible. A transitional object may increase security during hospitalization.

Toileting

Standard developmental counseling is advised. Regression may occur.

Discipline

Use normal patterns of discipline; it is important to maintain consistency for all siblings.

Child Care

Generally a small group setting is better than a large group to minimize exposure to infections. The caretaker should know the signs and symptoms that pose a concern.

Schooling

The child should return to school as soon as possible. Ongoing communication between primary care providers and teachers is nec-essary. Education of school staff and classmates is crucial. Assist the family in developing an individualized educational program (IEP). Periodically assess for school problems and learning disabilities. If the child is unable to participate in a regular school program, arrange for home tutoring.

Sexuality

Give support for altered body image. Assess for appropriate Tanner staging. Sperm banking may be an option before an adolescent male begins chemotherapy or radiation.

Transition into Adulthood

It is necessary to transition care from pediatric oncology center to adult oncology center knowledgeable on long-term survival of children with cancer.

Primary care providers may be of assistance in employment situations, if requested by client, by providing factual information concerning prognosis.

FAMILY CONCERNS

The family must deal with chronic uncertainty. Insurance and catastrophic financial effects are also concerns. Address needs of siblings.

REFERENCES

Alexander, S.W. et al (2002). Infectious complications in pediatric cancer patients. In P.A. Pizzo & D.G. Poplack (Eds.). *Principles and practice of pediatric oncology* (4th ed.). Philadelphia: Lippincott Williams & Wilkins, pp. 1239-1283.

American Academy of Pediatrics. (2000). In L.K. Pickering (Ed.). *2000 Red book: Report on the Committee on Infectious Diseases* (25th ed.). Elk Grove Village, Ill.: American Academy of Pediatrics.

American Academy of Pediatrics Section on Hematology/Oncology. (1997). Guidelines for the pediatric cancer center and role of such centers in diagnosis and treatment. *Pediatrics, 99,* 139-141.

Anghelescu, D. & Oakes, L. (2002). Working toward better cancer pain management for children. *Cancer Pract, 10*(suppl. 1), S52-S57.

Atkinson, W.L., Pickering, L.K., Schwartz, B., Weniger, B.G., Iskander, J.K., et al. (2002). General recommendations on immunization recommendations of the Advisory Committee on Immunization Practices (ACIP) and the American Academy of Family Physicians (AAFP). *MMWR Morb Mortal Wkly Rep, 51*(RR02), 1-36.

Bagnall-Reeb, H. & Perry, S. (2002). Surgery. In C.R. Baggott, K.P. Kelly, & D. Fochtman (Eds.). *Nursing care of children and adolescents with cancer* (3rd ed.). Philadelphia: W.B. Saunders, pp. 90-115.

Balis, F.M., Holcenberg, S.S., & Blaney, S.M. (2002). General principles of chemotherapy. In P.A. Pizzo & D.G. Poplack (Eds.). *Principles and practice of pediatric* oncology (4th ed.). Philadelphia: Lippincott Williams & Wilkins, pp. 237-308.

Benjamin, R.J. & Anderson, K.C. (2002). What is the proper threshold for platelet transfusion in patients with chemotherapy-induced thrombocytopenia? *Crit Rev Oncol Hematol, 42,* 163-171.

Berde, C.B., Billet, A.L., & Collins, J.J. (2002). Symptom management in supportive care. In P.A. Pizzo & D.G. Poplack (Eds.). *Principles and practice of pediatric oncology* (4th ed.). Philadelphia: Lippincott Williams & Wilkins, pp. 1301-1332.

Bleyer, W.A. (1997). Equal participation of minority patients in U.S. national pediatric cancer clinical trials. *J Pediatr Hematol Oncol, 19,* 423-427.

Bleyer, W.A. (2002). Cancer in older adolescents and young adults: Epidemiology, diagnosis, treatment, survival, and importance of clinical trials. *Med Pediatr Oncol, 38,* 1-10.

Chanock, S.J. et al. (2002). The other side of the bed: What caregivers can learn from listening to patients and their familes. In P.A. Pizzo & D.G. Poplack (Eds.). *Principles and practice of pediatric oncology* (4th ed.). Philadelphia: Lippincott Williams & Wilkins, pp. 1393-1409.

Cheung, N.K. & Rooney, C.M. (2002). Principles of immune and cellular therapy. In P.A. Pizzo & D.G. Poplack (Eds.). *Principles and practice of pediatric oncology* (4th ed.). Philadelphia: Lippincott Williams & Wilkins, pp. 381-408.

Cleary, K. & Nguyen, C. (2001). State of the art in surgical robotics: Clinical applications and technology challenges. *Computer Aided Surg, 6,* 312-328.

Crawford, J. & Lee, M.E. (2000). Recombinant human granulocyte colony-stimulating factor support of the cancer patient. In J.O. Armitage & K.H. Antman (Eds.). *Pharmacology, hematopoietins, stem cells* (3rd ed.). Philadelphia: Lippincott Williams & Wilkins, pp. 411-436.

Cripe, T.P. & Mackall, C.L. (2001). Exploiting genetic alterations to design novel therapies for cancer. *Hematol Oncol Clin North Am, 15,* 657-675.

Culy, C.R., Bhana, N., & Plosker, G.L. (2001). Ondansetron: A review of its use as an antiemetic in children. *Paediatr Drugs, 3,* 441-479.

DeSwarte-Wallace, J., Firouzbakhsh, S., & Finklestein, J.Z. (2001). Using research to change practice: Enteral feedings for pediatric oncology patients. *J Pediatr Oncol Nurs, 18,* 217-223.

Dodd, M.J., Larson, P.J., Dibble, S.L., Miaskowski, C., Greenspan, D., et al. (1996). Randomized clinical trial of chlorhexidine versus placebo for prevention of oral mucositis in patients receiving chemotherapy. *Oncol Nurs Forum, 23,* 921-927.

Dreyer, Z.E., Blatt, J., & Bleyer, A. (2002). Late effects of childhood cancer and its treatment. In P.A. Pizzo & D.G. Poplack (Eds.). *Principles and practice of pediatric oncology* (4th ed.). Philadelphia: Lippincott Williams & Wilkins, pp. 1431-1461.

Fielding, D. & Duff, A. (1999) Compliance with treatment protocols: Interventions for children with chronic illness. *Arch Dis Child, 80,* 196-200.

Golub, T.R. & Arceci, R.J. (2002) Acute myelogenous leukemia. In P.A. Pizzo & D.G. Poplack (Eds.). *Principles and practice of pediatric oncology* (4th ed.). Philadelphia: Lippincott Williams & Wilkins, pp. 545-589.

Gonzalez, R. et al (2002). Hematopoietic stem cell transplantation. In C.R. Baggott, K.P. Kelly, & D. Fochtman (Eds.). *Nursing care of children and adolescents with cancer* (3rd ed.). Philadelphia: W.B. Saunders, pp. 212-255.

Groll, A.H. et al. (2001). Management of specific infectious complications in children with leukemias and lymphomas. In C.C. Patrick (Ed.). *Clinical management of infections in immunocompromised infants and children.* Philadelphia: Lippincott Williams & Wilkins, pp. 111-143.

Gross, T.G., Egeler, R.M., & Smith, F.O. (2001) Pediatric hematopoietic stem cell transplantation. *Hematol Oncol Clin North Am, 15,* 795-808.

Gruber, W.C. (2001). Immunizations in the immunocompromised host. In C.C. Patrick (Ed.). *Clinical management of infections in immunocompromised infants and children.* Philadelphia: Lippincott Williams & Wilkins, pp. 511-536.

Guinan, E.C., Krance, R.A., & Lehmann, L.E. (2002). Stem cell transplantation in pediatric oncology. In P.A. Pizzo & D.G. Poplack (Eds.). *Principles and practice of pediatric oncology* (4th ed.). Philadelphia: Lippincott Williams & Wilkins, pp. 429-451.

Hensley, M.L., Schuchter, L.M., Lindley, C., Meropol, N.J., Cohen, G.I., et al. (1999). American Society of Clinical Oncology clinical practice guidelines for the use of chemotherapy and radiotherapy protectants. *J Clin Oncol, 17,* 3333-3355.

Higgins, K. & Brown, N. (2002). Treatment of acute promyelocytic leukemia with arsenic trioxide. *J Pediatr Oncol Nurs, 19,* 50.

Hobbie, W. et al. (2002). Care of survivors. In C.R. Baggott, K.P. Kelly, & D. Fochtman (Eds.). *Nursing care of children and adolescents with cancer* (3rd ed.). Philadelphia: W.B. Saunders pp. 426-464.

Holmes, F.A., Jones, S.E., O'Shaughnessy, J., Vukelja, S., George, T., et al. (2002). Comparable efficacy and safety profiles of once-per-cycle pegfilgrastim and daily injection filgrastim in chemotherapy-induced neutropenia: A multicenter dose-finding study in women with breast cancer. *Ann Oncol, 13,* 903-909.

Ivy, S.P. et al. (2002). Evolving molecular and targeted therapies. In P.A. Pizzo & D.G. Poplack (Eds.). *Principles and practice of pediatric oncology* (4th ed.). Philadelphia: Lippincott Williams & Wilkins, pp. 309-349.

Kostler, W.J., Hejna, M., Wenzel, C., & Zielinski, C.C. (2001). Oral mucositis complicating chemotherapy and/or radiotherapy: Options for prevention and treatment. *CA Cancer J Clin. 51,* 290-315.

Landis, S.H., Murray, T., Bolden, S., & Wingo, P.A. (1998). Cancer statistics. *CA Cancer J Clin, 48,* 6-30.

Link, M.P., Gebhardt, M.C., & Meyers, P.A. (2002). Osteosarcoma. In P.A. Pizzo & D.G. Poplack (Eds.). *Principles and practice of pediatric oncology* (4th ed.). Philadelphia: Lippincott Williams & Wilkins, pp. 1051-1089.

Look, A.T. & Kirsch, I.R. (2002). Molecular basis of childhood cancer. In P.A. Pizzo & D.G. Poplack (Eds.). *Principles and practice of pediatric oncology* (4th ed.). Philadelphia: Lippincott Williams & Wilkins, pp. 45-87.

Mandell, L.R., Kadota, R., Freeman, C., Douglass, E.C., Fontanesi, J., et al. (1999). There is no role for hyperfactionated radiotherapy in the management of children with newly diagnosed diffuse intrinsic brainstem tumors: Results of a Pediatric Oncology Group phase III trial comparing conventional vs. hyperfractionated radiotherapy. *Int J Radiat Oncol Biol Phys, 43,* 959-964.

Martinson, I.M., Kim, S., Yang, S.O., Cho, Y.S., Lee, J.S., et al. (1995). Impact of childhood cancer on Korean families. *J Pediatr Oncol Nurs, 12,* 11-17.

Mathijssen, R.H., Verweij, J., de Bruijn, P., Loos, W.J., & Sparreboom, A. (2002). Modulation of irinotecan (CPT-11) metabolism by St. John's wort in cancer patients. *Proc Am Assoc Cancer Res Abstract,* 2443.

McCullers, J.A. & Shenep, J.L. (2001). Assessment and management of suspected infection in neutropenic patients. In C.C. Patrick (Ed.). *Clinical management of infections in immunocompromised infants and children.* Philadelphia: Lippincott Williams & Wilkins, pp. 353-387.

Meistrich, M.L. & Byrne, J. (2002). Genetic disease in offspring of long-term survivors of childhood and adolescent cancer treated with potentially mutagenic therapies. *Am J Hum Genet, 70,* 1069-1071.

Moll, A.C. et al. (2001). Second primary tumor in hereditary retinoblastoma: A register-based study 1945-1997: Is there an age effect on radiation-related risk? *Opthamology, 108,* 1109-1114.

Murray, J.S. (1999). Attachment theory and adjustment difficulties in siblings of children with cancer. *Issues Ment Health Nurs, 21,* 149-169.

NACHRI. (2000). Home care requirements for children and adolescents with cancer. National Association of Children's Hospitals and Related Institutions (NACHRI) patient care oncology FOCUS group. *J Pediatr Oncol Nurs, 17,* 45-49.

Nagy, J.L., Adelstein, D.J., Newman, C.W., Rybicki, L.A., Rice, T.W., et al. (1999). Cisplatin ototoxicity: The importance of baseline audiometry. *Am J Clin Oncol, 22,* 305-308.

Neglia, J.P., Friedman, D.L., Yasui, Y., Mertens, A.C., Hammond, S., et al. (2001). Second malignant neoplasms in five-year survivors of childhood cancer: Childhood cancer survivor study. *J Natl Cancer Inst, 93,* 618-629.

Neuhouser, M.L., Patterson, R.E., Schwartz, S.M., Hedderson, M.M., Bowen, D.J., et al. (2001). Use of alternative medicine by children with cancer in Washington state. *Prev Med, 33,* 347-354.

Oeffinger, K.C. (2000). Childhood cancer survivors and primary care physicians. *J Fam Pract, 49,* 689-690.

Orudjev, E. & Lange, B.J. (2002). Evolving concepts of management of febrile neutropenia in children with cancer. *Med Pediatr Oncol, 39,* 77-85.

Overholser, C.D. (1999). Oral care for the cancer patient. In J. Klastersky, S.C. Schimpff, & H. Senn (Eds.). *Supportive care in cancer* (2nd ed.). New York: M. Dekker, pp. 229-251.

Pallasch, T.J., Gage, T.W., & Taubert, K.A. (1999). The 1997 prevention of bacterial endocarditis recommendations by the American Heart Association: Questions and answers. *J Calif Dent Assoc, 27,* 393-399.

Panzarella et al. (2002). Management of disease and treatment-related complications. In C.R. Baggott, K.P. Kelly, & D. Fochtman (Eds.). *Nursing care of children and adolescents with cancer* (3rd ed.). Philadelphia: W.B. Saunders, pp. 279-318.

Pollock, B., Krischner, J., & Vietti, T. (1991). Interval between symptom onset and diagnosis of pediatric solid tumors. *J Pediatr, 119,* 725-732.

Quinn, A.M. (2002). Cyberknife: A robotic radiosurgery system. *Clin J Oncol Nurs, 6,* 149-156.

Raetz, E.A., Moos, P.J., Szabo, A., & Carroll, W.L. (2001). Gene expression profiling methods and clinical applications in oncology. *Hematol Oncol Clin North Am, 15,* 911-930.

Rheingold, S.R. & Lange, B.J. (2002). Oncologic emergencies. In P.A. Pizzo & D.G. Poplack (Eds.). *Principles and practice of pediatric oncology* (4th ed.). Philadelphia: Lippincott Williams & Wilkins, pp. 1177-1203.

Rhodes, V.A. & McDaniel, R.W. (2001). Nausea, vomiting, and retching: Complex problems in palliative care. *CA Cancer Jr Clin, 51,* 232-248.

Richardson, R.C., Nelson, M.B., & Meeske, K. (1999). Young adult survivors of childhood cancer: Attending to emerging medical and psychosocial needs. *J Pediatr Oncol Nurs, 16,* 136-144.

Ries, L.A. et al. (Eds.). (1999). *Cancer incidence and survival among children and adolescents: United States SEER Program 1975-1995.* NIH Pub. No. 99-4649. Bethesda, Md.: National Cancer Institute, SEER Program.

Ries, L.A., Eisner, M.P., Kosary, C.L., Hankey, B.F., Miller, B.A., et al. (Eds). (2002). *SEER cancer statistics review, 1973-1999.* Bethesda, Md.: National Cancer Institute; Web site: http://seer.cancer.gov/csr/1973_1999/.

Rossetto, C.L. & McMahon, J.E. (2000). Current and future trends in transfusion therapy. *J Pediatr Oncol Nurs, 17,* 160-173.

Ruccione, K. (2002). Biologic basis of cancer in children and adolescents. In C.R. Baggott, K.P. Kelly, & D. Fochtman (Eds.). *Nursing care of children and adolescents with cancer* (3rd ed.). Philadelphia: W.B. Saunders, pp. 24-63.

Ruccione, K. & Kelly, K.P. (2000). Pediatric oncology nursing in cooperative group clinical trials comes of age. *Semin Oncol Nurs, 16,* 253-260.

Santacroce, S. (2002). Uncertainty, anxiety, and symptoms of posttraumatic stress in parents of children recently diagnosed with cancer. *J Pediatr Oncol Nurs, 19,* 104-111.

Sentivany-Collins, S. (2002). Treatment of pain. In C.R. Baggott, K.P. Kelly, & D. Fochtman (Eds.). *Nursing care of children and adolescents with cancer* (3rd ed.). Philadelphia: W.B. Saunders, pp. 319-333.

Shamberger, R.C., Jaksic, T., & Ziegler, M.M. (2002). General principles of surgery. In P.A. Pizzo & D.G. Poplack (Eds.). *Principles and practice of pediatric oncology* (4th ed.). Philadelphia: Lippincott Williams & Wilkins, pp. 351-367.

Sloper, P. (2000). Experiences and support needs of siblings of children with cancer. *Health Soc Care Community, 8,* 298-306.

Spinetta, J.J., Masera, G., Eden, T., Oppenheim, D., Martins, A.G., et al. (2002). Refusal, non-compliance, and abandonment of treatment in children and adolescents with cancer: A report of the SIOP working committee on psychosocial issues in pediatric oncology. *Med Pediatr Oncol, 38,* 114-117.

Stephenson, J. (2002). Cancer studies explore targeted therapy, researchers seek new prevention strategies. *JAMA, 287,* 3063-3067.

Stock, W. (2000). Outcomes of adolescents and young adults with ALL: A comparison of Children Cancer Group (CCG) and Cancer and Leukemia Group B (CALGB) regimens. *Blood, 96,* 467a (abstract 2009).

Tarbell, N.J. & Kooy, H.M. (2002). General principles of radiation oncology. In P.A. Pizzo & D.G. Poplack (Eds.). *Principles and practice of pediatric oncology* (4th ed.). Philadelphia: Lippincott Williams & Wilkins, pp. 369-380.

Thiele, C.J. & Kastan, M.B. (2002). Biology of childhood cancer. In P.A. Pizzo & D.G. Poplack (Eds.). *Principles and practice of pediatric oncology* (4th ed.). Philadelphia: Lippincott Williams & Wilkins, pp. 89-119.

Vietti, T.J. & Steuber, C.P. (2002). Clinical assessment and differential diagnosis of the child with suspected cancer. In P.A. Pizzo & D.G. Poplack (Eds.). *Principles and practice of pediatric oncology* (4th ed.). Philadelphia: Lippincott Williams & Wilkins, pp. 149-159.

Walker, C.L. et al. (2002). Family-centered psychosocial care. In C.R. Baggott, K.P. Kelly, & D. Fochtman (Eds.). *Nursing care of children and adolescents with cancer* (3rd ed.). Philadelphia: W.B. Saunders, pp. 365-390.

Ward, J.D. (2000). Pediatric cancer survivors: Assessment of late effects. *Nurse Pract, 25*(12), 18, 21-28, 35-39.

Weiner, S.L. et al. (2002). Pediatric cancer: Advocacy, insurance, education, and employment. In P.A. Pizzo & D.G. Poplack (Eds.). *Principles and practice of pediatric oncology* (4th ed.). Philadelphia: Lippincott Williams & Wilkins, pp. 1511-1526.

Zebrack, B.J., Zeltzer, L.K., Whitton, J., Mertens, A.C., Odom, L., et al. (2002). Psychological outcomes in long-term survivors of childhood leukemia, Hodgkin's disease, and non-Hodgkin's lymphoma: A report from the Childhood Cancer Survivor Study. *Pediatrics, 110*, 42-52.

18 Cerebral Palsy

Wendy M. Nehring

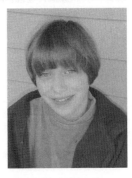

Etiology

Cerebral palsy, a condition first described by Dr. George Little in 1861, is an umbrella term used to define a group of nonprogressive disorders that cause aberrant movement and posture secondary to central nervous system (CNS) damage or insult in the early periods of brain development (Griffin et al, 2002; National Institute of Neurological Disorders and Stroke [NINDS], 2001). Cerebral palsy is described by both motor and anatomic groupings. Etiologically, it is a set of multifactorial disorders that are diverse in clinical presentation.

The classification system developed by Minear (1956) remains in use today. The four types of motor dysfunction seen in children with cerebral palsy are spastic, dyskinetic, ataxic, and mixed. Each type is then divided anatomically or by the number of extremities involved. Each category carries a different set of characteristics and prognoses (Box 18-1). Some health care professionals have started classifying cerebral palsy more succinctly according to the area of the brain affected (e.g., pyramidal [spastic] or extrapyramidal [primarily athetoid]) (Gupta & Appleton, 2001) or more broadly according to muscle behavior or movement (Pellegrino & Dormans, 1998).

Spastic

Spasticity describes the presence of increased muscle tone, which is noted through the passive range of motion of a joint. Recently, the Task Force on Childhood Motor Disorders (2001, p. 5) has emphasized the need to more accurately refer to spasticity as "upper motor neuron syndrome," although the term "spasticity" will be used in this chapter because it is more generally recognized at this time. Characteristics of spastic or pyramidal cerebral palsy include persistent primitive reflexes, exaggerated stretch reflexes, positive Babinski reflex, ankle clonus, and later development of contractures. This form of cerebral palsy is most distinctly divided by the extremities involved and affects approximately 70% to 80% of people with cerebral palsy. Damage occurs to the motor cortex and pyramidal tracts in the brain (Gersh, 1998a; Pellegrino & Dormans, 1998; Task Force on Childhood Motor Disorders, 2001).

Spastic diplegia affects all the extremities, but the lower extremities are affected more than the upper. Spastic diplegia is often seen in premature and low birth weight infants and is related to cerebral asphyxia with or without the presence of an intraventricular hemorrhage and hydrocephalus. In mild cases, the condition may not be recognized until the child is school aged. Spastic diplegia cerebral palsy occurs in 25% to 35% of the cases of cerebral palsy (Pellegrino & Dormans, 1998).

Spastic quadriplegia is characterized by a dysfunction of the four extremities—sometimes the legs are more affected—and often of the musculature surrounding the trunk and the mouth, pharynx, and tongue. In a few rare cases, three limbs can be affected (i.e., triplegia). Spastic quadriplegia is the most common form associated with cerebral palsy, however, and is diagnosed in premature and low birth weight infants who have had severe asphyxial insults. Medical complications, seizures, mental retardation, and sensory impairments are often associated with quadriplegic cerebral palsy. Quadriplegia occurs in 40% to 45% of the cases of cerebral palsy (Pellegrino & Dormans, 1998).

Spastic hemiplegia is characterized by a motor dysfunction on one side of the body with the upper extremity more affected than the lower extremity. This form of cerebral palsy is seen in low birth weight infants with a past episode of asphyxiation but can also result from a congenital vascular malformation or embolism causing postnatal brain damage. Periventricular leukomalacia is often found on a magnetic resonance image (MRI). Medical complications, sensory impairments, and growth retardation are often present. Spastic hemiplegia occurs in approximately 30% to 40% of all cases of cerebral palsy (Pellegrino & Dormans, 1998).

Double hemiplegia occurs when both sides of the body are affected and is caused by damage or insults to both hemispheres of the brain. The difference between this diagnosis and spastic quadriplegia is that the upper extremities are more affected than the lower.

Dyskinetic

Dyskinesia represents the second motor dysfunction group and is characterized by abnormal involuntary movements after the initiation of a voluntary movement (Raymond, 2002). Children with this form of cerebral palsy often display rigid muscle tone when awake and normal or decreased muscle tone when asleep. This aberrant positioning is a result of the inadequate regulation of muscle tone coordination by the CNS, which results from insult to the basal ganglia or extrapyramidal tracts. This category of cerebral palsy accounts for 10% to 15% of all cases of cerebral palsy.

The two forms of dyskinetic cerebral palsy are athetoid and dystonic (Pellegrino & Dormans, 1998). Athetoid cerebral palsy is a result of damage to the basal ganglia and is characterized by chorea (i.e., jerky, rapid, random movements) and athetosis (i.e., writhing, slow movements). Dystonic cerebral palsy is characterized by slow and twisting abnormal movements of the trunk or extremities that may involve abnormal posturing. In other words, with a voluntary change in position,

Classification System for Cerebral Palsy

Spastic—described by the extremities involved. Characterized by prolonged primitive reflexes, increased deep tendon reflexes (DTRs), rigidity, clonus, contractures, and scoliosis
  Diplegia—all extremities involved, lower > upper
  Quadriplegia—all extremities involved
  Hemiplegia—one side involved, upper > lower
  Double hemiplegia—both sides involved
Dyskinetic—characterized by abnormal voluntary movements
  Hyperkinetic, or choreoathetoid—large, jerky, and purposeless movements
  Dystonic—slow and twisting abnormal movements
Ataxic—described by the degree of muscle control, coordination of movements, and balance
Mixed—spasticity and dyskinesias can be present together

From National Institute of Neurological Disorders and Stroke. (2001). *Cerebral palsy: Hope through research*; Web site: www.ninds.nih.gov/health_and_medical/pubs/cerebral_palsyhtr.htm.

the extremity moved shifts into an abnormal position and stays in that position (Pellegrino & Dormans, 1998). The Task Force on Childhood Motor Disorders (2001) stated their preference for using "dystonic hypertonia" to describe this form of cerebral palsy.

Ataxic

The third motor dysfunction group of cerebral palsy is ataxia. Neurologic damage is present in the cerebellum. Ataxia includes a range of conditions marked by the degree of muscle tone and coordination of movements and balance. These conditions can range from ataxic to hypotonic to atonic. Children with ataxia walk with an unstable, wide-based gait and have some difficulty trying to move a hand or arm voluntarily or timing such movement. Increased or decreased muscle tone may be present (Pellegrino & Dormans, 1998). The incidence of this type of cerebral palsy is approximately 5% to 10% (NINDS, 2001; Pellegrino & Dormans, 1998).

Mixed

The final motor dysfunction group of cerebral palsy is the mixed group, in which more than one type of motor pattern is found as a result of many defects to various areas of the brain. The term "mixed" is also used when no one motor pattern is dominant. Spasticity and dyskinesia can exist either alone or together (Pellegrino & Dormans, 1998).

The etiology of cerebral palsy may be due to a number of risk factors. Sometimes a cause for the diagnosis of cerebral palsy is never clearly identified. The possible causes are delineated by the period of time when the insult to the brain may have occurred in a child's life. Most incidences of congenital cerebral palsy are unknown (NINDS, 2001). Table 18-1 lists the causes of cerebral palsy according to the following time periods: prenatal, labor and delivery, perinatal, childhood (i.e., postnatal), and other. During the prenatal period, both maternal and gestational risk factors are included. Noetzel and Miller (1998) ascertained that 75% to 90% of the etiology of cerebral palsy occurs between conception and delivery, and 10% to 25% occurs after delivery.

In the past, clinicians had often diagnosed cerebral palsy as a result of asphyxia when they did not know the cause. Today,

Causes of Cerebral Palsy

Time Period	Causes
Prenatal	**Maternal** Diabetes or hyperthyroidism Exposure to radiation or toxins Malnutrition Seizure disorder or mental retardation Infections Incompetent cervix Bleeding Polyhydramnios Genetic abnormalities Previous child with developmental disabilities Previous premature birth Previous fetal loss Medication use (e.g. thyroid, estrogen, progesterone) Inflammatory response Severe proteinuria **Gestational** Chromosomal abnormalities Genetic syndromes Teratogens Rh incompatibility infections Congenital malformations Fetal development abnormalities Problems in placental functioning Inflammatory response
Labor and delivery	**Labor and delivery complications** Premature delivery Prolonged rupture of membranes Fetal heart rate depression Abnormal presentations Long labor Preeclampsia Asphyxia
Perinatal	**Prematurity and associated problems** Sepsis and/or central nervous system (CNS) infection Seizures Intraventricular hemorrhage (IVH) Periventricular encephalomalacia (PVL) Meconium aspiration Days on mechanical ventilation Persistent pulmonary hypertension in newborn Intrauterine growth retardation Low birth weight
Childhood/postnatal	**Brain injury** Meningitis/encephalitis Toxins Traumatic brain injury Infections Stroke
Unknown	

Data from Griffin, H.D., Fitch, C.L., & Griffin, L.W. (2002). Causes and interventions in the area of cerebral palsy. *Infants and Young Children, 14*(3), 18-24; National Institute of Neurological Disorders and Stroke (NINDS). (2001). Cerebral palsy: Hope through research; Website: www.ninds.nih.gov/health_and_medical/pubs/cerebral_palsyhtr.htm; Dizon-Townson, D.S. (2001). "Preterm labour and delivery: A genetic predisposition. *Paediatr Perinat Epidemiol, 15* (suppl. 2), 57-62; MacLennan, A. (1999). A template for defining a causal relation between acute intrapartum events and cerebral palsy: International consensus statement. *B Med J, 319*, 1054-1060; Demott, K. (2001). E. coli infection quadruples risk of cerebral palsy. *OB/GYN News, 36*(18), 1; Schendel, D.E. (2001). Infection in pregnancy and cerebral palsy. *J Am Med Womens Assoc, 56*, 105-108.

asphyxia accounts for a very small percentage of cases of cerebral palsy. An international consensus statement has been written to outline specific criteria for a diagnosis of asphyxia (MacLennan, 1999).

Demott (2001) reported that *Escherichia coli* in the amniochorionic membranes of a very low birth weight (VLBW) infant multiplies the risk of cerebral palsy by four times. The presence of group B streptococcus triples the risk of cerebral palsy (Demott, 2001; Schendel et al, 2002). Chorioamnionitis was also found to be a strong risk factor for cerebral palsy and cystic periventricular leukomalacia in preterm and full-term infants (Wu & Colford, 2000). Additional risk factors include breech position, respiratory and vascular problems during labor and delivery, low Apgar scores, low birth weight, premature birth, maternal hyperthyroidism, newborn seizures, maternal proteinuria, maternal bleeding, abnormalities in the infant's nervous system (Moster et al, 2001; NINDS, 2001), and socioeconomic deprivation (Dolk et al, 2001).

It had been postulated that lower rates of cerebral palsy would result in mothers who received magnesium sulfate during pregnancy for tocolysis and preeclampsia. Recent clinical study has not found evidence for this finding. Instead, the risk appeared to be increased with the use of magnesium sulfate, and further study will serve to confirm the use of magnesium sulfate as a risk factor for cerebral palsy (Grether et al, 2000; Matsuda et al, 2000; Mittendorf et al, 2002). On the other hand, Gray and his colleagues (2001) found that the risk for cerebral palsy was lowered when corticosteroids were administered to mothers before the birth of their preterm (24 to 27 weeks' gestation) infant. Dosages are given to outweigh the risks.

Known Genetic Etiology

Cerebral palsy is rarely genetic, but a number of biochemical disorders and cerebral malformations may result in motor abnormalities. These conditions may be misdiagnosed as cerebral palsy, such as hypotonia, Duchenne muscular dystrophy, arginase deficiency, metachromatic leukodystrophy, adrenoleukodystrophy, heredity progressive spastic paraplegia, dopa-responsive dystonia, Lesch-Nyhan disease, Rett syndrome, ataxia telangiectasia, Niemann-Pick disease type C, and mitochondrial cytopathies (Gupta & Appleton, 2001; Raymond, 2002). On the other hand, some subtypes of cerebral palsy may be secondary to a genetic disorder, such as congenital ataxia and athetoid cerebral palsy. New knowledge in genetics may find a clearer genetic link in the etiology of cerebral palsy (Raymond, 2002).

Incidence and Prevalence

Approximately 10,000 infants born each year develop cerebral palsy (Centers for Disease Control and Prevention, National Center for Birth Defects and Developmental Disabilities, 2002). The incidence of cerebral palsy in the United States has remained steady or has slightly increased since 1970, mainly because of the decrease in incidence of kernicterus contrasted with the increase in very low birth weight and premature infants who survive (Lorenz et al, 1998). The incidence of cerebral palsy is increased with multiple births (Griffin et al, 2002).

The specific prevalence of cerebral palsy is 2 to 3 per 1000 live births, or 8000 to 12,000 children diagnosed each year with cerebral palsy (Schendel et al, 2002). Prevalence rates vary slightly in other countries: (1) Netherlands, 1977 to 1988, 1.51 per 1000 live births (Wichers et al, 2001); (2) Northern Ireland, 1981 to 1993, 2.24 per 1000 live births (Parkes et al, 2001); (3) northeastern England, 1970 to 1994, 1.6 to 2.3 per 1000 live births (Drummond & Colver, 2002); (4) four counties in England, 1984 to 1995, 2.2 per 1000 live births (Surman et al, 2002); and (5) Shiga Prefecture, Japan, 1977 to 1991, 1.34 per 1000 six-year-old children (Suzuki & Ito, 2002). Rates were higher in preterm and low birth weight infants. Recurrence risks are rare.

Clinical Manifestations at Time of Diagnosis

The three major elements leading to diagnosis of cerebral palsy are as follows: (1) a motor deficit with nonprogressive signs and symptoms, (2) failure of a child to reach normal motor milestones, and (3) CNS abnormality (Disabato, 2001). Diagnosis of cerebral palsy is based on an assessment of the child's developmental, functional, and physical abilities. If possible, medical history helps identify the cause of cerebral palsy. One or more forms of brain imagery are also done to aid in the diagnosis. When parents have related concerns, it is important for primary care providers to rule out other neurologic problems in conjunction with specialty consultations. The diagnosis of cerebral palsy is not given until after the child is 2 years of age because early muscle and motor tone abnormalities may signify another neurodevelopmental problem. Moreover, some children who first present with symptoms of cerebral palsy no longer have them after 24 months of age. This change is especially true in cases of prematurity, although other communication and learning problems may persist (Al-Sulaiman, 2001; NINDS, 2001).

Parents are often the first to discover a child's delayed or failed attainment of motor milestones at the appropriate time, or they may complain of difficulty in diapering their child. Other specific signs that may be noted by the parents or the clinician include poor head control and clenched hands after 3 months of age, no side protective reflexes after 5 months of age, extended Moro and atonic neck reflexes past 6 months of age, no parachute reflex after 10 months of age, crossing of the midline to reach objects before 12 months of age, hand preference before 18 months of age—sometimes as early as 6 months, and leg scissoring (Figure 18-1) in late infancy or the early toddler period. These signs can appear in one or both sides (NINDS, 2001). A more recently described sign of cerebral palsy in preterm infants is cramped synchronized general movements, which are noted by simultaneous contraction and relaxation of the muscles of the extremities in a "monotonous sequence" (Ferrari et al, 2002, p. 464). An assessment of normal and abnormal muscle tone is outlined in Box 18-2.

Clinical manifestations of cerebral palsy center on abnormal motor development, muscle tone, reflexes, and postures and are often associated with other disabilities (Disabato, 2001). Behavioral manifestations during infancy that may indicate cerebral palsy include irritability, a weak cry, poor sucking ability with tongue thrust, excessive sleep patterns, and little interest in surroundings. Infants may also sleep in a rag doll or

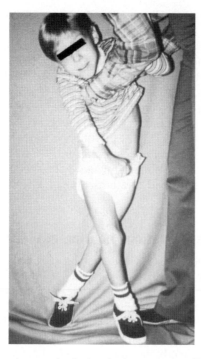

FIGURE 18-1 An example of scissoring in a young boy. (From Canale, S.T. & Beaty, J.H. [1995]. *Operative pediatric orthopaedics* [2nd ed.]. St. Louis: Mosby. Reprinted with permission.)

BOX 18-2

Assessment of Tone in Infants

NORMAL TONE
Infant moves well against gravity and lacks high- or low-tone characteristics.

LOW TONE
Infant lacks tone to move against gravity and resistance to passive movement; has low-tone postures (e.g., supine lying with arm abducted and/or legs abducted in a frogged position) or decreased movement.

HIGH TONE
Infant becomes stiff when moving against gravity; the neck or extremities resist passive movement; infant has hypertonic head reactions (e.g., hyperextension of the neck when rolling over and/or head pushing when supine or when pulled to sitting position); infants has high-tone posturing (e.g., increased extension of the head when supine lying, retracted shoulder girdle, lordosis of the back of extended lower extremities).

BOX 18-3

Clinical Manifestations of Cerebral Palsy

DELAYED GROSS MOTOR DEVELOPMENT
A universal manifestation
Delay in all motor accomplishments
Increases as growth advances
Delays more obvious as growth advances

ABNORMAL MOTOR PERFORMANCE
Very early preferential unilateral hand use
Abnormal and asymmetric crawl
Standing or walking on toes
Uncoordinated or involuntary movements
Poor sucking
Feeding difficulties
Persistent tongue thrust

ALTERATIONS OF MUSCLE TONE
Increased or decreased resistance to passive movements
Opisthotonic postures (exaggerated arching of back)
Feels stiff on handling or dressing
Difficulty in diapering
Rigid and unbending at the hip and knee joints when pulled to sitting position (an early sign)

ABNORMAL POSTURES
Maintains hips higher than trunk in prone position with legs and arms flexed or drawn under the body
Scissoring and extension of legs, with the feet plantar flexed in supine position
Persistent infantile resting and sleeping posture
Arms abducted at shoulders
Elbows flexed
Hands fisted

REFLEX ABNORMALITIES
Persistence of primitive infantile reflexes
   Obligatory tonic neck reflex at any age
   Nonpersistence beyond 6 mo of age
Persistence or hyperactivity of the Moro, plantar, and palmar grasp reflexes
Hyperreflexia, ankle clonus, and stretch reflexes elicited in many muscle groups on fast, passive movements

ASSOCIATED DISABILITIES*
Subnormal learning and reasoning (mental retardation in about two thirds of individuals)
Seizures
Impaired behavioral and interpersonal relationships
Sensory impairment (vision, hearing)

From Wong, D.L. et al. (2001). *Essentials of pediatric nursing* (6th ed.). St. Louis: Mosby. Reprinted with permission.
*May or may not be present.

---

floppy position or in an arched and extended position (i.e., opisthotonos). Later signs of abnormal mobility include "bunny hopping" (i.e., when crawling, the legs are brought forward together after the hands and arms are advanced) and "W sitting" (Pellegrino & Dormans, 1998). Children may also show signs of toe walking, crouched gait, foot deformity, flat foot, unequal leg length, or walking on the outer aspects of the feet. Box 18-3 summarizes the clinical manifestations of cerebral palsy.

Treatment

The goals of treatment of children with cerebral palsy are designed to maintain mobility and maximize joint range of motion, as well as to optimize muscle control and balance,

communication, and performance of activities of daily living. Treatment plans should be determined by the child's present and future health, developmental, and functional needs and goals and the parent's wishes if the child is too young to speak for himself or herself (Bottos et al, 2001; Gormley et al, 2001). A continuum of unfragmented care should prevail (Graveline et al, 2001). Box 18-4 summarizes the forms of treatment used in cerebral palsy. A developmental timeline for occupational, physical, and speech therapy, as well as orthotics, is included in Table 18-2 (Helsel et al, 2001).

BOX 18-4

Treatments for Cerebral Palsy

THERAPIES
Behavioral
Physical
Neuromuscular electrical stimulation
Occupational
Speech

ORTHOTIC DEVICES
Braces
Splints
Casting

ADAPTIVE EQUIPMENT
For functional use (e.g., eating utensils)
Switches
Computers
Boards
Scooters and tricycles
Wheelchairs

SURGERY
Orthopedic-corrective (e.g., tendon transfers, muscle lengthening)
Neurologic (e.g., neurectomies)
Selective dorsal rhizotomy

MEDICATIONS (FOR)
Spasticity
Pain
Constipation
Urinary tract infections
Upper respiratory infections
Decubitus ulcers
Other secondary complications and conditions

SPECIAL EDUCATION
Early intervention programs
Specialized learning programs and support services in school

TABLE 18-2

Developmental Timeline for Specific Therapies and Orthotics

Age	OT	PT	Speech	Orthotics
0-3 mo Hemiparetic, diparetic or tetraparetic not usually diagnosed Infant	Yes—developmental screening and follow-up treatment as needed Feeding addressed	Maybe—most likely involved if child has orthopedic issues	Probably not—only if severe oral motor deficit that may affect speech production	Probably not—may be involved if child has orthopedic issues
3-12 mo Infant	Yes—usually if hemiparetic or tetraparetic Fine motor development, feeding, ADL, cognitive and sensory issues	Yes—hemiparetic, diparetic, or tetraparetic Gross motor development, range of motion, etc.	Probably not—see above	Probably not—see above
1-3 yr Toddler	Yes—usually if hemiparetic or tetraparetic Usually outpatient Diparetics at times for visual motor or oral motor issues	Yes—hemiparetic, diparetic, or tetraparetic Usually outpatient	Yes—if tetraparetic Hemiparetic or diparetic if diaphragm involved or significant oral motor involvement Usually outpatient	Yes—may be for hemiparetic, diparetic, or tetraparetic as needed
3-6 yr Preschool	Yes—may also see diparetics from this age on for ADLs Outpatient and/or school	Yes—outpatient and/or school	Yes—outpatient and/or school	Yes—as needed
6-12 yr School years	Yes—usually school, but may also have outpatient postsurgical treatment for "tune-ups" and skills not related to school performance	Yes—see OT description for this age-group	Yes—usually school based May require additional therapy if augmentative communication system introduced	Yes—to update orthotics as needed for growth and development
12 yr–adult Adolescent to adulthood	Yes—may continue at school and/or out-patient for specific "tune-up" or functional independence issues, adaptive equipment, or postoperatively	Yes—may continue at school and/or outpatient for specific "tune-up" or functional independence issues, adaptive equipment, or postoperatively	Possibly—at school or to introduce and train with new augmentative communication device	Yes—generally to replace worn-out equipment or postoperatively

From Helsel, P., McGee, J., & Graveline, C. (2001). Physical management of spasticity. *J Child Neurol, 16,* 25.
OT, Occupational therapy; *PT,* physical therapy; *ADL,* activities of daily living.

Physical and Occupational Therapy

During infancy and toddlerhood, when most presumptive diagnoses take place, the first line of treatment involves physical and occupational therapy. The aim of these therapies is to enhance motor development, minimize the development of contractures, and prevent deterioration or weakening of the muscles (NINDS, 2001). For example, strength training has been used with good results (Damiano et al, 2002). Physical therapists have also used neuromuscular electrical stimulation in tandem with standard active and passive therapies to improve joint mobility, control muscle movement and strength, and reduce spasticity. Neuromuscular electrical stimulation has not been found useful for every muscle group but has been used successfully in muscle groups responsible for achieving task-oriented activities (Dali et al, 2002; Sommerfelt et al, 2001).

From the preschool years through adolescence, the aim of a physical and/or occupational treatment program is to help a child with cerebral palsy function optimally in the classroom. Gross motor skills, muscle control, balance, and coordination are needed for sitting and moving. Fine motor skills, muscle control, and coordination are needed for writing and holding materials. Motor, cognitive, and language skills also are needed for self-care activities. Bowel and bladder control and prevention of pressure ulcers are important to learn at this time. Independent ambulation may be decreased in adolescents using an orthotic device because of contractures, a lack of motivation, or weight gain, and they may choose to use a wheelchair to maximize their energy (Pellegrino & Dormans, 1998).

Other Therapies

Speech therapy should be recommended if an oromotor deficit exists. Augmentative communication devices may be warranted (Helsel et al, 2001).

Living with cerebral palsy may be frustrating and difficult for many children. Behavioral therapy or counseling may be needed at any point in a child's life (NINDS, 2001).

Orthotic Devices

Orthotic devices, which include braces and splints, usually accompany therapy when it alone no longer helps the child. Orthotic devices are used to provide stability to the joints, maintain the optimal range of motion of the joints, prevent the occurrence or progression of contractures, and control involuntary movements. The most common types of orthoses are the short arm or leg cast or splint, the hand splint, and the molded ankle-foot orthosis (MAFO), which is worn inside the shoe. Other types of adaptive equipment include devices for functional use (e.g., eating utensils), switches, computers, boards for positioning a child (e.g., on his or her side or in the prone or supine positions), scooters, tricycles, and wheelchairs. In severe cases, wheelchairs and gait trainers are constructed and molded for an individual child (Figure 18-2; Dursun et al, 2002; Teplicky et al, 2002; White et al, 2002). In each case, the orthosis is designed for a child and altered as the child grows or the condition changes.

Pharmacotherapy

Tilton & Maria (2001) wrote a consensus statement on pharmacotherapy for spasticity. Decision making in treatment

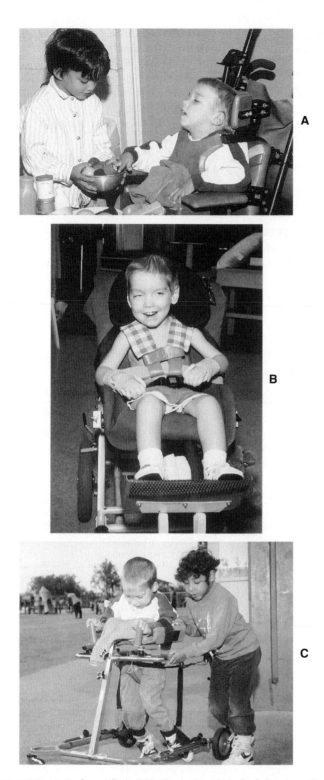

FIGURE 18-2 A and **B,** Individualized wheelchair. **C,** Gait trainer. (From Radcliffe, K.T. [1998]. *Clinical pediatric physical therapy.* St. Louis: Mosby. Reprinted with permission.)

approaches includes age, compliance, degree of spasticity, dosage, co-morbidity, costs, known adverse effects, and prior health and medication history. Dantrolene sodium (Dantrium), baclofen (Lioresal oral and intrathecal [after 4 years of age]), diazepam (Valium), phenol and alcohol blocks, and botulinum toxin A injections have been helpful in increasing function and reducing spasticity in general and for upper and lower extremities specifically (Albright et al, 2001; Autti-Ramo et al, 2001; Boyd et al, 2001; Edgar, 2001; Houltram et al, 2001; Koman et al, 2001; Linder et al, 2001; Love et al, 2001). Clinicians must choose muscles for injection in which resulting weakness will not inhibit function. Ambulation may also improve with continuous intrathecal baclofen infusion. This medication has been found to be most effective for spasticity in the lower extremities (Edgar, 2001). The effect of these drugs is individual, and continued study is needed to understand the most common adverse effects and long-term efficacy (Butler & Campbell, 2000). As stated below under Surgery, many researchers and experts in the field emphasize the use of multiple treatment modalities for the greatest effectiveness (Desloovere et al, 2001; Goldstein & Harper, 2001; Graham, 2001; Molenaers et al, 2001).

Pain management in cerebral palsy is discussed less frequently. Roscigno (2002) discussed the common medications used to reduce spasticity and addressed whether there is research evidence to determine if the pain associated with spasticity is decreased with the use of these medications. Intrathecal baclofen and botulinum toxin A are the only agents that have provided any evidence of pain relief. Additional research is needed (Nolan et al, 2000).

Medications are also prescribed for secondary conditions as they occur. These include treatment for constipation, urinary tract infections, upper respiratory infections, decubitus ulcers, and other secondary complications and conditions.

Surgery

Surgery for cerebral palsy is not usually an early choice of intervention. Both orthopedic and neurologic forms of surgery have been performed, but orthopedic surgery is not usually performed until after a child is 6 years old. A child attains independent ambulation by this age if independence is at all possible. Orthopedic surgery is performed to achieve greater leg movement and gait control, as well as to correct any extremity deformities. Orthopedic surgery is done to correct hip subluxation or dislocation and spinal deformities (e.g., scoliosis), to promote muscle balance and joint stabilization, to prevent contractures, and to reduce spasticity through muscle lengthening and tendon transfers (Boop et al, 2001; Flynn & Miller, 2002; Jacobs, 2001; NINDS, 2001). The child's degree of spasticity, size, and the effect of the spasticity on the child's life should be considered when determining surgical alternatives (Boop et al, 2001).

Selective dorsal rhizotomy is performed on many children with cerebral palsy. A meta-analysis of studies examining the effectiveness of selective dorsal rhizotomy, primarily in children with diplegic cerebral palsy, found that the surgery in combination with physical therapy is efficacious with a slight positive effect on gross motor function (McLaughlin et al, 2002). Over a 10-year period, 95% of subjects ($N = 208$) who had selective dorsal rhizotomy had improvement in passive range of motion, spasticity, and gait (Kim et al, 2001). Further study is needed to continue to look at the long-term effects of selective dorsal rhizotomy on the symptomatology of cerebral palsy, including its effects on quality of life and economic impact (Steinbok, 2001). In the meantime, the primary care

provider, surgeon, parents, and child should carefully discuss the risks and benefits.

Complementary and Alternative Therapies

Recent research evidence has found no significant gains from neurodevelopmental treatment (known also as the Bobath method, patterning, or NDT) or developmental skills (criterion-referenced) programs (Butler & Darrah, 2001; Mahoney et al, 2001). Therefore they should not be recommended.

The use of hyperbaric oxygenation to improve speech, attention, motor skills, and memory has recently been assessed in children with cerebral palsy. Results are preliminary and, to date, do not suggest significant improvements (Collet et al, 2001; Uszler et al, 2001).

Anticipated Advances in Diagnosis and Management

Computed tomography (CT), MRIs, and ultrasonography can be used to identify pathogenesis and to facilitate early diagnosis of cerebral palsy in low birth weight and premature infants (NINDS, 2001). Documentation of the effects of medications will further the continued efforts to improve the quality of life in children with cerebral palsy.

Associated Problems

Secondary conditions may be acute, chronic, or transitory and usually co-exist with cerebral palsy. These secondary conditions are listed in Box 18-5 (Bartlett & Palisano, 2000; NINDS, 2001). Plans for treatment, education, and habilitation must consider a child's individual presenting symptoms and complaints.

Cognitive Impairments

Learning disabilities or mental retardation frequently occurs in children with cerebral palsy. Mental retardation is usually most profound in children with spastic quadriplegia and least profound with hemiplegia, wherein more than 60% of the children have a normal intelligence quotient (IQ). Of children with spastic quadriplegia, diplegia, and extrapyramidal and mixed type of cerebral palsy, 50% to 60% also have mental retardation. Even if a child's IQ is normal, perceptual impairments and learning disabilities often exist. Any associated speech articulation problems, however, should not be misconstrued as mental retardation (Fennell & Dikel, 2001; Pellegrino & Dormans, 1998). Children with hemiplegia also have perceptual and attentional problems, with children with left hemiplegia experiencing more perceptual problems and inattention than children with right hemiplegia (Katz et al, 1998).

Seizures

Approximately 16% to as many as 94% of children with cerebral palsy will experience seizures. Seizures are most commonly seen in children with spastic quadriplegia and hemiplegia and are less common in children with dyskinesias and ataxia. Generalized tonic-clonic and minor motor types of seizures are the most common. Children with cerebral palsy who experience seizures usually also have intellectual disabilities. A genetic predisposition may also be present when

BOX 18-5

Problems Associated with Cerebral Palsy

COGNITIVE
Learning disabilities
Mental retardation

SEIZURE DISORDERS

LANGUAGE AND SPEECH DISORDERS
Articulation
Vocal strength and quality
Language processing

VISION
Refractive errors
Strabismus
Amblyopia
Cataracts
Retinopathy of prematurity
Cortical blindness
Homonymous hemianopsia (hemiplegia)

HEARING
Conductive
Sensorineural

OTHER SENSORY
Tactile hypersensitivity or hyposensitivity
Dyspraxia
Balance and movement problems
Proprioception difficulties
Stereognosis

MOTOR
Prolonged primitive reflexes
Absence of protective reflexes
Delayed motor milestones
Hip subluxation and dislocation
Scoliosis
Contractures

FEEDING AND EATING PROBLEMS
Chewing, sucking, and swallowing deficits
Drooling
Hypoxemia
Fatigue
Under weight or overweight
Gastroesophageal reflux
Aspiration

BOWEL
Constipation
Encopresis

URINARY
Bladder control
Urinary retention
Urinary tract infections

DENTAL
Malocclusions
Enamel defects and caries
Gum hyperplasia (with phenytoin)

PULMONARY
Respiratory infections
Pneumonia

SKIN
Decubitus ulcers
Latex allergy

BEHAVIORAL AND EMOTIONAL
Behavioral disorders
Attention deficit (hyperactivity) disorder, all forms
Self-injurious behaviors
Depression
Autism
Growth failure
Other

---

seizures and cerebral palsy are present in a child (Wallace, 2001). (See Chapter 25 for a further discussion of seizure disorders.)

Speech Impairments

The same muscle tone problems that make it difficult for children with cerebral palsy to move also create oromotor problems. Limitations in trunk movements and positioning may limit lung capacity, which is needed for strength in speaking both clearly and loudly. Problems in articulation, called dysarthrias, are caused by muscle tone deficiencies (NINDS, 2001). In recent years, computers and adaptive equipment (e.g., switches) have allowed individuals with speech problems to dramatically improve their communication (Figure 18-3).

Sensory Deficits

Vision. Children with cerebral palsy may develop a number of visual problems, including refractive error, strabismus, amblyopia, cataracts, retinopathy of prematurity, and cortical blindness. The majority of all children with cerebral palsy develop strabismus (Gersh, 1998b); about 75% develop some form of refractive errors (i.e., most often farsightedness); and approximately 25% with hemiplegia develop homonymous hemianopsia (the inability to see toward the affected side) (NINDS, 2001). Visual field size and binocular optokinetic nystagmus have been found in more than 50% of a sample of 47 children (Guzzetta et al, 2001).

Hearing. Children with cerebral palsy experience hearing impairments at a greater frequency than in the general population. The hearing loss is either sensorineural (i.e., damage to the auditory nerve and/or the inner ear) or, more commonly, conductive (i.e., as a result of anatomic abnormalities and/or frequent otitis media). Hearing impairments further add to speech and communication delays (NINDS, 2001).

Other Sensory Deficits. As a result of damage to the parietal lobe of the brain, children with cerebral palsy have deficits in other sensory functions. These deficits may include tactile hypersensitivity or hyposensitivity, dyspraxia (i.e., difficulty in

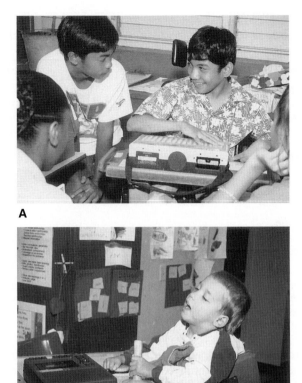

A

B

FIGURE 18-3 **A,** Child using an augmentative communication device. **B,** Child using a switch-activated tape player to sing along with music. (From Radcliffe, K.T. [1998]. *Clinical pediatric physical therapy.* St. Louis: Mosby. Reprinted with permission.)

using one's senses to plan movements), balance difficulties, and problems with proprioception, stereognosis, and movement (NINDS, 2001).

Motor Impairments

Successful attainment of motor milestones is always delayed in children with cerebral palsy. Some children's primitive reflexes persist and protective reflexes never develop, thus permanently blocking their ability to ambulate. Poor muscle tone and control often lead to secondary physical problems (e.g., hip dislocation, scoliosis, contractures), which create further motor impairment and other medical problems related to basic physiologic functioning. In the worst-case scenario, these impairments are life threatening.

Hip Subluxation and Dislocation, Scoliosis, and Contracture. Subluxation and dislocation of the hip are common in children with cerebral palsy. Subluxation occurs in approximately 25% of children with spastic cerebral palsy, and immobile children with spastic quadriplegia are especially at risk. Complications can include further motor impairment, positioning difficulties, pain, chronic arthritis, scoliosis, and hygienic concerns (Gersh, 1998b).

Scoliosis can result from unequal muscle tension resulting from the cerebral palsy or from poor posture or positioning in seating and recumbent positions. The degree of scoliosis

directly coincides with the amount of spasticity and neurologic damage present. The prevalence of scoliosis varies from 5% to 65% (Gersh, 1998b).

Shortening and misalignment of the muscles can be created by a constant pull of tight muscles or spasticity or by diminished muscle use, which may lead to contractures. Contractures in the lower extremities are most often seen in children with spastic quadriplegia and diplegia. Contractures in the upper extremities are most commonly found in children with spastic hemiplegia (Gersh, 1998b).

Feeding and Eating Problems

Feeding and eating difficulties are common in children with cerebral palsy, primarily as a result of orofacial muscle impairments. Compromised cardiopulmonary functioning, as well as poor muscle tone (i.e., either hypertonic or hypotonic) in the neck, shoulders, and trunk, can impede the process of eating. Specifically, muscle tone and function deficits create problems with sucking, chewing, swallowing, and aspiration. Increased drooling and gastroesophageal reflux may also occur. Feeding and eating disabilities are most often seen in children with the athetoid type of cerebral palsy. Early and severe feeding problems are a predictor for later growth, nutritional, and developmental outcomes. An interdisciplinary assessment is always warranted, and consideration of placement of a gastrostomy tube may be needed (Fung et al, 2002; Motion et al, 2002).

Bowel Problems

Constipation is a common and often chronic condition in children with cerebral palsy. Low muscle tone or spastic abdominal muscles can prevent contractility and pressure to adequately advance and empty the bowel contents. Further reasons for constipation include lack of exercise; inability to sense the signals of a bowel movement; painful defecations; inadequate fluid intake; a diet lacking in fruits, vegetables, and fiber; medications; a fear of toileting; poor positioning on the toilet; and behavior problems (Gersh, 1998b). Bowel incontinence, or encopresis, can also occur in cerebral palsy. Good dietary and bowel management is imperative.

Urinary Problems

Problems with bladder control and urinary retention that occur in cerebral palsy are often the result of neurologic insults (NINDS, 2001). Cognitive disabilities may reduce a child's ability to sense bladder fullness and signals to urinate. A combination of incomplete bladder emptying, infrequent voiding, severe fluid restriction, and urinary reflux increase the likelihood of frequent urinary tract infections, as do chronic constipation, improper perineal hygiene, and motor impairments. Overall, children with cerebral palsy are three times as likely to have urinary tract infections as the general population (Gersh, 1998b). Prompt treatment of urinary tract infections is imperative.

Dental Problems

Malocclusions commonly occur in children with cerebral palsy as a result of orofacial muscle tone deficiencies. An overbite or underbite can affect chewing and speech. Tooth enamel defects also occur frequently and if untreated may lead to dental caries.

Children who have seizures and take phenytoin (Dilantin) often experience hyperplasia (i.e., excessive growth of the gums). Problems with gum disease and oral hygiene can occur (Gersh, 1998b). Other medications taken for spasticity (e.g., sedatives, barbiturates) can reduce the amount of saliva, increasing the propensity for dental caries.

Pulmonary Effects

Alterations in positioning caused by abnormal muscle tone and spasticity, immobility, scoliosis, and contractures can affect pulmonary function and place children with cerebral palsy at a higher risk for respiratory infections (e.g., pneumonia). When respiratory infections occur, they often linger beyond the usual period because many children have difficulty coughing and blowing their nose. Aspiration and gastroesophageal reflux can also cause pneumonia. Knowing the warning signs of respiratory infection and pneumonia is important for health professionals and families because pneumonia is the leading cause of death in children with cerebral palsy (Reddihough et al, 2001). Children with severe dysphagia who show abnormal respiratory rates and fatigue during feeding are likely hypoxemic.

Skin Problems

Skin breakdown leading to raw and excoriated skin and decubitus ulcers is a common problem in children and adolescents with cerebral palsy—especially when mobility is compromised. Thorough skin assessment and protection of bony prominences while a child is seated or recumbent are necessary. Prompt and aggressive treatment of any evidence of skin breakdown is necessary. During infancy, when the child is in diapers, and later, in adolescence, when the child is menstruating, are times when vigilance is needed.

Latex Allergy

An association between cerebral palsy and latex allergy has recently been reported. Primary care providers should be mindful of the risk for anaphylaxis if a child has had repeated surgeries and ventriculoperitoneal shunts (Nolan et al, 2000).

Behavioral and Emotional Problems

As a result of exaggerated and prolonged existence of primitive reflexes—especially the startle reflex, infants and children with cerebral palsy overreact to the mildest amounts of stimulation. These children easily become tired and frustrated, and they may become demanding and uncooperative (Jacobs, 2001). Approximately 20% of children with cerebral palsy may also develop attention deficit hyperactivity disorder (Gersh, 1998a; see Chapter 12).

Prognosis

Prognosis, similar to treatment, depends on the type and severity of the cerebral palsy. In general, the more extremities involved, the more severe the involvement, and the greater the feeding and developmental disability, the worse the prognosis (Liptak et al, 2001; NINDS, 2001). On the other hand, increased quality of life, functional status, and formal and informal social supports enhance prognosis (Bjornson & McLaughlin, 2001; Robinson et al, 2001).

TABLE 18-3	
Prognosis for Independent Ambulation Based on Selected Motor Milestones	
Prognosis and Developmental Milestone	**Time (Mo)**
HEAD BALANCE	
Good	<9
Guarded	9-20
Poor	>20
SITTING	
Good	<24
Guarded	24-36
Poor	>36
GRAWLING	
Good	<30
Guarded	30-61
Poor	>61

From DePaz, A.C., Jr., Burnett, S.M., & Braga, L.W. (1994). Walking prognosis in cerebral palsy: A 22-year retrospective. *Dev Med Child Neurol, 36,* 130-134. Modified with permission.

Prognosis is also specifically discussed in terms of independent ambulation. If primitive reflexes are generally still present at 12 months of age and the protective reflexes are not yet present or the child has not walked by 6 to 7 years of age, the child will not ambulate independently (Pellegrino & Dormans, 1998). Table 18-3 gives locomotor prognoses based on attainment of selected motor milestones (DePaz et al, 1994).

Few studies have been completed on survival statistics for persons with cerebral palsy. Pharoah and Hutton (2002) found that mortality was affected by the degree of physical, sensory, and mental disability. Low birth weight was also a factor. Pneumonia was found to be the most common cause of death in persons with cerebral palsy living in Victoria, Australia between the years 1970 to 1995 (Reddihough et al, 2001). The presence of co-morbidities does appear to affect mortality.

PRIMARY CARE MANAGEMENT

Health Care Maintenance
Growth and Development

Growth retardation does not occur in all cases of cerebral palsy. Children who are nonambulatory or have spastic quadriplegia or seizures are shorter in height than peers of the same age (NINDS, 2001). Bone mineral density is decreased in children with cerebral palsy, resulting in osteopenia and a risk for fractures (Henderson et al, 2002; Tasdemir et al, 2001).

Obtaining accurate measurements for height and weight can be challenging if a child experiences motor difficulty and has contractures. When height cannot be measured in either a standing or recumbent position, the upper arm length (UAL) and lower leg length (LLL) measurements are adequate. Accurate measuring also monitors changes in spasticity, tone, contracture, and scoliosis. Triceps and subscapular skinfold thicknesses should also be obtained. The North American Growth in Cerebral Palsy Project's Web site (http://www.people. virginia.edu/~mon-grow/) lists full explanations for measuring each form of anthropometric techniques. Growth charts for children with cerebral palsy are anticipated in the next decade. Weight may be recorded from a standing position on a standardized scale or while the child is sitting or supine on a chair or hammock scale (e.g., Hosey). Primary care providers may most easily obtain an accurate weight by having a parent hold the child and step on the scale and then subtracting the parent's weight.

An interdisciplinary team is needed to longitudinally observe the development of a child with cerebral palsy. Periodic assessments of the child's mental, motor, language, self-care, and emotional development are warranted. Many general and specific screening instruments can be used by primary care providers and should be an important part of a child's care (see Chapter 2).

Assessment of a child's cognitive status is important because of the presence of mental retardation in many children with cerebral palsy, as well as physical limitations and speech and language problems that may make determining a child's true cognitive abilities difficult (Fennell & Dikel, 2001). Standardized intelligence tests for infants and children are appropriate, but someone experienced in examining children with motor and language delays should conduct this assessment.

Motor assessment is most often completed by the physical or occupational therapist. Videotaping a child's movements, in combination with computer gait analysis, has greatly enhanced the abilities of the physical therapist and physiatrist to plan and treat motor deficits and complications.

Speech and language problems can be screened by using, for example, the Preschool Language Scale or the Denver Articulation Screening Examination. There are also specific screening tools that assess a child's receptive and expressive language ability (see Chapter 2). Primary care providers must accurately assess parental reports of language skills, however, because parents often overestimate the number of spoken words by counting grunts and partial words. A speech therapist is the best person to assess language skills. Because of the many feeding and eating problems in infancy, a language assessment should be done in conjunction with a nutritional assessment when solid foods are introduced at about 6 months of age.

Self-care skills should be assessed throughout childhood and adolescence during history taking at each primary health care visit. This assessment can be done through an interview, a questionnaire, or a standardized test (e.g., Functional Independence Measure for Children [WeeFIM] or the Pediatric Evaluation of Disability Inventory). How quickly children adjust to a new communication strategy or device may indicate their cognitive level (Willard-Holt, 1998).

Emotional development is another important area for periodic assessment. Although there are a number of available instruments that measure self-concept and self-esteem, a good discussion with a trusted health professional is usually adequate for obtaining an understanding of how a child is coping at home, school, and other environments.

Diet

Undernutrition is most often seen during infancy in children with cerebral palsy. After any medical reasons for such difficulty are determined, further problems must be assessed.

Exercises to improve facial muscle tone can be initiated. If a child has trouble controlling the jaw or keeping the mouth closed, external assistance or supports can be applied. Children may also have oral tactile defensiveness and require a program of desensitization to different textures and a food plan developed around the foods that they will eat. Other children do not feel the food or drink in their mouths, so most of the food or liquid falls out of the mouth, creating skin problems. These children may also drool excessively.

Nutritional status often improves over time as a result of improved oromotor, gross motor, and fine motor skills; general improvement in health status; and better nutritional intake. Decreased independent mobility in late childhood and adolescence can even lead to a child being overweight (Anderson, 1998; Gersh, 1998b). This needs to be guarded against because becoming overweight can significantly affect motor performance and peer acceptance.

As a result of hypersensitivity, parents may need to try different nipples until one is found that the infant prefers. The size of the nipple hole may also need to be increased if thickened formula is prescribed. Motor problems may inhibit a child from being an independent feeder. Adaptive equipment can be designed for a growing child at each developmental stage. Most importantly, bottle feeding or baby foods should not be forced on an infant because there is a high risk for aspiration—a risk that is lifelong for children with severe cerebral palsy (Anderson, 1998). A nutritionist and an occupational therapist can suggest ways to help a child with oromotor difficulties and supplement the diet to ensure a child receives adequate calories (Anderson, 1998).

Some children with severe cerebral palsy may eventually need a feeding tube surgically inserted in the stomach. A child's oral feeding ability, degree of malnutrition, and health complications (i.e., respiratory distress) during feeding must be carefully assessed, however, before a permanent tube is placed. A temporary nasogastric tube can be prescribed during an acute illness. In any event, careful lifelong monitoring of a child's feeding abilities and nutritional status is critically important in cerebral palsy.

Safety

Children with motor impairments and seizure disorders are at increased risk for injury. Special concern should be taken when physical activities, car seats, and environmental surroundings are chosen for children with cerebral palsy. Children with cerebral palsy may not be restricted in the type of physical activity (e.g., canoeing), but adult supervision is needed. Seizure precautions and helmets may be necessary for children with seizure disorders. Car seats should be appropriately padded and positioned to protect a child's head—especially if head control is an issue. These precautions apply to any seating arrangement. A child's environment should be free of sharp edges in case of unexpected falls and roomy enough for the child to maneuver. If the child is in a wheelchair, the home environment should be wheelchair accessible. Some engineers are specially trained to suggest adaptations to homes, daycare settings, or schools to make them more wheelchair accessible. Home emergency plans should account for a child in a wheelchair, and local police and fire departments should be alerted.

Immunizations

Pertussis. Children with seizure disorders are at increased risk of seizure after receiving the pertussis vaccine. The risks and benefits of administering the pertussis vaccine when a child is at risk for seizures should be explained to the family, and the acellular form of the vaccine should be given in conjunction with tetanus and diphtheria (Committee on Infectious Diseases, 2000). Children with cerebral palsy who do not have seizures should maintain the regular schedule.

Measles. Children with a seizure disorder are also at risk for a seizure after receiving the measles vaccine in the form of the measles-mumps-rubella (MMR) vaccine. Because of the complications of measles, the high probability of contracting measles, and the unlikelihood of having a seizure after the immunization is administered, however, the standard schedule for measles vaccination should be followed (Committee on Infectious Diseases, 2000).

Chickenpox (Varicella). Children with cerebral palsy should be immunized against varicella. For children with severe cerebral palsy in whom complications of the disease could be life threatening, prophylactic treatment of varicella exposure in unimmunized children with oral acyclovir or varicella-zoster immunoglobulin should be recommended over the vaccine (Committee on Infectious Diseases, 2000).

Haemophilus Influenzae Type B. A 7-valent pneumococcal polysaccharide-protein conjugate vaccine (Prevnar, PCV7) is indicated for children with cerebral palsy and should be given according to the regular immunization schedule. This vaccination may be repeated after age 2 years if the child also has a chronic respiratory condition. The use of the 23-valent polysaccharide vaccine after age 2 years (PPV23; e.g., Pneumovax 23) may be warranted (Centers for Disease Control and Prevention, Advisory Committee on Immunization Practices, 2000).

Influenza Vaccine. Children with cerebral palsy are at risk for complications of influenza. Influenza vaccines and chemoprophylaxis should be given to children with cerebral palsy living in institutions during epidemics of influenza A (Committee on Infectious Diseases, 2000). Although the Committee on Infectious Diseases of the American Academy of Pediatrics does not recommend the influenza vaccine for all children with cerebral palsy, children who are severely affected and experience repeated respiratory infections would benefit from the yearly vaccine.

Other Immunizations. Children with cerebral palsy should receive immunizations for mumps, rubella, diphtheria, tetanus, pneumococcal infections, hepatitis B, and polio as recommended (Committee on Infectious Diseases, 2000). Hepatitis A vaccine should be given only if the child's place of residence is in a location of high incidence and community prophylaxis is being done (Centers for Disease Control and Prevention, Advisory Committee on Immunization Practices, 1999).

Screening

Vision. A pediatric ophthalmologist should annually assess the eyes of children with cerebral palsy because of the many types of visual impairments that may occur. Vision can also be screened each time the child comes for a primary care visit and a referral made to an ophthalmologist by the preschool years.

When performing a visual acuity test, children with motor problems may have difficulty showing which way an E points and those with speech problems may have difficulty naming the letters. Allen cards may be useful for screening.

Glasses often are prescribed for refractive errors. Contact lenses are contraindicated in children with cerebral palsy because their motor impairments inhibit placement and removal of the lenses. Glasses should be placed correctly on a child's face, and adaptive equipment (e.g., Velcro straps) may be recommended for comfortable and correct placement. Patching and surgery may be recommended for other vision complications associated with cerebral palsy (e.g., strabismus, amblyopia) (Gersh, 1998b).

Hearing. A pediatric audiologist should regularly check the hearing of a child with cerebral palsy. For specific diagnostic information, an audiologist will use a tympanometer and evoked response audiometry. An otolaryngologist also may assess hearing loss along with the audiologist (Gersh, 1998b).

Children with sensorineural hearing loss may be fitted with a hearing aid. A speech therapist may join the assessment team when the hearing aid is placed to facilitate language development through words or signs (Gersh, 1998b). Proper maintenance and use of hearing aids by children and families will help a child to optimally interact with the environment.

Dental. Children with cerebral palsy need a dentist who has experience with children with movement and motor disorders. The environment of the dentist's office must be accessible, with a chair that allows for easy transfer from a wheelchair if the child uses one. The chair must also protect fragile skin and support spastic extremities. Children with cerebral palsy should visit the dentist at least every 6 months and more often if a child also has a seizure disorder and is taking phenytoin (Dilantin) for the prevention or early treatment of gum hyperplasia (Gersh, 1998b). Sedation may be necessary for children with severe spasticity.

Malocclusions can be prevented through oromotor exercises to improve muscle tone around the oral cavity. An interdisciplinary team consisting of the nutritionist, occupational therapist, and speech-language pathologist can plan exercises to reduce the oral reflexes that can lead to development of overbites or underbites. This team can also address drooling problems and help a child to swallow saliva and keep the tongue in the mouth. If drooling persists, surgery may be warranted. Adaptive equipment (e.g., an altered toothbrush or a washcloth for washing the teeth) may be appropriate (Gersh, 1998b).

Blood Pressure. Routine screening is recommended.

Urinalysis. Routine screening is recommended.

Hematocrit. Routine screening is recommended.

Tuberculosis. Routine screening is recommended.

Condition-Specific Screening

Motor and Movement Problems. A motor assessment should be done at each primary care visit. Body alignment and positioning; passive and active range of motion; and signs of hip dislocation, spinal deformities, contractures, and movement patterns (e.g., gait disturbances) should be assessed and measured when appropriate (Blackman, 1997). Goniometric measurements of the joint mobility and motion of the knee and ankle can assist in screening for abnormalities in tone. Use of radiographs and MRIs may be needed for further diagnosis (NINDS, 2001). Palisano and his associates (1997) have developed a five-level classification system for gross motor function in children with cerebral palsy that is included in Box 18-6. Additional examination of the reliability and validity of the classification system for children under 2 years of age is needed. Reliability and validity are present over time in 1- to 12-year-olds (Wood & Rosenbaum, 2000). Correct management and follow-through by the child and family are necessary to prevent the development of further complications and can be useful in planning and evaluating interventions (Palisano et al, 2000).

Exercise should also be encouraged. Elements of flexibility, strength, endurance, and balance can be incorporated in an individualized physical fitness program (Preboth, 2000). Research is needed to better assess the benefits of exercise on blood pressure, cholesterol, mobility, and quality of life in children with cerebral palsy (Rimmer, 2001).

Common Illness Management

Differential Diagnosis

Fever. Children experience many febrile episodes in their lives as a result of the many viruses and bacteria that are present in their environment. Children with cerebral palsy are prone to respiratory and urinary tract infections and may also get gastrointestinal infections. In each of these infections, fever is usually an accompanying symptom. Children with cerebral palsy must be seen by a primary care provider if they are under 6 months of age, have had a fever over 38.6° C for 3 or more days without symptoms, appear acutely ill with undefined symptoms, or have had a seizure with a fever. A physical assessment and laboratory work need to be done by the primary care provider at this time for an accurate diagnosis and treatment.

Respiratory Tract Infections. Children with cerebral palsy are susceptible to upper and lower respiratory tract infections, namely, otitis media, sore throats, rhinorrhea, sinusitis, and influenza. Asthma is more prevalent in premature infants with cerebral palsy. Routine management of these problems is warranted with careful monitoring of the resolution of the infection. Sometimes these infections are not resolved with one round of antibiotics, and complications can occur (e.g., additional hearing loss from a case of otitis media). Referral to a specialist may be recommended.

Pain with an infection is difficult to assess in children with severe cerebral palsy. For example, the typical sign of pulling on the ear for an ear infection may not be present. Parents are often able to discern subtle signs in their child (e.g., increased irritability, decreased energy, less vocalizations, increased drooling) or to think that the child is just not acting like himself or herself. Children can also be asked "yes" or "no" questions to identify the source of pain. If a child uses a communication system, signs or symbols can be used to describe pain. Children's pain scales (e.g., the Wong Faces Scale) can be used by primary care providers to further assess a child's pain.

It is important to stress the high probability of pneumonia occurring after an initial upper respiratory infection or bout of influenza in children with severe cerebral palsy. Pneumonia can also be caused by aspiration and gastroesophageal reflux. Careful monitoring must be done to prevent a life-threatening situation. Children with cerebral palsy are unable to expectorate well and handle increased secretions. Dehydration can easily occur. Hospitalization may be suggested as a preventive measure to ensure close observation of any changes in a child's health status. If a child is being cared for at home, parents must understand the importance of the treatment plan and contact their clinician if the condition worsens.

Dermatology Issues. Skin problems arise from positioning in chairs and beds when bony prominences rubbing against hard surfaces occur. Decubitus ulcers can occur quickly, and vigilant skin management is warranted, especially in nonmobile children. Protection of the bony prominences with soft protective coverings is usually enough, but medical attention should be obtained for persistent areas of redness. Assess for latex allergy.

Urinary Tract Problems. Common problems are incontinence, urgency, frequency, and retention. Urinary tract infections also occur more frequently in children with cerebral palsy. The age of the child and any communication problems may impede obtaining detailed information on pain or other symptoms experienced by the child. A urinalysis and urine cultures must be ordered if there is any suspicion of a urinary tract infection or the cause of the fever or other symptoms cannot be identified. After one or two urinary tract infections have been diagnosed and treated in a child with cerebral palsy, the parents and primary care provider may be better able to identify the signs and symptoms associated with this condition in the child. This information is especially important in a child who is nonverbal and should be recorded in the child's chart for further reference.

Antibiotic therapy and additional comfort measures (e.g., increased fluid intake, perineal hygiene after voiding, increased rest, taking acetaminophen based on body weight) are recommended for urinary tract infections. Follow-up is imperative after a urinary tract infection and should include a urine culture 2 to 3 days after initiation and at the conclusion of antibiotic therapy to assess its effect. If recurrent urinary tract infections occur, referral to a pediatric urologist is recommended.

Gastrointestinal Problems. Parents may note that a child has abdominal pain, straining with hard stools, rectal bleeding, soiled underwear, and a distended, hard abdomen when constipated. Documenting the signs and symptoms of this problem in infants or nonverbal children is especially important. Increased fluids, exercise, and a healthy diet with additional fiber are recommended. A bowel management program designed by an interdisciplinary team may be needed if constipation is an ongoing problem. A program of stool softeners, laxatives, suppositories, and enemas can be prescribed, as well as suggestions for proper positioning and seating on the toilet. The effectiveness of the program should be closely monitored and recorded.

A pattern for bowel elimination should be initiated and maintained. Urinary tract infections and impactions are complications of chronic constipation. Constipation is a very difficult long-term problem to deal with when a child is immobile and has a poor appetite. Bowel management programs must be individualized and evaluated periodically.

BOX 18-6
Gross Motor Function Classification System

LEVEL I
Walks without restrictions, limitations in more advanced gross motor skills

Before 2nd birthday: Infants move in and out of sitting and floor sit with both hands free to manipulate objects. Infants crawl on hands and knees, pull to stand and take steps holding on to furniture. Infants walk between 18 mo and 2 yrs of age without the need for any assistive mobility device.

From age 2 to 4th birthday: Children floor sit with both hands free to manipulate objects. Movements in and out of floor sitting and standing are performed without adult assistance. Children walk as the preferred method of mobility without the need for any assistive mobility device.

From age 4 to 6th birthday: Children get into and out of, and sit in, a chair without the need for hand support. Children move from the floor and from chair sitting to standing without the need for objects for support. Children walk indoors and outdoors and climb stairs. Emerging ability to run and jump.

From age 6 to 12th birthday: Children walk indoors and outdoors and climb stairs without limitations. Children perform gross motor skills including running and jumping, but speed, balance, and coordination are reduced.

LEVEL II
Walks without assistive devices, limitations walking outdoors and in the community

Before 2nd birthday: Infants maintain floor sitting but may need to use their hands for support to maintain balance. Infants creep on their stomach or crawl on hands and knees. Infants may pull to stand and take steps holding onto furniture.

From age 2 to 4th birthday: Children floor sit but may have difficulty with balance when both hands are free to manipulate objects. Movements in and out of sitting are performed without adult assistance. Children pull to stand on a stable surface. Children crawl on hands and knees with a reciprocal pattern, cruise holding onto furniture, and walk using an assistive mobility device as preferred methods of mobility.

From age 4 to 6th birthday: Children sit in a chair with both hands free to manipulate objects. Children move from the floor to standing and from chair sitting to standing but often require a stable surface to push or pull up on with their arms. Children walk without the need for any assistive mobility device indoors and for sort distances on level surfaces outdoors. Children climb stairs holding onto a railing but are unable to run or jump.

From age 6 to 12th birthday: Children walk indoors and outdoors and climb stairs holding onto a railing but experience limitations walking on uneven surfaces and inclines and walking in crowds or confined spaces. Children have at best only minimal ability to perform gross motor skills, such as running and jumping.

LEVEL III
Walks with assistive mobility devices, limitations walking outdoors and in the community

Before 2nd birthday: Infants maintain floor sitting when the low back is supported. Infants roll and creep forward on their stomachs.

From age 2 to 4th birthday: Children maintain floor sitting often by "W-sitting" (sitting between flexed and internally rotated hips and knees) and may require adult assistance to assume sitting. Children creep on their stomach or crawl on hands and knees (often without reciprocal leg movements) as their primary methods of self-mobility. Children may pull to stand on a stable surface and cruise short distances. Children may walk short distances indoors using an assistive mobility device and adult assistance for steering and turning.

From age 4 to 6th birthday: Children sit on a regular chair but may require pelvic or trunk support to maximize hand function. Children move in and out of chair sitting using a stable surface to push on or pull up with their arms. Children walk with an assistive mobility device on level surfaces and climb stairs with assistance from an adult. Children frequently are transported when travelling for long distances or outdoors on uneven terrain.

From age 6 to 12th birthday: Children walk indoors or outdoors on a level surface with an assistive mobility device. Children may climb stairs holding onto a railing. Depending on upper limb function, children propel a wheelchair manually or are transported when travelling for long distances or outdoors on uneven terrain.

LEVEL IV
Self-mobility with limitations; children are transported or use power mobility outdoors and in the community

Before 2nd birthday: Infants have head control, but trunk support is required for floor sitting. Infants can roll to supine and may roll to prone.

From age 2 to 4th birthday: Children floor sit when placed but are unable to maintain alignment and balance without use of their hands for support. Children frequently require adaptive equipment for sitting and standing. Self-mobility for short distances (within a room) is achieved through rolling, creeping on stomach, or crawling on hands and knees without reciprocal leg movement.

From age 4 to 6th birthday: Children sit on a chair but need adaptive seating for trunk control and to maximize hand function. Children move in and out of chair sitting with assistance from an adult or a stable surface to push or pull up on with their arms. Children may at best walk short distances with a walker and adult supervision but have difficulty turning and maintaining balance on uneven surfaces. Children are transported in the community. Children may achieve self-mobility using a power wheelchair.

From age 6 to 12th birthday: Children may maintain levels of function achieved before age 6 or rely more on wheeled mobility at home, at school, and in the community. Children may achieve self-mobility using a power wheelchair.

LEVEL V
Self-mobility severely limited even with the use of assistive technology

Before 2nd birthday: Physical impairments limit voluntary control of movement. Infants are unable to maintain antigravity head and trunk postures in prone and sitting. Infants require adult assistance to roll.

From age 2 to 12th birthday: Physical impairments restrict voluntary control of movement and the ability to maintain antigravity head and trunk postures. All areas of motor function are limited. Functional limitations in sitting and standing are not fully compensated for through the use of adaptive equipment and assistive technology. At Level V, children have no means of independent mobility and are transported. Some children achieve self-mobility using a power wheelchair with extensive adaptations.

DISTINCTIONS BETWEEN LEVELS I AND II
Compared with children in Level I, children in Level II have limitations in the ease of performing movement transitions; walking outdoors and in the community; the need for assistive mobility devices when beginning to walk; quality of movement; and the ability to perform gross motor skills, such as running and jumping.

DISTINCTIONS BETWEEN LEVELS II AND III
Differences are seen in the degree of achievement of functional mobility. Children in Level III need assistive mobility devices and frequently orthoses to walk, while children in Level II do not require assistive mobility devices after age 4 yr.

DISTINCTIONS BETWEEN LEVELS III AND IV
Differences in sitting ability and mobility exist, even allowing for extensive use of assistive technology. Children in Level III sit independently, have independent floor mobility, and walk with assistive mobility devices. Children in Level IV function in sitting (usually supported), but independent mobility is very limited. Children in Level IV are more likely to be transported or use power mobility.

DISTINCTIONS BETWEEN LEVELS IV AND V
Children in Level V lack independence even in basic antigravity postural control. Self-mobility is achieved only if the child can learn how to operate an electrically powered wheelchair.

Drug Interactions

Medications may be prescribed to reduce spasticity. These medications should be used with caution if the adolescent with cerebral palsy is pregnant. Diazepam (Valium) and baclofen should be monitored closely if used in a child with a seizure disorder because seizure control could be altered. Dantrolene (Dantrium) and baclofen are also affected by the concurrent use of alcohol, so drinking should be strongly discouraged in the older adolescent. Dantrolene should also be discouraged if a degree of spasticity is needed for daily functioning. Adverse respiratory symptoms and bowel function should also be monitored when using Dantrolene (Wilson et al, 2003). No other specific drug interactions have been noted with medications used to treat spasticity. A discussion of the drug interactions for seizure medications is included in Chapter 25. The occurrence of constipation must be examined for its cause—whether because of diet or as a side effect of medications such as anticonvulsants or iron. Overall, drug interactions need to be assessed when a child with cerebral palsy is receiving multiple medications.

Developmental Issues

Sleep

A clinical manifestation of cerebral palsy in infancy is prolonged sleeping patterns interfering with nutritional intake and developmental stimulation. A variety of other sleeping problems may also exist with cerebral palsy, such as severe hypoxemia during sleep, which may require a sleep apnea monitor. A neutral body position (i.e., with the neck and head slightly flexed) is encouraged during sleep. Bolsters or wedges can be used to facilitate appropriate positions. A side-lying position should be used for children who drool so that excessive fluid can drain out of the mouth instead of down the throat, which may cause choking.

Toileting

If children with cerebral palsy are able to be toilet trained, then—like any other children—they will give their parents clues of their physical and neurologic readiness. The potty chair or toilet must adequately support the child's body and minimize the risk of skin breakdown from extended sitting. The child's feet must be able to touch the floor to assist the abdominal muscles in pushing. Special potty chairs can be made, or current chairs can be adapted with input from a physical or occupational therapist.

Discipline

Parents often discipline children who have special health and developmental needs differently from their siblings. As a result of their special needs and possible past health care emergencies, parents are often reluctant to discipline a child with cerebral palsy. Parents must be consistent when disciplining all their children; both parents should agree with the type of discipline; and the discipline should be developmentally appropriate for a child's mental age.

Child Care

Many child care programs today include children both with and without chronic conditions. Depending on the child's degree of functional and cognitive severity, parents may choose an early intervention or an inclusive child care program. Children enrolled in an early intervention program will have an individualized family service plan (IFSP) developed for the child's development and family support. In an inclusive child care program, the providers will need instruction by the parents or a member of the child's interdisciplinary health care team on the best approaches for care and development. Parents of a child with cerebral palsy must be aware that the risk for infection is greater in settings where children are together (e.g., in daycare) (Committee on Infectious Diseases, 2000) and that issues of safety and accessibility are also important to consider.

Schooling

Children with cerebral palsy may need to use different augmentative communication systems (e.g., communication boards, computers, keyboard voice synthesizers; Figure 18-3). Adaptive equipment for communicating, seating, writing, and reading may be needed and should be obtained. Occupational, physical, and speech therapy, as well as adaptive physical education, is often needed and individually planned for either group or individual sessions. An aide may be required to help a child with cerebral palsy with personal needs. A diagnosis of homonymous hemianopsia, in which the child can see straight ahead but not to the affected side, is important for a seating assignment in the front of the classroom (Gersh, 1998a; NINDS, 2001; Pellegrino & Dormans, 1998). Transportation to and from school, transfer needs between classrooms, and emergency health and safety plans must also be arranged with school personnel.

Along with an interdisciplinary health plan, which is mandatory for children with cerebral palsy, an accommodation plan or individualized educational plan (IEP) is also necessary, which may include physical, occupational, speech, and behavioral therapy and other formal and informal support services (Bartlett & Palisano, 2002). (See Chapter 5 for more information on daycare and school issues and needs.) Today most children with cerebral palsy participate in inclusive education. Special attention must be paid to a child's cognitive ability and social integration into the regular classroom by assisting the child with peer relationships and self-esteem. Primary care providers can assess the school situation, including safety, performance, ambulation, and fatigue issues during well-child visits.

During the junior high and high school years, children with cerebral palsy can be enrolled in vocational or college preparation programs, depending on career interests and the presence and degree of mental retardation. Adolescents with cerebral palsy may also experience renewed social problems during these years as they cope with adolescent self-esteem and contemplate life after school. Work and social opportunities are not as prevalent in the adult years as they are during childhood for individuals with special health and developmental needs. Adolescents often experience depression when faced with the stigma of their condition and rejection in social situations. School performance also may decrease. Parents and professionals should look for signs that might alert them to these psychosocial issues during adolescence and offer support and professional counseling where needed.

Sexuality

Social isolation, long-term low self-esteem, and a poor body image can affect the development of intimate relationships. Sexuality education can help the adolescent develop a positive self-esteem and body image. Role modeling and exposure to social situations can be planned and executed. During their adolescent years, children do not often discuss sexuality and their feelings with parents. Therefore peers, other adults, and support groups should be available to help adolescents with cerebral palsy with these issues. In some cases, referral to a sexuality counselor may be needed.

Female adolescents should begin to receive gynecologic care if they are sexually active. Because of spasticity, contractures, or poor muscle control, a woman's position for such an exam should be adapted; the Sims position is often better than the lithotomy position. The woman may also require assistance in positioning menstrual pads or tampons. An annual pelvic ultrasound can be done by the physician for baseline data. Pregnancy is possible for women with cerebral palsy.

Transition into Adulthood

The transition to adulthood in children with cerebral palsy must address medical care, equipment needs, communication, activities of daily life, mobility, nutrition, vocational decisions, transportation, housing, and social needs. Throughout life, optimal independence should be encouraged and learned helplessness avoided. Independence and self-advocacy should be stressed during the transitional period between adolescence and adulthood. Adolescents with cerebral palsy need to take an active role in choosing a primary care provider and health care interdisciplinary team. Their participation in decision making about dietary choices, medications, surgical interventions if needed, and adaptive equipment is important.

Vocational decisions should be discussed, and plans for successful employment should be determined. When deciding on a site for college or work, the physical layout, wheelchair accessibility, availability of personal aides, housing, and repair shop for wheelchairs and any other adaptive equipment must be considered and resources identified. Independence in the use of public transportation should be planned. Individuals with mild cerebral palsy may be able to drive. Independent living or assisted living arrangements must be discussed; and individuals should be placed on waiting lists early if living outside the home is desired because these lists are often years long. Social needs, including activities consistent with an individual's abilities, planned social programs, and opportunities to develop successful relationships, should be met. Most important, adolescents making the transition to adulthood must participate to the greatest possible extent in decisions about their lives.

Family Concerns and Resources

In incidences of mild cerebral palsy, the effects on the family may be minimal or nonexistent (see Chapter 4). Parents were most unhappy when they received the child's diagnosis close to the child's first birthday, when the child's prognosis for physical and mental development was poorer, and when the child was born with low birth weight and/or prematurely (33 weeks' gestation and less). A greater degree of unhappiness or dissatisfaction was related to maternal depression (Baird et al, 2000). Respite care is highly recommended to give families time away from the constant responsibilities of caring for a child with cerebral palsy. Social support, identification of and intervention with stressors, presence of parenting skills for caring for a child with special needs, and the use of early intervention programs are all very important for family well-being (Glasscock, 2000).

Grandparents are also affected. Grandparents of a child with a physical disability, especially the maternal grandmother, are an especially important support system (Findler, 2000).

There are no specific cross-cultural or religious concerns for children with cerebral palsy, although a stigma based on the diagnosis is attached to all families. The visibility of this condition may create more of a stigma in some cultures than in others, and in some cultures the child may be hidden from the outside world.

RESOURCES

A variety of local, state, and regional services for children with cerebral palsy exist. Appropriate resources and organizations are usually listed in the local yellow pages of the telephone directory under "Social Services and Organizations." Several books and organizations can also offer assistance to families and professionals:

Books

Campbell, S.K., vander Linden, D.W., & Palisano, R.J. (Eds.). (2000). *Physical therapy for children* (2nd ed.). Philadelphia: W.B. Saunders. (Available from W.B. Saunders, The Curtis Center, Independence Square West, Philadelphia, PA 19106.)

Dormans, J.P. & Pellegrino, L. (1998). *Caring for children with cerebral palsy.* Baltimore: Paul H. Brookes. (Available from Paul H. Brookes Publishing Co, PO Box 10624, Baltimore, MD 21285-0624.)

Geralis, E. (Ed.). (1998). *Children with cerebral palsy: A parent's guide.* Bethesda, Md.: Woodbine House. (Available from Woodbine House, 6510 Bells Mill Rd, Bethesda, MD 20817.)

Kennedy, M.A. (2001). *My perfect son has cerebral palsy: A mother's guide of helpful hints.* Bloomington, Ind.: 1stBooks Library. (Available from 1stBooks Library, 2595 Vernal Pike, Bloomington, IN 47404.)

Leonard, J.F., Myers, M.E., & Cadenhead, S.L. (1997). *Keys to parenting a child with cerebral palsy.* Hauppauge, N.Y.: Barrons Educational Series, Inc. (Available from Barrons Educational Series, Inc, 251 Wireless Blvd, Hauppauge, NY 11788.)

Miller, F. & Bachrach, S.J. (1998). Cerebral *palsy: A complete guide for caregiving.* Baltimore: Johns Hopkins University Press. (Available from Johns Hopkins University Press, PO Box 19966, Baltimore, MD 21211.)

Organizations

American Academy for Cerebral Palsy and Developmental Medicine
6300 North River Rd, Suite 727
Rosemont, IL 60018-4226
(847) 698-1635, (847) 823-0536 (fax)
woppenhe@ucla.edu, http://www.aacpdm.org

DisABILITY Information and Resources
http://www.makoa.org
Provides information on products, services, computer accessibility, home automation and environmental control, governmental and legislative disability information, legal advice and advocacy, sports, travel, recreation, and assistive technology

National Disability Sports Alliance (NDSA)
25 Independence Way
Kingston, RI 02881
(401) 792-7130, (401) 792-7132 (fax)
info@ndsaonline.org, http://www.ndsaonline.org

North American Growth in Cerebral Palsy Project
Department of Pediatrics
University of Virginia
2270 Ivy Rd
Charlottesville, VA 22903
(888) 4CP-GROW
4CP-GROW@virginia.edu;
http://www.people.virginia.edu/~mon-grow/healthcare/home.htm

UCP National
1660 L Street NW, Suite 700
Washington, DC 20036
(800) 872-5827 (national office), (202) 973-7197 (voice/tty), (202) 776-0414 (fax)
ucpnatl@ucp.org; http://www.ucpa.org

Summary of Primary Care Needs for the Child with Cerebral Palsy

HEALTH CARE MAINTENANCE

Growth and Development

Undernutrition in infancy often leads to growth retardation.

Different techniques should be used to get height, arm and leg lengths, and skinfold measurements.

Weights may be attained via standing or sitting scales or recumbent lifts.

Overweight conditions may occur in adolescence if mobility decreases.

Delayed development in motor and communication skills is common.

Development strengths and weaknesses must be assessed and recorded.

Mental retardation and seizure disorders inhibit intellectual development.

An exercise program may be individually developed.

Diet

Infants can have difficulty with sucking, swallowing, and chewing; so assessment should be done early.

Drooling and aspiration can also be problems.

Nutritional concerns may be lifelong, and placement of a gastrostomy tube may be warranted in severe cases.

Referral to a nutritionist is needed.

Safety

Children are at risk for injury as a result of spasticity, muscle control problems, delayed protective reflexes, and potential seizures.

Positioning and adaptive equipment are often required.

Immunizations

If the etiology for seizure activity is unknown, the pertussis vaccine may be deferred or an acellular vaccine used when age appropriate.

The measles and varicella vaccines should be given as scheduled.

Haemophilus influenzae type B (Hib) vaccine and other immunizations should be given as scheduled.

Children with cerebral palsy are at risk for complications of influenza and varicella.

Fever management is necessary to decrease the possibility of febrile seizures.

Screening

Vision. A pediatric ophthalmologist should be seen during infancy because of the likelihood of vision problems.

Vision should be checked for acuity, refractive errors, strabismus, retinopathy of prematurity, and cataracts.

Hearing. Referral to a pediatric audiologist may be necessary during infancy to check for hearing problems and loss.

Both sensorineural and conductive hearing loss is possible.

Routine screening for conductive hearing problems and loss should be done.

Dental. Children should be evaluated by a dentist experienced with children with motor problems every 6 months.

Proper dental hygiene is needed.

Administration of phenytoin may cause hyperplasia of the gums; proper preventive care and early treatment of this condition are important.

Blood Pressure. Routine screening is recommended.

Urinalysis. Routine screening is recommended.

A referral to a pediatric urologist may be needed if the child has chronic urinary tract infections.

Hematocrit. Routine screening is recommended.

Tuberculosis. Routine screening is recommended.

Condition-Specific Screening

A motor assessment, including assessment for scoliosis, hip dislocation, and contractures, should be done at every well-child visit.

COMMON ILLNESS MANAGEMENT

Differential Diagnosis

Fever Management of fever is routine.

Respiratory Tract Infections. Respiratory infections should be promptly treated. Pneumonia may be life threatening to children with severe cerebral palsy. Follow-up is important.

Urinary Tract Infections. Treatment for urinary tract infections should be prompt, and follow-up is essential. Urinary tract abnormalities may also be present.

Gastrointestinal Problems. Constipation is a long-term problem for many children. A bowel management program may be needed.

Drug Interactions

No medications are routinely prescribed, except if a seizure disorder is also present.

DEVELOPMENTAL ISSUES

Sleep Patterns

Correct positioning is needed during sleep because sleep apnea can occur.

Toileting

Adaptive equipment is often needed for correct positioning on the toilet. Bladder and bowel training may be delayed.

Discipline

It is important that consistent and age-appropriate discipline measures be taken.

Continued

Summary of Primary Care Needs for the Child with Cerebral Palsy—cont'd

Child Care

Careful planning must be undertaken in choosing the best child care arrangements, especially regarding issues of safety, accessibility, health care needs, and increased rates of infection.

Schooling

Use individualized educational plans (IEPs) and inclusive classrooms. Specialized services and therapies for each child must be procured. Adaptive equipment and computers enhance a child's ability to learn.

Behavioral and school problems can occur in adolescence as a result of poor esteem and body image.

Sexuality

Opportunities for social activities should be arranged. Transportation needs are important to consider.

Opportunities for same-sex and opposite-sex relationships are needed. Classes in social interaction and sexuality may be needed.

Gynecologic exams should begin for women with adaptations to the normal positioning.

Reproductive issues should be discussed.

Transition into Adulthood

A child's independence and self-advocacy should be promoted. Future residential and vocational plans need to be addressed.

FAMILY CONCERNS

Respite care meets a family's needs.

Effects on individual family members must be assessed and addressed. Special support groups are available for fathers and siblings.

Family stigmas may be perceived.

REFERENCES

Albright, A.L., Barry, M.J., Shafron, D.H., & Ferson, S.S. (2001). Intrathecal baclofen for generalized dystonia. *Dev Med Child Neurol, 43*, 652-657.

Al-Sulaiman, A. (2001). Electroencephalographic findings in children with cerebral palsy: A study of 151 patients. *Funct Neurol, 16*, 325-328.

Anderson, S. (1998). Daily care. In E. Geralis (Ed.). *Children with cerebral palsy: A parent's guide* (2nd ed.). Bethesda, Md.: Woodbine House, pp. 101-146.

Autti-Ramo, I., Larsen, A., Taimo, A., & von Wendt, L. (2001). Management of the upper limb with botulinum toxin type A in children with spastic type cerebral palsy and acquired brain injury: Clinical implications. *Eur J Neurol, 8*(suppl. 5), 136-144.

Baird, G., McConachie, H., & Scrutton, D. (2000). Parents' perceptions of disclosure of the diagnosis of cerebral palsy. *Arch Dis Child, 83*, 475-480.

Bartlett, D.J. & Palisano, R.J. (2000). A multivariate model of determinants of motor change for children with cerebral palsy. *Phys Ther, 80*, 598-614.

Bartlett, D.J. & Palisano, R.J. (2002). Physical therapists' perceptions of factors influencing the acquisition of motor abilities of children with cerebral palsy: Implications for clinical reasoning. *Phys Ther, 82*, 237-249.

Bjornson, K.F. & McLaughlin, J.F. (2001). The measurement of health-related quality of life (HRQL) in children with cerebral palsy. *Eur J Neurol, 8*(suppl. 5), 183-193.

Blackman, J.A. (1997). *Medical aspects of developmental disabilities in children birth to three* (3rd ed.). Gaithersburg, Md.: Aspen Publishers.

Boop, F.A., Woo, R., & Maria, B.L. (2001). Consensus statement on the surgical management of spasticity related to cerebral palsy. *J Child Neurol, 16*, 68-69.

Bottos, M., Feliciangeli, A., Sciuto, L., Gericke, C., & Vianello, A. (2001). Functional status of adults with cerebral palsy and implications for treatment of children. *Dev Med Child Neurol, 43*, 516-528.

Boyd, R.N., Morris, M.E., & Graham, H.K. (2001). Management of upper limb dysfunction in children with cerebral palsy: A systemic review. *Eur J Neurol, 8*(suppl. 5), 150-166.

Butler, C. & Campbell, S. (2000). Evidence of the effects of intrathecal baclofen for spastic and dystonic cerebral palsy. *Dev Med Child Neurol, 42*, 634-645.

Butler, C. & Darrah, J. (2001). Effects of neurodevelopmental treatment (NDT) for cerebral palsy: An AACPDM evidence report. *Dev Med Child Neurol, 43*, 778-790.

Centers for Disease Control and Prevention, Advisory Committee on Immunization Practices. (2000). Preventing pneumococcal disease among infants and young children. *MMWR Morb Mortal Wkly Rep, 49*(RR09), 1-38.

Centers for Disease Control and Prevention, Advisory Committee on Immunization Practices. (1999). Prevention of hepatitis A through active or passive immunization: Recommendations of the Advisory Committee on Immunization Practices (ACIP). *MMWR Morb Mortal Wkly Rep, 48*(RR12), 1-37.

Centers for Disease Control and Prevention, National Center for Birth Defects and Developmental Disabilities. (2002). *Cerebral palsy among children.* Atlanta: Author.

Collet, J-P, Vanasse, M.M., Amar, P., Goldberg, M., Lambert, J., et al. (2001). Hyperbaric oxygen for children with cerebral palsy: A randomized multicentre trial. *Lancet, 357*, 582-586.

Committee on Infectious Diseases. (2000). *2000 red book: Report of the committee on infectious diseases* (25th ed.). Elk Grove Village, Ill.: American Academy of Pediatrics.

Dali, C., Hansen, F.J., Pedersen, S.A., Skov, L., Hilden, J., et al. (2002). Threshold electrical stimulation (TES) in ambulant children with CP: A randomized double-blind placebo-controlled clinical trial. *Dev Med Child Neurol, 44*, 364-369.

Damiano, D.L., Dodd, K., & Taylor, N.F. (2002). Should we be testing and training muscle strength in cerebral palsy? *Dev Med Child Neurol, 44*, 68-72.

Demott, K. (2001). E. coli infection quadruples risk of cerebral palsy. *OB/GYN News, 36*(18), 1.

DePaz, A.C., Jr., Burnett, S.M., & Braga, L.W. (1994). Walking prognosis in cerebral palsy: A 22-year retrospective. *Dev Med Child Neurol, 36*, 130-134.

Desloovere, K., Molenaers, G., Jonkers, I., De Cat, J., De Borre, L., et al. (2001). A randomized study of combined botulinum toxin type A and casting in the ambulant child with cerebral palsy using objective outcome measures. *Eur J Neurol, 8*(suppl. 5), 75-87.

Disabato, J.A. (2001). The child with neuromuscular or muscular dysfunction. In D.L. Wong, M. Hockenberry-Eaton, D. Wilson, M.L. Winkelstein, & P. Schwartz. (Eds.). *Wong's essentials of pediatric nursing* (6th ed.). St. Louis: Mosby, pp. 1240-1260.

Dizon-Townson, D.S. (2001). Preterm labour and delivery: A genetic predisposition. *Paediatr Perinat Epidemiol, 15*(suppl. 2), 57-62.

Dolk, H., Pattenden, S., & Johnson, A. (2001). Cerebral palsy, low birthweight and socio-economic deprivation: Inequalities in a major cause of childhood disability. *Paediatr Perinat Epidemiol, 15*, 359-363.

Drummond, P.M. & Colver, A.F. (2002). Analysis by gestational age of cerebral palsy in singleton births in north-east England 1970-94. *Paediatr Perinat Epidemiol, 16*, 172-180.

Dursun, E., Dursun, N., & Alican, D. (2002). Ankle-foot orthoses: Effect on gait in children with cerebral palsy. *Disabil Rehabil, 24*, 345-347.

Edgar, T.S. (2001). Clinical utility of botulinum toxin in the treatment of cerebral palsy: Comprehensive review. *J Child Neurol, 16*, 37-46.

Fennell, E.B. & Dikel, T.N. (2001). Cognitive and neuropsychological functioning in children with cerebral palsy. *J Child Neurol, 16*, 58-63.

Ferrari, F., Cioni, G.E., Roversi, C., Bos, M.F., Paolicelli, A.F., et al. (2002). Cramped synchronized general movements in preterm infants as an early marker for cerebral palsy. *Arch Pediatr Adolesc Med, 156,* 460-468.

Findler, L.S. (2000). The role of grandparents in the social support system of mothers of children with a physical disability. *Fam Soc, 81,* 370-381.

Flynn, J.M. & Miller, F. (2002). Management of hip disorders in patients with cerebral palsy. *J Am Acad Orthop Surg, 10,* 198-209.

Fung, E.B., Samson-Fang, L., Stallings, V.A., Conaway, M., Liptak, G., et al. (2002). Feeding dysfunction is associated with poor growth and health status in children with cerebral palsy. *J Am Diet Assoc, 102,* 361-368.

Gersh, E. (1998a). What is cerebral palsy? In E. Geralis (Ed.). *Children with cerebral palsy: A parent's guide* (2nd ed.). Bethesda, Md.: Woodbine House, pp. 1-34.

Gersh, E. (1998b). Medical concerns and treatment. In E. Geralis (Ed.). *Children with cerebral palsy: A parent's guide* (2nd ed.). Bethesda, Md.: Woodbine House, pp. 61-100.

Glasscock, R. (2000). A phenomenological study of the experience of being a mother of a child with cerebral palsy. *Pediatr Nurs, 26,* 407-413.

Goldstein, M. & Harper, D.C. (2001). Management of cerebral palsy: Equinus gait. *Dev Med Child Neurol, 43,* 563-569.

Gormley, M.E., Jr., Krach, L.E., & Piccini, L. (2001). Spasticity management in the child with spastic quadriplegia. *Eur J Neurol, 8*(suppl. 5), 127-135.

Graham, H.K. (2001). Botulinum toxin type A management of spasticity in the context of orthopaedic surgery for children with spastic cerebral palsy. *Eur J Neurol, 8*(suppl. 5), 30-39.

Graveline, C., Helsel, P., McGee, J., & Maria, B.L. (2001). Consensus statement on the physical management of spasticity. *J Child Neurol, 16,* 64-65.

Gray, P.H., Jones, P., & O'Callaghan, M.J. (2001). Maternal antecedents for cerebral palsy in extremely preterm babies: A case-control study. *Dev Med Child Neurol, 43,* 580-585.

Grether, J.K., Hoogstrate, J., Walsh-Greene, E., & Nelson, K.B. (2000). Magnesium sulfate for tocolysis and risk of spastic cerebral palsy in premature children born to women without preeclampsia. *Am J Obstet Gynecol, 183,* 717-725.

Griffin, H.D., Fitch, C.L., & Griffin, L.W. (2002). Causes and interventions in the area of cerebral palsy. *Infants Young Child, 14*(3), 18-24.

Gupta, R. & Appleton, R.E. (2001). Cerebral palsy: Not always what it seems. *Arch Dis Child, 85,* 356-361.

Guzzetta, A., Fazzi, B., Mercuri, E., Bertuccelli, B., Canapicchi, R., et al. (2001). Visual function in children with hemiplegia in the first years of life. *Dev Med Child Neurol, 43,* 321-329.

Helsel, P., McGee, J., & Graveline, C. (2001). Physical management of spasticity. *J Child Neurol, 16,* 24-30.

Henderson, R.C., Lark, R.K., Gurka, M.J., Worley, G., Fung, E.B., et al. (2002). Bone density and metabolism in children and adolescents with moderate to severe cerebral palsy. *Pediatrics, 110;* Web site: http://www.pediatrics.org/cgi/content/full/110/1/e5.

Houltram, J., Noble, I., Boyd, R.N., Corry, I., Flett, P., et al. (2001). Botulinum toxin type A in the management of equinus in children with cerebral palsy: An evidence-based economic evaluation. *Eur J Neurol, 8*(suppl. 5), 194-202.

Jacobs, J.M. (2001). Management options for the child with spastic cerebral palsy. *Orthop Nurs, 20,* 53-62.

Katz, N., Cermak, S., & Shamir, Y. (1998). Unilateral neglect in children with hemiplegic cerebral palsy. *Percept Mot Skills, 86,* 539-550.

Kim, D.S., Choi, J.U., Yang, K.H., & Park, C.I. (2001). Selective posterior rhizotomy in children with cerebral palsy: A 10-year experience. *Childs Nerv Syst, 17,* 556-562.

Koman, L.A., Brashear, A., Rosenfeld, S., Chambers, H., Russman, B., et al. (2001). Botulinum toxin type A neuromuscular blockade in the treatment of equinus foot deformity in cerebral palsy: A multicenter, open-label clinical trial. *Pediatrics, 108,* 1062-1071.

Linder, M., Schindler, G., Michaelis, U., Stein, S., Kirschner, J., et al. (2001). Medium-term functional benefits in children with cerebral palsy treated with botulinum toxin type A: 1-year follow-up using gross motor function measure. *Eur J Neurol, 8*(suppl. 5), 120-126.

Liptak, G.S., O'Donnell, M., Conaway, M., Chumlea, W.C., Worley, G., et al. (2001). Health status of children with moderate to severe cerebral palsy. *Dev Med Child Neurol, 43,* 364-370.

Lorenz, J.M., Wolliever, D.E., Jetton, J.R., & Paneth, N. (1998). A quantitative review of mortality and developmental disabilities in extremely premature newborns. *Arch Pediatr Adolesc Med, 152,* 425-435.

Love, S.C., Valentine, J.P., Blair, E.M., Price, C.J., Cole, J.H., et al. (2001). The effect of botulinum toxin type A on the functional ability of the child with spastic hemiplegia: A randomized controlled trial. *Eur J Neurol, 8*(suppl. 5), 50-58.

MacLennan, A. (1999). A template for defining a causal relation between acute intrapartum events and cerebral palsy: International consensus statement. *BMJ, 319,* 1054-1060.

Mahoney, G., Robinson, C., & Fewell, R.R. (2001). The effects of early motor intervention on children with Down syndrome or cerebral palsy: A field-based study. *J Dev Behav Pediatr, 22,* 153-165.

Matsuda, Y., Kouno, S., Hiroyama, Y., Kuraya, K., Kamitomo, M., et al. (2000). Intrauterine infection, magnesium sulfate exposure and cerebral palsy in infants born between 26 and 30 weeks of gestation. *Eur J Obstet Gynecol Reprod Biol, 91,* 159-164.

McLaughlin, J., Bjornson, K., Temkin, N., Steinbok, P., Wright, V., et al. (2002). Selective dorsal rhizotomy: Meta-analysis of three randomized controlled trials. *Dev Med Child Neurol, 44,* 17-25.

Minear, W.L. (1956). A classification of cerebral palsy. *Pediatrics, 18,* 841-852.

Mittendorf, R., Dambrosia, J., Pryde, P.G., Lee, K.S., Gianopoulos, J.G., et al. (2002). Association between the use of antenatal magnesium sulfate in preterm labor and adverse health outcomes in infants. *Am J Obstet Gynecol, 186,* 1111-1118.

Molenaers, G., Desloovere, K., De Cat, J., Jonkers, I., De Borre, L., et al. (2001). Single event multilevel botulinum toxin type A treatment and surgery similarities and differences. *Eur J Neurol, 8*(suppl. 5), 88-97.

Moster, D., Lie, R.T., Irgens, L.M., Bjerkedal, T., & Markestad, T. (2001). The association of Apgar score with subsequent death and cerebral palsy: A population-based study in term infants. *J Pediatr, 138,* 798-803.

Motion, S., Northstone, K., Emond, A., Stucke, S., & Golding, J. (2002). Early feeding problems in children with cerebral palsy: Weight and neurodevelopmental outcomes. *Dev Med Child Neurol, 44,* 40-43.

National Institute of Neurological Disorders and Stroke (NINDS). (2001). Cerebral palsy: Hope through research; Web site: http://www.ninds.nih.gov/health_and_medical/pubs/.

Noetzel, M. & Miller, G. (1998). Traumatic brain injury as a cause of cerebral palsy. In G. Miller & J. Clark (Eds.). *The cerebral palsies: Causes, consequences, and management.* Boston: Butterworth-Heinemann.

Nolan, J., Chalkiadis, G.A., Low, J., Olesch, C.A., & Brown, T.C. (2000). Anaesthesia and pain management in cerebral palsy. *Anaesthesia, 55,* 32-41.

Palisano, R.J., Hanna, S.E., Rosenbaum, P.L., Russell, D.J., Walter, S.D., et al. (2000). Validation of a model of gross motor function for children with cerebral palsy. *Phys Ther, 80,* 974-985.

Palisano, R., Rosenbaum, P., Walter, S., Russell, D., Wood, E., et al. (1997). Development and reliability of a system to classify gross motor function in children with cerebral palsy. *Dev Med Child Neurol, 39,* 214-223.

Parkes, J., Dolk, H., Hill, N., & Pattenden, S. (2001). Cerebral palsy in Northern Ireland: 1981-93. *Paediatr Perinat Epidemiol, 15,* 278-286.

Pellegrino, L. & Dormans, J.P. (1998). Definitions, etiology, and epidemiology of cerebral palsy. In J.P. Dormans & L. Pellegrino (Eds.). *Caring for children with cerebral palsy: A team approach.* Baltimore: Paul H. Brookes, pp. 3-30.

Pharoah, P.O. & Hutton, J.L. (2002). Effects of cognitive, motor, and sensory disabilities on survival in cerebral palsy. *Arch Dis Child, 86,* 84-71.

Preboth, M. (2000). Fitness in persons with cerebral palsy. *Am Fam Physician, 61,* 2548.

Raymond, G.V. (2002). Abnormal mental development. In D.L. Rimoin, J.M. Connor, R.E. Pyeritz, & B.R. Korf (Eds.). *Emery and Rimoin's principles and practice of medical genetics* (4th ed.). New York: Churchill Livingstone, pp.1046-1065.

Reddihough, D.S., Baikie, G., & Walstab, J.E. (2001). Cerebral palsy in Victoria, Australia: Mortality and causes of death. *J Paediatr Child Health, 37,* 183-186.

Rimmer, J.H. (2001). Physical fitness levels of persons with cerebral palsy. *Dev Med Child Neurol, 43,* 208-212.

Robinson, G., Msall, M.E., Tremont, M.R., Fournier, M., & Taylor, M. (2001). Health status, functional limitations, family supports, and health related quality of life in children with cerebral palsy. *J Dev Behav Pediatr, 22,* 347.

Roscigno, C.I. (2002). Addressing spasticity-related pain in children with spastic cerebral palsy. *J Neurosci Nurs, 34,* 123-134.

Schendel, D.E. (2001). Infection in pregnancy and cerebral palsy. *J Am Med Wom Assoc, 56,* 105-108.

Schendel, D.E., Schuchat, A., & Thorsen, P. (2002). Public health issues related to infection in pregnancy and cerebral palsy. *Ment Retard Dev Disabil Res Rev, 8,* 39-45.

Sommerfelt, K., Markestad, T., Berg, K., & Saetesdal, I. (2001). Therapeutic electrical stimulation in cerebral palsy: A randomized, controlled, crossover trial. *Dev Med Child Neurol, 43,* 609-613.

Steinbok, P. (2001). Outcomes after selective dorsal rhizotomy for spastic cerebral palsy. *Childs Nerv Syst, 17,* 1-18.

Surman, G., Newdick, H., Marques, M., & Johnson, A. (2002). Cerebral palsy rates among very low birthweight babies fell in the early 1990s. *Arch Dis Child, 86,* A14.

Suzuki, J. & Ito, M. (2002). Incidence patterns of cerebral palsy in Shiga Prefecture, Japan, 1977-1991. *Brain Dev, 24,* 39-48.

Tasdemir, H.A., Buyukavci, M., Akcay, F., Polat, P., Yildiran, A., et al. (2001). Bone mineral density in children with cerebral palsy. *Pediatr Int, 43,* 157-160.

Task Force on Childhood Motor Disorders. (2001). Workshop on classification and definition of disorders causing hypertonia in childhood; Web site: http://www.ninds.nih.gov/news_and_events/.

Teplicky, R., Law, M., & Russell, D. (2002). The effectiveness of casts, orthoses, and splints for children with neurological disorders. *Infants Young Child, 15,* 42-51.

Tilton, A.H. & Maria, B.L. (2001). Consensus statement on pharmacotherapy for spasticity. *J Child Neurol, 16,* 66-67.

Uszler, J.M., Heuser, G.M., Lacroix, A., Tremblay, J., Lassonde, S.D., et al. (2001). Hyperbaric oxygenation for cerebral palsy. *Lancet, 357,* 2052.

Wallace, S.J. (2001). Epilepsy in cerebral palsy. *Dev Med Child Neurol, 43,* 713-717.

White, H., Jenkins, J., Neace, W.P., Tylkowski, C., & Walker, J. (2002). Clinically prescribed orthoses demonstrate an increase in velocity of gait in children with cerebral palsy: A retrospective study. *Dev Med Child Neurol, 44,* 227-232.

Wichers, M.J. van der Schouw, Y.T., Moons, K.G., Stam, H.J., & van Nieuwenhuizen, O. (2001). Prevalence of cerebral palsy in The Netherlands (1977-1988). *Eur J Epidemiol, 17,* 527-532.

Willard-Holt, C. (1998). Academic and personality characteristics of gifted children with cerebral palsy: A multiple case study, *Except Child, 65,* 37-50.

Wilson, B.A., Shannon, M.T., & Stang, C.L. (2003). *Nurse's drug guide 2003.* Upper Saddle River, N.J.: Prentice-Hall.

Wood, E. & Rosenbaum, P. (2000). The gross motor function classification system for cerebral palsy: A study of reliability and stability over time. *Dev Med Child Neurol, 42,* 292-296.

Wu, Y.W. & Colford, J.M., Jr. (2000). Chorioamnionitis as a risk factor for cerebral palsy: A meta-analysis. *JAMA, 284,* 1417-1429.

19 Cleft Lip and Palate

Ginny Curtin and Anne Boekelheide

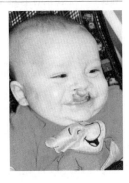

Etiology (Box 19-1)

The embryology of cleft lip with or without cleft palate is distinctly different from cleft palate alone. The cleft lip occurs when the median nasal and premaxillary prominences fail to fuse with the lateral maxillary prominences. The lip and alveolar ridge or primary palate is fully formed between 5 and 7 weeks of gestation. The presence of a cleft lip can hinder the closure of the palate. A cleft palate results from a failure of the palatine shelves to fuse between 6 and 12 weeks of gestation (Gorlin et al, 2001; Prescott et al, 2001).

Although the specific cause is usually unknown (Spritz, 2001), clefts can be divided into two categories: nonsyndromic and syndromic. The majority of clefts are nonsyndromic, meaning the cleft is not part of a pattern of malformation affecting other organs and systems. The term "multifactorial" (multiple genetic and environmental influences) is used to describe the etiology of nonsyndromic clefts. Examples of environmental factors that may increase the risk of a cleft occurring are maternal folic acid deficiency (Prescott et al, 2002) and teratogens such as maternal alcohol and tobacco use (Romitti et al, 1999); and folic acid antagonists and retinoic acid have been implicated but not definitively proven (Gorlin et al, 2001). A positive family history of oral facial clefts increases the incidence of nonsyndromic clefts.

A syndrome is a collection of two or more major anomalies that occur together. There are more than 350 syndromes that include oral facial clefts. Cleft palate alone is far more often associated with a syndrome than a cleft lip or cleft lip and palate (Gorlin et al, 2001).

Syndromic clefts can be grouped into categories based on the underlying etiology or defect. The first category would be single-gene disorders, such as Van der Woude syndrome. This condition is recognizable by the lower lip pits and has an autosomal dominant pattern of inheritance. Another category is chromosomal syndromes, such as velocardiofacial syndrome, which is a microdeletion of chromosome 22. This syndrome with velopharyngeal insufficiency or cleft palate is associated with cardiac malformation and developmental delay. There are also teratogenic syndromes that are caused by any agent that can adversely affect embryonic development. Examples of teratogenic syndromes include fetal alcohol syndrome and fetal hydantoin syndrome.

The fourth category of syndrome is actually called a sequence, such as holoprosencephaly (underdevelopment of the premaxilla and nasal septum, brain abnormalities) and Pierre Robin (U-shaped cleft palate, micrognathia [small lower jaw], glossoptosis [posteriorly rotated tongue]). Researchers postulated that in fetal development the micrognathia is the primary problem and the cleft palate is a result of the tongue being placed superiorly, obstructing the movement of the maxillary shelves in the midline. The suboptimal mandibular growth has been thought to be caused by a variety of factors. The factors vary from positional malformation in utero, intrinsic causes from chromosomal or teratogenic influences, neurologic or neuromuscular abnormalities inhibiting the tongue from normal movement into the floor of the mouth in utero, or connective tissue disorders (St. Hilaire & Buchbinder, 2000). Both holoprosencephaly and Pierre Robin sequence can have devastating consequences in the newborn period by interfering with the airway and normal swallowing.

Known Genetic Etiology

The knowledge of genetic etiology for syndromic clefts that include single-gene mutations and chromosomal abnormalities is more advanced than the understanding of the genetic causes for nonsyndromic clefts. Genetic influences are thought to play a major role, and recently there has been considerable effort to map and identify genes that constitute risk factors for nonsyndromic clefts (Spritz, 2001). In several studies, linkage and association analyses have suggested that several different genes are involved including those for transforming growth factor–alpha, transforming growth factor–beta$_{3a}$, retinoic acid receptor–alpha, BCL3, and MSX-1 (Kirschner & LaRossa, 2000). Animal models are an additional means of locating and testing candidate genes (Bender, 2000). As more is understood about the genetic influences on nonsyndromic clefts the question becomes more complex.

Incidence and Prevalence

Cleft lip and/or palate ranks among the most commonly occurring birth defects (Centers for Disease Control [CDC] National Center on Birth Defects and Developmental Disabilities). The generally accepted incidence rate of clefts worldwide is 1 in 700 births, although some ethnic differences exist (Murray, 2002). American Indians have an incidence of 3.6 in 1000 live births followed in descending order by Japanese, Chinese, whites, Hispanics, and blacks, with the lowest reported incidence of 0.3 in 1000. Incidence rates are based on varied reporting mechanisms, and problems occur with mixing together studies of live births, stillbirths, and spontaneous abortions. No registry or national database exists documenting cleft birth defects. Clefts may or may not be recorded when they are components of a known syndrome.

Etiology

Nonsyndromic—multifactorial
    Environmental
    Genetic
Syndromic
    Single-gene disorders
    Chromosomal abnormalities
    Teratogens
    Sequences

Clinical Manifestations at Time of Diagnosis

Cleft lip and palate—physical findings
Cleft palate—difficulty feeding because of infant's inability to create suction
Pierre Robin sequence—signs and symptoms of upper airway obstruction as a result of posterior position of tongue in the airway, micrognathia
Submucous cleft palate—nasal-sounding speech

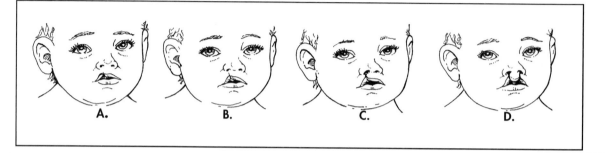

FIGURE 19-1 Varieties of lip clefts. **A, B,** and **C,** Unilateral, or one-sided, clefts in the lip and gum ridge. **D,** Bilateral, or two-sided, cleft. (From Moller, K.T., Starr, C.D., & Johnson, S.A. [1990]. *A parent's guide to cleft lip and palate.* Minneapolis: University of Minnesota Press. Modified with permission.)

Cleft lip and palate makes up approximately 50% of all oral facial clefts with a unilateral cleft lip occurring more often than a bilateral cleft lip. A left-sided cleft lip occurs twice as often as a right-sided cleft lip. Cleft lip alone makes up 25% of clefts and occurs more frequently in males with or without cleft palate. Females are affected more often with cleft palate alone.

Clinical Manifestations at Time of Diagnosis (Box 19-2)

Cleft lip is an obvious birth defect noted in the delivery room. It is described as unilateral or bilateral and incomplete or complete depending on whether the cleft extends into the nasal cavity (Figure 19-1). A microform cleft lip is characterized by very minor notching or the appearance of a well-healed surgical scar or "seam"; however, microform cleft lip is usually only described by a craniofacial team or plastic and reconstructive surgeon.

Cleft palate may involve the primary palate (lip and alveolus anterior to the incisive foramen) and the secondary palate (hard and soft palates) (Figure 19-2). A submucous cleft palate is characterized by a notch at the posterior spine of the hard palate, translucence at the midline, or bifid uvula.

No standard classification system to describe cleft palate exists (Kirschner & LaRossa, 2000); clinicians draw a diagram or use physical descriptors to define tissue deficiencies (Millard, 1980, 1993; Figure 19-3).

Infants with cleft palate only should be examined carefully for other anomalies, and as previously mentioned, all infants with clefts need a physical examination by a dysmorphologist (Willner, 2000). Some clefts of the palate are not detected by the staff in the delivery room. Infants who are unable to

successfully breast feed, are unable to "latch on," or exhibit difficulties with bottle feedings such as prolonged (greater than 30 to 45 minutes) feeding times should be reexamined carefully for the presence of a cleft. Even a small cleft of the soft palate usually produces ineffective sucking as a result of the infant's inability to create a vacuum to draw the milk out of the nipple (Curtin, 1990). The mother may initially report that the baby will nurse for 45 minutes yet does not seem satisfied. The mother's breasts may still feel engorged at the end of a feeding, and there is never a feeling that the breast is empty of milk. Frequent snacking usually results; however, urine output is inadequate and the baby continues to be fussy. After approximately 4 to 5 days of this feeding behavior, the infant becomes sleepier and lethargic and exhibits signs of dehydration, including weight loss (Livingstone et al, 2000). For some bottle-fed infants, the parents report that it may take more than 1 hour for the infant to consume 1 oz of formula. It is at this time that a palatal cleft may be noted. Somnolent, dehydrated 4-day-old infants may be hard to examine because they are resistant to opening their mouth. Insertion of a water-moistened gloved finger may be useful in examining palatal integrity (American Cleft Palate–Craniofacial Association, 2000).

Pierre Robin sequence often has a rather benign presentation with the findings of cleft palate, glossoptosis, and micrognathia (Box 19-3). Airway obstruction may not become evident until the infant is 2 weeks of age or until the first upper respiratory tract infection. Therefore it is prudent to observe these infants closely during the first months of life and consider a baseline pediatric pulmonary evaluation within the first weeks of life. The infants are able to maintain adequate oxygen and carbon dioxide saturations initially after birth, but they can tire over time with increased work of breathing. As infants grow,

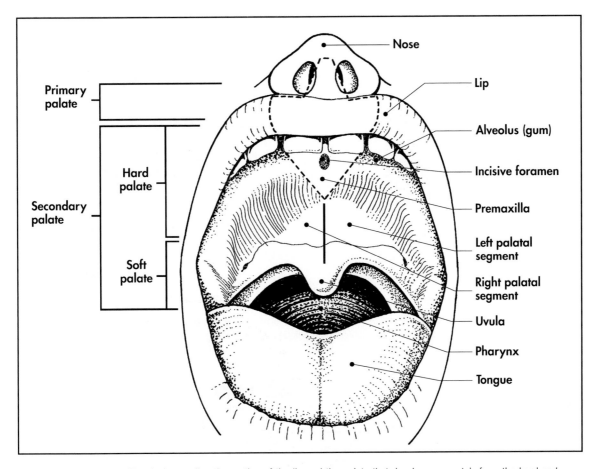

FIGURE 19-2 The dashes outline the portion of the lip and the palate that develops separately from the hard and soft palates. Unilateral clefts of the lip occur on one side or the other along the dotted line through the lip and possibly the palate. Bilateral cleft of the lip occurs on both sides of the incisive foramen and includes the prolabium (i.e., the part of the lip attached to the premaxilla). (From Berkowitz, S. [1994]. *The cleft palate story.* Chicago: Quintessence Publishing Co., Inc. Modified with permission.)

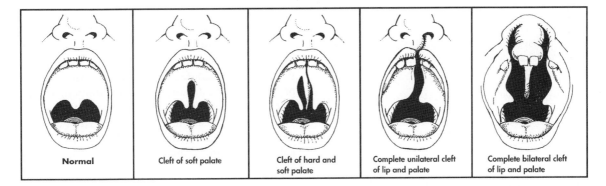

FIGURE 19-3 Types and examples of clefts. (From Lynch, J.I., Brookshire, B.L., & Fox, D.R. [1993]. *A curriculum for infants and toddlers with cleft palate.* Austin, Tex.: Pro-Ed, Inc. Modified with permission.)

the size of the airway cannot accommodate their body's demand for more oxygen. There is increased respiratory effort demonstrated by retractions, nasal flaring, and stridor. With increased effort the muscles of the tongue and nasopharynx or larynx collapse especially during sleep when the muscles of the upper airway are relaxed. The tongue is retropositioned in the mandible, and the infant has difficulty expiring carbon dioxide, which particularly occurs when the baby is placed supine and also during sleep when the ventilatory effort is diminished (Figure 19-4). When this occurs there is complete or partial obstruction of the airway, and although it appears that the child is breathing, there are only intermittent breath sounds to auscultation. Oxygen saturation can drop and CO_2 levels rise, necessitating treatment (Myer et al, 1998).

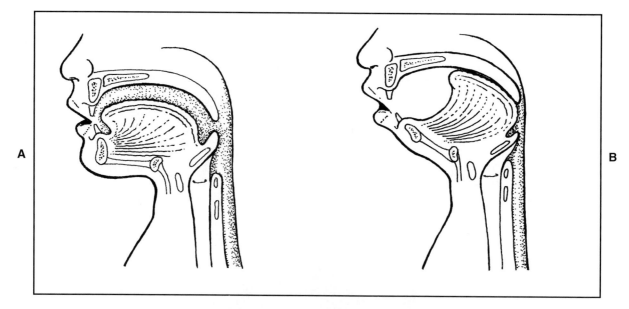

FIGURE 19-4 Pierre Robin sequence. Anatomic features of larynx. **A,** Normal. **B,** Mandibular hypoplasia. Note that posterior placement of tongue makes larynx appear more anteriorly situated than normal.

BOX 19-3

Findings Apparent in Infants with Pierre Robin Sequence

Increasing levels of carbon dioxide when measured serially as a result of carbon dioxide retention from intermittent upper airway obstruction with retropositioning of the tongue.

Transient oxygen desaturations measured by pulse oximetry accompanied by increased work of breathing with chest wall retractions and gasping sounds as the tongue blocks the upper airway. These episodes usually self-correct within a short time as the infant repositions the tongue forward; however, the frequency may increase as the infant tires.

Difficulty during feedings, especially when the nipple is removed from the mouth and the infant is still swallowing residual milk. The tongue becomes retropositioned easily without the stimulus of the nipple to move it forward. Gagging sounds may be heard and become worse with supine positioning.

Deceleration on the growth curve despite adequate intake of formula or expressed breast milk. This should signal a possible worsening respiratory status.

From Monasterio, F.O., Drucker, M., Molina, F., & Ysunza, A. (2002). Distraction osteogenesis in Pierre Robin sequence and related respiratory problems in children. *J Craniofac Surg, 13,* 79-83; Sidman, J.D., Sampson, D., & Templeton, B. (2001). Distraction osteogenesis of the mandible for airway obstruction in children. *Laryngoscope, 111,* 1137-1146. Reprinted with permission.

The presentation of a child with a submucous cleft palate is more elusive. The observation of a posterior notch in the nasal spine at the juncture of the hard and soft palates along with a translucence of the soft palate is unusual unless there are clinical symptoms to warrant closer physical examination of the soft palate. There may or may not be a bifid uvula, which can also be a normal variant, and a short soft palate with muscle separation in the midline. Submucous cleft palate is frequently undetected until the preschool years when the speech is unintelligible secondary to velopharyngeal insufficiency (Gorlin et al, 2001).

BOX 19-4

Treatment

Establishment of adequate feeding
Airway management for infants with Pierre Robin sequence
Plastic surgery and oral-maxillofacial reconstruction
Otolaryngology management
Audiology and speech pathology treatment
Dental/orthodontic care

Children who have nasal-sounding speech for all sounds should have a more detailed examination of their velopharyngeal mechanism. This nasal tone is often not noted until age 3 to 5 years. When the submucous cleft palate is found, then a primary care provider may retrospectively find a predictable history of nasal regurgitation of fluids, inability to breast feed in infancy, initial feeding problems, slow weight gain, and prolonged bottle-feeding times. In addition, a child may have a history of frequent episodes of serous and acute otitis media as a result of eustachian tube dysfunction associated with the cleft palate (Aniansson et al, 2002). Only submucous cleft palates that are symptomatic require intervention (Ysunza et al, 2001).

Treatment

Goals of Treatment and/or Team Care (Box 19-4)

Goals of treatment are (1) to achieve optimum growth and function in speech, hearing, dental, and psychosocial development and (2) to achieve optimal esthetic repair. The American Cleft Palate–Craniofacial Association believes that every individual with cleft lip or cleft palate is best served by the multidisciplinary coordinated approach offered by a cleft palate or craniofacial team (see Resources at the end of this chapter for listings). Parents may contact the team independently, or contact can be facilitated by their primary health care provider.

Newborns should be referred to a team before discharge from the birthing hospital. Older children can and should be referred for team consultation because management occurs over the first 18 years of life. The team must include a qualified speech pathologist, an orthodontist, and a plastic surgeon. Other specialties on a cleft palate team often include audiology, otolaryngology, dental specialties (e.g., pediatric dentistry, prosthodontics, oral and maxillofacial surgery), genetics/dysmorphology, genetic counseling, nursing, social work, psychology, and pediatrics. Teams that care for children with more complex craniofacial deformities may also include members from anesthesia, neurosurgery, ophthalmology, radiology, and psychiatry.

Initial management of a newborn with a cleft involves diagnosis clarification (i.e., rule out associated syndromes), psychosocial support for the grieving family of the child with a congenital birth defect, feeding issues, and airway management for infants with Pierre Robin sequence.

Establishment of Adequate Feeding

The goal of feeding is to maintain optimum nutrition using a technique that is as normal as possible. Infants with an isolated cleft lip or a cleft lip and alveolus (gum) do not generally experience any feeding difficulties. Infants with cleft palate, on the other hand, require some minor adaptations to establish effective feeding. Generating intraoral negative pressure is necessary to draw milk out of a nipple, and an infant with a cleft palate is unable to accomplish this because of the air leak through the nose. There is generally no problem with the infant's ability to swallow. Despite "noisy" feeding sounds there is no increased risk of aspiration pneumonia in infants with cleft palate. Therefore the feeding technique must deliver the milk into the oral cavity so the baby can swallow it normally.

Although infants with a cleft lip or cleft lip and alveolus may be able to breast feed with minor positioning modifications, infants with cleft palate are rarely able to breast feed owing to the inability to create a vacuum. The simplest adaptation is to use a large soft nipple with a fast flow of milk or open a standard nipple hole with a cross cut. This does not always deliver adequate milk in a 30-minute feeding. Therefore bottles that can be squeezed or have a one-way flow valve are used to increase the volume of milk flowing into the baby's mouth.

One of the more common feeding devices used is the Mead Johnson Cleft Lip and Palate Nurser (Figure 19-5), which has a soft plastic compressible bottle and a cross-cut nipple that is slightly longer and narrower than regular nipples. The nipple, however, is not the crucial element of this device, as evidenced by some infants' preference for an orthodontic type of nipple that is also effective. The orthodontic nipple is useful in large clefts because it can span the distance between the edges of the cleft. This large nipple can provide some tongue stabilization during the sucking process, and its single hole provides a faster flow of milk. The soft plastic bottle allows the parent to control the rate of milk delivered, with rhythmic squeezing of the bottle timed to the infant's cues of swallowing. The nipple should be aimed at the parts of the palate that are intact to take advantage

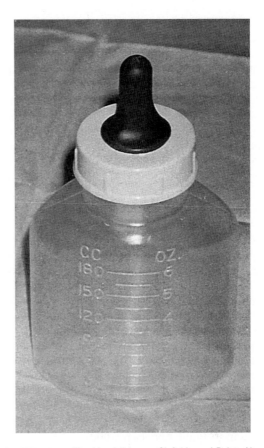

FIGURE 19-5 The Mead Johnson Cleft Lip and Palate Nurser.

of any possible nipple compression between the tongue and the palate.

Alternatives to the Mead Johnson nurser are available but are more costly and complicated without being more effective in establishing feeding. The Medela Company distributes a Haberman feeder, which provides milk flow when the nipple is manually compressed by the feeder or when the infant's gums apply pressure to the plastic nipple. There are varying flow rates and also a one-way valve between the nipple and bottle to decrease the chances of air ingestion with milk.

A less expensive (than the Haberman feeder) and simpler one-way valve system is the Pigeon nipple. It is commercially available (see Resources) with instructions for use available in English or Japanese. The nipple is made of soft, easily compressible, nonlatex isoprene and has a one-way valve that fits into the nipple assembly. Therefore the milk only flows into the mouth, not back into the bottle when the baby compresses the nipple.

The Ross cleft palate nipple is intended for postoperative feeding and is not appropriate for newborns because the flow rate is too fast. Likewise, the Lamb nipple is an outdated device that is bulky and causes gagging.

Whatever feeding method is chosen, there are principles or guidelines most effective in achieving appropriate weight gain. The family needs personalized teaching within the first week of life regarding assessment, feeding methodology, and evaluation of response to feeding by a practitioner experienced in management of infants with clefts (American Cleft

Palate–Craniofacial Association, 2000). Ideally this practitioner should be a member of a cleft palate or craniofacial team. Consistency with a chosen technique for a minimum of 24 hours is important to allow both parent and infant to adapt. Continuous switching of nipples is confusing. Feedings should last no longer than 30 to 45 minutes, and the frequency should not be less than every 2½ to 3 hours. These guidelines promote conservation of energy and decreased caloric expenditure during the feeding process. It is helpful for the parents to know how many ounces their child needs each day to grow normally. A quick easy guide is a minimum of 2 oz of milk per 1 lb of baby's weight every 24 hours. Therefore a 7-lb baby will need 14 oz each day.

Infants who have Pierre Robin sequence require a careful airway assessment, and effective airway management strategies must be in place before addressing feeding issues. These strategies may include placing a tracheostomy for severe upper airway obstruction, lip-tongue placation, or prone positioning. A feeding specialist in conjunction with a craniofacial team will develop the feeding plan for oral feeding with or without a nasogastric tube or gastrostomy tube.

The use of feeding appliances or acrylic prosthetic devices varies across the United States. These devices assist the infant with a cleft by creating a barrier over the palatal cleft to enable the baby to then compress a nipple against a hard surface. This device may be useful in feeding but does not enable an infant to successfully breast feed, and bottle feeding can be established without it (Prahl-Andersen, 2000).

Surgical Reconstructive Management

There is a frequent misconception that cleft lip or palate or both are merely surgical problems that are corrected in early childhood when the lip and palatal defects are closed. Parents who are very eager for the surgical repairs soon learn of the multidisciplinary rehabilitative services that must be coordinated with the surgeries. Specific timing of surgery also depends on the child's health and development.

Surgical Reconstruction of a Cleft Lip. Surgical repair of cleft lip is generally done between 3 and 5 months of age. Many surgeons use the rule of 10s—10 weeks of age, hemoglobin level of 10 g/dl, and 10 lb in body weight—in planning the repair. Occasionally if the cleft is very wide, especially in a unilateral defect, a surgical cleft lip adhesion is done at about 1 month of age to better approximate the lip tissue in preparation for the definitive procedure at the usual age. Some centers are preparing the lip before surgery by moving the premaxilla into a better position with simple taping techniques or a more precise movement with orthodontic appliances (Peterson-Falzone et al, 2001).

Postoperative management for an infant with cleft lip has changed dramatically in recent years. Unrestricted breast or bottle feeding immediately after surgery has been shown to decrease the length of hospital stay, increase oral intake, and improve parental satisfaction without negatively affecting suture line integrity (Boekelheide et al, 1992). Surgery can be performed on an outpatient basis with the infant discharged with elbow restraints. Parents are instructed to clean the suture line with normal saline followed by application of petroleum jelly or antibiotic ointment for 1 to 2 weeks. Pain management is usually adequate with oral acetaminophen.

Secondary lip revisions may be necessary before beginning school or during the school-age years. A nasal repair during the toddler years to lengthen the columella (soft tissue from nasal tip to nostril sill area) is frequently indicated for children with bilateral clefts.

Surgical Reconstruction of a Cleft Palate. Surgical repair of a cleft palate is usually done between 9 and 18 months of age. This is timed to provide the reconstructed palate needed for speech development (Figure 19-6). The repair is most commonly done at one time in one stage. The postoperative management usually dictates a 1- or 2-night hospital stay for airway monitoring and establishing adequate oral hydration. The use of elbow restraints and avoidance of straws and utensils for feeding for 2 weeks are routine. The use of bottles 24 to 48 hours after palatal surgery is variable depending on the center. Cup feeding is taught for liquids and blenderized solid food. Some centers use mist tents or supplemental humidity for 1 night to liquefy dried bloody nasal and oral secretions. Good pain management usually requires a parenteral narcotic (e.g., morphine sulfate) with an enteral analgesic (acetaminophen) on the day of surgery. On the first postoperative day an enteral narcotic analgesic (e.g., acetaminophen with codeine elixir) is substituted for the parenteral narcotic. Regularly scheduled analgesia around the clock after surgery optimizes the success of oral feeding. Infants may require pain management at home with acetaminophen (with or without codeine) for up to 2 weeks after surgery.

Secondary palatal surgery may be recommended by the speech pathologist in order to address persistent nasal speech after a period of speech therapy. The procedures may lengthen the palate (i.e., Furlow palatoplasty), create a smaller space in all dimensions (i.e., sphincter pharyngoplasty), or create a flap of tissue in the middle (i.e., pharyngeal flap) with two side ports to produce velopharyngeal sufficiency or closure during speech. This secondary palatal surgery is done for children of preschool age in order to achieve clear speech before school entry (Sie et al, 2001). This procedure is also used in school-aged children who develop nasal speech after the adenoid pad involutes.

Repair of the bony defect along the gum or alveolar ridge is timed according to dental development and eruption of secondary teeth (Berkowitz, 1996). Roots of the teeth need to be anchored on bone, and generally iliac crest cancellous bone is harvested and packed into the alveolar cleft defect. This surgical procedure is usually done at 7 to 9 years of age. Dietary restrictions and the use of blenderized food for 2 weeks by cup are indicated. Once the bone has healed it is possible to use implants to replace missing teeth in the alveolar cleft.

Nasal reconstructive surgery (i.e., rhinoplasty) is done when full growth has been attained (i.e., after menstruation in females and the growth spurt in males). Some teens also require midface oral and maxillofacial surgery to address facial imbalances as a result of growth disturbance from the clefting that cannot be completely corrected by orthodontics.

Otolaryngology Treatment

Otolaryngology management involves monitoring persistent serous otitis media and frequently placement of ventilation tubes in the tympanic membranes (Muntz, 1993). Ventilation tubes should be considered if there is fluid in the middle ear

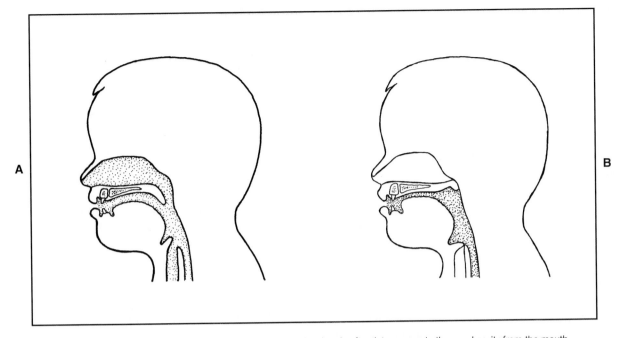

FIGURE 19-6 Anatomy of the roof of the mouth. The hard and soft palates separate the nasal cavity from the mouth. **A,** Soft palate open. Muscles relax for breathing and making certain speech sounds. **B,** Soft palate closed. Muscles in the soft palate and throat seal off the nasal cavity for swallowing foods and liquids and making certain speech sounds. (From Mead Johnson & Co. [1997]. *Looking forward: A guide for parents of the child with cleft lip and palate.* Evansville, Ind.: Author. Modified with permission.)

space at the time of any other surgical procedures (i.e., cleft lip or palate repair). Because of the high incidence of middle ear problems, some centers favor placement of ventilation tubes at the time of surgical palate repair for all children. Following placement of the tubes, some otolaryngologists advise the use of silicone ear plugs while bathing and swimming to prevent water from entering the middle ear; however, updated research supports use of earplugs only for diving to depths of 6 feet or greater or in the case of recurrent otorrhea (Lee et al, 1999; Salata & Derkay, 1996).

A small percentage of children have chronic eustachian tube dysfunction after 5 years of age and may require multiple replacements of ventilating tubes to maintain normal hearing through the school-aged years. The indication for tubes may be recurrent or persistent serous otitis media or severe retraction of the tympanic membrane in which there is little air present in the middle ear space, resulting in an increased risk for cholesteatoma. The tympanic membranes may be very scarred or weak and thin, which may result in persistent perforation of the tympanic membrane after extrusion of the ventilating tube. This membrane does not need to be patched surgically on an urgent basis if the hearing is not negatively affected because the perforation is functioning like a patent ventilating tube. When the child is a teenager, it may be patched when the eustachian tube functioning improves and there are no recurrent infections (Muntz, 1993).

Audiology and Speech Pathology Treatment
Diagnostic audiologic evaluation and management are an integral component of the treatment plan for infants and children with cleft palate. Speech and language development is similarly monitored and therapy provided as appropriate (see Associated Problems).

Dental and Orthodontic Treatment
Dental care should begin early (i.e., at 2 to 3 years of age) to preserve the health of the primary dentition. Children with bilateral or unilateral clefts of the alveolar ridge require considerable orthodontic management (Prahl-Andersen, 2000).

A child with a cleft palate alone requires regular pediatric dental care and orthodontic services. The anterior and lateral palatal growth may be restricted—especially if the cleft extends into the hard bony palate. Cleft palate repair in infancy creates scarring along areas that normally experience significant growth during childhood. As a result, a palatal expansion appliance may be necessary in order to achieve adequate dental occlusion.

Children with Pierre Robin sequence who have micrognathia in infancy usually experience catch-up mandibular growth during the first year of life. Sometimes, however, children may need orthodontic management to deal with dental crowding as a result of the small mandible.

Complementary and Alternative Therapies
Parents frequently ask the plastic surgeon if there are complementary or alternative therapies to reduce the visibility of the scar on the lip following cleft lip surgery. Some surgeons routinely cover the incision with paper tape or Steri-strips until the wound is completely healed. This acts to stabilize the adjoining tissue, decreasing the stress on the incision with movement

from crying or smiling. Another therapy that has been used is a silicone patch over the incision. There are also creams and ointments with vitamin E that do no harm as long as the wound has healed before it is applied; however, the effectiveness in reducing scar formation has not been substantiated. The act of massaging cream on the lip may break down some of the scar-forming fibrinogen and soften the area; however, it is difficult to get an infant to hold still for a lip massage.

Anticipated Advances in Diagnosis and Management

There has been a recent focus on fetal surgery for cleft lip and palate repair (Wagner & Harrison, 2002). Proposed advantages of such surgical intervention include decreased scar formation in fetal wound healing; decreased potential costs as a result of less need for extensive postoperative care, orthodontia, and speech therapy; and minimized psychologic trauma associated with facial deformity. This type of surgical repair has been done in the laboratory in fetal mice, rabbits, sheep, and monkeys. Currently, nonlethal conditions such as cleft lip and palate are not repaired in humans because of the high surgical risks. The potential risks to the mother and the early fetus are considerable and probably do not justify the intervention. Endoscopic techniques may reduce the risks of surgery in the future (Wagner & Harrison, 2002). Obvious limitations to this treatment modality include accurate prenatal diagnosis through ultrasound, which would capture some infants with cleft lip but would not include those with a cleft palate only. Nonetheless, the current research will be beneficial for an increased understanding of craniofacial development and effects of management on wound healing.

Prenatal diagnosis of a cleft lip with ultrasonography is becoming more common as the technique and interpretation are perfected. It is important to define any other anomalies, such as those found with a chromosomal syndrome, which have a much different prognosis than an isolated cleft of the lip, which may or may not include a cleft of the palate as well. Families need to obtain accurate diagnostic information with follow-up genetic counseling when a prenatal diagnosis is made. Realistic and accurate preparation by the craniofacial center with emphasis on the first year of life management issues is helpful for the couple referred from the obstetric ultrasound screening process (Jones, 2002).

Potential advances in the management of children with cleft lip and palate include genetic testing to identify the genes that are transformed when an infant has a clefting disorder (Murray, 2002). Further research regarding the effects of maternal vitamin deficiencies and environmental factors on gene transformation may provide clues into preventive measures that may be used during pregnancy (Prescott et al, 2002).

Recently, surgical techniques that lengthen the mandible have been introduced to avoid a tracheostomy for infants with significant upper airway obstruction caused by Pierre Robin sequence. The technique is known as distraction osteogenesis and is usually undertaken only at major craniofacial centers with experienced surgeons and neonatal intensive care personnel (Denny & Kalantarian, 2002; Monasterio et al, 2002; Sidman et al, 2001). Distraction osteogenesis was pioneered by

orthopedic surgeons in such procedures as long bone lengthening when a child has a leg length discrepancy. An osteotomy is created on both sides of the mandible, and hardware is attached to the bony fragments and serially expanded with an appliance at the same time as the mandible is regenerating new bony growth. Lengthening the mandible in this way draws the tongue forward and out of the airway. The enthusiasm for this new intervention must be tempered with the concerns for tooth buds that may be in the path of the distraction hardware. This procedure requires a complete otolaryngology evaluation to determine the level of obstruction (i.e., the tongue may not be the only source of the obstruction).

Associated Problems (Box 19-5)
Audiology and Otolaryngology

Infants and children with an isolated cleft lip or cleft lip and alveolus generally do not have abnormal hearing at a rate above the general population. Infants and children with cleft palate, however, have significant hearing and middle ear problems. Audiology testing is appropriate in children with cleft palate to monitor the degree of conductive hearing loss in order to guide the clinician in providing appropriate interventions and documenting the effectiveness of management. Hearing can be tested in newborns in the nursery by a screening known as algorithm auditory brainstem response screening (AABR), or otoacoustic emissions (American Cleft Palate–Craniofacial Association, 2000). If an infant does not pass the hearing screen, it is appropriate to proceed with more complex testing known as auditory brainstem response (ABR) testing, which monitors the sensorineural auditory system.

Children who are at least 6 to 9 months of age may be tested by behavioral audiologic testing. This type of testing requires some degree of cooperation and is done when an infant can sit and respond to sounds. These findings should ideally correlate with the physical examination by the otolaryngologist so a combined approach to management can then be devised.

The dynamic functioning of the eustachian tube, which serves as the communication link between the middle ear space and the back of the throat, is controlled by the palatal musculature. The child with cleft palate has abnormal placement and underdevelopment of palatal musculature. As a result the eustachian tube functions poorly. When a child develops an upper respiratory tract infection, fluid can accumulate in the middle ear space. This fluid usually drains into the oral cavity when the infection and swelling of the eustachian tube subside (Figure 19-7). In a child with cleft palate, however, the eustachian tube may only rarely open, and as a result the fluid remains behind the tympanic membrane on a long-term basis.

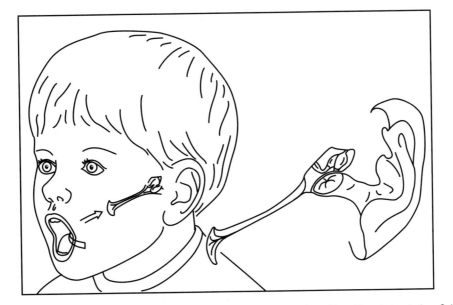

FIGURE 19-7 Ear–eustachian tube relationship and proximity to the palate. (From Ross Laboratories, Columbus, Ohio.) Reprinted with permission.

Infants and children with cleft palate have up to a 90% incidence of developing chronic serous otitis media associated with eustachian tube dysfunction.

Monitoring children with ear tubes in place is usually done every 6 months and more frequently as necessary for blocked, infected, or prematurely extruded tubes. It is especially important to monitor for the presence of middle ear fluid and resultant conductive hearing loss in children who are rapidly acquiring speech and language skills and are already challenged by the cleft palate, which makes this acquisition more difficult.

Many parents query the primary care provider as to why the eustachian tube dysfunction continues after the surgical repair of the cleft palate. Even though palatal tissue is restored closer to normal, the dynamic mechanisms that control the influence of the palatal musculature on eustachian tube function are not normalized.

Speech Pathology

Children with cleft lip only usually do not have significant speech articulation problems. These children may only require short-term therapy that focuses on bilabial sounds found in *m* and *b* and *p*, which require competent lip closure. Children with clefts of the alveolus have additional challenges with anterior sounds as well as with managing air leakage from the front of the gums into the anterior nasal cavity before the alveolar bone graft surgery (Peterson-Falzone et al, 2001).

Children with clefts of the palate have problems with speech articulation trying to correct the nasal air escape (Witt & D'Antonio, 1993). The goal of palate surgery is to create a normally functioning palate before the emergence of compensatory mechanisms. The speech pathologist should meet the parents before surgery to explain normal speech and language development. Families must be taught the fact that babies need to receive speech input directed at them and need to reciprocate in a turn-taking fashion with the use of body language and

prespeech babbling behavior. Anticipatory guidance is standard practice for such families.

Following surgical closure of the cleft palate, the speech pathologist evaluates the success of the surgery. If formal speech therapy is needed it can begin with children as young as 2 years of age. Without this intervention, these children can become frustrated in their inability to expand in expressive speech and language skills and may develop behavioral responses such as temper tantrums in order to communicate. In addition, the child is unable to communicate even simple desires to strangers who are unfamiliar with their speech repertoire.

Ongoing monitoring and parental guidance on a 6-month basis with the speech pathologist are appropriate during the toddler and preschool years. At some point during this time, the speech pathologist may determine that the child could benefit from regular speech therapy services. For children under 3 years of age, therapy may be provided by an infant development program that has specific speech therapy services or a speech pathologist who is community or hospital based. After 3 years of age, the child usually receives speech therapy that is provided by the local school district. An individualized education program (IEP) is necessary for this isolated service because it is a component of special education services. The speech pathologist at the craniofacial or cleft palate center should continue to monitor progress every 6 to 12 months and provide feedback and suggestions to the speech pathologist providing the therapy.

The desired outcome following cleft palate surgery and speech therapy is clear articulation by 4 years of age. Although many variables have been studied, including type of cleft, age of surgical repair, type of surgical technique used, initiation time, and length of speech therapy services, no one factor has been determined to provide the desired outcome (Peterson-Falzone et al, 2001). Rather, it is a combination of factors that produces the optimal outcome.

Children who do not have clear speech development by 4 years of age may require secondary surgical palatal treatment—ideally before school entry. This surgery is particularly helpful if the articulation of sounds is good but there is persistent nasal air emission as a result of a deficiency of palatal tissue or a palate that has inadequate motion. If secondary surgical or prosthetic management is done, follow-up speech therapy is usually needed to obtain maximum benefit from the intervention. It is not unusual for school-aged children to receive speech therapy during school, especially because they receive active orthodontic services that may further challenge speech articulation.

Dental and Orthodontic Problems

Some children with a cleft alveolus have missing or supernumerary teeth. Care should be taken not to remove these teeth because they maintain alveolar bone mass in a dental arch that is deficient in bone at the area of the cleft. Children often develop a crossbite from surgical closure of the palate causing collapse of the arches. The crossbite does not always need to be corrected in primary dentition, but some pediatric dentists do offer early interceptive orthodontic treatment. Children may also have delayed dental eruption (Pham et al, 1997).

At 5 to 7 years of age, it is appropriate for a child with an alveolar cleft to have an orthodontic consultation, baseline records (e.g., photographs, dental study models, radiographs, examination), and a treatment plan. Initial management focuses on expansion of the maxillary arch with a fixed active appliance in preparation for surgical grafting with iliac crest donor bone. The orthodontist usually indicates the appropriate time to perform the bone graft procedure. Following the grafting procedure, the expectation is that adjacent teeth will erupt into the arch. Missing teeth may be replaced by implants (Kearns et al, 1997) or prosthetics.

Orthodontic management is usually done in phases and may have periods of rest when the teeth are held in place by a passive retention type of appliance. The timing and phase of intervention depend on the maxillary and mandibular growth that occurs into the teen years. It is not uncommon for orthodontic management to span a period of 10 years. Compliance with the recommended regimen is crucial because active movement of teeth depends on keeping frequent appointments, maintaining appliances, and practicing good oral hygiene. Maintaining regular pediatric dental care services during the orthodontic treatment is also important.

Psychosocial Adjustment to a Physical Deformity

Parents of the infant with a cleft are the first clients for the long-term psychosocial management of the child. According to observations, families who positively accommodate to their child's chronic condition have children who appear to cope at a higher level than parents who exhibit negative adaptive behaviors. The degree of clefting is not predictive of the level of psychosocial functioning (Endriga & Kapp-Simon, 1999).

The first questions parents ask the primary care provider after the birth of a child with cleft lip or palate are "How did this happen?" and "Did I do something wrong?" (Bender,

2000). The parents should be reassured that clefts can occur in the healthiest of pregnancies; therefore they should not blame themselves. The birth of an infant with a facial malformation is a constant reminder of the physical condition. Bonding and attachment activities are related to the infant's face, and it takes some time to adjust and positively regard an abnormal face (Endriga & Kapp-Simon, 1999). Most families learn over time to appreciate their infant's own personality and special way of expressing a "wide smile." Some families have a secondary grief reaction once the child's lip is repaired and express that they "miss the cleft" (Curtin, 1990). A second adjustment to the "new" face is necessary and may take 1 to 2 weeks after surgery. Parents do not regret deciding to have the lip repair done, but rather, it is a normal adjustment. Parents are reassured when the team providers give them anticipatory guidance about their feelings. The feelings of grief commonly experienced by parents at the birth of their child with a cleft can resurface at times of stress, such as hospitalization, initiation of speech, dental eruption, and school entry. It is important for parents to recognize that everyone copes with grief differently and not to expect other family members to be feeling the same emotions at the same time.

The health care provider can model acceptance of the child and encourage the parents to support the interests and talents their child exhibits in areas such as music, art, sports, or academia. One technique parents can use to communicate their acceptance of their child with a cleft is to incorporate stories about the child's adventures as a baby going to the hospital for the lip surgery with a positive outcome. That way the cleft is part of the child and the outcome is due to their innate characteristics.

Children in the preschool years gain an increased understanding of their birth defect as they develop a sense of self-awareness and experience teasing from peers. Simple explanations about the cleft can be reviewed, and strategies for deflecting the teasing can be suggested. School-aged children may need support from counselors, school personnel, and their family to promote a positive self-image and to cope with teasing. Teenagers are able to articulate their wishes and priorities in treatment planning and should participate in the decision-making process. Teenagers also have increased self-image concerns and may benefit from counseling services.

Prognosis

The long-term prognosis for children with nonsyndromic cleft lip and palate is excellent. The goals of team management are to achieve good speech articulation, functional dental occlusion, normal hearing acuity, an acceptable appearance, and a positive self-regard. In addition, children with Pierre Robin sequence have a goal of achieving adequate airway function. They are generally cared for in tertiary medical centers with cleft-craniofacial teams that work with pediatric pulmonary or pediatric otolaryngology specialists to achieve adequate airway function.

Prognosis for development can vary from normal for a child with a nonsyndromic cleft to severely delayed for a child with a chromosomal defect causing the cleft. Therefore all infants with cleft lip and palate need to be examined by a geneticist or dysmorphologist before surgery (American Cleft Palate–Craniofacial Association, 2000; Willner, 2000).

PRIMARY CARE MANAGEMENT

Health Care Maintenance

Growth and Development

Growth and development are not affected in children with a nonsyndromic cleft lip and palate. In the past, infant feeding devices used to provide nutrition for neonates with a cleft palate were suboptimal. With the evolution of the squeeze bottle and the proliferation of team care and trained professionals to provide teaching, this aspect of management has been simplified. In addition, current postoperative feeding routines are simpler and hospital stays are shorter, which all contribute to a more normalized nutritional status.

Infants with cleft lip and palate are expected to grow along the same parameters as infants without clefts. Once the feeding method has been taught by a member of the cleft-craniofacial team, the primary care provider will monitor the child's growth. All children with craniofacial abnormalities should be referred to a pediatric endocrinologist if short stature (other than constitutional) is identified (Cunningham & Jerome, 1997). Children who have a known syndrome may have growth and developmental problems related to the syndrome.

Occasionally infants with clefts do not grow along the expected norms. There may be extenuating psychosocial factors that challenge the parent or caretaker in feeding the infant. Initially an observation and review of the feeding method should be pursued along with a 24- to 72-hour diet record. Serial weight checks can provide both parental and health care provider reassurance. For the infant with Pierre Robin sequence, deceleration on the growth curve should prompt a careful reassessment of respiratory status and the probable finding of some degree of upper airway obstruction.

Diet

Mothers of infants with cleft palate can provide expressed breast milk for their children. Hospital-grade electric pumps work the best and can be rented from a lactation consultant who is trained to provide education and support regarding long-term pumping and storage of breast milk. Most mothers use a double pumping system attachment to decrease the amount of time spent pumping milk. Mothers with low income may be able to procure an electric pump from their local Women, Infants, and Children (WIC) agency.

Mothers who are pumping breast milk four to six times per day in addition to bottle feeding the milk six to eight times per day need support and assistance from others. It is important to balance the needs of the mother and the family with the needs of the infant with a cleft in such a way that the mother not only feels encouraged to continue but also feels support if she decides to discontinue pumping. Mothers who are able to persevere with providing their infant expressed breast milk will be encouraged by a study that linked breast milk intake to a decreased incidence of otitis media specifically in infants with clefts (Aniansson et al, 2002; Paradise et al, 1994).

Upright positioning of the infant during feeding will decrease the amount of nasal regurgitation. Parents should be reassured that a small amount of nasal regurgitation is expected and should be handled by simply wiping the nose of the infant with a cloth rather than interpreted as a signal of a problem. Cleansing of the nose and mouth with water or a cotton-tipped applicator or bulb syringe is not necessary because the mouth is self-cleaning and the nasal secretions and milk will drain by gravity. The parent may need to be reassured about the anatomy of the cleft palate. The oral cavity and nasal cavity are continuous, and the parent may have an unspoken fear that the feeding will hurt the infant or that the nasal turbinates and the vomer represent brain tissue that can be injured with feeding. It is not unusual to see an ulcer on the vomer (bottom of nasal septum seen near the middle of the open cleft palate). This is caused by suckling or bottle feeding and goes away as the tissue toughens.

The primary care provider can offer anticipatory guidance by discouraging the use of bottles—especially when filled with formula, milk, or juice in bed. This practice causes baby bottle caries. The supine position favors accumulation of the fluid into the middle ear space when the eustachian tube is open in a population that is already at risk for recurrent otitis media.

For an infant who is 4 to 6 months old, introduction of solid foods and progression to table foods is sequenced the same as for infants without clefts. There may be some nasal regurgitation as the infant learns this new skill. Varying textures can sometimes alleviate this issue. Some parents require extra encouragement to proceed with the introduction of solid foods by spoon. Delayed initiation of this normal developmental skill can create negative feeding behaviors and may interfere with the normal oral motor development necessary in producing pre-speech sounds. Using a bottle type of infant feeders or enlarging nipple holes to accommodate solid foods also delays normal development. Messy spoon feedings are expected, and nasal reflux of solids should be handled calmly. Infants and children have only minor dietary restrictions. Some tricky foods for a child with an unrepaired cleft palate include peanut butter, soft cheese, and sweets, which are all gummy in texture. Avoiding foods that are a choking risk, such as peanuts, popcorn, and pellet candy, is advised because these foods can lodge in the nasal cavity. Parents are very concerned with future speech development in their infant with a cleft palate and therefore may respond to solid food progression as an aid toward a speech goal.

Safety

In addition to routine anticipatory guidance on safety issues, the child may have some restrictions during the first 2 to 4 weeks following reconstructive surgical procedures. Elbow restraints are generally used for 1 to 2 weeks after reconstructive surgery in the infant and toddler. Older preschool children may especially need these restraints, which are referred to as "reminders," at naptime and bedtime.

Dietary restrictions that are recommended postoperatively (e.g., avoidance of utensils, straws, and textured foods) are generally only necessary for about 2 weeks after surgery to allow for nontraumatic healing of the oral tissues. Some families may actually need to be encouraged and reassured to advance to soft foods 2 weeks after the surgery and an unrestricted diet 1 month after the surgery.

Youngsters need to avoid contact sports for 6 weeks after alveolar bone grafting procedures, nasal reconstruction, and midface jaw procedures to prevent disruption of the surgery before bone healing.

Infants with Pierre Robin sequence who require prone positioning for adequate respiration may need a car safety bed rather than a car seat when traveling in an automobile; these beds are available commercially (see Resources at the end of this chapter).

Immunizations

Infants and children with cleft lip and palate should receive all routine immunizations at the ages recommended by the American Academy of Pediatrics. A planned surgical procedure is not a rationale for deferring routine immunizations; the child is better protected within the hospital setting when immunization status is current. Administration of immunizations within 24 hours of a planned surgical procedure is not advisable because a low-grade fever following vaccine administration may preclude surgery. Administration of the measles-mumps-rubella (MMR) or varicella vaccine within 1 week before scheduled surgery is not recommended for similar reasons. Administration of the pneumococcal vaccine is advocated for this population because of its protective effect in preventing some of the episodes of acute otitis media, although admittedly the vaccine's prime target is the more life-threatening meningitis risk (Overturf, 2000).

Screening

Vision. Routine vision screening is recommended. Children with cleft palate alone should have a pediatric ophthalmology dilated examination at approximately 1 year of age and again before school entry at age 4 or 5 years to screen for Stickler syndrome, which is associated with myopia and sometimes leads to retinal detachment.

Hearing. A high index of suspicion and prompt referral to an audiologist and otolaryngologist should be made if the child does not pass an audiologic screening in the school-age years. Detailed audiologic testing (as previously described) is done by the specialty center in the early years of life.

Dental. Routine screening is recommended for a child with an isolated cleft lip. Dental and orthodontic care is indicated for children with clefts of the alveolar ridge or the secondary palate. A pediatric dental provider is strongly advised—even if the family needs to travel some distance to obtain the service. The primary care provider should promote good oral hygiene practices, including initiation of tooth brushing or cleansing with a rough face cloth with eruption of the first tooth. Parents must be counseled on the hazards of baby-bottle tooth decay (Bian et al, 2001).

Dental eruption may be slightly delayed in a child with a cleft. Many families believe that once their child starts orthodontic care they no longer need to see the regular pediatric dentist. However, dental cleanings and topical fluoride treatment are actually even more important during active orthodontic management.

Blood Pressure. Routine screening is recommended.
Hematocrit. Routine screening is recommended.

Urinalysis. Routine screening is recommended.
Tuberculosis. Routine screening is recommended.

Common Illness Management
Differential Diagnosis

Fever. The parents of a child with a cleft are alerted to the increased incidence of middle ear disease. The presence of a fever, increased irritability, tugging at the ears, and asking family members to repeat verbalizations all signal the need to have the ears examined for acute or serous otitis media.

Children with cleft palate are defined as an outlying population by the current American Academy of Pediatrics (AAP) recommendations regarding middle ear disease, favoring ongoing monitoring of serous otitis media rather than aggressive surgical management (Otitis Media Guideline Panel, 1994). Primary care providers are advised to refer these children to the otolaryngologist for a microscopic office examination if they have persistent (i.e., 3 months or longer) middle ear fluid or recurrent (i.e., every 1 to 2 months) acute otitis media. Management of acute otitis media is with the usual oral antibiotics. Prompt management is indicated for acute otitis media rather than the "watch and wait" approach currently in practice in the healthy child population because of the frequency of otitis media and the deleterious effects on hearing in an at-risk population. Prophylactic antibiotic use is not recommended because of development of resistant pathogens (Bluestone, 1998) as well as its ineffectiveness in the management of chronic serous otitis media—the main problem in children with cleft palate.

Otolaryngology practitioners favor an adenoidectomy procedure for children with chronic serous otitis media requiring more than one set of middle ear ventilation tubes. This procedure is specifically not indicated for children with cleft palate because all available tissue in the nasopharynx is important in the development of clear speech without excess nasality. However, an adenoidectomy may be indicated in a child with a cleft palate who experiences sleep apnea.

Drug Interactions

Medications are not required as part of the normal treatment regimen.

Developmental Issues
Sleep Patterns

Infants and children with a unilateral cleft lip usually have a deviated nasal septum that causes noisy breathing during upper respiratory tract infections but does not negatively affect air exchange.

Children who have secondary palatal surgery to address nasal speech have a smaller upper airway space in the nasopharynx. These children are particularly at risk for sleep state upper airway obstruction during the first 6 weeks following surgery when local edema is present. Symptoms may include chest wall retractions with or without partial ventilation, irregular snoring with pauses greater than 15 to 20 seconds, diaphoresis, nighttime waking—especially after an apnea episode, daytime somnolence, and enuresis (Sirois et al, 1994). The child's symptoms should be reported to the specialty center physician, who may be a pediatric pulmonologist or oto-laryngologist. The severity of the symptoms will be assessed, and medical management (e.g., steroid administration or in-patient observation) may be warranted. The surgical procedure rarely needs to be revised because the symptoms are usually temporary and the desired outcome is to provide a decreased nasal airflow during speech without negatively affecting the ventilatory capabilities.

An infant with Pierre Robin sequence may have a disrupted sleep experience as a result of sleep state obstructive apnea. Careful history taking, evaluation, and management by the pediatric pulmonologist or otolaryngologist are appropriate.

Sleep patterns are usually disrupted following hospitalizations. Families should be told of this probable change in sleeping pattern at both the preoperative and postoperative visits.

Toileting

There is no physiologic effect on toileting. The psychologic impact of stressful surgeries and hospitalization experiences can temporarily delay acquisition of toileting skills or result in regression of recently acquired skills.

Discipline

Parents of children with a congenital birth defect often feel guilty that they "caused" the problem in some way. This feeling can then translate into an altered perception of the child as being special and requiring extra attention to overcompensate for the guilt. In addition, parents are very saddened to learn of the initial surgeries that their child will require and the long-term management. Many parents report that they wish the treatment could be done on them rather than on the child. Because the initial surgeries are done in infancy, the psychologic burden is thrust on the parents.

Parents must be encouraged to return to the infant's or child's normal routine following hospitalizations (Strauss, 2001). A routine is reassuring for the child and promotes normalcy and an earlier return to normal behavior. Parents who focus exclusively on the needs of the infant or child who is sick and cater to every whim soon find that this is not functional or pleasant for the child or the family. Symptoms of this phenomenon include the following: no structured feeding or meal routine; irregular nap times; nighttime waking; nighttime feedings; co-sleeping in the parental bed (only if this is not the family's usual practice); excessive fussiness, irritability, or clinginess; loss of previously achieved developmental milestones; and inability to get along with others (Elmendorf et al, 1993). These are all normal reactions to a stressful experience such as a hospitalization but usually do not persist beyond 2 to 6 weeks after a 24- to 48-hour hospital stay. Parents can benefit from anticipatory guidance and encouragement to promote normalcy, which initially may appear harsh and unsympathetic. When it is presented as comforting for the child, however, most parents embrace the concept.

Issues of discipline arise again when a child with a cleft lip or palate enters school, especially if the child appears very different from peers and is teased. Overprotectiveness and lack of appropriate limits can actually exacerbate these problems. The child and family can often benefit from short-term counseling regarding self-image concerns and development of skills to cope with teasing from others.

Child Care

Child care in a group daycare setting can be stressful for parents of a child who is at risk for frequent ear infections. For this reason, some parents choose a setting with a more limited number of children—especially during the winter months.

Once children are old enough to attend a Head Start program or structured preschool, they should. Such programs can be helpful as an adjunct to speech therapy because a child's peers will promote expressive language development. Peers usually do not understand the elaborate gesturing system and mono-syllabic vocalizations that substitute for expressive language and may encourage children to expand their repertoire by modeling.

Schooling

Children with cleft palate are eligible for special education services (i.e., speech therapy) under the Individuals with Disabilities Education Act (IDEA), Public Law 101-476 (see Chapter 5). Parents should request in writing a speech evaluation focused on articulation when a child is 2 years 9 months of age. It is helpful if the parents provide medical information and any prior speech evaluations.

Peer teasing can occur as a child progresses through school because of speech and facial appearance issues (Millard & Richman, 2001). Some parents and children use the "class presentation" approach to explain the cleft, and teachers can incorporate this into their lesson plans about differences among people. A child rarely reports teasing and ridicule so severe that school phobia and frequent absences become an issue. It is important to query parents about these issues at primary care visits and offer supportive services and coordinated efforts between the primary care providers and the school system.

Children with cleft lip and palate may have learning disabilities, particularly in the areas affected by expressive language, such as reading problems (Endriga & Kapp-Simon, 1999). Children who have an isolated cleft palate that is part of a syndrome may have a lower intellectual potential that is specifically associated with the syndrome. These children should be evaluated by special education professionals as appropriate.

Sexuality

No special sexual problems are associated with cleft lip and palate. The obvious concerns about self-image may be exaggerated during adolescence.

When discussing reproductive issues, the risks of recurrence for clefting must be addressed. The rates quoted for nonsyndromic clefts are between 2% and 7% (Gorlin et al, 2001), depending on previous family history and the severity of the cleft. A bilateral cleft lip is rare and more severe than a unilateral one and also has a slightly higher risk of recurrence. Other factors, such as gender, influence the recurrence risk as well. A complete family history and physical examination of an affected individual by a geneticist and genetic counselor are necessary to provide the most accurate information.

Women with increased risk for having a child with a cleft are eligible for a detailed ultrasound that has a better resolution of the facial features than a traditional ultrasound. Women of childbearing age are counseled to take increased folic acid and a multivitamin supplement 3 months before conception and during the first trimester in the hope of reducing the recurrence risk of a cleft condition (Prescott et al, 2002).

Transition into Adulthood

State funding for care of children with cleft lips and palates is available to financially eligible children up to age 21 years. Most individuals are able to complete the orthodontic and oral-maxillofacial surgical procedures by this age. Problems are encountered if there were treatment lapses or delays during crucial stages of dental development or orthodontic management that necessitated restarting the treatment. In addition, orthodontic interventions are effective during active treatment, and then the position of the teeth and the occlusion are often maintained with removable appliances (e.g., a retainer worn at night). Adolescents and their families often do not appreciate the need for these appliances, so relapse occurs. If relapse occurs before the insurance is terminated, some active management can be reinitiated. Otherwise, young adults must usually pay for these services as out-of-pocket expenses. It is difficult for young adults to gain third-party payment for follow-up lip or nasal surgery because such procedures are considered to be cosmetic to insurance carriers even though the treatment is for reconstruction of a congenital birth defect.

Family Concerns and Resources

Parents of children with a cleft lip worry about their child's physical attractiveness to others, especially strangers. Parents are sensitive to the reactions and comments of professionals and their family and look at others' facial and emotional reactions when viewing their baby with a facial deformity. Fears of feeding or hurting the face and the mouth and concern that the cleft extends into the brain are common. Demonstrating feeding techniques and promoting normal infant care routines provide opportunities for learning and allaying anxieties.

It is beneficial to recommend that parents photograph their infant with a facial cleft. The provider can discuss with parents the usefulness of retaining a photograph that will be available for the child to view when older. If the parents are resistant, stating that they prefer to forget this time of sadness and wish to defer picture taking until after cleft lip repair, it may be prudent for a professional working with the family to take a photograph to keep in the infant's chart.

Families may verbalize concerns regarding oral, auditory, and dental problems in their child. These concerns and consequent stressors recur over time with multiple hospitalizations, tooth eruption, initial speech, school entry, and adolescent self-image concerns.

Orthodontic services are a crucial component of the rehabilitation process and are covered by the local state and federal funding programs for children with birth defects if a family is financially eligible. Families who do not meet the financial eligibility often find this care very expen-sive. Many insurance companies do not authorize treatment by nonmedical providers who render services such as dental, orthodontic, or prosthetic care as well as speech and psychologic care.

Special cultural issues that affect families who have a child with a cleft lip and palate are mostly concerned with the etiology of the cleft condition. Superstitions about why clefts occur often originate in a family's country of origin. Hispanic and Filipino cultural folklore believes that clefting is related to the lunar cycle. A lunar eclipse or a crescent moon during a woman's pregnancy predisposes her unborn child to clefts. Some Asian cultural folklores relate construction, cutting, a fall, or moving the mother's bed during pregnancy with birth defects—especially clefting. In Chinese culture the center of a person's face is very important and integral to that person's being (i.e., instead of the heart, which is common in Western culture). This view has implications for a cleft lip and palate deformity in its central location.

Most young parents acknowledge that such beliefs are part of cultural folklores and are explanations that their parents and grandparents provided for the untoward events that happened during a pregnancy. Trying to disprove these theories is unnecessary, especially because the etiology of clefts is unknown. It is more useful to focus on the common feeling of paternal and maternal guilt associated with a birth defect and work through the grief process over time.

Some families bring with them extreme fears of surgery and hospitalization, but fear usually seems to be experience related (i.e., a relative who died after a surgical procedure) rather than related to a specific cultural framework. The concept of health care in general, especially preventive health care (e.g., the routine dental care or anticipatory guidance needed to prevent speech articulation problems), is unfamiliar to some families. The very idea of seeking nonemergent health care services is particularly unknown in families who originate from other countries outside the United States that do not have many health care resources.

RESOURCES

About Face-USA
PO Box 737
Warrington, PA 18976
(888) 486-1209
www.aboutfaceusa.org
Provide newsletter, information, and support

American Cleft Palate–Craniofacial Association (ACPA)
104 South Estes Dr, Suite 204
Chapel Hill, NC 27514
(919) 933-9044; (919) 933-9604 (fax)
Cleftline: 1-800-24-CLEFT
cleftline@aol.com, www.cleft.com
Referral to local cleft-craniofacial team; written pamphlets and fact sheets in English and Spanish; distribution of document; "Parameters for Evaluation and Treatment" (4/00)

Changing Faces
www.changingfaces.co.uk
Support organization and publisher of child and adult books and material on the emotional and social aspects of living with a facial difference

Children's Medical Ventures
5 Technology Dr
Wallingford, CT 06492
(888) 766-8443
Hospital ordering: (800) 377-3449
www.childmed.com
Specialty feeding products, cleft palate nipple (Pigeon nipple)

Cleft lip and palate: Critical elements of care (1st ed.), Seattle, 1997, Children's Hospital and Regional Medical Center
(206) 527-5709, ext. 1

COSCO
Columbus, IN
(800) 468-0174
Dream Ride infant car bed/car seat: car safety bed for infants with Pierre Robin sequence who require prone positioning

Let's Face It
(360) 676-7325
www.faceit.org
Comprehensive guide to support and information on craniofacial anomalies

Mead, Johnson & Co., Nutritional Division
Evansville, IN 47721-0001
(812) 429-5000
1-800-BABY123
Free booklet for cleft lip and palate nursers, "Your cleft lip and palate child: A basic guide for parents"

Medela, Inc
4610 Prime Parkway
McHenry, IL 60050-7005
(800) 435-8316; (816) 362-1166
For breast pump rentals and Haberman feeders

Wide Smiles
PO Box 5153
Stockton, CA 95205-0153
(209) 942-2912
www.widesmiles.org

Books for Parents

Berkowitz, S. (1994). *The cleft palate story*. Chicago: Quintessence Publishing.

Charkins, H. (1996). *Children with facial difference: A parent's guide*. Bethesda, Md.: Woodbine House.

Moller, K.T., Starr, C.D., & Johnson, S.A. (1990). *A parent's guide to cleft lip and palate*. Minneapolis: University of Minnesota Press.

Videocassettes for Parents

"Feeding the Newborn with a Cleft Palate"
Hospital for Sick Children–Cleft Lip and Palate Program
555 University Ave
Toronto, Ontario M5G1X8
(416) 813-7490; (416) 813-6637 (fax)

"Teasing and How to Stop It"
British Columbia's Children's Hospital
4480 Oak St
Vancouver, BC V6H 3V4
(604) 875-2345

"Understanding Cleft Lip and Palate—A Guide for New Parents"
Foundation for Faces of Children
258 Harvard St, #367
Brookline, MA 02446
Excellent videotape for new parents in the nursery; free and in English and Spanish

Summary of Primary Care Needs for the Child with Cleft Lip and Palate

HEALTH CARE MAINTENANCE
Growth and Development

Expectations for physical growth and development are the same as those for the noncleft population.
Syndromic clefts may be associated with developmental delay.

Diet
Use of squeeze bottle, cleft palate nurser, or special nipples enhances bottle feeding. Provision of expressed breast milk with use of an electric pump is desirable in infants with cleft palate.
Introduction of solids by spoon is possible at the same time as in unaffected infants.
Gummy or sticky foods or foods that can cause choking should be avoided.

Safety
Elbow restraints are needed following surgical procedures.
Avoidance of utensils, straws, and textured foods is recommended for approximately 2 wk after surgical procedures to allow for nontraumatic oral healing.
Contact sports should be avoided for 6 wk after surgeries.
Prone positioning for infants with Pierre Robin sequence may require car safety bed vs. car seat.

Immunizations
All routine immunizations should be given on schedule.
May elect not to administer DaPT within 24 hr of a surgical procedure and MMR/varicella 1 wk before a surgery.
Administer pneumococcal vaccine as additional protective effect in preventing otitis media.

Screening
Vision. Routine screening is recommended.
Children with isolated cleft palate or Pierre Robin sequence need a dilated eye examination by a pediatric ophthalmologist at 1 yr of age and 4 to 5 yr of age to rule out myopia, which is found in Stickler syndrome.
Hearing. Audiology screening for children with cleft lip and alveolus is recommended with the same guidelines as for the unaffected population.
Ongoing close monitoring for conductive hearing loss in children with cleft palate is required because of eustachian tube dysfunction.
Dental. Screening for milk bottle caries is important to preserve dentition and prevent alveolar bone loss.
Routine pediatric dental care is given for children with cleft lip. In addition, children with cleft alveolus and palate need an orthodontic evaluation by age 5 to 7 yr.
Blood pressure. Routine screening is recommended.
Hematocrit. Routine screening is recommended.
Urinalysis. Routine screening is recommended.
Tuberculosis. Routine screening is recommended.

COMMON ILLNESS MANAGEMENT
Differential Diagnosis
Fever. Rule out acute otitis media. Chronic serous otitis media or recurrent acute otitis media must be aggressively treated.
Drug interactions. There are no drug interactions.

Continued

Summary of Primary Care Needs for the Child with Cleft Lip and Palate—cont'd

DEVELOPMENTAL ISSUES

Sleep Patterns

Unilateral cleft lip and palate and deviated septum result in noisy breathing especially with upper respiratory infection.

There is an increased risk of sleep state obstructive apnea following secondary palatal surgical procedures.

Disruption of sleep patterns may occur following surgical procedures and hospitalization.

Signs of sleep state obstructive apnea require careful pulmonary evaluation and management in infants with Pierre Robin sequence.

Toileting

Temporary regression may occur following surgical procedure and hospitalization.

Discipline

Discipline expectations are normal, with allowances during hospitalizations and 1 to 2 wk after surgery.

Overprotectiveness or lack of limit setting may result if family pities child.

Child Care

Child care may need to be in a smaller group setting during winter months because of increased risk of otitis media.

Speech therapy sessions need to be coordinated with child care arrangements.

Schooling

Speech therapy begins at age 3 yr for children with cleft palate, they require an individualized education program (IEP). They may also require assistance with expressive language development.

Peer teasing may negatively impact performance.

Teasing may occur because of lip, nose, and dentition appearance or speech articulation problems.

Sexuality

Genetic counseling is recommended to discuss recurrence risks.

It is recommended that women of childbearing age take folic acid to hopefully reduce recurrence risk of clefts.

During pregnancy a detailed ultrasound is available to ascertain whether the fetus has a cleft lip.

Transition into Adulthood

Treatment plan should be completed by age 21 yr.

There is difficulty in procuring third-party payment for any orthodontic, oral-maxillofacial, or plastic surgical services in adulthood.

Family Concerns

There is heightened awareness of physical appearance.

Presurgical photographs are important.

Speech, audiology, and dental issues are challenging for families.

Cultural superstitions are common regarding the etiology of clefts.

Multiple surgical procedures during childhood are stressful for families.

REFERENCES

American Cleft Palate–Craniofacial Association. (2000). *Parameters for evaluation and treatment of patients with cleft lip/palate or other craniofacial anomalies. Official publication of the American Cleft Palate–Craniofacial Association* (revised edition).Chapel Hill, N.C.: Author.

Aniansson, G., Svensson, H., Becker, M., & Ingvarsson, L. (2002). Otitis media and feeding with breast milk of children with cleft palate. *Scand J Plast Reconstr Surg Hand Surg, 36*(1), 9-15.

Bender, P.L. (2000). Genetics of cleft lip and palate. *J Pediatr Nurs, 15,* 242-249.

Berkowitz, S. (1996). Secondary alveolar bone grafting: After lip and palate closure. In S. Berkowitz (Ed.). *Cleft lip and palate* (vol. I and II). San Diego: Singular Publishing Group, pp. 103-113.

Bian, G. et al. (2001). Caries experience and oral health behavior in Chinese children with cleft lip and/or palate. *Pediatr Dent, 23*(5), 431-434.

Bluestone, C.D. (1998). Role of surgery for OM in the era of resistant bacteria. *Pediatric Infect Dis J, 17*(11), 1090-1098.

Boekelheide, A. et al. (1992). *Comparison of postsurgical feeding techniques following cleft lip repair on suture line integrity, volume of oral fluid intake and length of hospital stay: A multicenter study.* Presented at the American Cleft Palate–Craniofacial Association Annual Meeting, Portland, Ore.

Centers for Disease Control and Prevention (CDC) National Center on Birth Defects and Developmental Disabilities; Web site: www.cdc.gov/ncbddd/bd/faq1.htm.

Charkins, H. (1996). *Children with facial differences: A parent's guide.* Bethesda, Md.: Woodbine House.

Cunningham, M.L. & Jerome, J.T. (1997). Linear growth characteristics of children with cleft lip and palate. *J Pediatr, 131*(5), 707-711.

Curtin, G. (1990). The infant with cleft lip or palate: More than a surgical problem. *J Perinat Neonatal Nurs, 3,* 80-89.

Denny, A. & Kalantarian, B. (2002). Mandibular distraction in neonates: A strategy to avoid tracheostomy. *Plast Reconstr Surg, 109*(3), 896-906.

Elmendorf, E.N., D'Antonio, L.L., & Hardesty, R.A. (1993). Assessment of the patient with cleft lip and palate—a developmental approach. *Clin Plast Surg, 20,* 607-621.

Endriga, M.C. & Kapp-Simon, K.A. (1999). Psychological issues in craniofacial care, state of the art. *Cleft Palate Craniofac J, 36*(1), 3-11.

Gorlin, R.Y., Cohen, M.M., & Hennekam, R.C. (2001). Orofacial clefting syndromes: General aspects. In R.Y. Gorlin, M.M. Cohen, & R.C. Hennekam (Eds.). *Syndromes of the head and neck* (4th ed.). New York: Oxford University Press, pp. 850-876.

Jones, M.C. (2002). Prenatal diagnosis of cleft lip and palate: Detection rates, accuracy of ultrasonography, associated anomalies, and strategies for counseling. *Cleft Palate Craniofac J, 39*(2), 169-173.

Kearns, G., Perrott, D.H., Sharma, A., Kaban, L.B., & Vargervik, K. (1997). Placement of endosseous implants in grafted alveolar clefts. *Cleft Palate Craniofac J, 34*(6), 520-525.

Kirschner, R.E. & LaRossa, D. (2000). Cleft lip and palate. *Otolaryngol Clin North Am, 33*(6), 1191-1215.

Lee, D., Youk, A., & Goldstein, N.A. (1999). A meta-analysis of swimming and water precautions. *Laryngoscope, 109*(4), 536-540.

Livingstone, V.H. et al. (2000). Neonatal hypernatremic dehydration associated with breast-feeding malnutrition: A retrospective survey. *CMAJ, 162*(5), 647-652.

Millard, D.R. (1980). *Cleft craft: The evolution of its surgery. The unilateral deformity* (vol. 1). *Bilateral and rare deformities* (vol. 2). *Alveolar and palatal deformities* (vol. 3). Boston: Little, Brown, & Co.

Millard, D.R. (1993). Introduction, clefts 1993, past, present and future. *Clin Plast Surg, 20,* 597-598.

Millard, T. & Richman, L.C. (2001). Different cleft conditions, facial appearance, and speech: Relationship to psychological variables. *Cleft Palate Craniofac J, 38*(1), 68-75.

Moller, K.T., Starr, C.D., & Johnson, S.A. (1990). *A parent's guide to cleft lip and palate.* Minneapolis: University of Minnesota Press.

Monasterio, F.O., Drucker, M., Molina, F., & Ysunza, A. (2002). Distraction osteogenesis in Pierre Robin sequence and related respiratory problems in children. *J Cranfac Surg, 13,* 79-83.

Muntz, H.R. (1993). An overview of middle ear disease in cleft palate children. *Facial Plast Surg, 9,* 177-180.

Murray, J.C. (2002). Gene/environment causes of cleft lip and/or palate. *Clin Genet, 61*(4), 248-256.

Myer, C.B. et al. (1998). Airway management in Pierre Robin sequence. *Otolaryngol Head Neck Surg, 118,* 630-635.

Otitis Media Guideline Panel. (1994). Quick reference guide for clinicians managing otitis media with effusion in young children. *J Am Acad Nurse Pract, 6*(10), 493-499.

Overturf, G.D. (2000). American Academy of Pediatrics Committee on Infectious Diseases technical report: Prevention of pneumococcal infections, including the use of pneumococcal conjugate and polysaccharide vaccines and antibiotic prophylaxis. *Pediatrics, 106,* 367-376.

Paradise, J.L., Elster, B.A., & Tan, L. (1994). Evidence in infants with cleft palate that breast milk protects against otitis media. *Pediatrics, 94,* 853-860.

Peterson-Falzone, S., Hardin-Jones, M., & Karnell, M. (2001). *Cleft palate speech* (3rd ed.). St. Louis: Mosby.

Pham, A.N., Seow, W.K., & Shusterman, S. (1997). Developmental dental changes in isolated cleft lip and palate. *Pediatr Dent, 19*(2), 109-113.

Prahl-Andersen, B. (2000). Dental treatment of predental and infant patients with clefts and craniofacial anomalies. *Cleft Palate Craniofac J, 37*(6), 528-532.

Prescott, N.J., Natalie, J., & Malcolm, S. (2002). Folate and the face: Evaluating the evidence for the influence of folate genes on craniofacial development. *Cleft Palate Craniofac J, 39*(3), 327-331.

Prescott, N.J., Winter, R.M., & Malcolm, S. (2001). Non-syndromic cleft lip and palate: Complex genetics and environmental effects. *Ann Hum Genet, 65*(pt. 6), 505-515.

Romitti, P.A., Lidral, A.C., Munger, R.G., Daack-Hirsch, S., Burns, T.L., et al. (1999). Candidate gene for non-syndromic cleft lip and palate and maternal cigarette smoking and alcohol consumption: Evaluation of gentotype-environment interactions from a population-based case-control study of orofacial clefts. *Teratology, 59*(1), 39-50.

Salata, J.A. & Derkay, D.S. (1996). Water precautions in children with tympanostomy tubes. *Arch Otolaryngol Head Neck Surg, 122*(3), 276-280.

Sidman, J.D., Sampson, D., & Templeton, B. (2001). Distraction osteogenesis of the mandible for airway obstruction in children. *Laryngoscope, 111,* 1137-1146.

Sie, K.C., Tampakopoulou, D.A., Sorom, J., Gruss, J.S., & Eblen, L.E. (2001). Results with Furlow palatoplasty in management of VPI. *Plast Reconstr Surg, 108,* 17-25.

Sirois, M., Caouette-Laberge, L., Spier, S., Larocque, Y., & Egerszegi, E.P. (1994). Sleep apnea following a pharyngeal flap: A feared complication. *Plast Reconstr Surg, 93*(5), 943-947.

Spritz, R.A. (2001). The genetics and epigenetics of orofacial clefts. *Curr Opin Pediatr, 13*(6), 556-560.

Strauss, R.P. (2001). "Only skin deep": Health, resilience, and craniofacial care. *Cleft Palate Craniofac J, 38*(3), 226-230.

St. Hilaire, H. & Buchbinder, D. (2000). Maxillofacial pathology and management of Pierre Robin sequence. *Otolaryngol Clin North Am, 33*(6), 1241-1258.

Wagner, W. & Harrison, M.R. (2002). Fetal operations in the head and neck area: Current state. *Head Neck, 24*(5), 482-490.

Willner, J.P. (2000). Genetic evaluation and counseling in head and neck syndromes. *Otolaryngol Clin North Am, 33*(6), 1159-1169.

Witt, P.D. & D'Antonio, L.L. (1993). Velopharyngeal insufficiency and secondary palatal management—a new look at an old problem. *Clin Plast Surg, 20,* 707-721.

Ysunza, A., Pamplona, M.C., Mendoza, M., Molina, F., Martinez, P., et al. (2001). Surgical treatment of submucous cleft palate: A comparative trial of two modalities for palatal closure. *Plast Reconstr Surg, 107*(1), 9-14.

20 Congenital Adrenal Hyperplasia

Erin Powell Alving and Daniel F. Gunther

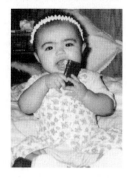

Etiology

The adrenal glands are small triangular organs located at the top of each kidney. They are divided into two major components: the adrenal medulla, which is in the center of the gland, and the adrenal cortex, which surrounds the medulla.

The adrenal cortex synthesizes mineralocorticoids (mainly aldosterone), glucocorticoids (primarily cortisol), and androgens (male hormones) through three separate metabolic pathways (Figure 20-1). Cortisol, aldosterone, and adrenal androgens play a crucial role in maintaining homeostasis by helping to regulate the body's blood pressure; glucose, sodium, and water levels; sexual development; and other metabolic processes (New, 1995; Speiser, 2001). Cortisol is particularly crucial in mediation of the body's response to stress.

Congenital adrenal hyperplasia (CAH) is caused by a deficiency of one of the enzymes used by the adrenal cortex to produce cortisol from cholesterol—a five-step conversion process. Inherited defects have been described in all five enzymes, but in more than 90% of cases the defect is in the enzyme 21-hydroxylase (Levine, 2000). Other enzyme defects are rare and are not discussed here.

Adrenal production of glucocorticoids is regulated by a feedback system to the hypothalamus and pituitary gland (Figure 20-2). The hypothalamus secretes corticotropin-releasing factor (CRF), which causes the pituitary gland to produce adrenocorticotropic hormone (ACTH), which in turn stimulates the adrenals to produce cortisol. Cortisol feeds back to the hypothalamus and pituitary, reducing release of CRH and ACTH and thus the level of adrenal stimulation. In CAH the "block" at 21-hydroxylase leads to decreased cortisol production, which means less feedback and therefore ever-increasing stimulation of the adrenals by ACTH, causing hypertrophy of the gland. Since the androgen pathway is "upstream" of the block, androgens (dehydroepiandrosterone [DHEA], androstenedione) are overproduced, like a river overflowing its banks.

In severe cases of CAH, where the 21-hydroxylase enzyme is completely, or nearly completely, inactive, these high levels of androgens lead to in utero virilization of females, causing them to be born with ambiguous genitalia (Figure 20-3). Males are generally normal in appearance. Without treatment in the first several weeks after birth, the lack of cortisol and aldosterone can result in salt loss, hypovolemic shock, and death—so-called adrenal crises.

Classification

The hallmarks of CAH are an ever-present risk of developing adrenal crises in times of stress and the progressive virilization of both boys and girls in childhood and throughout life. The severity of both problems differs in individuals according to the severity of the 21-hydroxylase enzyme defect. Traditionally, CAH has been broadly divided into three categories based on severity and timing of presentation:

- *Classical salt wasting.* These children are the most severely affected. Females present with ambiguous genitalia at birth, and both males and females will present with salt-wasting adrenal crises in the first several weeks of life. Death will result without treatment.
- *Classical non–salt wasting.* This type is sometimes called "simple virilizing." Females will present with varying degrees of genital virilization, but both males and females do not manifest life-threatening salt wasting.
- *Nonclassical.* This type is also called "late onset" or "cryptic." These less severely affected individuals make up the majority of those with CAH. Girls do not have ambiguous genitalia at birth. The manifestations can be quite variable, ranging from young children presenting with pubic hair and advanced bone age to hirsutism and menstrual irregularities in adult women. Both males and females may have problems with infertility.

This classification system is somewhat arbitrary and even misleading in the sense that it suggests a qualitative difference among the groups. In reality, there is a continuum of severity, from mild to severe, based on the specific combination of 21-hydroxylase gene defects. The term "non–salt wasting" should be used with caution since it is now well appreciated that all affected children are salt wasters to some extent (Frisch et al, 2001).

Known Genetic Etiology

The gene that codes for the 21-hydroxylase enzyme *(CYP21)* is located on the short arm of chromosome 6, adjacent to the major histocompatibility complex (HLA class I and II). In addition to the active gene there is a "pseudogene" that flanks it. The active gene and pseudogene are capable of swapping genetic material through a process called gene conversion. It is this conversion that accounts for the frequency of mutations in the active gene (Wedell et al, 1994). A small number of these gene conversions account for the majority of cases of 21-hydroxylase CAH. Six of the most common mutations totally inactivate the gene ("null" mutations). Other mutations attenuate the enzyme to variable extents but do not completely inactivate it, allowing for some cortisol and aldosterone production.

CAH is an autosomal recessive disease—two defective genes must be inherited (one from the mother, one from the

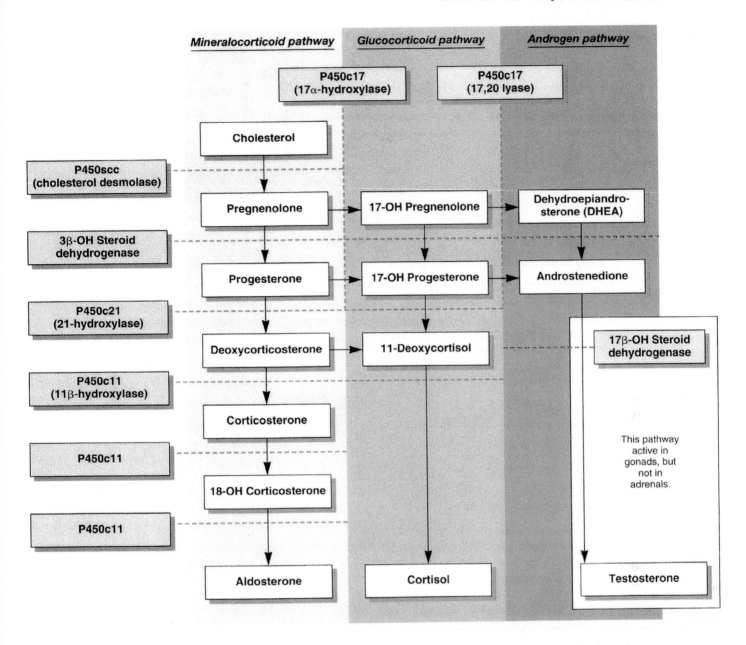

FIGURE 20-1 Adrenal steroid pathway for mineralocorticoids, glucocorticoids, and androgens. (From Gunther, D.G. & Bukowski, T.P. [1998].Congenital adrenal hyperplasia: A spectrum of disorders. *Contemporary Urology, 11*[1], 54. Reprinted with permission.)

father) for the disease to become manifest. Most children with CAH are compound heterozygotes, having inherited a different mutation from each of their parents. If a "null" mutation is inherited from both parents the child will be severely affected (classical salt wasting). If two mild defects are inherited, the child will be mildly affected (nonclassical). Those that inherit a "null" mutation from one parent and a less severe mutation from the other, will fall somewhere in between (Gunther & Bukowski, 1999; Miller, 1994).

Incidence and Prevalence

More than 8 million newborns worldwide have been screened for classical 21-hydroxylase deficiency CAH. Screening reports from Brazil, Canada, France, Germany, Israel, Italy, Japan, New Zealand, Portugal, Saudi Arabia, Scotland, Spain, Sweden, Switzerland, and the United States show incidences ranging from 1:5000 live births in Saudi Arabia to 1:23,000 live births in New Zealand (Pang & Shook, 1997). The overall incidence of classical 21-hydroxylase deficiency is estimated to be 1:15,000 live births worldwide (Speiser, 2001), although some isolated populations (e.g., the Yu'pik-speaking Eskimos of Alaska) have an extraordinarily high incidence of CAH—as many as 1 in 282 (Trautman et al, 1996). Two thirds to three fourths of cases are the salt-losing form (New, 1998).

The incidence of nonclassical CAH is even higher—1:1000 in diverse white populations. Haplotype studies suggest that 3.7% of Ashkenazi Jews and 1.9% of Hispanics may be

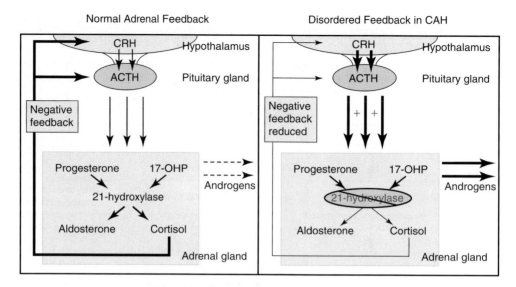

FIGURE 20-2 Hypothalamic/pituitary/adrenal feedback loop in normal subjects and in those with CAH. Note that in CAH corticotrophin-releasing hormone (CRH) and adenocorticotropic hormone (ACTH) are increased because of decreased cortisol feedback. This leads to adrenal gland hypertrophy and a build-up of "upstream" steroids—progesterone and 17-hydroxyprogesterone (17-OHP), which are then shunted toward androgen production.

BOX 20-1

Clinical Manifestations at Time of Diagnosis

Virilization
Elevated serum 17-OHP (hydroxyprogesterone)
Electrolyte changes

BOX 20-2

Signs and Symptoms of Acute Adrenal Insufficiency

Nausea or vomiting
Pallor
Cold, moist skin
Weakness
Dizziness or confusion
Rapid heart rate
Rapid-breathing
Abdominal, back, or leg pain
Dehydration
Hypotension

---

affected. Blacks have a relatively low incidence. It is estimated that nonclassical 21-hydroxylase deficiency CAH is the most common autosomal recessive disease in humans (Levine, 2000). Overall prevalence rates are not reported.

Clinical Manifestations at Time of Diagnosis (Box 20-1)

Virilization

Nearly all female infants with CAH will have some virilization apparent on physical examination at birth (Figure 20-3). The findings range from a mildly enlarged clitoris to complete fusion and rugae of the labia with a male-appearing phallus. The scale of virilization developed by Prader is useful in staging the degree of virilization (Figure 20-4). Unfortunately, severely virilized female infants may go undiagnosed because they are mistaken for cryptorchid males with hypospadias or micropenis, although virilization to that extent (Prader stage 5) is rare. Because the most common cause of ambiguous genitalia is CAH, it should be high on the clinician's index of suspicion during the work-up (Levine, 2000). In karyotype-proven females (46,XX) who have normal müllerian structures (ovaries, fallopian tubes, uterus) and no history of maternal exposure to exogenous androgens, the diagnosis is nearly certain (Gunther & Bukowski, 1999). Male newborns with CAH look normal and cannot be reliably identified by physical

examination, although the penis may be slightly enlarged and genital pigmentation mildly increased (Speiser, 2001).

Elevated Serum 17-OHP

Newborns with either form of classical CAH will have significantly elevated 17-hydroxyprogesterone (17-OHP) levels by 24 to 36 hours of age. False-positive results are possible, however, in premature or low birth weight infants (Pang & Shook, 1997).

Electrolyte Changes

Newborns with salt-losing CAH will have elevated activity levels of plasma renin at birth but normal electrolytes generally (Pang, 1997). If salt-losing CAH is not diagnosed and replacement therapy is not started at birth, both male and female infants will have symptoms of acute adrenal insufficiency and a salt-losing crisis within the first few weeks of life. These symptoms include failure to thrive, weakness, vomiting, and dehydration (Speiser, 2001; Box 20-2). Unfortunately these symptoms are nonspecific and usually prompt a work-up for sepsis, pyloric stenosis, or severe malabsorption. Hyponatremia combined

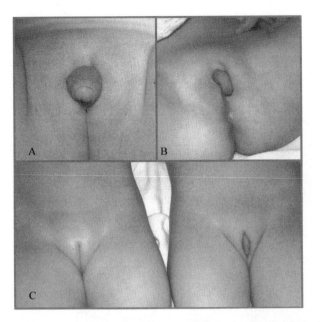

FIGURE 20-3 Examples of ambiguous genitalia in, **A,** a female infant with CAH and, **B,** a toddler with CAH. **C,** Three-year-old fraternal twins, one with CAH and the other unaffected, highlight the difference in clitoral development.

BOX 20-3
Treatment

Glucocorticoid replacement
Mineralocorticoid replacement
Sodium chloride supplementation (salt-losing infants)
Stress treatment
Gender assignment and genital surgery

---

with hyperkalemia is a hallmark of adrenal insufficiency, which will help differentiate it from other causes of dehydration. Children not as severely affected (simple virilizers, nonclassical) may go undiagnosed for years. These children still have an impaired ability to withstand stress, so even minor illnesses, especially febrile illnesses, may cause excessive weakness, pallor, hypotension, and prolonged convalescence. Severe stressors (e.g., surgery, a fractured bone) can trigger acute adrenal insufficiency, with extreme weakness, abdominal pain, vomiting, dehydration, hypotension, and—if not adequately treated—vascular collapse and death (Levine, 2000).

Treatment (Box 20-3)

It was not until the 1950s that an understanding of the metabolic defect in CAH led to the current concept of replacement therapy, and it was another decade before adequate therapy was routinely used (Merke et al, 2002). A basal, replacement dose of hydrocortisone is intended to suppress ACTH stimulation of the adrenals and the resultant overproduction of adrenal androgens. The goals of treatment are to prevent acute adrenal insufficiency, prevent further virilization, achieve normal growth and adult stature, achieve normal fertility, normalize blood pressure, and achieve electrolyte homeostasis (Gunther & Bukowski, 1999).

Glucocorticoid Replacement

In both salt-losing and non–salt-losing CAH, glucocorticoids (usually hydrocortisone tablets) are given as a replacement for cortisol. Determining an optimal replacement dose is crucial to minimize side effects while achieving desired therapeutic effects. Excessive hydrocortisone dosage can lead to obesity, stunted linear growth, and signs of Cushing syndrome (e.g., truncal obesity, striae, bruising, hirsutism, muscle weakness, hypertension) (Speiser, 2001). Inadequate dosage puts a child at risk for acute adrenal insufficiency and allows excessive androgen production, which causes virilization and accelerates growth and advancement of bone age. A common regimen is 10 to 15 mg/m^2/day of hydrocortisone divided into three doses given orally every 8 hours, but there is considerable disagreement on the optimal dosage regimen (New, 1998; Speiser, 2001).

Hydrocortisone oral suspension (Cortef) was voluntarily recalled by the manufacturer in July 2001 (Merke & Cutler, 2001). Consequently, hydrocortisone is no longer available in a liquid preparation.

Historically more potent glucocorticoids such as prednisone and dexamethasone have not been widely used in young children because of concerns about overtreatment. However, recently it has been suggested that cautious use of dexamethasone may provide a once per day dosing option for even young children without adversely affecting growth (Rivkees & Crawford, 2000). Older adolescents and adults frequently use these agents for replacement and find the once or twice daily administration more manageable (Speiser, 2001).

Mineralocorticoid Replacement

Salt-losing CAH requires mineralocorticoid replacement with fludrocortisone (Florinef) in addition to glucocorticoid therapy (New, 1998). Even children with non–salt-wasting CAH have mild impairment of aldosterone synthesis, as evidenced by elevated plasma renin activity, even though such impairment may not be apparent clinically. Many practitioners now advocate adding fludrocortisone to the treatment regimen of all children with CAH. This may normalize the plasma renin activity levels and may permit a reduction of the hydrocortisone dose and improve linear growth (Lim et al, 1995; Speiser, 2001). The usual dose of fludrocortisone is 100 µg orally per day. Higher doses may be necessary in infants and sometimes adolescents (Speiser, 2001). Doses do not need to be increased in times of stress. Sodium chloride supplementation, 3 to 5 mEq/kg/day, may be required in infants if salt loss exceeds salt intake in spite of mineralocorticoid therapy (Lim et al, 1995).

Treatment in Times of Stress

The basal steroid dose should be tripled during the acute phase of an illness (e.g., temperature >38.4° C or >101.1° F, vomiting, malaise) or other times of stress, such as a serious accident, a broken bone, or significant pain. A return to basal dose does not require prolonged tapering and should be accomplished as soon as the acute stress is resolved (Levine, 2000).

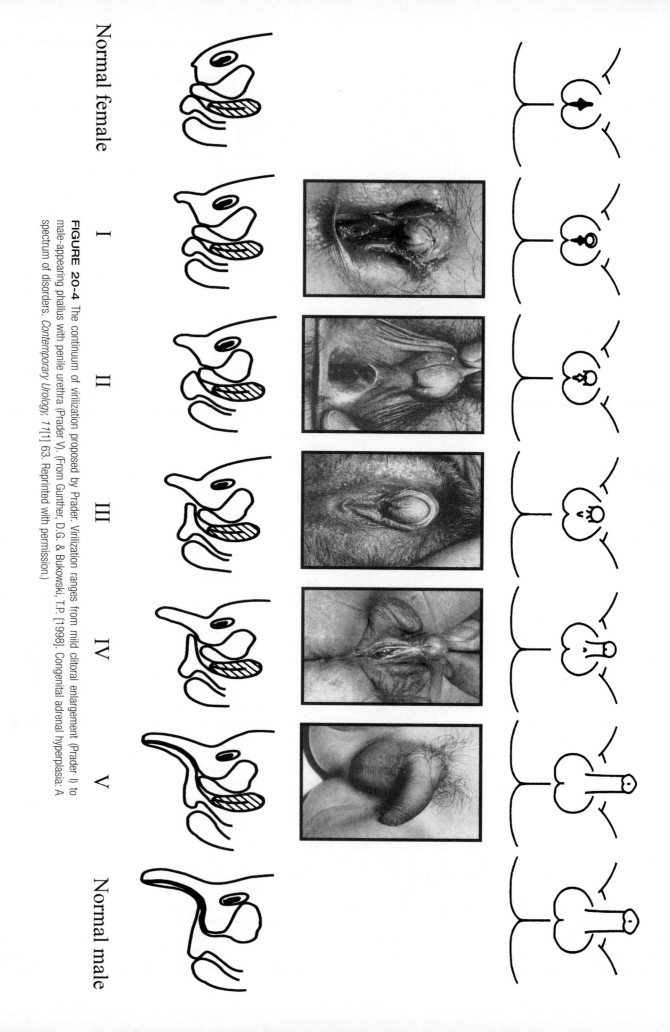

FIGURE 20-4 The continuum of virilization proposed by Prader. Virilization ranges from mild clitoral enlargement (Prader I) to male-appearing phallus with penile urethra (Prader V). (From Gunther, D.G. & Bukowski, T.P. [1998]. Congenital adrenal hyperplasia: A spectrum of disorders. *Contemporary Urology, 11*[1] 63. Reprinted with permission.)

Normal female I II III IV V Normal male

If a child vomits more than once, the stress is severe, or the child does not respond to oral treatment, injectable hydrocortisone (Solu-Cortef) may be given in equivalent doses to oral. Parents should have injectable hydrocortisone on hand, know the indications for using it, and learn how to prepare and give an intramuscular (IM) injection. Steroids can also be given intravenously (IV) (Solu-Cortef, Solu-Medrol) during acute stress or at the time of surgery. *If the necessity of giving emergency treatment is uncertain, there is no physical harm in treating suspected acute adrenal insufficiency. In such situations it is always best to err on the side of prompt, aggressive treatment.*

Gender Assignment and Genital Surgery

Conventionally, females with CAH are raised as females in all but the most severe cases and most girls with CAH experience virilization to an extent that surgical correction seems reasonable. This has been standard practice for many years and remains so today. Recently, however, some long-standing basic assumptions about gender and genitalia are being increasingly questioned.

Assignment of the female gender for chromosomal females seems sensible given that müllerian structures (uterus, fallopian tubes, ovaries) are intact and fertility is preserved. Most girls with CAH seem satisfied with their gender of rearing and there is little gender dysphoria in most reports (Zucker et al, 1996). However, there has been increasing consideration for the effect of prenatal exposure to high-level androgens and how this may affect development. Recognition that virilizing effects on the brain play a role in gender identification and "masculinized" behavior has led some to contend that severely virilized girls (Prader stage 5) should be raised as males (Diamond & Sigmundson, 1997; Meyer-Bahlburg, 2001). Clearly, gender assignment in the realm of ambiguous genitalia is an ongoing ethical debate, calling for continued long-term follow-up studies. To date little scientific data support any one position and the predominant standard of care is to raise these children as girls, consistent with their chromosomal gender (Gunther & Bukowski, 1999).

Surgical techniques to create functional and more normal-appearing genitalia (feminizing genitoplasty) have advanced significantly in recent years. Experienced surgeons are now able to successfully reduce the size of the clitoris while preserving sensation and erectile function and achieving a good cosmetic result (Figure 20-5). Clitorectomy, once the standard of care for clitiromegaly, is no longer acceptable practice. Vaginoplasty separates the single urogenital sinus into a separate urethra and vagina. There can be varying degrees of difficulty with the vaginoplasty, and a variety of techniques are used for the reconstruction depending on the stage of virilization and the nature of the anatomy (Gunther & Bukowski, 1999).

The timing of surgery is still a matter of debate. Feminizing genitoplasty often requires more than one procedure (e.g., clitoral reduction, separation of the fused labia, correction of a urogenital sinus, vaginoplasty). Most surgeons now advocate initial correction before 2 years of age with subsequent refinement in adolescence if necessary to accommodate intercourse (Bailez et al, 1992; Donahoe & Gustafson, 1994; Premawardhana et al, 1997).

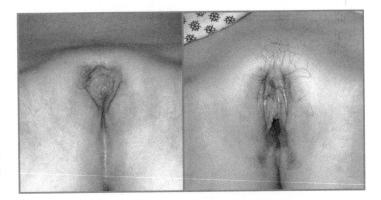

FIGURE 20-5 A 5-year-old girl before (left) and after (right) feminizing genitoplasty by a skilled pediatric urologist. Note the reduction in clitoral size and construction of a labia minora and vaginal introitus. (From Gunther, D.G. & Bukowski, T.P. [1998]. Congenital adrenal hyperplasia: A spectrum of disorders. *Contemporary Urology, 11*[1], 63. Reprinted with permission.)

Outcomes depend greatly on the the skill of the urologist. Having an experienced urologist perform these procedures is crucial to obtaining a good cosmetic result and reducing the risk of urinary incontinence (Gunther & Bukowski, 1999; Schnitzer & Donahoe, 2001). Families opting for surgery should carefully inquire into the surgeon's level of experience, how many procedures of this kind he or she has done in the past, and what the outcomes have been.

Feminizing genitoplasty has also recently become more controversial. For many years it was thought axiomatic that normal-appearing genitalia are crucial for the formation of proper gender identity—for both child and parents (Wilson & Reiner, 1998); but over the last several years this assumption has been called into question by some who see feminizing genitoplasty as a mutilating procedure that often leads to both physical and psychologic scarring (Daaboul & Frader, 2001). Intersex advocacy groups, such as the Intersex Society of North America, maintain that intersex is an anatomic variation from the standard male and female types and that these individuals must be treated with respect for their autonomy and self-determination (Fausto-Sterling, 2000). These groups advocate early psychologic counseling and support in lieu of surgery, until these children are old enough to decide whether to have their genitalia altered. Unfortunately, few long-term follow-up studies of intersex individuals exist to support either position and the debate to this point has generated more heat than light.

Complementary and Alternative Therapies

There are currently no known complementary or alternative therapies for treatment of CAH.

Anticipated Advances in Diagnosis and Management

Newborn Screening

Currently 13 countries and 31 US states routinely screen neonates for CAH using 17-hydroxyprogesterone levels on dried filter paper (National Newborn Screening and Genetics Resource Center, 2002). This has resulted in early diagnosis and associated reductions in morbidity and mortality. Improvements in assay types and reference ranges for low birth weight and preterm infants have contributed to more accurate newborn screening for CAH. Although false-positive results in preterm and low birth weight infants are still problematic, this issue is being addressed through the continued refinements of newborn screening (Therrel, 2001).

Prenatal Diagnosis and Treatment

Recent advances have been made in prenatal diagnosis and prenatal treatment of CAH. Prenatal diagnosis can be made in the first trimester by HLA typing or DNA analysis performed by chorionic villus sampling (CVS) at or after 9 weeks' gestation. Virilization of female fetuses with CAH can be prevented or reduced by administering dexamethasone to mothers during pregnancy, which crosses the placenta to suppress the fetal adrenals. Dexamethasone therapy must be started before genital formation begins at about 8 weeks' gestation. Because a prenatal diagnosis of CAH is not available in the early weeks of pregnancy, the treatment initially includes both affected and unaffected fetuses.

Although initial attempts at prenatal dexamethasone treatment have shown some favorable outcomes and appear to have no complications for infants, results have been variable in preventing virilization. Maternal side effects can also be significant, and long-term effects on growth and psychomotor development in treated children are unknown. More experience is warranted to establish a standard of treatment with prenatal dexamethasone, and long-term studies on growth and psychomotor development of treated children are also necessary.

Improved Medical Therapies

There is an ongoing search for improved treatment regimens that achieve the therapeutic goals while reducing or eliminating undesirable side effects. Current management of CAH often involves choosing between the effects of excess cortisol and the effects of excess androgen because extraphysiologic doses of hydrocortisone are required to fully suppress adrenal androgen overproduction (VanWyk & Gunther, 1996).

One promising solution to this dilemma is reducing the dose of hydrocortisone to physiologic levels and adding flutamide and testolactone to the treatment regimen (Merke et al, 2002). Flutamide is an antiandrogen that is able to block the effects of androgen excess. Testolactone is an aromatase inhibitor that blocks the conversion of androgen to estrogen, which may help improve final height because of estrogen's role in accelerated advancement of bone age (Merke et al, 2002). A reduced, physiologic dose of hydrocortisone eliminates the side effects of hypercortisolism. Preliminary results of a long-term National Institutes of Health (NIH) study have shown normalized growth velocity and bone maturation in the experimental group using this regimen after 2 years (Merke et al, 2000). One obvious drawback of this regimen is that it increases the complexity of treatment, which may lead to decreased adherence to the regimen. Recently introduced androgen blockers and aromatase inhibitors that are given only once daily may help in compliance.

Another area of research is focusing on corticotropin-releasing hormone (CRH) receptor antagonists as a new approach to CAH treatment. Preliminary studies in rats have shown that a prototype CRH receptor antagonist, antalarmin, effectively decreases ACTH and cortisol secretion without causing adrenal insufficiency. Adrenal size is reduced with chronic treatment and is well tolerated. Once toxicology studies are complete, this therapy can be studied in humans (Merke et al, 2002, Merke & Cutler, 2001).

Adrenalectomy

Some clinicians have suggested adrenalectomy as a way of simplifying and improving the management of CAH (Meyers & Grua, 2000; Ritzen & Wedell, 1996; VanWyk & Gunther, 1996). The rationale for adrenalectomy is that it eliminates the need to suppress adrenal androgens, so lower doses of glucocorticoids can be used, reducing the side effects of overtreatment. Proponents of adrenalectomy restrict its use to individuals with a complete absence of 21-hydroxylase, because they are the most difficult to manage and have the lowest final heights (Ritzen & Wedell, 1996; VanWyk & Gunther, 1996). Adrenalectomy as a treatment for severe salt-losing CAH is still considered experimental although more reports are appearing in the literature (Gmyrek et al, 2002).

Advances in Genetic Treatment

Gene therapy is not currently an option for management of CAH although features of the genetic component of this disorder may facilitate gene therapy in the future. Preliminary studies using mouse models have been promising. Once a viral vector specific to the adrenals is developed, gene therapy may be a viable option (Merke & Cutler, 2001).

Associated Problems

The problems associated with CAH are limited in children receiving appropriate therapy. However, primary care providers must be aware of the potential for acute adrenal insufficiency, growth disorders, virilization, and problems surrounding issues of sexuality (Box 20-4).

Acute Adrenal Insufficiency

Children with CAH may develop acute adrenal insufficiency with any significant illness or injury because they lack the ability to produce increased amounts of cortisol as part of the body's normal stress response.

Accelerated Growth and Bone Age

Excessive androgen production results in accelerated linear growth and rapidly advancing bone age in children with CAH who are inadequately treated or undiagnosed. These children may be taller than their peers initially but end up shorter than most as adolescents and adults because of premature closure of the epiphyses. Even if properly managed, the majority of people with CAH will have a shorter final adult height than predicted from mean parental height. Although glucocorticoids reduce adrenal androgen secretion, dosing to maintain physiologic levels can be difficult, and excessive levels can suppress growth. Use of antiandrogens or aromatase inhibitors may improve height outcomes for these children, although no data on final adult height are yet available for these experimental therapies (Migeon & Wisniewski, 2001).

Virilization

Male sexual differentiation in newborn boys with CAH is essentially normal. However, the female fetus with virilizing CAH is exposed to high levels of androgens starting at 7 weeks' gestation. This prevents the formation of separate vaginal and urethral canals, resulting in a single urogenital sinus. The clitoris becomes enlarged, and in severe cases there is rugation and fusion of the labial folds. If untreated or insufficiently treated, boys and girls will develop pubic hair and apocrine body odor by school age. Boys can have an adult-size penis without testicular enlargement and girls continue to have clitoral growth. If the treatment continues to be suboptimal by puberty, females develop acne, hirsutism, poor breast development, and ovarian dysfunction with irregular menstrual periods. Adolescent males may develop adrenal rest tumors (Levine, 2000; Speiser, 2001).

Problems with Sexual Development

Most children with consistently well-controlled CAH will have normal onset and progression of puberty (Lim et al, 1995). Some children, however, may enter puberty prematurely. The onset of precocious puberty is believed to be caused by the "priming" of the pubertal timing system by chronically high androgen levels, triggering the complex—and poorly understood—system of pubertal development (Pescovitz et al, 1984). Children who do experience precocious puberty can be successfully treated with gonadotropin-releasing hormone (GnRH) analogs (Dacou-Voutetakis & Karidis, 1993). GnRH analogs are available as subcutaneous (SC) injections given daily (e.g., leuprolide acetate [Lupron]), IM injections given every 4 weeks (e.g., leuprolide acetate [Lupron Depot Ped]), and intranasal spray (e.g., nafarelin [Synarel]) given four times per day.

The occurrence of precocious puberty not only increases the complexity, expense, and burden of a family's medical regimen but also increases psychosocial stresses. Children with precocious puberty are faced with physical sexual development before they are developmentally and emotionally ready, as well as with teasing and sexual harassment. These children are also at increased risk for sexual abuse (Jackson & Ott, 1990). Parents of a child with precocious puberty must meet with school and daycare personnel to ensure that teasing and sexual harassment are not tolerated. Children must be taught how to maintain their "sexual boundaries" (i.e., what kind of remarks, activities, or touching are "OK" and "not OK") and where to go for help.

Reduced Fertility

Women with CAH have decreased fertility rates compared with unaffected women. By adolescence, females with inadequately treated CAH or undiagnosed nonclassical CAH may have late menarche, menstrual irregularity, and hirsutism caused by androgen excess (Speiser, 2001). Females with the salt-wasting form are more likely to have an inadequate vaginal introitus, impairing sexual activity and their ability to conceive (Lo & Grumbach, 2001). Even when adequately managed, women with CAH have higher than normal levels of circulating progestational hormones for significant periods of time, which may have the effect of an endogenous "mini pill" that suppresses fertility (Helleday et al, 1993). Despite these factors, many women with CAH are able to conceive and carry a pregnancy to term. Those that are diagnosed early, have had consistent adherence to medical therapy, and are of non–salt-wasting status have the best potential for pregnancy (Lo & Grumbach, 2001; Speiser, 2001).

Testicular Masses

Activation of ectopic adrenal tissue, usually found on the testes, can result in adrenal rest tumors in males with CAH. These tumors respond to ACTH stimulation and grow, often resulting in oligospermia and infertility (Avila et al, 1996). Identification of testicular masses in men with CAH as adrenal rest tissue is important, because the treatment is glucocorticoid therapy rather than surgery (the treatment of choice for testicular neoplasms) (Merke et al, 2002).

Congenital Anomalies

The incidence of congenital anomalies associated with CAH is not thought to be significantly increased over that of the general population. Although there have been reports of an increased incidence of upper urinary tract abnormalities associated with CAH, these have not been clearly established (Bacon et al, 1990).

Prognosis

The major risk for children with CAH is death from an unrecognized salt-losing crisis early in infancy or from inadequately treated acute adrenal insufficiency during stress. Screenings of individuals with a family history of CAH for the carrier state, prenatal screenings, and routine neonatal screenings have the potential to greatly reduce the number of children who die of CAH (Therrell, 2001). CAH screening is now included in the newborn screening programs of 31 US states, and other states are considering adding it to their programs (National Newborn Screening and Genetics Testing Center, 2002). Nearly all female infants with CAH have morbidity associated with prenatal virilization and the surgical procedures necessary to correct it. If prenatal treatment of female fetuses to prevent virilization becomes available as a standard treatment, it should have a substantial effect on reducing the morbidity in girls with CAH.

PRIMARY CARE MANAGEMENT

Health Care Maintenance

Growth and Development

Because abnormal linear growth is an indication of inappropriate treatment or poor compliance, careful monitoring of growth is essential. Linear growth should be measured every 1 to 4 months for infants and every 3 to 6 months for children older than 2 years of age. These measurements should be done carefully, using an infantometer for lengths and a stadiometer for heights. The standard scale-mounted measuring device is not accurate enough to detect slight variations in growth. Measurements should be plotted on a standardized growth chart and assessed for changes in growth rate (e.g., an increase or decrease in percentile).

Poor Growth. Linear growth is acutely sensitive to excessive levels of hydrocortisone; therefore any decrease in height percentile on the growth chart should prompt a reassessment of the hydrocortisone dosage. A child's hydrocortisone therapy will occasionally be increased based on a high laboratory 17-OHP result when the result was high because of acute illness, stress from an unusually traumatic venipuncture, or frequently missed hydrocortisone doses before sampling. To avoid unnecessary and possibly harmful increases in hydrocortisone doses, clinicians must rule out these other causes of high 17-OHP values before increasing medication doses. Clinicians can do this by taking a careful history and comparing the prescribed dose of hydrocortisone with the established dose ranges. The primary care provider may be in a position to identify the problem and should contact the endocrinologist with this information.

Another cause of poor linear growth in children with CAH is chronically inadequate mineralocorticoid levels (Migeon & Wisniewski, 2001). A plasma renin activity level that is abnormally high indicates that a child needs additional mineralocorticoid or dietary sodium. A careful history and comparison with established dose ranges will determine if this problem is one of compliance or inadequately prescribed doses.

A child with poorly controlled CAH, or one who was not diagnosed until preschool or school age, may have early cessation of growth because of premature closure of the epiphyses. If such premature closure is suspected, radiographic studies of bone age should be done to assess skeletal maturity.

Excessive Growth. Inadequate hydrocortisone replacement will cause excessive androgen synthesis by the adrenals, resulting in accelerated linear growth. An elevated serum 17-OHP level or clinical findings of increased virilization (e.g., pubic and axillary hair, oily skin, acne, enlargement of the phallus) confirm the cause of excessive growth. Clinicians must be careful to assess whether the inadequate hydrocortisone replacement is secondary to an inappropriately prescribed dose or to poor adherence.

Excessive Weight Gain. Glucocorticoid replacement therapy—even at doses within the accepted therapeutic range—has been associated with obesity (Cornean et al, 1998). Clinicians must closely monitor weight gain, avoid overtreatment with glucocorticoids, and encourage good dietary and activity habits to reduce any tendency toward obesity.

Development. Children with CAH who are diagnosed in infancy or very early in childhood and receive consistently adequate treatment should develop normally (Lim et al, 1995). However, if the diagnosis of CAH is not made until late childhood, the child will be much taller and more mature looking than peers. Because of their mature physical appearance, people may expect these children to have the emotional maturity and behavior of older children. This expectation may lead to frustration for all concerned, inappropriate demands and punishment, and the creation or exacerbation of behavior problems.

When these children stop growing early because of premature epiphyseal closure, they will go from being the tallest to the shortest children in their peer group. Short stature has an effect on behavior and social relationships and probably has an even greater effect on someone who spent early childhood as the tallest person in any group of peers (Holmes et al, 1986; Young-Hyman, 1986).

Parents, school personnel, child care workers, and others who regularly interact with these children should be given clear, frequently reinforced guidelines on age-appropriate expectations to avoid demanding too much of tall but immature children or too little of short adolescents.

Diet

The main modification to a normal diet is an allowance for adequate sodium intake. Although an appropriate dose of mineralocorticoid prevents significant sodium depletion in children with salt-losing CAH, these children should be offered salty foods and allowed to salt their food to taste. This recommendation also applies to children with non–salt-losing CAH because they may have a mild salt deficit when compared with unaffected children. As mentioned previously, good dietary habits are essential to reduce the tendency to gain excessive weight (Cornean et al, 1998). The advice of a dietitian can be helpful in identifying "nutritionally dense" foods that meet a child's dietary needs without excessive calories.

Safety

Children with CAH are not physically impaired or at increased risk for any of the usual physical hazards of childhood, but they are at risk for having their special needs neglected when away from home. Injuries such as a broken bone may not be recognized as potentially life-threatening events. Teachers, child care personnel, coaches, and others in regular contact with the child should have written information describing the condition and the need for prompt treatment in an emergency. The child should wear a Medic-Alert bracelet with this information on it.

The decision of whether to keep injectable hydrocortisone at school or daycare depends on the situation and must be made on a case-by-case basis. Factors to consider are as follows: (1) Can the primary care provider or emergency department be reached in 5 to 10 minutes? (2) Is a parent always available at short notice? (3) Are there trained personnel at the site who are willing to give an IM injection? (4) Does the child engage in activities with a high risk of serious injury?

If injectable hydrocortisone is kept at school or daycare, the most convenient preparation is the 100-mg Solu-Cortef Mix-O-Vial (Pharmacia & Upjohn), which is easy to use and store. Written indications for use and dosage should be provided by the endocrinologist.

Participation in sports is a normal part of childhood and should be encouraged; however, if possible, children with CAH should be directed toward activities with a low risk of serious injury (e.g., swimming, track, tennis). Minor injuries (e.g., bruises, mild or moderate sprains, abrasions) are not cause for special concern. If these children are involved in high-risk sports (e.g., football), parents should meet with the coach to explain their child's special needs in an emergency, as well as provide appropriate written materials, instructions, and authorization for treatment. A parent or team clinician should ideally be present and have hydrocortisone for IM injection on hand during competition. Their presence should be mandatory if the activity takes place more than 15 minutes away from a source of emergency care.

Immunizations

Children with CAH are not immunosuppressed and should receive all standard immunizations at the usual ages. There is currently no recommendation for or against giving additional immunizations (e.g., pneumococcal, influenza), but the benefits of immunity to these diseases must be weighed against the possibility of adverse reactions to the vaccine. In weighing these factors, many clinicians believe that giving additional immunizations is worthwhile to reduce the risk of acute adrenal insufficiency triggered by illness.

It is not necessary to increase the basal dose of hydrocortisone before immunizations are given unless there is a history of adverse reactions to previous immunizations with that vaccine. A common but discretionary recommendation is to give a child acetaminophen a few hours before giving an immunization that is likely to produce a rapid-onset febrile reaction and continue it for 24 to 48 hours afterward.

For new vaccines or new combinations of vaccines, the package insert should be referred to for information on the type and timing of possible reactions and families should be counseled to observe their child closely on the days when reactions are likely to occur (e.g., 5 to 12 days after measles vaccination).

Stress doses of hydrocortisone should be given if a child develops a temperature of more than 38.4° C or is fussy or lethargic after an immunization. Any immunization reaction should be documented so that stress doses of hydrocortisone can be given before subsequent immunizations with the same vaccine.

Screening

Vision. Routine screening is recommended.
Hearing. Routine screening is recommended.
Dental. Routine screening is recommended.
Blood Pressure. Blood pressure should be checked at each primary care visit, which requires special equipment (e.g., a Dinamap [Critikon]) for infants. Every effort should be made to relax and quiet children so that readings are accurate.

Elevated blood pressure in a quiet child may indicate excessive mineralocorticoid or hydrocortisone dosage, whereas low blood pressure may indicate an inadequate mineralocorticoid or hydrocortisone dosage. Either situation should prompt an evaluation of the replacement therapy regimen and compliance.

Hematocrit. Routine screening is recommended.
Urinalysis. Routine screening is recommended.
Tuberculosis. Routine screening is recommended.

Condition-Specific Screening

Serum 17-OHP. Primary care providers may want to order additional screening tests to more closely monitor the adequacy of replacement therapy in children who have difficulty with compliance. The serum 17-OHP level is widely accepted as a measure of hydrocortisone therapy, even though it has the disadvantage of being influenced by temporary stress (e.g., traumatic venipuncture), the length of time since the last hydrocortisone dose, and diurnal fluctuations. To help evaluate the significance of 17-OHP results, clinicians should note on the specimen the time of day (i.e., preferably morning) and the time of the last dose of hydrocortisone. Androstenedione and testosterone levels can be evaluated along with 17-OHP to monitor adequacy of hydrocortisone therapy. Some clinicians rely on 24-hour urinary 17-ketosteroid and pregnanetriol levels to monitor hydrocortisone therapy because of the lack of short-term fluctuations, despite the difficulty in collecting a 24-hour specimen. Serum 17-OHP levels should be no more than three times above normal (i.e., preferably less than 200 ng/dl). Urinary 17-ketosteroid and pregnanetriol levels should also be in the normal to near-normal range for age, as should plasma renin activity. Specimens ordered by the primary care provider should be coordinated with the endocrinologist and sent to the same laboratory to ensure consistency.

Plasma Renin Activity. Mineralocorticoid therapy is monitored by measuring plasma renin activity level. The primary care provider who is monitoring 17-OHP levels should include a plasma renin activity assay for individuals with salt-losing CAH.

Bone Age. The frequency of radiographic studies of bone age depends on the clinical course. Bone-age evaluations are not helpful in newborns. Initial bone age should be determined early in childhood (i.e., at 2 to 3 years of age or at the time of diagnosis if the diagnosis is delayed) and can be used as a baseline for future studies. If a child is growing normally and has consistently acceptable 17-OHP and plasma renin activity levels, routine screening should not be necessary more than every few years.

If a child has growth acceleration, physical findings of increased virilization, or consistently high 17-OHP laboratory results, bone age should be determined to further assess the effects of androgen excess. If bone age is accelerated, this finding can be used to help impress on the family the serious and permanent consequences of poor adherence. All bone-age studies should ideally be read by the same person to avoid inconsistencies in interpretation.

Common Illness Management

Children with CAH are not immunosuppressed and their susceptibility to common childhood illnesses is no different from that of their peers; it is their ability to withstand the stress of illness that is impaired. During periods of illness, these children must be observed closely; consultation with an endocrinologist is necessary if a child shows any signs or symptoms of acute adrenal insufficiency (Box 20-2).

The primary care provider caring for a child with CAH should keep injectable hydrocortisone in the office for emergencies. The most commonly used preparation is the 100-mg Solu-Cortef Mix-O-Vial (Pharmacia & Upjohn) because of its long shelf life and convenience (e.g., it does not require refrigeration). When reconstituted by rotating and depressing the plunger-stopper, it contains 100 mg of hydrocortisone in 2 ml and can be given IM or IV.

In addition to a Medic-Alert bracelet or necklace, the child and family should carry written materials (e.g., a wallet card) stating the diagnosis, stress dose of hydrocortisone, indications for administering the stress dose, and the name and telephone number of the endocrinologist. This emergency information should be updated regularly.

Upper Respiratory Infections and Allergies

If the symptoms are mild and the child does not have fever or marked malaise, no specific treatment or increase in basal dose of hydrocortisone is necessary for upper respiratory infections or allergies. Parents should watch for worsening of symptoms, fever, or unusual lethargy; and school-aged children should know to report these symptoms to their teacher and contact their parents. If symptoms worsen or complications develop, children should be promptly treated with a stress dose of hydrocortisone and seen by the primary care provider for assessment and specific therapy for the illness.

Acute Illnesses

Any known or suspected bacterial illness (e.g., acute otitis media, urinary tract infection, streptococcal pharyngitis, cellulitis) should be treated aggressively with the appropriate antibiotic and stress doses of hydrocortisone during the acute phase of the illness if fever, pain, and malaise are present. When the diagnosis is uncertain or there is a significant risk for secondary infections or complications (e.g., a suspicious but not clearly inflamed tympanic membrane, viral pneumonia, prolonged or marked nasal congestion in a child with a history of frequent acute otitis media or sinusitis), it is wise to treat the child with antibiotics rather than wait for the situation to worsen. The child must be observed closely, with an initial office visit for diagnosis and assessment of the child's overall condition and daily telephone progress reports until the acute phase of the illness has passed. Follow-up office visits should be scheduled as for any other child.

Fever

Although fever is a physiologic response to illness, it is also a stress. Therefore fever in a child with CAH should be treated with acetaminophen in the recommended dose for age. Stress doses of hydrocortisone should be given. It is important to advise families that reducing the fever does not cure the illness and that other treatments (e.g., antibiotics, stress doses of hydrocortisone) should continue to be given as directed. The child must be observed closely (i.e., as described for bacterial and viral illnesses) until the illness has resolved.

Vomiting

If a child with CAH vomits once but otherwise appears well, three times the usual oral dose of hydrocortisone should be given about 20 minutes later, and the child should be closely observed. If a child appears weak or lethargic after vomiting once or vomits more than once, the family should give injectable hydrocortisone IM and contact the endocrinologist immediately. If family members are not able to give injectable

hydrocortisone, they must immediately take the child to the nearest emergency room to receive parenteral hydrocortisone and appropriate fluid and electrolyte therapy because this can be a life-threatening situation. The emergency room staff should contact the endocrinologist but should not delay hydrocortisone therapy while awaiting consultation. A wallet card or other written information on the child's diagnosis, emergency treatment, and endocrinologist can facilitate prompt and appropriate care.

Injury

A child with a significant injury (e.g., fracture, concussion, injury from an automobile accident) should immediately be given hydrocortisone IM and evaluated further for acute adrenal insufficiency at an emergency room. Emergency room personnel should contact the endocrinologist but not delay hydrocortisone therapy while awaiting consultation.

Acute Adrenal Insufficiency

Acute adrenal insufficiency is a life-threatening situation. Symptoms of acute adrenal insufficiency include weakness, nausea, abdominal discomfort, vomiting, dehydration, and hypotension. Any of these signs or symptoms in a child with CAH should be presumed to indicate acute adrenal insufficiency and be treated with hydrocortisone IV or IM at three to five times the basal dose. This administration should be done at home—or in the primary care setting if the child is there—instead of delaying initial treatment until the child arrives at an emergency room.

The diagnosis of acute adrenal insufficiency can be confirmed by laboratory values showing hyponatremia and hyperkalemia. Although consultation with an endocrinologist should be sought, treatment should not be delayed.

An IM injection of hydrocortisone or IV therapy in an emergency room is a frightening experience that no one wants to go through unnecessarily. In this type of situation, however, it is always best to err on the side of aggressive treatment.

Drug Interactions

Families are often afraid of giving their child steroids because of negative publicity in the popular press. It is important to stress to families that the hydrocortisone and fludrocortisone medications their child takes for CAH are replacing substances normally produced in the body and that the recommended doses are calculated to match normal blood levels as closely as possible. This is very different from taking high doses of glucocorticoids to treat inflammatory diseases. Families may have read stories of athletes having severe side effects from using steroids to increase muscle mass, so they should be told that anabolic steroids are completely different from hydrocortisone in actions and side effects. Replacement therapy for CAH is also an entirely different situation from taking a foreign substance such as an antibiotic. Because the medications for CAH replace hormones normally present in the body, concern about using other medications is limited to their effect on the absorption or rate of metabolism (Box 20-5).

Barbiturates (e.g., phenobarbital [Donnatal], phenytoin [Dilantin], rifampin [Rifadin, Rifamate, Rimactane]) increase the rate of metabolism of glucocorticoids. Therefore children

BOX 20-5
Drug Interactions

Barbiturates
Phenytoin
Rifampin

with CAH who are taking any of these medications for more than a few weeks may require a higher than usual dose of hydrocortisone for adequate cortisol replacement (Bello & Garrett, 1999). A serum 17-OHP level done approximately 2 weeks after the start of any of the medications listed here will show if an adjustment in the hydrocortisone dose is necessary. Short-term use of barbiturates perioperatively or prophylactic use of rifampin for *Haemophilus influenzae* meningitis should not require a change in hydrocortisone dose.

Antibiotics, decongestants, antihistamines, cough preparations, analgesics, antipyretics, and topical preparations have no unusual adverse effects.

Developmental Issues

Sleep Patterns

Children with CAH do not differ from their peers in their sleep patterns or needs. Unusual fatigue may indicate an illness or inadequate cortisol replacement and should be evaluated.

Toileting

Children who have obvious virilization of their external genitalia should be given privacy when using the toilet to avoid teasing. The initial corrective surgery for girls who experience virilization is usually done at an early age to avoid problems related to looking different. Although boys who experience excessive virilization may have some regression in pubic hair and penile size once they establish consistently adequate treatment, they will be noticeably different from their peers until adolescence. These children are otherwise no different in toileting readiness or skills than their peers and are not unusually prone to constipation, incontinence, enuresis, polyuria, or other disorders related to toileting.

Discipline

Children with CAH should be expected to behave appropriately for their age. The only special consideration has to do with children who appear older than their actual age. Parents, teachers, and others must be given clear guidelines on appropriate expectations for a child's developmental stage if it is different from his or her appearance.

Another area that raises disciplinary issues is compliance with taking medication, especially during toddlerhood and adolescence when children struggle with issues of dependency and autonomy. Parents should be advised from the beginning to use a matter-of-fact approach and avoid negotiating something that is nonnegotiable. During infancy and early school years, parents have full responsibility for giving medications. As children mature and are able to assume more responsibility, parents

should encourage their child's active participation (e.g., by remembering when it is "pill time," marking off the calendar for each dose, or filling a pillbox). Adolescents should have the primary responsibility for taking the medication with the parents offering support. Using a watch with a beeper is helpful for adolescents, as is a pillbox, which also provides an unobtrusive way for a parent to see if the medication disappears on schedule.

Clinicians can help make older children and adolescents aware of the consequences of poor adherence by pointing out signs of virilization to girls and slowed growth to both genders and emphasizing that it is within their power to "get back to normal." The risks of acute adrenal insufficiency and impaired fertility associated with poor adherence should also be discussed with adolescents, again with emphasis that such things are avoidable.

An adolescent will occasionally choose to make adherence to medications the focus of serious rebellion. Every effort should be made to explain the purpose and necessity of medication, and counseling should promptly be sought if the problem is severe or chronic.

Child Care

Parents should meet with child care personnel before enrollment to explain their child's special needs. Child care personnel do not require detailed knowledge of CAH but should be given a clear explanation that a child has a metabolic disorder that requires simple but important treatment.

Written information for the child care center should include written authorization to give hydrocortisone orally with instructions on the dose, time, and purpose; instructions on when to call parents, the telephone numbers where they can be reached, and what symptoms or events require emergency care; where to take the child for care; authorization for treatment; and the name and telephone number of the primary care provider and endocrinologist. It is neither necessary nor desirable to have special rules or restrictions on activities at school or child care for children with CAH. The usual policies on safety and appropriate play are sufficient to avoid serious injury.

Because hydrocortisone is usually given every 8 hours, many children will need at least one dose while at daycare. Mineralocorticoid is given once daily to children with salt-losing CAH and can be administered at home. Although most child care providers are conscientious, they may occasionally miss or delay doses of hydrocortisone if they do not understand its importance or are distracted by other demands on their attention. A routine that ties medication time to a regular activity (e.g., rest period or story time) can be established, or the child can wear a watch programmed to beep at the desired time. A letter from the primary care provider or the endocrinologist is helpful in making this invisible condition real to the people caring for these children.

Schooling

Children with CAH may have more absences than usual because of their need for close observation at home during acute illnesses. Concerns about excessive absences should be brought to the attention of the primary care provider, who can assess their appropriateness. Legitimate absences include any illness that would keep other children at home. In addition, symptoms such as a scratchy throat and malaise that might be ignored in other children should be initially observed at home.

Studies of cognitive abilities and school function in children with CAH have shown inconsistent results. Although earlier studies found normal or above normal cognitive function in individuals with CAH (Ehrhardt & Baker, 1977; Galatzer & Laron, 1989; Nass & Baker, 1991), later studies have found an increased prevalence of cognitive impairment or learning disabilities (Helleday et al, 1994; Plante et al, 1996).

Although it is not possible to identify what influence CAH itself has on cognitive and educational function with the information currently available, it is clear that acute CAH crises have a deleterious effect. Not surprisingly, children who had episodes of acute adrenal insufficiency with hypoglycemia or convulsions have a significantly higher prevalence of learning difficulties than children—with or without CAH—who did not experience such events (Donaldson et al, 1994). Because hypoglycemia and convulsions are associated with learning difficulties, these findings may represent a complication of poor management rather than the biochemical abnormality inherent in CAH. A child with CAH who has had severe hypoglycemia and convulsions should be assessed for learning difficulties and referred for special education intervention if indicated.

Sexuality

Virilization is nearly always present at birth in infant girls. Because genital surgery is nearly always needed and considerable attention is paid to genital examination during clinic visits, these girls get the message that there is something "wrong" with them and that it has to do with their genitalia. It is important to reassure these girls that they have all the normal female organs, hormones, and chromosomes and that any surgeries are simply to correct a cosmetic mistake that happened before they were born. The consensus statement on 21-hydroxylase deficiency from the Lawson Wilkins Pediatric Endocrine Society and the European Society for Paediatric Endocrinology (LWPES/ESPE CAH Working Group, 2002) recommends eliminating the previous practice of frequent genital examinations in females unless there is concern about poor control or to assess pubertal progression.

Children with CAH should be regularly evaluated for premature sexual development in order to determine the adequacy of therapy. Clinicians should include appropriate counseling regarding sexual development to the child and family.

Menstrual irregularities caused by androgen excess are common in adolescent girls with CAH. Androgen excess can also cause hirsutism and acne in children and adolescents of either gender and may contribute to impaired fertility (Lo & Grumbach, 2001; Speiser, 2001).

Although many observers have noted "tomboyish" behavior (e.g., rough and tumble play) or "increased activity levels" in girls with CAH, most early studies are difficult to interpret because of small sample size, lack of data on adequacy of treatment, and lack of control groups (Ehrhardt & Baker, 1977; Galatzer & Laron, 1989; Hines & Kaufman, 1994; Hochberg et al, 1987; Money et al, 1984). Stereotyping behavior as "masculine" or "feminine" also remains controversial. Some recent studies using better methodology have shown significant differences in the gender-stereotypic activities and sexual behaviors of girls and women with CAH and those of their unaffected sisters. Investigators attribute these differences to prenatal exposure to high levels of adrenal androgens (Berenbaum, 1999; Berenbaum et al, 2000; Dittmann et al, 1990, 1992; Zucker et al, 1996). The data suggest that, compared with their unaffected sisters, more women with CAH delay or fail to establish intimate heterosexual relationships (Dittmann et al, 1992; Kuhnle et al, 1995). However, the data are conflicting on whether there is an increased prevalence of homosexual orientation among women with CAH (Dittmann et al, 1992; Kuhnle et al, 1995). Prenatal androgen exposure is considered to be a predisposing—rather than a causative—factor in gender behavior, and all aspects of psychosocial development must be considered in the care of girls with CAH (Dittmann et al, 1992). Primary care providers must use caution when interpreting these data and base discussions of sexuality on an individualized assessment of each child and family.

Women with CAH—particularly those with the salt-losing form—may not have an adequate introitus for comfortable sexual function, in spite of surgical intervention (Lo & Grumbach, 2001). In addition, women who become pregnant may require cesarean delivery because of a small birth canal (Lo & Grumbach, 2001). One study evaluated fertility in eight women with CAH who were diagnosed early, were generally compliant with treatment, had an introitus that was adequate for intercourse, and were sexually active (Premawardhana et al, 1997). Five of the eight women conceived (i.e., three of this five had salt-wasting CAH and two had non–salt-wasting CAH), for an overall fertility rate of slightly greater than 60%. It is important to note that a significant number of women had successful pregnancies in spite of late diagnosis and treatment of CAH, inadequate reconstruction of the introitus, and poor compliance with replacement therapy (Lo & Grumbach, 2001).

Promising developments that may improve sexual function for women with CAH include better surgical techniques for clitoroplasty and vaginoplasty (Gunther & Bukowski, 1999), as well as prenatal treatment to prevent virilization of affected female fetuses (New, 2001). Males with CAH generally do not have problems with sexual function or fertility, although prolonged androgen excess can eventually result in infertility (New, 1995). When children with CAH reach adolescence, their primary care provider or endocrinologist should discuss with them the availability and purpose of genetic counseling, screening for carriers, and prenatal and neonatal diagnosis. Because CAH is an autosomal recessive trait, children must receive an abnormal gene from each parent to have the disorder; if one parent has CAH and the other is not a carrier, their children will not have CAH. All unaffected children with a parent with CAH will be carriers of the trait.

Transition into Adulthood

As children with CAH approach adulthood, the primary care provider needs to help their families identify an internist or family practice provider to assume primary care responsibilities. If a child has had specialty care through a pediatric endocrinologist, the transition must also be made to adult endocrine care; the pediatric endocrinologist usually has a list of names available. Counseling for early prenatal care (i.e., prenatal screening, diagnosis, and potential treatment) should be provided as well.

Unfortunately, insurance may become a problem when children reach an age when they are no longer covered by government-sponsored insurance for children with disabilities or their parents' insurance. Medicaid—for those who meet the criteria—and group insurance through employment—for those with medical benefits—will cover care for CAH. Information about other programs and resources can be sought from county social services agencies, health departments, and state insurance commissions.

Family Concerns and Resources

The parents of an infant girl with CAH must cope with the effect of ambiguous genitalia and of possibly a delayed or even incorrect gender assignment. The initial explanations and reassurances that health care personnel give to the family must be both sensitive and accurate to prevent serious misperceptions of the child's condition and prognosis. Discussions with parents should focus on listening to the parents' concerns and reinforcing the normality of their daughter's internal female organs and chromosomes and explaining that the appearance of the external genitalia is correctable and the underlying condition treatable.

People tend to blame the occurrence of an abnormality in a baby on something the mother or father did. It is important to discuss this issue with the parents and the extended family and to repeatedly reinforce the lack of fault. Even after the best of explanations and reassurances, these families continue to have much anxiety and guilt about their child's condition, so constant reinforcement and support are necessary.

Families must be taught to be assertive in communicating the urgency of their child's need for hydrocortisone to health care personnel who are not familiar with the child or CAH. Unfortunately, treatment is commonly delayed because of a lack of understanding of the implications of acute illness in children with CAH. Primary care providers can help avoid delays in treatment by alerting other health care personnel (e.g., call group, emergency room staff) to a child's special needs. The endocrinologist should be consulted for any questions about treatment. In addition, the child should wear a Medic-Alert bracelet or necklace, and the family should carry written information on the child's condition (e.g., wallet card) to facilitate prompt treatment.

Parents have initial difficulty believing the seriousness of CAH unless the diagnosis was made during an episode of acute adrenal insufficiency. Once parents experience the rapidity with which their child can change from being robustly healthy to being deathly ill, they may be fearful of future episodes. It is difficult for these parents to find a balance between protecting their child from serious harm and allowing the child to have an active, normal life. This balance must be assessed at each primary care visit by asking about the child's social and academic progress, outside interests and activities, and special concerns. Any problem areas should then be discussed.

Children with CAH may experience emotional disturbances related to multiple factors involved in having this chronic condition. Such factors include being concerned about sexuality and fertility, being perceived and treated as different by others, including their parents, receiving mixed or confusing messages from health care personnel, being overprotected by their parents, and dealing with their own fears related to life-threatening crises they may have experienced. Psychotherapy is indicated for significant emotional disturbance and behavioral problems. Newborn siblings should be screened for CAH, and if the screening results are positive, confirming tests should be done. If the diagnosis of CAH is confirmed, treatment can be immediately initiated in order to prevent an adrenal crisis (Brosnan et al, 1998; Pang, 1997). Because non–salt-wasting CAH can present with virilization or accelerated growth, all older siblings with these findings should be screened.

Although prenatal diagnosis and treatment are still being refined, they should be discussed in detail with parents. Testing for the carrier state is also available and should be explained to unaffected siblings and other first-degree relatives.

The effect of CAH on a family varies with their cultural beliefs about the cause of congenital disorders and their attitudes toward sexuality. Primary care providers must determine what these beliefs are in order to provide sensitive and successful care to the child and family. Families will usually tell providers their beliefs if asked.

Individuals from cultures in which sexual topics are not openly discussed can be expected to have difficulty asking questions about CAH. Primary care providers and endocrinologists are faced with the challenge of presenting information on a sensitive subject without offending a family's values. It may be helpful to have a male health care provider speak to the men in the family and a female provider speak separately to the women in the family.

RESOURCES

Informational Pamphlets for Patients and Families

"Congenital Adrenal Hyperplasia" by Sharon Connaughty (1996)
Available from:
Patient/Parent Education Department of British Columbia's Children's Hospital
4480 Oak St
Vancouver, British Columbia, V6H 3V4

"Congenital Adrenal Hyperplasia" by Songya Pang
Available from:
The Magic Foundation
1327 N. Harlem Ave
Oak Park, IL 60302
(708) 383-0808; (708) 383-0899 (fax); (800) 3MAGIC 3 (parent help line)
http://www.magicfoundation.org

"Congenital Adrenal Hyperplasia Due to 21 Hydroxylase Deficiency: A Guide for Patients and Their Families"
Available on-line from the Division of Pediatric Endocrinology at Johns Hopkins Children's Center:
www.hopkinsmedicine.org/pediatricendocrinology/cah
Recommended by the Lawson Wilkins Pediatric Endocrine Society and the European Society for Paediatric Endocrinology
Downloadable version available

"Hormones and Me: Congenital Adrenal Hyperplasia (CAH)," a 29-page booklet for families of children with CAH
Available from:
Serono Symposia Australia: Unit 3-4
25 Frenchs Forest Rd East
Frenchs Forest NSW 2086, Australia

"Your Child with Congenital Adrenal Hyperplasia"
Available from the Royal Children's Hospital, Melbourne:
www.rch.unimelb.edu.au/cah_book
Recommended by the Lawson Wilkins Pediatric Endocrine Society and the European Society for Paediatric Endocrinology
Downloadable version available

Pamphlets with Medication Information

"Guidelines for the Child Who Is Cortisol Dependent" (provides parents with information on cortisone replacement and illness management)
"How to Mix and Inject Injectable Hydrocortisone" (gives parents a clear description of this procedure)
"Congenital Adrenal Hyperplasia" (explains CAH and its management)
All available from:
Department of Education
University of Wisconsin Hospital
600 Highland Ave
Madison, WI 53792

"The Hydrocortisone/Florinef Handout," a concise 2-page handout for parents that includes information on illness management
Available from:
Pediatric Endocrinology, CB 7220, Burnett-Womack
University of North Carolina at Chapel Hill
Chapel Hill, NC 27599

"Medication Instructions for Patients with Congenital Adrenal Hyperplasia: Instructions for Families"
Available from:
Pediatric Endocrinology Nursing Society
PO Box 2933
Gaithersburg, MD 20886-2933
www.pens.org
Also describes dosages

Organizations

CARES (Congenital Adrenal Hyperplasia Research, Education, and Support) Foundation Inc.
Nonprofit organization formed in 2001 to educate the public, physicians, and legislators about CAH and to provide support to families of children with CAH
CARES Web site provides useful information about CAH and links to other related sites:
www.caresfoundation.org

National Adrenal Diseases Foundation (NADF)
Nonprofit organization dedicated to providing support, information, and education to individuals having Addison disease as well as other diseases of the adrenal glands

Erin A. Foley, MPH, President/Director
National Adrenal Diseases Foundation
505 Northern Bvd
Great Neck, NY 11021
(516)487-4992
www.medhelp.org/nadf/

Pediatric Endocrinology Nursing Society (PENS)
PO Box 2933
Gaithersburg, MD 20886-2933
www.pens.org
Organization with professional members in many regions who are willing to speak to parent, school, professional, or other groups

Products

Medic-Alert bracelets and necklaces (recommended for all children with CAH)
Available from:
Medic-Alert Foundation
PO Box 1009
Turlock, CA 95381-1009
www.medicalert.org (in the United States) or www.medicalert.ca (in Canada)

Acknowledgment The authors gratefully acknowledge the contribution of Betty Flores and Judy Ruble, the authors of this chapter in previous editions.

Summary of Primary Care Needs for the Child with Congenital Adrenal Hyperplasia

HEALTH CARE MAINTENANCE

Growth and Development

If CAH is diagnosed in infancy and adequately and consistently treated, growth and development are normal.

Accelerated linear growth occurs if CAH is inadequately treated.

Accelerated bone age advancement and early closure of epiphyses with reduced final adult height will occur if CAH is inadequately treated.

Stunted linear growth will occur if CAH is overtreated with hydrocortisone.

Precocious puberty may occur with improved treatment.

Diet

Children should be allowed to salt food to taste and eat salty foods.

Good dietary and activity habits are necessary to counteract the tendency for hydrocortisone therapy to promote excessive weight gain.

Safety

These children have no increased susceptibility to injury.

There is a risk of acute adrenal insufficiency with a serious injury (e.g., fracture, concussion).

A Medic-Alert bracelet or necklace should be worn and written information should be carried stating the diagnosis, stress dosage of hydrocortisone, and the name and telephone number of the endocrinologist.

Immunizations

Routine immunizations are recommended.

Giving additional vaccines (e.g., pneumococcal, influenza) is discretionary.

Increased stress doses of hydrocortisone are not prophylactically necessary unless the child has a history of previous adverse reaction to the vaccine.

Give increased stress dose of hydrocortisone for immunization reactions involving fever, unusual malaise, and lethargy.

Giving acetaminophen before immunization with likelihood of febrile reaction is discretionary.

Summary of Primary Care Needs for the Child with Congenital Adrenal Hyperplasia—cont'd

HEALTH CARE MAINTENANCE—cont'd

Screening

Vision. Routine screening is recommended.

Hearing. Routine screening is recommended.

Dental. Routine screening is recommended.

Blood Pressure. Blood pressure should be checked at each visit (including infants). Children with abnormal findings should be referred to an endocrinologist.

Hematocrit. Routine screening is recommended.

Urinalysis. Routine screening is recommended.

Tuberculosis. Routine screenings is recommended.

Condition-Specific Screening

Screening serum 17-OHP levels or 24-hour urine pregnanetriol values may be indicated and should be coordinated with the endocrinologist.

Checking plasma renin activity levels may be indicated and should be coordinated with the endocrinologist.

Bone age should be checked every 2 to 3 years or more often if there are indications of androgen excess.

COMMON ILLNESS MANAGEMENT

If the child has nausea or vomiting; pallor; cold moist skin; weakness; dizziness or confusion; rapid heart rate; rapid breathing; abdominal, back, or leg pain; dehydration; or hypotension, then acute adrenal insufficiency should be ruled out.

A temperature greater than 101.1° F (38.4° C), significant malaise, pain, lethargy, or persistent vomiting (regardless of cause) should be covered by stress doses of hydrocortisone in addition to appropriate specific therapy.

If the child has hypertension, excessive dietary sodium intake and/or overtreatment with mineralocorticoids or glucocorticoids should be ruled out.

If the child has hypotension, inadequate mineralocorticoid and/or glucocorticoid dosage should be ruled out.

Drug Interactions

Long-term use of barbiturates, phenytoin, or rifampin increases the rate of metabolism of glucocorticoids. Adjustments in dosage may be required.

DEVELOPMENTAL ISSUES

Sleep Patterns

Unusual fatigue or lethargy may indicate the need for increased doses of hydrocortisone.

Toileting

There is no impairment in readiness or functioning. Children with obvious virilization should be allowed privacy.

Discipline

Expectations are normal based on age and developmental level.

Physical appearance may differ from age and developmental level, leading to inappropriate expectations.

Child Care

Child care providers must be aware of special needs with illness and injury and the importance of routine and stress medication.

Schooling

Children with CAH who have a history of acute adrenal insufficiency and/or hypoglycemic seizures should be assessed for learning difficulties.

School personnel should be aware of special needs of the child's illness and injury.

Sexuality

Virilization of infant girls requires surgical correction.

Inadequate treatment results in continued virilization, acne, hirsutism, menstrual irregularities, infertility in girls, and—eventually—impairment of fertility in boys.

Most children will be fertile.

Transition into Adulthood

Transition to providers of adult primary care and endocrine care should be accomplished.

Source of medical insurance must be identified.

FAMILY CONCERNS

Rapid onset of acute adrenal insufficiency is possible.

Appropriate emergency treatment may be delayed because of health care providers' lack of awareness or knowledge of CAH.

The normality of girls should be stressed.

Others in the family may be affected (e.g., siblings, children of affected child). Genetic counseling, prenatal screening, diagnosis, and treatment are available.

Family members may have difficulty speaking openly about sexuality and genitalia.

REFERENCES

Avila, N., Premkumar, A., Shawker, T., Jones, J., Laue, L., et al. (1996). Testicular adrenal rest tissue in congenital adrenal hyperplasia: Findings at Gray-scale and color Doppler. *US Radiology, 198*, 99-104.

Bacon, G. et al. (1990). *A practical approach to pediatric endocrinology* (3rd ed.). Chicago: Year Book Medical Publishers.

Bailez, M.M., Gearhart, J.P., Migeon, C., & Rock, J. (1992).Vaginal reconstruction after initial construction of the external genitalia in girls with salt-wasting adrenal hyperplasia. *J Urol, 148*, 680-682.

Bello, C. & Garrett, S. (1999). Therapeutic issues in oral glucocorticoid use. *Lippincott's Primary Care Practice, 3*(3), 333-344.

Berenbaum, S. (1999). Effects of early androgens on sex-typed activities and interests in adolescents with congenital adrenal hyperplasia. *Horm Behav, 35*, 102-110.

Berenbaum, S., Duck, S., & Bryk, K. (2000). Behavioral effects of prenatal versus postnatal androgen excess in children with 21-hydroxylase-deficient congenital adrenal hyperplasia. *J Clin Endocrinol Metab, 85*, 727-733.

Brosnan, C.A., Brosnan, P., Therrell, B.L., Slater, C.H., Swint, J.M., et al. (1998). A comparative cost analysis of newborn screening for classic congenital adrenal hyperplasia in Texas. *Public Health Rep, 113*(2), 170-178.

Cornean, R., Hindmarsh, P., & Brook, C. (1998). Obesity in 21-hydroxylase deficient patients. *Arch Dis Child, 78*, 261-263.

Daaboul, J. & Frader, J. (2001). Ethics and the management of the patient with intersex: A middle way. *J Pediatr Endocrinol, 14*(9), 1575-1583.

Dacou-Voutetakis, C. & Karidis, N. (1993). Congenital adrenal hyperplasia complicated by central precocious puberty: Treatment with LHRH-agonist analog. *Ann NY Acad Sci, 687*, 250-254.

Diamond, M. & Sigmundson, H.K. (1997). Management of intersexuality: Guidelines for dealing with persons with ambiguous genitalia. *Arch Pediatr Adolesc Med, 151*, 1046-1050.

Dittmann, R., Kappes, M., & Kappes, M. (1992). Sexual behavior in adolescent and adult females with congenital adrenal hyperplasia. *Psychoneuroendocrinology, 17*, 153-170.

Dittmann, R.W., Kappes, M.H., Kappes, M.E., Borger, D., Meyer-Bahlburg, H.F., et al. (1990). Congenital adrenal hyperplasia I: Gender-related behavior and attitudes in female patients and sisters. *Psychoneuroendocrinology, 15*, 401-420.

Donahoe, P. & Gustafson, M. (1994). Early one-stage surgical reconstruction of the extremely high vagina in patients with congenital adrenal hyperplasia. *J Pediatr Surg, 29*(2), 352-358.

Donaldson, M.D., Thomas, P.H., Love, J.G., Murray, G.D., McNinch, A.W., et al. (1994). Presentation, acute illness, and learning difficulties in salt wasting 21-hydroxylase deficiency. *Arch Dis Child, 70*, 214-218.

Ehrhardt, A. & Baker, S. (1977). Males and females with congenital adrenal hyperplasia: A family study of intelligence and gender-related behavior. In P. Lee, L. Plotnick, & A. Kowarski (Eds.). *Congenital adrenal hyperplasia.* Baltimore: University Park Press.

Fausto-Sterling, A. (2000, July/August). The five sexes, revisited. *The Sciences.*

Frisch, H., Battelino, T., Schober, E., Baumgartner-Parzer, S., Nowotny, P., et al. (2001). Salt wasting in simple virilizing congenital adrenal hyperplasia. *J Pediatr Endocrinol, 14*(9), 1649-1655.

Galatzer, A. & Laron, Z. (1989). The effects of prenatal androgens on behavior and cognitive functions. In M. Forest (Ed.). *Androgens in childhood.* Karger & Basel.

Gmyrek, G.A., New, M.I., Sosa, R.E., & Poppas, D.P. (2002). Bilateral laparoscopic adrenalectomy as a treatment for classical congenital adrenal hyperplasia attributable to 21-hydroxylase deficiency. *Pediatrics, 109*(2), E28.

Gunther, D. & Bukowski, T. (1999). Congenital adrenal hyperplasia: A spectrum of disorders. *Contemp Urol, 11*(1), 52-69.

Helleday, J., Bartfai, A., Ritzen, E.M., & Forsman, M. (1994). General intelligence and cognitive profile in women with congenital adrenal hyperplasia (CAH). *Psychoneuroendocrinology, 19*(4), 343-356.

Helleday, J., Siwers, B., Ritzen, E.M., & Carlstrom, K. (1993). Subnormal androgen and elevated progesterone levels in women treated for congenital virilizing 21-hydroxylase deficiency. *J Clin Endocrinol Metab, 76*(4), 933-936.

Hines, M. & Kaufman, F. (1994). Androgen and the development of human sex-typical behavior: Rough-and-tumble play and sex of preferred playmates in children with congenital adrenal hyperplasia (CAH). *Child Dev, 65*, 1042-1053.

Hochberg, Z., Gardos, M., & Benderly, A. (1987). Psychosexual outcome of assigned females and males with 46XX virilizing congenital adrenal hyperplasia. *Eur J Pediatr, 146*, 497-499.

Holmes, C., Karlsson, J., & Thompson, R. (1986). Longitudinal evaluation of behavior patterns in children with short stature. In B. Stabler & L. Underwood (Eds.). *Slow grows the child.* Hillsdale, N.J.: Lawrence Erlbaum Assoc.

Jackson, P. & Ott, M. (1990). Perceived self-esteem among children diagnosed with precocious puberty. *J Pediatr Nurs, 5*, 190-203.

Kuhnle, U., Bullinger, M., & Schwartz, H. (1995). The quality of life in adult female patients with congenital adrenal hyperplasia: A comprehensive study of the impact of genital malformations and chronic disease on female patients' life. *Eur J Pediatr, 154*, 708-716.

Levine, L.S. (2000). Congenital adrenal hyperplasia. *Pediatr Rev, 21*(5), 159-170.

Lim, Y., Batch, J., & Warne, G. (1995). Adrenal 21-hydroxylase deficiency in childhood: 25 years' experience. *J Paediatr Child Health, 31*(3), 222-227.

Lo, J. & Grumbach, M. (2001). Pregnancy outcomes in women with congenital virilizing adrenal hyperplasia. *Endocrinol Metab Clin North Am, 30*(1), 207-229.

LWPES/ESPE CAH Working Group. (2002). Consensus statement on 2-hydroxylase deficiency from the Lawson Wilkins Pediatric Endocrine Society and the European Society for Paediatric Endocrinology. *J Clin Endocrinol Metab, 87*(9), 4048-4053.

Merke, D., Bornstein, S., Avila, N., & Chrousos, G. (2002). Future directions in the study and management of congenital adrenal hyperplasia due to 21-hydrocylase deficiency. *Ann Intern Med, 136*(4), 320-334.

Merke, D. & Cutler, G. (2001). New ideas for medical treatment of congenital adrenal hyperplasia. *Endocrinol Metab Clin North Am, 30*(1), 121-135.

Merke, D., Keil, M., Jones, J., Fields, J., Hill, S., et al. (2000). Flutamide, testolactone, and reduced hydrocortisone dose maintain normal growth velocity and bone maturation despite elevated androgen levels in children with congenital adrenal hyperplasia. *J Clin Endocrinol Metab, 85*(3), 1114-1120.

Meyer-Bahlburg, H. (2001). Gender and sexuality in classic congenital adrenal hyperplasia. *Endocrinol Metab Clin North Am, 30*(1), 155-171.

Meyers, R. & Grua, J. (2000). Bilateral laparoscopic adrenalectomy: A new treatment for difficult cases of congenital adrenal hyperplasia. *J Pediatr Surg, 35*(11), 1586-1590.

Migeon, C. & Wisniewski, A. (2001). Congenital adrenal hyperplasia owing to 21-hydroxylase deficiency: Growth, development, and therapeutic considerations. *Endocrinol Metab Clin North Am, 30*(1), 193-206.

Miller, W.L. (1994). Genetics, diagnosis, and management of 21-hydroxylase deficiency. *J Clin Endocrinol Metab, 78*(2), 241-246.

Money, J., Schwartz, M., & Lewis, V. (1984). Adult erotosexual status and fetal hormonal masculinization and demasculinization: 46XX congenital virilizing adrenal hyperplasia and 46XY androgen-insensitivity syndrome compared. *Psychoneuroendocrinology, 9*, 405-414.

Nass, R. & Baker, S. (1991). Learning disabilities in children with congenital adrenal hyperplasia. *J Child Neurol, 6*, 306-312.

National Newborn Screening and Genetics Resource Center. (2002). US national screening status report; Web site: http://genes-r-us.uthscsa.edu/index.htm.

New, M. (1995). Congenital adrenal hyperplasia. In L. DeGroot et al. (Eds.). *Endocrinology* (3rd ed.). Philadelphia: W.B. Saunders.

New, M. (1998). Diagnosis and management of congenital adrenal hyperplasia. *Annu Rev Med, 49*, 311-328.

New, M. (2001). Prenatal treatment of congenital adrenal hyperplasia. *Endocrinol Metab Clin North Am, 30*(1), 1-13.

Pang, S. (1997). Congenital adrenal hyperplasia. *Endocrinol Metab Clin North Am, 26*(4), 853-891.

Pang, S. & Shook, M. (1997). Current status of neonatal screening for congenital adrenal hyperplasia. *Curr Opin Pediatr, 9*(4), 419-423.

Pescovitz, H. et al. (1984). True precocious puberty complicating congenital adrenal hyperplasia: Treatment with a luteinizing hormone-releasing hormone analog. *J Clin Endocrinol Metab, 58*(5), 857-861.

Plante, E., Boliek, C., Binkiewicz, A., & Erly, W.K. (1996). Elevated androgen, brain development and language/learning disabilities in children with congenital adrenal hyperplasia. *Dev Med Child Neurol, 38*, 423-437.

Premawardhana, L.D., Hughes, I.A., Read, G.F., & Scanlon, M.F. (1997). Longer term outcome in females with congenital adrenal hyperplasia (CAH): The Cardiff experience. *Clin Endocrinol, 46*(3), 327-332.

Ritzen, E. & Wedell, A. (1996). Adrenals of patients with severe forms of congenital adrenal hyperplasia do more harm than good! *J Clin Endocrinol Metab, 81*(9), 3182-3184.

Rivkees, S. & Crawford, J. (2000). Dexamethasone treatment of virilizing congenital adrenal hyperplasia: The ability to achieve normal growth. *Pediatrics, 106*(4), 767-773.

Schnitzer, J. & Donahoe, P. (2001). Surgical treatment of congenital adrenal hyperplasia. *Endocrinol Metab Clin North Am, 30*(1), 137-154.

Speiser, P. (2001). Congenital adrenal hyperplasia owing to 21-hydrocylase deficiency. *Endocrinol Metab Clin North Am, 30*(1), 31-59.

Therrell, B. (2001). Newborn screening for congenital adrenal hyperplasia. *Endocrinol Metab Clin North Am, 30*(1), 15-30.

Trautman, P.D., Meyer-Bahlburg, H.F., Postelnek, J., & New, M.I. (1996). Mothers' reactions to prenatal diagnostic procedures and dexamethasone treatment of congenital adrenal hyperplasia. *J Psychosom Obstet Gynaecol, 17*(3), 175-181.

VanWyk, J. & Gunther, D. (1996). The use of adrenalectomy as a treatment for congenital adrenal hyperplasia. *J Clin Endocrinol Metab, 81*(9), 3180-3182.

Wedell, A., Thlen, A., Ritzen, E., Stengler, B., & Luthman, H. (1994). Mutational spectrum of the steroid 21 hydroxylase gene in Sweden: Implications for genetic diagnosis and association of disease manifestation. *J Clin Endocrinol Metab, 78*(5), 1145-1152.

Wilson, B.E. & Reiner, W.G. (1998). Management of intersex: A shifting paradigm. *J Clin Ethics, 9*(4), 360-368.

Young-Hyman, D. (1986). Effects of short stature on social competence. In B. Stabler & L. Underwood (Eds.). *Slow grows the child.* Hillsdale, N.J.: Lawrence Erlbaum Assoc.

Zucker, K.J., Bradley, S.J., Oliver, G., Blake, J., Fleming, S., et al. (1996). Psychosexual development of women with congenital adrenal hyperplasia. *Horm Behav, 30*, 300-318.

21 Congenital Heart Disease

Elizabeth H. Cook and Sarah S. Higgins

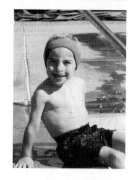

Etiology

Congenital heart disease (CHD) is a grouping of anatomic defects that results from abnormal development of the heart and related structures that is present—although not always manifested—at birth. At least one third of the infants born with CHD will become critically ill within the first year of life and require surgery or interventional cardiac catheterization (Craig et al, 2001).

A full understanding of the etiology of CHD is a rapidly growing (although still limited) field. Traditional thinking was that the majority of congenital heart defects had a multifactorial cause, in which there was interplay of a genetic predisposition for abnormal cardiac development with an environmental trigger (e.g., a virus or maternal ingestion of certain drugs) at the vulnerable time of cardiac development. As more information about genetic (see Known Genetic Etiology) and environmental effects on the developing heart is discovered, more specific identification of cause is being determined.

Cardiac development occurs between day 18 and day 45 of gestation (Artman, Mahoney, & Teitel, 2002). Maternal exposure to teratogens during cardiac development of the fetus may result in heart defects. The fetus is vulnerable to cardiac teratogens from 2 to 10 weeks of gestation (Reiss, 2001). This exposure may be from a maternal infection, a maternal health condition, or maternal ingestion of drugs (Table 21-1).

Physiology of Congenital Heart Disease

CHD is commonly categorized as acyanotic or cyanotic, depending on the hemodynamic changes that occur as a result of the specific heart anomaly. In acyanotic heart disease, the systemic circulation is not exposed to unoxygenated blood; in cyanotic heart disease, unoxygenated blood mixes in the systemic circulation (Figure 21-1, p. 384). A brief description of the intracardiac pressure-flow relationship may clarify this classification of CHD.

Depleted of oxygen, blood returns to the heart from the venous system and enters the right atrium. From the right atrium, blood flows through the tricuspid valve into the right ventricle, where it is pumped through the pulmonary arteries into the lungs to pick up oxygen. Therefore the oxygen saturation in the right side of the heart is low (i.e., approximately 70%). The pressure in the right-sided circulation is also relatively low (i.e., approximately 25/2 mm Hg in the right ventricle and 25/10 mm Hg in the pulmonary arteries).

The blood that enters the left atrium from the lungs is rich in oxygen, with the oxygen saturation reaching 95% to 100%. The blood flows through the mitral valve into the left ventricle, where it is pumped into the systemic circulation via the aorta. Blood in the left ventricle is under high pressure (e.g., approximately 100/5 mm Hg), as is that in the aorta (i.e., approximately 100/60 mm Hg).

Because the pressure in the left side of the heart is greater than that in the right side, blood flows from the left to the right side of the heart if there is an abnormal connection between the two sides. This flow is called left-to-right shunting. Because of the significant difference in left- and right-sided oxygen saturations, heart defects that cause left-to-right shunting are acyanotic. Left-to-right shunts commonly cause overcirculation of the lungs and may result in congestive heart failure (CHF).

Cyanosis usually results from one or both of the following physiologic problems: (1) right-to-left shunting, which results from obstruction of blood flow to the lungs plus an intracardiac communication; or (2) intracardiac mixing of oxygenated and deoxygenated blood. Figure 21-2 on pp. 385-387 summarizes and illustrates the most common defects. Additional information on cardiovascular disorders in children can be found in Craig et al (2001).

Known Genetic Etiology

As more diagnostic chromosomal tests are available, the genetic basis of CHD is becoming clearer. Approximately 10% of children with CHD demonstrate a known associated chromosomal abnormality (Lewin, 2000). For some cardiac conditions (i.e., hypertrophic cardiomyopathy, long QT syndrome, Marfan syndrome, supravalvular aortic stenosis), single-gene mutations responsible for specific defects have been mapped or identified.

Many defects are associated with a syndrome in which other systems also are affected (Table 21-1). One of the most common genetic associations with CHD is Down syndrome; more than 40% of children with Down syndrome have a heart defect (see Chapter 24) (Lewin, 2000). Other syndromes that do not have an identified chromosomal defect (e.g., asplenia syndrome, VACTERL* syndrome) often have CHD as one of many anomalies.

Incidence and Prevalence

CHD generally occurs in approximately 0.8% to 1% of live births (Clark, 2001), making it one of the most common birth defects. The incidence of specific heart defects is shown in

---

*VACTERL syndrome refers to a constellation of abnormalities of the vertebrae, anus, cardiovascular system, trachea, esophagus, renal system, and limb buds.

TABLE 21-1
Conditions Commonly Associated with Cardiac Malformations

Condition	Associated Defect
INFANT SYNDROME	
Genetic Disorders	
Trisomy 13	ASD, VSD, TOF
Trisomy 18	VSD, PDA, PS
Trisomy 21	AVSD, VSD, ASD
Turner syndrome (XO)	COTA, ASD, AS, bicuspid aortic valve
DiGeorge/velocardiofacial syndrome (deletion 22q11)	Interrupted aortic arch, TOF, truncus arteriosus, ASD, VSD
Marfan syndrome	Great artery aneurysms, aortic insufficiency, mitral regurgitation
Noonan syndrome	PS, ASD
William syndrome	Supravalvular subaortic stenosis, branch pulmonary artery stenosis
Ellis–van Creveld syndrome	ASD, single atrium
Genetic Disorder Not Identified	
Osteogenesis imperfecta	Aortic valve disease
Holt-Oram syndrome	ASD, VSD, single atrium
Cri du chat syndrome	VSD, PDA, ASD
Treacher Collins syndrome	VSD, PDA, ASD
Asplenia syndrome	VSD, single ventricle, common AV valve, TGA
VACTERL syndrome	TOF, VSD
MATERNAL CONDITION	
Rubella	PDA, ASD, VSD, peripheral pulmonary stenosis
Diabetes	TGA, VSD, COTA, ASD, HLHS, cardiomyopathy
Lupus erythematosus	Heart block
Phenylketonuria	TOF, VSD, COTA, HLHS
MATERNAL INGESTION	
Alcohol	VSD, PDA, ASD, pulmonary atresia, DORV, TOF
Amphetamines	VSD, PDA, ASD, TGA
Cocaine	VSD, ASD, congenital complete heart block
Hydantoin	PS, AS, COTA, PDA, VSD, ASD
Lithium	Ebstein anomaly
Retinoic acid	VSD, varied CHD
Sex hormones	VSD, TGA, TOF
Thalidomide	TOF, truncus arteriosus, VSD, ASD
Trimethadione	ASD, PDA, VSD
Valproic acid	TOF, VSD, AS, PDA
Warfarin	TOF, VSD

Data from Allen, H.D. et al. (eds.) (2001). *Moss and Adams' heart disease in infants, children, and adolescents including the fetus and young adult* (6th ed.). Philadelphia: Lippincott, Williams & Wilkins. Reprinted with permission.
AS, Aortic stenosis; *ASD,* atrial septal defect; *AVSD,* atrioventricular septal defect; *COTA,* coarctation of the aorta; *HLHS,* hypoplastic left heart syndrome; *PDA,* patent ductus arteriosus; *PS,* pulmonary stenosis; *TGA,* transposition of the great arteries; *TOF,* tetralogy of Fallot; *VACTERL,* a constellation of abnormalities of the vertebrae, anus, cardiovascular system, trachea, esophagus, renal system, and limb buds; *VSD,* ventricular septal defect; *DORV,* double outlet right ventricle.

TABLE 21-2
Incidence of Specific Heart Defects

Defect	CHD (%)	Prevalence (per 10,000 live births)
Ventricular septal defect (VSD)	15-25	15.57
Tetralogy of Fallot (TOF)	10	2.6
Pulmonary stenosis (PS)	8-12	3.78
Coarctation of the aorta (COTA)	8-10	1.39
Patent ductus arteriosus (PDA)	5-10*	0.88
Atrial septal defect (ASD)	5-10	2.35
Transposition of the great arteries (TGA)	5	2.64
Aortic stenosis (AS)	3-6	0.81
Atrioventricular septal defect (AVSD)	2	3.27
Tricuspid atresia (TA)	1-3	3.6
Pulmonary atresia (PA)	1-2	5.8
Hypoplastic left heart syndrome (HLHS)	1-2	1.78
Total anomalous pulmonary venous return (TAPVR)	1	0.66
Ebstein anomaly	<1	0.52
Truncus arteriosus	<1	0.69

Data from Park, M.K. (2002). Pediatric cardiology for practitioners (4th ed.). St. Louis: Mosby; Clark, E.B. (2001). Etiology of congenital cardiovascular malformations: Epidemiology and genetics. In H.D. Allen et al. (Eds.). *Moss and Adams' heart disease in infants, children, and adolescents including the fetus and young adult* (6th ed.). Philadelphia: Lippincott, Williams & Wilkins.
*Excluding premature.

BOX 21-1
Clinical Manifestations at Time of Diagnosis

CONGESTIVE HEART FAILURE
Tachypnea
Tachycardia
Hepatomegaly
Dyspnea
Pale, cool mottled skin
Periorbital edema
Persistent, dry cough
Poor feeding; failure to thrive
Easily fatigued
Diaphoresis

HYPOXEMIA AND CYANOSIS
Blue coloration of lips, gums, nail beds, around eyes and mouth, skin, and mucous membranes
Slowed growth
Decreased activity
Polycythemia

chromosomal abnormality, the recurrence risk of the heart lesion is related to the recurrence risk of the syndrome. With left-sided defects (e.g., hypoplastic left-sided heart syndrome, aortic valve abnormalities) the rate of another defect of the same spectrum recurring may be as high as 18% (Clark, 2001; Park, 2002).

Clinical Manifestations at Time of Diagnosis

The clinical presentation of a child with CHD varies depending on the specific defect. Symptoms usually relate to the degree of CHF or cyanosis (Box 21-1).

Table 21-2. Gender distribution is equal for CHD as a whole, but boys tend to have a higher incidence of some severe defects (e.g., transposition of the great arteries, left-sided heart defects).

The risk of CHD recurring in the same family depends on several factors. The odds for recurrence are greatest if the mother or full sibling—instead of the father or half-sibling—has the heart defect. If the defect is part of a syndrome or

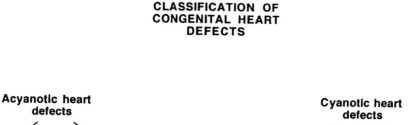

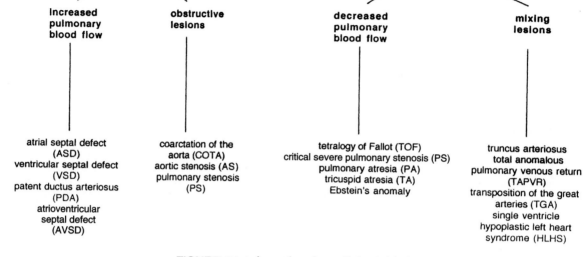

FIGURE 21-1 Acyanotic and cyanotic heart defects.

Congestive Heart Failure

CHD is the most common cause of CHF in children, and many cases occur within the first year of life. CHF occurs when there is a strain on the myocardium from pressure or volume overload that is severe enough to reduce cardiac output to a level insufficient to meet the body's metabolic demands. Symptoms of CHF result from the decreased cardiac output and the body's compensatory mechanisms, which include cardiac hypertrophy, cardiac dilation, and stimulation of the sympathetic nervous system. Initially the compensatory mechanisms serve to improve cardiac performance. Over time, however, these compensatory mechanisms may actually exacerbate the decreased cardiac output. Infants with CHF are tachypneic, dyspneic, tachycardic, pale, cool, mottled, diaphoretic, and easily fatigued. Additional symptoms include periorbital edema, hepatomegaly, and a persistent cough. A history of difficult feeding and decreased food intake is a classic sign of CHF. Therefore growth failure is a common consequence of CHF in infancy and childhood (Abad-Sinden & Sutphen, 2001; Leitch, 2000).

Clinical manifestations of CHF depend on the severity of the defect and pulmonary vascular resistance. CHF is manifested in neonates with a severe cardiac defect (e.g., transposition of the great arteries, hypoplastic left-sided heart syndrome, critical aortic stenosis, total anomalous pulmonary venous return, especially with pulmonary venous obstruction) or large left-to-right shunts in a premature infant (e.g., patent ductus arteriosus [PDA], ventricular septal defect [VSD], atrioventricular septal defect [AVSD]). Premature infants with a left-to-right shunt may develop symptoms of CHF earlier than term infants

because their pulmonary vascular resistance drops faster than that of term infants. Infants with defects causing moderate left-to-right shunts (e.g., moderate VSD) do not usually develop symptoms until 4 to 8 weeks of age, when the high pulmonary vascular resistance of the fetal period becomes low enough to cause increased pulmonary blood flow. The onset of symptoms is usually gradual; tachypnea, changes in feeding patterns, and poor weight gain are often early clues. Children with small VSDs, small PDAs, or atrial septal defects (ASDs) generally are asymptomatic.

Hypoxemia and Cyanosis

Hypoxemia is the presence of an arterial oxygen saturation that is below normal. Cyanosis is the blue coloration of the skin and mucous membranes caused by deoxygenated hemoglobin. This coloration is usually seen in the lips, gums, and nail beds and around the eyes and mouth. Cyanosis is difficult to detect in children with dark skin pigmentation and is best perceived by observing mucous membranes and nail beds in natural light. Children with cyanosis often have slowed growth, although they are not usually poor feeders. Polycythemia occurs in children who are chronically hypoxemic, because the body attempts to increase its oxygen-carrying capacity. Toddlers who are cyanotic (most commonly seen in children requiring staged repair of a complex lesion) usually limit their activity but still become easily fatigued and breathless if running, climbing stairs, or playing for long periods of time. Increasing cyanosis may be subtle and difficult to discern; monitoring increasing

Text continued on p. 388.

ACYANOTIC HEART DEFECTS

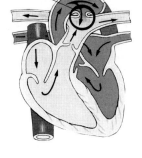

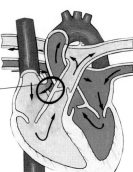

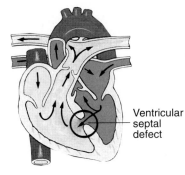

Patent Ductus Arteriosus

Failure of the fetal artery connecting the aorta and pulmonary artery to close within the first few weeks of life. The continued patency of this vessel allows blood to flow from the higher-pressure aorta to the lower pressure pulmonary artery, causing left-to-right shunting. The additional blood is recirculated through the lungs and returns to the left atrium and ventricle. The effect of this altered circulation is increased workload on the left side of the heart, increased pulmonary vascular congestion, and potentially increased right ventricular pressure and hypertrophy. Congestive heart failure is common.

Atrial Septal Defect

Abnormal opening between the atria, allowing blood from the higher pressure left atrium to flow into the slightly lower pressure right atrium. This volume is well tolerated by the right ventricle because the shunt is under low pressure and pulmonary vascular changes occur only after several decades if the defect is unrepaired. Patients are often asymptomatic. Spontaneous closure of the defect may occur, usually within the first year of life.

Ventricular Septal Defect

Abnormal opening between the left and right ventricles. A left to right shunt is caused by the flow of blood from the high pressure left ventricle to the lower pressure right ventricle. The high pressure of the flow into the right ventricle and pulmonary arteries frequently causes congestive heart failure and may cause increased pulmonary vascular resistance if the defect is unrepaired. Many ventricular septal defects close spontaneously, usually within the first year of life.

Atrioventricular Septal Defect

Incomplete fusion of the endocardial cushions. Consists of a low atrial septal defect that is continuous with a high ventricular septal defect and a single, large central atrioventricualr valve that allows blood to flow between all of chambers of the heart, though flow is generally from left to right. Once pulmonary vascular resistance drops, there is significant left-to-right shunting. The resultant pulmonary vascular engorgement predisposes the child to the development of early and severe congestive heart failure.

FIGURE 21-2 Congenital heart defects. (From Wong, D.L. et al [Eds.]. [2003]. Wong's nursing care of infants and children [7th ed.]. St. Louis: Mosby. Modified with permission.)   *Continued*

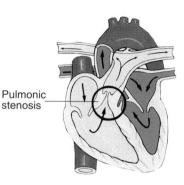

Pulmonic Stenosis

Narrowing at the entrance of the pulmonary artery. Resistance to blood flow causes right ventricular hypertrophy and decreased pulmonary blood flow. **Pulmonary atresia** is the extreme form of pulmonary stenosis, in that there is no flow from the right ventricle to the pulmonary arteries. Aortopulmonary collateral arteries may develop to perfuse the lungs. Clinical manifestations depend on the severity of the stenosis or atresia, from asymptomatic in mild disease to severely cyanotic in critical pulmonary stenosis or pulmonary atresia.

Coarctation of the Aorta

Localized narrowing of the aorta near the insertion of the ductus arteriosus, resulting in increased pressure proximal to the defect (head and upper extremities) and decreased pressure distal to the obstruction (body and lower extremities). Onset of clinical symptoms relates to the severity of the coarctation. In infants, if the defect is severe, perfusion to the descending aorta may be compromised and congestive heart failure may develop from the increased pressure in the ventricle. Children with mild to moderate coarctation may go undiagnosed until school age, when a discrepancy in upper vs. lower extremity blood pressure is discovered.

Aortic Stenosis

Narrowing of the outflow tract of the aorta. May be valvar (most common) in which the valve cusps are malformed, subvalvar in which there is muscular or fibrous area below the valve, or supravalvar (rare) in which there is narrowing above the valve. Aortic stenosis causes resistance to blood flowing through the left ventricle, decreased cardiac output, left ventricular hypertrophy, and pulmonary vascular congestion. The hemodynamic consequences of this may be pulmonary artery hypertension.

CYANOTIC HEART DEFECTS

Tetralogy of Fallot

Includes four defects: ventricular septal defect, pulmonic stenosis, overriding aorta, and right ventricular hypertrophy. The altered hemodynamics vary widely, depending on the degree of pulmonic stenosis and size of ventricular septal defect. Some infants are cyanotic at birth; others have mild cyanosis which progresses as the pulmonic stenosis increases. As the right ventricular pressure increases from increasing right ventricular outflow tract obstruction, the shunting may become right to left, causing acute episodes of cyanosis and hypoxia, called blue spells or tet spells.

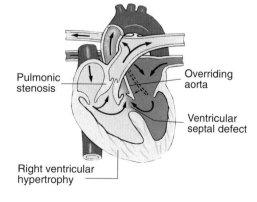

FIGURE 21-2, cont'd.

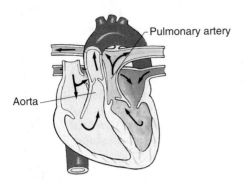

Transposition of the Great Arteries

The pulmonary artery leaves the left ventricle, and the aorta leaves from the right ventricle. Associated defects such as atrial septal defect, ventricular septal defect, or patent ductus arteriosus must be present to permit blood to enter the systemic circulation and/or pulmonary circulation for mixing of saturated and desaturated blood. Infants with minimal communication between the systemic and pulmonary circuits are severely cyanotic at birth as the patent ductus arteriosus closes. Infants with a large communication will be less severely cyanotic but have symptoms of congestive heart failure.

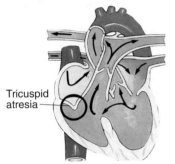

Tricuspid Atresia

Failure of the tricuspid valve to develop; consequently there is no communication between the right atrium and ventricle. It is often associated with pulmonic stenosis and transposition of the great arteries. The right ventricle is frequently hypoplastic. Blood flows through an atrial septal defect or a patent foramen ovale to the left side of the heart and through a ventricular septal defect to the right ventricle and out to the lungs. There is complete mixing of oxygenated and deoxygenated blood in the left side of the heart, resulting in systemic desaturation.

Truncus Arteriosus

Failure of normal septation and division of the embryonic bulbar trunk into the pulmonary artery and aorta, resulting in a single vessel that overrides both ventricles. Blood from both ventricles mixes in the common great artery, causing desaturation and hypoxemia. Blood ejected from the heart flows preferentially into the lower-pressure pulmonary arteries, causing increased pulmonary blood flow and decreased systemic blood flow. Pulmonary vascular disease develops early in the unrepaired child.

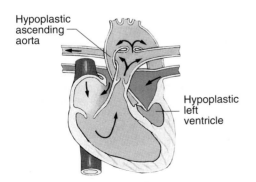

Hypoplastic Left Heart Syndrome

Underdevelopment of the left side of the heart, resulting in a hypoplastic left ventricle and aortic atresia. Most blood from the left atrium flows across the patent foramen ovale into the right atrium, to the right ventricle, and out the pulmonary artery. The descending aorta receives blood from the patent ductus arteriosus supplying systemic blood flow. The amount of blood flow to the pulmonary and systemic circulations depends on a delicate balance between the pulmonary and systemic vascular resistances. As the ductus arteriosus closes deterioration is rapid with cyanosis and decreased cardiac output.

FIGURE 21-2, cont'd.

hemoglobin may facilitate the determination of progressive hypoxemia.

Treatment

Early Corrective Surgery

The natural history of some congenital heart defects (e.g., small VSD, ASD) is such that spontaneous closure of the defect may occur, avoiding intervention. These children have few if any symptoms. Most lesions, however, require surgery. For most defects, an echocardiogram provides all the information needed to perform surgery (Kimball & Meyer, 2001). For some cardiac defects, however, cardiac catheterization, perfusion scan, or magnetic resonance imaging (MRI) may also be performed before surgery to determine the precise anatomy and physiology of a child's heart. As techniques in surgical intervention, cardiopulmonary bypass, cardiac preservation, and postoperative care are refined, the trend in treating children with CHD is toward definitive repair at a very young age (frequently early infancy). Early corrective surgery decreases the negative consequences of long-standing hypoxemia, myocardial strain, and pulmonary overcirculation.

Interventional Cardiac Catheterization

For an increasing number of defects, interventional cardiac catheterization has replaced surgery as the treatment of choice. Some forms of aortic and pulmonary valvular or vascular stenosis can be repaired through balloon valvuloplasty and angioplasty. Vascular stents can be placed within the vessel to maintain the patency of stenosed vessels in conjunction with balloon angioplasty. Closure of PDAs, septal defects, and unnecessary collateral blood vessels is being performed via placement of various occlusive devices within the defect (Bridges et al, 2001; Uzark, 2001). Clinical results of PDA closure with transcatheter coils are comparable to surgical closure, with no significant long-term complications and a significant decrease in cost (Prieto et al, 1998).

In addition, electrophysiologic studies are used in conjunction with cardiac catheterization to identify cardiac arrhythmias, evaluate the effectiveness of certain drugs under controlled circumstances, and abolish or ablate the accessory pathway causing the arrhythmia (Hanisch, 2001). Catheter therapy has now been applied to cure or modify most pediatric arrhythmias including atrioventricular (AV) node reentry tachycardia, ectopic atrial tachycardia, and some forms of ventricular tachycardia (Saul, 2001). Implantable pacemaker/cardioverter–defibrillators (ICDs) may be indicated for children with long QT syndrome, cardiomyopathy, ventricular tachycardia, and sudden cardiac death (Hanisch, 2001). The broad field of therapeutic cardiac catheterization has become a valuable tool in managing many children with CHD.

Staged Corrective Surgery

There is a population of children with complex CHD (e.g., children with single-ventricle physiology) for whom staged repair is the treatment of choice. The child may undergo one or multiple palliative procedures as a neonate or infant followed by definitive repair after infancy. In these children, symptoms of cyanosis and CHF may exist until the definitive repair is performed, sometimes into toddlerhood.

Control of Congestive Heart Failure

Control of CHF (Box 21-2) is usually achieved with the use of diuretics and inotropes (e.g., digoxin, angiotensin converting enzyme [ACE] inhibitors). Because failure to thrive is a common complication of CHF (alone or in combination with cyanosis), feeding support is also a priority in management. Support may include methods of decreasing fatigue during feeding, increasing the caloric concentration of formula, or providing gavage feeding.

Infants who are cyanotic also require monitoring for progressive cyanosis, anemia, and dehydration. Parents of children who are cyanotic must learn to identify increasing blueness and cyanotic spells. Infants awaiting surgery are closely followed by a cardiologist to manage CHF or cyanosis and to time surgery.

Prevention of Pulmonary Hypertension

Crucial factors in determining the timing of surgery include preventing irreversible pulmonary hypertension and the development of aortopulmonary collateral vessels, as well as maintaining adequate ventricular function. Large left-to-right shunts rarely cause irreversible changes in the pulmonary vasculature before 12 months of age. Once these irreversible changes occur, however, surgery is contraindicated and the child becomes progressively cyanotic.

To aid the cardiologist in following the progress of the child's disease, communication between the cardiologist and the primary care provider is important. Signs or symptoms of increasing tachycardia, tachypnea, decreasing feeding, slowed weight gain, hepatomegaly, worsening perfusion, or increased cyanosis should be reported to the cardiologist.

Complementary and Alternative Therapies

Parents of children with CHD need to be cautioned about utilizing complementary therapies since some may interfere with medications used to manage heart conditions. Products containing gingko interact with warfarin (Coumadin). Herbal and dietary supplements have not undergone the rigorous review of the Food and Drug Administration (FDA). Because there is no standardization related to dosage, side effects, and drug interactions with herbal products, their use is not recommended.

BOX 21-2

Treatment

Surgery—neonatal/infant corrective or staged corrective surgery for complex defects; infant or early childhood repairs for less complex defects
Interventional cardiac catheterization
Electrophysiologic studies; ablation
Implantable pacemaker/cardioverter/defibrillator
Control congestive heart failure (CHF)
    Support feeding
    Monitor for worsening cyanosis, anemia, and dehydration
Prevent pulmonary hypertension

Anticipated Advances in Diagnosis and Management

Many aspects of pediatric cardiology will continue to benefit from the advances in technology, genetics, and research. The ability to diagnose CHD by echocardiogram has expanded beyond major centers through teleechocardiography. The FDA has recently approved the first ASD closure device, and further advances in devices and techniques associated with interventional cardiac catheterization continue to expand treatment options for children with CHD. Fetal surgery and interventional cardiac catheterization both show promise in preventing minor defects in utero from developing into critical ones once the heart is fully formed and the child is born.

Refinements in surgical techniques continue to improve outcomes, particularly for children with complex disease. Early results with the total cavopulmonary anastomosis Fontan procedure (used for single-ventricle type of defects) show a decreased mortality and improved clinical status as compared with the more traditional Fontan procedure (Marcelletti et al, 2000). Tissue engineering of prosthetic valves and conduits has great potential to create devices with the ability to grow with the child (Walters, 2000). This technique would be a major breakthrough for pediatric cardiac surgery, in which a significant proportion of surgeries are performed to replace devices children have "outgrown."

Clinical electrophysiology (i.e., including pacemaker therapy) is another growing field. Rhythm control—whether accomplished via advanced antiarrhythmic drugs, ablative therapy, or implantable devices—continues to evolve as more clinical experience is gained, new technologies are refined, and adult treatments are adapted for use in children.

Associated Problems (Box 21-3)

Hematologic Problems

Children with cyanotic heart disease develop polycythemia to increase the oxygen-carrying capacity of the blood. If the hematocrit reaches 65% or higher, there is a marked increase in the viscosity of the blood, resulting in an increased tendency for thrombus formation (Park, 2002). Bleeding disorders are also seen in children with polycythemia, most commonly thrombocytopenia and defective platelet aggregation, but also prolonged prothrombin time and partial thromboplastin time and lower levels of factors V and VIII. These children may bruise easily or develop petechiae, gingival bleeding, or epistaxis (Park, 2002).

Anemia can be a special problem in children with CHD. In children with existing CHF, decreased hemoglobin may exacerbate myocardial strain. Therefore children with an acyanotic heart defect should have a hemoglobin level within the normal range for their age. Supplemental iron may be prescribed if their hemoglobin falls below normal levels or after surgery if their hemoglobin falls as a result of blood loss. In cyanotic infants, iron deficiency anemia has been associated with cerebral venous thrombosis (Park, 2002). Children who are cyanotic with a low hematocrit may exhibit hypoxic spells more readily than if the oxygen-carrying capacity of the blood were normal. Cyanosis will not be as obvious in children with anemia as in children with normal or elevated hemoglobin.

It is important for children with cyanosis who have a low hematocrit to receive iron therapy. It is equally important to monitor their response to the therapy in order to prevent the hematocrit from rising to undesirably high levels, thus increasing blood viscosity. Adequate hydration must be maintained in children with cyanotic heart disease to avoid increased hemoconcentration. Problems associated with fever and exposure to hot weather can cause excessive perspiration; vomiting and diarrhea can cause dehydration. The problem of dehydration can be exacerbated if any of these conditions causing excessive volume loss occur in an infant or child who is receiving diuretic therapy.

Infectious Processes

Children with significant heart defects are at high risk for developing a variety of infections. Recurrent respiratory tract infections are especially common in children with lesions causing increased pulmonary blood flow. Infections can significantly affect a child's health in the following ways: (1) severe respiratory tract infections can exacerbate hypoxemia in cyanotic children; (2) fever can increase metabolic rate and oxygen demands, thus precipitating myocardial decompensation; (3) dehydration in a child with polycythemia can lead to thrombus formation; and (4) electrolyte imbalances from vomiting, diarrhea, or fever can impact cardiac performance or lead to digoxin toxicity in the child receiving dioxin.

Children with asplenia syndrome (i.e., a condition that includes absence of the spleen and complex cardiac defects) are extremely susceptible to bacteremia with an associated high mortality. *Streptococcus pneumoniae* and *Haemophilus influenzae* type B are the most common pathogens. Routine pneumococcal and Hib immunizations are recommended (see Immunizations). Daily antimicrobial prophylaxis against pneumococcal infections should be strongly considered for children younger than 5 years of age with asplenia syndrome. Some experts continue prophylaxis throughout childhood and into adulthood in particularly high-risk clients with asplenia.

BOX 21-3
Associated Problems

Hematologic
   Polycythemia
   Bleeding disorders
   Anemia
Infectious processes
   Respiratory tract infections
   Bacteremia
Infective endocarditis
Central nervous system (CNS) complications
   Brain abscess
   Cerebrovascular accident (CVA)
Arrhythmias/heart block
Failure to thrive
Slowed development
Vulnerable child syndrome

Recommended treatment for prophylaxis is oral penicillin V 125 mg twice daily for children under 5 years and 250 mg twice daily for children 5 years and older (Committee on Infectious Diseases, 2000a). Recently, the percentage of pneumococcal organisms that show some degree of resistance to penicillin has increased. Therefore close observation and prompt intervention for symptoms of infection are critical.

Infective Endocarditis

Endocarditis may occur because of blood-borne bacteria that lodge on damaged, synthetic, or abnormal heart valves, prosthetic material, or the endocardium near congenital anatomic defects. In the long term, individuals with the following conditions constitute the greatest risk: (1) rigid prosthetic—especially left-sided valves; (2) prosthetic conduits, such as the Fontan type of operations; (3) complex cyanotic heart defects; and (4) surgically constructed systemic-to-pulmonary shunts (Dajani and Taubert, 2001). Endocarditis may occur if prophylaxis precautions are not followed during most dental procedures and surgical or invasive procedures involving mucosal surfaces or contaminated tissues. Most cases of endocarditis, however, are not attributable to an invasive procedure (Box 21-4; Dajani et al, 1997). In the past, *Streptococcus viridans, Staphylococcus aureus*, and enterococcus accounted for approximately 90% of the cases. Recently there has been an increase in the incidence of endocarditis caused by organisms such as fungi, *Haemophilus*, & *Actinobacillus* (Park, 2002). The current recommendation for prophylaxis for dental, oral, respiratory tract, or esophageal procedures is amoxicillin (i.e., 50 mg/kg for children; 2.0 g for adults) given orally 1 hour before the procedure (Box 21-5).

Central Nervous System Complications

In children with cyanosis caused by right-to-left intracardiac shunting, the normally effective phagocytic filtering action of the pulmonary capillary bed is bypassed. As a result, these children are at increased risk for brain abscess, most commonly after 2 years of age. Infants who are cyanotic with iron deficiency anemia are prone to develop cerebrovascular accidents. A possible explanation for this finding is that relative anemia secondary to cyanosis leads to increased blood viscosity and increased coagulability and thus venous thrombosis (Park, 2002). In addition, intracardiac thrombus from cardiac catheterization or surgery may embolize, leading to a cerebrovascular accident.

Arrhythmias

Rhythm disturbances can occur in children with CHD as a direct result of the cardiac defect, electrolyte imbalances, medications, or surgical repair. Atrial arrhythmias are more

---

BOX 21-4

Infective Endocarditis Prophylaxis*

CARDIAC CONDITIONS

Endocarditis prophylaxis recommended for the following:

High-risk category
  Prosthetic cardiac valves
  Previous history of bacterial endocarditis
  Complex cyanotic heart defects (e.g., transposition, tetralogy of Fallot [TOF], single type of ventricle defect)
  Surgically constructed systemic-to-pulmonary shunts or conduits
Moderate-risk category
  Most other congenital cardiac defects (i.e., other than those listed here)
  Rheumatic and other acquired valvular dysfunction
  Mitral valve prolapse with valvular regurgitation
  Hypertrophic cardiomyopathy

Endocarditis prophylaxis not recommended for the following:

Negligible-risk category (no greater risk than the general population)
  Isolated secundum atrial septal defect
  Surgical repair without residua beyond 6 mo of secundum atrial septal defect (ASD), ventricular septal defect (VSD), or patent ductus arteriosus (PDA)
  Physiologic, functional, or innocent heart murmurs
  Mitral valve prolapse without valvular regurgitation
  Previous Kawasaki disease without valvular dysfunction
  Previous rheumatic fever without valvular dysfunction
  Intravascular and epicardial cardiac pacemakers and implanted defibrillators
  Previous coronary artery bypass graft surgery

PROCEDURES FOR WHICH ENDOCARDITIS PROPHYLAXIS IS RECOMMENDED

Dental procedures known to induce gingival or mucosal bleeding, including professional cleaning

Tonsillectomy and/or adenoidectomy
Surgical procedures that involve intestinal or respiratory mucosa
Bronchoscopy with rigid bronchoscope
Sclerotherapy for esophageal varices
Esophageal stricture dilation
Endoscopic retrograde cholangiography with biliary obstruction
Biliary tract surgery
Cystoscopy
Urethral dilation
Prostate surgery
Urethral catheterization if urinary tract infection is present

PROCEDURES FOR WHICH ENDOCARDITIS PROPHYLAXIS IS NOT RECOMMENDED

Dental procedures not likely to cause gingival bleeding (e.g., simple adjustment of orthodontic appliances or fillings above the gum line, restorative dentistry)
Shedding of deciduous teeth
Insertion of tympanostomy tubes
Bronchoscopy with flexible bronchoscope, with or without biopsy[†]
Endotracheal intubation
Transesophageal echocardiography[†]
Cardiac catheterization
Implanted cardiac pacemakers or defibrillators
Endoscopy with or without gastrointestinal biopsy[†]
Cesarean delivery
Uncomplicated vaginal delivery[†]
Vaginal hysterectomy[†]
In the absence of infection for urethral catheterization, uterine dilation and curettage, therapeutic abortion, sterilization procedures, or insertion or removal of intrauterine devices

From Dajani, A.S. (1997). Prevention of bacterial endocarditis: Recommendations by the American Heart Association. *Circulation, 96,* 358-366. Modified with permission.
*This box lists common pediatric conditions and procedures but is not meant to be all-inclusive.
[†]Prophylaxis is optional for high-risk patients.

common than ventricular rhythm disturbances in children. In infants and children who have not had cardiac surgery, there is an increased incidence of supraventricular tachycardia with Ebstein anomaly, tricuspid atresia, hypertrophic cardiomyopathy, and double-outlet right ventricle (Van Hare, 1999). Anatomically corrected transposition of the great arteries (L-TGA) is a rare congenital heart defect that may also lead to supraventricular tachycardia (SVT) or varying degrees of heart block (Park, 2002).

Postoperatively, disturbances in atrial rhythms may be seen in children after surgical manipulation of the atrium (e.g., the Fontan procedure, repair of total anomalous pulmonary venous return [TAPVR], ASD repair, Mustard or Senning procedure). Intraarterial baffling procedures (e.g., the Mustard procedure) for transposing the great arteries have essentially been replaced by arterial switch procedures in part because of the incidence of arrhythmias in more than 50% of children and adolescents. Both atrial and ventricular arrhythmias are a growing problem in adolescents and young adults with CHD with associated increasing morbidity and mortality (Warnes et al, 2001). Postoperative second- or third-degree heart block may occur in surgeries involving the ventricular septum (e.g., repair of VSD, AV canal repair, tetralogy of Fallot [TOF] repair) or with

---

BOX 21-5
Endocarditis Prophylaxis Recommendations

For dental, oral, respiratory tract, or esophageal procedures:

For most patients: amoxicillin, 50 mg/kg (max 2.0 g) orally 1 hr before procedure.

For patients unable to take oral medications: ampicillin, 50 mg/kg (max 2.0 g) IM or IV 30 min before procedure.

For patients allergic to amoxicillin, ampicillin, and/or penicillin: clindamycin, 20 mg/kg (maximum 600 mg) orally 1 hr before procedure *or* cephalexin* or cefadroxil,* 50 mg/kg (max 2.0 g) orally 1 hr before procedure *or* azithromycin or clarithromycin, 15 mg/kg (max 500 mg) orally 1 hr before procedure.

For patients allergic to amoxicillin, ampicillin, and/or penicillin who are unable to take oral medications: clindamycin, 20 mg/kg (max 600 mg) IV 30 min before the procedure *or* cefazolin, 25 mg/kg (max 1.0 g) IM or IV 30 min before the procedure.

For gastrointestinal and genitourinary tract procedures:

For high-risk patients: ampicillin, 50 mg/kg (max 2.0 g) IM or IV, plus gentamicin, 1.5 mg/kg (120 mg) IM or IV within 30 min before procedure; then ampicillin, 25 mg/kg (max 1 g) IM or IV, or amoxicillin, 25 mg/kg (max 1 g) orally 6 hr after initial dose.

For high-risk patients allergic to ampicillin and/or amoxicillin: vancomycin, 20 mg/kg (max 1.0 g) IV over 1 to 2 hr plus gentamicin, 1.5 mg/kg (max 120 mg) IM or IV; complete injection and/or infusion within 30 min of starting procedure.

For moderate-risk patients: amoxicillin, 50 mg/kg (max 2.0 g) orally 1 hr before procedure *or* ampicillin, 50 mg/kg (max 2.0 g) IM or IV within 30 min of starting procedure.

For moderate-risk patients allergic to ampicillin and/or amoxicillin: vancomycin, 20 mg/kg (max 1.0 g) IV over 1 to 2 hr; complete the infusion within 30 min of starting procedure.

From Dajani, A.S. (1997). Prevention of bacterial endocarditis: Recommendations by the American Heart Association. *Circulation, 96,* 358-366. Modified with permission.
IM, Intramuscular; *IV,* intravascular.
*Cephalosporins should not be used in patients with immediate type of hypersensitivity reactions to penicillins.

---

subaortic resection and aortic valve replacement. In addition, children who have had a complete repair of TOF can develop ventricular ectopy, which can infrequently lead to sudden death (Hanisch, 2001).

Digoxin toxicity generally manifests as atrioventricular block, but it can also produce a wide variety of arrhythmias (Artman, 2001). A low serum potassium concentration potentiates the effects of digoxin. A child receiving a non–potassium-sparing diuretic (e.g., furosemide [Lasix]) without potassium replacement may be at particular risk of digoxin toxicity. A therapeutic digoxin level is generally 1.0 to 2 ng/ml, although toxicity has been seen at lower levels and may not be seen at higher levels in some infants. A sound rule is to assume that an arrhythmia noted in a child receiving digoxin therapy is caused by digoxin until proved otherwise. If extra beats or an abnormal rhythm—including bradycardia and tachycardia—is identified by the primary care provider, an electrocardiogram should be obtained and the child should be referred to the cardiologist for further evaluation as soon as possible.

Failure to Thrive

Growth failure has frequently been observed in children with CHD. The decreased growth is usually more pronounced in weight than in height. CHF is one of the most potent factors in the development of failure to thrive because of inadequate caloric intake secondary to tachypnea, malabsorption, and the relative hypermetabolism associated with CHF and pulmonary hypertension (Ackerman et al, 1998; Leitch, 2000). A new onset of slowed growth is particularly important to recognize because it may suggest significant hemodynamic compromise, necessitating an alteration in the drug regimen or surgery. Corrective surgery, particularly in infancy, generally restores a normal growth pattern and energy expenditure (Leitch, Karn, Ensing, & Denne, 2000). Weight usually improves more quickly than height. Palliative surgery generally improves growth, although not to the same degree as corrective surgery. As the age of corrective surgery decreases the recovery of height, weight, and head circumference improves. There are also some syndromes associated with CHD (e.g., Turner syndrome, Down syndrome) that display slowed growth independent of a heart defect.

Slowed Development

The majority of children with CHD show normal outcomes; however, as a group they tend to have more neurodevelopmental problems. Those at highest risk are children with complex cardiac anatomy necessitating deep hypothermic circulatory arrest as a neonate in surgery and children with single-ventricle physiology, particularly hypoplastic left heart syndrome (Forbess et al, 2000; Mahle, 2001; O'Brien & Boisvert, 2001; Uzark et al, 1998; Wernovsky et al, 2001). The effects of cyanosis on intelligence quotient (IQ) have suggested that children who are cyanotic may have a lag in intellectual development. Several factors may contribute to this neurodevelopmental delay, including a decrease in the child's ability to physically interact with the environment, parental overprotection, and prolonged hospitalization and illness (Mahle, 2001; Wray & Sensky, 1999). In addition, there is a relatively high incidence of microcephaly and neurologic abnormalities in children with hypoplastic left heart syndrome (Limperopoulos et al, 1999; Mahle, 2001). Analysis of children with cyanotic heart disease reveals no significant correlation between IQ or visual motor integration ability and degree of hypoxemia or age of repair (Uzark et al, 1998; Wray & Sensky, 1999). However, delays in speech and fine motor skills have frequently been observed, and learning disabilities are common (Bellinger et al, 2000).

CHF and cyanosis may significantly affect gross motor development. Children with CHD may sit, crawl, and walk much later than their peers. Parental overprotection and lack of activity may also contribute to delayed development (Mahle, 2001; Smith, 2001).

Vulnerable Child Syndrome

Although overprotection may generally be a problem for children with a chronic condition, children with a heart defect are at high risk for overprotection and altered parent-infant attachment (Wray & Sensky, 1999). Parental anxiety can occur as a result of the disturbing array of clinical symptoms and feeding problems of a child with CHF or cyanosis, the fear of a sudden catastrophic event, and the paradox of becoming attached while dealing with fears about a child's vulnerability and potential death (Carey, 1999; Clark & Miles, 1999; Hinoki, 1998). The mere presence of the defect unrelated to the severity of the heart disease, however, can produce severe anxiety leading to overprotection and placement of inappropriate limits on a child (Morelius et al, 2002). Social adjustment and the development of independence are challenges for children from school age to adolescents and may be related to parental overprotection (Kao et al, 2000; Tong et al, 1998). Because overprotection may delay development in children with existing physical impediments to development, primary care providers should be aware of feelings of vulnerability in parents and children and reinforce the importance of treating these children normally.

Prognosis

The prognosis for children with CHD is good for the majority of lesions. Only the most complex defects require multiple surgeries. Most children have had definitive repair by their first year. Improved preoperative diagnosis, medical management, and surgical technique have contributed to the significant decrease in surgical mortality of almost all congenital cardiac defects to approximately 5% (American Heart Association [AHA], 2000a; McElhinney & Wernovsky, 2001; Van Arsdell et al, 2000; Walters, 2000). The notable exception is hypoplastic left heart syndrome (HLHS), which has a hospital mortality of approximately 15% to 37%, depending on the institution (Daebritz, 2000; Walters, 2000). HLHS is also unique in its late hospital mortality. Whereas posthospital survival is excellent for most forms of CHD, approximately 10% to 20% of infants with HLHS who survive the first-stage Norwood procedure die within the first year of life (McElhinney & Wernovsky, 2001). The majority of children after surgery require long-term follow-up for potential problems related to myocardial changes, ventricular failure, deteriorating or outgrown prosthetic materials, electrophysiologic sequelae, and infective endocarditis.

PRIMARY CARE MANAGEMENT

Health Care Maintenance

Growth and Development

Significant delays in both height and weight are seen in children with symptomatic CHD (Abad-Sinden & Sutphen, 2001; Leitch, 2000). Height is generally not affected as much as weight, and head circumference should not affected. If growth is slowed to a point where a child's growth curve flattens, the child should be referred to the cardiologist for an evaluation of worsening CHF. Because growth of a child with well-controlled CHF may still be slow, it is important to look at trends of weight gain, as well as make comparisons with the norms.

In assessing the developmental and emotional status of children with CHD, primary care providers must take into account factors such as preexisting neurologic abnormalities, hypoxemia, CHF, extended hospitalization, parental overprotection, and physical incapacity. Preoperatively, infants with CHF are often too exhausted to pass all the developmental tasks in screening tests. If a child is developing at a slower but progressive rate, referral for additional developmental testing is not immediately warranted. If there appear to be significant alterations in the level of alertness or if there is no progress in mastering developmental tasks, further assessment is advised. If CHD is part of a syndrome that involves developmental delay, referral and enrollment in an infant-stimulation program would be important.

Infants and children who have been hospitalized may display developmental regression as an adaptation to the stress of hospitalization. Parents may note that after surgery there are disturbances in their child's patterns of sleep, feeding, behavior, toilet training, and speech. Although this regression can be very troublesome for parents, it is a common response to the stress of hospitalization. It usually resolves within a few weeks and does not warrant further developmental follow-up. If there are other neurologic symptoms, such as change in level of consciousness, seizures, or weakness, the child should be examined and referred as needed.

When discussing developmental concerns with parents, the practitioner should help the parents normalize their responses to their child with a chronic condition. Primary care providers can guide parents in treating their child normally by reinforcing that children who are symptomatic will limit themselves naturally.

Diet

Feeding is often a major problem for children with CHD, particularly if they have a complex defect or are experiencing CHF. During feeding, symptomatic infants often have difficulty coordinating sucking, swallowing, and breathing. The distribution of calories in these infants is similar to the recommended dietary allowances, but the caloric needs of symptomatic infants with failure to thrive are about 150 kcal/kg/day (Abad-Sinden & Sutphen, 2001; Leitch, 2000). If infants are not adequately gaining weight, their caloric intake may need to be increased by concentrating breast milk or formula. Concentrating the breast milk or formula to 24 to 30 calories per ounce will elevate the total calories without increasing the total volume. If breast milk or formula is concentrated by adding powder formula to breast milk or decreasing the amount of water added to powder or concentrate, the increased renal solute load the infant receives must be considered. An alternative is to add low-osmolarity glucose polymers or oils to standard formulas to increase the caloric density. A diet providing increased carbohydrates and fats may lead to increased retention of nitrogen for growth. Consulting a nutritionist and the cardiologist is advised if nutritional manipulations are used.

Breast-feeding of children with even a hemodynamically significant heart defect is not contraindicated if growth is adequate. Breast milk is the best source of nutrition for infants with a chronic illness, such as CHD (Committee on Nutrition, 1999). The physiologic stress of breast-feeding is actually less than the stress related to bottle feeding (Marino et al, 1995). Methods to decrease the work of feeding during breast or bottle feeding include holding infants at a 45-degree angle to minimize tachypnea, feeding them for no longer than 40 minutes at a time to minimize fatigue, allowing them to develop their own rhythm of feeding and resting, and following their cues for hunger, satiety, and tiring.

A child with complex disease or CHF may not gain weight despite aggressive feeding and breast milk or formula concentration. Such children may need gavage feedings to minimize the calories used with feeding. Using a pacifier during gavage feeding helps an infant develop a strong suck, facilitates the transition to oral feeding after surgery, and promotes future language development.

Parents often need a tremendous amount of support for feeding a child with CHD. Children with symptomatic CHD and tachypnea have difficulty consuming enough calories to satisfy hunger and may be irritable. Both infants and mothers may contribute to a less than optimal feeding situation. Infants with CHD give fewer feeding cues and respond less to caregivers, and mothers of infants with CHD may exhibit less fostering behavior (e.g., eye contact, smiling, cuddling) during feeding. Parents may also feel the pressure of getting a child to gain weight for surgery. In addition, a parent's self-esteem may be tied to the feeding and growth of the child. Primary care providers should stress to parents that feeding can be a positive time for bonding and nurturing. Ongoing support includes teaching the parents to be sensitive to the infant's cues for hunger, satiety, and distress; pointing out the positive aspects of the child; and reinforcing feeding skills. Through feeding, the parent and child are developing their relationship. A primary care provider who understands the potential problems of feeding can be instrumental in fostering a positive feeding relationship by providing support and counseling.

Safety

In addition to standard safety precautions, children with CHD have unique safety needs. For example, digoxin elixir has a pleasant taste and attractive color, which increase the potential for accidental ingestion by the child or siblings. Therefore safe storage and administration of medications are essential. Marking a syringe at the correct dose, giving paper instructions on medication administration, and allowing parents to practice drawing the medication will help ensure the safe use of all medications.

Electrical safety is critical for children with permanent pacemakers. An electric shock may irreparably damage the pacemaker, requiring immediate surgical replacement. There is no risk of electromagnetic interference between a permanent pacemaker and common household items, such as electrical appliances, radios, cellular phones, or electronic equipment. Both microwave ovens and pacemakers have filtering systems that prevent interference with the pacemaker's function. Large magnets placed directly over the pacemaker will temporarily change its function; therefore MRI is contraindicated for children with a permanent pacemaker. Metal detectors should also be avoided because they have an electromagnetic field that may temporarily alter a pacemaker's function, as well as set off the alarm as a result of the metal in the pacemaker. Small magnet toys, however, will not alter a pacemaker's function. A pacemaker identification card or letter from the primary care provider should be sufficient to allow a child to avoid metal detectors or airport security.

Children with permanent pacemakers or receiving anticoagulants for prosthetic valves can maintain most normal activities. They should be counseled to avoid contact sports (e.g., football, boxing, karate), which could damage the pacemaker or cause excessive bleeding (American College of Cardiology and American College of Sports Medicine, 1994). Older children with pacemakers and children taking anticoagulants should wear Medic-Alert bracelets for emergencies.

Travel may need to be altered for children with CHD. Altitudes of 5000 feet or higher are not recommended for children with moderate to severe pulmonary hypertension, severe CHF, or significant hypoxemia (i.e., PO_2 of 50 mm Hg). These children may require precautions to fly on an airplane because cabin pressure is usually equivalent to an altitude of 5000 to 7500 feet. Supplemental oxygen can be supplied by the airlines to increase the inspired oxygen to 20%.

Training parents of children with CHD in cardiopulmonary resuscitation (CPR) may be effective and particularly warranted for certain problems. Suggesting CPR training to parents as a skill that is worthwhile for any parent to know can allay potential concerns about the importance of learning CPR. The American Red Cross or the American Heart Association may offer CPR training to families.

Immunizations

The standard immunization protocol, including the heptavalent pneumococcal conjugate vaccine (PCV7) and influenza vaccine, is recommended for children with CHD (Committee on Infectious Diseases, 2000a). A significant percentage of children with CHD, however, are behind in their immunization schedule. The timing of immunizations in children having heart surgery requires several considerations. Immunizations should not be given before cardiac catheterization or surgery because a fever would delay the procedure. Measles vaccine has been shown to cause a significant increase in the rate of thrombocytopenia, which could exacerbate the decreased platelet count and function seen after cardiopulmonary bypass. In addition, blood transfusion may affect immune response to vaccines for several weeks. Salicylates are commonly used to control postoperative inflammatory reactions or for platelet inhibition; however, their use is not recommended for 6 weeks after the varicella vaccine (Smith, 2001). After surgery, immunizations should be delayed approximately 6 weeks so that a fever from an immunization is not confused with a postoperative infection.

Children with hemodynamically significant CHD may be more susceptible to complications of influenza and should receive the influenza vaccine yearly in the autumn beginning at 6 months of age. The recommended dosage is 0.25 ml from 6 to 35 months and 0.5 ml thereafter. Two doses administered at least 1 month apart are recommended for children receiving the vaccine for the first time (Committee on Infectious Diseases, 2000b). For children with asplenia or hemodynamically significant CHD who have received the full complement of the PCV7 vaccine, an additional dose of 0.5 ml given intramuscularly is recommended at 2 to 5 years of age (Committee on Infectious Diseases, 2000a).

Screening

Vision. Routine screening is recommended.

Hearing. Routine screening is recommended.

Dental. Dental care should be meticulously followed to prevent caries and gum disease, which may predispose a child to bacteremia if left untreated. Most children with CHD need endocarditis prophylaxis before all dental procedures except simple adjustment of braces and shedding of deciduous teeth (Boxes 21-4 & 21-5; Dajani et al, 1997). Because oral procedures (e.g., dental cleaning, drilling at the gum level, pulling a permanent tooth) produce a higher inoculum of bacteria over a longer period of time than the shedding of deciduous teeth, antibiotic coverage is recommended for these procedures. The specific regimen depends on the type of defect, the procedure being performed, and the child's sensitivity to penicillin. The child's cardiologist should communicate this information to the dentist and primary care provider. Wallet-size cards that outline specific prophylactic regimens are available from the American Heart Association.

Blood Pressure. Blood pressure should be obtained in upper and lower extremities for children with preoperative or postoperative repair of the aorta to identify discrepancies in pressure readings that may indicate progression of the heart defect. A child who has had a Blalock-Taussig shunt procedure to increase blood flow to the lungs or a subclavian flap repair of coarctation of the aorta will have a diminished or absent pulse in the upper extremity on the side of the surgical scar.

Hematocrit. A rise in hemoglobin and hematocrit may indicate progressive hypoxemia in the child with a cyanotic heart defect. Further, because of the problems associated with anemia in the child with cyanosis or CHF, hemoglobin and hematocrit levels should be checked regularly. Iron supplementation should be prescribed if the hemoglobin level is low for a child's specific condition. Because the child's cardiologist will be checking these values periodically, communication with the cardiologist may save a child the pain and expense of repeated laboratory tests.

Urinalysis. Routine screening is recommended.

Tuberculosis. Routine screening is recommended.

Condition-Specific Screening

Drugs and Electrolytes. Infants and children taking digoxin or Coumadin may need to have serum blood levels measured periodically. If the child is taking diuretics, electrolytes may be routinely monitored by the cardiologist and may need to be checked if the child develops gastroenteritis.

Common Illness Management
Differential Diagnosis

Children with CHD may be susceptible to common pediatric problems that can be more severe than in children with structurally normal hearts. Therefore it is important for primary care providers to know the common problems that can lead to serious complications. It is equally important, however, that they treat these children normally and look for common, uncomplicated problems. Families need reinforcement that these children are normal but have special medical needs. Children who have had heart surgery are often scared or hesitant of examinations, particularly of their chest. If the child's trust is gained before the examination, visits will be less stressful for the child and more productive for the primary care provider (Box 21-6).

Fever. Although febrile illnesses can have serious consequences in children with CHD, an acute fever may also be caused by a common, uncomplicated childhood illness. Primary care providers should investigate and treat fever the same way they would for any child the same age while being

---

BOX 21-6

Differential Diagnosis

FEVER
Focus found: common intercurrent illness unrelated to CHD postoperatively vs. **Wound infection:** wound erythema, drainage
   Postpericardiotomy syndrome: pericardial friction rub, malaise, chest pain
   Infective endocarditis: malaise, anorexia, night sweats, new murmur

RESPIRATORY COMPROMISE
Upper or lower respiratory infection (URI or LRI): fever, productive cough, infiltrates on chest radiograph vs. **Congestive heart failure (CHF):** poor feeding, sweating, dry cough, cardiomegaly
Respiratory syncytial virus

GASTROINTESTINAL SYMPTOMS
Acute gastroenteritis vs. digoxin toxicity
   Worsening CHF
   Acute vs. digoxin worsening

NEUROLOGIC SYMPTOMS
Brain abscess
Cerebrovascular accident (CVA)

CHEST PAIN
Musculoskeletal problems, pulmonary conditions vs. cardiac etiology

SYNCOPE
Autonomic nervous system, seizures, hyperventilation vs. cardiac abnormalities

mindful of the more serious possibilities. The long-term use of antibiotics without a diagnosis just because the child has CHD is not warranted and will put the child at risk of developing infections from resistant organisms.

A fever within a few weeks after heart surgery may be a sign of an operative infection or postpericardiotomy syndrome (i.e., an inflammatory reaction of the pericardial sac after heart surgery). A careful and complete examination is necessary to identify a source of infection. If no focus of infection (e.g., otitis media, pharyngitis) is found, the primary care provider should obtain a complete blood count (CBC) with differential and a blood culture and should refer the child to the cardiologist or surgeon. In addition, if there are any signs of a superficial surgical wound infection, the child should be referred to the cardiologist or surgeon. Postpericardiotomy syndrome should be suspected by the presence of a fever the first week after surgery, with a pericardial friction rub, chest pain, malaise, irritability, or enlargement of the cardiac silhouette on a chest radiograph. It is seen fairly frequently after surgery in which the pericardium has been opened but is rarely seen in children younger than 2 years of age (Rheuban, 2001; Wernovsky et al, 2001). The condition is usually self-limited and treatment consists of antiinflammatory agents (aspirin, nonsteroidal antiinflammatory agents, or occasionally steroids) and rest.

A fever will increase the metabolic demands and thus the work of the heart. It is therefore important to evaluate a febrile child with symptomatic CHD for the development or worsening of CHF. Children with asplenia must be seen by the primary care provider immediately on developing a fever for a complete work-up to identify the cause and initiate antibiotic therapy.

Infective Endocarditis. Primary care providers should be alert to signs of endocarditis in children with CHD who have a sustained, unexplained fever because symptomatology may be nonspecific and insidious. Fever may be associated with decreased activity, anorexia, malaise, night sweats, petechiae, splenomegaly, or a new murmur. Children with an unexplained fever and any of these symptoms should be referred to their cardiologist for evaluation, including an echocardiogram, to look for vegetations within the heart. Blood cultures should be drawn before initiating antibiotics. Over one half of the cases of pediatric infective endocarditis occur in children at least 10 years of age (Dajani & Taubert, 2001). Children who have palliative systemic-to-pulmonary shunts, who have prosthetic valves, and who have had a previous episode of infective endocarditis are at high risk (Dajani et al, 1997). Parental knowledge of measures to prevent endocarditis is limited. Therefore primary care providers must reinforce instructions on endocarditis prophylaxis at each visit.

Respiratory Infection. Children with CHD—particularly those with a defect causing left-to-right shunting—may have frequent or significant upper and lower respiratory infections. It is important to evaluate the degree of respiratory compromise compared with the child's baseline respiratory status. If there is an increase in respiratory effort or the presence of adventitious breath sounds, a chest radiograph should be obtained to rule out pneumonia or worsening CHF. Infiltrates evident by radiograph, fever, and productive cough could indicate a lower respiratory infection. Cardiomegaly, poor feeding, sweating, and a

dry cough would indicate CHF and require referral to the cardiologist. The primary care provider should have follow-up contact with a family 24 hours after initial contact to evaluate the child's progress.

Respiratory Syncytial Virus. Respiratory syncytial virus (RSV) can have especially serious effects in a child with symptomatic CHD. In addition, performing cardiac surgery in a child still recuperating from RSV can increase the risk of postoperative complications, particularly pulmonary hypertension (Khongphatthanayothin et al, 1999). Since there is no RSV vaccine approved for use in children with CHD, the family must be instructed in ways to prevent the spread of infection to their infant or child (e.g., hand washing, avoiding ill contacts), particularly around the time of surgery.

Gastrointestinal Symptoms. Vomiting or anorexia may occur secondary to gastroenteritis, worsening CHF, or digoxin toxicity. If the history and physical findings are not compatible with more common causes of gastrointestinal (GI) symptoms, a child must be evaluated for other symptoms of CHF and a serum digoxin level obtained.

Excessive fluid losses from vomiting, diarrhea, or anorexia can lead to dehydration and thrombus formation in children who are cyanotic and polycythemic. Replacement fluids or consultation with the cardiologist to hold diuretic therapy may be necessary until the GI disturbance is resolved.

Neurologic Symptoms. A child with unexplained fever, headache, focal neurologic signs, or seizures must be immediately referred to a medical center because of the risk of a brain abscess (most common in children <2 years of age) or cerebrovascular accident (CVA) (most common in children >2 years of age).

Chest Pain. Only a very small percentage of children complaining of chest pain have symptoms caused by significant cardiovascular abnormality (Driscoll, 2001). The most common cause of chest pain is conditions involving the musculoskeletal structures of the chest wall (e.g., costochondritis, idiopathic chest wall pain, trauma, muscle strain, sickle cell–related chest-wall bone pain). Less common causes include asthma, pneumonia, and gastroesophageal reflux. Cardiac etiologies of chest pain include pericarditis, aortic stenosis, obstructive hypertrophic cardiomyopathy, coronary artery ischemia, or arrhythmias (i.e., particularly in toddlers unable to differentiate pain from unusual sensations of arrhythmias). The mean age of children complaining of chest pain is 12 to 14 years.

Critical components in a child's history that may clarify the cause can be determined with the following questions: (1) Is the chest pain related to exercise, eating, or breathing? (2) Is there related lightheadedness or syncope? (3) Are there any other serious medical problems? (4) Is there unusual stress at home or school? (5) Is there a family history of sudden death or heart disease? (6) Did the child experience recent physical trauma or new physical activity? The practitioner should be concerned if the chest pain is associated with symptoms such as syncope, lightheadedness, or dyspnea. A careful history and physical examination can usually differentiate benign conditions from dangerous ones. An electrocardiogram and referral to a cardiologist should occur if the primary care provider identifies chest pain in conjunction with syncope, dizziness, easy fatigue, palpitations, exertion, drug use, fever, or associated medical problems (e.g., lupus erythematosus, diabetes, Marfan syndrome, Kawasaki disease).

Syncope. Syncope is the transient loss of consciousness, usually from decreased cerebral blood flow. The most common causes of syncope in pediatrics involve the autonomic nervous system. These conditions may be caused by emotional stress, breath holding, hypovolemia, or anemia. Other causes include arrhythmias, seizures, pulmonary hypertension, hypercyanotic spells, or psychogenic reaction (often with hyperventilation). As with chest pain, a thorough history and physical examination are critical. Particular attention should be paid to the activity and position of the child before the event, as well as associated symptoms. Syncope during or following activity warrants special attention because it may be a marker for sudden death (Scott, 2001). Family history of syncope, seizures, deafness, sudden death, or long QT syndrome should be noted. Physical examination should concentrate particularly on neurologic and cardiovascular systems. Diagnostic work-up may include an electrocardiogram (ECG), and referral to a cardiologist may be recommended for further evaluation (i.e., including an exercise test and tilt-table test).

Drug Interactions

Children with CHF or arrhythmias often receive combinations of digoxin, diuretics, and other medications. The addition of any drug to a child's regimen when he or she is receiving cardiac medications should receive close attention and consultation with a pharmacist or cardiologist if there are questions about interaction.

Co-administration of digoxin and quinidine (Cin-Quin), verapamil (Calan, Isoptin), or amiodarone (Cordarone) may elevate digoxin plasma concentrations (Trujillo and Nolan, 2000). Aminoglycosides can affect renal function and alter excretion of digoxin. Children with severe CHF may require medications (e.g., captopril [Capoten] or enalapril [Vasotec]) to decrease resistance to left ventricular ejection (i.e., afterload), thus decreasing the workload on the heart. These drugs may increase serum potassium; therefore if a child is taking a potassium-sparing diuretic (e.g., spironolactone [Aldactone]) along with captopril, serum potassium should be checked periodically. The combination of adenosine (Adenocard) and carbamazapine (Tegretol) may act synergistically and cause heart block. Concurrent use of clonidine (Catapres) and verapamil (Calan, Isoptin) may lead to severe hypotension and AV block.

There are many well-documented interactions between cardiac and psychotropic drugs; consultation with the cardiologist would be vital before beginning this class of drug.

Warfarin (Coumadin) may be used in children with a propensity for clotting (i.e., those with prosthetic valves or pulmonary hypertension). When a child is taking warfarin, bleeding status is checked by periodic measurement of prothrombin time (PT) and International Normalized Ratio (INR). These values can be altered with concomitant use of warfarin and many medications (i.e., erythromycin). Any time a child receiving warfarin requires antibiotics or other medications, the primary care provider should consult with the cardiologist before administering them to prevent possibly altering the INR. There is no interaction with warfarin and immunizations.

When advising parents on the use of over-the-counter (OTC) medications for their child, the practitioner should stress the importance of using the simplest preparation of medication and avoiding multiple ingredient products if possible. Decongestants, sympathomimetics, and drugs containing caffeine should be avoided in a child with a rapid heart rhythm (e.g., supraventricular tachycardia, atrial fibrillation) or hypertension because they may exacerbate tachyarrhythmias or increase blood pressure. Aspirin may be used in children requiring mild anticoagulation (i.e., after the Fontan procedure) or with postpericardiotomy syndrome. It should be avoided for 3 weeks before surgery because of its anticoagulant properties, and it should be avoided altogether in children receiving warfarin (Coumadin). It is important for the primary care provider to counsel parents to read labels of OTC medications because they may contain aspirin. Nonsteroidal antiinflammatory drugs (NSAIDs) can decrease the effectiveness of beta-blockers and ACE inhibitors (Smith, 2001). The primary care provider may be monitoring certain drug levels (digoxin, antiarrhythmics) or response to drugs (INR in the child taking anticoagulants) in close association with the cardiologist.

Developmental Issues

Sleep Patterns

Infants with CHF who are tachypneic may be unable to satisfy their hunger and thus have a difficult time sleeping through the night. Referral to the cardiologist is advised if a child's respiratory status is deteriorating to the point of interfering with feeding and sleeping. When discussing sleep with parents, primary care providers should ask them where the child sleeps. Parents may be keeping the child in their bed because of fears about their child's stability. Primary care providers should reinforce the stability of a child to help parents deal with their anxiety. The transition to the child's bed should not occur when the child's routine or security has been disrupted (e.g., around the time of hospitalization or surgery).

Toileting

Children receiving diuretic therapy may have difficulty with toilet training. If a child is receiving diuretics for a short period of time, parents may want to delay toilet training until the medication has been discontinued. If a child is receiving long-term diuretic therapy, the timing of the diuretic may need to be adjusted to facilitate toilet training. Toilet training, as with other developmental milestones, may be affected by the regression frequently seen after a child has been hospitalized.

Discipline

Behavioral expectations of children with CHD should be similar to those for children without a heart defect. It is not uncommon for parents to overprotect and pamper children with CHD. The diagnosis of CHD may cause changes in a family's approach and attitudes toward discipline, not only to the child with the disease but also to the healthy siblings. Primary care providers can play a key role in reinforcing the importance of setting limits and disciplining children as if there were no heart disease, as well as helping to normalize family dynamics in light of the risk of overprotection.

On the other hand, infants with CHF who are irritable, hard to console, and difficult to feed may present a very stressful situation for parents. Primary care providers must be aware of family stressors and infant characteristics that may lead to abuse of a child with a chronic condition.

Child Care

Some parents choose to stop working when they have a child with a cardiac condition, but many do not. Child care is necessary for most families. Several factors that must be balanced when parents are deciding to return to work include the following: (1) the financial and emotional need to return to work; (2) parental anxiety about leaving the child; (3) the increased incidence of infection for children in child care and the effect of infection on a child's cardiovascular status; and (4) parental confidence in a child care provider's ability to recognize symptoms, give medications properly, and respond to emergencies appropriately.

Before surgery or cardiac catheterization, parents may be counseled to take their child out of child care to avoid exposure to infections that would cancel the procedure. Children with asplenia or DiGeorge syndrome are at the highest risk of infection. For these children who are prone to infection, home or small group daycare is advised. For 6 weeks after surgery, parents should limit activities that stress the child's sternum (e.g., climbing, pulling, heavy lifting, rough playing, or lifting the child under the arms). Parents must communicate these restrictions to the child care provider to see if it is realistic or safe for the child to return to daycare before normal activity is allowed. Primary care providers can play a key role in educating child care providers about a child's condition, as well as in reinforcing activity limits—and lack of limits.

Schooling

Most school-aged children with CHD can attend school with their peers, although children with complex heart disease are at risk for having learning disabilities ranging from attention disorders to visual-perceptual problems, speech delays, and IQ/performance discrepancies (Bellinger et al, 2000, Forbess et al, 2000). Since learning problems may be more subtle than a significant decrease in IQ, the practitioner should be particularly alert to signs of learning disabilities. Special education is often warranted for children with CHD. Missed school is often related to hospitalization, recuperation from surgery, and visits to the cardiologist. Primary care providers can play an important role in assessing the need for home or in-hospital schooling for prolonged absences and facilitating services. Absenteeism may also be associated with parental perception of a child's vulnerability and their lack of control over improving their child's health status.

As children enter junior high and high school, they may have body image concerns related to their scar, small stature, or ability to keep up with peers. Parents often underestimate their child's activity tolerance, and adolescents with heart disease may have a distorted conception of their disease and their abilities and limitations related to physical activity (Canobbio, 2001). The American Heart Association (AHA, 2000b) recommends a combination of moderate and vigorous physical activity for adults and children to decrease the long-term risks of

developing stroke, coronary artery disease, hypertension, and obesity. Specific to CHD, detailed recommendations have been established for determining the level of activity related to each congenital cardiac lesion, arrhythmia, or acquired heart disease (American College of Cardiology and American College of Sports Medicine, 1994). The issue in prescribing specific activities to children with congenital heart disease is that it is hard to quantify the degree of myocardial demand for specific activities related to the hemodynamic consequences of specific defects and each repair (Canobbio, 2001). Because of this potential problem, children should generally be encouraged to participate in physical activity to their tolerance based an individualized plan formulated from discussions with the child, primary care provider, cardiologist, parents, and school professionals.

A standard letter of recommendations for activity (Figure 21-3) will clarify expectations and limits so that children can participate in physical activities to their highest potential. The cardiologist may perform stress testing to develop an individualized activity plan. This information should be relayed to the primary care provider. An ongoing discussion with parents and children will reinforce the realistic goals for activity and help prevent overprotection.

Sexuality

Technologic and surgical advances have enabled the majority of young women with CHD to reach childbearing age. Many can successfully carry a pregnancy through delivery. A woman with complex congenital heart defects, however, warrants a careful evaluation of maternal and fetal risk (Canobbio, 2001). The increased risk of CHD in the offspring of individuals with CHD should be discussed with a cardiologist or a genetic counselor before conception if possible.

The issues of contraception and safety of pregnancy must be discussed with parents before their daughter becomes an adolescent, as well as when she is in early adolescence. Communication with the cardiologist will give the primary care provider critical information about a girl's risk factors for contraception and pregnancy given her particular physical status.

Because of the problem with estrogen-containing oral contraceptives and thromboembolism, oral contraceptives are not recommended for women who are cyanotic and those with right-to-left shunts, pulmonary vascular disease, or prosthetic valves or conduits (Canobbio, 2001). Implanted contraceptive agents, such as medroxyprogesterone acetate (Depo-Provera) or levonorgestrel (Norplant), are suitable for these women (Daniels et al, 2001). Because of the potential for cervicitis and subsequent bacteremia, intrauterine devices (IUDs) are contraindicated in women at risk for developing infective endocarditis (Conobbio, 2001; Daniels et al, 2001). Barrier methods (e.g., condoms, diaphragms with spermicidal cream) are safe methods of birth control from a cardiac standpoint but are not as effective in preventing pregnancy. For women at very high risk for cardiac compromise with pregnancy, surgical sterilization should be discussed. The social, emotional, and ethical considerations regarding sterilization make it a very controversial topic that should be discussed at length with the young woman and possibly her family. Tubal ligation in women with long-standing pulmonary hypertension leading to Eisenmenger

**RECOMMENDATIONS FOR PHYSICAL ACTIVITY IN SCHOOL
FOR CHILDREN WITH HEART DISEASE**

DATE_____

To Whom it May Concern:

_____ is a patient of mine for a congenital heart condition. The following recommendations are guidelines for physical activity in school. The child's cardiac diagnosis is
_____
_____.

_____(1) May participate in the entire physical education program, including varsity competitive sports without any restriction.

_____(2) May participate in the entire physical education program EXCEPT for varsity competitive sports where there is strenuous training and prolonged physical exertions, such as football, hockey, wrestling, soccer, basketball, etc. Less strenuous sports such as baseball and golf are acceptable at varsity level. All activities during the regular physical education program are acceptable.

_____(3) May participate in the physical education program except for restrictions from all varsity sports and from excessively stressful activities such as rope climbing, weight lifting, sustained running (i.e., laps) and fitness testing. MUST be allowed to stop and rest when tired.

_____(4) May participate only in mild physical activities such as walking, golf, and circle games.

_____(5) Restricted from the entire physical education program.

_____(6) Additional remarks: (see other side)

_____(7) Duration of recommendations: _____

If there are any additional questions about these recommendations, please contact me.

Sincerely,

_____ (cardiologist's signature)

FIGURE 21-3 Sample letter of recommendation for activity.

syndrome carries with it a high surgical risk and should not be performed unless absolutely necessary. If tubal ligation is recommended, it is best to wait, if possible, until young adulthood when a woman has gained maturity and can participate in the decision.

Experts often look at a client's cardiovascular status based on the New York Heart Association (NYHA) Functional Classification to determine the relative risk of pregnancy. Adolescents with mild heart disease that has not been operated on or those with well-repaired cardiac defects (NYHA class I or II) are generally at no higher risk from pregnancy than the general population (Canobbio, 2001). Adolescents in class III or above with CHF need special attention during pregnancy. Pregnancy in adolescents with pulmonary vascular disease carries a high risk for morbidity and mortality and may need to be terminated for the safety of the mother (Canobbio, 2001; Daniels et al, 2001). It is important for primary care providers to discuss the risks of pregnancy with the cardiologist so that the recommendation can be reinforced to the adolescent. A multidisciplinary approach involving the cardiologist, the high-risk obstetrician, and the primary care provider should be used for adolescents with CHD who are pregnant.

Transition into Adulthood

There are approximately 800,000 adults with CHD in the United States (Warnes et al, 2001). Adolescents or adults with surgically treated CHD are generally classified according to their postoperative clinical status: category I—complete repair, asymptomatic; category II—palliation/complete repair, asymptomatic; category III—repair with residual defects, minimal; and category IV—palliation/inoperable, moderate to severe symptoms. Problems requiring long-term follow-up include electrophysiologic sequelae, prosthetic materials, and infective endocarditis (Perloff, 1991). Additional long-term postoperative concerns include ventricular failure, which is particularly problematic after intraarterial baffling procedures, and systemic-to-pulmonary shunts in functional single ventricles. Myocardial ischemia and fibrosis in open-heart repairs can affect the long-term performance of the myocardium.

Specific issues for adolescents with CHD as they transition into adult health care include (1) lack of confidence in the care given to them from unknown providers, (2) fear of future invasive procedures, (3) insecurity about their ability to advocate for themselves, and (4) inadequate education about their condition and the specific details of immediate and long-term care needs (Higgins and Tong, 2003). A lack of knowledge about endocarditis prophylaxis in many adolescents and adults with CHD underscores the importance of repetitive patient education in this area at every follow-up clinic visit (Veldtman et al, 2001).

Transitioning the care of the adolescent with CHD into adulthood was the focus of the 32nd Bethesda Conference (Webb and Williams, 2001), convened by the American College of Cardiology. Three areas of recommendations reported were as follows: (1) organizing the care for adults with CHD, (2) improving access to care, and (3) addressing the special needs of adults with congenital heart problems. A recommendation for the delivery of care to adolescents and adults with CHD was to establish adult congenital heart disease regional centers. These centers would include a multidisciplinary team of pediatric and adult cardiologists, congenital heart surgeons, and advanced practice nurses who would coordinate care (Landzburg et al, 2001).

Recommendations were further made to develop a structured plan for the adolescent transitioning from a pediatric cardiology setting into an adult cardiology practice. This plan includes a "health care passport" designed to accompany the adolescent into the new cardiology setting. The specific "passport" information includes the adolescent's diagnosis, surgical procedures, medications with side effects, endocarditis prophylaxis, exercise prescription, contraception, frequency of medical follow-up, and insurance coverage (Foster et al, 2001).

Facilitating the effective coordination of care from pediatric to adult health care is central to the successful long-term management of an increasing number of children surviving CHD. Management of these individuals by a core interdisciplinary team with expertise in congenital heart conditions, as well as the social and psychologic impact of growing up with CHD, is paramount throughout their adulthood (Higgins and Tong, 2003).

Family Concerns and Resources

The family of a child with CHD may have ongoing concerns about symptoms, feeding problems, sudden death, finances, and the long-term physical and emotional effects of multiple surgeries. When parents are counseled about symptoms, it is important that primary care providers convey that the parents will be watching for trends over time rather than minute by minute. Reinforcing the fact that parents become the experts in observing their child for changes decreases their feelings that only health care providers can adequately monitor their child.

Some parents of children with CHD believe that their primary care provider is unable to meet many of their child's illness needs, whereas other parents of adolescents with mild heart disease would prefer to see their primary care provider for all routine health care needs and many cardiovascular health needs (Kao et al, 2000; Miller et al, 2000). Parental information needs related to caring for their infant after cardiac surgery are significant, and the parent's level of understanding may be limited. A review of postoperative instructions by the primary care provider and ongoing, careful evaluation of the child will help solidify the parent's knowledge base and reinforce the health care provider's position as a valuable asset to the child's care.

The insurability of a child with heart disease depends on the particular defect and repair. As children become older, they often lose their parents' coverage and have difficulty obtaining insurance as adults (Foster et al, 2001). Parents must investigate the options for extended coverage of the child on their health insurance plan well before the policy's coverage expires for the child. Depending on their parents' income, children with CHD may qualify for the supplemental public insurance.

Parents may also be concerned about the occurrence of CHD in subsequent children. The cardiologist or genetic counselor should advise a family about specific risks to future children; and the primary care provider should reinforce this information and support the family in their decision making. Early prenatal diagnosis of CHD is possible through ultrasound of the fetal heart (i.e., fetal echocardiogram).

Parent support groups are valuable resources and provide an important network for families who are coping with anxieties related to caring for a child with CHD. Newsletters and special interest groups often develop from parent networking (see section on organizations at the end of this chapter). The primary care provider should contact the local American Heart Association (AHA) or the pediatric cardiology department to see if such groups exist. Written information on many aspects of CHD is also available through the AHA. Public health or home health nursing may be an additional source of support, especially for families learning to identify symptoms, give multiple medications, provide adequate nutrition to a newly diagnosed infant with CHD, or care for a child with complex home care needs. Summer camps for children with CHD are available in several locations across the United States.

The Internet has a wealth of information about heart defects, surgical procedures, and support for families of children with heart defects. Parents should be advised to use Web sites from the American Heart Association (AHA) and medical centers with pediatric cardiology subspecialty departments for medical information regarding their child's disease. Other Web sites may be valuable for support and information sharing to help families cope with the stressors of having a child with CHD.

Informational Materials

The following resource booklets and pamphlets are available for families through the local or national chapter of the AHA (this is not a complete listing of resources):

"If Your Child Has a Heart Defect—A Guide for Parents"
"Feeding Infants with Heart Disease—A Guide for Parents"
"Dental Care for Children with Heart Disease"
"Abnormalities of Heart Rhythm—A Guide for Parents"
"Caring for a Child with a Heart Condition—A Guide for Parents" [San Francisco chapter]
"Marfan's Syndrome"
"Kawasaki's Disease"
"Coumadin"
"AHA Scientific Statement: Guidelines for Parent Support Groups" (1998)

Organizations

This list is by no means complete but will provide information as well as links to other resources. There are many on-line and in-person parent support groups and child/family resources across the United States.

American Heart Association
National Center
7272 Greenville Ave
Dallas, TX 75231
www.americanheart.org

Children's Health Information Network
1561 Clark Dr
Yardley, PA 19067
www.tchin.org

Summary of Primary Care Needs for the Child with Congenital Heart Disease

HEALTH CARE MAINTENANCE

Growth and Development

Significant delays in weight and height are common in children with symptomatic CHD preoperatively; corrective surgery improves growth.

Intellectual development is not significantly impaired by CHD; cyanosis, parental overprotection, and congestive heart failure (CHF) may contribute to delayed development.

Neurologic abnormalities may occur in children with CHD.

Diet

Feeding is a major problem for children with CHD—especially for a child with CHF; required daily allowances are normal, but caloric needs may be higher.

Breast-feeding is encouraged if growth is adequate.

Parents may need to concentrate formula or breast milk if growth is inadequate. Gavage feeding may be necessary to conserve energy.

Parents should be taught methods to decrease work of feeding.

Feeding is a major source of stress for parents, who will need much support.

Safety

Safe storage of medications is critical.

For the child with a pacemaker, electrical safety is critical. There is no risk of damage with usual household appliances, including microwaves. Children with pacemakers should not have magnetic resonance images (MRIs) and should avoid metal detectors and wear a Medic-Alert bracelet.

Children taking anticoagulants or with permanent pacemakers should avoid contact sports.

Air travel and altitude may need to be limited depending on the defect.

Cardiopulmonary resuscitation training for parents is warranted for certain defects.

Immunizations

Standard immunization protocol is recommended; delay should occur only around cardiac catheterization or surgery.

With complex, cyanotic, or symptomatic CHD, influenza and pneumococcal vaccines are recommended.

With asplenia syndrome, daily antimicrobial prophylaxis and pneumococcal vaccine are recommended for children. Reimmunization once after 2 years is recommended.

Screening

Vision. Routine screening is recommended.

Hearing. Routine screening is recommended.

Dental. Dental care is important to prevent caries, which predispose a child to bacteremia and endocarditis. Endocarditis prophylaxis is recommended for all dental procedures except routine adjustment of braces and shedding of deciduous teeth (Boxes 21-4 and 21-5).

Blood Pressure. Check blood pressure in all four extremities for children with aortic abnormalities preoperatively and postoperatively. Children with a Blalock-Taussig shunt or subclavian flap repair of coarctation of the aorta will have low or absent blood pressure values in the arm on the side of surgery.

Hematocrit. A rise in hematocrit may indicate worsening cyanosis. Anemia is problematic in children with CHF or cyanosis. Monitor hemoglobin levels closely in coordination with the cardiologist.

Urinalysis. Routine screening is recommended.

Tuberculosis. Routine screening is recommended.

Condition-Specific Screening

Serum levels of digoxin, warfarin, and diuretics may need to be monitored.

Complete blood counts (CBCs) and electrolytes are also monitored frequently before surgery.

COMMON ILLNESS MANAGEMENT

Differential Diagnosis

Fever. Postoperatively rule out (1) wound infection and (2) postpericardiotomy syndrome. If no focus is found, obtain a CBC and blood culture and consult with the cardiologist. The child with asplenia with fever must be seen immediately. Fever may worsen CHF.

Infective Endocarditis. Symptoms are often vague; a high level of suspicion is needed for diagnosis. It is rarely seen in children less than 2 years of age. The child should be referred to the cardiologist for evaluation.

Refer to the cardiologist if fever, malaise, anorexia, splenomegaly, or night sweats are present.

Respiratory Infection. Frequent or significant upper and lower respiratory infections may occur; rule out CHF or pneumonia. Respiratory syncytial virus (RSV) can cause significant morbidity.

Gastrointestinal Symptoms. Rule out digoxin toxicity and CHF; excessive fluid losses are dangerous in children who are cyanotic or taking diuretics and digoxin.

Neurologic Symptoms. Cyanotic children are at increased risk for brain abscess (if >2 years) or cerebrovascular accident (if <2 years); unexplained fever, headaches, seizures, or focal neurologic signs require immediate referral to a medical center.

Summary of Primary Care Needs for the Child with Congenital Heart Disease—cont'd

Children with CHD are at increased risk of neurologic abnormalities (e.g., seizures, muscle tone abnormalities, motor asymmetry).

Chest Pain. Most chest pain is caused by noncardiac problems. Careful history and physical examination usually differentiate benign from dangerous conditions.

Syncope. There are many cardiac and noncardiac causes for syncope.

Close attention should be paid to head, eyes, ears, nose, and throat to rule out vestibular disease.

An electrocardiogram may be useful to rule out cardiac causes.

Drug Interactions

The addition of any drug to a child's regimen should be preceded by consultation with a pharmacist or cardiologist.

Accurate administration of digoxin is critical. Many medications can alter plasma levels of digoxin.

Potassium levels need to be monitored in children taking diuretics and digoxin.

Aminoglycosides may decrease renal function and increase the digoxin level.

Digoxin or anticoagulant dosages may need to be monitored.

Children taking warfarin may have prothrombin time (PT) and International Normalized Ratio (INR) altered when given antibiotics.

Interactions between antiarrhythmia drugs and psychotropic drugs may occur.

Decongestants are not recommended for children with rapid heart arrhythmias or hypertension.

DEVELOPMENTAL ISSUES

Sleep Patterns

Children may have difficulty sleeping through the night if they are tachypneic and unable to satisfy their hunger.

Toileting

Toilet training children receiving diuretics may be difficult.

Discipline

Normal behavior should be expected from children regardless of CHD. Parents often overprotect and pamper children with CHD.

Infants with CHF may be irritable and hard to console. The stress and coping of caregivers must be assessed.

Child Care

The child care provider must understand medications, be able to recognize symptoms, and know emergency procedures.

Infants with DiGeorge syndrome or asplenia syndrome are prone to infection, so home daycare or small-group daycare is recommended.

Vigorous activity should be limited for 6 weeks after surgery.

Schooling

Learning disabilities are common in children with CHD. Children may need home tutoring around hospitalization and surgery time.

Children may develop self-image concerns about their scar, ability to keep up with peers, and small stature.

The American Heart Association (AHA) publishes guidelines for activity limits based on each defect. Generally, children limit themselves. Children who have a pacemaker or are taking anticoagulants should avoid rough contact sports.

Parents frequently underestimate their child's activity tolerance.

Sexuality

Oral contraceptives are not recommended for individuals with pulmonary hypertension, cyanotic CHD, or prosthetic valves.

An intrauterine device is not recommended for individuals at risk for developing endocarditis.

An individual's heart defect and functional ability (i.e., as assessed by the cardiologist) determine risks associated with pregnancy; teens need early and thorough counseling.

Transition into Adulthood

Late postoperative concerns include arrhythmias, ventricular failure, myocardial ischemia, prosthetic failure, thromboembolism, and infective endocarditis.

Adolescents and adults with CHD should be followed in adult congestive heart disease regional centers. Individuals should be given a health care passport.

FAMILY CONCERNS

Families have ongoing concern about symptoms, multiple surgeries, and sudden death.

Children and adults with CHD have difficulty finding insurance coverage.

Parents may be concerned that CHD will occur in subsequent children and may want genetic counseling; prenatal diagnosis of CHD is possible through fetal echocardiography.

REFERENCES

Abad-Sinden, A. & Sutphen, J.L. (2001). Growth and nutrition. In H.D. Allen et al. (Eds.). *Moss and Adams' heart disease in infants, children, and adolescents including the fetus and young adult* (6th ed.). Philadelphia: Lippincott Williams & Wilkins.

Ackerman, I.L., Karn, C.A., Denne, S.C., Ensing, G.J., & Leitch, C.A. (1998). Total but not resting energy expenditure is increased in infants with ventricular septal defects. *Pediatrics, 102,* 1172-1177.

American College of Cardiology and American College of Sports Medicine. (1994). 26th Bethesda conference recommendations for determining eligibility for competition in athletes with cardiovascular abnormalities. *J Am Coll Cardiol, 24,* 845-899.

American Heart Association, Inc. (2000a). Congenital cardiovascular disease statistics; Web site: http://www.americanheart.org/children.

American Heart Association, Inc. (2000b). Exercise (physical activity) and children; Web site: http://www.americanheart.org/children.

Artman, M. (2001). Pharmacologic therapy. In H.D. Allen et al. (Eds.). *Moss and Adams' heart disease in infants, children, and adolescents including the fetus and young adult* (6th ed.). Philadelphia: Lippincott, Williams & Wilkins.

Artman, M., Mahoney, L., & Teitel, D.F. (2002). Molecular and morphogenetic cardiac embryology: Implications for congenital heart disease. In M. Artman et al. (Eds.). *Neonatal cardiology.* New York: The McGraw-Hill Companies.

Bellinger, D.C. et al. (2000). Eight-year neurodevelopmental status: The Boston circulatory arrest study. *Circulation, 102*(suppl. 2), II-497 (abstract).

Bridges, N.D. et al. (2001). Cardiac catheterization, angiography and intervention. In H.D. Allen et al. (Eds.). *Moss and Adams' heart disease in infants, children, and adolescents including the fetus and young adult* (6th ed.). Philadelphia: Lippincott, Williams & Wilkins.

Canobbio, M.M. (2001). Health care issues facing adolescents with congenital heart disease. *J Pediatr Nurs, 16,* 363-370.

Carey, L.K. (1999). *Parenting young children with congenital heart disease.* PhD manuscript, Marquette University.

Clark E.B. (2001). Etiology of congenital cardiovascular malformations: Epidemiology and genetics. In H.D. Allen et al. (Eds.). *Moss and Adams' heart disease in infants, children and adolescents including the fetus and young adult* (6th ed.). Philadelphia: Lippincott, Williams & Wilkins.

Clark, S.M. & Miles, M.S. (1999). Conflicting responses: The experiences of fathers of infants diagnosed with severe congenital heart disease. *J Soc Pediatr Nurs, 4,* 7-14.

Committee on Infectious Diseases. (2000a). Policy statement: Recommendations for the prevention of pneumococcal infections, including the use of pneumococcal conjugate vaccine (Prevnar), pneumococcal polysaccharide vaccine, and antibiotic prophylaxis. *Pediatrics, 106,* 362-366.

Committee on Infectious Diseases. (2000b). *Report of the committee on infectious diseases* (25th ed.). Elk Grove Village, Ill.: American Academy of Pediatrics.

Committee on Nutrition. (1998). *Pediatric nutrition handbook* (4th ed.). Elk Grove Village, Ill: American Academy of Pediatrics.

Craig, J. et al. (2001). Cardiovascular critical care problems. In M.A. Curley & P.A. Moloney-Harmon (Eds.). *Critical care nursing of infants and children* (2nd ed.). Philadelphia: W.B. Saunders.

Daebritz, S.H. (2000). Results of Norwood stage I operation: Comparison of hypoplastic left heart syndrome with other malformations. *J Thorac Cardiovasc Surg, 119,* 358-367.

Dajani, A.S. & Taubert, K.A. (2001). Infective endocarditis. In H.D. Allen et al. (Eds.). *Moss and Adams' heart disease in infants, children, and adolescents including the fetus and young adult* (6th ed.). Philadelphia: Lippincott Williams & Wilkins.

Dajani, A.S., Taubert, K.A., Wilson, W., Bolger, A.F., Bayer, A., et al. (1997). Prevention of bacterial endocarditis: Recommendations by the American Heart Association. *Circulation, 96,* 358-366.

Daniels, C.J. et al. (2001). Adolescent and young adult cardiology. In H.D. Allen et al. (Eds.). *Moss and Adams' heart disease in infants, children, and adolescents including the fetus and young adult* (6th ed.). Philadelphia: Lippincott, Williams & Wilkins.

Driscoll, D.J. (2001). Chest pain in children and adolescents. In H.D. Allen et al. (Eds.). *Moss and Adams' heart disease in infants, children, and adolescents including the fetus and young adult* (6th ed.). Philadelphia: Lippincott, Williams & Wilkins.

Forbess, J.M. et al. (2000). Neurodevelopmental outcomes in children following the Fontan operation. *Circulation, 102*(suppl. 2), II-743 (abstract).

Foster, E., Graham, T.P., Jr., Driscoll, D.J., Reid, G.J., Reiss, J.G., et al. (2001). Task force 2: Special health care needs of adults with congenital heart disease. *J Am Coll Cardiol, 37,* 1176-1183.

Hanisch, D. (2001). Pediatric arrhythmias. *J Pediatr Nurs, 16,* 351-362.

Higgins, S.S. & Tong, E. (2003). Transitioning adolescents with congenital heart disease into adult health care. *Progress in Cardiovascular Nursing, 18*(2), 93-98.

Hinoki, K.W. (1998). Congenital heart disease: Effects on the family. *Neonatal Netw, 17*(5), 7-10.

Kao, Y. et al. (2000). Life adjustment of school-aged children with congenital heart disease after corrective surgery. *Journal of Nursing (Chinese), 47*(1), 43-55.

Khongphatthanayothin, A., Wong, P.C., Samara, Y., Newth, C.J., Wells, W.J., et al. (1999). Impact of respiratory syncytial virus infection on surgery for congenital heart disease: Postoperative course and outcome. *Crit Care Med, 27,* 1974-1981.

Kimball, T.R. & Meyer, R.A. (2001). Echocardiography. In H.D. Allen et al. (Eds.). *Moss and Adams' heart disease in infants, children, and adolescents including the fetus and young adult* (6th ed.). Philadelphia: Lippincott, Williams & Wilkins.

Landzburg, M.J. et al. (2001). Task force 4: Organization of delivery systems for adults with congenital heart disease. *J Am Coll Cardiol, 37,* 1187-1193.

Leitch, C.A. (2000). Growth, nutrition and energy expenditure in pediatric heart failure. *Prog Pediatr Cardiol, 11*(3), 195-202.

Leitch, C.A., Karn, C.A., Ensing, G.J., & Denne, S.C. (2000). Energy expenditure after surgical repair in children with cyanotic congenital heart disease. *J Pediatr, 137*(3), 381-385.

Lewin, M.B. (2000). The genetic basis of congenital heart disease. *Pediatr Ann,* 468-480.

Limperopoulos, C., Majnemer, A., Shevell, M.I., Rosenblatt, B., Rohlicek, C., et al. (1999). Neurologic status of newborns with congenital heart defects before open heart surgery. *Pediatrics, 103,* 402-408.

Mahle, W.T. (2001). Neurologic and cognitive outcomes in children with congenital heart disease. *Curr Opin Pediatr, 13,* 482-486.

Marcelletti, C.F. et al. (2000). Revision of previous Fontan connections to total extracardiac cavopulmonary anastomosis: A multicenter experience. *J Thorac Cardiovasc Surg, 119,* 340-346.

Marino, B.L., O'Brien, P., & LoRe, H. (1995). Oxygen saturations during breast and bottle feedings in infants with CHD. *J Pediatr Nurs, 10,* 360-364.

McElhinney, D.B. & Wernovsky, G. (2001). Outcomes of neonates with congenital heart disease. *Curr Opin Pediatr, 13,* 104-110.

Miller, M.R., Forest, C.B., & Kan, J.S. (2000). Parental preferences for primary and specialty care collaboration in the management of teenagers with congenital heart disease. *Pediatrics, 106*(2), 264-269.

Morelius, E. et al. (2002). Parental stress in relation to the severity of congenital heart disease in the offspring. *Pediatr Nurs, 28*(1), 28-34.

O'Brien, M.P. & Boisvert, J.T. (2001). Current management of infants and children with single ventricle anatomy. *Pediatr Nurs, 16*(5), 338-350.

Park, M.K. (2002). *Pediatric cardiology for practitioners* (4th ed.). St. Louis: Mosby.

Perloff, J.K. & Koos, B. (1998). *Pregnancy and CHD.* In J.K. Perloff (Ed.). *CHD in adults* (2nd ed.). Philadelphia: W.B. Saunders.

Perloff, S.K. (1991). CHD in adults: A new cardiovascular subspecialty. *Circulation, 84,* 1881.

Prieto, L.R., DeCamillo, D.M., Konrad, D.J., Scalet-Longworth, L., & Latson, L.A. (1998). Comparison of cost and clinical outcome between transcatheter coil occlusion and surgical closure of isolated patent ductus arteriosus. *Pediatrics, 101,* 1020-1024.

Reiss, R.E. (2001). Maternal diseases and therapies affecting the fetal cardiovascular system. In H.D. Allen et al. (Eds.). *Moss and Adams' heart disease in infants, children, and adolescents including the fetus and young adult* (6th ed.). Philadelphia: Lippincott, Williams & Wilkins.

Rheuban, K.S. (2001). Pericardial disease. In H.D. Allen et al. (Eds.). *Moss and Adams' heart disease in infants, children, and adolescents including the fetus and young adult* (6th ed.). Philadelphia: Lippincott, Williams & Wilkins.

Saul, J.P. (2001). Electrophysiologic therapeutic catheterization. In H.D. Allen et al. (Eds.). *Moss and Adams' heart disease in infants, children, and adolescents including the fetus and young adult* (6th ed.). Philadelphia: Lippincott, Williams & Wilkins.

Scott, W.A. (2001). Syncope and the assessment of the autonomic nervous system. In H.D. Allen et al. (Eds.). *Moss and Adams' heart disease in infants, children, and adolescents including the fetus and young adult* (6th ed.). Philadelphia: Lippincott, Williams & Wilkins.

Smith, P. (2001). Primary care in children with congenital heart disease. *J Pediatr Nurs, 16,* 308-319.

Tong, E.M., Sparacino, P.S., Messias, D.K., Foote, D., Chesla, C.A., et al. (1998). Growing up with congenital heart disease: The dilemmas of adolescents and young adults. *Cardiol Young, 8,* 303-309.

Trujillo, T.C. & Nolan, P.E. (2000). Antiarrhythmic agents: Drug interactions of clinical significance. *Drug Saf, 26,* 509-532.

Uzark, K. (2001). Therapeutic cardiac catheterization for congenital heart disease—a new era in pediatric care. *Journal of Pediatric Nursing, 16,* 300-307.

Uzark, K., Lincoln, A., Lamberti, J.J., Mainwaring, R.D., Spicer, R.L., et al. (1998). Neurodevelopmental outcomes in children with Fontan repair of functional single ventricle. *Pediatrics, 101,* 630-633.

Van Arsdell, G.S., McCrindle, B.W., Einarson, K.D., Lee, K.J., Oag, E., et al. (2000). Interventions associated with minimal Fontan mortality. *Ann Thorac Surg, 70,* 568-574.

Van Hare, G. (1999). Supraventricular tachycardia. In P.C. Gillette & A.J. Garson (Eds.). *Clinical pediatric arrhythmias* (2nd ed.). Philadelphia: W.B. Saunders.

Veldtman, G.R. et al. (2001). Illness understanding in children and adolescents with heart disease. *West J Med, 174,* 171-175.

Walters, H.L. (2000). Congenital heart surgical strategies and outcomes: HEARTS. *Pediatr Ann, 29,* 489-497.

Warnes, C.A., Liberthson, R., Danielson, G.K., Dore, A., Harris, L., et al. (2001). Task force 1: The changing profile of congenital heart disease in adult life. *J Am Coll Cardiol, 37,* 1170-1175.

Webb, G.D. & Williams, R.G. (2001). Care of the adult with congenital heart disease. *J Am Coll Cardiol, 37.*

Wernovsky, G. et al. (2001). Intensive care. In H.D. Allen et al. (Eds.). *Moss and Adams' heart disease in infants, children, and adolescents including the fetus and young adult* (6th ed.). Philadelphia: Lippincott, Williams & Wilkins.

Wong, D.L. (2003). The child with cardiovascular dysfunction. In D.L. Wong et al. (Eds.). *Wong's nursing care of infants and children* (7th ed.). St. Louis: Mosby.

Wray, J. & Sensky, T. (1999). Controlled study of preschool development after surgery for congenital heart disease. *Arch Dis Child, 80,* 511-516.

22 Cystic Fibrosis

Ann H. McMullen and Elizabeth A. Bryson

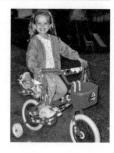

Etiology

Cystic fibrosis (CF), a condition characterized by complex multisystem involvement, is the most common life-shortening genetic illness among white children, adolescents, and young adults. Significant advances in genetic and biomedical research have been made over the past 15 years that have influenced health professionals' understanding of the condition and its cause, clinical management, and approaches to detection. Although still without cure, CF is no longer considered a terminal childhood disease but a chronic illness with a median life expectancy of 33 years of age today (Cystic Fibrosis Foundation [CFF], 2002b). Experts expect that further advances in CF will extend the median life expectancy and the quality of life of affected individuals in the future.

Known Genetic Etiology

After a succession of scientific breakthroughs in genetics, in 1989 the CF gene was isolated on the long arm of chromosome 7, which encodes a protein product (i.e., cystic fibrosis transmembrane conductance regulator [CFTR]) (Rommens et al, 1989). More than 1000 unique mutations in the CFTR gene have been reported, the most common of which is the delta F508 mutation, which accounts for 70% of CF alleles. CF genetic mutations have been divided into five classes based on their influence on CFTR manufacture and function at the cellular level. These defects include lack of CFTR production, trafficking, conductance and regulation problems, and reduction in synthesis of the protein (Moss, 2001). The specific class of defect may in part explain the phenotypic expression of the disease; however, the variability in expression is probably complicated by factors such as multiple person-environment interactions and the presence of other gene modifiers (Doull, 2001; Tsui & Durie, 1997). Significant scientific inquiry is underway to further understand the CFTR defect and to develop therapeutic pharmacologic approaches to change its function at the cellular level.

Although identifying the relationship among specific mutations and defects in CFTR function is important, so also is an understanding of how abnormal CFTR function produces the clinical picture of persistent respiratory infection and inflammation. At this time, this relationship and the host responses to infection and inflammation are not fully understood. For example, why is the CF airway such an inviting environment for bacterial colonization; and what factors contribute to the damage and deterioration of lung parenchyma from host response to the bacteria? Current research is targeted at control of the inflammatory process and understanding and changing the airway environment that fosters colonization and infection (Moss, 2001).

At least one function of CFTR appears to be as a chloride ion channel regulated by cyclic adenosine monophosphate (AMP) (Ramsey, 1993). An impermeability to chloride ions, as well as increased sodium reabsorption, leads to decreased water movement across cell membranes. This defect causes secretions to become viscous and less well hydrated and lumen of airways and ducts to be obstructed (Cutting, 1994; Davis, 2001). The pathogenesis of an ion-transport defect leads to pathologic sequelae of mucus-obstructing ducts in various body organs. Progressive pathologic changes are produced in nearly every organ of the body. The most consistent changes occur in the exocrine glands (e.g., pancreatic acini, bile ducts and gallbladder, prostatic glands, salivary and lacrimal glands, mucous glands of the tracheobronchial tree, upper respiratory tract and intestinal wall, sweat glands) (Rosenstein, 1998). Table 22-1 is an overview of cystic fibrosis that delineates organ system pathogenesis, clinical manifestations, and treatment.

Incidence and Prevalence

The transmission of CF follows an autosomal recessive mode with an incidence in whites of approximately 1 in 3300. The incidence in other races is lower: in blacks, it is about 1 in 17,000; in Asians, it is about 1 in 32,000; and in Hispanics, it is about 1 in 8000. Occurrence is possible in any race, however. With a gene frequency in whites of approximately 1 in 29, it is estimated that for 1 in 400 to 500 couples, both partners are carriers of this recessive trait, with a subsequent 1 in 4 risk of bearing an affected child with each pregnancy (Hamosh et al, 1998; Brown & Schwind, 1999). The Cystic Fibrosis National Registry reported about 23,000 individuals living with cystic fibrosis in the United States in 2001 with approximately 1000 new diagnoses during that year (CFF, 2002b).

Clinical Manifestations at Time of Diagnosis

The pathophysiologic hallmarks of CF are as follows: (1) pancreatic enzyme deficiency from duct blockage by viscous mucus; (2) progressive chronic obstructive lung disease associated with viscous infected mucus and subsequent interstitial destruction; and (3) sweat gland dysfunction, resulting in abnormally high sodium and chloride concentrations in the sweat (Davis, 2001).

There are three common clinical presentations (Box 22-1). The first is meconium ileus in neonates, which occurs in 7% to 10% of newly diagnosed infants. The occurrence of meconium

TABLE 22-1

Overview of Cystic Fibrosis

System	Pathogenesis	Clinical Manifestations	Complications	Management
Sweat glands	Abnormal electrolytes	High rate of salt loss; salt depletion	Heat prostration	Dietary salt replacement, sweat test
Lungs	Thick, tenacious mucus	Cough; decreased exercise tolerance	Infection	Chest physiotherapy (CPT): postural drainage, cupping/vibration; alternative methods of CPT
	Mucous plugging	Air trapping: increased anteroposterior chest diameter	Fibrosis, bronchiectasis	Antibiotics: oral, intravenous, aerosolized
	Obstruction	Hyperresonance	Atelectasis	Bronchodilators
	Decreased mucociliary clearance	Wheezing, fine and coarse crackles, clubbing	Hypoxia, respiratory failure	DNase
			Pneumothorax	Antiinflammatories
			Hemoptysis	Ibuprofen
			Cor pulmonale	Cromolyn sodium
			Allergic bronchopulmonary aspergillosis	Inhaled steroids
			Failure to thrive (increased energy expenditure)	Oral corticosteroids
			Hypertrophic osteoarthropathy	High-calorie diet
Upper airway	Viscous mucus	Chronic sinusitis	Obstruction, mouth breathing	Decongestants (inter-mittent use)
		Nasal polyposis		Nasal cromolyn sodium or corticosteroids
				Antibiotics
				Surgery
Gastrointestinal (GI) tract	Inspissated tenacious meconium	No passage of meconium	Obstruction: meconium ileus	Enema, surgery
	Maldigested food and viscous mucus in gut	Abdominal distention	Distal ileal obstruction syndrome (DIOS)	Pancreatic enzymes
		Cramping abdominal pain	Fecal mass in colon	Dietary changes to avoid constipation
			Volvulus, intussusception	Laxatives
				Gastrografin with Tween 80 enema or Go-LYTELY; Miralax
Pancreas	Viscous secretions obstructions, fibrosis	Maldigestion; bulky, foul-smelling stools	Pancreatitis	Enzyme replacement
	Abnormal electrolytes	Fat malabsorption (including fat-soluble vitamins)	Fibrosis	Antacids
	Suboptimal enzyme function		Failure to thrive	H$_2$ antagonists
			Delayed maturation	High-energy diet
			Rectal prolapse	Normal fat intake
				Concentrated dietary supplements
				Aggressive nutritional supplementation
			Vitamin deficiency	Vitamin supplement
			Glucose intolerance	Insulin preferred; oral hypoglycemics may be used
Biliary	Obstruction	Subclinical cirrhosis	Cirrhosis	Ursodiol (Actigall)
	Fibrosis		Portal hypertension	Cholecystectomy
			Cholelithiasis	
Salivary glands	Abnormal electrolyte concentrations	Probably not clinically significant		
Reproductive tract	Abnormal viscous secretions	Male: obliteration of vas deferens, sterility		Genetic and reproductive counseling
		Female: thick vaginal and decreased cervical secretions		

ileus should be presumed to be CF until testing confirms or rules out the diagnosis. Meconium plug syndrome—although less frequently associated with the diagnosis of CF—should also raise the primary care provider's suspicion.

The second common clinical presentation is failure to thrive with malabsorption as a result of lost or diminished exocrine pancreatic function, which occurs in 80% to 90% of children with CF. These children exhibit varying degrees of weight loss or poor growth patterns, usually in the presence of a normal to voracious appetite; frequent foul-smelling, greasy, bulky stools; rectal prolapse (i.e., in 25% of children); and a protuberant belly with decreased subcutaneous tissue in the extremities.

The third common clinical presentation is the occurrence of chronic or recurrent upper and lower respiratory infections. Manifestations include the following: nasal polyps, chronic sinusitis, recurrent pneumonia and bronchitis, bronchiectasis, and atelectasis. Children with these manifestations have a chronic cough that persists after a respiratory infection and may

---

BOX 22-1

Clinical Manifestations at Time of Diagnosis

Meconium ileus in the neonate
Malabsorption with failure to thrive
Chronic or recurrent upper and/or lower respiratory infections

---

BOX 22-2

Progressive Changes in the Clinical Picture of Cystic Fibrosis

I. Early
   A. Dry, hacking, nonproductive cough
   B. Increased respiratory rate
   C. Decreased activity
II. Moderate
   A. Increased cough, increased sputum production
   B. Rales, musical rhonchi, scattered or localized wheezes
   C. Repeated episodes of respiratory tract infection
   D. Signs of obstructive lung disease
      1. Increased anteroposterior diameter
      2. Depressed diaphragm
      3. Palpable liver border
   E. Decreased appetite
   F. Failure to gain weight or grow, or weight loss
   G. Decreased exercise tolerance
III. Advanced
   A. Chronic, paroxysmal, productive cough
   B. Increased respiratory rate, shortness of breath on exertion, orthopnea, dyspnea
   C. Diffuse and localized fine and coarse crackles
   D. Signs of severe obstructive lung disease
      1. Marked increase in anteroposterior diameter (barrel chest, pigeon breast)
      2. Limited respiratory excursion of thoracic cage
      3. Depressed diaphragm
      4. Hyperresonance over entire chest
      5. Decreased ventilation, persistent hypoxemia
   E. Noisy respirations
   F. Marked decrease in appetite
   G. Muscular weakness
   H. Cyanosis
   I. Digital clubbing
   J. Rounded shoulders
   K. Fever, tachycardia, toxicity
   L. Hemoptysis
   M. Pneumothorax
   N. Lung abscess
   O. Signs of cardiac failure (cor pulmonale, edema, enlarged tender liver)
   P. Bone pain and osteoarthropathy

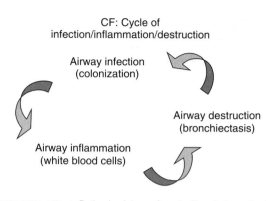

FIGURE 22-1 Pathophysiology of cystic fibrosis lung disease.

BOX 22-3

Indications for Sweat Testing

Pulmonary
Chronic cough
Recurrent or chronic pneumonia
Staphylococcal pneumonia
Recurrent bronchiolitis
Atelectasis
Hemoptysis
Mucoid *Pseudomonas* infection

Gastrointestinal
Meconium ileus, neonatal jaundice
Steatorrhea, malabsorption
Rectal prolapse
Childhood cirrhosis (portal hypertension or bleeding esophageal varices)
Hypoprothrombinemia beyond newborn period

Other
Family history of cystic fibrosis
Failure to thrive
Salty sweat, salty taste when kissed, salt frosting of skin
Nasal polyps
Heat prostration, hyponatremia, and hypochloremia, especially in infants
Pansinusitis
Azoospermia
Digital clubbing
Recurrent pancreatitis

Modified from Ewig, J.M. (1997). Cystic fibrosis. In R.A. Hoekelman (Ed.). *Primary pediatric care* (3rd ed.). St. Louis. Mosby.

---

become paroxysmal and productive, provoking choking and vomiting. Auscultatory findings may include fine crackles and expiratory wheezes—particularly in the upper lobes and right middle lobe. Some children, however, have no findings on auscultation. Infants may have recurrent episodes of wheezing and tachypnea. *Staphylococcus aureus*, which is often seen initially, and subsequently *Pseudomonas aeruginosa* and *Haemophilus influenzae* are frequent isolates in a respiratory tract culture. Fungi—including *Candida albicans* and *Aspergillus fumigatus*—are also often cultured from the respiratory tract (Colin

& Wohl, 1994). Early roentgenographic changes include air trapping and peribronchial thickening, followed by atelectasis, infiltrates, and hilar adenopathy (Rosenstein & Langbaum, 1984; Schwartz, 1987). Without treatment, these early signs and symptoms progress and complications occur (Colin & Wohl, 1994). Box 22-2 and Figure 22-1 summarize the clinical progression of changes in CF lung disease.

Although these presentations are most common, CF's multisystem involvement (Table 22-1) may lead to the presentation of variable and subtle symptoms, possibly leading to diagnostic delays and creating an anxious and difficult period for the family and the primary care provider. Manifestations may be minimal or absent during childhood. In 2001, 10% of new diagnoses were made in individuals over 10 years of age (CFF, 2002b). Diagnostic delays may be decreased if primary care providers maintain a high level of suspicion of the various symptoms associated with CF. See Box 22-3 for indications for sweat testing, which is the gold standard test for diagnosing CF.

Diagnosis

Diagnosis of CF requires a positive sweat test in the presence of (1) clinical symptoms consistent with CF, (2) a family history of CF, or (3) a positive neonatal screening test. Sweat testing is done by pilocarpine iontophoresis with quantitative analysis of sweat sodium and chloride. Sweat should only be collected and assayed through a qualified laboratory. All the 117 regional CF centers certified by the CF Foundation have clinical chemistry laboratories that meet specifications for the accuracy and reliability of sweat tests. Sweat sodium and chloride concentrations above 60 mmol/L collected on two separate occasions are consistent with a diagnosis of CF. A value of 40 to 60 mmol/l is considered borderline and should be repeated (NCCLS, 2000; Rosenstein & Cutting, 1998). Adequate quantities of sweat may be difficult to obtain from infants under 4 weeks of age, so CF centers may elect to obtain deoxyribonucleic acid (DNA) mutation analysis to help with early diagnosis in these infants when sweat collections yield an inadequate quantity. Once the diagnosis has been established in a child, all siblings should be sweat tested. In a small number of individuals with clinical symptoms suggestive of CF, the sweat test may be borderline or even high normal. In these situations, the primary care provider should consult with CF specialty providers who can use expanded laboratory criteria and methods (e.g., identifying CF mutations by DNA analysis and abnormal bioelectric properties of nasal epithelium) to diagnose CF (Rosenstein & Cutting, 1998; Stern & Orenstein, 1998; Wilmott, 1998).

Genetic Testing

The effect of genetic discoveries on understanding etiology and pathophysiology is only beginning to unfold whereas approaches to detection are changing and reflect new technologic advances. Carrier screening is available and reliable for siblings and family members of a child with CF whose deletions have been identified. Appropriate studies of DNA deletion and linkage analysis are highly complex, and any family member contemplating such a screening should be referred to a regional CF center with a pediatric genetics center for counseling.

Prenatal diagnosis is available to parents of a child affected with CF and other at-risk couples. As a result, increasing numbers of at-risk families are using these diagnostic resources and confronting the ethical dilemma of having a therapeutic abortion vs. continuing the pregnancy. Such decision making occurs while the science of treatment is advancing and clinicians observe the variability of the phenotypic expression of CF in an individual child. Chorionic villus sampling (CVS) at 8 to 10 weeks' gestation or amniocentesis at 12 to 16 weeks' gestation may provide information on CF mutations in the fetus. Wertz and associates (1992) surveyed parents of childbearing age who had a child with CF about their attitudes on prenatal diagnosis. Almost one half of the couples surveyed desired more children and intended to use prenatal diagnosis. Of those who expected to use prenatal diagnosis, 44% would carry a fetus found to have CF to term, 28% would abort, and 28% were undecided. Prenatal diagnosis services, along with related counseling, are an area of specialization and should be coordinated by the regional CF center (Fernbach & Thomson, 1992; Shapiro & Seilheimer, 1994).

Heterozygote (carrier) detection of the general population is technically possible and being implemented. Specialized genetic laboratories now offer screening for up to 86 of the most common CF mutations, which account for about 85% to 90% of mutant CF genes in North America. In a study to determine receptivity of prenatal care providers and their patients to carrier testing for CF, Loader and colleagues (1996) found the acceptance rate among pregnant women to be 57%. In 1997, the National Institutes of Health (NIH) convened a Consensus Development Conference on Cystic Fibrosis. The conference recommended that genetic screening for CF mutations be offered not only to high-risk individuals but also to any couple planning a pregnancy or seeking prenatal care. The American College of Medical Genetics and the American College of Obstetricians and Gynecologists now support offering carrier screening to these individuals and have adopted standards and guidelines for implementation of this program. As population-based carrier screening programs are being developed, many issues have not been completely addressed, such as the anticipated burden of widespread screening on existing genetic counseling resources, the limitation of options available to at-risk couples who undergo testing during pregnancy, the large number of mutations and the absence of guidelines for developing an appropriate mutation test panel, and numerous other issues (Grody et al, 2001; Brown & Schwind, 1999).

Neonatal screening of immunoreactive trypsinogen (IRT)—although possible—is controversial because of the high number of false-positive results. The test accuracy is increased, however, when coupled with DNA testing for gene mutations. Statewide screening programs in Colorado and Wisconsin have been in place for over a decade and are addressing the dilemma of the benefits of early diagnosis vs. the cost of testing newborns and educating and counseling the family (Shapiro & Seilheimer, 1994). More recently, additional states have begun screening programs. There is growing evidence that early diagnosis of CF is beneficial in the area of improved growth and nutrition. Screening could also be potentially beneficial by allowing the couple the ability to obtain genetic counseling before a subsequent pregnancy and in eliminating parental frustration and anxiety often associated with diagnosis in the symptomatic child. As more targeted therapies are developed, early diagnosis may become even more beneficial to a child. No national consensus on screening, however, has yet been achieved (Rock, 1997; Young et al, 2001).

Treatment

Nutritional Management

Pancreatic Enzyme Supplementation. The principal treatment for the resulting malabsorption in cystic fibrosis is oral pancreatic enzyme replacement (Box 22-4). Enteric coating of enzyme preparations decreases the likelihood of inactivation by gastric acid, and doses may be adjusted to achieve weight gain and one or two formed stools per day. Concerns have been raised, however, by reports of colonic strictures in children with CF (Borowitz et al, 1995). These strictures have occurred in children under 12 years of age receiving enzyme doses of more than 6000 lipase units/kg/meal. Current recommendations are that pancreatic enzyme doses should be reduced to the lowest

BOX 22-4
Treatment

NUTRITION
Pancreatic enzyme replacement
High-calorie diet
Vitamin, mineral, and NaCl replacement

RESPIRATORY
Antimicrobials
Airway clearance
    Chest physiotherapy
    Active cycle of breathing
    Forced expiration
    Positive expiratory pressure
    Airway oscillation
    Exercise
Bronchodilators
Antiinflammatory therapy
Dornase alfa (rhDNAse)
Bilateral lung transplantation

TABLE 22-2
Factors Contributing to a Poor Response to Pancreatic Enzyme Therapy

Enzyme factors	Outdated prescription
	Enzymes not stored in cool place
Dietary factors	Excessive juice intake
	Parental perception that enzymes are not needed with milk or snacks
	"Grazing" eating behavior
	High-fat fast foods
Poor adherence to prescribed enzyme regimen	Toddler's willful refusal
	Chaotic household, multiple meal givers
	Anger or desire to be "normal"
	Teenage girls' desire to be slim
Acid intestinal environment	Poor dissolution of enteric coating
	Microcapsule contents released all at once
Concurrent gastrointestinal disorder	Biliary disease, cholestasis, Crohn disease, and others

From Drucy, S. et al. (1995). Use of pancreatic enzyme supplements for patients with cystic fibrosis in the context of fibrosing colonopathy, *J Pediatr, 127*, 681-684.

effective dose without altering a child's diet. Dosing guidelines of 1000 to 2000 lipase units/kg/meal are now used by most CF centers as a safe range. The safety of doses between 2500 and 6000 lipase units/kg/meal is not known, and such doses should be used with caution (Borowitz et al, 1995; Fitzsimmons et al, 1997).

Children often experience continued problems with malabsorption despite reasonable coverage with enzymes. Table 22-2 lists factors that contribute to a poor response to pancreatic enzyme therapy. Initial assessment and intervention should address adherence, enzyme storage, and a child's eating habits (e.g., small frequent snacks without taking enzymes). Neutralizing gastric acid with antacids or inhibiting its production with histamine-receptor antagonists may improve the efficacy of the enzyme preparation. If the problem persists, consultation with the CF center may be helpful.

High-Calorie Diet. Caloric and protein requirements are increased in children with CF because of malabsorption related to pancreatic insufficiency, inadequate enzyme supplementation, and progressive pulmonary disease. Most authorities agree that these children have a basal energy requirement that is 25% to 50% greater than the usual recommended daily allowance for energy intake (Erdman, 1999). Experts in CF nutrition (CFF, 2001a) note the following:

There are three specific times when special attention should be focused on growth and nutritional status within the scope of usual clinical care: (1) the first 12 months after diagnosis of CF; (2) birth to 12 months of age for infants diagnosed prenatally or at birth, until a normal pattern of growth (head circumference, weight and length) is clearly established; and (3) the peripubertal growth period (girls about 9 to 16, and boys about 12 to 18 years of age).

The goal of focused interventions during these periods is to establish and support normal growth and development during periods of physiologic stress from growth and disease process.

With progression of pulmonary disease, children usually have long-term weight and nutrition problems as a result of their increased pulmonary energy requirements. Children with CF should optimally maintain a weight-height index greater than or equal to 90%. However, evidence is growing that children maintained at more than 96% of their ideal weight for height have much better long-term outcomes (CFF, 1997, 2001a). Calories are encouraged in both complex carbohydrates and fats. Dietary fat is the highest density source of calories and also improves the palatability of foods and maintains normal essential fatty acid status. Ways to maximize calories are found in Box 22-5. When an individual has difficulty with certain high-fat foods, these may be limited; however, children should generally be encouraged to cover high-fat intake with additional enzymes. Aggressive nutritional supplementation (i.e., oral, enteral, parenteral) is routinely used for children with weight loss problems and growth delay despite a reasonable intake. Early short-term studies documented improved weight gain and stabilization of pulmonary function with this approach (Levy et al, 1985; Soutter et al, 1986). Later studies documented decreased mortality, improved growth, and—for some individuals—a decreased rate of pulmonary decline (Dalzell et al, 1992; Steinkamp & von der Hardt, 1994). However, long-term studies using appropriate control group methodology have not been done. Nutritional status and pulmonary function as well as quality of life, adverse effects, cost, and adherence would be important outcomes for evaluation (Conway, Morton, & Wolfe, 2002).

Vitamin, Mineral, and NaCl Replacement. Optimal dietary intake also includes attention to fat-soluble vitamins, essential fatty acids, calcium, iron, zinc, and sodium. Because fat malabsorption is particularly problematic in CF and deficiencies in fat-soluble vitamins have been reported, CF centers recommend a standard age-appropriate dose of non–fat-soluble multivitamins plus supplementation of vitamins A, D, E, and K at an age-appropriate dose. Consultation with the CF center nutritionist can be helpful in establishing the appropriate doses of vitamins. Water-miscible preparations combining the fat-soluble vitamins A, D, E, and K are available, providing the convenience of

BOX 22-5

Maximizing Calories for the Healthy Individual with Cystic Fibrosis

Adding Calories to Foods

Add fats such as butter, gravy, cheese, or dressings to starches, fruits, and vegetables.

Use whipped cream on fruits and desserts.

Make "super" milk: ½ cup whole milk + ½ cup half & half.

Flavor milk with syrups or powders (chocolate, strawberry, etc.) or add whole-milk yogurt to milk.

Add eggs to hamburger meat or casseroles (never serve raw eggs).

Use extra salad dressing; avoid low-calorie or reduced-calorie dressings.

Serve gravies and cheese sauces.

High-Calorie Foods and Snacks*

Full-fat ice cream, puddings

Cookies and milk

Cheese or peanut butter crackers

Muffins or bagels with cream cheese or butter

Cheese breadsticks

Chips and dip

French fries

Whole-milk yogurt

Egg salad, tuna salad, cheese or avocado slices with crackers

Trail mixes, nuts, and granola (after the age of 2 yr)

Cold cuts, pizza

Fresh vegetables with salad dressing or dip

*Assess age appropriateness, especially with respect to choking risk in young children, before recommending.

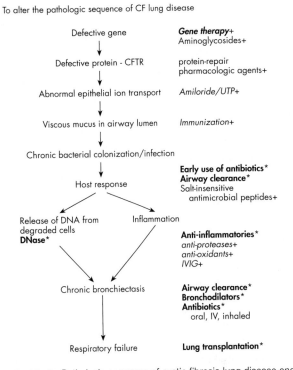

FIGURE 22-2 Pathologic sequence of cystic fibrosis lung disease and the therapies used.

supplementation with a single vitamin preparation for most children (CFF, 1997, 2001a; Erdman, 1999).

There is a high prevalence of osteopenia and osteoporosis in children and adults with CF (Bhuhikanok et al, 1998), and CF nutritionists recommend the dietary intake of calcium for the general population be emphasized in CF. The use of biphosphonates in CF has been shown to be effective in increasing bone density in small studies, but larger clinical trials are needed (Brenckmann & Papaioannou, 2001).

Respiratory Management

Interventions are designed to interrupt the cascade of pathophysiologic phenomena by either preventing the development of abnormal airway secretions and lung infections or treating the existing infection and inflammation (Figure 22-2). Progressive lung disease is the major cause of morbidity and mortality in CF. The pathophysiologic basis of CF lung disease is impaired mucociliary clearance of dehydrated mucus followed by endobronchial infection. Children with CF become chronically colonized with gram-negative organisms that may be quantitatively decreased with antimicrobial therapy but cannot be eradicated. The respiratory tract environment in CF that promotes bacterial growth is not fully understood, and there is widespread controversy over the optimal approach to the long-term treatment of sequelae to this bacterial growth. General agreement exists, however, that bacterial infection—especially from *Pseudomonas aeruginosa* and other gram-negative bacilli with their virulence factors—and the intense host inflammatory response to infection (i.e., antibody response and neutrophil influx) lead to chronic bronchiectasis (Figure 22-2). CF centers

recognize that antimicrobial therapy is of primary importance in decreasing the rate of this deterioration and has played a significant role in the increased survival of individuals with CF (Denton & Wilcox, 1997; Marshall & Samuelson, 1998; Weiner, 2002).

Antibiotic/Microbial Therapy. Pulmonary exacerbations often follow mild viral illnesses, particularly upper respiratory tract infections. It has been hypothesized that viruses may suppress host defenses, although this mechanism has not been clearly proven (Prober, 1991; Rosenfeld & Ramsey, 1992). It can be argued that an early course of oral antibiotic therapy should be used with viral illness symptoms to prevent exacerbation of the bacterial pulmonary infection during the viral illness. Continuous oral antibiotic coverage to reduce the frequency of exacerbations in young children, however, has more recently been questioned. In a multicenter trial of continuous *Staphylococcus* prophylaxis with cephalexin vs. a placebo over a 5- to 7-year period, there were no differences in the pulmonary and nutritional outcomes of each group; but the group treated with antibiotics had a higher rate of *Pseudomonas aeruginosa* colonization (Ramsey, 1996).

Traditional concerns about the development of resistant organisms with overuse of antibiotics must be balanced against the concern for progressive bronchiectasis and parenchymal damage. The initial choice of antibiotic and dose should provide broad-spectrum coverage (i.e., specifically for *Staphylococcus aureus, Streptococcus pneumoniae,* and *Haemophilus* species). Accurate identification of pathogens with appropriate antibiotic sensitivity testing is important to successful treatment of infections (Weiner, 2002). Further considerations in children whose pulmonary infections do not respond to initial therapy include antibiotic resistance, lack of adherence, or abnormal pharmacokinetics (Lees, 2000; Ramsey, 1996).

Aerosolization delivers high concentrations of antibiotics to the site of infection while decreasing the risk of systemic absorption and toxicity. This approach has been used most effectively as suppressive therapy in individuals chronically colonized with *Pseudomonas aeruginosa.* Aminoglycosides and colistin (Coly-Mycin M Parenteral) have been the most consistent choices; and high-dose tobramycin has been the most extensively studied antibiotic for nebulization. High-dose tobramycin used as suppressive therapy twice daily every other month has been associated with slowed decline of pulmonary function, improved quality of life, and improved weight gain (Moss et al, 1999; Nickerson et al, 1999; Quittner & Buu, 2002). Because of the potential for developing resistant strains of *Pseudomonas* species, the clinical expertise of the CF team is recommended in selecting appropriate individuals for therapy and in monitoring their therapy (Marshall & Samuelson, 1998).

When oral and aerosolized antibiotics do not control pulmonary exacerbations, intravenous antibiotics may be necessary. A pulmonary and nutritional "tune-up" or "clean-out" may be initiated in the hospital or home. These 2-week (or longer) courses of therapy allow the CF center team to employ more aggressive strategies to contain infection and supplement nutrition. Such strategies include using intravenous antibiotics (i.e., often an aminoglycoside with either a semisynthetic penicillin or third-generation cephalosporin), as well as increased pulmonary toilet, physical therapy, exercise, and nutritional support measures. Intravenous antibiotics are chosen for their effectiveness in treating *Pseudomonas aeruginosa*, which is less responsive to oral therapy. Quinolone antibiotics are currently the only available oral preparations that effectively treat *Pseudomonas* species; and of these, ciprofloxacin (Cipro) has been the most extensively studied in CF. Because of the lack of data on side effects in children, quinolones have not been approved by the Food and Drug Administration (FDA) for use in individuals under 18 years of age. In clinical trials of Cipro in children with CF, however, the antibiotic was well tolerated and without reports of side effects. Many CF centers use it judiciously in children. Clinicians should be aware that *Pseudomonas aeruginosa* rapidly develops resistance to oral quinolones; frequent use and use in more severely affected individuals are often associated with a suboptimal response (Marshall & Samuelson, 1998).

Airway Clearance. Other pulmonary therapeutic interventions are aimed at relief of bronchial obstruction through clearance of pulmonary secretions. Chest physical therapy (e.g., postural drainage and cupping and/or clapping and/or vibration two to four times per day) has been effective and has been standard therapy for years. Other techniques of airway clearance have been developed for school-aged children and adolescents; such techniques include active cycle of breathing (ACB) and forced expiration technique (FET), autogenic drainage (AD), positive expiratory pressure (PEP), and airway oscillation (e.g., Flutter device, mechanical percussor, vest). The common advantage of these techniques is that they allow the child independence in clearing the airway of mucus. Cumulative data of short-term trials indicate that airway clearance, whatever the specific technique, when compared with no airway clearance is associated with improved outcomes; however, more definitive long-term studies that compare the effectiveness of specific therapies remain to be done (Davidson & McIlwaine, 1995; van der Schans et al, 2002).

Routine chest therapy is recommended for all children with pulmonary involvement; the specific regimen recommended for an individual with CF should be made by the CF center's physician and respiratory or physical therapist. Exercise (i.e., particularly an aerobic conditioning program) is also encouraged because it positively influences general health, cardiopulmonary and musculoskeletal function, and airway clearance (DeJong et al, 1994; Loutzenhiser & Clark, 1993). A recent 3-year home-based exercise intervention demonstrated a slowing of decline in forced vital capacity (FVC) and forced expiratory volume (FEV; Accurso, 1995) as well as an improved sense of well-being in the intervention group (Schneiderman-Walker et al, 2000).

Reactive airways disease (RAD) may result from chronic inflammation and infection. Bronchodilators are often used if a clinical response can be observed or if a beneficial response of a more than 10% increase in forced vital capacity in 1 second (FVC_1) after bronchodilator use is shown by pulmonary function testing (Pattishall, 1990; Ramsey, 1996). Many children with CF use an aerosolized bronchodilator before chest physical therapy. Nebulized hypertonic saline has also been shown to improve mucociliary clearance in small clinical trials. Routine use of this therapy awaits further large clinical trials (Wark & McDonald, 2002). Acetylcysteine (Mucomist), which is a mucolytic agent, and expectorants have no clear effectiveness; in fact, acetylcysteine may irritate the respiratory tract (Rosenstein, 1999).

Antiinflammatory Therapy. Children with CF mount an intense inflammatory response to chronic bronchial infection, which contributes to parenchymal destruction and disease progression. Konstan and associates (1994) reported that adolescents and adults with mild CF lung disease who appeared clinically healthy were found to have evidence of bacterial infection and significant local inflammatory response on bronchoalveolar lavage. Even bronchoalveolar lavage fluid from infants has been shown to have increased DNA levels, which is an early marker for inflammation (Kirchner et al, 1993).

Clinicians have long recognized the clinical efficacy of antiinflammatory therapy and have used short courses of oral and inhaled corticosteroids, as well as cromolyn sodium, in reactive airway disease associated with CF. Findings of small studies have supported these practices; but large, long-term trials are needed to determine the specific use of both short courses of oral corticosteroids and long-term use of inhaled steroids (Konstan, 1998). In a large clinical trial of the long-term use of systemic corticosteroids, participants had improved lung function but developed significant side effects, namely, cataracts, growth retardation, and glucose abnormalities (Rosenstein & Eigen, 1991). Inhaled corticosteroid use has increased significantly over the past 10 years, and preliminary results in small studies suggest that they may improved pulmonary function. However, their role in management awaits further investigation (Rosenstein, 1999). In the mid 1990s, Konstan and colleagues (1995) reported that long-term use of high-dose ibuprofen by preadolescents with mild lung disease was associated with a slower rate of progression of lung disease over a 4-year period. Ibuprofen use requires serum drug levels to be monitored so that therapeutic doses can be established (Konstan, 1998). Individuals most likely to benefit from this therapy should be selected and their ibuprofen regimen monitored by the CF center team.

Recombinant Human Dornase Alfa (rhDNAse). Pharmacotherapies that clear airways of thick, tenacious secretions may indirectly improve inflammation. In 1994, the FDA approved aerosolized recombinant human dornase alfa (rhDNAse), a breakthrough in new CF pharmacotherapy. Dornase alfa cleaves extracellular DNA, which is present in high concentrations in purulent CF airway mucus, and reduces its viscosity to a more liquid form (Hubbard et al, 1992). Studies have shown its efficacy in improving pulmonary function as well as decreasing the frequency of hospitalizations, school or work absenteeism, and CF-related symptoms in individuals with mild to moderate pulmonary disease (i.e., FVC >40% of predicted). Side effects were limited to upper airway irritation (i.e., resulting in hoarseness, rash, chest pain, conjunctivitis) and were usually mild and transient (Accurso, 1995; Hodson, 1995; Shak, 1995). Serial pulmonary function testing and clinical markers of morbidity should be used to monitor children started on dornase alfa. Initial studies documented that ongoing efficacy was based on daily use (Ramsey, 1993). Recently, Quan and colleagues (2001) reported that young children with mild disease on dornase alfa had better pulmonary outcomes and fewer pulmonary exacerbations over the 96-week study period than did those on placebo. The effectiveness of dornase alfa in CF over the long term may well be in preventing early disease progression.

Bilateral lung transplantation has emerged as a viable therapeutic option for individuals with end-stage CF lung disease. As of 2001, estimates of overall 5-year survival after transplantation are approximately 50%. Improved surgical techniques and antirejection drugs have had—and will continue to have—a marked impact on survival statistics. The biggest impediment to more widespread use of this intervention is the critical shortage of suitable organ donors (CFF, 2002a; Yankaskas & Mallory, 1998). Although this procedure offers hope to individuals with end-stage disease and their families, it also presents them with significant psychosocial and financial challenges. Because the waiting time before transplant is increasing, referral should be made when the clinical course predicts length of survival to be about 2 years. Because such complex decisions are involved, consideration of transplantation, individual and family counseling, and referral for evaluation should be coordinated through the CF center.

Anticipated Advances in Management
Pharmacologic Advances

New breakthroughs in pharmacologic interventions that focus on the treatment of CF lung disease, which is the major determinant of morbidity and mortality in CF, are currently being tested. Four of the more promising areas of research are as follows:

1. Modulation of salt and water transport in CF airway epithelium: initial studies of aerosolized amiloride and uridine triphosphate (UTP) showed success in stimulating chloride secretion and inhibiting sodium absorption in the airway epithelium of children with CF, leading to more hydrated airway mucus. Multicenter trials are under way (Knowles et al, 1995; Moss, 2001; Rubin, 1999).
2. Interruption of the neutrophil-mediated inflammatory cascade with agents such as antiproteases, pentoxifylline, and intravenous immune globulin (Moss, 2001; Rubin, 1999): An observation has also been made that macrolides, used with some success to treat diffuse panbronchiolitis, a rare lung disease that resembles CF, may have an antiinflammatory effect in CF. Pilot studies in small samples have demonstrate improvement in symptoms and pulmonary function. Clinicians await results from larger, controlled trials currently in progress (Jaffe & Bush, 2001).
3. Novel therapeutic approaches directed at the common defects of CFTR (e.g., protein-repair therapy): These approaches include the use of aminoglycosides, phenylbutyrate, CPX, genistein, melrinone, and gene therapy (Doull, 2001). Gene therapy, however, has received the most attention by the lay CF community. The first human trial of gene therapy for CF was initiated at the NIH in April of 1993 (Wilson, 1994). The goal of this therapy is to insert coding for normal CFTR protein in airway epithelial cells. For all these therapies, clinical studies of safety, efficacy, and methodology are in progress in research centers across the United States. Individuals with CF, their families, and their health care providers ultimately hope that gene therapy and other therapeutic approaches will eventually be collectively realized in a cure for CF (Albelda et al, 2000; Rubin, 1999; Zeitlin, 1998).
4. A number of promising therapies being used in clinical care: for example, early evidence of improved growth and clinical status with the use of growth hormone and megestrol acetate in CF in small samples has been reported (Hardin et al, 2001; Marchand et al, 2000). These therapies are experimental and should only be considered in consultation with the CF team and subspecialists in endocrinology.

Associated Problems (Box 22-6)
Salt Depletion: Hyponatremia and Dehydration

Children with CF have abnormal sodium and chloride loss in their sweat and are therefore at risk for dehydration secondary to electrolyte imbalance. Risk factors include hot weather, febrile illnesses with or without vomiting and diarrhea, and strenuous physical activity. Excessive salt loss may lead to listlessness, vomiting, heat prostration, and dehydration. Infants are at particular risk because of the low salt content of breast milk, commercial infant formulas, and infant foods. Prevention includes supplementing salt in infant formulas with sodium, at least 4 mEq/kg/day, and adding salt to an older child's diet (CFF, 2001a; Wagner & Sherman, 1997).

Associated Problems

Salt depletion
Rectal prolapse
Nasal polyps and parasinusitis
Distal ileal obstruction syndrome (DIOS)
Hemoptysis
Gastroesophageal reflux
Cystic fibrosis–related diabetes mellitus
Other serious complications

Rectal Prolapse

Rectal prolapse, which can occur in as many as 20% to 25% of individuals with CF (Littlewood, 1992), may be the presenting symptom and may occur only once or be a recurrent problem. Initiation of appropriate enzyme replacement or adjustment of enzyme dosage often prevents its recurrence. Persistent or recurrent prolapse may rarely require surgical intervention (Borowitz, 1994). The first episode of rectal prolapse is frightening for both parents and child, and its reduction usually requires both immediate guidance (i.e., via phone) and assistance in the primary care provider's office or emergency department.

If a child experiences recurrent episodes of rectal prolapse, parents may learn to manually reduce a prolapse. With the child lying on his or her side, a parent (i.e., using a glove and lubricant jelly) is usually able to gently invert the mucosa through the rectal opening.

Nasal Polyps and Parasinusitis

Nasal polyps occur in 10% of children with CF and, if found on physical examination of any child, should raise the suspicion of CF. The upper respiratory tract (i.e., including sinuses) is lined with respiratory epithelial cells similar to the lining in the lungs and is therefore also affected by CF pathology. Sinuses are often chronically infected, producing symptoms, such as frontal headaches, tenderness on palpation, purulent nasal discharge, and postnasal discharge, that further contribute to the chronic cough. Treatment includes extended use of antibiotics and nasal cromolyn sodium or steroids, as well as intermittent use of nasal decongestants. Children may also find warm mist and saline nasal rinses to be comfort measures; some CF clinicians and otolaryngologists recommend sinus irrigations with saline. Surgical interventions for polyposis and sinusitis are sometimes necessary and are usually followed by stringent postsurgical nasal and/or sinus hygiene regimens (Stern, 1998).

Distal Ileal Obstruction Syndrome and/or Constipation

Although the prevalence of distal ileal obstruction syndrome (DIOS) is higher in adolescents and young adults, young children with CF are also at risk for developing total or partial intestinal obstruction. Constipation is often the result of a combination of malabsorption (i.e., from inadequate pancreatic enzyme doses or failure to take enzymes), decreased intestinal motility, and abnormally viscous intestinal secretions. DIOS is seen when intestinal contents accumulate at the ileocecum. Abdominal cramping with either diarrhea or the absence of stool and anorexia occurs. A stool mass may be palpable in the right lower quadrant. If the obstruction becomes complete, vomiting and increased pain and distention occur. Appendicitis, intussusception, and volvulus occur more frequently in children with CF and must be considered. A plain abdominal film may help to confirm the diagnosis of DIOS. Contrast enemas (e.g., meglumine diatrizoate [Gastrografin] with Tween 80) may be both diagnostic and therapeutic and are the treatment of choice for children with complete obstruction. Children with partial obstruction may be treated with polyethylene-glycol solutions (Golytely, Colyte) or Gastrografin given orally or by nasogastric tube (Borowitz, 1994; Davis, 2001). Miralax, a newer polyethylene glycol product, has proved useful in early intervention of a partial obstruction. Follow-up should include long-term use of some combination of stool softener, mild stimulant, and bulk laxative, as well as the addition of bulk to the diet, consistent enzyme use, and exercise.

Hemoptysis

It is not uncommon in CF for blood-streaked sputum and small quantities of bright red blood to be expectorated from the lungs. Although initially alarming to the child and family, this bleeding is usually self-limited. Bleeding reflects increased bronchial infection, inflammation, and irritation, which require more aggressive treatment. Initiation or change of antibiotic therapy should be considered in addition to increasing routine pulmonary toilet. Massive hemoptysis (i.e., usually 240 ml/24 hr), however, requires immediate referral to the CF center team for management.

Gastroesophageal Reflux

Heartburn and regurgitation are reported by more than 20% of individuals with CF, although the frequency with which reflux exacerbates pulmonary disease is unknown. Reflux is probably related to chest hyperinflation and increased abdominal pressure from coughing. Infants presenting with failure to thrive and regurgitation and older children with dysphagia and epigastric pain should be evaluated for reflux and treated appropriately (Orenstein & Orenstein, 1998). In addition to pharmacologic management with a histamine-receptor antagonist and motility agent, dietary measures and an upright position after feedings and/or meals should be instituted. Postural drainage should always be done before feedings and/or meals (Rosenstein, 1999).

CF-Related Diabetes Mellitus (CFRD)

The prevalence of CF-related diabetes is increasing as individuals with CF live longer. It is the leading co-morbidity in cases reported in the 2001 National Registry (CFF, 2002b). CFRD results from both insulin deficiency and resistance, and its management is complicated by the high-caloric requirements of the illness (Rosenecker et al, 2001). CF centers routinely screen for CFRD and have well-developed guidelines for treatment, including nutritional management. The primary care provider should maintain a high suspicion for glucose intolerance, particularly in the adolescent and in children with more severe

BOX 22-7
Serious Complications of Cystic Fibrosis

Colonization with highly resistant bacteria and other organisms
Cor pulmonale
Massive hemoptysis
Pneumothorax
Hypertrophic pulmonary osteoarthropathy
Liver disease including portal hypertension
Gallbladder disease
Allergic bronchopulmonary aspergillosis (ABPA)
Pancreatitis

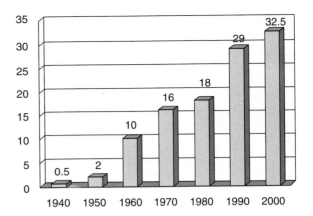

FIGURE 22-3   Median survival age: 1940 to 2000. (Data from Cystic Fibrosis Foundation. [2001]. Patient Registry 2001 Annual Report, Bethesda, Md: Author.)

disease; when CFRD is suspected, consultation with the CF center is strongly recommended.

Other Serious Complications

Cystic fibrosis is a multisystem condition with an increased rate of complications and morbidity with age and disease progression. The complications listed in Box 22-7 are more serious and usually require the expertise of the CF center team. Primary care providers must recognize the early signs and symptoms of these complications so that timely referral for evaluation and treatment is possible.

Colonization with *Burkholderia cepacia* has emerged as a perplexing problem in some CF centers. This organism is highly resistant to antibiotic therapy and has been implicated in the rapid progression of lung disease. Other resistant organisms, particularly *Stenotrophomonas maltophilia*, are also becoming more prevalent in the CF population. Following an extensive review of the evidence, a multidisciplinary team of experts in CF microbiology and clinical care has made evidence-based recommendations for prevention of cross-infection among individuals with CF. These guidelines, which recommend minimizing close contact among CF patients, are rapidly becoming the standard of care in CF centers throughout North America (CFF, 2001b).

Prognosis

Despite 40 years of remarkable progress and a recent surge of new approaches to treatment, CF remains a progressive disease without cure. The median survival age is over 30 years (Figures 22-3 and 22-4), and survival has markedly increased over the past 20 years. This change is likely a result not only of an improved understanding of pathophysiology and treatment but also of an appreciation and detection of the milder phenotypic expressions of the disease. With continued improvement in survival, CF is becoming a long-term condition of children, adolescents, and a growing population of adults (CFF, 2002a).

PRIMARY CARE MANAGEMENT

Health Care Maintenance
Growth and Development

The achievement of adequate nutrition and normal growth in children with cystic fibrosis is a continual challenge for heath

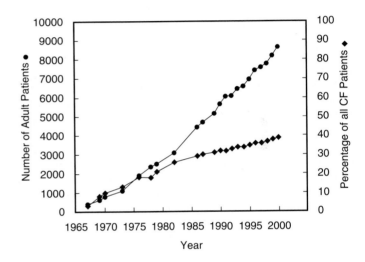

FIGURE 22-4   Adults with cystic fibrosis, 1965 to 2000. (Data from Cystic Fibrosis Foundation. [2001]. Patient Registry 2001 Annual Report, Bethesda, Md: Author.)

care providers. Malnutrition and growth retardation are common complications of CF and may be presenting clinical signs both in infancy and early adolescence; but catch-up growth is often observed after diagnosis and initiation of pulmonary and nutritional therapy (Anthony et al, 1999). Nutritional growth retardation is a significant independent prognostic indicator of survival as highlighted in the longitudinal analysis of the National CF Registry data (Beker et al, 2001; Shepard, 2002). Other organic causes of malnutrition can be present and contribute to the need for increased caloric needs, such as CF-related diabetes, reflux, and hepatobiliary disease (Anthony et al, 1999).

It is important to detect suboptimal growth of children with CF early so appropriate intervention strategies can be taken. First, adequate surveillance of growth by appropriate measurement and plotting of head circumference, weight, length or height, and body mass index (BMI) at routine visits is essential (Erdman, 1999). Head circumference should be measured with a nonstretchable tape with the infant lying down. Weight should be measured on an electronic digital scale with infants unclothed and minimal clothing without any shoes for older children. For length, the infant should be measured on a length board until 24 months of age and then on a stadiometer after 2 years of age for the most accurate height. It is important to plot the measurements using the recent 2000 Centers for Disease Control growth charts for appropriate age and gender. The CF center will do specific growth measurements such as anthropometric measurements (triceps skinfold thickness, mid-arm circumference) and lab assessment annually (CFF, 2001a).

Pubertal development is often delayed with the mean age of menarche being 14.5 years for females (Moshang & Holsdw, 1980) and a 2- to 4-year lag for males (Robbins & Ontjes, 1999). This delay is usually related to poor nutritional status and growth retardation rather than a primary endocrine disorder (Johannesson et al, 1997). Primary care providers may be able to help adolescents understand that this delay is not unusual or unexpected and that sexual development—although delayed—will occur. Pubertal development of individuals with CF can be assessed by a standardized method of self-assessment (Morris & Udry, 1980) or physical examination using Tanner stages starting at age 9 years for girls and 12 years for boys (CFF, 2001a; Tanner, 1962).

Studies demonstrate that this period of pubertal growth is critical to achieving peak bone mass and adult bone health (Bailey et al, 1999; Bhuhikanok et al, 1998). Bone health can be evaluated by history, physical examination, and laboratory and radiologic assessment and is important for those individuals with CF who have specific risk factors, such as long-term use of corticosteroids, poor nutrition, and delayed pubertal development. Primary care providers should communicate these concerns to the CF care team so the appropriate evaluation can be done (CFF, 2001a).

Diet

The goal of nutritional therapy in children with CF is to promote normal growth. Their diet is usually a well-balanced, high-protein diet with unrestricted fat that provides 100% to 150% of the recommended daily allowance (RDA) of calories (Orenstein, 2003; Rosenstein, 1999). Each individual with CF has a unique set of nutritional problems depending on age and disease progression. It is important to remember that the nutritional intervention must be individualized and take into account the child's age, severity of lung disease, degree of maldigestion and malabsorption, dietary preferences, and financial resources (Erdman, 1999).

In infancy, breast-feeding should be continued whenever possible for the immunologic, nutritional, and emotional advantages it offers. Conventional formulas with appropriate enzyme supplementation can also meet the nutritional needs of infants but often a caloric density greater than the standard 20 kcal/oz may be needed. This can be achieved by concentrating the formula, fortifying the breast milk, or adding fat and/or carbohydrates. Either breast milk or formula should be given until 12 months of age, at which time an infant with CF who has maintained normal growth can switch to whole milk. The primary care provider can also provide guidance on the introduction of solid foods at 4 to 6 months according to the recommendations of the American Academy of Pediatrics for individuals with uncomplicated CF (CFF, 2001a).

As toddlers and preschoolers experience developmentally appropriate changes in eating patterns, parents are often anxious about providing adequate food intake to maintain the child's well-being and growth. Maintaining growth at this developmental stage can be achieved by routinely adding calories to table foods with fats such as butter, sour cream, cheese, peanut butter, and whole milk. In toddlers, self-feeding skills begin to develop as do eating problems. Primary care providers can help parents understand how to provide appropriate nutritious foods, set limits for mealtimes, and encourage the child's feeding autonomy. Parents should avoid mealtime battles, force feeding, and grazing behavior (CFF, 2001a; Erdman, 1999). In a study of families of toddlers with CF, Powers and associates (2002) found that toddlers with CF and healthy peers did not differ on the rate of mealtime behaviors (i.e., amount of talking or reinforcements given), but they differed on the types of strategies used to manage meals. Research also demonstrated that toddlers with CF were not getting the CF dietary recommendations for calories and that parents may need additional support in learning how to manage their child's mealtime behavior.

School-aged children with CF need to have a basic understanding about their disease, including the importance of good nutrition and enzyme therapy. This age-group presents additional nutritional challenges that include taste fatigue with oral nutritional supplements, resistance to taking enzymes in the presence of peers, and decreased time to complete treatments (CFF, 2001a).

The adolescent period is a time of increased energy requirements resulting from changes in lifestyle and increased physical activity along with the potential progression in lung disease. All these factors increase the need for calories at a time when there can be denial about one's disease, poor adherence, rebellion, and altered body perceptions, especially in females (Erdman, 1999; Lai et al, 1998). During this developmental stage it is vital that dietary intake, growth velocity, and nutritional status are monitored every 3 months by either the CF care center or the primary care provider (CFF, 2001a). To be most effective, nutritional interventions to increase caloric needs should be planned with the teenagers themselves, not the parents. Adolescents are most receptive to the idea that the nutritional interventions will promote pubertal development, muscular strength, and energy rather than improving their CF and weight gain.

Parents often have questions about enzyme supplementation doses. Enzymes are given with each meal and most snacks except those that have very little or no fat. Enzymes are also necessary with breast milk and any of the predigested formulas. Doses are adjusted by the CF care team according to the growth curve, stool pattern, and signs of malabsorption (i.e., abdominal cramping, flatulence). The enzyme beads should not be chewed or crushed; destroying the enteric coating inactivates the enzymes and may excoriate the oral mucosa (CFF, 2001a). For infants and younger children who cannot swallow the enzyme capsule, it can be opened and the beads mixed with applesauce or other nonalkaline food that can be consumed immediately. Finally, generic enzymes are not bioequivalent to proprietary, and this should be investigated whenever one is demonstrating signs of malabsorption or growth failure (Hendeles et al, 1990).

Primary care providers should remember that nutritional issues in children with CF are unique and may not respond to the traditional interventions. Whenever difficult nutritional problems arise, the multidisciplinary team at the CF centers should be consulted.

Safety

In addition to age-appropriate anticipatory guidance about safety issues, primary care providers should emphasize safe storage and handling of the large quantities of medications often used by children with CF. Keep medications out of reach, and use safety caps on all medications (World Health Organization [WHO], 1994). The issue of accidental ingestion of pancreatic enzymes by another child may arise because ample supplies of these enzymes are often available at mealtimes in the home and carried by the child for use. Enzymes are not likely to be harmful if small quantities are ingested; they are activated in the small intestine and excreted in stool (*Physicians' Desk Reference*, 2002).

Many of the antibiotics that individuals with CF take for an exacerbation or on a long-term basis will alter the skin's tolerance for sun exposure. It is important for all children to use sunscreen, but for those who are taking antibiotics such as ciprofloxacin, avoidance of the sun and artificial ultraviolet light is recommended.

Hand hygiene is a part of education by primary care providers for all children whether they have a chronic disease or not because it is the single most important practice to prevent transmission of infectious agents. Hand hygiene includes cleaning one's hands with soap and water or waterless antiseptic hand rubs. For a child with CF, this is extremely important for the routine times such as before and after eating and toileting as well as when exposed to other individuals with CF. A recent CFF consensus document on infection control for individuals with CF (CFF, 2001b) discusses the multiple studies that have documented the transmission of CF pathogens from patient to patient and stresses the importance of minimizing the exposure of the child with CF to another person with CF.

Immunizations

Infants and children with CF should receive all routine immunizations at the ages recommended by the American Academy of Pediatrics (AAP) (AAP, 2000) and the Centers for Disease Control and Prevention (CDC). In a few instances the CF team may recommend a brief delay in order to stabilize an acute pulmonary or nutritional problem, but there is no evidence to support delay of routine immunizations (Orenstein et al, 2002).

Immunization with an annual influenza vaccine is also recommended, following CDC guidelines for the type and dose of vaccine for all children with CF who are 6 months and older. It should be administered during the autumn of each year before the start of the influenza season. For those children with CF who are taking high doses of corticosteroids for a prolonged period, influenza administration should be deferred temporarily (AAP, 2000). It is also important for primary care providers to encourage all household contacts to also be immunized against influenza to help reduce the individual's risk of exposure (Orenstein et al, 2002).

Since respiratory syncytial virus (RSV) can be a risk to a person with CF, RSV immunization is an appealing notion, but the safety and efficacy of passive immunization with intravenous immunoglobulins or monoclonal antibody have not been demonstrated to be routinely useful in CF (CFF, 2001b; Orenstein et al, 2002). Research is needed in this area.

Routine immunization with the new heptavalent pneumococcal conjugate vaccine is recommended in infancy as per the American Academy of Pediatrics guidelines (AAP, 2000). Although there has been some discussion about the need for immunization of individuals with CF with the 23-valent pneumococcal polysaccharide vaccine (Burns, 2000), it is recommended by the Advisory Committee on Immunization Practices (ACIP) of the CDC for all persons 2 years of age and older who have chronic pulmonary disease. Since adverse reactions to the immunization are mild and a pneumococcal infection to an individual with CF could be life threatening, it would be prudent to immunize according to the Committee on Infectious Diseases (AAP, 2000).

Screening

Vision. Routine screening is recommended. A pediatric ophthalmologist should monitor steroid-dependent children annually for early detection of cataracts or glaucoma.

Hearing. Routine screening is recommended. Children should be monitored by an audiologist for occurrence of high-frequency hearing loss after every two to four courses of intravenous aminoglycosides or 180 accumulated days of aerosolized aminoglycoside (CFF, 1997).

Dental. Routine screening is recommended. Precautions for the use of tetracycline before permanent tooth formation are advised. Orthodontia work can cause some difficulty in eating, and nutritional supplements may need to be added if there is growth failure.

Hematocrit. Routine screening is recommended. Anemia may result from other organic causes, such as protein deficiencies or chronic infection, and further studies may be warranted to differentiate between iron deficiency and anemia of chronic illness (CFF, 2001a, 2001c).

Blood Pressure. Blood pressure should be measured at every visit because of possible hypertension from corticosteroids.

Tuberculosis. Routine screening is no longer recommended for all children, only those who are at increased risk of acquiring tuberculosis infection and disease. Although active disease caused by *Mycobacterium tuberculosis* is probably no more prevalent in individuals with CF than in the general population, recent reports have documented the presence of atypical mycobacteria in individuals with CF as high as 12.5% (Oliver et al, 2000).

Condition-Specific Screening

Pulmonary function testing (PFT) is used to measure lung function and is routinely performed in children over 5 years of age at every CF center visit and hospitalization. PFTs and chest roentgenography monitor the progression of pulmonary disease and identify acute problems.

Other screenings routinely performed at CF center visits include sputum cultures with antibiotic sensitivities; blood and urine assays of liver and renal function; complete blood counts; and serum and anthropometric measures of nutritional status. Depending on the individual's age, medications, and disease progression, more intensive laboratory monitoring may be indicated (CFF, 2001c).

Primary care providers and the CF care team should communicate their findings of each visit including the physical examination and any laboratory and radiologic assessment to all health care providers. This will not only provide continuity of care but also eliminate the repetition of screening evaluations and lab work since many of the routine screening tests recommended by the American Academy of Pediatrics may also be part of the annual screening that is done by the CF care centers (i.e., urinalysis, hematocrit, etc).

Common Illness Management

Differential Diagnosis

Symptoms associated with common pediatric illnesses may also be symptoms specific to CF, and questions about their cause and management often arise. Parents often need to hear that their child will develop common, minor childhood illnesses and will usually respond to routine management. Parents should be reassured that the CF center team is available to the primary care provider whenever questions about the cause and treatment of an acute illness arise. Thorough history taking and examination not only are necessary for primary care providers to make a differential diagnosis but also are reassuring to parents and the child (Box 22-8).

Gastrointestinal Symptoms. Abdominal pain is a relatively common complaint in individuals with CF and can be caused by a variety of conditions, not all which are related to CF. Diarrhea, constipation, and abdominal cramping may be presenting complaints of a partial or complete intestinal obstruction. A history of intermittent cramping pain and changes in stool pattern in the absence of other acute gastrointestinal and systemic symptoms is suggestive of distal ileal obstruction syndrome (DIOS). Abdominal pain may also be suggestive of gallstones or pancreatitis, and a careful pain history is essential. Appendicitis, intussusception, peptic ulcer disease, fibrosing colonopathy, necrotizing enterocolitis (for those taking antibiotics), and volvulus should always be in the differential diagnosis (Borowitz et al, 1995; Orenstein, 2003). Children who have gastrointestinal symptoms that coincide with those of others with whom they have had close contact and that suggest infectious causes not related to CF should be treated

appropriately. Finally, children with CF have an increased prevalence of gastroesophageal reflux disease (GERD), which can be manifested by regurgitation, esophagitis, feeding refusal, cough, weight loss, esophageal ulcerations, and blood loss in older patients (Gaskin, 1988; Rosenfeld & Ramsey, 1999). In treating GERD in infants, one can first try conservative measures, including the use of the prone position, avoidance of head-down positioning for chest physical therapy, and thickening formula feeds. The administration of prokinetic agents to increase lower esophageal sphincter tone and promote gastric emptying may be indicated in those who do not respond to conservative measures (Orenstein, 2003).

Fever. Fever associated with a CF pulmonary exacerbation is a relatively uncommon presentation (Ewig & Martinez, 2001), and evaluation of fever in children with CF should elicit the same broad-based approach used with other children. An initial brief febrile period with a viral illness can be anticipated in children with CF and symptomatically treated per usual practice protocols. When a viral illness exacerbates lower respiratory tract symptoms—as often occurs with upper respiratory tract infections, an increase in airway clearance techniques and a 2- to 4-week course of oral or aerosolized antibiotics are usually recommended (Rosenstein, 1999). Prevention of hyponatremia and dehydration during febrile illness includes adding salt to a child's intake, increasing fluids, and reviewing warning signs of dehydration with parents. When a rehydration solution is indicated, electrolyte-balanced clear liquids (e.g., Pedialyte) may be used. One must also evaluate the fever that could be symptomatic of influenza. In younger children and infants, the manifestations are similar to common respiratory viral illnesses, whereas older children may have additional complaints of headache, chills, myalgia, and malaise (Cherry, 1999). Approved treatment of influenza includes one of the recommended antiviral drugs, such as amantadine or rimantadine, which should be initiated within 48 hours of onset of illness (AAP, 2000).

Chest Pain. Children with lung disease occasionally complain of chest pain. These complaints should always be evaluated because of the potential occurrence of pneumothorax. Complaints associated with pneumothorax are typically an abrupt onset of sharp pain unilaterally followed by dull aching and accompanied by profound shortness of breath and activity intolerance. This complication, confirmed by physical examination and chest roentgenogram, is best managed at the regional CF center following local emergency stabilization as indicated.

Other causes of chest pain include musculoskeletal strains, especially from prolonged paroxysmal coughing episodes. These chest pains are usually bilateral, not associated with dyspnea and reproduced by palpation. This pain usually responds to rest and antiinflammatory agents. Chest pain, especially during pulmonary exacerbations, can be pleural inflammation. This type of chest pain increases with deep breaths and is not reproducible on palpation. Since this chest pain is usually secondary to underlying infection, treatment should include an increase in airway clearance, antibiotics, and nonnarcotic analgesics (Orenstein et al, 2002). Some children and adolescents with CF experience midline chest and epigastric burning related to gastroesophageal reflux (GER) and

---

BOX 22-8

Differential Diagnosis

Gastrointestinal symptoms: Common vs. distal ileal obstruction syndrome (DIOS); rule out appendicitis, volvulus, intussusception, gallstones, pancreatitis

Fever: Viral illness with exacerbation of chronic infection

Chest pain: Pneumothorax vs. muscle pull vs. gastroesophageal reflux (GER)

Cough: Sinusitis vs. lower respiratory tract exacerbation

Wheezing: Heightened bronchial reactivity caused by chronic infection and inflammation

esophagitis (CFF, 1991; Schidlow et al, 1993). If antacids are not effective, the CF center team should be consulted regarding the use of histamine-receptor antagonists and proton pump inhibitors.

Cough. The respiratory tract is almost always involved in CF, even in those children who present early in life. The most prominent feature of pulmonary involvement is a chronic cough. Initially, the cough can be dry, but as the disease progresses or in an acute exacerbation, it becomes paroxysmal and productive. An increase in cough is always of significance and requires intervention even if the chest is clear to auscultation (Orenstein et al, 2002). Nighttime coughing and/or wheezing may develop and can be associated with reactive airway disease, increased pulmonary infection and inflammation, or postnasal discharge from sinusitis or rhinitis (Ewig & Martinez, 2001; Rosenstein, 1999). Delineating a clear cause can be challenging. Both antibiotic therapy and initiation of or increase in the use of aerosolized bronchodilators and antiinflammatory agents may be helpful. Cough suppressants are generally contraindicated and should only be used after consultation with the CF center team. A trial of decongestants may be useful. Antihistamines may be used when allergy plays a role in symptomatology, but primary care providers should be aware that antihistamines might increase the viscosity of mucus, inhibiting its mobilization.

Wheezing. Wheezing is a common manifestation of CF—particularly in infancy—that is most often attributed to heightened bronchial reactivity from chronic infection and inflammation. This often makes it difficult to distinguish airway symptoms caused by infection from those caused by asthma. One who has recurrent wheezing, not just a cough, a family history of asthma, a personal history of atopy and responses to antiasthma medications is most likely to have asthma (Balfour-Lynn, 2002). Bronchodilators have been used in individuals with CF for many years and can increase airflow significantly in those who also have asthma although responses typically vary over time and with degree of illness (Ewig & Martinez, 2001; Orenstein, 2003; Rosenstein, 1999). In children with CF where clinical data support the diagnosis of asthma, inhaled corticosteroids should be the first-line prophylaxis, but doses should not escalate (Balfour-Lynn, 2002). It is imperative that antibiotics also be used during acute asthma exacerbations if there is underlying respiratory infection. Finally there are other underlying causes of wheezing that should be included in the differential diagnosis, including foreign body aspiration especially in toddlers, allergic bronchopulmonary aspergillus, other medications that could induce bronchospasm (i.e., aerosolized colistin or tobramycin), GER, and RSV infection (Stern, 1998).

Drug Interactions

Although very few drug interactions have been studied specifically in individuals with CF, primary care providers should be cognizant that certain drugs commonly used to manage CF lung disease may interact with other medications. With the use of corticosteroids, there is an increased risk for gastrointestinal ulceration if the child with CF is also taking high-dose nonsteroidal antiinflammatory drugs, such as ibuprofen. Itraconazole and ketoconazole can decrease the clearance of corticosteroids; decrease the absorption of antacids, cimetidine, ranitidine, and famotidine; and interact with phenytoin (Smith et al, 1999). Children taking ciprofloxacin, an antibiotic that is used frequently in CF, should be advised not to take antacids, zinc, or calcium supplements concurrently. For those individuals who have had a lung transplant, antirejection medications, such as cyclosporine, have multiple drug interactions and the primary care provider should consult the transplant center before prescribing any new medications. The use of herbal supplements has been increasing in the general population as well as in individuals with CF. A detailed medication history including herbal supplements and over-the-counter medications can help alleviate potential drug interactions. Health care providers should provide education about the medications that are prescribed.

Primary care providers routinely include anticipatory guidance about substance abuse to children, adolescents, and parents. The harmful effect of tobacco smoke, both active and passive, has been well documented in reports such as *Tobacco or Health* from the World Health Organization in the early 1990s. Smoking has been implicated in heart disease, lung cancer, and respiratory disease (WHO, 1994). Children who have a chronic respiratory disease such as CF are most vulnerable to passive smoking. Although many of the studies examining the effects of smoking on children with CF in the 1990s found contradictory evidence because of small samples and subtle changes, studies of the normal population demonstrated that multiple medical conditions increased the morbidity and mortality of passive smoke exposure (Verma et al, 2002).

Verma and associates reviewed the literature on the effects of active smoking in CF and found that even though the age of onset was often later for children with CF, 21% had tried smoking, 11% were smoking, and 20% had tried other substances, including marijuana. For those persons with CF who actively smoked, there was a dose-dependent relationship between the number of cigarettes smoked and the severity of the disease (Rubin & Rosenstein, 1990; Verma et al, 2002). Education about the harmful effects of smoking and referral to smoking cessation programs should be provided and reinforced by primary care providers.

Alcohol can have detrimental effects on anyone who abuses it, but it can be worse for someone with CF. Malnutrition is a common complication of CF, and alcohol in excess can worsen one's nutritional status. It can also increase the risk for liver damage to those with CF who have already had the potential for hepatobiliary disease. Alcohol use in individuals taking nonsteroidal antiinflammatories or corticosteroids can greatly increase the risk for gastrointestinal ulceration and bleeding.

Developmental Issues
Sleep Patterns

Sleep patterns may be altered with an acute exacerbation or with gradual progression of disease that increases cough and/or can decrease oxyhemoglobin saturation (Milross et al, 2001). Nighttime coughing can interfere with the child's sleep, as well as that of family members. Children with CF also have a busy morning routine, which requires early rising for school-aged children and adolescents to get in their multiple medications and treatments. They are often more vulnerable to fatigue because of their increased basal metabolic rate. Difficulty falling asleep and remaining asleep are associated somatic symptoms of depression. Several studies have examined sleep quality and found individuals with CF to have symptoms of obstructive sleep apnea, snoring, attention deficit, and hyperactivity (Akanli & Wheeler-Dobrota, 2002; Naqvi et al, 2002). Although sleep requirements are not necessarily greater in these children, sleep should not be reduced. All health care providers should include a detailed sleep history as part of their evaluation. It is also important to help families maintain a consistent bedtime ritual that is appropriate for their child's developmental level. When a child with CF is hospitalized, family members should be encouraged to bring transitional objects (i.e., blankets, stuffed animals, music) from home to help them sleep.

Toileting

As in other children, toilet training should proceed when cues of developmental readiness are noted in a child. Many children with CF, however, continue to have stools more than once per day and may have some abdominal cramping before stooling, even with adequate enzyme therapy. These problems may impede the child's interest in toileting, and parents should allow for this delay.

Even though enzymes improve digestion of nutrients, some maldigested food passes through the intestine. As a result, stools may be excessive, urgent, and malodorous and an embarrassment for children and adolescents. Parents, teachers, and friends' parents should be aware of the need for privacy during toileting.

Stress urinary incontinence has been recognized in adolescents and adults and more recently has been studied in children with CF. One recent survey (Moraes et al, 2002) demonstrated stress urinary incontinence in 14% of 6- to 17-year-olds, more commonly in females. Urinary leakage was usually associated with laughing, coughing, sneezing, pulmonary exacerbations (Judi & Connett, 2002), and daily airway clearance and exercise (Nixon et al, 2001). Trials of Kegel exercises to strengthen the pelvic floor have been successful. Although urinary incontinence is a fairly new area of study, it is a problem that can cause anxiety and psychosocial issues in individuals with CF.

Discipline

From the time of diagnosis, parents of children with CF not only grieve the loss of a healthy child but also feel guilty about their genetic contribution. Parents struggle to redefine a future for their child and family. The primary care provider can provide ongoing support and counseling during this difficult adjustment period especially since he or she often already has an established relationship with the parents and/or child.

Improved medical treatments have increased life expectancy for those with CF but also increased the time and complexity of the daily home regimen. This time commitment of daily therapy may not only create conflicts between parents and children but also be viewed by siblings as an inequity in parental attention. There have been reports of enuresis, headaches, depression, abdominal pain, and poor school performances in siblings of children with chronic illness (Bryon, 1999). Conscious efforts by parents to give individual attention to each child may prevent feelings of jealousy and guilt. Coyne (1997) identified effective parental coping strategies, including assigning meaning to the illness, sharing the burden, and incorporating therapy in a schedule. Helping parents to set limits and encourage similar responsibilities for the child with CF and siblings makes it easier for them to maintain consistency in family life.

Parents of adolescents with CF are often frustrated and anxious about disease progression, particularly when they have difficulty maintaining their child's adherence to the treatment program on one hand and seek to promote independence on the other. Factors influencing adherence with CF regimens included inadequate knowledge and psychosocial difficulties (Angst, 2002). Normal adolescent behavior (i.e., testing limits, perceiving themselves as invincible, taking risks) is complicated by the chronicity and morbidity of CF. It is those therapies that are burdensome and do not result in any clear-cut short-term benefit (e.g., airway clearance) that are missed as compared with treatments such as aerosols or enzymes that have a more immediate consequence that may be felt if they were not done. Parents who begin to transfer responsibility for management of their CF to their child beginning in their early school years often report fewer problems in adolescence. Adolescents with CF may also be more adherent if allowed to control parts of their treatment regimen, such as which type of airway clearance or at what time to do it. Encouraging school-aged children and adolescents to participate actively in clinic visits by asking and answering the questions and involving them in decision making is essential to their development of accountability and independence. Behavioral contracts may be useful tools for families and health care providers who are experiencing more problems with an adolescent (D'Angelo & Lask, 2001).

Part of every visit should be dedicated to psychosocial issues, such as discipline and coping of the child with CF and the rest of the family. Referral for individual and family counseling may be necessary to assist with the particular challenges that arise.

Child Care

Parents of children with CF often struggle with child care issues, especially at the time of diagnosis. Certain factors should be remembered when health care providers assist parents in making the appropriate choice for child care. First, the financial needs of the family are critical to determine what type of child care they can afford. Second, one must examine what is available to families in their area—private home or a licensed child care center. Ideally, the best child care setting would be in the child's own home or in another home setting with few children since this decreases exposure to viral illnesses. Whatever setting is selected, it is important to address any guilt feelings parents have about placing their child with CF in child care. When a child care program has been selected, child care providers should be specifically educated on issues such as (1) the child's individual nutritional and pulmonary treatment program; (2) the child's chronic cough and lack of contagion; and (3) methods to prevent the spread of viral illness in the setting. (See the educational materials at the end of this chapter.)

Schooling

School officials, including principals, teachers, coaches, and the school nurse, should be educated about several issues with the child with CF in the school setting. (See educational resources at the end of the chapter). First, the child will need to take medications during school, including enzymes with lunch and snacks and at times, inhalers, aerosols, and/or antibiotics. It is helpful if the school can allow the older child to carry his or her medications instead of going to the office. This allows the child to participate in all activities and to educate peers about his or her treatments for CF.

A student with CF may be fatigued because of malnutrition, early morning treatments, and, as the disease progresses, interruption of sleep from coughing. Education of the school personnel about altering the school day schedule or establishing an individualized educational plan (IEP) to fit the individual needs of the student can help keep a child in school. Home instruction may be necessary for the child who is too ill, but these children will still need the social interaction that friends can provide.

Coughing is another school issue that is often misunderstood by the school personnel and classmates. Children with CF are encouraged to cough, because it is the body's way of clearing secretions. It is important for these students to be given the privacy, if needed, to cough and not suppress it. Classmates and their families should understand that the cough is not contagious.

The most sensitive school issue for children with CF is related to their bowel movements, which can be foul smelling, excessive, and urgent. The student needs extra restroom privileges and preferably the use of a private restroom (i.e., teachers' lounge or nurse's office).

Full participation in school activities including gym is desirable for most children with CF. How much the student can participate in physical education will depend on the severity of CF and how the student is feeling that day. It is important to remind both the student and the teacher that children with CF lose an abnormally high amount of salt through their sweat and this can cause an increased risk of dehydration, electrolyte imbalance, and even heat prostration. Thus the student should be encouraged to carry water or sports drinks and eat salty snacks when exercising, especially during hot weather (Brascia & Flynn, 2001).

Children with CF do not evidence impairment in their intellectual/academic performance when compared with their peers. Problems in school performance are more likely related to absenteeism as a result of physical illness, fatigue, or psychologic reactions to the disease (i.e., lowered self-esteem, depression) (Morris et al, 2002). Further evaluation may be necessary to determine the cause of poor school performance so that the appropriate interventions can be prescribed.

Sexuality

The majority of male adults with CF (98%) have obstruction or absence of the vas deferens resulting in azoospermia and sterility. A sperm count is recommended for purposes of counseling (Rosenstein, 1999). Male adolescents and young adults need reassurance that this condition does not indicate impotence, that it will not diminish their ability to have normal sexual relations, and that they can possibly father children through in vitro fertilization (IVF). Health care providers do need to educate teens about the use of condoms to decrease the risk of sexually transmitted diseases despite the fact that they may be sterile.

Although fertility in females with CF is decreased because of thickened cervical mucus, many women are still able to have children (Ewig & Martinez, 2001). In contemplating pregnancy, women with CF need to be counseled as to the potential risk to themselves, the genetic risk and health of their offspring, and the challenges of child care responsibilities in light of deteriorating health and shortened life expectancy (Rosenstein, 1999). Contraception alternatives for adolescent and young adult women with CF can be a sensitive issue to discuss for both the health care provider and the individual, but contraception needs to be assessed at regular visits. A variety of contraceptive methods have been used in females with CF, and the results are similar to those of the general population. Oral contraceptives have been reported to have side effects of headaches, heartburn, and breakthrough bleeding; and their effectiveness may be decreased when certain antibiotics are taken at the same time. Because of the comparative risk of pregnancy, many CF center providers recommend oral contraceptives or another form of birth control after fully discussing these issues with a young woman. Reproductive issues in CF should be managed in consultation with the CF center team and its high-risk obstetrician/gynecologist consultant.

Frequent antibiotics can cause fungal vaginitis in women with CF. This presents with vaginal itching, irritation, discomfort, and pain with urination and intercourse. Conventional treatment with antifungal cream or suppositories can be used, but many women need oral antifungal agents (Sawyer, 2001).

Transition into Adulthood

Advances in CF treatment have led to improved outcomes and greater life expectancy. In most regional CF centers, by the year 2006, 50% of the population will be over the age of 18 years (CFF, 2002c). Transition programs that move adolescents into the care of adult providers have been developed in most CF centers. These programs feature a committed team of adult providers who have developed expertise in CF care and become jointly involved with pediatric providers in delivering care during adolescence. The timing of transition to the adult programs has usually been between 18 and 21 years of age although some may be ready earlier than 18 years and others who are in the terminal phase of their disease may never be transitioned. Preparation of the adolescent for transition to adult care begins by increasing independence early in adolescence. This begins by maximizing opportunities for independence, including prompting responsibility for the adolescents' own daily medical regimen and educating them on communicating with their health care team (i.e., calling for prescription refills, being seen in the examination room alone, discussing their concerns). Some adolescents and their families may find this transition difficult because of the long-established relationship they have had with the pediatric CF center and their primary care providers. For others, it is seen as a significant "rite of passage" into adulthood (Yankaskas & Fernald, 1999).

Family Concerns and Resources

Families who deal with CF have a multitude of special concerns, including the stress of its prognosis, the added financial burden of medical care, and the maintenance of family life despite the uncertainty of exacerbations, hospitalizations, and disease progression. A myriad of studies in the past 10 years have examined how families, including mothers, fathers, and well siblings, cope with CF in their family member. It is remarkable how well the majority of them adjust, and the incidence of depression is low (Bluebond-Langner, 1996; Orenstein, 2003). Families who are dealing with CF, like any chronic condition, need and appreciate the consistency and open communication that they develop with health care professionals. The health care team should be sensitive to the individual needs of each family member and the coping mechanisms they embrace. From the time of diagnosis, through the first hospitalization and the progression of the disease, questions should be answered honestly and directly but within a framework of cautious optimism (Rosenstein, 1999). CF is a complex disease and needs the support of the multidisciplinary team including not only those health care providers at the CF center but also the home care team, community support groups, and primary care provider.

Care for children with CF is a significant burden on families, especially with the advent of additional treatment options and improved life expectancy. This coincides with increasing medical costs and shrinking insurance benefits. Families often need assistance with unraveling prescription coverage, bills, government benefits, appeals, and referrals. The social worker at the CF center is often the best person to assist the families in the jargon used in insurance matters such as co-pay, deductible, authorization, PPO (preferred provider organization), HMO (health maintenance organization), and POS (point of service; see Chapter 8). It is also the CF center staff who can guide the families to additional resources such as the state-funded program for the medically handicapped that is offered in most states for children with chronic diseases such as CF. Health care providers can be strong advocates in helping children with CF and their families with financial planning issues.

Another issue that health care professionals may encounter in dealing with children with CF is cultural diversity. Although CF is primarily found in whites of Northern European descent, it is not unusual to find CF in children who are black, Hispanic, or Asian. In different parts of the United States, there have been religious groups such as the Amish, Mennonites, Ashkenazi Jews, and Jehovah's Witnesses that each has their own set of beliefs that can alter the care the health care professionals provide. Education about the particular group's beliefs and culture is important in understanding how a trusting relationship can be formed with these families.

Despite all the advances in the diagnosis and treatment of CF that have been made over the past few decades, the median age of survival is about 33 years old according to the 2001 CFF

Registry Data (CFF, 2001c). Children with CF still face end-of-life issues, and most will die from respiratory failure. Mechanical ventilation for respiratory failure in individuals with CF has generally been ineffective and is usually not recommended unless there is clearly a reversible component. More recently, noninvasive positive pressure ventilation has been used in end-stage CF primarily in those individuals awaiting lung transplantation. Care provided at the end of life is often a mix of preventive, therapeutic, and palliative treatments depending on values and preferences of both the individual with CF and the family (Tonelli, 1998). Together primary care providers and the CF care team can help prepare individuals with CF and their families for the types of decisions they will face at the end of life.

Community Resources

The CF Foundation (CFF) is a national organization that was formed in 1955 by a committed group of parents whose children had CF. It now operates as a nonprofit, voluntary health organization that funds CF research, supports CF centers, provides training for medical professionals, and educates the public about CF. The mission of the CFF is to develop treatments and a cure for CF while continually working toward improving the quality of life for individuals with CF and their families. A network of local chapters in the United States raises money to support CF programs and research through a variety of fundraising events (Beall, 1999). Involvement in the local fundraising events helps give families an opportunity to participate in the fight for a cure for this dreadful disease.

There are 117 regional CF centers in the United States that offer a multidisciplinary team approach in the care and management of cystic fibrosis and are accredited by the CF Foundation. The CFF has a Therapeutic Development Program that is an innovative resource for drug development from the discovery phase through several stages of evaluation and involves a network of eight CF care centers throughout the United States (Beall, 1999). The foundation has also supported the development of CF clinical practice guidelines, which are written guidelines based on the best available scientific information and supplemented by clinical experience and expert consensus. These clinical practice guidelines can provide education to health care professionals and improve quality of care (McColley, 2002). Parents of children with CF should be encouraged to establish an ongoing relationship with a regional CF center accredited by the CFF.

Years ago, the primary care provider might not have been involved in the care of the child with CF. Today, with the increasing number of newly diagnosed patients with CF (many later in life) and the ongoing education of medical professionals, primary care providers are an integral part of the health care team. Together, each health care provider brings a unique emphasis and expertise to a complex disease.

Educational Materials

A vast array of educational materials has been published recently. These resources are in the forms of videos, pamphlets, books, CD-ROMs, and Web sites. The Cystic Fibrosis

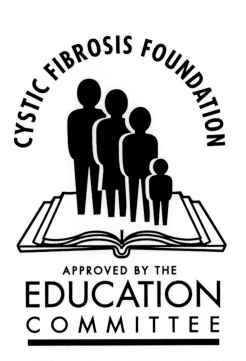

FIGURE 22-5 Cystic Fibrosis Foundation Education Committee logo. Those educational materials that have been reviewed and approved by the CF Education Committee will have their logo. (Reprinted with permission from the Cystic Fibrosis Foundation.)

Foundation, with the help of many CF health care professionals, has organized the materials into a large resource guide that is available by contacting the CF Foundation via mail, phone, fax, or E-mail.

The Cystic Fibrosis Foundation
6931 Arlington Rd
Bethesda, MD 20814
(301) 951-4422 or (800) FIGHT CF (344-4823)
Fax: (301) 951-6378
E-mail: info@cff.org

In 2000, the CFF formed an education committee whose mission was to improve the understanding and knowledge for patients and families about CF and to standardize the education materials available for people with CF. Those educational materials that have been reviewed and approved by the CF Education Committee will have their logo (Figure 22-5).

There are numerous other educational materials published by pharmaceutical companies, hospitals, universities, and individuals. Below are just a few of the resources that are available and are used frequently by CF care teams:

Advocacy Manual: A Clinician's Guide to the Legal Rights of People with Cystic Fibrosis
Manual with current information about health insurance, education, employment, and government benefit programs for people with CF.
Available from CF Foundation

"Can We Talk? My Sibling Has CF," pamphlet for well siblings about CF
Available from:
Solvay Pharmaceuticals
901 Sawyer Rd
Marietta, GA 30062

"Catch All the Sites: Your Cystic Fibrosis Web Site Guide," pamphlet with a listing of Web sites that are applicable for patients, families, and health care professionals
Available from:
Digestive Care, Inc
1120 Win Dr
Bethlehem, PA 18017-7059
(610) 882-5950

"Cystic Fibrosis in the Classroom: The Problems, the Needs, the Solutions," pamphlet for school personnel about having students with CF
Available from Digestive Care, Inc

Cystic Fibrosis: A Guide for Patient & Family, very comprehensive book for patients and families
Available from:
Lippincott-Raven Publishers
227 East Washington Square
Philadelphia, PA 19106

Cystic Fibrosis: The Impact of Nurses on Patient Management, excellent self-study guide for nurses
2003 from Genentech, Inc., South San Francisco, California

Fat and Loving It!!!, a recipe book with nutritional tips for patients with CF and great cooking ideas
Available from Digestive Care, Inc
Fitting Cystic Fibrosis into Life Every Day, a CD/ROM for 10- to 15-year-olds about CF, including information on IVs and radiology
Available from:
STARBRIGHT Foundation
11835 West Olympic Blvd
Los Angeles, CA 90064
(310) 479-1212

An Introduction to Cystic Fibrosis for Patients and Families (English and Spanish), excellent book and video for newly diagnosed; currently being revised
Available Fall 2003 from the CF Foundation

"Jeremy Bishop Explains CF: Children's Guide for Learning about CF," pamphlet and video that are appropriate for school-aged children with CF
Available from Axcan Scandipharm Inc

Mallory's 65 Roses, delightful book for children with CF ages 3 to 6 years old
Available from:
Axcan Scandipharm Inc
22 Inverness Center Parkway
Birmingham, AL 35242
(800) 615-4393

"Nutrition and Cystic Fibrosis: Changes Through Life," "Nutrition for Teens with Cystic Fibrosis," "Nutrition for Your Child (Four to Seven) with Cystic Fibrosis," "Nutrition for your Toddler (One to Three) with Cystic Fibrosis," "Nutrition for Your Infant (Birth to One) with Cystic Fibrosis," pamphlets with great nutritional age-appropriate tips
Available from CF Foundation

Psychosocial Aspects of Cystic Fibrosis, detailed book for health care professionals on a myriad of psychosocial issues of people with CF and their families
Available from Oxford University Press

Acknowledgement The authors are especially grateful for the thoughtful review of this chapter by Dr. John McBride. Dr. McBride is Associate Chair of Pediatrics at the Children's Hospital Medical Center of Akron and a Pediatric Pulmonologist at the Robert T. Stone M.D. Respiratory Center at the medical center.

Summary of Primary Care Needs of the Child with Cystic Fibrosis

HEALTH CARE MAINTENANCE

Growth and Development

Malnutrition and growth retardation are common complications. Catch-up growth can be achieved with proper nutritional therapy and treatment for pulmonary complications.

Adequate surveillance of growth is essential.

Pubertal development often is delayed—mean age of menarche for females is 14.5 years, and there is a 2- to 4-year lag for males.

Assessment of bone health is essential, especially for those with specific risk factors.

Diet

Goal is to promote normal growth. Fortified breast milk is recommended in infancy.

Diet is a well-balanced, high-protein diet with unrestricted fat that promotes 100% to 150% of recommended daily allowances (RDAs).

Nutritional issues correlate with age of the child and severity of disease.

Pancreatic enzyme replacement and vitamin supplementation are necessary in most children with CF.

Consultation with a nutritionist is recommended to maintain and improve growth.

Safety

Safe storage of multiple medications is emphasized.

Sunscreen should be used or the sun should be avoided when the child is taking antibiotics.

Hand hygiene for routine times, such as before and after eating, as well as with exposure to others with CF, is emphasized.

Immunizations

All routine immunizations should generally be given on schedule, including heptavalent pneumococcal vaccine.

Influenza vaccine should be given annually per Centers for Disease Control and Prevention (CDC) guidelines to child and family members.

Respiratory syncytial virus (RSV) immunizations are routinely used in CF.

23-Valent pneumococcal polysaccharide vaccine should be administered to all persons 2 years and older.

Screening

Vision. Routine screening is recommended.

Hearing. Routine screening is recommended. An auditory screen for high-frequency hearing loss should be done with aminoglycoside therapy.

Dental. Routine care is recommended.

Hematocrit. Routine screening is recommended with full review of iron status as indicated.

Blood Pressure. Measure at every visit.

Tuberculosis. Screen only those who are at increased risk of acquiring TB.

Condition-Specific Screening

Pulmonary function tests (PFT), chest roentgenography, sputum culture with antibiotic sensitivities, blood and urine assays of liver and renal function, complete blood counts, and serum and anthropometric measures of nutritional status are monitored at routine CF center visits.

COMMON ILLNESS MANAGEMENT

Differential Diagnosis

Abdominal Pain. Rule out distal ileal obstruction syndrome (DIOS), gallstones, pancreatitis, appendicitis, intussusception, Pelvic inflammatory disease in young women, fibrosing colonopathy, and volvulus.

Fever and Viral Illness. Prevention of hyponatremia and dehydration is emphasized. Influenza vaccine is given if indicated.

Chest Pain. Rule out pneumothorax, gastroesophageal reflux disease (GERD), musculoskeletal strain, and pleural inflammation.

Cough/Wheezing. Differentiation among asthma, exacerbation of CF, rhinitis, and/or sinusitis will help select treatment.

Tobacco Smoke. Those with chronic respiratory disease are most vulnerable to passive smoke. Education about harmful effects of smoking is imperative to those with CF.

Alcohol. Detrimental effects will occur if alcohol is abused, especially since people with CF have increased liver disease and malnutrition.

Drug Interactions/Substance Abuse

Corticosteroids. Increased risk for gastrointestinal ulceration with high-dose nonsteroidal antiinflammatory drugs, such as ibuprofen, itraconazole, and ketoconazole can decrease clearance of steroids.

Ciprofloxacin. Avoid antacids, zinc, or calcium supplements concurrently.

Herbal Supplements. Many can have potential side effects and/or interactions.

DEVELOPMENTAL ISSUES

Sleep Patterns

Sleep patterns may be altered with acute exacerbation or progression of disease because of increased cough and decreased oxyhemoglobin saturation.

Early morning routines may require adjustment of bedtime.

Difficulty falling asleep may be a sign of depression.

Snoring may be related to sleep apnea.

Toileting

Delayed bowel training may occur secondary to increased frequency of stools and associated abdominal cramping.

Provide privacy for toileting.

Stress urinary incontinence has been found in adolescents with CF.

Discipline

Expectation should be normal with allowances during periods of acute illnesses.

Summary of Primary Care Needs of the Child with Cystic Fibrosis—cont'd

Discipline—cont'd

Encourage independence in CF management with child/adolescent having some control over treatment choices.

Individual and family counseling may be indicated.

Child Care

Assist parents in making appropriate child care choices and educational providers.

Home and small daycare programs are recommended to reduce viral exposure.

Daycare workers need information on CF.

Schooling

Education of school officials is imperative.

Allow child to carry his or her own enzymes if possible.

School schedule may need to be altered as disease progresses.

Provide privacy for coughing episodes and toileting.

School performance may be affected by fatigue and coughing related to impending pulmonary exacerbation.

CF does not affect one's intellectual/academic performance.

Sexuality

Sperm count is recommended for males.

Education about sexually transmitted diseases (STDs) is needed.

Females contemplating pregnancy need counseling regarding their own and their child's risks.

Frequent antibiotics can cause fungal vaginitis.

Transition into Adulthood

Prepare for transition by increasing independence in adolescence.

Identify knowledgeable adult providers.

FAMILY CONCERNS

Despite a multitude of special concerns, including the stress of its prognosis, financial burden, and uncertainty of illness, most families adjust well.

Provide open and honest communication.

Provide multidisciplinary team support.

Cultural issues of minorities and subpopulations include religious beliefs, financial issues, and use of alternative therapies.

End-of-life care often is a mix of preventive, therapeutic, and palliative treatments.

REFERENCES

Accurso, F.J. (1995). Aerosolized dornase alfa in cystic fibrosis patients with clinically mild disease. *Dornase Alfa Clinical Series, 2*(1), 1-6.

Akanli, L. & Wheeler-Dobrota, N. (2002). Cystic fibrosis and sleep related problems. *Pediatr Pulmonol, 371*(suppl. 23), 305.

Albelda, S., Wiewrodt, R., & Zuckerman, J.B. (2000). Gene therapy for lung disease: Hype or hope? *Ann Intern Med, 132*(8), 649-660.

American Academy of Pediatricians. (2000). *Red book: Report of the committee on infectious diseases* (25th ed.). Elk Grove Village, Ill.: AAP Publication.

Angst, D. (2002). Working with families to enhance adherence. *Pediatr Pulmonol,* suppl. 22, 143-144.

Anthony, H., Paxton, S., Catto-Smith, A., & Phelan, P. (1999). Physiological and psychosocial contributors to malnutrition in children with cystic fibrosis: Review. *Clin Nutr, 18*(6), 327-335.

Bailey, D., McKay, H., Mirwald, R., Crocker, P., & Faulkner, R. (1999). A six-year longitudinal study of the relationship of physical activity to bone mineral accrual in growing children: The University of Saskatchewan bone mineral accrual study. *J Bone Miner Res, 14,* 1672-1679.

Balfour-Lynn, I. (2002). Asthma in CF: Corticosteroids. *Pediatr Pulmonol,* suppl. 23, 101-102.

Beall, R. (1999). The cystic fibrosis foundation. In J. Yankaskas & M. Knowles (Eds.). *Cystic fibrosis in adults.* Philadelphia: Lippincott-Raven Publishers, pp. 477-483.

Beker, L., Russek-Cohen, E., & Fink, R. (2001). Stature as a prognostic factor in cystic fibrosis survival. *J Am Diet Assoc, 101,* 438-442.

Bhuhikanok, G., Wang, M-C., Marcus, R., Harkins, A., Moss, R., et al. (1998). Bone acquisition and loss in children and adults with cystic fibrosis: A longitudinal study. *J Pediatr, 133,* 18-27.

Bluebond-Langner, M. (1996). *In the shadow of illness.* Princeton, N.J.: Princeton University Press.

Borowitz, D. (1994). Pathophysiology of gastrointestinal complications of cystic fibrosis. *Semin Respir Crit Care Med, 15*(5), 391-401.

Borowitz, D.S., Grand, R.J., & Durie, P.R. (1995). Use of pancreatic enzyme supplements for patients with cystic fibrosis in the context of fibrosing colonopathy. *J Pediatr, 127,* 681-684.

Brascia, T. & Flynn, K. (2001). *Cystic fibrosis in the classroom* (pamphlet). Bethlehem, Pa.: Digestive Care, Inc.

Brenckmann, C. & Papaioannou, A. (2001). Biphosphonates for osteoporosis in people with cystic fibrosis. *Cochrane Database Syst Rev,* no. 3.

Brown, T. & Schwind, E.L. (1999). Update and review: Cystic fibrosis. *J Genet Couns, 8*(3), 137-162.

Bryon, M. (1999). Siblings and CF: When should we be worried? *Pediatr Pulmonol, 18*(2), 161-163.

Burns, J. (2000, October 16). Personal communications. The CF Foundation, Bethesda, Md.

Cherry, J. (1999). Influenza viruses. In J. McMillian (Ed.). *Oski's pediatrics* (3rd ed.). Philadelphia: Lippincott, Williams & Wilkins, pp. 1089-1091.

Colin, A.A. & Wohl, M.E. (1994). Cystic fibrosis. *Pediatr Rev, 15*(5), 192-200.

Conway, S.P., Morton, A., & Wolfe, S. (2002). Enteral tube feeding for cystic fibrosis. *Cochrane Database Syst Rev,* CF001198.

Coyne, I. (1997). Chronic illness: The importance of support for families caring for a child with cystic fibrosis. *J Clin Nurs, 6*(2), 121-129.

Cutting, G.R. (1994). Genotype defect: Its effect on cellular function and phenotypic expression. *Semin Respir Crit Care Med, 15*(5), 356-363.

Cystic Fibrosis Foundation. (2002a). *Adult care consensus,* Bethesda, Md. Author.

Cystic Fibrosis Foundation. (1997). *Clinical practice guidelines,* Bethesda, Md. Author.

Cystic Fibrosis Foundation. (1991). *Consensus on gastrointestinal problems in CF,* Bethesda, Md. Author.

Cystic Fibrosis Foundation. (2001b). *Infection control consensus,* Bethesda, Md. Author.

Cystic Fibrosis Foundation. (2001a). *Nutrition consensus,* Bethesda, Md. Author.

Cystic Fibrosis Foundation. (2002b). *Patient registry 2001 annual report,* Bethesda, Md. Author.

Cystic Fibrosis Foundation. (2001c). *Preventive maintenance care for the patient with cystic fibrosis,* Bethesda, Md. Author.

Cystic Fibrosis Foundation. (2002c, October). Bethesda, Md. Personal communication.

Dalzell, A.M., Shepherd, R.W., Dean, B., Cleghorn, G.J., Holt, T.L., et al. (1992). Nutritional rehabilitation in cystic fibrosis: A 5-year follow-up study. *J Pediatr Gastroenterol Nutr, 15*(2), 141-145.

D'Angelo, S. & Lask, B. (2001). Approaches to problems of adherence. In M. Bluebond-Langerner, B. Lask, & D. Angst (Eds.). *Psychosocial aspects of cystic fibrosis*. London: Arnold Press & New York: Oxford University Press.

Davidson, A.G. & McIlwaine, M. (1995). Airway clearance techniques in cystic fibrosis. *New Insights into Cystic Fibrosis, 3*(1), 6-11.

Davis, P.B. (2001) Cystic fibrosis. *Pediatr Rev, 22*(8), 257-263.

DeJong, W. et al. (1994). Effect of a home exercise training program in patients with cystic fibrosis. *Chest, 105*(2), 463-468.

Denton, M. & Wilcox, M.H. (1997) Antimicrobial treatment of pulmonary colonization and infection by *Pseudomonas aeruginosa* in cystic fibrosis patients. *J Antimicrob Chemother, 40*, 468-474.

Doull, I. (2001). Recent advances in cystic fibrosis. *Arch Dis Child, 85*, 62-66.

Erdman, S. (1999). Nutritional imperatives in cystic fibrosis therapy. *Pediatr Ann, 28*(2), 129-136.

Ewig, J. & Martinez, J. (2001). Cystic fibrosis. In Hoekelman, R.A. (Ed.). *Primary pediatric care* (4th ed.). St. Louis: Mosby.

Fernbach, S.D. & Thomson, E.J. (1992). Molecular genetic technology in cystic fibrosis: Implications for nursing practice. *J Pediatr Nurs, 7*(1), 20-25.

Fitzsimmons, S.C., Burkhart, G.A., & Borowitz, D. (1997). High-dose pancreatic enzyme supplements and fibrosing colonopathy in children with cystic fibrosis. *N Engl J Med, 336*, 1283-1289.

Gaskin, K. (1988). The impact of nutrition in cystic fibrosis: A review. *J Pediatr Gastroenterol Nutr, 7*(suppl. 1), S12-S17.

Grody, W.W., Cutting, G.R., Klinger, K.W., Richards, C., Watson, M.S., et al. (2001). Laboratory standards and guidelines for population-based cystic fibrosis carrier screening. *Genet Med, 3*(2), 149-154.

Hamosh, A., Fitz-Simmons, S.C., Macek, M., Jr., Knowles, M.R., Rosenstein, B.J., et al. (1998). Comparison of the clinical manifestations of cystic fibrosis in African Americans and Caucasians. *J Pediatr, 132*, 255-259.

Hardin, D.S., Ellis, K.J., Dyson, M., Rice, J., McConnell, R., et al. (2001). Growth hormone decreases protein catabolism in children with cystic fibrosis. *J Clin Endocrinol Metab, 86*, 4424-4428.

Hendeles, L., Dorf, A., Stecenko, A., & Weinberger, M. (1990). Treatment failure after substitution of generic pancrelipase capsules. *JAMA, 236*, 2459-2461.

Hodson, M.E. (1995). Aerosolized dornase alfa (rhDNase) for therapy of cystic fibrosis. *Am J Respir Crit Care Med, 151*, S70-S74.

Hubbard, R.C., McElvaney, N.G., Birrer, P., Shak, S., Robinson, et al. (1992). A preliminary study of aerosolized recombinant human deoxyribonuclease I in the treatment of cystic fibrosis. *N Engl J Med, 326*(12), 812-815.

Jaffe, A. & Bush, A. (2001). Cystic fibrosis: Review of the decade. *Monaldi Arch Chest Dis, 56*(3), 240-247.

Johannesson, M., Gonlieb, C., & Hjelte, L. (1997). Delayed puberty in girls with cystic fibrosis despite good clinical status. *Pediatrics, 99*(1), 20-34.

Judi, M. & Connett, G. (2002). Stress incontinence problems in the pediatric population. *Pediatr Pulmonol, 399*(suppl. 23), 101-102.

Kirchner, K.K. et al. (1993). Increased DNA levels in bronchoalveolar lavage fluid obtained from infants with cystic fibrosis. *Pediatr Pulmonol*, suppl. 9, 288.

Knowles, M.R., Olivier, K., Noone, P., & Boucher, R.C. (1995). Pharmacologic modulation of salt and water in the airway epithelium in cystic fibrosis. *Am J Respir Crit Care Med, 151*, S65-S69.

Konstan, M.W. (1998). Therapies aimed at airway inflammation in cystic fibrosis. *Clin Chest Med, 19*(3), 505-513.

Konstan, M.W., Hilliard, K.A., Norvell, T.M., & Berger, M. (1994). Bronchoalveolar lavage findings in cystic fibrosis patients with stable, clinically mild lung disease suggest ongoing infection and inflammation. *Am J Respir Crit Care Med, 150*, 448-454.

Konstan, M.W., Byard, P.J., Hoppel, C.L., & Davis, P.B. (1995). Effect of high dose ibuprofen in patients with cystic fibrosis. *N Engl J Med, 332*(13), 848-854.

Lai, H., Kosorrok, M., Sondel, S., Chen, S., Fitzsimmons, S., et al. (1998). Growth status in children with cystic fibrosis based on the National Cystic Fibrosis Patient Registry data: Evaluation of various criteria used to identify malnutrition. *J Pediatr, 132*, 478-485.

Lees, C.M. (2000). The current management of cystic fibrosis. *Int J Clin Pract, 54*(3), 171-179.

Levy, L.D., Durie, P.R., Pencharz, P.B., & Corey, M.L. (1985). Effects of long-term nutritional rehabilitation on body composition and clinical status in malnourished children and adolescents with cystic fibrosis. *J Pediatr, 107*, 225-230.

Littlewood, J.M. (1992). Gastrointestinal complications. *Br Med Bull, 48*, 847-859.

Loader, S., Caldwell, P., Kozyra, A., Levenkron, J.C., Boehm, C.D., et al. (1996). Cystic fibrosis carrier population screening in the primary care setting. *Am J Hum Genet, 59*(1), 234-247.

Loutzenhiser, J.K. & Clark, R. (1993). Physical activity and exercise in children with cystic fibrosis. *J Pediatr Nurs, 8*, 112-119.

Marchand, V., Baker, S.S., Start, T.J., & Baker, R.D. (2000). Randomized, double-blind, placebo-controlled pilot trial of megestrol acetate in malnourished children with cystic fibrosis. *J Pediatr Gastroenterol Nutr, 31*, 264-269.

Marshall, B.C. & Samuelson, W.M. (1998). Basic therapies in cystic fibrosis: Does standard therapy work? *Clin Chest Med, 19*(3), 487-504.

McColley, S. (2002). Clinical practice guidelines: Do they improve quality of care? *Pediatr Pulmonol, 399*(suppl. 23).

Milross, M., Piper, A., Grunstein, R., Sullivan, C., & Bye, P. (2001). Non-invasive ventilation and sleep-disordered breathing in cystic fibrosis—challenges and options. *Pediatr Pulmonol, S18.4*, 173-175.

Moraes, T., Carpenter, S., & Taylor, L. (2002). Cystic fibrosis and incontinence in children. *Pediatr Pulmonol, 398*(suppl. 23), 315.

Morris, K., Ryan, C., Williams, T., Gardner, W., & Orenstein, D, (2002). Neuropsychological correlates of CF in adolescence. *Pediatr Pulmonol, 492*(suppl. 23), 349.

Morris, N. & Udry, J. (1980). Validation of a self-administered instrument to assess stage of adolescent development. *J Youth Adolesc, 9*, 271-280.

Moshang, T. & Holsdw, D., Jr. (1980). Menarchal determinants in cystic fibrosis. *Am J Dis Child, 134*, 1139-1142.

Moss, R.B. (2001, January 15). New approaches to cystic fibrosis. *Hosp Pract*, 25-37.

Moss, R.B. et al. (1999). Who benefits more? An analysis of FEV_1 and weight in adolescents (age 13-17) CF patients using TOBI™ (tobramycin solution for inhalation). Presented at 1999 North American Cystic Fibrosis Conference, October 7-10, Seattle.

Naqvi, S., Sawnani, H., Vlasic, V., Mack, C., Legendre, C., et al. (2002). Sleep complaints and sleep quality in patients with cystic fibrosis. *Pediatr Pulmonol*, no. 370, suppl. 23, 305.

NCCLS document C34-A2. (2000). Sweat testing: Sample collection and quantitative analysis: Approved guideline (2nd ed.). Wayne, Pa.: Author.

Nickerson, B. et al. (1999, October 7-10). Safety and effectiveness of 2 years of treatment with TOBI (tobramycin solution for inhalation) in CF patients. Presented at 1999 North American Cystic Fibrosis Conference, Seattle.

Nixon, G., Glazner, J., Martin, J., & Sawyer, S. (2001). Urinary incontinence in female adolescents with cystic fibrosis. *Pediatr Pulmonol*, 503.

Oliver, K., Handler, A., Less, J., Tudor, G., & Knowles, M. (2000). Clinical impact of nontuberculous mycobacteria on the course of cystic fibrosis lung disease: Results of a multicenter nested cohort study. *Pediatr Pulmonol*, suppl. 20, 102-103.

Orenstein, D. (2003). Cystic fibrosis. In *Rudolph's pediatrics* (21st ed.). New York: McGraw-Hill.

Orenstein, S.R. & Orenstein, D.M. (1998). Gastroesophageal reflux and respiratory disease in children. *J Pediatr, 112*, 847-858.

Orenstein, D., Winnie, G., & Altman, H. (2002). Cystic fibrosis: A 2002 update. *J Pediatr, 140*, 156-164.

Pattishall, E.N. (1990). Longitudinal response of pulmonary function to bronchodilators in cystic fibrosis. *Pediatr Pulmonol, 9*, 80-85.

Physicians' desk reference. (2002). Montvale, N.J.: Medical Economics Co.

Powers, S., Patton, S., Byars, K., Mitchell, M., Maynard, M., et al. (2002). Parent and child mealtime behaviors in families of toddlers with cystic fibrosis. *Pediatr Pulmonol Suppl, 23*, 346.

Prober, C.G. (1991). The impact of respiratory viral infections in patients with cystic fibrosis. *Clin Rev Allergy Immunol, 9*(1), 87-102.

Quan, J.M., Tiddens, H.A., Sy, J.P., McKenzie, S.G., Montgomery, M.D., et al. (2001). A two-year randomized, placebo-controlled trial of dornase alfa in young patients with cystic fibrosis with mild lung function abnormalities. *J Pediatr, 139*, 813-820.

Quittner, A.L. & Buu, A. (2002). Effects of tobramycin solution for inhalation on global ratings of quality of life in patients with cystic fibrosis and *Pseudomonas aeruginosa* infection. *Pediatr Pulmonol, 33*, 269-276.

Ramsey, B.W. (1996). Management of pulmonary disease in patients with cystic fibrosis. *N Engl J Med, 335*(3), 179-188.

Ramsey, B.W. (1993). A summary of the results of the phase III multicenter clinical trial: Aerosol administration of recombinant human Dnase reduces the risk of respiratory tract infection and improves pulmonary function in patients with cystic fibrosis. *Pediatr Pulmonol,* (suppl. 9), 152-153.

Robbins, M. & Ontjes, D. (1999). Endocrine and renal disorders. In J. Yankaskas & M. Knowles (Eds.). *Cystic fibrosis in adults.* Philadelphia: Lippincott-Raven Publishers.

Rock, M.J. (1997) Controversies in newborn screening: The Wisconsin experience. *New Insights into Cystic Fibrosis, 5*(2), 1-6.

Rommens, J.M., Iannuzzi, M.C., Kerem, B., Drumm, M.L., Melmer, G., et al. (1989). Identification of the cystic fibrosis gene: Chromosome walking and jumping. *Science, 245,* 1059-1065.

Rosenecker, J., Eichler, I., Barmier, H., & von der Hardt, H. (2001). Diabetes mellitus and cystic fibrosis: Comparison of clinical parameters in patients treated with insulin versus oral glucose-lowering agents. *Pediatr Pulmonol, 32,* 351-355.

Rosenfeld, M. & Ramsey, B. (1992). Evolution of airway microbiology in the infant with cystic fibrosis: Role of nonpseudomonal and pseudomonal pathogens. *Semin Respir Infect, 7,* 158-167.

Rosenstein, B. (1999). Cystic fibrosis. In J. McMillian (Ed.) *Oski's pediatrics* (3rd ed.). Philadelphia: Lippincott, Williams & Wilkins.

Rosenstein, B.J. & Cutting, G.R. (1998). The diagnosis of cystic fibrosis, a consensus statement. *J Pediatr, 132,* 589-595.

Rosenstein, B.J. & Eigen, H. (1991). Risks of alternate-day prednisone in patients with cystic fibrosis. *Pediatrics, 87,* 245-246.

Rosenstein, B.J. & Langbaum, T.S. (1984). Diagnosis. In L.M. Taussig (Ed.). *Cystic fibrosis.* New York: Theime Stratton, Inc.

Rubin, B. & Rosenstein, B. (1990). Exposure of children with cystic fibrosis to environmental tobacco smoke. *N Engl J Med, 323,* 782-788.

Rubin, B.K. (1999). Emerging therapies for cystic fibrosis lung disease. *Chest, 115,* 1120-1126.

Sawyer, S. (2001). Sexual and reproductive health in CF: Don't ask, won't tell. *Pediatr Pulmonol, 22,* 113-114.

Schidlow, D.V., Taussig, L.M., & Knowles, M.R. (1993). Cystic Fibrosis Foundation consensus conference report on pulmonary complications of cystic fibrosis. *Pediatr Pulmonol, 15*(3), 187-198.

Schneiderman-Walker, J., Pollock, S.L., Corey, M., Wilkes, D.D., Canny, G.J., et al. (2000). A randomized controlled trial of a 3-year home exercise program in cystic fibrosis. *J Pediatr, 136*(3), 304-310.

Schwartz, R.H. (1987). Cystic fibrosis. In R.H. Hoekelman (Ed.). *Primary pediatric care* (3rd ed.). St. Louis: Mosby.

Shak, S. (1995). Aerosolized recombinant human Dnase I for the treatment of cystic fibrosis. *Chest, 107*(2), 65S-70S.

Shapiro, S.K. & Seilheimer, D.K. (1994). Screening for cystic fibrosis: Clinical issues and genetic counseling implications. *New Insights into Cystic Fibrosis, 2*(1), 6-11.

Shepard, R. (2002). Achieving genetic potential for nutrition and growth in cystic fibrosis. *J Pediatr, 140*(4), 393-395.

Smith, A., Cohn, M., & Ramsey, B. (1999). Pharmacotherapy. In J. Yankaskas & M. Knowles (Eds.). *Cystic fibrosis in adults.* Philadelphia: Lippincott-Raven Publishers, pp. 345-364.

Soutter, V.A. et al. (1986) Chronic undernutrition/growth retardation in cystic fibrosis. *Clin Gastroenterol, 15*(1), 137-155.

Steinkamp, G. & von der Hardt, H. (1994). Improvement of nutritional status and lung function after long-term nocturnal gastrostomy feeding in cystic fibrosis. *J Pediatr, 124,* 244-249.

Stern, R.C. (1998). Sinus disease in CF: Current concepts. *New Insights into Cystic Fibrosis, 6*(1), 1-5.

Stern, R. & Orenstein, D. (1998). Inpatient treatment of cystic fibrosis pulmonary disease. In *Treatment of the hospitalized cystic fibrosis patient.* New York: Basel, Hong Kong, pp. 79-133.

Tanner, J. (1962). *Growth at adolescence* (2nd ed.). Oxford: Blackwell Scientific Publications.

Tonelli, M. (1998). End-of-life care in cystic fibrosis. *Curr Opin Pulmonary Med,* no. 4, 332-336.

Tsui, L.C. & Durie, P.R. (1997) What is a CF diagnosis?—genetic heterogeneity. *New Insights into Cystic Fibrosis, 5*(1), 1-5.

van der Schans, C., Prasad, A., & Main E. (2002). Chest physiotherapy compared to no chest physiotherapy for cystic fibrosis. In *The Cochrane Library, Issue 3,* Oxford: The Cochrane Database of Systemic Review.

Verma, A., Clough, D., McKenna, D., & Dodd, M. (2002). *Pediatr Pulmonol,* suppl. 22, 143-144.

Wagner, M. & Sherman, J. (1997). Cystic fibrosis and the general pediatrician. *Contemp Pediatr,* 328-336.

Wark, P.A. & McDonald V. (2002). Nebulised hypertonic saline for cystic fibrosis. (Cochrane Review). *The Cochrane Library, Issue 1,* Oxford: The Cochrane Database of Systemic Review.

Weiner, D.J. (2002). Respiratory tract infections in cystic fibrosis. *Pediatr Ann, 31*(2), 116-123.

Wertz, D.C. et al. (1992). Attitudes toward abortion among parents of children with cystic fibrosis. *Am J Public Health, 81,* 992-996.

Wilmott, R.W. (1998). Making the diagnosis of cystic fibrosis. *J Pediatr, 132,* 563-565.

Wilson, J.M. (1994). Cystic fibrosis: Strategies for gene therapy. *Semin Respir Crit Care Med, 15*(5), 439-445.

World Health Organization. (1994). *Tobacco or health: A global status report.* Geneva, Switzerland: Author.

Yankaskas, J. & Fernald, G. (1999). Adult social issues. In J. Yankaskas & M. Knowles (Eds.). *Cystic fibrosis in adults.* Philadelphia: Lippincott-Raven Publishers, no. 22, pp. 465-476.

Yankaskas, J.R. & Mallory, G.B., Jr. (1998). Lung transplantation in cystic fibrosis: Consensus conference statement. *Chest, 113*(1), 217-226.

Young, S., Kharrazi, M., Pearl, M., & Cunningham, G. (2001). Cystic fibrosis screening in newborns: Results from existing programs. *Curr Opin Pulm Med, 7,* 427-433.

Zeitlin, P.L. (1998). Therapies directed at the basic defect in cystic fibrosis. *Clin Chest Med, 19*(3), 515-525.

23 Diabetes Mellitus (Types 1 and 2)

Elizabeth A. Boland and Margaret Grey

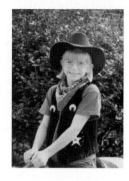

Etiology

Diabetes mellitus was first described in the Egyptian *Ebers Papyrus* in 1500 BC. Type 1, or insulin-dependent, diabetes mellitus, most commonly occurs in young people and is characterized by beta-cell failure. In type 2, or non–insulin-dependent, diabetes mellitus, individuals are often overweight and usually more than 30 years of age, overproduce insulin, and have a receptor-site defect. In recent years, however, type 2 diabetes has become increasingly common in children and youth, with up to 40% of new cases of diabetes under the age of 20 years old being type 2 (American Diabetes Association [ADA], 2000; Fagot-Campagna et al, 2000). Individuals with type 2 diabetes can often be treated orally with hypoglycemic agents, but those with type 1 diabetes must be treated with insulin.

Known Genetic Etiology

The cause of type 1 diabetes is unknown, but many factors have been hypothesized to contribute. It is clear that type 1 diabetes is an autoimmune disease. In autoimmunity, "self" antigens are no longer recognized as such, so a self-destructive process occurs. Islet cell antibodies can be detected in a majority of individuals newly diagnosed with type 1 diabetes, and evidence of an autoimmune response may be present up to 9 years before the onset of clinical symptoms (Bingley et al, 1993). Genetic susceptibility is a necessary precursor to the development of type 1 diabetes. Certain histocompatibility leukocyte antigen (HLA) genes are thought to play a role in the genetic inheritance of the tendency to develop type 1 diabetes. Individuals with type 1 diabetes have an increased frequency of HLA genes B8, B15, DR3, and DR4. The HLA-DR genes are known to be associated with autoimmunity. Evidence of autoimmunity is necessary but not sufficient for the development of type 1 diabetes. It is hypothesized that without genetic susceptibility, other factors will not initiate the autoimmune process. Other factors (e.g., host and environmental factors) may influence the development of the illness because the concordance rate is only 50% in identical twins. Such factors include age, race, stress, and infectious agents (Leslie & Elliot, 1994).

The genetic and pathologic processes leading to the development of type 2 diabetes are multiple and poorly defined. There is an interplay of genetic and environmental factors, with a significant hereditary component that appears to be polygenic. Although genetic predisposition exists, the following factors are associated with high risk: obesity—especially central obesity, sedentary lifestyle, diet high in fat and low in fiber, minority group, family history of type 2 diabetes, insulin resistance, puberty, and female gender (Fagot-Campagna et al,

2000; Pihoker et al, 1998). Those most likely to be affected include Native American, black, and Hispanic children (Fagot-Campagna et al, 2000). Peripheral insulin resistance is the primary metabolic defect associated with type 2 diabetes and is associated with hyperinsulinemia, glucose intolerance and dyslipidemia. Insulin resistance is also associated with acanthosis nigricans, a thickening and darkening of skin usually seen on the neck and axilla. Insulin resistance is considered an independent risk factor for the development of type 2 diabetes, hypertension, and atherosclerosis. The combination of obesity, insulin resistance, hypertension, dyslipidemia, and atherosclerosis is known as the insulin resistance syndrome, the metabolic syndrome, or syndrome X (Haffner, 1997; Reaven, 1993). In addition, insulin resistance is associated with polycystic ovary disease and is thereby associated with infertility.

Although the problem of insulin resistance and its relationship to obesity and other co-morbid conditions has been well established in adults, it is only recently that it has been described in substantial numbers of youth. A recent study of obese minority youth ages 5 to 10 years demonstrated a significant relationship between obesity and the presence of the insulin resistance syndrome, particularly in black girls (Young-Hyman et al, 2001). A comparison of type 1 and type 2 diabetes is shown in Box 23-1.

BOX 23-1

Comparison of Type 1 and Type 2 Diabetes in Youth

	Type 1 Diabetes	Type 2 Diabetes
Age	Throughout childhood	Puberty
Onset	Acute, severe	Mild to severe, often insidious
Insulin secretion	Very low	Variable
Insulin dependence	Permanent	Decreased
Genetics	Polygenic	Polygenic
Race/ethnic distribution	All (low frequency in Asians)	Blacks, Hispanics, Asians, Native Americans
Frequency (of all diabetes in children and youth)	60%-70%	30%-40%
Association		
Obesity	No	Strong
Acanthosis nigricans	No	Yes
Autoimmunity	Yes	No

Incidence and Prevalence

Type 1 diabetes mellitus is the most common metabolic disorder of childhood, affecting 0.17% of individuals younger than 20 years of age, or about 127,000 children in the United States (ADA, 2002b). Overall, the annual incidence of type 1 diabetes in the United States is approximately 18 new cases per 100,000 people under the age of 20 years, with a peak incidence at about 10 to 12 years of age in girls and 12 to 14 years in boys.

The true incidence and prevalence of type 2 diabetes in children are unknown. There have been no population-based studies to determine the true rate in the childhood population, but the prevalence has been estimated at between 2 and 50 per 1000 in various populations (Fagot-Campagna et al, 2000). Nonetheless, it is known that the incidence is on the rise, and because the disease is often silent, as many as twice the number of children diagnosed with type 2 may have the disease. In a recent report, Sinha and colleagues (2002) demonstrated that in a multiethnic cohort of obese children and adolescents who underwent oral glucose tolerance tests, 25% of the obese children and 21% of the obese adolescents had impaired glucose tolerance, and 4% had silent type 2 diabetes. The average age

of onset of type 2 diabetes in youth is 12 to 14 years, but cases have been reported in children as young as 5 years of age (Glaser, 1997).

Clinical Manifestations at Time of Diagnosis

Despite the fact that the autoimmune process may be long-standing before the diagnosis of type 1 diabetes is made, the signs and symptoms of type 1 diabetes are usually present for a short time. Once the autoimmune process has destroyed enough of the pancreatic beta, or islet, cells to produce clinical evidence of illness, the classic symptoms (i.e., polydipsia, polyuria, polyphagia) of diabetes occur. As shown in Figure 23-1, the lack of insulin production leads to disturbances in metabolism of carbohydrate, protein, and fat.

The hormone insulin, produced by the pancreatic beta cells (i.e., islets of Langerhans), is responsible for the use of glucose in the cell. In the absence of insulin, there are three general alterations, as follows: (1) reduced entry of glucose into the cell; (2) unavailability of carbohydrate as a substrate for energy needs; and (3) the cell's use of alternate substrates (i.e., fatty acids derived from adipose stores and amino acids from body

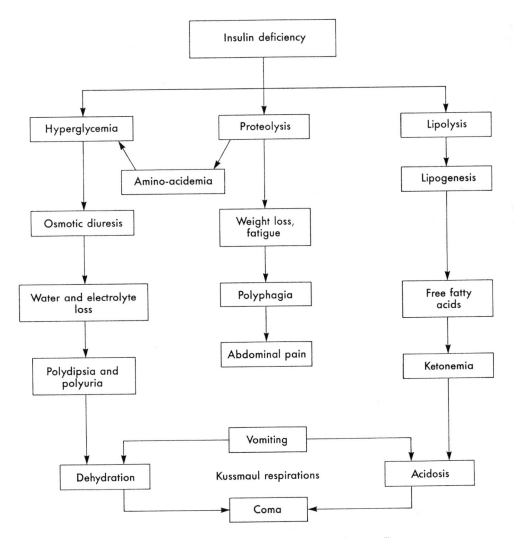

FIGURE 23-1 Signs and symptoms of type 1 diabetes mellitus.

BOX 23-2

Diagnostic Criteria

Classic symptoms of diabetes, including polydipsia, polyuria, polyphagia, and weight loss with random plasma glucose >200 mg/dl, *or*

Fasting plasma glucose level >126 mg/dl, *or*

One oral glucose tolerance test (OGTT) with the 2-hour plasma glucose >200 mg/dl, using 1.75 g/kg to maximum of 75-g glucose load

Data from American Diabetes Association. (2002). Clinical practice recommendations 2002. *Diabetes Care, 23*(suppl. 1), S5-S20.

protein). Thus when there is lack of insulin, glucose cannot be used in the cell for energy, and hyperglycemia results. The extraordinary concentration of glucose in the blood promotes an osmotic diuresis, so that large amounts of urine are produced. This osmotic diuresis is responsible for the symptom of polyuria, and as the body struggles to maintain homeostasis, polydipsia ensues.

If glucose is not available as a source of energy, alternative sources must be used. The body relies on lipolysis, as well as proteolysis. When this occurs, polyphagia becomes prominent as the body tries to avoid starvation. If these symptoms go uncorrected, the hyperglycemia and ketonemia secondary to increased lipolysis will progress to severe levels, and diabetic ketoacidosis will occur.

Unlike type 1 diabetes, the primary defect in type 2 diabetes is peripheral insulin resistance, with obesity and sedentary lifestyle contributing to its development. Initially, there is a compensatory increase in insulin secretion (Ferranninni & Camastra, 1998). There is also a decrease in the first-phase insulin response, and a state of chronic hyperglycemia ensues. In addition, there is inappropriate hepatic gluconeogenesis, causing fasting hyperglycemia. This further worsens peripheral insulin resistance and beta-cell dysfunction. Most affected individuals have marked peripheral insulin resistance with serum insulin levels high but insufficient to maintain normoglycemia (Callahan & Mansfield, 2000). Pancreatic beta-cell function eventually declines, and insulin secretion decreases. Because the onset of type 2 diabetes is gradual and insidious compared with type 1 diabetes, the disease may go undetected for months or years. Clinical manifestations that suggest type 2 diabetes include obesity and acanthosis nigricans, in addition to polydipsia and polyuria.

High-risk youth (those who are obese and have additional risk factors for type 2 diabetes, including a family history of type 2 diabetes) should be screened every 2 years beginning at age 10 years or at the onset of puberty if it occurs before age 10 years with a fasting plasma glucose or an oral glucose tolerance test. The criteria for diagnosis of diabetes are shown in Box 23-2. The child who meets the criteria for impaired glucose tolerance (or prediabetes) should be referred for intensive lifestyle management to prevent type 2 diabetes from developing. If symptoms of diabetes occur, they will be similar to those in type 1, including polyphagia, polydipsia, and polyuria.

The diagnosis of diabetes is easily established. Any children with the classic symptoms should have their levels of blood and urinary glucose and urine ketones determined. If the blood glucose level is more than 200 mg/dl, and symptoms of diabetes are present, the diagnosis of type 1 diabetes is established.

Alternatively, if fasting blood glucose (i.e., no calories in 8 hours before the test) is greater than or equal to 126 mg/dl or the 2-hour plasma glucose level is greater than or equal to 200 mg/dl on a glucose tolerance test, then the diagnosis is established (ADA, 2002a). The diagnosis of impaired glucose tolerance, or prediabetes, is established when there is an intermediate stage between normal glucose metabolism and diabetes. This stage includes people who have fasting glucose levels above 100 mg/dl but below 126 mg/dl (ADA, 2002a).

Type 2 diabetes can usually be differentiated from type 1 at diagnosis by the presence of obesity. In addition, insulin and C-peptide levels are elevated and there is an absence of antibodies to the pancreatic islet cell (antiinsulin, antityrosine phosphatases IA-2 and IA-2 [Borg et al, 2001], antiglutamic acid decarboxylase [GAD] antibodies) (ADA, 2002b). Further, separation of acute-onset diabetes with ketosis or frank ketoacidosis from insiduous-onset diabetes and cases of nonketotic severe hyperglycemia can be helpful. The child with new-onset diabetes whose glucose is above 750 to 1000 mg/dl in the absence of significant ketosis or ketoacidosis is unlikely to have type 1 diabetes.

Treatment

Type 1

Diabetes Control and Complications Trial (DCCT). The DCCT was a multicenter, randomized clinical trial designed to compare intensive diabetes therapy with conventional therapy to determine its effects on the development and progression of early vascular and neurologic complications of type 1 diabetes (DCCT Research Group, 1993a). A total of 1441 people aged 13 to 39 years with type 1 diabetes—726 of whom had no retinopathy at baseline and 715 of whom had mild retinopathy—were randomly assigned to intensive or conventional therapy. Intensive therapy consisted of insulin pump therapy (otherwise known as continuous subcutaneous insulin infusion [CSII]) or three or more injections per day of insulin with frequent blood glucose monitoring, with monthly visits and frequent telephone contacts; conventional therapy comprised one or two insulin injections per day. The goals of intensive therapy were to reduce glucose to the normal range and keep glycosylated hemoglobin in the normal range.

After 6.5 years, the study was terminated because the results were so impressive; in the group without retinopathy, the risk for developing it decreased 76% with intensive therapy, and in the secondary prevention group, the progression of retinopathy was slowed by 54%. Further, microalbuminuria was reduced by 39%, albuminuria by 54%, and clinical neuropathy by 60%. Intensive therapy, however, was associated with a twofold to threefold increase in severe hypoglycemia and clinically significant weight gain. Based on these findings, the researchers and the American Diabetes Association (ADA) recommended that for individuals with type 1 diabetes, "a primary treatment goal should be blood glucose control at least equal to that achieved in the intensively treated cohort" (ADA, 1993).

Among the 1441 people in the DCCT (1994) were 195 adolescents (i.e., 13 to 17 years of age at entry), 125 with no retinopathy and 70 with mild retinopathy. Because adolescents face unique issues compared with adult subjects with regard to

Treatment

TYPE 1
Insulin to achieve near-normal blood glucose
Diet sufficient for growth
Monitoring of blood sugars at least 4 times daily
Glycosylated hemoglobin to assess overall control

TYPE 2
Weight loss and maintenance
Diet lower in fat and calories
Decreased sedentary activity
Insulin or metformin

TABLE 23-1
Types and Actions of Insulin Preparations

Class/name	Approximate Action Curves (hr)		
	Onset	Peak	Duration
QUICK ACTING			
Insulin lispro	0.25	1	2-4
Insulin aspart	10-20 min	1-3	3-5
RAPID ACTING			
Regular	0.5-1	2-4	4-6
INTERMEDIATE ACTING			
NPH	1.5-2	6-12	18-24
Lente	1.5-2	6-12	16-24
LONG ACTING			
Ultralente	4-8	10-20	16-24
Glargine	1-2	None	24

diabetes, data on these subjects were analyzed separately. In contrast to the larger study group, the adolescents took longer to attain near-normal glycosylated hemoglobin (i.e., 6 to 12 months vs. 6 months at nadir). Nevertheless, similar positive results of intensive treatment were also found within this group: the risk of retinopathy, retinopathy progression, microalbuminuria, and clinical neuropathy decreased by 53% to 70%. Thus the DCCT Research Group (1994) recommends that most teens with diabetes be treated with intensive therapy because the potential for reduction of long-term complications was substantial. The research group also noted that the adolescents in the DCCT were the most difficult to manage and required the most time of the treatment team, but that the potential savings in suffering and long-term costs to young people with type 1 diabetes were considered worth the investment of treatment resources.

Since the release of the results of the DCCT, many diabetes providers recommend intensive therapy regimens to achieve the goals of treatment (i.e., to return the blood glucose levels to near normal and to prevent complications for most young people with diabetes) (Box 23-3) (ADA, 1999). The ADA (2002a) guidelines recommend the blood glucose level be normalized using intensive treatment regimens as the goal of treatment for children and adolescents. Insulin doses are often adjusted according to frequent blood glucose monitoring (i.e., at least four times per day), monitored dietary intake, and anticipated exercise. Treatment goals may be slightly more relaxed in children under 7 years of age because of the risk of severe hypoglycemia. The concern with severe hypoglycemia in young children is the effect of lowered blood sugar on brain development and functioning. These regimens require frequent and careful monitoring by the diabetes team (i.e., physician, nurse, dietitian, behaviorist) and are difficult to accomplish in a primary care setting.

Insulin Therapy. There are multiple approaches to providing insulin to children and adolescents with type 1 diabetes. The appropriate regimen should be determined by the child and the family. The available types of insulin shown in Table 23-1 can be combined to create a regimen that fits the child's lifestyle and the provider's and family's goals. Most children use genetically engineered human insulin preparations.

Insulin replacement results in a dramatic reversal of the disease symptoms. At diagnosis, most children are hospitalized—in part for correction of the metabolic derangement but

also for education in the management of the condition. Once any acidosis is corrected, subcutaneous treatment with insulin is the mainstay of therapy. Most children's diabetes is adequately controlled on an initial regimen of two injections of insulin per day: one before breakfast and one before the evening meal. These injections usually consist of rapid-acting and intermediate-acting insulin. Based on the blood glucose response, the dose is titrated to achieve blood glucose levels as close to normal as possible.

Shortly after the diagnosis is made, many children experience a sharp reduction in the insulin requirement. Commonly, the doses of rapid insulin are sharply reduced or discontinued during this time. Many children are well managed with two injections of intermediate-acting insulin, and some may not even require an evening injection. The insulin requirement eventually returns, and children should be cautioned that this "honeymoon period" (the duration of which is quite variable) does not indicate that the diabetes has gone away. Once destruction of the beta cells is complete—usually within 2 years of diagnosis—most children will require insulin replacement of approximately 1 unit/kg of body weight/day, although 2 or more units/kg of body weight may be necessary, particularly in adolescents.

Once the honeymoon is over, it is difficult to achieve optimal metabolic control without using intensive insulin regimens. Intensive regimens consist of three or more daily injections or the use of an insulin pump. Multiple daily injection (MDI) regimens usually consist of rapid or quick-acting insulin (regular, aspart, or lispro) before meals with intermediate insulin (NPH or Lente) or long-acting (Ultralente) insulin twice per day. Recently, a new, long-acting, 24-hour insulin called glargine was approved for children 6 years or older. This is a clear, peakless, basal insulin that is usually taken once per day. It cannot be mixed with other insulins and therefore needs to be taken as a separate injection. When glargine is used, quick-acting insulin is taken before each meal and large snack, based on the carbohydrate amount in the meal. Such regimens more closely mimic the body's normal response to a carbohydrate meal.

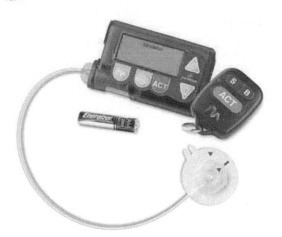

FIGURE 23-2 Example of an insulin pump used for continuous subcutaneous insulin infusion. (Courtesy of Medtronic MiniMed, Sylmar, Calif.)

Insulin pump therapy or CSII is the other option for intensive therapy (Figure 23-2). The pumps are battery powered and are about the size of a pager. A reservoir containing quick-acting insulin is inserted into the pump and connects to fine tubing that is connected to an infusion set that is inserted into the hip or the abdomen area every other day. There are multiple different infusion sets available for people to use. Many of the sets are inserted at a 90-degree angle, and others can be inserted at a 30- to 45-degree angle, which seems to work better for very young children and those with very little subcutaneous fat. These infusion sets are inserted with a spring-loaded device, making insertion quite easy for the parent or older child. They also have "quick-release" or disconnect mechanisms, allowing the pump to be easily removed for bathing or sports, while leaving the catheter in place under the skin.

The pump delivers small amounts of rapid-acting insulin at a basal rate that can be varied throughout the 24-hour day based on personal needs, and larger bolus doses are programmed in by the child or family to cover all meals and snacks. Bolus doses are varied based on the amount of carbohydrate in the planned meal or snack, current blood glucose level, and any anticipated exercise.

Over the past few years there have been many improvements in insulin pumps. They are smaller, the programming is simpler, they have more alarms, and some pumps have a "child lock" feature that can be set by parents to prevent younger children from inadvertently giving themselves an insulin dose. Although insulin pumps were used infrequently by children in the past, many more pediatric providers are recommending CSII therapy for children and adolescents. An earlier report in adolescents (Boland et al, 1999) showed that adolescents who used insulin pumps were able to achieve better metabolic control than those on multiple daily injection (MDI) regimens (glycosylated hemoglobin [Hb A_{1c}] levels 7.5% vs. 8.3%). Most impressive, the rate of severe hypoglycemia was 50% lower with CSII compared with MDI regimens. A later report by Ahern and colleagues (2002) demonstrated that pump treatment can be both safe and successful in the treatment of children with diabetes of all ages. These authors described the clinical outcomes of 161 children (26 preschoolers, 76 school-agers, 59 adolescents) who had used CSII for at least 12 months. There was a significant and consistent reduction in mean Hb A_{1c} (by 0.6% to 0.7%) and a 32% decrease in severe hypoglycemic events. Other reports in very young children have found that the use of CSII can greatly reduce the incidence of severe hypoglycemia (Tubiana-Rufi et al, 1996) and can also result in improved diabetes control and greater parent satisfaction (Buckingham et al, 2001) in this challenging age-group.

Diet and Exercise. Because replacement of insulin is not perfect, regulation of both diet and exercise helps to minimize variation in blood glucose levels. Routine exercise should be encouraged for all children, including those with type 1 diabetes. However, insulin doses often have to be adjusted, or an extra snack may be necessary to help prevent hypoglycemia that can occur with prolonged activity (see physical activity discussion under Primary Care Management).

Children with type 1 diabetes—unlike individuals with type 2 diabetes—are often slender. Therefore the goal of dietary therapy is to provide sufficient calories for normal growth and development. A meal plan based on an individual's usual intake pattern is used to integrate insulin therapy into typical eating and exercise patterns. Such a meal plan helps avoid hyperglycemia, prevent hypoglycemia, and maintain metabolic balance. Consistent with the current recommendations of the American Academy of Pediatrics, American and Canadian Diabetes Associations, and the American Dietetic Association, a meal plan should comprise 55% to 60% carbohydrate, 10% to 20% protein, and 10% to 20% fats, with less than 10% saturated fats. As discussed in the section below on diet, carbohydrate counting is an approach that allows for more flexibility in dietary management.

Daily caloric requirements can be estimated to be 1000 calories for the first year of life with approximately 100 calories added each year until age 10 to 12 years. Thereafter, unless they are exceptionally active on a regular basis, females may need their total calories reduced to the common adult level of 1400 to 1600 calories daily. Males, however, will continue to need approximately 2000 calories daily. Shortly after diagnosis, children may need an additional 200 to 700 kcal/day to make up the negative energy balance at diagnosis.

Glucose Monitoring. Maintenance of near-normal or normal blood glucose levels requires constant self-monitoring. Self-monitored blood glucose (SMBG) levels allow people with diabetes to have more precision in monitoring than with urine testing. Glucose is not found in the urine until the blood glucose level rises above the renal threshold (i.e., usually about 180 mg/dl). The goal of therapy is to maintain blood glucose levels from 80 to 120 mg/dl before meals and 100 to 140 mg/dl at bedtime (ADA, 2002a). Therefore self-monitoring of blood glucose levels lets children know exactly what the blood glucose level is at any moment and adjust the dose of insulin in response to their actual blood glucose level.

Most children are advised to test their blood at least four times daily, at various times throughout the day, and when symptoms are present. The results of SMBG testing are used to identify asymptomatic hypoglycemia, determine patterns in insulin action, and appropriately alter the insulin dose. For example, if a child consistently has high blood glucose levels before lunch, the morning intermediate-acting insulin (i.e.,

NPH or Lente) is increased to prevent this effect. If the child is using a glargine regimen, then the morning rapid-acting insulin may need to be increased to normalize the lunch values.

Monitoring by the Diabetes Treatment Team. Children and adolescents with diabetes are evaluated every 3 months by the diabetes treatment team. Quarterly visits correspond to the rate at which the glycosylated hemoglobin levels can be expected to change. Glycosylated hemoglobin (Hb A_{1c}) is a measure of the attachment of glucose to the circulating hemoglobin molecule. In individuals without diabetes, glycosylated hemoglobin comprises 3% to 6% of the total hemoglobin; those with diabetes, however, have levels in excess of 6% that vary in proportion to the blood glucose levels. The glycosylated hemoglobin level reflects the average blood glucose level over the most recent 3 months because the life span of the hemoglobin molecule is approximately 90 to 120 days. This level is not affected by short-term fluctuations and is considered to be an objective and accurate measure of long-term diabetes control (ADA, 2002a; Goldstein et al, 1995).

Type 2

Initial Treatment. At diagnosis, youth with type 2 diabetes may present with diabetic ketoacidosis, but it is much less common than with diabetes 1. They may need insulin initially to correct the metabolic derangement at diagnosis. Treatment with insulin, as with type 1, rapidly improves the symptoms of diabetes.

Lifestyle Intervention. The cornerstone of treatment for type 2 diabetes in youth, however, is intensive lifestyle intervention that focuses on decreasing adiposity, increasing activity, and behavioral adjustment. Demonstrable improvement in insulin sensitivity occurs with modest weight loss (Ludwig & Ebbeling, 2001). It is believed that modest weight loss or weight maintenance as a child grows, with improvement in physical fitness, can delay or prevent the need for pharmacologic treatment. Unfortunately, there have been few large-scale studies of this approach in children and adolescents. Trials on the reduction of obesity in children and youth suggest that interventions that incorporate nutritional counseling with a focus on decreasing fat and caloric density (Epstein et al, 1985; Stolley & Fitzgibbon, 1997), physical activity to increase lean muscle mass and decrease adiposity (Epstein et al, 1985; McMurray et al, 2000), and behavioral modification with goal setting and problem solving (Grey et al, 2002b) are more likely to succeed. Physical activity that decreases sedentary behavior and encourages aerobic activity is favored, especially activity that can be sustained over the long term. Long-term treatment is often necessary and difficult.

Pharmacologic Treatment. If lifestyle intervention fails, pharmacologic treatment is necessary. At one time, insulin was the only choice, but treatment with insulin was often counterproductive, since insulin promotes fat metabolism and children often gained more weight. Recently, metformin has been evaluated for safety and efficacy in children (Jones et al, 2002), and it has recently been approved for use in children (Jones, 2002). Metformin improves metabolic control by reducing hepatic glucose production, increasing insulin sensitivity, and reducing intestinal glucose absorption, without increasing insulin secretion. Metformin has been found to significantly improve

metabolic control compared with placebo, and it does not have a negative effect on body weight or lipid profiles. Further, adverse events (mostly gastrointestinal symptoms, especially diarrhea) were consistent with adverse events reported with adults (Jones et al, 2002).

Once there is beta-cell failure in late type 2 diabetes, metformin will no longer be effective, and insulin becomes the only effective treatment. As with type 1 diabetes, all treatments must be monitored with blood glucose monitoring and quarterly glycosylated hemoglobin and weight measurements.

Complementary and Alternative Therapies

Type 1. Although insulin is necessary for the treatment of type 1 diabetes , there is some suggestion that additional behavioral biofeedback assisted relaxation may help improve glucose control (McGrady et al, 1991). The rationale behind this is that stress in itself can raise glucose levels, and therefore therapies aimed at decreasing stress may help overall glucose control.

Type 2. Whereas complementary therapies such as hypnosis are commonly used by adults with diabetes to achieve weight loss, there is little in the literature about their use in children and adolescents. The mineral chromium has been studied in adults for weight loss and control of type 2 diabetes with mixed results (Althius et al, 2002), but there have not been studies in children. Families also may resort to fad diets, such as the Atkins diet, in an attempt to help their children with type 2 diabetes lose weight.

Anticipated Advances in Diagnosis and Management

The Diabetes Prevention Trial—Type 1 (DPT-1) is currently being conducted in the United States. All consenting first-degree relatives of people with type 1 diabetes are being screened to see if they are at risk for developing the disease in the next 5 years. Any relatives who test positively are asked to have more specific testing, including glucose tolerance testing and HLA typing. Individuals found to be at significant risk of developing type 1 diabetes are asked to participate in a randomized clinical trial to determine if small doses of Ultralente insulin, administered twice daily for a total dose of 0.25 units/ kg/day, will prevent onset of the disease. Individuals found to be at a smaller risk for the development of type 1 diabetes are asked to participate in a randomized trial to determine if oral insulin will prevent the onset of diabetes. The trial was based on animal and human studies with small samples that suggest that small doses of insulin may protect the pancreatic beta cells from the destruction associated with type 1 diabetes by preventing the autoimmune process from proceeding. The study group recently reported their results for the parenteral insulin study (Diabetes Prevention Trial—Type 1 Diabetes Study Group, 2002); parenteral insulin at these doses did not prevent or delay the onset of type 1 diabetes. The oral insulin study is still under way.

In addition, researchers are developing artificial insulin delivery systems and transplantation of beta cells as new methods of treatment. The artificial insulin delivery systems will improve on the CSII by incorporating a feedback loop that will alter the insulin delivered according to the blood glucose level. Transplantation of beta cells or the whole pancreas results in a cure for people with diabetes who are already taking immunosuppressants for previous organ transplants (Sutherland & Gruessner, 1997). The remaining challenge is to prevent autoimmune destruction of these cells in individuals who are not immunosuppressed. More recently, there has been success with islet cell transplantation for people with labile diabetes (Edmonton protocol). These people received immunosuppressive therapy as well, and insulin independence was obtained for 11 of 12 adults studied (Ryan et al, 2001). Further research to determine effective, safe immunosuppressive therapies is needed, since islet cell transplantation may indeed be an eventual cure for type 1 diabetes.

New insulin delivery systems are also being tested. Data from a recent trial of inhaled insulin presented at the ADA meeting in 2002 suggested that adults and adolescents can achieve control similar to conventional therapy with a regimen of inhaled insulin with meals and intermediate-acting insulin to cover nighttime insulin needs (Skyler, 2002). Implantable insulin pumps that deliver insulin intraperitoneally have also been used in adults but not yet in children (Dunn et al, 1997).

One of the most exciting areas of new research in diabetes treatment has been in continuous glucose sensor technology. Two different devices that measure interstitial glucose continuously have been approved by the US Food and Drug Administration (FDA). The first to be approved was the Continuous Glucose Monitoring System (CGMS) developed by Medtronic MiniMed. The CGMS sensor is a platinum electrode inside a semipermeable matrix containing glucose oxidase. The sensor is inserted through a needle into the subcutaneous tissue in the abdominal or buttocks area, using a spring-loaded device, and then the needle is removed. The glucose oxidase in the sensor catalyzes the oxidation of glucose in the interstitial fluid, generating an electric current. A thin cable carries the current to a pager-size monitor. The monitor analyzes data every 10 seconds and reports average values every 5 minutes. The sensor readings are calibrated against four finger stick measurements that are entered into the meter by the individual. The CGMS does not give the person immediate glucose readings. Instead, sensor values are stored and later downloaded to a computer for analysis by the clinician once the sensor has been removed.

The other FDA-approved glucose sensor device is the Glucowatch Biographer developed by Cygnus. It looks like a watch and is worn on the forearm, 3 or more inches from the wrist or elbow joint. An adhesive pad incorporating two hydrogel disks attaches the device to the skin. Each disk is the size of a dime (Tamada et al, 1999). A triple A battery from the biographer sends a small current through the disks to pull glucose from the interstitial fluid underneath the skin. The glucose in the interstitial fluid is then measured. The maximal current used is very small. The biographer model most recently approved by the FDA for both children and adults (Glucowatch 2 Biographer) gives up to six readings per hour for 13 hours. Individuals can read glucose values displayed on the biographer. It also has a high- and low-glucose alarm that can be set by the user for certain glucose levels of their choice (e.g., less than 70 mg/dl and/or more than 300 mg/dl). A 2-hour warm-up time followed by a single glucose meter value is needed to calibrate the device. People who wear the biographer may develop erythema

and a localized skin reaction to the adhesive used to secure the watch to the skin or to the hydrogel pads themselves.

Although the accuracy of the biographer has been established (Garg et al, 1999), FDA approval does not allow for immediate changes in therapy to be made based on the biographer results. Instead, a finger stick glucose measurement should be done when alarms go off.

The ability to continuously monitor glucose levels, particularly at night, will enable clinicians to maximize the benefits of insulin delivery systems, allowing for safer therapy for children. For example, use of the CGMS in more than 50 well-controlled children and adolescents revealed unexpected nighttime hypoglycemia and postprandial hyperglycemia (Boland et al, 2001). These occurrences had not been depicted with routine glucose monitoring. Further, devices with both hyperglycemic and hypoglycemic alarms will allow clinicians to better use intensive therapy in children while minimizing the risks of hypoglycemia. Even more exciting is the possibility of combining sensor technology with insulin pump delivery systems. We may finally be at the threshold of the development of a true artificial pancreas, something that has been anticipated for more than 25 years (Albisser et al, 1974).

New pharmacologic treatments for type 2 diabetes are currently being evaluated in children. Another class of insulin sensitizers, the glitizones, has not yet been evaluated for safety and efficacy in children but are expected to be soon. Further, advances in the treatment of obesity will likely affect treatment for type 2 diabetes in children and adolescents as well.

Associated Problems (Box 23-4)
Diabetic Ketoacidosis and Hypoglycemia

Figure 23-1 shows the physiologic process that results in diabetic ketoacidosis (DKA) when there is a lack of insulin. Any potential stressor (e.g., illness, fever, injury, psychosocial stress) can increase the risk of metabolic derangement caused by disturbances in counterregulatory hormones and lead to DKA. Thus any stressor in a child with diabetes must be managed with care.

BOX 23-4
Associated Problems

	Type 1	Type 2
Diabetic ketoacidosis	Yes	Yes
Nonketotic severe hyperglycemia	No	Yes
Hypoglycemia	Yes, in both when Rx with insulin	
Monilial vaginitis	Yes, in both if poorly controlled	
Cardiovascular complications:		
Hyperlipidemia	Yes	Common
Hypertension	Yes	Common
Complications associated with:		
Renal failure	Yes	Yes
Eye degeneration	Yes	Yes
Neuropathies	Yes	Yes
Polycystic ovary syndrome	No	Yes
Depression/psychosocial problems	Yes	Yes

Comparison of Hyperglycemia and Hypoglycemia

DIABETIC KETOACIDOSIS (HYPERGLYCEMIA)
Slow onset
Increased thirst and urination
High blood and urine glucose levels
Urinary ketones
Weakness and abdominal pain
Heavy, labored breathing
Anorexia
Nausea and vomiting
Candidal infections

HYPOGLYCEMIA
Rapid onset
Excessive sweating
Fainting
Headache
Trembling and shaking
Hunger
Unable to wake
Irritability
Personality change

It should be noted that children with type 2 diabetes can present with DKA, but once the diabetes has stabilized after diagnosis, DKA is rare in these children. What can occur is nonketotic severe hyperglycemia (HGNK). HGNK is usually associated with significant dehydration and is characterized by very high plasma glucose levels (>750 mg/dl) without ketosis or ketoacidosis. Treatment with intravenous hydration and insulin is required.

Children with well-controlled diabetes will occasionally experience episodes of hypoglycemia, especially when treated with insulin. Because the symptoms of hyperglycemia and hypoglycemia can sometimes be confused, they are compared in Box 23-5. Hypoglycemia may be caused by too much insulin, too little food, too much exercise, or a combination of these. Although hypoglycemia is easily treated, prevention is the best approach. Again, SMBG determination is helpful. With SMBG testing, children can identify patterns of lower blood glucose levels that may indicate periods of increased risk. During these periods, the insulin dose can be altered to prevent the hypoglycemia. If a child anticipates unusual physical activity, both insulin and diet can be adjusted to prevent low glucose levels. Hypoglycemia can occur with the sulfonylureas, an older treatment for type 2 diabetes. Changing to metformin is associated with a lower incidence of hypoglycemia in people with type 2 diabetes.

Hypoglycemia presents particular problems at different ages. Infants and toddlers are unable to express the feelings associated with hypoglycemia, so they must be observed for listlessness, sleepiness, or irritability. Parents should be instructed that unusual behavior at any time is an indication for blood glucose levels to be measured. If the result is less than 70 mg/dl, a conscious infant should be given 2 to 4 oz of sweet liquids or a small amount of cake frosting and an unconscious or convulsing infant should be given 0.25 to 0.5 ml of glucagon

by injection. Older children can be taught the symptoms of hypoglycemia and how to prevent its occurrence. They should also be instructed to carry high-sugar foods with them at all times. All children with diabetes should wear medical identification so that they can be diagnosed and treated appropriately if they lose consciousness while away from home. In the DCCT, intensive regimens were associated with a threefold increase in the incidence of severe hypoglycemia (DCCT Research Group, 1995), so extra care must be taken by children on intensive regimens.

Some substances can increase the likelihood of hypoglycemia. Adolescents need to know that alcohol augments the glucose-lowering effects of insulin and that the symptoms of alcohol intoxication and hypoglycemia are similar. Low blood glucose levels can increase the body's sensitivity to alcohol, and many experimenting teenagers have found themselves in the emergency room with profound hypoglycemia. Stimulants such as amphetamines and cocaine may increase metabolism and decrease appetite, so hypoglycemia may occur.

Candidal Infections

Once healthy girls are toilet trained, monilial infections of the perineum are rare until adolescence, when the effects of estrogen on the vagina provide a potential environment for growth of *Candida*. Hyperglycemia also leads to increased glucose levels in vaginal secretions, which provides an ideal medium for *Candida*. Thus girls with poorly controlled diabetes are at increased risk for monilial vaginitis; any complaint of vaginal discharge and itching should be investigated with a potassium hydroxide preparation and treated appropriately.

Cardiovascular Complications

Hyperlipidemia and hypertension are common in youth with type 2 diabetes. Blood pressure should be obtained at every quarterly visit and recorded. Blood lipids (total cholesterol, low-density lipoproteins [LDL], high-density lipoproteins [HDL], triglycerides) should be measured yearly in all youths with type 2 diabetes. Although there have been few studies of children with type 2 diabetes and hyperlipidemia, aggressive treatment is recommended.

Polycystic Ovaries

Insulin resistance and type 2 diabetes are also associated with polycystic ovary syndrome in girls. This disorder is associated with increased ovarian or adrenal androgen production. Symptoms include menstrual irregularities and evidence of hyperandrogenism, especially hirsutism. Girls with polycystic ovary disease should be referred to a reproductive endocrinologist for follow-up. Treatment with low-dose birth control pills along with insulin sensitizers may be necessary.

Long-Term Complications

Little has been known until recently about the long-term complications of type 2 diabetes in youth. Unfortunately, recent data suggest that complications follow the same rapid trajectory as in adults. This risk is true because those with type 2 diabetes also have hyperinsulinemia and obesity, both risk factors for cardiovascular disease. Dean & Flett (2002) recently reported that in a population of Native American young people who developed type 2 diabetes in youth, complications such as renal disease, microvascular and macrovascular disease, and retinopathy were already present when the youths were in their early 20s. Thus the recommendations of the United Kingdom Prospective Diabetes Study (UKPDS) (Clarke et al, 2001) to aggressively treat both glucose control and blood pressure control are accepted as the current standards for management of type 2 diabetes in youth.

Depression and Other Psychosocial Complications

For the most part, it is accepted that type 1 diabetes is a risk factor for adolescent psychiatric disorder (Kovacs et al, 1997). Approximately three times more adolescents with diabetes have psychiatric disorders than their age-mates, with rates as high as 33% (Blanz et al, 1993). This increased morbidity is primarily associated with the incidence of major depression (approximately 27.5%) and generalized anxiety disorder (18.4%), rather than psychiatric behavioral disorders (Kovacs et al, 1997). A substantial number of adolescents with diabetes consider suicide after the onset of the disease. The rate of suicidal ideation has been found to be higher than would be expected (26.4%), but in contrast, the number of suicide attempts was only 4.4%, a rate comparable to the general population of adolescents (Goldston et al, 1997). In addition, adolescents who have recurrent DKA may be more likely to have psychiatric disorders, especially anxiety and depression, than those without recurrent hospitalization (Liss et al, 1998).

Whereas a smaller percentage of adolescents with diabetes manifest significant psychiatric problems, many have difficulty in psychosocial adjustment. The presence of diabetes in adolescence may hinder normal adolescent development by limiting the development of independence. One study examined the personal meaning and perceived impact of diabetes on 54 adolescents and found that youths felt that diabetes controlled or limited their freedom and independence (Kyngas & Barlow, 1995). Girls have been found to report more symptoms of anxiety and depression related to these restrictions and to be in worse metabolic control than boys (LaGreca et al, 1995). Interventions such as coping skills training (Grey et al, 2000) and parent-child conflict reduction (Anderson et al, 1999) may be helpful in reducing these problems. Appropriate referral to behavioral treatment should not be delayed if problems in adjustment are suspected.

Obesity in youth is associated with body dissatisfaction and lower self-esteem (Caldwell, Brownell & Wilfley, 1997; Strauss, 2000), altered body image (Kolody & Sallis, 1995; Thompson et al, 1995), decreasing preference for physical activity (Kolody & Sallis, 1995), self-efficacy for activity (Kolody & Sallis, 1995), and depression (Falkner et al, 2001). Although studies of the psychosocial consequences of type 2 diabetes in youth are just beginning, there is every reason to believe that the consequences of type 2 will be similar to those found in type 1 and in obesity.

Prognosis

Diabetes is the sixth leading cause of death in the United States (ADA, 2002b). Children with diabetes at the age of 10 years can expect to live until the age of 54 years, but their peers without diabetes can expect to live to the age of 72 years (ADA, 2002b). For the most part, this early mortality is a result of the long-term complications of the illness. However, because diabetes treatment and technology continue to improve, and because people with diabetes are managed more aggressively since the DCCT was completed, there is hope that children diagnosed after DCCT will have fewer long-term complications and therefore may have a better prognosis.

Complications can range from asymptomatic mild proteinuria to blindness, renal failure, painful neuropathies, cardiovascular disease, and death. Hyperglycemia is a necessary—but not sufficient—factor for the development of complications. In addition to hyperglycemia, genetic factors seem to influence the development of complications. Epidemiologic evidence suggests that the prevalence of microvascular complications is relatively high in the general population with diabetes, with approximately 40% of affected individuals experiencing renal failure and 50% having diabetic retinopathy after 15 years (ADA, 2002b). Although the DCCT showed that improvement in metabolic control to near normal levels delays the onset or progression of complications, complications were not eliminated. It is clear, however, that the better the metabolic control, the better the chance of avoiding complications.

PRIMARY CARE MANAGEMENT

Health Care Maintenance
Growth and Development

Because type 1 diabetes is a metabolic disorder affecting carbohydrate metabolism, growth and sexual development may be slowed. Children and adolescents whose diabetes is less well controlled may fail to grow normally. Therefore accurate measurement of height and weight and comparison with growth norms are imperative.

Even when children have normal linear growth, there may be delays in the onset and progression of puberty if glycemic control is inadequate. At each visit, Tanner stages should be assessed and recorded. Any deviation from the normal pattern should be investigated. In girls, menarche may be delayed. Loss of regular menses once cycling has been established may indicate a further degeneration in diabetic control and should be investigated.

Obesity can occur in children and adolescents with type 1 diabetes, especially in those on intensive regimens. In the DCCT, intensive therapy was associated with a 73% higher risk of becoming overweight (DCCT Research Group, 1995). Management of this obesity should be done carefully, with attention to the need to maintain self-monitoring, because glucose levels may change dramatically when a weight loss diet is followed.

Adolescents who manipulate weight by overeating or reducing or omitting insulin are another concern. Some adolescent girls with type 1 diabetes engage in insulin withholding to maintain body shape or lose weight (Pollock et al, 1995). Researchers have studied the incidence of eating disorders in adolescents with type 1 diabetes with conflicting results. Some have found that adolescents with diabetes are at higher risk for eating disorders than those without diabetes (Polonsky et al,

TABLE 23-2
Dietary Exchange System

Food Exchange	Approximate Content in g/Serving			
	Calories	Carbohydrate	Protein	Fat
Fruit	60	12	0	0
Starch	68	15	2	0
Milk				
Whole	170	12	8	10
Skim	90	12	8	Trace
Meat				
Lean	55	0	7	3
Medium fat	75	0	7	5
High fat	95	0	7	8
Fat	45	0	0	5
Free	0	Negligible	0	0

1994), but others have not found differences between the two groups of adolescents (Striegel-Moore et al, 1992). Nevertheless, alterations in insulin dosage may affect an adolescent's ability to grow and develop normally and should be considered in evaluation of children with growth difficulties.

In type 2 diabetes, obesity is often associated with early puberty as well as accelerated linear growth. Height and weight should be measured at each visit and body mass index (BMI) calculated. BMI should be plotted and followed as an indicator of the effectiveness of treatment. Tanner staging should be completed at each visit, and unusually rapid progression should be noted and a referral made.

Diet

Although insulin therapy is the cornerstone of treatment for type 1 diabetes, a dietary plan is important in maintaining near-normoglycemia without wide swings in blood glucose levels. Long-term adherence to the dietary plan is probably the most difficult aspect of management for families.

Many meal plans are based on the exchange system. Current exchange lists can be obtained from the ADA (see Resources at the end of this chapter), but the basic components are listed in Table 23-2. There are six food groups, including a "free" group. Within the groups, the nutritional composition of a serving of different foods is relatively constant. For example, in the starch category, one exchange is one slice of bread, 1/2 cup of white rice, or one medium baked potato. This system helps families learn portion sizes and healthy childhood nutrition.

All dietary management plans for type 1 diabetes have the goal of providing adequate calories and nutrients for normal growth and maintaining blood glucose as normal as possible. The consistency of daily intake with regular meals and snacks is important. Families, in consultation with the diabetes team, should select the appropriate meal plan because they are in the best position to judge the approach that will work. Imposing a rigid approach on an unwilling family only leads them to deviate from the diet. In addition, most children will not adhere without question to a diet perceived as different from that of peers. Thus primary care providers must be understanding in their approach and work with families to ensure as much dietary consistency as possible.

The two approaches to dietary management most commonly used with children are the ADA exchange lists and carbohydrate counting. With the ADA exchange lists, the goal is for children to have adequate calories for growth that are distributed appropriately over the day and through the food groups. This dietary plan should be developed with the child and parents so that usual routines and favorite foods can be incorporated.

Carbohydrate counting is used most frequently by those on intensive regimens (DCCT Research Group, 1993b). This method provides more flexibility in the diet by providing for varying amounts of carbohydrates at meals and snacks with appropriate coverage with rapid-acting insulin. Protein and fat intake is not controlled, but efforts to stay within low-fat guidelines are encouraged. For example, adolescents who choose to eat a second sandwich at lunch (i.e., 30 g extra carbohydrate in the bread) may need to take 5 to 10 units of rapid-acting insulin before the meal, depending on their regimen.

The wide availability of artificially sweetened foods and drinks has eased some of the difficulties children with diabetes faced in following the meal plan. Parents sometimes express concern, however, that extensive use of artificial sweeteners will be problematic for their children. There are three nonnutritive sweeteners approved for use by the FDA in the United States: saccharine, aspartame, and acesulfame K. For these and all other additives, the FDA determines an acceptable daily intake (ADI; i.e., the amount that can be safely consumed on a daily basis over a person's lifetime without any adverse effects), which includes a 100-fold safety factor. Average intake is actually much less than the acceptable daily intake. For example, the average aspartame consumption in the general population (i.e., including children) is 2 to 3 mg/kg/day or approximately 4% of the US ADI of 50 mg/kg.

As noted above, dietary management is the cornerstone of treatment for type 2 diabetes. A multidisciplinary approach involving dietary modification, increased physical activity, decreased sedentary time, and behavioral therapy offers the best hope for a successful outcome. Traditional dietary approaches have emphasized individualization and reduction in dietary fat intake. In addition, reducing calories from sodas and fruit drinks can be helpful. Often the dietary approach is based on the same exchange system described above, with reductions of 200 to 500 calories per day to achieve weight loss.

Physical activity is to be encouraged for all children. Regular exercise and active participation in organized sports have positive effects on both the psychosocial and physical well-being of children with type 1 diabetes. Parents and their children should be advised that different types of exercise may have different effects on blood glucose levels. For example, sports that involve short bursts of activity may increase glucose levels, whereas a more prolonged activity is more likely to decrease blood glucose levels. Parents and their children also need to be warned that a prolonged session of physical activity during the day may lead to hypoglycemia while the child is sleeping during the night, and therefore an extra bedtime snack or a change in the evening insulin may be necessary.

For children with type 2 diabetes, physical activity is strongly encouraged to enhance weight management. Activities that decrease sedentary behavior and increase aerobic capacity

(McMurray et al, 2000) have been demonstrated to lower insulin and glucose levels. Further, physical activity should be aimed at establishing life-long habits, rather than participation in youth sports alone. Encouraging families to participate in activities together may help to establish an exercise habit.

Safety

The safety issues faced by families with a child or adolescent with diabetes are twofold. As discussed earlier, hypoglycemia is a significant risk for all affected children receiving insulin, so families and others in a child's social sphere should be prepared to respond appropriately. Children should wear medical identification so proper treatment can be instituted quickly. Older children need to know how to prevent severe hypoglycemia, especially when exercising. Children should be taught to eat a snack of complex carbohydrate and protein (i.e., peanut butter and crackers) before exercise, to avoid injecting insulin into an exercising muscle, and to carry glucose with them at all times. Further, the use of uncooked corn starch in convenient snack bars (i.e., Extend Bar) has been advocated for a preexercise snack or a bedtime snack by some diabetes clinicians. The rationale for this is that uncooked corn starch is a complex carbohydrate that is slowly hydrolyzed by the enzyme amylase so that it is slowly absorbed by the gastrointestinal tract. When traveling or on school day trips, children or their parents should carry the supplies with them—not in checked baggage—and always have food available in case a meal is delayed. Airlines require insulin and syringes to be carried in the box with the pharmacy label to bring them on board an airplane.

Parents or caretakers of children with type 1 diabetes must learn to treat episodes of severe hypoglycemia with glucagon. Glucagon is the antagonist hormone to insulin and releases glycogen from the liver. When a child or adolescent cannot take sugar by mouth, glucagon is administered by intramuscular injection to rapidly raise the blood glucose level. The dose for infants or toddlers is 0.5 mg (0.5 ml), and the dose for older children is 1 mg (1.0 ml).

Another important safety issue is the proper disposal of syringes. Children and parents must be taught the importance of proper disposal of syringes to reduce the risk of injury to themselves and others.

For youths with type 2 diabetes taking oral medications, care should be taken to ensure that medications are taken as prescribed. As with all medications, safety containers should be used so that young children do not accidentally ingest them. Should an accidental ingestion occur, children should be watched for hypoglycemia and a poison control center should be contacted.

Immunizations

Children and adolescents with diabetes should follow the immunization schedule—including vaccines for hepatitis A and B and varicella—recommended by the American Academy of Pediatrics. Children with diabetes are potentially at an increased risk for developing complicated influenza illness; therefore they may benefit from yearly influenza vaccination after the age of 6 months (American Academy of Pediatrics, 2002). Some providers also recommend that youths with diabetes receive the pneumococcal vaccine, but with improved metabolic control, there is less risk for infection.

Screening

Vision. Vision screening is particularly important in children with diabetes because visual problems are common. A small number of children develop cataracts early in the course of the illness; therefore observing the normalcy of the red reflex during the ophthalmic examination is very important. Fluctuations in blood glucose levels can also affect visual acuity. Children experiencing hypoglycemia may complain of visual disturbances, and those with hyperglycemia may also complain of blurred vision. Thus it is important to relate the results of routine visual screening to the level of metabolic control, because improvement in metabolic control may improve the results of the visual testing.

Parents and children are often most concerned about the risk of diabetic retinopathy. Retinopathy of diabetes is the leading cause of blindness. Therefore the ADA (2002b) recommends that funduscopic examination be performed in individuals with diabetes at each primary care visit. Further, an annual examination with dilation by a pediatric ophthalmologist is recommended for children over 12 years of age who have had diabetes for at least 5 years. Since type 2 diabetes may have been present for some time before it is diagnosed, dilated retinal examination should be done at the time of diagnosis and then yearly.

Hearing. Routine screening is recommended.

Dental. Routine screening is recommended. If metabolic control is poor, children may experience increased dental caries and gingivitis because of increased glucose in saliva. Thus those with poorer control should have frequent dental screening and appropriate treatment.

Blood Pressure. Screening should be performed at each visit. Hypertension has been reported in up to 45% of all individuals with diabetes. Thus the ADA (2002a) recommends that orthostatic measurements be performed and recorded routinely. Aggressive blood pressure control may significantly improve the long-term outcome for youths with both type 1 and type 2 diabetes. Current treatment guidelines suggest that the use of angiotensin converting enzyme (ACE) inhibitors to achieve and maintain normotension may improve the risk for microvascular kidney complications (Clarke et al, 2001).

Hematocrit. Routine screening is recommended.

Urinalysis. Screening is performed yearly, with examination for levels of ketones, glucose, and protein. After 5 years of type 1 diabetes or after puberty, total urinary protein excretion should be measured yearly by the microalbuminuria method to screen for renal complications. If proteinuria is detected, serum creatinine clearance or blood urea nitrogen concentration should be measured and glomerular filtration assessed. In youth with type 2 diabetes, screening should be done at diagnosis and yearly thereafter.

Tuberculosis. Routine screening is recommended.

Condition-Specific Screening

Lipids. Individuals with both type 1 and type 2 diabetes are at risk for disorders of lipid metabolism, and these disorders may increase the risk of macrovascular complications. Children

Differential Diagnosis

Stressors, including illness, can lead to diabetic ketoacidosis (DKA).
Illness requires "sick day" management.
It is important to maintain hydration during illness.
Vaginal discharge may be candidal infection.
Skin manifestations may require referral.
Weight loss may indicate poor metabolic control.
Gastroparesis may be the cause of prolonged vomiting.

Indications for Evaluation by a Health Care Provider

Vomiting for more than 6 hours or more than 5 diarrheal stools in 1 day
Any change in mental status
Syncope
Temperature >38.9° C (102° F) for 12 hours
Blood glucose levels more than 400 mg/dl twice
Moderate or high ketone levels that do not decrease with extra insulin intake
Dysuria or other symptoms of urinary tract infection
Decreased urinary output

with type 1 diabetes should be screened with blood lipid profiles yearly after puberty. If a child has other risk factors or has type 2 diabetes, lipid screening should begin earlier, as is true for children without diabetes.

Thyroid. Because type 1 diabetes is an autoimmune disease, it is associated with other autoimmune diseases—especially Hashimoto thyroiditis. Children and adolescents who show any change in growth pattern or develop signs and symptoms of hypothyroidism (e.g., fatigue, dry skin, constipation) or hyperthyroidism (e.g., heat intolerance, tremor, diarrhea) should be tested with thyroid function studies (i.e., triiodothyronine, thyroxine, and thyroid-stimulating hormone levels).

Common Illness Management

Differential Diagnosis (Box 23-6)

Management of Vomiting and Diarrhea and Prevention of Diabetic Ketoacidosis. Provided that their diabetes is under reasonable metabolic control, children and adolescents with diabetes are not at higher risk than their peers for most common infectious diseases of childhood. Because any stressor may lead to DKA in a child with type 1 diabetes, infections and other stressors must be managed with care.

Regardless of the insult, there are several important principles for management. The need to continue to take insulin even when unable to eat a normal diet is of utmost importance because the excess of counterregulatory hormones released in response to the stressor will more than offset the decreased oral intake. Thus even though dietary intake may be decreased, insulin requirement may be increased.

The principles of management include monitoring parameters of control, maintaining hydration, preventing hypoglycemia, and preventing DKA or HGNK. For these principles to work effectively, it is imperative that the child and family know that any illness or insult involving fever, gastrointestinal symptoms, congestion in the head or chest, or urinary symptoms should be managed as a sick day. Once a day is identified as a sick day, the usual rules for self-monitoring are altered to reflect the need for closer monitoring. Blood glucose levels should be tested every 1 to 4 hours, and individuals with blood glucose levels greater than 200 mg/dl should test their urine for ketones. Blood glucose levels of more than 400 mg/dl on two determinations and moderate or high ketone levels in the urine that do not decrease with additional insulin should be viewed as an indication that the child should be seen and evaluated by either the primary care provider or the specialist.

Maintaining hydration is important to help clear extra glucose and ketones, and hydration must be carefully monitored if vomiting or diarrhea is present. If children cannot eat their usual diet, a large fluid intake should be maintained. In adolescents, this amount should be more than 8 oz of fluid hourly. Such fluids should contain adequate amounts of carbohydrate (i.e., 50 to 75 g in 6 to 8 hours) to maintain the usual caloric intake. Children often drink regular (i.e., not diet) sodas or flavored gelatin water or suck on ice pops when ill. If a child is vomiting or has diarrhea, broth or electrolyte solutions help replace sodium losses.

A child with type 1 may need additional insulin to prevent DKA, and a child with type 2 may need insulin to treat DKA or to prevent HGNK. If the blood glucose level is greater than 300 mg/dl, the family should generally administer the usual dose of insulin and add up to 20% of the total daily dose as rapid-acting insulin every 4 hours. Such management should be undertaken in careful consultation with the child's diabetes team. Recent studies have shown that treatment with the rapid-acting insulin lispro during ketosis and hyperglycemia may result in quicker correction than with conventional rapid-acting insulin (Attia et al, 1998).

Box 23-7 lists the indications for which children or adolescents should be seen and evaluated. Most important is the need for children with any alteration in mental status to be evaluated. Primary care providers should never assume that sleepiness in children with diabetes is merely the result of the fatigue associated with an illness.

Vaginal Discharge. Young women with diabetes are prone to candidal infections when glucose control is inadequate. Treatment with an antifungal agent is warranted in young girls if vaginal discharge with itching exists without evidence of other sexual activity. If there has been sexual contact of any kind, the vagina should be examined, and testing for other infections (e.g., *Chlamydia*) should be performed.

Other Skin Manifestations. Children and adolescents with diabetes may develop skin lesions associated with diabetes (e.g., necrobiosis diabeticorum). If these scaly lesions develop—usually on extensor surfaces—treatment by a dermatologist is warranted.

Acanthosis Nigricans. Acanthosis nigricans is a marker for insulin resistance. If acanthosis is present, the child should be referred for oral glucose tolerance testing and appropriate treatment. Girls with polycystic ovary disease are often hirsute.

Referral to a reproductive endocrinologist and treatment with low-dose estrogen birth control pills will often correct the hirsutism.

Weight Loss. The most common cause of weight loss in youth with type 1 diabetes is worsening metabolic control. Therefore evaluation of weight loss should include assessment of overall glucose control. If control is inadequate and attempts to improve control are not successful, then deliberate withholding of insulin for weight control should be investigated. Individuals with diabetes may also develop bulimic characteristics as a method of weight control, but vomiting and abdominal distress in youth with long-standing diabetes may also be a symptom of diabetic gastroparesis. Evaluation for gastroparesis includes radiographic gastric emptying studies that should be done under the direction of a specialist.

Drug Interactions

Many over-the-counter medications and antibiotics contain glucose, and some contain alcohol or traces of gluconeogenic substances, such as sorbitol or glycerine (Kumar et al, 1991). In the amounts usually ingested, these compounds may raise blood glucose levels slightly but should not markedly impair metabolic control.

Developmental Issues

Sleep Patterns

Children with diabetes who are in good control should have no problems sleeping. Those who are hyperglycemic overnight, however, will have difficulty sleeping because of the recurrent need to urinate. This problem can be managed by improving metabolic control.

Nighttime hypoglycemia is a concern of parents of children receiving insulin. A child may not wake with the usual early signs and symptoms, and the first sign may be a severe event with nightmares or seizures. Therefore it is important to prevent nighttime hypoglycemia by appropriately adjusting the evening insulin dose and offering a bedtime snack with carbohydrate and protein or fat. Parents should also be instructed in the use of the counterregulatory hormone glucagon in case the child is not able to be aroused.

Nightmares are common in young children and may be caused by hypoglycemia. Parents should determine the blood glucose level before assuming the cause of a nightmare. If the cause is hypoglycemia, treatment includes administration of glucose. If the nightmares are not related to hypoglycemia, appropriate comfort measures should be instituted. Prevention is the key, however, and significant nighttime hypoglycemia is to be avoided as much as possible by careful adjustment of diet and insulin.

Toileting

Several issues related to toileting are important in the management of diabetes in children. Many children have secondary enuresis at the time of diagnosis. It is important to tell children who were previously dry that diabetes is the cause of their enuresis and that the enuresis should remit when the diabetes is adequately controlled. Enuresis can occur, however, with well-controlled diabetes. Other methods of diagnostic

confirmation and treatment should be explored with these families.

Although testing urine for glucose is not as critical to management as it was before SMBG testing was available, urinary ketone levels are important indicators of status when a child with type 1 diabetes is ill. Parents should know how to obtain such samples from infants and toddlers. Cotton balls tucked into a diaper can provide an adequate sample for use on a dipstick to determine ketone levels in children who are not yet toilet trained. Urine is readily obtainable when a child uses a potty chair during toilet training. When children move onto the bathroom commode, parents needs to teach them to urinate into a paper cup so that the urine can be tested. If taught when a child is feeling well, this task can be made into a game so that, when necessary, the behavior has been learned.

Discipline

Although the issues related to discipline of a child with diabetes are not different from those of all children with a chronic condition, parents of children with diabetes report that their second most common concern in raising the child is discipline (Hodges & Parker, 1987). Parents most often worry that a hypoglycemic episode will be missed by attributing the unruly behavior to lack of discipline. It is appropriate for parents to test the blood glucose level at any time hypoglycemia is suspected. Then if the result is within the normal range, the child can be appropriately disciplined. Blood testing should be performed in a matter of fact way, so that children do not misinterpret the test as a punishment. Some parents also worry that the stress of imposed discipline will raise the blood glucose level because of the presence of counterregulatory hormones. Although severe stressors may increase blood glucose levels, no evidence suggests that usual disciplinary measures increase blood glucose levels or worsen diabetic control. Indeed, some authors (Grey & Tamborlane, in press) have suggested that parents who set reasonable limits for their children are more likely to have children in good metabolic control.

Child Care

Toddlers and preschoolers with diabetes benefit from the socialization of preschool programs. They do not need specialized medical daycare. Preschool teachers should be informed of parental expectations, such as blood glucose testing and insulin administration. Snack and lunch intake is very important, so preschool teachers must be aware of the child's need to eat and what should be served at each mealtime. They should be aware of appropriate food substitutions when food is refused. All caregivers should be told how to manage symptoms of hypoglycemia. Emergency telephone numbers should always be available and should include telephone numbers of the parents, another emergency contact, the primary care provider, and the diabetes specialists.

Parents of children with diabetes often express concerns about the abilities of baby sitters or daycare workers to manage a young child's type 1 diabetes. Parents of young children can begin by leaving the child for only short periods of time, thus reassuring themselves that the sitter can successfully care for the child. Clear instructions on the child's diet and management of hypoglycemia should be provided in writing. Parents should be encouraged to train sitters in blood glucose monitoring and recognition of hypoglycemic symptoms.

Schooling

Children whose diabetes is adequately controlled should attend school regularly and participate in any activities for which they are otherwise suited. Parents should be encouraged to inform the school nurse and the child's teachers when the diabetes is diagnosed. It is important that school personnel are knowledgeable about the child's care so that hypoglycemia or illness can be appropriately managed. The need for other involvement (e.g., SMBG testing or injections) depends on the child's usual regimen. For youths with type 2 diabetes, the school can be invaluable in providing support and follow-up in a weight loss program.

With older children, providers need to work with the child, family, and school personnel to arrange a school schedule that fits the child's diabetes regimen. For example, a child who has had regular and NPH insulin at 7:00 AM should probably have a snack before a gym class that precedes a late lunch period. Arrangements must be made so that the child can always have access to glucose-containing foods or tablets in case of a hypoglycemic episode. The child should always have food available on field trips. A sack lunch with all food groups serves nicely as a substitute if a meal is unexpectedly delayed.

Sports are also encouraged. For youths with type 1 diabetes, coaches should be aware of the diabetes and keep foods containing glucose on hand. Depending on the degree of exercise on extra-activity days, the insulin dose may be lowered or the diet increased or both in an attempt to prevent hypoglycemia. Hypoglycemia following exercise may occur up to 12 hours after the event, so children should be carefully monitored when any new activity is undertaken. Children should be advised that insulin is absorbed more rapidly from exercising muscle; therefore if a muscle is to be exercised, insulin should be injected in another site. For example, if a child will run track, the insulin could be administered in the arm or the abdomen instead of the leg. For youths with type 2 diabetes, physical activity is crucial to improving outcomes. These youths should be encouraged to participate fully in physical activities in the school and at home.

Children with type 1 or type 2 diabetes whose diabetes is in poor control may experience difficulties in school performance. Because hypoglycemia can cause a child to lose the ability to concentrate when the blood glucose level is low, learning can be a problem. When the blood glucose level is consistently too high, many children experience difficulties in concentration and grades may suffer. Thus any child with diabetes whose school performance changes should be carefully assessed for alterations in metabolic control. Unless there are other problems, children with diabetes should not require special education or an individual learning plan. Indeed, several class action suits have been brought against school districts that required otherwise well children with diabetes to attend special education classes.

Because children and adolescents with diabetes are encouraged to participate fully in sports and other activities, they may be encouraged to go to camp as well. There are specialized camps for children with diabetes, which may help young people to learn about their diabetes and meet peers who also have diabetes. Children and adolescents with diabetes may also safely attend regular camps. Whether the camp is diabetes specific or not, care should be taken to adjust the insulin dose and food intake to account for the markedly increased physical activity at camp. Extra blood glucose monitoring may be necessary.

As with all children with long-term conditions, emphasis should be on the normality of the child—not the diabetes. Such an approach helps to minimize the sense of being different that is experienced by all affected children.

Sexuality

Achievement of normal growth and development is a goal of therapy for type 1 diabetes. If the diabetes is adequately controlled, sexual development should be normal. If sexual development is delayed, however, normal concerns about self-adequacy and physical adequacy may be amplified. Primary care providers need to monitor secondary sexual development carefully in children with diabetes, and any deviation from normal should be investigated. Tightening the metabolic control often improves growth. If not, the cause should be investigated.

All sexually active teenagers need information about birth control. Such information is especially important for those with type 1 and type 2 diabetes because the risks for complications of pregnancy are at least five times greater than the already high risk for adolescents. Because of the risk for acquired immunodeficiency syndrome (AIDS), many providers are encouraging condoms over all other birth control methods. Unfortunately, as with all teenagers, proper and consistent use of condoms is variable. Other barrier methods (e.g., diaphragms, foams, creams) may also be used by those with diabetes but share the same disadvantages as condoms and do not prevent sexually transmitted diseases.

Teenagers who are willing to use contraceptives often find using the birth control pill acceptable. Earlier versions of the combination pill (i.e., containing both estrogen and progesterone) carried risks for cerebral ischemia, myocardial infarction, and rapid progression of retinopathy and were not recommended for adolescents with diabetes. Newer low-dose estrogen combination pills, however, seem to be reasonably well tolerated and are the oral contraceptive of choice. These medications are also used to treat amenorrhea associated with polycystic ovary disease in youth with type 2 diabetes.

Although avoidance of adolescent pregnancy is clearly preferred for youth with type 1 or type 2 diabetes, some teenagers express the desire to become pregnant. It has been clearly demonstrated, however, that pregnancy outcomes can be dramatically improved if euglycemia is maintained both in the months preceding conception and throughout the pregnancy. Therefore female adolescents at risk for pregnancy or contemplating pregnancy should be counseled about pregnancy outcomes and helped to achieve better metabolic control.

Male adolescents often express concern about the well-known complication of impotence in adult men. Impotence is thought to be a result of both vascular and neurologic compromise in those with long-standing diabetes. Fortunately, impotence caused by diabetes is very rare in adolescence, so most of these individuals can be reassured.

Transition into Adulthood

The challenges of making the transition into adulthood may be more complex for adolescents with type 1 diabetes because of the extraordinary demands of disease self-management on the client and the family. Wysocki & associates (1992) found that older adolescents had worse adjustment to diabetes and metabolic control than younger children. In addition, difficulties in adjustment in early adolescence tended to persist into young adulthood. Further, other studies have suggested that young adults with type 1 diabetes have more difficulty with vocational adjustment and marital relationships (Bryden et al, 2001) than other young adults. Thus the care provided during this crucial time may be important for long-term quality of life.

Wysocki & associates (1992) also found that adolescents who were better adjusted had better metabolic control in early adulthood. This finding suggests that the care provided in early adolescence with attention to improving psychosocial adjustment is just as important as providing quality transitional care. Little empiric work on the provision of care in the transition from adolescence to adulthood has been accomplished, but Court (1993) surveyed adolescents on their views about the transfer process from pediatric to adult care. Court found that adolescents value continuity of care by a provider they trust, as well as expect confidentiality and privacy, informality, and waiting rooms tailored to their needs. In addition, young adults and late adolescents may be less capable of insulin self-regulation than providers assume. Therefore transition to adult care must be designed to respect the wishes of these young people and to support their assumption of self-care and development in their vocational and social roles. Grey and colleagues (2002a) have recently reported that youth receiving intensive insulin treatment have better metabolic control and quality of life in young adulthood than was found in studies conducted before the release of the DCCT findings.

Another concern of young adults is the increasing risk of complications. One study (Dunning, 1995) found that concerns about complications were common among young adults with diabetes and included concerns about eye disease, pregnancy and childbirth, hypoglycemia, and loss of independence. It is clear that these young people need help implementing intensive regimens and self-care management styles that will help to delay complications.

Studies of youth with type 2 diabetes transitioning to young adulthood are just beginning. Little is known about their care requirements or the process of transition.

Family Concerns and Resources

Families of children with type 1 diabetes worry about the appropriate assumption of self-care because of its importance in preventing long-term complications. Recommendations for understanding the levels at which children should assume various self-care activities are available. There is, however, broad disagreement among professionals as to the appropriate age for management of skills (Wysocki et al, 1990), and some clinicians fear that a too-early assumption of self-management is associated with poorer psychologic and metabolic outcomes. Therefore decisions about the assumption of self-care activities should be made with the family, child, and providers working together. Until more data on the effect of assuming self-care at different ages are available, providers' strict regulation of such activities may be unwarranted.

In studies of parental concerns in type 1 diabetes (Hauenstein et al, 1989; Hodges & Parker, 1987), several issues are prominent. First is the adherence to the diabetes regimen—especially diet and the assumption of self-care. Second is the question of genetics and inheritance. In addition, psychosomatic issues may be of particular importance to families dealing with diabetes because poorly functioning families have been shown to be associated with poorer metabolic control (Kovacs et al, 1989). Parents frequently also express concerns about long-term complications and the risk of hypoglycemia. As noted earlier, the risk of severe hypoglycemia is three to four times greater in children on intensive treatment regimens. Parents may be more concerned about their child participating in sports, going on field trips, or spending the night at a friend's house if he or she is on an intensive treatment regimen.

Guilt is often of concern to parents of children with diabetes, particularly because the disease is inherited. Families must be provided with appropriate genetic counseling so that they are aware of the risks to other family members and to offspring of the individual with diabetes. Such information often helps to assuage the guilt present at diagnosis because the risk for first-degree relatives is low. The sibling of a child with type 1 diabetes has about a 5% to 10% risk, and an offspring of one parent with diabetes has about a 1% to 2% risk as compared with a 0.05% risk for the general population. The risk for type 2 diabetes is higher in families, with the risk as high as 50%.

Considerable attention has been paid to family problems and their effect on metabolic control in children with diabetes. Studies of the influence of family life on diabetes control have been inconclusive (Kovacs et al, 1989). Some families, however, exhibit psychosomatic characteristics that clearly have an adverse effect on the child with diabetes. Such families should be referred for family therapy.

Social issues (e.g., cultural differences) may also influence adaptation to diabetes in youth, but little work on these questions has been done with adolescents with type 1 diabetes. Delameter & associates (1999) found that minority children and adolescents had worse metabolic control than white children. Differences in metabolic control among these families may be because of cultural dietary factors (e.g., eating more foods that affect blood glucose swings or participating in less exercise). Because eating behaviors and participation in sports may be influenced by cultural values, families should be assessed for their beliefs and values about food and exercise.

Although some of these family issues may also be true for youth with type 2 diabetes, there has been no research on these families. There are, however, studies that deal with the profound influence of the family on dietary and activity levels. Based on a comprehensive review of the literature on family determinants of health behavior, Sallis & Nadler (1988) concluded that physiologic and behavioral risk factors for chronic conditions such as obesity and hypertension, as well as behavioral patterns related to dietary intake and physical activity, are clustered within families. Several studies have shown that having more than one overweight parent is closely tied to youthful obesity (Fisher & Birch, 1995; Klesges et al, 1995; Whitaker et al, 1997). Moreover, parents exert a powerful influence on their children's health behaviors, including those behaviors that put youth at risk for type 2 diabetes. Youths' dietary and activity patterns have been linked to the family environment (Dowda et al, 2001; Dunning, 1995; Fisher & Birch, 1995). In particular, parental control of the youth's diet and the parents' own eating behaviors have been associated with excess body fat in youth.

RESOURCES

Two national organizations provide help for families coping with diabetes in a child: the American Diabetes Association (ADA) and the Juvenile Diabetes Research Foundation International (JDRFI) (see the list of organizations that follows). The ADA is the largest such organization, composed of both lay individuals and professionals. The ADA supports research, education, fund raising, and camps, as well as provides lobbying efforts related to diabetes. It publishes several pamphlets and books for families to use in understanding diabetes. At the local level, many affiliates provide support and educational programs for families and children. The ADA deals with all types of diabetes, not only type 1 diabetes.

Research toward a cure for type 1 diabetes is the primary focus of the JDRFI. The organization does provide some support for families, but its major effort is devoted to fund raising for research to find a cure for type 1 diabetes. Some families find that working toward a cure helps deal with the illness in their family.

Organizations

American Diabetes Association
1660 Duke St
Alexandria, VA 22314
(800) ADA-DISC
www.diabetes.org

Juvenile Diabetes Research Foundation
120 Wall St
New York, NY 10005-4001
(800) 533-CURE
www.jdrf.org

Relevant Web Sites

CDC Diabetes Home Page
www.cdc.gov

Children with Diabetes
www.childrenwithdiabetes.com

Diabetes Book Store
www.DiabetesBookstore.com

Diabetes Monitor
www.diabetesmonitor.com

Health; diseases and conditions; diabetes
www.yahoo.com/Health/Diseases_and_Conditions/Diabetes/

Insulin Pumpers
www.insulin-pumpers.org/

KidsRPumping
www.members.aol.com/CamelsRFun/index.html/

National Institute of Diabetes and Digestive and Kidney Disease (NIDDK)
www.niddk.nih.gov

News and Chat Groups

www.jdrf.org

Access to chat room links are available on this site.

Summary of Primary Care Needs for the Child with Diabetes Mellitus (Types 1 and 2)

HEALTH CARE MAINTENANCE

Growth and Development

Height and weight are normal in type 1 unless diabetes control is less than adequate.

Secondary sexual development may be delayed.

Rapid weight gain may require intervention.

Weight loss usually indicates poor control or insulin omission.

Weight and body mass index (BMI) must be elevated in type 2.

Secondary sexual development may be accelerated in type 2 diabetes with hirsutism if polycystic ovaries are present.

Diet

Maintenance of normoglycemia is critical.

Stress the importance of regular distribution of meals and snacks.

In type 1, sufficient calories for growth are paramount.

In type 2, reduction in calories and fat is a cornerstone of treatment to reduce BMI.

Physical activity is encouraged in type 1 with modification of insulin as needed.

Increasing aerobic capacity and decreasing sedentary behaviors are the focus in children with type 2 diabetes.

Safety

Prevent hypoglycemia with careful monitoring; be sure a glucose source is always available.

Dispose of syringes properly.

Use glucagon for severe hypoglycemic episodes.

Safely store oral medications.

A medical identification bracelet should be worn to ensure appropriate prompt treatment.

Immunizations

Routine immunizations are recommended.

Yearly influenza vaccine is recommended.

Screening

Vision. Check red reflex and perform funduscopic examination at each visit.

A thorough pediatric ophthalmologic examination every 5 years is advised and a yearly examination is advised for children with diabetes for >5 years. In type 2 diabetes, examination should occur at diagnosis and yearly.

Cataracts are possible at diagnosis.

Continued

Summary of Primary Care Needs for the Child with Diabetes Mellitus (Types 1 and 2)—cont'd

Screening—cont'd

Hearing. Routine screening is recommended.

Dental. Routine screening is recommended. Poor metabolic control can lead to increased cavities and gingivitis.

Blood Pressure. Blood pressure and orthostatic variation should be checked at each visit. Hypertension should be aggressively managed.

Hematocrit. Routine screening is recommended.

Urinalysis. Perform urinalysis yearly for ketones, glucose, and protein determinations; after 5 years screen for microalbuminuria yearly. Youths with type 2 diabetes should be screened at diagnosis and yearly.

Tuberculosis. Routine screening is recommended.

Condition-Specific Screening

Lipid screening should be done yearly after puberty or earlier if other risk factors are present.

Hemoglobin A_{1c} is checked every 3 months by the diabetic team.

Perform thyroid function studies if a change in growth patterns occurs or symptoms of hypothyroidism develop.

Perform other studies as indicated.

COMMON ILLNESS MANAGEMENT

Differential Diagnosis

Illness requires "sick day" management.

It is important to maintain hydration during illness.

It is most important to evaluate for hypoglycemia with changes in mental status.

Candidal vaginal infections are more common in adolescent females.

Skin lesions must be evaluated.

Weight loss in type 1 diabetes and weight gain in type 2 diabetes may indicate poor metabolic control.

Diabetic gastroparesis may cause vomiting or abdominal pain.

Drug Interactions

Beware that many over-the-counter (OTC) medications and antibiotics contain glucogenic substances or alcohol.

DEVELOPMENTAL ISSUES

Sleep Patterns

Prevention of nighttime hypoglycemia is important.

Nightmares may be the result of hypoglycemia.

Toileting

Enuresis may be present when control is poor.

Measurement of urinary ketones is important when blood glucose levels are high or when the child is ill.

Discipline

Unruly behavior may be caused by hypoglycemia.

The potential for conflict over diet, blood testing, and insulin administration should be recognized.

Stress associated with discipline should not elevate blood glucose.

Child Care

Teachers and baby sitters need training in management of dietary needs and hypoglycemia.

Schooling

Full attendance and participation are expected.

School personnel must be aware of the child's special needs.

If metabolic control is poor, performance may be affected.

Sexuality

If diabetes is adequately controlled, sexual development should be normal.

Pregnancy prevention is very important because of combined risks of diabetes and adolescent pregnancy.

Low-dose estrogen combination oral contraceptives are recommended because of the risk for complications with birth control pills or oral contraceptives containing estrogen.

Pregnancy outcomes are dramatically improved if euglycemia is maintained preceding and during pregnancy.

Impotency caused by long-term vascular and neurologic compromise is a rare problem during adolescence.

Type 2 diabetes is associated with polycystic ovary syndrome.

Depression and psychosocial adjustment problems may be present.

Transition into Adulthood

Challenges in the transition to adulthood may be more complex for adolescents with type 1 diabetes because of the extraordinary demands of the disease self-management.

Vocational adjustment and marital relationships may be more difficult for some young adults with type 1 diabetes than others.

If adjustment is better in early adolescence, young adults are more likely to have better adjustment and metabolic control.

FAMILY CONCERNS

Assumption of self-care activities and adherence to the regimen are prime concerns.

Parents often experience guilt about the inheritance of type 1 diabetes.

Psychosomatic families may have more problems with diabetic management.

Minority children and children from single-parent homes are at highest risk for poor metabolic control.

Minority children and adolescents tend to have worse metabolic control than white children and adolescents. Differences in metabolic control may be from cultural dietary factors or participation in less exercise, both of which may be influenced by cultural values.

Food preferences and adiposity are associated with family eating and activity patterns. Families should be encouraged to adopt healthy eating and activity behaviors.

Depression, anxiety, and psychosocial difficulties are not uncommon in children and adolescents with diabetes.

REFERENCES

Ahern, J.H. et al. (2002). Insulin pump therapy in pediatrics: A therapeutic alternative to safely lower HbA1c levels across all age groups. *Pediatr Diabetes*, 10-15.

Albisser, A.M., Leibel, B.S., Ewart, T.G., Davidovac, Z., Botz, C.K., et al. (1974). Clinical control of diabetes by the artificial pancreas. *Diabetes, 23*, 397-404.

Althius, M.D., Jordon, N.E., Ludington, E.A., & Wittes, J.T. (2002). Glucose and insulin responses to dietary chromium supplements: A meta-analysis. *Am J Clin Nutr, 72*, 148-155.

American Academy of Pediatrics. (2002). Summaries of infectious diseases. In G Peter (Ed.). *Red book: Report of the committee on infectious diseases* (27th ed.). Elk Grove Village, Ill.: Author.

American Diabetes Association. (2000). Type 2 diabetes in children and adolescents. *Diabetes Care, 23*, 381-389.

American Diabetes Association. (1993). Position statement: Implications of the Diabetes Control and Complications Trial. *Diabetes, 42*, 1555-1558.

American Diabetes Association. (1999). Clinical practice recommendations 1999. *Diabetes Care, 22*(suppl. 1), S1-S114.

American Diabetes Association. (2002a). Clinical practice recommendations. *Diabetes Care, 25*(suppl. 1).

American Diabetes Association. (2002b). Diabetes facts; Web site: www.diabetes.org.

Anderson, B.J., Brackett, J., Ho, J., & Laffel, L.M. (1999). An office-based intervention to maintain parent-adolescent teamwork in diabetes management. *Diabetes Care, 22*, 713-721.

Attia, N., Jones, T.W., Holcombe, J., & Tamborlane, W.V. (1998). Comparison of human regular and lispro insulins after interruption of continuous subcutaneous insulin infusion and the treatment of acutely decompensated IDDM. *Diabetes Care, 21*, 817-821.

Bingley, P.J., Bonfacio, E., & Gale E.A.M. (1993). Can we really predict IDDM? *Diabetes, 42*, 213-220.

Blanz, B.J., Rensch-Riemann, B.S., Fritz-Sigmund, D.I., & Schmidt, M.H. (1993). IDDM is a risk factor for adolescent psychiatric disorders. *Diabetes Care, 16*, 1579-1587.

Boland, E.A., Grey, M., Oesterle, A., Fredrickson, L., & Tamborlane, W.V. (1999). Continuous subcutaneous insulin infusion: A new way to lower risk of severe hypoglycemia, improve metabolic control, and enhance coping in adolescents with type 1 diabetes. *Diabetes Care, 22*, 1779-1784.

Boland, E.A. et al. (2001). Limitations of conventional methods of self-monitoring of blood glucose: Lessons learned from three days of continuous glucose sensing in pediatric patients with type 1 diabetes. *Diabetes Care, 24*, 1858-1862.

Borg, H., Gottsater, A., Landin-Olsson, M., Fernlund, P., & Sundkvist, G. (2001). High levels of antigen-specific islet antibodies predict future beta-cell failure in patients with onset of diabetes in adult age. *J Clin Endocrinol Metab, 86*, 3032-3038.

Bryden, K.S., Peveler, R.C., Stein, A., Neil, A., Mayou, R.A., et al. (2001). Clinical and psychological course of diabetes from adolescence to young adulthood: A longitudinal cohort study. *Diabetes Care, 24*, 1536-1540.

Buckingham, B.A. et al. (2001). Continuous subcutaneous insulin infusion (CSII) in children under five years of age. *Diabetes, 50*(suppl. 2), A107.

Caldwell, M.B., Brownell, K.D., & Wilfley, D.E. (1997). Relationship of weight, body dissatisfaction, and self-esteem in African American and white female dieters. *Int J Eat Disord, 22*, 127-130.

Callahan, S.T. & Mansfield, M.J. (2000). Type 2 diabetes in adolescents. *Curr Opin Pediatr, 12*, 310-315.

Clarke, P., Gray, A., Adler, A., Stevens, R., Raikou, M., et al. (2001). United Kingdom Prospective Diabetes Study: Cost-effectiveness analysis of intensive blood-glucose control with metformin in overweight patients with type II diabetes. *Diabetologia, 44*, 298-304.

Court, J.M. (1993). Issues of transition to adult care. *J Pediatr Child Health, 29*(suppl. 1), S53-S55.

DCCT Research Group. (1993a). The effect of intensive treatment of diabetes on the development and progression of long-term complications in insulin-dependent diabetes mellitus. *N Engl J Med, 329*, 435-459.

DCCT Research Group. (1993b). Expanded role of the dietitian in the DCCT: Implications for clinical practice. *J Am Diet Assoc, 93*, 758-767.

DCCT Research Group. (1994). Effect of intensive diabetes treatment on the development and progression of long-term complications in adolescents with insulin-dependent diabetes mellitus: DCCT. *J Pediatr, 125*, 177-188.

DCCT Research Group. (1995). Adverse events and their association with treatment regimens in the diabetes control and complications trial. *Diabetes Care, 18*, 1415-1427.

Delamater, A.M., Shaw, K.H., Applegate, E.B., Pratt, I.A., Eidson, M., et al. (1999). Risk for metabolic control problems in minority youth with diabetes. *Diabetes Care, 22*, 700-705.

Dean, H.C. & Flett, B. (2002). Natural history of type 2 diabetes diagnosed in childhood: Long-term follow-up in young adult years. *Diabetes, 51*, A24.

Diabetes Prevention Trial—Type 1 Diabetes Study Group. (2002). Effects of insulin in relatives of patients with type 1 diabetes mellitus. *N Engl J Med, 346*, 1685-1691.

Dowda, M., Answorth, B.E., Addy, C.L., Saunders, R., & Riner, W. (2001). Environmental influences, physical activity, and weight status in 8- to 16-year olds. *Arch Pediatr Adolesct Med, 155*, 711-717.

Dunn, F.L., Nathan, D.M., Scavini, M., Selam, J.L., & Wingrove, T.G. (1997). Long-term therapy of IDDM with an implantable insulin pump: The Implantable Insulin Pump Trial Study Group. *Diabetes Care, 20*, 59-63.

Dunning, P.L. (1995). Young-adult perspectives of insulin-dependent diabetes. *Diabetes Education, 21*, 58-65.

Epstein, L.H. et al. (1985). A comparison of lifestyle exercise, aerobic exercise, and calisthenics on weight loss in obese children. *Behav Ther, 16*, 345-356.

Fagot-Campagna, A., Pettitt, D.J., Engelgau, M.M., Burrows, N.R., Geiss, L.S., et al. (2000). Type 2 diabetes among North American children and adolescents: An epidemiologic review and a public health perspective. *J Pediatr, 136*, 664-672.

Falkner, N.H., Neumark-Sztainer, D., Story, M., Jeffery, R.W., Beuhring, T., et al. (2001). Social, educational, and psychological correlates of weight status in adolescents. *Obes Res, 9*, 32-42.

Ferranninni, E. & Camastra, S. (1998). Relationship between impaired glucose tolerance, non-insulin dependent diabetes mellitus and obesity. *Eur J Clin Invest, 28*(suppl. 2), 3-7.

Fisher, J. & Birch, L. (1995). Fat preferences and fat consumption of 3- to 5-year old children are related to parental adiposity. *J Am Diet Assoc, 95*, 759-764.

Garg, S.K., Potts, R.O., Ackerman, N.R., Fermi, S.J., Tamada, J.A., et al. (1999). Correlation of fingerstick blood glucose measurements with the Glucowatch Biographer glucose results in young subjects with type 1 diabetes. *Diabetes Care, 22*, 1708-1714.

Glaser, N.S. (1997). Non-insulin-dependent diabetes mellitus in childhood and adolescence. *Pediatr Clin North Am, 44*, 307-333.

Goldstein, D.E., Little, R.R., Lorenz, R.A., Malone, J.I., Nathan, D., et al. (1995). Tests of glycemia in diabetes. *Diabetes Care, 18*, 896-909 (technical review).

Goldston, D.B., Kelley, A.E., Reboussin, D.M., Daniel, S.S., Smith, J.A., et al. (1997). Suicidal ideation and behavior and noncompliance with the medical regimen among diabetic adolescents. *J Am Acad Child Adolesc Psychiatry, 36*, 1528-1536.

Grey, M., Boland, E.A., Davidson, M., Li, J., & Tamborlane, W.V. (2000). Coping skills training has long-lasting effects on metabolic control and quality of life in adolescents on intensive therapy. *J Pediatr, 137*, 107-113.

Grey, M. et al. (2002). Preventing type 2 diabetes in high risk youth: Results of a pilot study. *Diabetes, 64*, A66.

Grey, M., Insabella, G., & Knafl, G. (2002). Intensive therapy and the transition to young adulthood. *Diabetes, 64*, A66-A67.

Grey, M. & Tamborlane, W.V. (in press). Behavioral and family aspects of the treatment of children and adolescents with type 1 diabetes. In D. Porte, R. Sherwin, & A.D. Baron (Eds.) *Ellenberg and Rifkin's diabetes mellitus* (6th ed.), New York: McGraw-Hill.

Haffner, S.M. (1997). Impaired glucose tolerance, insulin resistance, and cardiovascular disease. *Diabetic Med, 14*(suppl. 3), S12-S18.

Hauenstein, E.J., Marvin, R.S., Snyder, A.L., & Clarke, W.L. (1989). Stress in parents of children with diabetes mellitus. *Diabetes Care, 12*, 18-23.

Hodges, L.C. & Parker, J. (1987). Concerns of parents with diabetic children. *Pediatr Nurs, 13*, 22-24.

Jones, K.L. (2002). Treatment of type 2 diabetes mellitus in children. *JAMA, 287*, 716.

Jones, K.L., Arslanian, S., Peterokova, V.A., Park, J.S., & Tomlinson, M.J. (2002). Effect of metformin in pediatric patients with type 2 diabetes: A randomized controlled trial. *Diabetes Care, 25*, 89-94.

Klesges, R., Klesges, L., Eck, L., & Shelton, M. (1995). A longitudinal analysis of accelerated weight gain in preschool children. *Pediatrics, 95*, 126-130.

Kolody, B. & Sallis, J. F. (1995). A prospective study of ponderosity, body image, self-concept, and psychological variables in children. *J Dev Behav Pediatr, 16*, 1-5.

Kovacs, M., Goldston, D., Obrosky, D.S., & Bonar, L.K. (1997). Psychiatric disorders in youth with IDDM: Rates and risk factors. *Diabetes Care, 20*, 36-44.

Kovacs, M., Goldston, D., Obrosky, D.S., & Bonar, L.K. (1989). Family functioning and metabolic control of school-aged children with type 1 diabetes, *Diabetes Care, 12*, 409-414.

Kumar, A., Weatherly. M., & Beaman, D.C. (1991). Sweeteners, flavorings, and dyes in antibiotic preparations. *Pediatrics, 87*, 352-360.

Kyngas, H. & Barlow, J. (1995). Diabetes: An adolescent's perspective. *J Adv Nurs, 22*, 941-947.

LaGreca, A.M. et al. (1995). Adolescents with diabetes: Gender differences in psychosocial functioning and glycemic control. *Child Health Care, 24*, 61-78.

Leslie, D.G. & Elliot, R.G. (1994). Early environmental events as a cause of IDDM: Evidence and implications. *Diabetes, 43*, 843-850.

Liss, D.S., Waller, D.A., Kennard, B.D., McIntire, D., Capra, P., et al. (1998). Psychiatric illness and family support in children and adolescents with diabetic ketoacidosis: A controlled study. *J Am Acad Child Adolesc Psychiatry, 37*, 536-544.

Ludwig, D.S. & Ebbeling, C.B. (2001). Type 2 diabetes mellitus in children: Primary care and public health considerations. *JAMA, 286*, 1427-1430.

McGrady, A., Bailey, B.K., & Good, M.P. (1991). Controlled study of biofeedback-assisted relaxation in type 1 diabetes. *Diabetes Care, 14*, 360-365.

McMurray, R.G., Bauman, M.J., Harrell, J.S., Brown, S., & Bangdiwala, S.I. (2000). Effects of improvement in aerobic power on resting insulin and glucose concentrations in children. *Eur J Appl Physiol, 81*, 132-139.

Pihoker, C., Scott, C.R., Lensing, S.Y., Cradock, M.M., & Smith, J. (1998). Non-insulin dependent diabetes mellitus in African-American youth of Arkansas. *Clin Pediatr (Phila), 37*, 97-102.

Pollock, M., Kovacs, M., & Charron-Prochownik, D. (1995). Eating disorders and maladaptive dietary/insulin management among youths with childhood-onset insulin dependent diabetes mellitus. *Am Acad Child Adolesc Psychiatr, 34*, 291-296.

Polonsky, W.H., Anderson, B.J., Lohrer, P.A., Aponte, J.E., Jacobson, A.M., et al. (1994). Insulin omission in women with IDDM. *Diabetes Care, 17*, 1178-1185.

Reaven, G.M. (1993). Role of insulin resistance in human disease (syndrome X): An expanded definition. *Annu Rev Med, 44*, 121-131.

Ryan, E.A., Lakey, J.R., Rajotte, R.V., Korbutt, G.S., Kin, T., et al. (2001). Clinical outcomes and insulin secretion after islet transplantation with the Edmonton protocol. *Diabetes, 50*, 710-719.

Sallis, J. & Nadler, P. (1988). Family determinants of health behavior. In D. Gochman (Ed.). *Health behavior: Emerging research perspectives*. New York: Plenum.

Sinha, R., Fisch, G., Teague, B., Tamborlane, W.V., Banyas, B., et al. (2002). Prevalence of impaired glucose tolerance among children and adolescents with marked obesity. *N Engl J Med, 346*, 802-810.

Skyler, J.S., for the Exubera Phase III Study Group. (2002). Efficacy and safety of inhaled insulin (Exubera) compared to subcutaneous insulin therapy in an intensive insulin regimen in patients with type 1 diabetes: Results from a 6-month, randomized comparative trial. *Diabetes, 47*(suppl. 1), A134.

Stolley, M.R. & Fitzgibbon, M.L. (1997). Effects of an obesity prevention program on the eating behavior of African American mothers and daughters. *Health Educ Behav, 24*, 152-164.

Strauss, R.S. (2000). Childhood obesity and self-esteem. *Pediatrics, 105*, E15-E25.

Striegel-Moore, R.H., Nicholson, T.J., & Tamborlane, W.V. (1992). Prevalence of eating disorder symptoms in preadolescent and adolescent girls with type 1 diabetes, *Diabetes Care, 15*, 1361-1368.

Sutherland, D.E.R. & Gruessner, R.W.G. (1997). Current status of pancreas transplantation for the treatment of type 1 diabetes mellitus, *Clin Diabetes,* 152-156.

Tamada, J.A., Garg, S., Jovanovic, L., Pitzer, K.R., Fermi, S., et al. (1999). Non-invasive glucose monitoring: Comprehensive clinical results. *JAMA, 282*, 1839-1844.

Thompson, J.K., Coovert, M.D., Richards, K.J., Johnson, S., & Cattarin, J. (1995). Development of body image, eating disturbance, and general psychological functioning in female adolescents: Covariance structure modeling and longitudinal investigations. *Int J Eat Disord, 18*, 221-236.

Tubiana-Rufi, N., de Lonlay, P., Bloch, J., & Czernichow, P. (1996). Remission of severe hypoglycemia incidents in young diabetic children treated with subcutaneous infusion. *Arch Pediatr Adolesc Med, 3*, 969-976.

Whitaker, R., Wright, J., Pepe, M., Seidel, K., & Dietz, W. (1997). Predicting obesity in young adulthood from childhood and parental obesity. *N Engl J Med, 337*, 869-873.

Wysocki, T., Meinhold, P., Cox, D.J., & Clarke, W.L. (1990). Survey of diabetes professionals regarding developmental changes in diabetes self-care. *Diabetes Care, 13*, 65-68.

Wysocki, T., Hough, B.S., Ward, K.M., & Green, L.B. (1992). Diabetes mellitus in the transition to adulthood: Adjustment, self-care, and health status. *Dev Behav Pediatr, 13*, 194-201.

Young-Hyman, D., Schlundt, D.G., Herman, L., De Luca, F., & Counts, D. (2001). Evaluation of insulin resistance syndrome in 5- to 10-year old overweight/obese African American children. *Diabetes Care, 24*, 1359-1364.

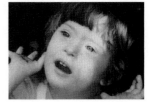

24 Down Syndrome

Wendy M. Nehring

Etiology

Down syndrome, which was first described by Jean Etienne Esquirol in 1838 and promulgated by John Langdon Down in 1866, is a condition that is associated with a recognizable phenotype and limited intellectual endowment because of extra chromosome 21 material. It is the most frequent autosomal chromosomal anomaly and the primary chromosomal cause of mental retardation. Chromosome 21 was the initial chromosome to be completely mapped with the deoxyribonucleic acid (DNA) sequence fully determined (Hattori et al, 2000). This chromosome contains 127 genes, 59 pseudogenes, and 98 predicted genes. The exact band of chromosomal material implicated in Down syndrome has been isolated and has been designated the "Down syndrome critical region" located at 21q22 to qter. However, even though the genes of this chromosome have been identified, until the function of each of the genes is understood, the pathology of Down syndrome remains unknown (Tolmie, 2002).

Known Genetic Etiology

Nondisjunction. Nondisjunction of chromosome 21 is responsible for the majority of cases of trisomic Down syndrome, with approximately 90% of maternal meiotic origin, and this form is not inherited (Hassold & Sherman, 2000). Nondisjunction (i.e., the uneven division of chromosomes) can occur during anaphase 1 or 2 in meiosis (i.e., reduction and division of germ cells) or in anaphase of mitosis (i.e., somatic cell division). In nondisjunction, the pair of chromosomes fails to separate and migrate properly during cell division. When this occurs in meiosis, the haploid number for the respective daughter cells is unequal. If the cell receiving 24 rather than 23 chromosomes is fertilized, a trisomic zygote results (Figure 24-1).

Factors found to influence maternal nondisjunction are maternal age (Tolmie, 2002), earlier menopause, lower numbers of oocytes (Kline et al, 2000), presence of identified gene polymorphisms involved in folate metabolism (Hobbs et al, 2000; O'Leary et al, 2002), and/or repeated presence of mDNA deletion mutations (Schon et al, 2000).

The recurrence risk for nondisjunction Down syndrome is approximately 1%. For older mothers, the risk is 1% plus the percentage of risk for chronologic age (Tolmie, 2002).

Mosaicism, while associated with fewer phenotypic features and defined by the presence of a percentage of cell lines with trisomy 21, is also most often caused by maternal meiotic nondisjunction (Figure 24-1). Mitotic nondisjunction is found in a lower percentage of cases (Tolmie, 2002).

Translocation. In Down syndrome caused by translocation (~5% of cases), there are also three copies of chromosome 21. The third copy does not occur independently, however, but is attached to another chromosome—usually to one of the D or G group. Robertsonian translocations, where the long arms of chromosome 21 attach to the long arms of chromosome 14, 21, or 22, are the most common translocations, although other forms can occur (Tolmie, 2002).

The total chromosome count in Down syndrome is 46, even though material for 47 chromosomes is present. Although the phenotype for Down syndrome caused by translocation is the same as that for nondisjunction, the inheritance pattern is quite different. With translocation, the disorder may recur in future pregnancies. If one parent has 45 chromosomes—including a translocation of chromosome 21, the gametes produced could result in a trisomic zygote. Although six combinations are theoretically possible, three are nonviable. Of the three that are viable, one is normal (i.e., N = 46), one results in a balanced translocation (i.e., N = 45), and one is an unbalanced translocation resulting in Down syndrome (i.e., N = 46) (Figure 24-2). The recurrence risk for a second child with translocation Down syndrome (usually 14; 21) is approximately 10% at the lowest probable maternal age and very low for the mother older than 35 years. If the translocation carrier is the father, the risk is approximately 5% (Aitken et al, 2002; Tolmie, 2002). If the translocation involves both copies of chromosome 21 (21;21), the recurrence risk is 100% (Aitken et al, 2002).

A variety of hypotheses as to the cause of Down syndrome have been offered over the years, including the following: (1) a genetic predisposition to nondisjunction; (2) autoimmunity; (3) hormonal alterations in aging women; (4) viral disease; (5) environmental and chemical factors such as irradiation before conception, smoking, and drug exposure; (6) consanguinity; (7) gestational diabetes; and (8) frequency of coitus (Chen et al, 1999; Narchi & Kulaylat, 1997). No one factor has been confirmed, although new genetic findings suggest that the cause is probably multifactorial.

Incidence and Prevalence

The prevalence rate for Down syndrome is 1 in 650 to 1000 live births, with the incidence rate dropping to approximately 1 in 800 live births, although this figure could be underestimated because of increased median maternal birth age (Aitken et al, 2002). Prenatal diagnosis of women of advanced maternal age explains this difference over time. Prevalence rates vary by inheritance pattern. Nondisjunction is found in the majority of Down syndrome conceptions. Approximately 90% of these

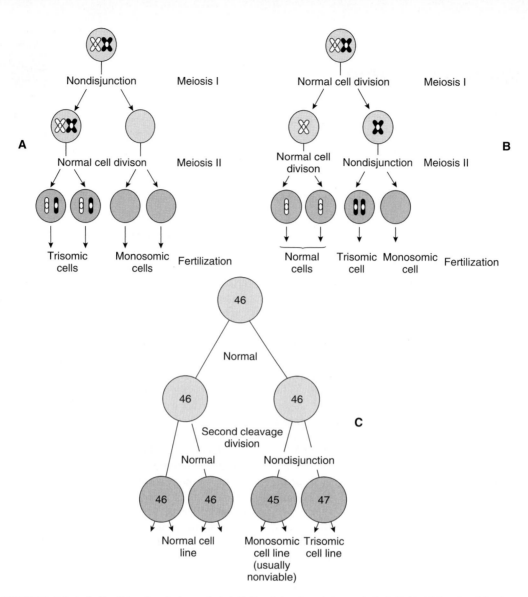

FIGURE 24-1 **A**, Nondisjunction during meiosis I. **B**, Nondisjunction during meiosis II. **C**, Nondisjunction following fertilization, during mitosis, resulting in mosaicism. (From Wong, D.L. et al. [1999]. *Whaley & Wong's nursing care of infants & children* [6th ed.] St. Louis: Mosby. Reprinted with permission.)

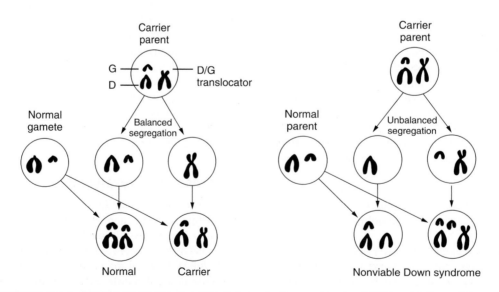

FIGURE 24-2 Possible zygotes from the union of a somatically normal carrier of D/G translocation and a genetically and somatically normal individual. (From Wong, D.L. et al. [1999]. *Whaley & Wong's nursing care of infants & children* [6th ed.]. St. Louis: Mosby. Reprinted with permission.)

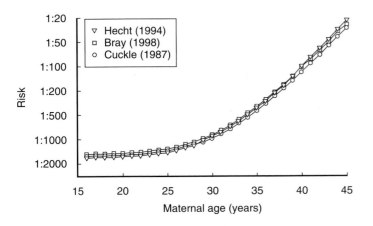

FIGURE 24-3 Age-specific risks for Down syndrome from three different studies. (From Aitken, D.A., et al. [2002]. Prenatal screening for neural tube defects and aneupoidy. In D.L. Rimoin et al. [Eds.]. *Emory and Rimoin's principles and practices of medical genetics* [4th ed.]. New York: Churchill Livingstone, pp. 763-801. Reprinted with permission.)

cases are of maternal meiotic causation, with 75% of this number occurring at maternal meiosis I. Only about 8% of total cases of nondisjunction are of paternal origin. Translocation occurs in about 5% of cases, and mosaicism occurs in approximately 2% of cases (Roizen, 1997; Tolmie, 2002).

Down syndrome caused by translocation is independent of parental age. The incidence is also stable across age cohorts, although one third of the cases of translocation Down syndrome are inherited from parents (Tolmie, 2002).

For women in their early 20s, the incidence of having a child with Down syndrome is approximately 1 in every 2000 births. The incidence rises gradually until maternal age surpasses 35 years and then climbs to approximately 42 in every 1000 live births for 45-year-old women (Hecht & Hook, 1996). Advanced paternal age (i.e., age 55 years and older) has also been shown to affect the incidence of nondisjunction Down syndrome (Tolmie, 2002). Although the extra chromosome is paternal in origin, nondisjunction still occurs after fertilization. Because the overwhelming percentage of cases of Down syndrome is caused by nondisjunction, parental age directly affects the overall incidence (Figure 24-3).

Down syndrome is found in all races and ethnic groups. Although the incidence rates of Down syndrome vary little among whites, blacks, and Hispanic infants born to mothers under 35 years of age, rates are significantly higher in Hispanic infants and moderately higher in black infants born to mothers over 35 years of age. Differences in these rates may reflect differences in early prenatal care, prenatal diagnosis, and views on abortion (Khoshnood et al, 2000).

Clinical Manifestations at Time of Diagnosis

Down syndrome is most often diagnosed immediately after birth as a result of its distinctive phenotype. In infants of color or those born very prematurely, diagnosis may be delayed because the clinical features may not be as clearly recognized. Although more than 50 physical characteristics can be identified at birth (Box 24-1), no one feature is considered diagnostic. Features vary in their expression and are not always present.

Some of the most commonly associated features, however, include generalized hypotonia, brachycephaly, epicanthal folds, palpebral fissures, single transverse palmar creases, incurved fifth finger, neck skinfold, and widely spaced first and second toes.

A variety of congenital anomalies are commonly associated with Down syndrome. Congenital cardiac disease is seen in approximately 16% to 62% of children with Down syndrome, with endocardial cushion defects accounting for about 25% to 30% and septal defects making up another 32% to 40% of cardiac malformations (Kriss, 1999; Saenz, 1999; Tolmie, 2002). Gastrointestinal (GI) malformations are seen in 2% to 15% of children with Down syndrome; among the most common problems are duodenal or esophageal atresia, congenital megacolon (Hirschsprung disease), imperforate anus, tracheoesophageal fistula, and pyloric stenosis (Kriss, 1999; Saenz, 1999; Tolmie, 2002). Anomalies can usually be surgically corrected in the neonatal period. Although many children experience total correction of the anomaly, others will experience untoward sequelae throughout their lives.

Treatment

No treatment can eliminate the chromosomal defect that causes Down syndrome. Extensive interdisciplinary services and research over the last 40 years have, however, transformed society's view of children with Down syndrome and accepted treatment protocols. Accepted approaches include genetic counseling, prompt referral for surgical correction of congenital anomalies, prevention of secondary conditions, enrollment in an early intervention program, and inclusion from preschool through high school (ages 3 to 21 years; Box 24-2).

Genetic Counseling

Validation of Down syndrome and its genotype by chromosomal analysis via karyotype should be considered for all affected children during the neonatal period (American Academy of Pediatrics [AAP], Committee on Genetics, 2001; Saenz, 1999; Tolmie, 2002). Although this validation will not affect a child's treatment or prognosis, it has significant implications for the genetic counseling of family members. Because translocation is the cause of about 5% of cases, parents and siblings must be tested to determine their carrier status, as well as have the risk of recurrence in future pregnancies carefully explained to them.

Surgery

Surgical corrections of most major cardiac, GI, and genitourinary anomalies are now performed routinely, although not without risk. The risk for upper airway compromise during and after surgery is increased in Down syndrome because of clinical features such as subglottic stenosis, smaller mid and lower face skeleton, adenoid and tonsil volume, tracheal stenosis, hypotonia, and a narrow nasopharyngeal inlet. Atlantoaxial instability also poses a surgical risk, although if cervical spine radiographs are normal, any neck flexion or extension during the surgical period does not pose a problem (Todd et al, 2000). Further, postextubation stridor (Shott, 2000) and apnea (Uong et al, 2001) are common, and a longer hospital stay is recommended for children with Down syndrome. Specifically, perioperative and late cardiac mortality is only associated with

BOX 24-1

Clinical Manifestations in Down Syndrome

SKULL
False fontanel
Flat occipital area
Brachycephaly
Separated sagittal suture
Hypoplasia of midfacial bones
Reduced interorbital distance
Underdeveloped maxilla
Obtuse mandibular angle

EYES
Oblique narrow palpebral fissures
Epicanthal folds
Brushfield spots
Strabismus
Nystagmus
Myopia
Hypoplasia of the iris

EARS
Small, shortened ears
Low and oblique implantation
Overlapping helices
Prominent antihelix
Absent or attached earlobes
Narrow ear canals
External auditory meatus
Structural aberrations of the ossicles
Stenotic external auditory meatus

NOSE
Hypoplastic
Flat nasal bridge
Anteverted, narrow nares
Deviated nasal septum

MOUTH
Prominent, thickened, and fissured lips
Corners of the mouth turned downward
High-arched, narrow palate
Shortened palatal length
Protruding enlarged tongue
Papillary hypertrophy (early preschool)
Fissured tongue (later school years)
Periodontal disease
Partial anodontia
Microdontia
Abnormally aligned teeth
Anterior open bite
Mouth held open

NECK
Short, broad neck
Loose skin at nape

CHEST
Shortened rib cage
Twelfth rib anomalies
Pectus excavatum or carinatum
Congenital heart disease

ABDOMEN
Distended and enlarged abdomen
Diastasis recti
Umbilical hernia
Muscle tone and musculature
Hyperflexibility
Muscular hypotonia
Generalized weakness
Integument
Skin appears large for the skeleton
Dry and rough
Fine poorly pigmented hair

EXTREMITIES
Short extremities
Partial or complete syndactyly
Clinodactyly
Brachyclinodactyly

Upper Extremities
Short broad hands
Brachyoclinodactyly
Single palmar transverse crease
Incurved short fifth finger
Abnormal dermatoglyphics

Lower Extremities
Short and stubby feet
Gap between first and second toes
Plantar crease between first and second toe
Second and third toes grouped in a forklike position
Radial deviation of the third to the fifth toe

PHYSICAL GROWTH AND DEVELOPMENT
Short stature
Increased weight in later life

OTHER FINDINGS SEEN IN NEWBORNS
Enlarged anterior fontanel
Delayed closing of sutures and fontanels
Open sagittal suture
Nasal bone not ossified, underdeveloped
Reduced birth weight

complete atrioventricular septal defect (Reller & Morris, 1998).

In addition to life-saving surgeries, some children with Down syndrome also undergo plastic surgery to alter their phenotypic appearance. As these children continue to become more integrated into society, they may be stigmatized because of their physiognomy. Some parents, concerned about their child's social acceptance, seek plastic surgery for the child (e.g., partial glossectomies, neck resections, Silastic implants for the chin and nose, and reconstruction of dysplastic helices). Better articulation of speech, less mouth breathing, fewer and less severe upper respiratory tract infections, and improved mastication and swallowing may be realized, especially if a pathologic condition exists that warrants corrective surgery. The degree of success, however, may be small or nonexistent. There are surgical risks, surgery is expensive, and it is most often not covered by insurance. Any parents and/or children with Down syndrome wanting to undergo plastic surgery should talk at length with their primary care provider and surgeon before the procedure so that they understand the risks (Aylott, 1999; Jones, 2000).

Prevention and Treatment of Secondary Conditions

Children with Down syndrome are susceptible to a number of secondary conditions, including but not limited to feeding problems, vision and hearing abnormalities, constipation, upper respiratory infections, thyroid disorders, and skin problems (Box 24-3). Regular visits to the primary health care provider and a Down syndrome clinic, if available, and comprehensive anticipatory guidance can help to prevent these problems. If they do occur, intervention and treatment can begin early. Referring the family to a support group composed of other families with a child with Down syndrome can also provide a means for information and support to prevent such conditions.

Complementary and Alternative Therapies

Early Intervention. Infant stimulation programs and continued early childhood education are designed to optimize a child's rate of development and minimize the amount of developmental lag that will occur between children with Down syndrome and their developmentally normal peers. Specific therapeutic exercises are devised to stimulate an infant's cognitive, social, motor, and language domains. These exercises are incorporated in the Individualized Family Service Plan (IFSP) that is mandated by IDEA (Public Law 105-17). Researchers have found motor and cognitive improvement in infants after their participation in an early intervention program (AAP, Committee on Genetics, 2001). Parents are usually taught these skills by special education teachers, physical therapists, occupational therapists, and speech pathologists so that therapy can be conducted at home. Timing seems to be a critical factor, however, with earlier interventions correlated with greater developmental gains. These children will later be referred to a specialized program designed to continue these intervention strategies and then integrated into generic child care or school (see Chapter 5).

Inclusion. In the 1990s, the term "inclusion" replaced the earlier term of "mainstreaming" when referring to public school services for the child with intellectual disabilities. With inclusion, the child aged 3 to 21 years is included in the regular classroom, including preschool programs, under IDEA (see Chapter 5).

Numerous other approaches (e.g., patterning, cell therapy, megavitamin therapy, administration of butoctamide hydrogen succinate) designed to improve the developmental outcomes of these children have been tried. Unfortunately, the results of these interventions have been disappointing. The drug piracetam, which some consider to be a cognitive enhancer, has received the most attention of late. Lobaugh and his associates (2001) found no significant improvements in cognitive functioning in a small sample of children with Down syndrome after taking piracetam for 4 months. In fact, aggressiveness was found in 22% of the sample. Piracetam should not be used for the purpose of raising the child's intelligence (Holmes, 1999).

Human growth hormone (hGH) therapy for children with Down syndrome is investigational and controversial. Children with Down syndrome should be treated with hGH only if they are deficient in this hormone because an increase in brain growth stimulated by hGH has not been found to increase cognitive function, gross motor development, or craniofacial development. Many ethical issues about its usage exist, such as the following: What are the goals of treatment? How are the children being evaluated? What are the parents' roles in treatment decisions? When is such treatment appropriate when its scientific efficacy is unfounded? How will this child benefit from being taller? Is the discomfort associated with the therapy warranted? Who will pay for the therapy? Moreover, hGH therapy has been associated with leukemia. The benefits of this therapy are not significant nor do they outweigh the risks (Anneren et al, 1999, 2000; Carlstedt et al, 1999; Lantos, 2000).

Anticipated Advances in Diagnosis and Management

Advances in Knowledge of Genetic Etiology or Treatment

Maternal age has been the traditional screening risk factor for Down syndrome. Researchers and health professionals are calling for a screening policy based on statistical modeling and decision analysis (i.e., using financial and human factors) (Cuckle, 1998; Serra-Prat et al, 1998). Pregnant women must be aware of the screening options available to them (i.e., biochemical screening, ultrasound, chorionic villi sampling, amniocentesis) based on maternal age. A variety of serum markers have been studied for their use in detecting Down syndrome. Their values may vary in the first and second trimesters, affecting the optimal time for screening. Multimarker serum screening enhances accuracy of detection. Multimethod screening (e.g., biochemical screening and ultrasound) is most efficacious (Aitken et al, 2002). Ultrasound measurement of nuchal translucency has not been consistently developed, and its technique has not been standardized for consistent results in all settings. Research on the use of multiplex fluorescent polymerase chain reaction (PCR) amplification for the prenatal diagnosis of trisomy 21 is being done and may be the screening technique of the near future (Blake et al, 1999).

Associated Problems (Box 24-3)

Mental Retardation

The intellectual capabilities of children with Down syndrome vary dramatically. Most of these children are moderately retarded (i.e., intelligence quotient [IQ] of 40 to 55, standard

BOX 24-3
Associated Problems

Mental retardation
Cardiac defects
Gastrointestinal tract anomalies
Musculoskeletal and motor abilities
Immune system deficiency
Hearing loss
Growth retardation
Altered respiratory function
Thyroid dysfunction
Malignancies
   Leukemia
   Testicular germ cell
Celiac disease
Vision problems
Sleep-disordered breathing
Skin conditions
Dental changes
Seizure disorders

deviation [SD] of 15), but a small percentage are either mildly affected (i.e., IQ of 56 to 69, SD of 15) or severely impaired (i.e., IQ of 39, SD of 15). For a few children, their IQs are not consistent with a diagnosis of mental retardation (AAP, Committee on Genetics, 2001). Known correlates to the intelligence and adaptive behavior skills of children are their physical condition, home environment, and individualized early intervention (AAP, Committee on Genetics, 2001; Hauser-Cram et al, 1999). Unfortunately, cognitive function often deteriorates with age, and significant losses in intelligence, memory, and social skills are seen earlier (i.e., often by age 40 years) than in persons without Down syndrome (Lott & Head, 2001).

Mental retardation may also be accompanied by behavior disorders, such as social withdrawal, noncompliance, inattention, and thought disorder (Coe et al, 1999). Depression, autistic-like behavior, and psychotic episodes have been reported. Neurologic deterioration, disturbed family life, and stress associated with inclusion may affect the mental health of children with Down syndrome. Normal childhood and adolescent stressors are also of concern. For example, adolescents with Down syndrome often desire to date other adolescents of normal intelligence. When they are rejected, along with their inability to drive to social events, adolescents with Down syndrome often become depressed.

Cardiac Defects

Approximately 16% to 62% of children with Down syndrome have congenital heart defects. In order of decreasing frequency, the most common heart anomalies include atrioventricular septal defect (i.e., endocardial cushion defect and atrioventricular canal defect), ventricular septal defect, patent ductus arteriosus, and atrial septal defect (see Chapter 21). Other heart or cardiac-associated conditions that may occur in Down syndrome include tetralogy of Fallot, polycythemia, pulmonary artery hypertension (Kriss, 1999; Saenz, 1999), and pulmonary vascular obstructive disease, which can progress to congestive heart failure and death (Suzuki et al, 2000). Researchers are currently examining a genetic link to cardiac heart defects and

Down syndrome and have proposed that an allele from three grandparents (heterotrisomy) can lead to ventricular septal defects (Baptista et al, 2000).

Children with Down syndrome and cardiac defects requiring surgery also are at risk for developing subacute bacterial endocarditis (Cohen, 1999). In addition, children with Down syndrome who do not have congenital heart disease are at risk for developing mitral valve prolapse with age; by the end of adolescence, mitral valve prolapse has been detected in more than 50% of the individuals tested (Tolmie, 2002). The use of echocardiography and a cardiac evaluation during the newborn period has greatly enhanced detection rates, early management, and survival rates (AAP, Committee on Genetics, 2001; Amark & Sunnegardh, 1999).

Gastrointestinal Tract Anomalies

Common congenital GI tract anomalies include tracheoesophageal fistula, Hirschsprung disease, pyloric stenosis, duodenal atresia, annular pancreas, aganglionic megacolon, and imperforate anus, with duodenal atresia and Hirschsprung disease occurring most commonly (Kriss, 1999; Saenz, 1999; Tolmie, 2002). Increased prevalence of cholelithiasis in the first 2 years of life in children with Down syndrome has also been noted (Toscano et al, 2001). Most of these anomalies require immediate surgical correction and careful follow-up throughout life.

Musculoskeletal and Motor Abilities

Orthopedic problems are second only to cardiac defects as a cause of morbidity in Down syndrome. Flaccid muscle tone and ligamentous laxity occur to some extent in all children with Down syndrome, possibly because of an intrinsic defect in their connective tissue. Among these conditions are pes planus, patellar subluxation, scoliosis, dislocated hips, atlantoaxial subluxation, joint and muscle pain, and rapid muscle fatigue. These problems may occur throughout a child's life, and the primary care provider should carefully screen for them at each visit.

Surgical correction may be indicated for patellar hypermobility with subluxation, scoliosis, or dislocated hips. Although the incidence of congenital dislocated hip in children with Down syndrome is similar to that of unaffected peers, approximately 1 in 20 will acquire dislocated hips between the time they learn to walk and the end of their school-aged period.

Another significant disorder associated with Down syndrome is atlantoaxial instability. Atlantoaxial instability results from a "loose joint" between C1 and C2 and increased space between the atlas and odontoid process and affects approximately 13% of children with Down syndrome (Cohen, 1998; Pueschel, 1998). At least 98% to 99% of affected children are asymptomatic. Subluxation or dislocation may result; and early manifestations may include neck pain, torticollis, deteriorating gait, or changes in bowel or bladder function. If left untreated, symptoms may progress to frank neurologic findings associated with spinal cord compression. The atlantodens interval may change over time in a small percentage of children (i.e., generally narrowing but occasionally widening) (Tseng & Cheng, 1998). Secondary to the numerous studies done on atlantoaxial instability, other cervical spinal abnormalities (e.g., degenerative disk diseases including premature arthritis and spondylosis) have been noted (Angelopoulou et al, 1999; Bosma et al, 1999).

Immune System

Children with Down syndrome have altered immune function. Immune system deficits directly contribute to the increased incidence and severity of numerous other conditions, including—but not limited to—periodontal disease, respiratory problems, thyroid disorders, lymphocytic thyroiditis, leukemia, diabetes mellitus, alopecia areata, adrenal dysfunction, vitiligo, and joint problems (Smith, 1995). Premature aging, also present in Down syndrome, may be the result of altered immune function (Holland, 2000; Lin et al, 2001). Insulin-dependent diabetes mellitus (IDDM) also occurs in 1 in 250 children with Down syndrome, which is more than twice the rate in the general population (Pueschel et al, 1999).

Hearing Loss

The incidence of hearing loss in children with Down syndrome is approximately 40% to 75%. Structural deviations of the skull, foreface, external auditory canal, middle and inner ears, and throat accompanied by eustachian tube dysfunction are associated with congenital and acquired hearing loss that can be sensorineural or conductive or both and occur unilaterally or bilaterally (Tolmie, 2002). The immune deficiency present in children with Down syndrome also affects recurrent ear infections (Cohen, 1999). Hearing loss may greatly affect speech and cognitive development if not treated promptly and correctly.

Growth Retardation

At birth, infants with Down syndrome weigh less, are typically shorter, and have smaller occipital-frontal circumferences than unaffected children. The velocity of linear growth is also reduced, with the most marked reductions between 6 and 24 months of age. This reduction in velocity recurs during adolescence, when the growth spurt—which is less vigorous than would normally be expected—occurs earlier in adolescents with Down syndrome (Tolmie, 2002). Other causes for the reduction in linear growth may be congenital heart disease, hypothalamic dysfunctions, thyroid disorders, and/or nutrition problems, and each should be evaluated if suspected (Cohen, 1999).

Children with Down syndrome tend to be overweight. Beginning around 2 years of age, these children often have untoward weight gain that persists throughout their lives. For virtually every age, more than 30% of children with Down syndrome are above the 85th percentile for weight/height ratios, but some researchers have found this percentage to be as high as 50%. Children of school age show the greatest propensity for weight/height percentile gain (Cohen, 1999). Significant differences have been seen between the growth parameters of children with Down syndrome—with and without congenital heart defects, with the severity of growth delay correlating to the severity of disease (i.e., especially during infancy before cardiac surgery) (Cousineau & Lauer, 1995).

Respiratory Functioning

Combined with a compromised immune system, pulmonary hypertension and hyperplasia, fewer alveoli, a decreased alveolar blood capillary surface area, and associated upper airway obstruction (e.g., lymphatic hypertrophy in the Waldeyer ring) predispose children with Down syndrome to respiratory tract infections, as well as high-altitude pulmonary edema (Durmowicz, 2001). If recurrent severe respiratory tract infections occur, they will have a significant effect on a child's development.

Thyroid Dysfunction

Thyroid dysfunction in Down syndrome is commonly associated with autoimmune dysfunction (Tolmie, 2002) and is usually an acquired rather than a congenital condition. The prevalence of thyroid dysfunction may reach 20% in adults. Specifically, congenital hypothyroidism has an incidence of 1 in 141 infants with Down syndrome, which is 28% higher than that of the general population. Subclinical hypothyroidism is seen in 30% to 50% of school-aged children with Down syndrome (Roizen, 1997). Graves disease, goiter, chronic lymphocytic thyroiditis, and hypothyroidism occur most often. Although thyroid dysfunction may remain subclinical for an extended period, alterations in thyroid-stimulating hormone and thyroid-binding globulin may be seen (Foley, 1995).

Malignancies

Leukemia. Children with Down syndrome are 18 to 20 times more likely to acquire leukemia than children without Down syndrome (Kriss, 1999; Tolmie, 2002), although the reasons for this predisposition to leukemia in Down syndrome is unknown (Lange, 2000). One form of leukemia, transient leukemia (TL), occurs most often in infants with Down syndrome (~10%). This form of leukemia occurs during the newborn period and disappears within the first 3 months. In approximately 20% to 30% of these cases, the child develops acute megakaryoblastic leukemia (AMKL) before age 4 years (Al-Kasim et al, 2002; Taub, 2001). Low-dose cytarabine (Ara-C), an antimetabolite chemotherapy drug, has been used successfully to treat TL (Al-Kasim et al, 2002), although carefully determined dosages should be made since children with Down syndrome tend to experience more severe treatment toxicities and have been shown to be more sensitive to cytarabine and methotrexate (MTX) (Taub, 2001).

The overall incidence of AMKL in children with Down syndrome is approximately 500 times greater than in children without Down syndrome, but children with Down syndrome who acquire AMKL have a better prognosis and respond to treatment better than other children. AMKL primarily occurs in children with Down syndrome before the age of 4 years (Zipursky et al, 1999). The lethal form of AMKL appears with telomerase activity present, whereas in the benign form, it is not found (Holt et al, 2002).

Children with Down syndrome with acute myeloid leukemia (AML) appear to have a better clinical outcome than children without Down syndrome with AML. Researchers hypothesize that this difference is due to a higher sensitivity to the chemotherapy drugs (Zwaan et al, 2002).

Acute lymphatic leukemia (ALL) also occurs at a higher rate (i.e., almost 10 times greater than that in the general population) in children with Down syndrome. ALL occurs most often after the age of 4 years (Lange et al, 1998; Zipursky, 1996).

Testicular Germ Cell Tumors. The incidence of testicular germ cell tumors may be increased in males with Down syndrome. More study is needed, however, to understand this trend (Hasle, 2001).

Celiac Disease

The frequency of celiac disease in children with Down syndrome is 4% to 17%; in the general population, celiac disease generally occurs in 1 in 2000 live births (Hansson et al, 1999; Zachor et al, 2000). Screening has been successfully done with the antiendomysium antibody of the immunoglobulin A class (IgA AEA). Researchers recommend screening all individuals with Down syndrome and performing a small bowel biopsy for diagnosis (Csizmadia et al, 2000; Zachor et al, 2000). Csizmadia and her colleagues (2000, p. 260) suggest screening begin between 1.1 and 3.2 years with typing for "DQA1*0501 and DQB*02 alleles" followed by IgA determinations and repeated annually if there is no diagnosis.

Vision Problems

The increased prevalence of numerous ocular deviations is associated with Down syndrome. The most commonly occurring abnormalities are, in order of decreasing frequency, slanted palpebral fissures, spotted irises, refractive errors, strabismus, nystagmus, cataracts, blepharitis, pseudopapilledema, and keratoconus (Tolmie, 2002). Degree of strabismus is correlated with severity of intellectual disability (Merrick & Koslowe, 2001). A significant loss in visual acuity will result if many of these conditions are not diagnosed and treated in early childhood. Moreover, visual problems—especially refractive errors—increase with age (Tsiaras et al, 1999) and may interfere with cognitive development.

Sleep-Disordered Breathing

Anatomic and physiologic differences (e.g., midfacial hypoplasia, glossoptosis) predispose children with Down syndrome to obstructive sleep apnea and other sleep-disordered breathing problems (Levanon et al, 1999). Problems frequently diagnosed included hypoventilation (81%), obstructive sleep apnea (63%), desaturation (56%), and multiple abnormalities (63%). Levanon and colleagues found significant sleep fragmentation with frequent shifts from deeper to lighter non–rapid eye movement stages. Age, obesity, and cardiac disease did not affect the incidence of these problems.

Skin Conditions

Several skin conditions—most of an immune origin—are common in individuals with Down syndrome. These conditions include atopic dermatitis, cheilitis, seborrheic dermatitis, ichthyosis, and vitiligo (Roizen, 1997).

Dental Changes

Children with Down syndrome seem to develop caries less often than unaffected children. Numerous other dental problems (e.g., bruxism, malocclusion, defective dentition, microdontia, periodontal disease), however, are more prevalent in these children because of anatomic anomalies of the oral cavity and immunologic dysfunction. The average age of the first tooth eruption in children with Down syndrome is 13 months (Bell et al, 2002; Roizen, 1997; Tolmie, 2002). Of particular significance is juvenile periodontitis, which occurs in approximately 100% of children with Down syndrome. This disease progresses rapidly and may even be noted in deciduous dentition (Cichon et al, 1998). Poor dental care alone does not account for juvenile periodontitis; the altered immune function in conjunction with the extensive gingival inflammation of children with Down syndrome is thought to also be responsible (Amano et al, 2000). Mouth breathing and consumption of a diet high in soft foods—two common occurrences in children with Down syndrome—also contribute to their dental problems.

Seizure Disorders

Children with Down syndrome have an increased frequency of seizure disorders, with approximately 5% to 10% of these children being diagnosed with epilepsy (Tolmie, 2002). Structural differences and biochemical changes associated with Down syndrome have been implicated, although this has not been confirmed. The distribution of the onset of seizures is bimodal, occurring before age 3 years and after 13 years. Of the affected children, 40% begin to have seizures (i.e., generally infantile spasms and generalized tonic-clonic seizures) before 1 year of age. The prognosis of infantile spasms in children with Down syndrome is better than in the general population (Roizen, 1997). The onset of seizures again peaks in adults in their 30s, with tonic-clonic seizures and partial simple and partial complex seizures being the most common. Seizures in adulthood can be indicative of Alzheimer disease (Tolmie, 2002) (see Chapter 25).

Prognosis

Because Down syndrome is associated with numerous anatomic and physiologic aberrations, life expectancy is reduced, with approximately a 10% mortality rate in the first year of life that rises to 15% by 10 years of age (Leonard et al, 2000). The number and severity of congenital anomalies significantly decrease life expectancy for some of these children. Premature aging and a high incidence of Alzheimer disease may reduce life expectancy for adults. With correct medical, educational, and social interventions, most individuals live well into adulthood and have satisfying, productive lives. Today, the median age for death in a review of death certificates for Caucasians with Down syndrome from 1983 to 1997 was 49 years. The median age was less for persons with Down syndrome of other races. Primary causes of death were congenital heart disease, dementia, hypothyroidism, and leukemia (Yang et al, 2002). Successful outcomes seem to depend heavily on the early interventions children and their families receive. If children with Down syndrome are to reach their full potential, aggressive, interdisciplinary management is paramount.

PRIMARY CARE MANAGEMENT

Health Care Maintenance

Primary care providers are encouraged to consult the "Health Care Guidelines for Individuals with Down Syndrome: 1999 Revision" (Cohen, 1999) (Figures 24-4 and 24-5) and the

Name: _____   **Birthday:** _____

Medical Issues	At Birth or at Diagnosis	6–mo	1	1–1/2	2	2–1/2	3	4	5	6	7	8	9	10	11	12
Age, in years																
Karotype & Genetic Counseling	_____															
Usual Preventative Care	_____	___	___	___	___	___	___	___	___	___	___	___	___	___	___	___
Cardiology	Echo															
Audiologic Evaluation	ABR or OAE	___	___	___	___	___	___	___	___	___	___	___	___	___	___	___
Ophthalmologic Evaluation	Red reflex	___	___		___		___	___	___	___	___	___	___	___	___	___
Thyroid (TSH & T$_4$)	State screening	___	___		___		___	___	___	___	___	___	___	___	___	___
Nutrition	_____	___	___	___	___	___	___	___	___	___	___	___	___	___	___	___
Dental Exam[1]					___	___	___	___	___	___	___	___	___	___	___	___
Celiac Screening[2]					___											
Parent Support	_____	___	___	___	___	___	___	___	___	___	___	___	___	___	___	___
Developmental & Educational Services	Early Intervention	___	___	___	___	___	___	___	___	___	___	___	___	___	___	___
Neck X-rays & Neurological Exam[3]							X-ray	___	___	___	___	___	___	___	___	___
Pneumococcal Conjugate Vaccine Series		_____														

Instructions: Perform indicated exam/screening and record date in blank spaces. The grey or shaded boxes mean no action is to be taken for those ages.

[1]Begin Dental Exams at 2 years of age, and continue every 6 months thereafter.
[2]IgA antiendomysium antibodies and total IgA.
[3]Cervical spine x-rays: flexion, neutral and extension, between 3-5 years of age. Repeat as needed for Special Olympics participation. Neurological examination at each visit.

FIGURE 24-4 Down Sydrome Health Care Guidelines (1999 revision) Record Sheet #1: Birth to Age 12 Years. (From *Down Syndrome Quarterly, 4,* no. 3. [1999, September]. Reprinted with permission.)

Name: _____   Birthday: _____

Age, in years								
Medical Issues	13	14	15	16	17	18	19	20-29
Usual Preventative Care	___	___	___	___	___	___	___	___
Audiologic Evaluation	___	___	___	___	___	___	___	___
Ophthalmologic Evaluation	___	___	___	___	___	___	___	___
Thyroid (TSH & T$_4$)	___	___	___	___	___	___	___	___
Nutrition	___	___	___	___	___	___	___	___
Dental Exam[1]	___	___	___	___	___	___	___	___
Parent Support	___	___	___	___	___	___	___	___
Developmental & Educational Services	___	___	___	___	___	___	___	___
Neck X-rays & Neurological Exam[2]	___	___	___	___	___	___	___	___
Pelvic exam[3]				___	___	___	___	___
Assess Contraceptive Need[3]				___	___	___	___	___

Instructions: Perform indicated exam/screening and record date in blank spaces. The grey or shaded boxes mean no action is to be taken for those ages.

[1]Begin dental exams at 2 years of age, and continue every 6 months thereafter.
[2]Cervical spine x-rays: flexion, neutral and extension, between 3-5 years of age. Repeat as needed for Special Olympics participation. Neurological examination at each visit.
[3]If sexually active.

FIGURE 24-5 Down Sydrome Health Care Guidelines (1999 revision) Record Sheet #2: 13 Years to Adulthood. (From *Down Syndrome Quarterly, 4,* no. 3. [1999, September]. Reprinted with permission.)

"Health Supervision Guidelines for Children with Down Syndrome" (AAP, Committee on Genetics, 2001).

Growth and Development

Evaluating the growth of children with Down syndrome is a detailed process. When linear growth is assessed, primary care providers must take into account the variations in velocity. Whereas growth adequacy is often determined by maintaining a particular percentile rank, variations in growth velocity affect the growth curves of these children during early childhood. Growth velocities for children with and without Down syndrome are similar during the school-aged period, however, and stability is then seen in percentile curves.

Measurements should be plotted on both the National Center for Health Statistics (NCHS) growth charts and growth charts with specific norms for children with Down syndrome (Figures 24-6 to 24-11). The NCHS growth charts allow children with Down syndrome to be compared with their chronologic-age peers and also provide a frame of reference for parents. The weight/height percentiles on the NCHS growth charts are independent of a child's age and are also useful in determining appropriate weight in children before adolescence. The specialty charts, in which all percentiles for stature are less than their analogous percentiles on the NCHS charts, provide an excellent reference point for comparing growth among children with Down syndrome and determining those at risk for failure

Boys with Down Syndrome:
Physical Growth: 1 to 36 Months

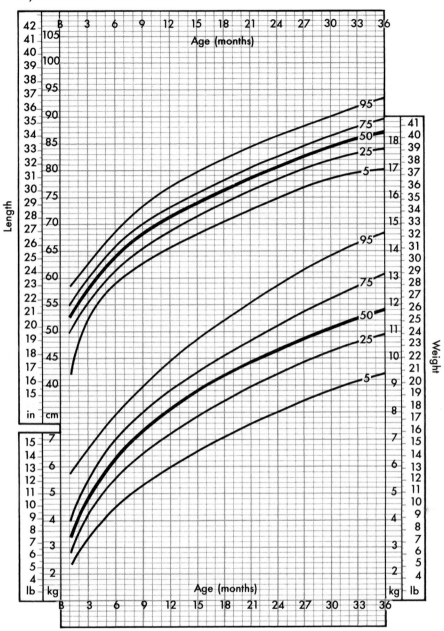

FIGURE 24-6 Boys with Down syndrome: physical growth: 1 to 36 months. This graph is based on data from the Developmental Evaluation Clinic of the Children's Hospital, Boston; The Child Development Center of Rhode Island Hospital; and the Clinical Genetics Service of the Children's Hospital of Philadelphia (supported by March of Dimes grant 6-449).

to thrive or obesity. The methodology used in obtaining the growth charts for children with Down syndrome has been questioned, but it is recommended that these charts be consulted until future charts are available (Cohen & Patterson, 1998).

Because inappropriate growth and excessive weight gain have ramifications for motor performance and social acceptance for children with Down syndrome, yearly assessments are required. Interventions for weight management may be introduced as necessary. Caloric reduction and increased exercise

incorporated into a behavior management program are likely to be the most effective approach to decrease cardiovascular risk factors of obesity, hypertension, and being sedentary (Pastore et al, 2000).

Children with Down syndrome have the most difficulty with language development, especially with expressive language. They often do not speak their first word until 24 months of age (Chapman & Hesketh, 2000). Encouragement of nonverbal communication skills (e.g., taking turns with toys and social interaction between parents and the child) facilitates the

Girls with Down Syndrome:
Physical Growth: 1 to 36 Months

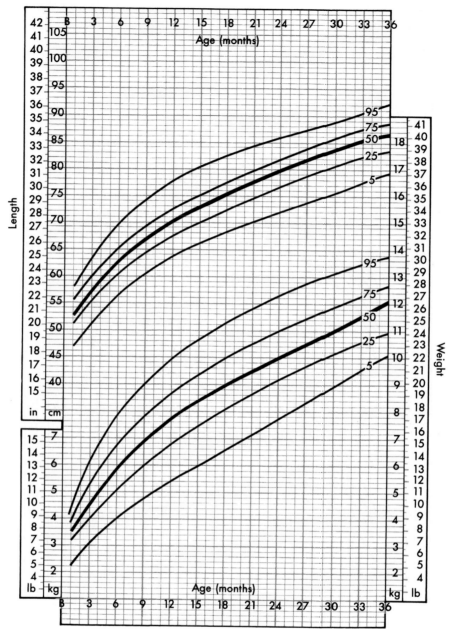

FIGURE 24-7 Girls with Down syndrome: physical growth: 1 to 36 months. This graph is based on data from the Developmental Evaluation Clinic of the Children's Hospital, Boston; The Child Development Center of Rhode Island Hospital; and the Clinical Genetics Service of the Children's Hospital of Philadelphia (supported by March of Dimes grant 6-449).

development of verbal language development (Stoel-Gammon, 2000).

Children with Down syndrome will pass through the normal developmental milestones but at a much slower rate than expected. The primary care provider can assist in a child's development by referring the family to an early intervention program as soon as possible after the child's birth. As the child grows older, a variety of activities that are known to assist in development (e.g., Special Olympics, summer camp) can be encouraged. If a child has significant congenital anomalies, program personnel will need guidance as to the intensity of activity the child is allowed. A child's progress should be carefully documented on standardized developmental schedules (Figure 24-12, p. 460) at each primary care visit. Since Down syndrome is associated with global development delay, most children with Down syndrome will have intelligence quotients (IQs) below the second standard deviation on standardized tests, such as the Wechsler Intelligence

Boys with Down Syndrome:
Physical Growth: 2 to 18 Years

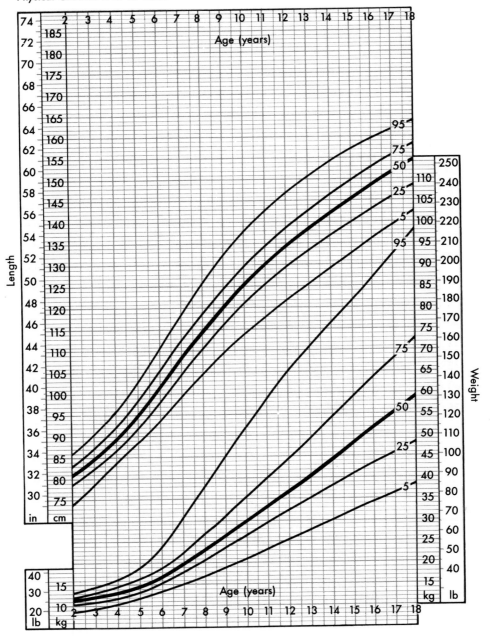

FIGURE 24-8 Boys with Down syndrome: physical growth: 2 to 18 years. This graph is based on data from the Developmental Evaluation Clinic of the Children's Hospital, Boston; The Child Development Center of Rhode Island Hospital; and the Clinical Genetics Service of the Children's Hospital of Philadelphia (supported by March of Dimes grant 6-449).

Scale for Children–Revised or the Bayley Scales of Infant Development.

Diet

Among the most significant concerns are feeding difficulties in young children and obesity in older children. Feeding problems may be encountered because of the disproportionately large tongues, muscle flaccidity, poor coordination, significantly delayed social maturation, thyroid or pituitary disorders, and

congenital heart disease found in children with Down syndrome.

For infants, breast-feeding should be encouraged. The immunogenic qualities of breast milk offer additional protection against upper respiratory tract infections and other illnesses. The extra effort required of infants who are breast feeding also helps them to develop orofacial muscles and tongue control and promotes greater jaw stability. Breast feeding may take longer at first, and mothers will need

Girls with Down Syndrome:
Physical Growth: 2 to 18 Years

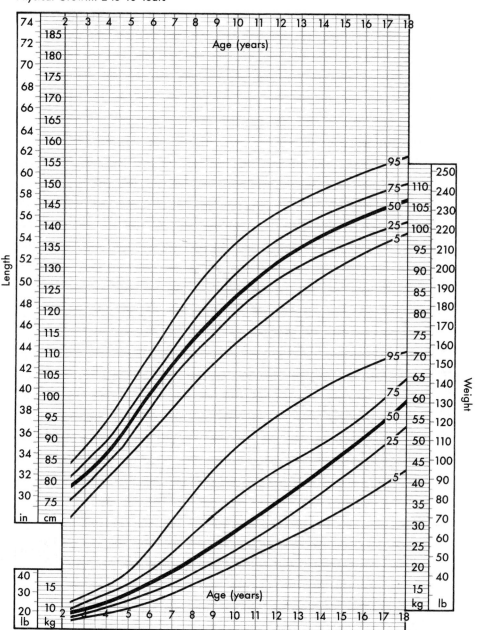

FIGURE 24-9 Girls with Down syndrome: physical growth: 2 to 18 years. This graph is based on data from the Developmental Evaluation Clinic of the Children's Hospital, Boston; The Child Development Center of Rhode Island Hospital; and the Clinical Genetics Service of the Children's Hospital of Philadelphia (supported by March of Dimes grant 6-449).

to be encouraged in their efforts. The LaLeche League of America has material on breast feeding infants with Down syndrome.

Blended and chopped foods and shallow-bowl, latex-covered spoons may help children who are learning to eat solids. If significant problems (e.g., aspiration) occur, an occupational therapist or other developmental therapist should be consulted in designing an individualized feeding program (Saenz, 1999).

There are no routine dietary restrictions for older children. Care should be taken to avoid excessive caloric intake if inappropriate weight gain is a problem. A balanced diet, a program of physical exercise, and vitamin and mineral supplementation are recommended as necessary (Saenz, 1999).

The only dietary restriction for children with Down syndrome is for those diagnosed with celiac disease. These children must be on a gluten-free diet to relieve symptoms and protect against future malignancy (Book et al, 2001).

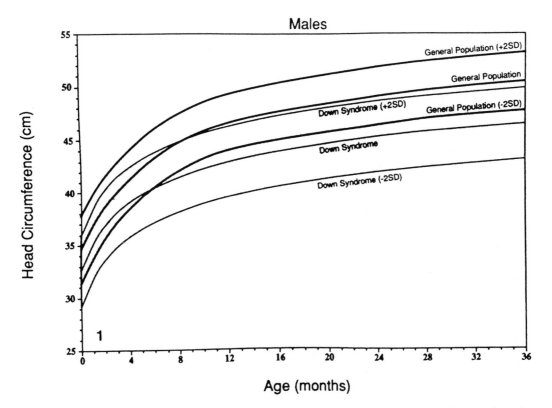

FIGURE 24-10 Head circumference growth curves for males with Down syndrome compared with those for males in the general population. (From Palmer, C.G. et al. [1992]. Head circumference of children with Down syndrome 0 to 36 months. *Am J Med Genet, 42,* 61-67. Reprinted with permission.)

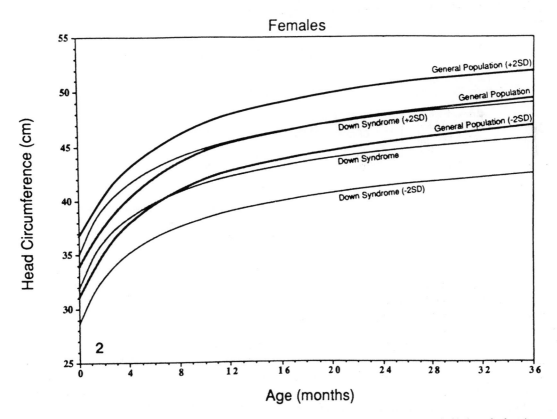

FIGURE 24-11 Head circumference growth curves for females with Down syndrome compared with those for females in the general population. (From Palmer, C.G. et al. [1992]. Head circumference of children with Down syndrome 0 to 36 months. *Am J Med Genet, 42,* 61-67. Reprinted with permission.)

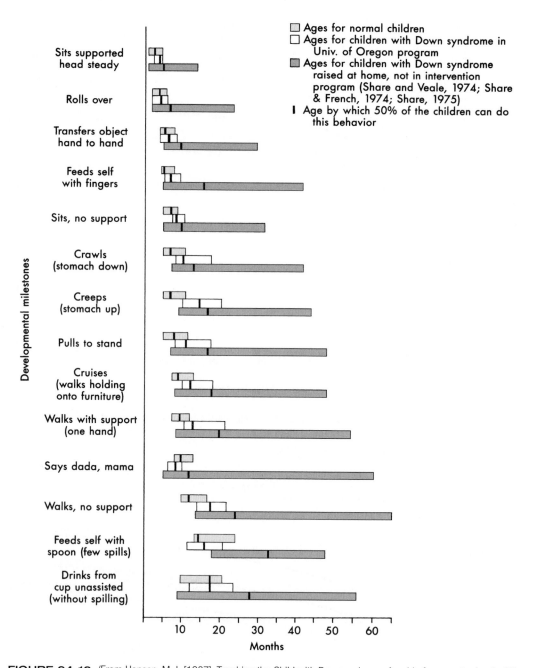

FIGURE 24-12 (From Hanson, M.J. [1987]. Teaching the Child with Down sydrome: A guide for parents. Austin, TX: Pro-Ed. Reprinted with permission.)

Safety

Safety issues for children with Down syndrome are the same as for their developmental, not chronologic, peers. Primary care providers must adjust their normal schedule for providing anticipatory guidance to the development of children with Down syndrome. If information is given too far in advance of a child's developmental progression, parents may forget or find the information to be a painful reminder that their child is progressing more slowly than unaffected children.

Children with Down syndrome are more likely to sustain joint injuries as a result of their musculoskeletal problems. For children with atlantoaxial instability or those who have not yet been adequately evaluated, contact sports, somersaults, or other activities that may result in cervical injury should be restricted. Documentation that the child is not in danger of subluxation may be required for children participating in the Special Olympics.

Immunizations

Children with Down syndrome tend to develop autoantibodies at a higher frequency than the general population, which is possibly due to accelerated aging of their immune system. More research is needed on this topic to further understand how and why this development occurs. As a result of the development of autoantibodies, additional immunizations may be necessary because these children are at high risk for infection. In areas endemic for specific diseases, antibody titer levels may be assessed to determine a child's immune status (Tolmie, 2002).

There are, however, no contraindications for immunizations for children with Down syndrome. If they have a cell-mediated disorder, live-viral vaccines are contraindicated. In most cases, the national immunization schedule should be followed (Committee on Infectious Diseases, 2000).

A 7-valent pneumococcal polysaccharide-protein conjugate vaccine (Prevnar, PCV7) is indicated for children with Down syndrome and should be given according to the regular immunization schedule. This vaccination may be repeated after age 2 years if the child also has an immunocompromising condition, such as leukemia, or a chronic cardiac or respiratory condition. The use of the 23-valent polysaccharide vaccine after age 2 years (PPV23; e.g., Pneumovax 23) may be warranted (Centers for Disease Control and Prevention, Advisory Committee on Immunization Practices, 2000).

Yearly immunoprophylaxis for influenza should also be considered for all children over 6 months of age. In cases of recurrent infections, antiviral medications (e.g., amantadine) may be considered to prevent the occurrence of influenza (Saenz, 1999).

Hepatitis A vaccination should not be given to children with Down syndrome unless warranted because their place of residence has a high incidence rate and community prophylaxis is being done (Centers for Disease Control and Prevention, Advisory Committee on Immunization Practices, 1999).

Screening

Vision. Because of the large number of ocular defects associated with Down syndrome, all children should be evaluated by an ophthalmologist by 6 months of age and every 2 years to assess for strabismus and cataracts. Early referral is critical considering the synergistic effects that diminished vision and hearing have on development. Significant visual impairment is usually preventable because the conditions common in Down syndrome (e.g., strabismus, myopia) are treatable (Committee on Genetics, 2001; Cohen, 1999). Future screening recommendations should be determined in conjunction with the ophthalmologist according to the status of the child's eyes. At minimum, the primary care provider should screen for visual problems at each well-child visit. Such screening should include testing acuity, examining the red reflex and optic fundi, and checking alignment and oculomotor functions. Because children with Down syndrome may have difficulty using a Snellen or lazy E chart, acuity screening performed with the Titmus picture test, Teller acuity cards, or Allen picture cards will yield more valid results.

Many children with Down syndrome have difficulty keeping their glasses in place, so parents should be counseled that purchasing glasses with lightweight plastic lenses and using an elastic strap around the child's occiput to secure them will help correct this problem. Contact lenses are not routinely recommended but may be appropriate for children with keratoconus.

Hearing. Because good hearing is a requisite for cognitive, social, and language development and because these children are at high risk for conductive hearing loss, careful assessment is necessary. The health care provider should use the smallest size speculum (2 mm) for the examination because of typically tiny ear openings. It is recommended that all infants be evaluated for auditory brainstem responses (ABR) or otoacoustic emission (OAE) during the first 3 months of life (Committee on Genetics, 2001). Behavioral audiograms should take place every 6 months until the child is 3 years of age and yearly thereafter (Cohen, 1999). If the external ear orifice is stenotic or there are other difficulties that preclude adequate pneumootoscopic examination, alternate methods of evaluation must be used. Tympanometry provides one useful adjunct to assessment but is not reliable in children under 1 year of age. Because of the importance of early intervention, infants between 9 and 12 months of age should be referred for microotoscopy if examination is difficult. The accumulation of cerumen leading to impacted canals is common; removal of cerumen every 6 months is recommended for children with this problem. When middle ear disease occurs, it deserves aggressive intervention and close follow-up if further developmental insult is to be prevented. Therefore a hearing evaluation by an otolaryngologist should take place every 6 months until the child is 3 years old and then on an annual basis (Committee on Genetics, 2001; Cohen, 1999).

If hearing aids are required, those that fasten onto the earpiece of eyeglasses may be better than ear molds. Hearing aids dependent on ear molds are hard to fit for children who are just beginning to wear them. These children often do not like the increased sound. Parents may need help finding methods (e.g., behavior management) to help improve their child's compliance for leaving the hearing aid in place. Parents must also be cautioned to devise mnemonic cues for remembering to change the batteries routinely because it is unlikely that their child will be able to realize that the hearing aid is malfunctioning.

Dental. Because of the extremely high prevalence of dental problems in young children, aggressive dental care is necessary. Primary care providers must document and carefully observe the dental problems of these children. All children with Down syndrome should be evaluated before the age of 18 months by a dentist or pedodontist skilled in caring for children with developmental disabilities. Locating such dentists is often difficult for parents, and specific referrals to professionals may be warranted.

Good dental hygiene—including twice daily brushing and flossing—is indicated to reduce the amount of periodontal disease. If good dental hygiene is difficult to achieve, using a Water Pik or an electric toothbrush should be considered. Effective tooth-brushing techniques may be difficult to achieve because of the child's limited manual dexterity, enlarged tongue, and small mouth. Close supervision is required, and independent tooth brushing and mouth care may not be feasible until the child is at least of preschool age.

Weaning children from a bottle by 18 months and diets that contain low-sugar, crunchy foods (e.g., fresh vegetables) also help deter dental deterioration and should be encouraged. In areas where the water supply is nonfluoridated, fluoride supplementation should be initiated. If periodontal disease is severe, chemical plaque control may be necessary. For children with congenital heart disease, prophylactic antibiotics should accompany all dental interventions (Cohen, 1999) (see Chapter 21).

Blood Pressure. Routine screening is recommended. If there is a history of cardiac disease or a positive family history of cardiac disease or hypertension, more careful assessment is required. A cardiac evaluation, including an echocardiogram, however, is warranted during infancy to rule out congenital heart disease or cardiac defects (AAP, Committee on Genetics, 2001; Cohen, 1999).

Hematocrit. Routine screening is recommended.

Urinalysis. Routine screening is recommended.

Tuberculosis. Routine screening is recommended. No special precautions must be taken unless the child is or has been institutionalized.

Condition-Specific Screening (Box 24-4)

Thyroid Dysfunction. Because the abnormalities seen in Down syndrome are similar to some seen in thyroid dysfunction, it is difficult to diagnose thyroid problems by clinical examination. Thyroid-stimulating hormone levels (TSH, T_4) should be assessed at 6 and 12 months of age and annually thereafter (Committee on Genetics, 2001; Cohen, 1999). If there are any signs or symptoms suggestive of thyroid dysfunction, a complete thyroid panel should be drawn.

Atlantoaxial Instability. Primary care providers must appraise the risk of atlantoaxial subluxation for all children with Down syndrome who are planning to engage in physically active exercise or the Special Olympics or who are to undergo surgical or rehabilitative procedures (Cohen, 1999). Currently, the need for cervical spine radiographic studies in children with Down syndrome is controversial (Tolmie, 2002).

Hip Dislocation. Assessing hip stability through age 10 years is indicated because early detection (i.e., before the dislocation is fixed and acetabular dysplasia occurs) allows for optimal surgical correction. Early presenting signs of habitual dislocation are an increasing limp, decreasing activity, and an audible click. Pain does not usually occur unless the dislocation is acute. In older children, radiographic studies may be necessary for assessment.

Mitral Valve Prolapse. Screening should begin in adolescence. Echocardiographic evaluations are recommended before surgical or dental procedures (Cohen, 1999).

Celiac Disease. Although screening is not mandatory for individuals with Down syndrome, increased attention has been brought to the incidence of celiac disease in persons with Down syndrome. IgA-antiendomysium antibodies (EMA) and total IgA have been found to be good immunologic markers in screening for this disease (Cohen, 1999; Csizmadia et al, 2000; Zachor et al, 2000).

Common Illness Management
Differential Diagnosis (Box 24-5)

Immune Dysfunction. The significant changes in the immune systems of children with Down syndrome have significant implications for primary care providers. Specifically, all infections must be treated aggressively because negative sequelae are more likely to develop. The incidence of many autoimmune diseases (i.e., including insulin-dependent diabetes mellitus and chronic arthritis) is also much greater in this population. If a child exhibits signs and symptoms compatible with a diagnosis of any of these diseases, a thorough evaluation is indicated. Parents must be educated about the signs and symptoms of conditions and the need to seek medical advice promptly (see Chapters 23 and 31).

Upper Respiratory Tract Infections. Children with Down syndrome are prone to upper respiratory tract infections. These infections should be managed aggressively because untoward sequelae—including otitis media and pneumonia—are apt to develop. Children with congenital heart disease should be examined at the first signs of illness because these children are more likely to develop secondary problems and parents may confuse an upper respiratory tract infection with early congestive heart failure. These children may also need to be given subacute bacterial endocarditis prophylaxis (see Chapter 21).

Behavioral Changes. Behavioral changes may be caused by a variety of physiologic and psychologic problems, including the following: (1) thyroid dysfunction, (2) obstructive sleep apnea, (3) neurodegeneration (primarily in older individuals), (4) declining physical competence (e.g., congestive heart failure), (5) disturbed home environment, and (6) overstimulation. Interventions must be cause specific. Trials with stimulants, antidepressants, or antipsychotic drugs may be indicated in some cases after a thorough evaluation, although diagnosis of mental illness should not be given based solely on the fact that the child has Down syndrome.

Gastrointestinal Symptoms. Because pyloric stenosis and Hirschsprung disease are more common in children with Down syndrome, primary care providers should carefully pursue reports of persistent vomiting, constipation, or chronic diarrhea in infants. Constipation, a common problem, may also be related to inadequate peristalsis, poor diet, lack of exercise, or thyroid dysfunction. The cause of constipation must clearly be assessed so that the correct interventions are initiated.

Leukemia. Children with Down syndrome acquire leukemia 18 to 20 times as often as other children. Easy bruising, unusual pallor, or listlessness must be fully evaluated. Parents must be alerted to immediately seek health care for their child if any of these signs or symptoms develops.

Drug Interactions

Because children with Down syndrome are at risk for health problems affecting any organ or system of their body, they may often be taking medications. It is important that family members understand how to administer the medications, what the side effects are, and to report any allergic reactions to the primary care provider. Over-the-counter medications are often ineffective (e.g., with skin problems), and prescription medications may be needed.

Developmental Issues

Sleep Patterns

Sleep disorders are uncommon in children with Down syndrome, with the exception of obstructive sleep apnea and related conditions. Anatomic and immunologic differences predispose school-aged children in particular to this condition. The primary care provider should have a high index of suspicion if the child has a history of snoring, restless sleep, abnormal sleep positions, being awake for hours during the night, night terrors, or daytime somnolence, as well as if failure to thrive, pulmonary hypertension, or behavioral problems are present. Referral to a sleep laboratory for periodic overnight polysomnography evaluation is warranted (AAP, Committee on Genetics, 2001; Cohen, 1999). Surgical treatment can range from tonsillectomy and adenoidectomy to a combination of skeletal and soft tissue alterations (Lefaivre et al, 1997).

Toileting

The median age for toilet training children with Down syndrome is approximately 36 months. Parents must be advised of this to reduce frustrations associated with unrealistic expectations. Routine toilet training techniques are effective. It takes longer, however, to train a child with Down syndrome, and additional positive reinforcement is necessary.

Children with Down syndrome may experience constipation secondary to their generalized muscle flaccidity and low activity levels. Dietary corrections, occasional use of bulk laxatives, and increases in exercise can alleviate this problem.

Discipline

Children with Down syndrome are usually not more difficult to discipline than other children. Parents must be encouraged to remember that discipline needs to be appropriate for the child's developmental, not chronologic, age. Children with Down syndrome should not receive special compensation just because they have Down syndrome. Parental expectations should be consistent, and limits should be set for all children in the family. Behavior management programs can be developed for specific discipline problems when a child has not been responsive to the parents' usual methods.

Child Care. Daycare should provide appropriate social, cognitive, and physical stimulation for a child with Down syndrome. When selecting the type of daycare setting, parents should be encouraged to consider the child's personality and medical needs as well as their own philosophy about inclusion. Many generic daycare centers include children with Down syndrome into their programs and are sufficiently staffed to provide an excellent experience for these children. If a child has significant medical problems, specialized daycare, which is often available through the school system, may be a better option. If a child is highly susceptible to infections, a home care setting (i.e., with fewer than six children) is recommended. Primary care providers should be aware of resources in their community to assist parents with daycare placement. Local parent groups for children with Down syndrome, as well as the local affiliates of the Arc of the United States and other specialty agencies, may also help with placement.

Schooling

A variety of options—from total inclusion to residential placement—for academic placement exist. If circumstances permit, children with Down syndrome do best in an environment fully integrated with nondisabled peers. Children with Down syndrome, however, need support from their families while they deal with being exceptional and with social pressures from peers. Parents and teachers working together to create a supportive environment can ensure that a child has some social and academic successes. Otherwise, the child may become frustrated and demoralized, which can lead to disruptive behavior and poor self-esteem.

Families may need assistance in choosing the school setting they deem most appropriate for their child. Primary care providers can be instrumental in helping families locate appropriate community services to assist in educational placement. All children with Down syndrome are eligible for educational provisions under Public Law 105-17 (IDEA) (see Chapter 5). Parents should be encouraged to contact their social worker or local office of mental retardation shortly after the child's birth so that they can receive the educational, vocational, and supportive services for which the child is eligible.

Sexuality

Pubertal changes in adolescents with Down syndrome occur at approximately the same time as in their unaffected peers. Accompanying these physical changes, adolescents will have social interests and biologic drives similar to those of their chronologic-age peers and must be given the opportunity to participate in social activities with their peers. For parents who are highly protective, the social education and sexual education that must accompany their child's increasing independence are often difficult and sensitive issues (AAP, Committee on Genetics, 2001; Cohen, 1999). Primary care providers need to help parents recognize their responsibility in ensuring that children can handle themselves in a socially and sexually appropriate manner.

Individualized instruction about self-care skills, biologic changes, social implications, and contraception is paramount to minimizing both the appearance of sexual impropriety and the risk of being sexually exploited. Routine pelvic examination is not recommended for females who are not sexually active; and the young woman, her parents, and the primary care provider should discuss the frequency of this examination (Cohen, 1999). Genetic counseling for both the parents and the child is necessary. Although men are virtually always sterile, women are capable of reproducing. Planned Parenthood, the Arc of the United States, and parent support groups offer printed and audiovisual materials specifically designed for use with these families.

The age at onset of menses for females is similar to that of their mothers. Handling pubertal changes is difficult for some female adolescents. Family members must be helped to recognize the behavior changes that may be related to normal hormonal cycles. For those women who are menstruating and are unable to manage their own hygienic care, parents and other caregivers must follow Universal Precautions.

Primary gonadal insufficiency may be present in males and is evidenced by small testes, a concentration of serum follicle-stimulating hormone, and a negative correlation between testicular volume and luteinizing hormone level (Tolmie, 2002). Some parents may request that their daughter with Down syndrome be sterilized. The right to procreative choice is protected by law, and statutes regarding sterilization vary greatly from state to state. Primary care providers are strongly suggested to consult their state office of mental retardation for current guidelines because sterilization is illegal in some jurisdictions. If sterilization is to be pursued, the adolescent must participate in the decision to the extent possible (Committee on Bioethics, 1999).

Transition into Adulthood

The life expectancy for individuals with Down syndrome has increased dramatically with most living well into middle age, creating the need to address independent living, sexuality, vocational choices, and health maintenance in adulthood and older adulthood.

Individuals with Down syndrome vary in their abilities to live independently; some require ongoing, consistent supervision, and others merely need minimal guidance with complex tasks. Most individuals remain at home until a crisis forces different arrangements. Because individuals with Down syndrome often have aged parents, families can help plan for a smooth transition to a different living situation within the context of normal development. For example, some parents may help their son or daughter move to a group home at about the same age as their other children left for college. Recreational activities, such as bowling, swimming, and dancing, are encouraged because they promote social relationships and physical fitness. Registering to vote is also an important function of adulthood.

Vocational choices are directed by an individual's cognitive abilities, social skills, and adaptive abilities. Many persons with Down syndrome can seek competitive employment in custodial work, offices, housekeeping, restaurants, landscaping, or other occupations where the required skills are not too difficult and are fairly repetitive, and there is ongoing supervision. The skills necessary to survive in the work force (e.g., basic money management, telling time, using public transportation) must be mastered before such positions are sought. For others, working in sheltered workshops is a better option because this type of job requires fewer adaptive abilities.

Generally, the overall health of most individuals with Down syndrome is good. Premature aging may occur as early as the 20s with dental changes often seen first. Dermatologic, thyroid, cardiac, and sensory problems are the most troublesome and worsen with age. Changes in mental health may also be a concern after children complete formal schooling at 21 years of age. Depression and dementia are the most common psychiatric disorders seen in Down syndrome and constitute part

of the behavioral phenotype of Down syndrome (Chapman & Hesketh, 2000). This prevalence may be a result of decreased social opportunities and lack of readily available transportation. Perhaps of greatest concern is Alzheimer disease, which occurs in a sizable proportion of adults with Down syndrome over 40 years of age (Lott & Head, 2001). The actual percentage differs among studies, but the minimum percentage is generally considered to be 25%. The incidence rises as the person ages. IQ levels and adaptive functioning also decline over time. Further longitudinal study of adults with Down syndrome—especially documentation of health status changes—is warranted.

Family Concerns and Resources

Parents of children with Down syndrome will experience joy and pride in their child, although they will be faced with many challenges throughout their child's life. Most parents meet these challenges with resilience and adaptive functioning (Roach et al, 1999). For some parents, however, raising these children can become overwhelming. Locating and coordinating acceptable medical, educational, and ancillary personnel may produce stress. Primary care providers may be of tremendous assistance to the families in identifying appropriate resources (e.g., respite care) and helping parents become their child's best lifelong advocate. Mothers in particular may find it difficult to balance their time and responsibilities among their children and spouse.

Although many concerns are similar for all families who have a child with special needs, one notable issue for families of children with Down syndrome is the need for long-range planning. Most children with Down syndrome may never become totally self-sufficient, and families must plan for a child's lifetime through, for example, estate planning and custody arrangements. They must also enroll an adult child to receive Supplemental Security Income (SSI) (see Chapter 8). Other children with Down syndrome, however, may marry and live semiindependent lives. The degree of the child's limitations, the internal strengths of the family, and the support from extended family and community networks all affect a family's adjustment.

RESOURCES

Caring for a child with Down syndrome is a complex task because of the physical, cognitive, and social concerns that must be addressed. Additional resources for professionals and parents of children with Down syndrome are given here.

Informational Materials

Bruni, M. (1998). *Fine motor skills in children with Down syndrome: A guide for parents and professionals*. Bethesda, Md.: Woodbine House.
Available from:
Woodbine House
6510 Bells Mill Rd
Bethesda, MD 20817

Cohen, W.I., Nadel, L., & Madnick, M.E. (Eds.). (2002). *Down syndrome: Visions for the 21st century*. New York: John Wiley & Sons.
Available from:
John Wiley & Sons
111 River St
Hoboken, NJ 07030

Hassold, T.J. (1999). *Down syndrome: A promising future, together.* New York: Wiley-Liss.
Available from:
Wiley-Liss, Inc
605 Third Ave
New York, NY 10158-0012

Kumin, L. (1994). *Communication skills in children with Down syndrome: A guide for parents.* Bethesda, Md.: Woodbine House.
Available from:
Woodbine House
6510 Bells Mill Rd
Bethesda, MD 20817

Oelwein, P.L. (1995). *Teaching reading to children with Down syndrome: A guide for parents and teachers.* Bethesda, Md.: Woodbine House.
Available from:
Woodbine House
6510 Bells Mill Rd
Bethesda, MD 20817

Pueschel, S.M. (Ed.). (2000). *A parents guide to Down syndrome: Toward a brighter future* (2nd ed.). Baltimore: Paul H. Brookes.
Available from:
Paul H Brookes Publishing Co
PO Box 10624
Baltimore, MD 21285-0624

Pueschel, S.M. & Sustrova, M. (Eds.). (1997). *Adolescents with Down syndrome: Toward a more fulfilling life.* Baltimore: Paul H. Brookes.
Available from:
Paul H Brookes Publishing Co
PO Box 10624
Baltimore, MD 21285-0624

Rondal, J., Perera, J., & Nadel, L. (Eds.). (1999). *Down syndrome: A review of current knowledge.* London: Whurr Publishers, Ltd.
Available from:
Whurr Publishers, Ltd
19b Compton Terrace
London, England, N1 2UN

Stray-Gundersen, K. (Ed.). (1995). *Babies with Down syndrome: A new parents guide* (3rd ed.). Bethesda, Md.: Woodbine House.
Available from:
Woodbine House, Inc
6510 Bells Mill Rd
Bethesda, MD 20817

Van Dyke, D.C. et al (Eds.). (1995). *Medical and surgical care for children with Down syndrome: A guide for parents.* Bethesda, Md.: Woodbine House.
Available from:
Woodbine House
6510 Bells Mill Rd
Bethesda, MD 20817

Winders, P.C. (1997). *Gross motor skills in children with Down syndrome: A guide for parents and professionals.* Bethesda, Md.: Woodbine House.
Available from:
Woodbine House
6510 Bells Mill Rd
Bethesda, MD 20817

Organizations

The Arc of the United States
1010 Wayne Ave, Suite 650
Silver Spring, MD 20910
(301) 565-3842; (301) 565-3843 (fax)
info@thearc.org; http://www.thearc.org

Canadian Down Syndrome Society
811-14 Street NW
Calgary, Alberta, Canada T2N 2A4
(403) 270-8500; (403) 270-8291 (fax)
dsingo@cdss.ca; http://www.cdss.ca

The Commission on Mental and Physical Disability Law
American Bar Association
740 15th St, NW
Washington, DC 20005
(202) 662-1570; (202) 662-1032 (fax)
cmpdl@abanet.org; http://www.abanet.org/disability

National Down Syndrome Congress
1370 Center Drive, Suite 102
Atlanta, GA 30338
(800) 232-6372 (NDSC); (770) 604-9500 (fax)
info@ndsccenter.org; http://www.ndsccenter.org

National Down Syndrome Society
666 Broadway, 8th Floor
New York, NY 10012-2317
(800) 221-4602; (212) 979-2873 (fax)
Info@ndss.org; http://www.ndss.org/

Summary of Primary Care Needs for the Child with Down Syndrome

HEALTH CARE MAINTENANCE
Growth and Development

Children usually have a shorter stature and increased weight (after infancy).

Occipitofrontal circumference may be decreased.

Children should have height and weight measured at each visit and plotted on NCHS growth charts and growth charts for children with Down syndrome. Caloric reduction and increased exercise are recommended.

Virtually all children will have mental retardation and global developmental delay.

Expressive language problems are common.

Normal progression of developmental milestones occurs but at slower rate.

Early intervention programs are recommended for older children.

Virtually all children will have hypotonia and joint laxity. Obesity compounds these complications.

Cognitive function often deteriorates with age.

Diet. Breast feeding is encouraged in infancy.

Feeding support is needed in infancy to ensure adequate weight gain.

Diets may need to be tailored to help correct constipation or obesity.

Vitamin and mineral supplementation is often recommended. Potential for aspiration is a concern.

Safety. Anticipatory guidance needs to be based on a child's developmental—not chronologic—age.

There is increased incidence of musculoskeletal and/or joint injuries from laxity.

Atlantoaxial instability is a hazard and must be ruled out before active sports programs or surgery.

Continued

Summary of Primary Care Needs for the Child with Down Syndrome—cont'd

Growth and Development—cont'd

Immunizations. Routine immunizations are recommended.

Immunity may not be conferred from immunizations because of a compromised immune system. Titer analysis during outbreaks of communicable diseases is recommended.

Pneumococcal polysaccharide and influenza immunoprophylaxis should be considered.

Screening

Vision. The incidence of ocular defects is high. All infants should be evaluated by an ophthalmologist by 6 months of age and at 2 years.

Acuity and alignment testing and examination of the red reflex and optic fundi should be done at each visit.

Hearing. Anatomic abnormalities of ears are common. Auditory brainstem response testing is recommended by 3 months of age. Evaluation by specialist recommended every 6 months until age 3 years and then annually.

Otoscopy and tympanometry should be performed at each visit.

Cerumen impaction and otitis media are common.

Of these children, 40% to 75% have hearing loss. Many will require hearing aids.

Dental. Dental screening should be done a minimum of every 6 months from age 18 months because of the high incidence of periodontal disease.

Good dental hygiene is important. If not in water, fluoride is recommended.

Children with congenital heart disease (CHD) may require antibiotic prophylaxis to prevent endocarditis.

Blood Pressure. Routine screening is recommended.

A full cardiac evaluation with echocardiogram should be done in infancy.

Hematocrit. Routine screening is recommended.

Urinalysis. Routine screening is recommended.

Tuberculosis. Routine screening is recommended.

Condition-Specific Screening

Obtain karyotype in neonatal period.

Thyroid-stimulating hormone levels should be checked at 6 and 12 months of age and yearly thereafter.

Atlantoaxial instability risk should be assessed before surgery or athletic involvement.

Screening for hip dislocation is necessary through age 10 years or whenever a gait abnormality occurs.

Screening for mitral valve prolapse should start in adolescence.

Screening for celiac disease with IgA-antiendomysium antibodies of the immunoglobulin A class should be considered.

COMMON ILLNESS MANAGEMENT

Differential Diagnosis

Immune Dysfunction. Children with Down syndrome are more susceptible to infections and autoimmune disorders.

Upper Respiratory Tract Infections. Upper respiratory tract infections are often associated with otitis media and pneumonia and should be managed aggressively, especially when a child has CHD.

Behavioral Changes. Thyroid dysfunction, obstructive sleep apnea, neurodegeneration, declining adaptive functioning, disturbed home environment, overstimulation, and attention deficit hyperactivity disorder (ADHD) should be ruled out.

Gastrointestinal Symptoms. Pyloric stenosis, Hirschsprung disease, inadequate peristalsis, and thyroid dysfunction should be ruled out.

Constipation is a common problem and may be due to decreased peristalsis, poor diet, lack of exercise, or thyroid dysfunction.

Leukemia. Unusual pallor, easy bruising, and listlessness should be fully evaluated.

Drug Interactions

Children may be taking different medications for different conditions, so primary care providers should be aware of drug interactions and side effects.

DEVELOPMENTAL ISSUES

Sleep Patterns

Obstructive sleep apnea may occur; it is a problem of primarily school-aged children. Surgical intervention may be necessary. Refer for periodic overnight polysomnography if history warrants further assessment.

Toileting

Delayed bowel and bladder training may occur as a result of developmental lag; constipation is common because of low activity level, decreased peristalsis, and poor diet.

Discipline

Discipline must be developmentally appropriate; behavior management programs are often successful.

Child Care

Small group daycare lessens the risk of repeated infections.

Children may be eligible for special programs through Public Law 105-17 (IDEA); infants up to 3 years of age may be eligible for early intervention programs.

Schooling

Children and youth are eligible for special education services under programs most commonly used.

Summary of Primary Care Needs for the Child with Down Syndrome—cont'd

DEVELOPMENTAL ISSUES—cont'd

Sexuality

Sex education must be taught so that children with Down syndrome are not abused and do not display inappropriate sexual behaviors.

Girls may need assistance with menstrual hygiene.

Boys are usually infertile, but girls may be fertile.

Transition into Adulthood

Emphasis should be on independent living, vocational skills, and health maintenance.

Mental health problems (e.g., depression, Alzheimer disease) may be problematic.

FAMILY CONCERNS

Special family concerns may include long-term care and prolonged adaptation to the diagnosis.

REFERENCES

Aitken, D.A., Crossley, J.A., & Spencer, K. (2002). Prenatal screening for neural tube defects and aneuploidy. In D.L. Rimoin, J.M. Connor, R.E. Pyeritz, & B.R. Korf (Eds.). *Emery and Rimoin's principles and practices of medical genetics* (4th ed.). New York: Churchill Livingstone.

Al-Kasim, F., Doyle, J.J., Massey, G.V., Weinstein, H.J., & Zipursky, A. (2002). Incidence and treatment of potentially lethal diseases in transient leukemia of Down syndrome: Pediatric oncology group study. *J Pediatr Hematol Oncol, 24,* 9-13.

Amano, A., Kishima, T., Kimura, S., Takiguchi, M., Ooshima, T., et al. (2000). Peridontopathic bacteria in children with Down syndrome. *J Periodontol, 71,* 249-255.

Amark, K. & Sunnegardh, J. (1999). The effect of changing attitudes to Down's syndrome in the management of complete atrioventricular septal defects. *Arch Dis Child, 81,* 151-154.

Angelopoulou, N., Souftas, V., Sakadamis, A., & Mandroukas, K. (1999). Bone mineral density in adults with Down's syndrome. *Eur Radiol, 9,* 648-651.

Anneren, G., Tuvemo, T., Carlsson-Skwirut, C., Lonnerholm, T., Bang, P., et al. (1999). Growth hormone treatment in young children with Down's syndrome: Effects on growth and psychomotor development. *Arch Dis Child, 80,* 334-338.

Anneren, G., Tuvemo, T., & Gustafsson, J. (2000). Growth hormone therapy in young children with Down syndrome and a clinical comparison of Down and Prader-Willi syndromes. *Growth Horm IGF Res,* suppl. B, S87-S91.

Aylott, J. (1999). Should children with Down's syndrome have cosmetic surgery? *Br J Nurs, 8,* 33-38.

Baptista, M.J., Fairbrother, U.L., Howard, C.M., Farrer, M.J., Davies, G.E., et al. (2000). Heterotrisomy, a significant contributing factor to ventricular septal defect associated with Down syndrome? *Hum Genet, 107,* 476-482.

Bell, E.J., Kaidonis, J., & Townsend, G.C. (2002). Tooth wear in children with Down syndrome. *Aust Dent J, 47,* 30-35.

Blake, D., Tan, S.L., & Ao, A. (1999). Assessment of multiplex fluorescent PCR for screening single cells for trisomy 21 and single gene defects. *Mol Hum Reprod, 5,* 1166-1175.

Book, L., Hart, A., Black, J., Feolo, M., Zone, J.J., et al. (2001). Prevalence and clinical characteristics of celiac disease in Down's syndrome in a US study. *Am J Med Genet, 98,* 70-74.

Bosma, G.P., van Buchem, M.A., Voormolen, J.H., van Biezen, F.C., & Brouwer, O.F. (1999). Cervical spondylarthrotic myelopathy with early onset in Down's syndrome: Five cases and a review of the literature. *J Intellect Disabil Res, 43,* 283-288.

Carlstedt, K., Anneren, G., Huggare, J., Modeer, T., & Dahllof, G. (1999). The effect of growth hormone therapy on craniofacial growth and dental maturity in children with Down syndrome. *J Craniofac Genet Dev Biol, 19,* 20-23.

Centers for Disease Control and Prevention, Advisory Committee on Immunization Practices. (2000). Preventing pneumococcal disease among infants and young children. *MMWR Morb Mortal Wkly Rep, 49*(RR09), 1-38.

Centers for Disease Control and Prevention, Advisory Committee on Immunization Practices. (1999). Prevention of hepatitis A through active or passive immunization: Recommendations of the Advisory Committee on Immunization Practices (ACIP). *MMWR Morb Mortal Wkly Rep, 48*(RR12), 1-37.

Chapman, R.S. & Hesketh, L.J. (2000). Language, cognition, and short-term memory in individuals with Down syndrome. *Downs Syndr Res Pract, 7,* 1-15.

Chen, C.L., Gilbert, T.J., & Daling, J.R. (1999). Maternal smoking and Down syndrome: The confounding effect of maternal age. *Am J Epidemiol, 149,* 442-446.

Cichon, P., Crawford, L., & Grimm, W.-D. (1998). Early-onset periodontitis associated with Down's syndrome: A clinical interventional study. *Ann Periodontol, 3,* 370-380.

Coe, D.A., Matson, J.L., Russell, D.W., Slifer, K.J., Capone, G.T., et al. (1999). Behavior problems of children with Down syndrome and life events. *J Autism Dev Disord, 29,* 149-156.

Cohen, W. (1998). Atlantoaxial instability. What's next? *Arch Pediatr Adolesc Med, 152,* 119-122.

Cohen, W.I. (Ed.). (1999). Health care guidelines for individuals with Down syndrome: 1999 Revision. *Down Syndr Q, 4,* 1-16.

Cohen, W.I. & Patterson, B. (1998). News from the Down syndrome medical interest group. *Down Syndr Q, 3*(3), 15.

Committee on Bioethics. (1999). Sterilization of minors with developmental disabilities. *Pediatrics, 104,* 337-347.

Committee on Genetics. (2001). Health supervision guidelines for children with Down syndrome. *Pediatrics, 107,* 442-448.

Committee on Infectious Diseases. (2000). *2000 Red book: Report of the Committee on Infectious Diseases* (25th ed.). Elk Grove Village, Ill.: American Academy of Pediatrics.

Cousineau, A.I. & Lauer, R.M. (1995). Heart disease and children with Down syndrome. In D.C. Van Dyke, P. Mattheis, S.S. Eberly, & J. Williams (Eds.). *Medical and surgical care for children with Down syndrome: A guide for parents.* Bethesda, Md.: Woodbine House.

Csizmadia, C.G., Mearin, M.L., Oren, A., Kromhaut, A., Crusius, J.B., et al. (2000). Accuracy and cost-effectiveness of a new strategy to screen for celiac disease in children with Down syndrome. *J Pediatr, 137,* 756-761.

Cuckle, H. (1998). Rational Down syndrome screening policy. *Am J Public Health, 88,* 558-559.

Durmowicz, A.G. (2001). Pulmonary edema in 6 children with Down syndrome during travel to moderate altitudes. *Pediatrics, 108,* 443-447.

Foley, T.P., Jr. (1995). Thyroid conditions and other endocrine concerns in children with Down syndrome. In D.C. Van Dyke, P. Mattheis, S.S. Eberly, & J. Williams (Eds.). *Medical and surgical care for children with Down syndrome: A guide for parents,* Bethesda, Md.: Woodbine House.

Hansson, T., Anneren, G., Sjoberg, O., Klareskog, K., & Dannaeus, A. (1999). Celiac disease in relation to immunologic serum markers, trace elements, and HLA-DR and DQ antigens in Swedish children with Down syndrome. *J Pediatr Gastroenterol Nutr, 29,* 286-292.

Hasle, H. (2001). Pattern of malignant disorders in individuals with Down's syndrome. *Lancet Oncol, 2,* 429-436.

Hassold, T. & Sherman, S. (2000). Down syndrome: Genetic recombination and the origin of the extra chromosome 21. *Clin Genet, 57,* 95-100.

Hattori, M., Fujiyama, A., Taylor, T.D., Watanabe, H., Yada, T., et al. (2000). The DNA sequence of human chromosome 21: The chromosome 21 mapping and sequencing consortium. *Nature, 405,* 311-319.

Hauser-Cram, P., Warfield, M.E., Shonkoff, J.P., Krauss, M.W., Upshur, C.L., et al. (1999). Family influences on adaptive development in young children with Down syndrome. *Child Dev, 70,* 979-989.

Hecht, C.A. & Hook, E.B. (1996). Rates of Down syndrome at live birth at one-year maternal age intervals in studies with apparent close to complete ascertainment in populations of European origin: A proposed revised rate schedule for use in genetic and prenatal screening. *Am J Med Genet, 62,* 376-385.

Hobbs, C.A., Sherman, S.L., Yi, P., Hopkins, S.E., Torfs, C.P., et al. (2000). Polymorphisms in genes involved in folate metabolism as maternal risk factors for Down syndrome. *Am J Hum Genet, 67,* 623-630.

Holland, A.J. (2000). Ageing and learning disability. *Br J Psychiatry, 176,* 26-31.

Holmes, L.B. (1999). Concern about piracetam treatment for children with Down syndrome. *Pediatrics, 103,* 1078.

Holt, S.E., Brown, E.J., & Zipursky, A. (2002). Telomerase and the benign and malignant megakaryoblastic leukemias of Down syndrome. *J Pediatr Hematol Oncol, 24,* 14-17.

Jones, R.B. (2000). Parental consent to cosmetic facial surgery in Down's syndrome. *J Med Ethics, 26,* 101-102.

Khoshnood, B., Pryde, P., & Wall, S. (2000). Ethnic differences in the impact of advanced maternal age on birth prevalence of Down syndrome. *Am J Public Health, 90,* 1778-1781.

Kline, J., Kinney, A., Levin, B., & Warburton, D. (2000). Trisomic pregnancy and earlier age at menopause. *Am J Hum Genet, 67,* 395-404.

Kriss, V.M. (1999). Down syndrome: Imaging of multiorgan involvement. *Clin Pediatr (Phila), 38,* 441-449.

Lange, B. (2000). The management of neoplastic disorders of haematopoiesis in children with Down's syndrome. *Br J Haematol, 110,* 512-524.

Lange, B.J., Kobrinsky, N., Barnard, D.R., Arthur, D.C., Buckley, J.D., et al. (1998). Distinctive demography, biology, and outcome of acute myeloid leukemia and myelodysplastic syndrome in children with Down syndrome: Children's cancer group studies 2861 and 2891. *Blood, 91,* 608-615.

Lantos, J.D. (2000). Growth hormone therapy for Prader-Willi and Down syndromes: A post-modern medical dilemma. *Growth Horm IGF Res,* suppl. B, S93-S94.

Lefaivre, J.F., Cohen, S.R., Burstein, F.D., Simms, C., Scott, P.H., et al. (1997). Down syndrome: Identification and surgical management of obstructive sleep apnea. *Plast Reconstr Surg, 99,* 629-637.

Leonard, S., Bower, C., Petterson, B., & Leonard, H. (2000). Survival of infants born with Down's syndrome: 1980-1996. *Paediatr Perinat Epidemiol, 14,* 163-171.

Levanon, A., Tarasiuk, A., & Tal, A. (1999). Sleep characteristics in children with Down syndrome. *J Pediatr, 134,* 755-760.

Lin, S.J., Wang, J.Y., Klickstein, L.B., Chuang, K.P., Chen, J.Y., et al. (2001). Lack of age-associated LFA-1 up-regulation and impaired ICAM-1 binding in lymphocytes from patients with Down syndrome. *Clin Exp Immunol, 126,* 54-63.

Lobaugh, N.J., Karaskov, V., Rombough, V., Rovet, J., Bryson, S., et al. (2001). Piracetam therapy does not enhance cognitive functioning in children with Down syndrome. *Arch Pediatr Adolesc Med, 155,* 442-448.

Lott, I.T. & Head, E. (2001). Down syndrome and Alzheimer's disease: A link between development and aging. *Ment Retard Dev Disabil Res Rev, 7,* 172-178.

Merrick, J. & Koslowe, K. (2001). Refractive errors and visual anomalies in Down syndrome. *Downs Syndr Res Pract, 6,* 131-133.

Narchi, H. & Kulaylat, N. (1997). High incidence of Down's syndrome in infants of diabetic mothers. *Arch Dis Child, 77,* 242-244.

O'Leary, V.B., Parle-McDermott, A., Molloy, A.M., Kirke, P.N., Johnson, Z., et al. (2002). MTRR and MTHFT polymorphism: Link to Down syndrome? *Am J Med Genet, 107,* 151-155.

Pastore, E., Marino, B., Calzolari, A., Digilio, M.L., Giannotti, A., et al. (2000). Clinical and cardiorespiratory assessment in children with Down syndrome without congenital heart disease. *Arch Pediatr Adolesc Med, 154,* 408-410.

Pueschel, S.M. (1998). Should children with Down syndrome be screened for atlantoaxial instability? *Arch Pediatr Adolesc Med, 152,* 123-125.

Pueschel, S.M., Romano, C., Failla, P., Barone, C., Pettinato, R., et al. (1999). A prevalence study of celiac disease in persons with Down syndrome residing in the United States of America. *Acta Paediatr, 88,* 953-956.

Reller, M.D. & Morris, C.D. (1998). Is Down syndrome a risk factor for poor outcome after repair of congenital heart defects? *J Pediatr, 132,* 738-741.

Roach, M.A., Orsmond, G.I., & Barratt, M.S. (1999). Mothers and fathers of children with Down syndrome: Parental stress and involvement in childcare. *Am J Ment Retard, 104,* 422-436.

Roizen, N.J. (1997). Down syndrome. In M.L. Batshaw (Ed.). *Children with disabilities* (4th ed.). Baltimore: Paul H. Brookes.

Saenz, R.B. (1999). Primary care of infants and young children with Down syndrome. *Am Fam Physician, 59,* 381-390, 392, 395.

Schon, E.A., Kim, S.H., Ferreira, J.C., Magalhaes, P., Grace, M., et al. (2000). Chromosomal non-disjunction in human oocytes: Is there a mitochondrial connection? *Hum Reprod,* suppl. 2, 160-172.

Serra-Prat, M., Gallo, P., Jovell, A.J., Aymerich, M., & Estrada, M.D. (1998). Trade-offs in prenatal detection of Down syndrome. *Am J Public Health, 88,* 558-559.

Shott, S.R. (2000). Down syndrome: Analysis of airway size and a guide for appropriate intubation. *Laryngoscope, 110,* 585-592.

Smith, C.S. (1995). Immune system concerns for children with Down syndrome. In D.C. Van Dyke, P. Mattheis, S.S. Eberly, & J. Williams (Eds.). *Medical and surgical care for children with Down syndrome: A guide for parents.* Bethesda, Md.: Woodbine House.

Stoel-Gammon, C. (2000). Down syndrome phonology: Developmental patterns and intervention strategies. *Downs Syndr Res Pract, 7,* 1-17.

Suzuki, K., Yamaki, S., Miori, S., Murakami, Y., Mori, K., et al. (2000). Pulmonary vascular disease in Down's syndrome with complete atrioventricular septal defect. *Am J Cardiol, 86,* 434-437.

Taub, J.W. (2001). Relationship of chromosome 21 and acute leukemia in children with Down syndrome. *J Pediatr Hematol Oncol, 23,* 175-178.

Todd, N.W., Holt, P.J., & Allen, A.T. (2000). Safety of neck rotation for ear surgery in children with Down syndrome. *Laryngoscope, 110,* 1442-1445.

Tolmie, J.L. (2002). Down syndrome and other autosomal trisomies. In D.L. Rimoin, J.M. Connor, R.E. Pyeritz, & B.R. Korf (Eds.). *Emery and Rimoin's principles and practices of medical genetics* (4th ed.). New York: Churchill Livingstone.

Toscano, E., Trivellini, V., & Andria, G. (2001). Cholelithiasis in Down's syndrome. *Arch Dis Child, 85,* 242-243.

Tseng, S.H. & Cheng, Y. (1998). Occiput-cervical fusion for symptomatic atlantoaxial subluxation in a 32-month-old child with Down syndrome: A case report. *Spinal Cord, 36,* 520-522.

Tsiaras, W.G., Pueschel, S., Keller, C., Curran, R., & Giesswein, S. (1999). Amblyopia and visual acuity in children with Down's syndrome. *Br J Ophthalmol, 83,* 1112-1114.

Uong, E.C., McDonough, J.M., Tayag-Kier, C.E., Zhao, H., Haselgrove, J., et al. (2001). Magnetic resonance imaging of the upper airway in children with Down syndrome. *Am J Respir Crit Care Med, 163,* 731-736.

Yang, Q., Rasmussen, S.A., & Friedman, J.M. (2002). Mortality associated with Down's syndrome in the USA from 1983 to 1997: A population-based study. *Lancet, 359,* 1019-1025.

Zachor, D.A., Mroczek-Muselman, E., & Brown, P. (2000). Prevalence of celiac disease in Down syndrome in the United States. *J Pediatr Gastroenterol Nutr, 31,* 275-279.

Zipursky, A. (1996). The treatment of children with acute megakaryoblastic leukemia who have Down syndrome. *Pediatr Hematol Oncol, 18,* 10-12.

Zipursky, A., Brown, E.J., Christensen, H., & Doyle, J. (1999). Transient myeloproliferative disorder (transient leukemia) and hematologic manifestations of Down syndrome. *Clin Lab Med, 19,* 157-167.

Zwaan, C.M., Kaspers, G.J., Pieters, R., Hahlen, K., Janka-Schaab, G.E., et al. (2002). Different drug sensitivity profiles of acute myeloid and lymphoblastic leukemia and normal peripheral blood mononuclear cells in children with and without Down syndrome. *Blood, 99,* 245-251.

25 Epilepsy

Joan Blair and Janice Selekman

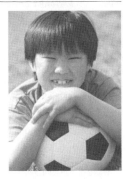

Etiology

Epilepsy is a chronic condition defined by the repeated occurrence of unprovoked seizures, separated by more than 24 hours (Clark & Wilson, 1997; Hauser, 2001). Seizures occur as the manifestation of abnormal, excessive, hypersynchronous discharges of neuronal activity in the brain (American Epilepsy Society [AES], 2000; Hauser, 2001). Clinically, they are sudden paroxysmal changes in neurologic functioning, causing alteration of motor, behavior, and/or autonomic functions (Upadhyay et al, 2001). Seizures are further characterized as epileptic and nonepileptic. Epileptic seizures are those associated with corresponding electrographic activity in the brain (Upadhyay et al, 2001). They arise either from a general dysfunction of the biochemical mechanisms of the brain (generalized seizures) or from distinct areas of the brain (localization-related seizures) (Leppik, 2001). Nonepileptic seizures, conversely, are clinical events that do not correspond to electrographic activity (Upadhyay et al, 2001). They can be a response to a physiologic event, such as fever, toxins, or hypoxia, or a reaction to some type of psychic stressor (psychogenic seizures) (Leppik, 2001).

The International League Against Epilepsy (ILAE) developed a classification of epileptic seizures in 1969, revised it in 1981 (Table 25-1), and updated the classification in 1989 to add epileptic syndromes (Box 25-1) (Engel, 2001). The epilepsies are classified according to seizure type and electroencephalogram (EEG) findings (partial or generalized seizures) or according to etiology (idiopathic [primary], cryptogenic, or symptomatic [secondary] epilepsy). The epilepsy syndrome can also be subdivided anatomically into localization-related or generalized epileptic syndromes (Dreifuss, 1992).

BOX 25-1

International League Against Epilepsy Classification of Epilepsies and Epileptic Syndromes

1. Localization-related (i.e., focal, local, partial) epilepsies and syndromes
1.1 Idiopathic (with age-related onset)
    The following syndromes are established but more may be identified in the future:
    Benign childhood epilepsy with centrotemporal spike
    Childhood epilepsy with occipital paroxysms
    Primary reading epilepsy
1.2 Symptomatic
    Chronic progressive epilepsia partialls continua of childhood (i.e., Kojewnikow's syndrome)
    Syndromes characterized by seizures with specific modes of precipitation
1.3 Cryptogenic
    Presumed to be symptomatic, etiology unknown
2. Generalized epilepsies and syndromes
2.1 Idiopathic (with age-related onset; listed in order of age)
    Benign neonatal familial convulsions
    Benign neonatal convulsions
    Benign myoclonic epilepsy in infancy
    Childhood absence epilepsy (i.e., pyknolepsy)
    Juvenile absence epilepsy
    Juvenile myoclonic epilepsy (i.e., impulsive petit mal)
    Epilepsy with grand mal seizures on wakening
    Other generalized idiopathic epilepsies not already defined
    Epilepsies with seizures precipitated by specific modes of activation
2.2 Cryptogenic or symptomatic (in order of age)
    West syndrome (e.g., infantile spasms, Blitz-Nick-Salaam Krampfe)
    Lennox-Gastaut syndrome
    Epilepsy with myoclonic-astatic seizures
    Epilepsy with myoclonic absences

2.3 Symptomatic
2.3.1 Nonspecific etiology
    Early myoclonic encephalopathy
    Early infantile epileptic encephalopathy with suppression burst
    Other symptomatic generalized epilepsies not already defined
2.3.2 Specific syndromes
    Epileptic seizures may complicate many disease states; under this heading are diseases in which seizures are the presenting or predominant feature
3. Epilepsies and syndromes undetermined—whether focal or generalized
3.1 With both generalized and focal seizures
    Neonatal seizures
    Severe myoclonic epilepsy in infancy
    Epilepsy with continuous spike-waves during slow-wave sleep
    Acquired epileptic aphasia (i.e., Landau-Kleffner syndrome)
    Other undetermined epilepsies not already defined
3.2 Without unequivocal generalized or focal features; all cases with generalized tonic-clonic seizures in which clinical EEG findings do not permit classification as clearly generalized or localization related (e.g., in many cases of sleep–grand mal) are considered not to have unequivocal generalized or focal features
4. Special syndromes
4.1 Situation-related seizures (e.g., Gelegenheit-sanfalle)
    Febrile convulsions
    Isolated seizures or isolated status epilepticus
    Seizures occurring only when there is an acute metabolic or toxic event caused by such factors as alcohol, drugs, eclampsia, nonketotic, hyperglycemia

Adapted from the commission on Classification and Terminology of the International League Against Epilepsy (1989). Proposal for revised classification of epilepsies and epileptic syndromes. *Epilepsia, 30*(4), 389-399.

TABLE 25-1

International Classifications of Epileptic Seizures

I. Partial (Focal, Local) Seizures

Partial seizures are those in which the first clinical and electroencephalographic (EEG) changes generally indicate initial activation of a system of neurons limited to part of one cerebral hemisphere. A partial seizure is classified primarily on the basis of whether or not consciousness is impaired during the attack. When consciousness is not impaired, the seizure is classified as a simple partial seizure. When consciousness is impaired, the seizure is classified as a complex partial seizure. Impairment of consciousness may be the first clinical sign, or simple partial seizures may evolve into complex partial seizures. In patients with impaired consciousness, aberrations of behavior (i.e., automatisms) may occur. A partial seizure may not terminate but instead progress to a generalized motor seizure. Impaired consciousness is defined as the inability to respond normally to exogenous stimuli by virtue of altered awareness and/or responsiveness.

There is considerable evidence that simple partial seizures usually have unilateral hemispheric involvement and rarely have bilateral hemispheric involvement; complex partial seizures, however, often have bilateral hemispheric involvement.

Partial seizures can be classified into one of the following three fundamental groups:

- Simple partial seizures
- Complex partial seizures:
  With impairment of consciousness at onset
  Simple partial onset followed by impairment of consciousness
- Partial seizures evolving to generalized tonic-clonic convulsions:
  Simple evolving to generalized tonic-clonic convulsions
  Complex evolving to generalized tonic-clonic convulsions (including those with simple partial onset)

Clinical Seizure Type	EEG Seizure Type

A. Simple partial seizures (consciousness not impaired)
    1. With motor signs
      (a) Focal motor without march
      (b) Focal motor with march (jacksonian)
      (c) Versive
      (d) Postural
      (e) Phonatory (vocalization or arrest of speech)
	Local contralateral discharge starting over the corresponding area of cortical representation (not always recorded on the scalp)

2. With somatosensory or special-sensory symptoms (e.g., simple hallucinations: tingling, light flashes, buzzing)
      (a) Somatosensory
      (b) Visual
      (c) Auditory
      (d) Olfactory
      (e) Gustatory
      (f) Vertiginous	

3. With autonomic symptoms or signs (including epigastric sensation, pallor, sweating, flushing, piloerection, and pupillary dilation)	

4. With psychic symptoms (i.e., disturbance of higher cerebral function); these symptoms rarely occur without impairment of consciousness and are much more commonly experienced as complex partial seizures
      (a) Dysphasic
      (b) Dysmnesic (e.g., déjà vu)
      (c) Cognitive (e.g., dreamy states, distortions of time sense)
      (d) Affective (e.g., fear, anger)
      (e) Illusions (e.g., macropsia)
      (f) Structured hallucinations (e.g., music, scenes)	

B. Complex partial seizures (with impairment of consciousness; may sometimes begin with simple symptoms)
    1. Simple partial onset followed by impairment of consciousness
      (a) With simple partial features, followed by impaired consciousness
      (b) With automatisms
    2. With impairment of consciousness at onset
      (a) With impairment of consciousness only
      (b) With automatisms
	Unilateral or, frequently, bilateral discharge; diffuse or focal in temporal or frontotemporal regions

C. Partial seizures evolving to secondarily generalized seizures (may be generalized tonic-clonic, tonic, or clonic)
    1. Simple partial seizures *(A)* evolving to generalized seizures
    2. Complex partial seizures *(B)* evolving to generalized seizures
    3. Simple partial seizures evolving to complex seizures evolving to generalized seizures
	Discharges listed above become secondarily and rapidly generalized

II. Generalized Seizures (Convulsive or Nonconvulsive)

Generalized seizures are those in which the first clinical changes indicate initial involvement of both hemispheres. Consciousness may be impaired, which may be the initial manifestation. Motor manifestations are bilateral. The ictal EEG patterns are initially bilateral and presumably reflect neuronal discharge that is widespread in both hemispheres.

TABLE 25-1
International Classifications of Epileptic Seizures—cont'd

Clinical Seizure Type	EEG Seizure Type

A. Absence seizures
  1. Typical absence seizures
    (a) Impairment of consciousness only
    (b) With mild clonic components
    (c) With atonic components
    (d) With tonic components
    (e) With automatisms
    (f) With autonomic components (*b-f* may be used alone or in combination)
	Usually regular and symmetric 3-Hz, but may be 2- to 4-Hz, spike–and–slow-wave complexes; may have multiple spike–and–slow-wave complexes; abnormalities bilateral

2. Atypical absence seizures, which may have:
    (a) Changes in tone that are more pronounced than in absence
    (b) Onset and/or cessation that is not abrupt
	EEG more heterogeneous; may include irregular spike–and–slow wave complexes, fast activity or other paroxysmal activity; abnormalities bilateral but often irregular and asymmetric

B. Myoclonic seizures (single or multiple myoclonic jerks)	Polyspike and wave or sometimes spike and wave or sharp and slow waves
C. Clonic seizures	Fast activity (e.g., ≥10 c/sec) and slow waves; occasional spike-and-wave patterns
D. Tonic seizures	Low voltage fast activity, a fast rhythm of 9-10 c/sec or more, decreasing in frequency and increasing in amplitude
E. Tonic-clonic seizures	Rhythm at ≥10 c/sec, decreasing in frequency and increasing in amplitude during tonic phase, interrupted by slow waves during clonic phase
F. Atonic seizures (astatic) (combinations of the above may occur, e.g., *B* and *F*, *B* and *D*)	Polyspikes and waves or flattening or low-voltage fast activity

III. Unclassified Epileptic Seizures
These include all seizures that cannot be classified because of inadequate or incomplete data and some that defy classification in hitherto described categories. They include some neonatal seizures (e.g., rhythmic eye movements, chewing, swimming movements).

IV. Addendum
Repeated epileptic seizures occur under a variety of circumstances:
1. As fortuitous attacks, coming unexpectedly and without any apparent provocation
2. As cyclic attacks, at more or less regular intervals (e.g., in relation to the menstrual cycle or the sleep-waking cycle)
3. As attacks provoked by nonsensory factors (e.g., fatigue, alcohol, emotion) or sensory factors, (i.e., sometimes referred to as "reflex seizures")
The term "status epilepticus" is used whenever a seizure persists for a sufficient length of time or is repeated often enough that recovery between attacks does not occur. Status epilepticus may be divided into partial (e.g., jacksonian) or generalized (e.g., absence status or tonic-clonic status). When very localized motor status occurs, it is referred to as "epilepsia partialis continua."

Adapted from Proposal for revised clinical and electroencephalographic classification of epileptic seizures. The Commission on Classification and Terminology of the International League Against Epilepsy. (1981): *Epilepsia, 22,* 489-501.

BOX 25-2
Underlying Causes of Epilepsy

Symptomatic epilepsies
  No immediate cause for the seizure
  Prior insult to brain or static encephalopathy present
Idiopathic epilepsies
  Benign course
  Presumed genetic origin
Cryptogenic epilepsies
  No identifiable cause
  Presumed underlying pathologic cause that could be detected with improved diagnostic techniques

Box 25-2 depicts the underlying causes of epilepsy grouped into the three classifications by the ILAE. Symptomatic epilepsies reveal no immediate cause for the seizure, but there has been a prior insult to the brain (i.e., asphyxia, severe electrolyte disturbance, stroke, meningitis, trauma, vascular lesion, central nervous system [CNS] degenerative conditions) or an encephalopathy that is static (i.e., cerebral palsy, mental retardation) (Hauser, 2001; Shinnar, 1999). Idiopathic epilepsies consist of a mostly benign course of epilepsy with a presumed genetic origin, such as in benign rolandic epilepsy and childhood absence epilepsy. In cryptogenic epilepsies, no cause is identified, but there is presumed to be an underlying pathologic cause that could be detected with improved diagnostic techniques (Shinnar, 1999; Steinlein, 1999).

The molecular genetic studies of the epilepsies began in the 1980s, and the first gene for an idiopathic epilepsy was discovered in 1995 (Berkovic & Ottman, 2000). In addition, the concept of channelopathies has come to the forefront with the discovery of the dysfunction of ion channels as a cause of the idiopathic epilepsies. This can be seen in the autosomal dominant nocturnal frontal lobe epilepsy (ADNFLE), where mutations in the neuronal nicotinic acetylcholine receptor alpha$_4$- and beta$_2$-subunit genes have been identified as a cause for the syndrome (Kaneko et al, 2002a, 2002b).

Single-gene defects can contribute to a variety of epilepsy phenotypes. An example of this is generalized epilepsy with febrile seizures plus (GEFS+). A sodium channel mutation (a single-gene defect) may be associated with simple febrile seizures and then later progress to afebrile seizures or a more severe epilepsy phenotype (Berkovic & Ottman, 2000). However, idiopathic epilepsies are rarely inherited as single-gene disorders. Instead they are more often complex genetic diseases, with multiple genes being simultaneously involved (Kaneko et al, 2002a; Serratosa, 1999). Abnormalities in different genes and different mutations (genetic heterogeneity) may cause the same epilepsy phenotype (Berkovic & Ottman, 2000; Kaneko et al, 2002b). This can be seen in benign familial neonatal convulsions (BFNCs), where two potassium channel genes (KCNQ2 and KCNQ3) are responsible for the majority of individuals with this disorder (Berkovic & Ottman, 2000). Other genetic or environmental factors may have some influences on the epilepsy phenotype as well (Kaneko et al, 2002b; Serratosa, 1999). The variability in GEFS+ is probably a result of modifying genes in addition to environmental factors (Berkovic & Ottman, 2000).

Incidence and Prevalence

The cumulative incidence of epilepsy is approximately 1% in children through 15 years of age, determined by several population-based studies (Shinnar, 1999). The incidence rates for epilepsy in the United States are 30 to 60 cases per 100,000 (Annegers, 1997; Shinnar, 1999). In the United States, the overall prevalence of active epilepsy is 1.5 million, with the prevalence in children ages 5 to 14 years being 150,000 to 325,000 (Shinnar, 1999). The incidence seems highest in Italy and Scandinavia, intermediate in Japan and the United States, and lowest in Canada and the United Kingdom (Hauser, 2001). The incidence of epilepsy also varies with age. The incidence is highest in the first year of life with approximately 100 cases per 100,000 children. Incidence falls after age 1 year; however, the rate of the fall varies. For example, in Canada, the incidence stays rather constant from ages 1 through 10 years, and in early adolescence it drops by approximately 50% to equal the incidence in the adult years. In developing countries, the incidence seems to be lower in early childhood compared with adolescence. In contrast, the incidence in developed countries is higher in the first decade of life compared with the second decade. In regard to gender, the incidence seems to be slightly higher in males, except in Scandinavia, where the incidence is higher in females (Hauser, 2001).

In the United States, 120,000 children under the age of 18 years seek medical attention for a newly diagnosed seizure each year. This is approximately 40% of all those people (children and adults) who seek medical attention yearly for a newly diagnosed seizure. Of these cases, 75,000 to 100,000 are for evaluation of febrile seizures, which are the most common type of seizures in children. In addition, approximately 20,000 to 45,000 children are diagnosed as having epilepsy each year. In the United States, 5 to 6 years of age is the median age of seizure onset (Shinnar & Pellock, 2002). In recent years there seems to be some evidence that the incidence of epilepsy has declined over the past 2 decades, possibly because of improved diagnosis, vaccinations for meningitis, improved neonatal care, and the use of child safety seats and bicycle helmets (Shinnar, 1999; Shinnar & Pellock, 2002). Although many people with epilepsy reach remission, many go on to have active epilepsy. The majority of adults with active epilepsy had a childhood onset (Shinnar & Pellock, 2002).

Previously, it was believed that childhood epilepsies were mostly generalized. However, with the development of the International Classification of Epileptic Seizures and Epileptic Syndromes by the ILAE (Engel, 2001) and more population-based studies, this has not been found to be true (Shinnar & Pellock, 2002). The incidence of localization-related seizures (partial with or without secondary generalization) remains approximately 20/100,000 from infancy through age 65 years and then sharply increases. New cases of partial epilepsy rise with age. Myoclonic seizures are most common in the first year of life, occurring in about 46/100,000, but then the incidence declines rapidly to about 14/100,000 by 2.5 years of age and continues to rapidly decline. The incidence of generalized tonic-clonic seizures is approximately 15/100,000 in the first year of life and then drops to 10/100,000 in children ages 10 to 14 years. These rates remain constant until they again rise in people over 65 years of age. Absence seizures, whether accompanied by generalized tonic-clonic seizures or not, have an incidence of 11/100,000 from ages 1 through 10 years. The onset of absence seizures is uncommon after 14 years of age (Annegers, 1997).

Most epilepsies in childhood are benign, and most catastrophic secondarily generalized epilepsies begin in infancy (Camfield & Camfield, 2002). Certain events, such as brain tumors, brain traumas, CNS infections, and cerebrovascular disease, greatly increase the risk of epilepsy. In addition, neurologic events from birth such as cerebral palsy (CP) and mental retardation (MR) are associated with a high incidence of epilepsy. About 15% to 30% of new cases of epilepsy in children are associated with neurologic problems from birth, CP, MR, or a combination (Hauser, 2001; Shinnar & Pellock, 2002).

Epilepsy as a result of brain tumors occurs in children, but the incidence is highest in the 25- to 64-year age-group. In regard to head traumas, children who have had a severe head trauma with or without early seizures (occurring within 1 week to 1 month after the incident) have a 10% risk of developing posttraumatic epilepsy. The incidence of epilepsy after a CNS infection is highest in children, with a second peak noted in the elderly. Seizures secondary to cerebrovascular disease can occur in children; however, they are most common in people 45 to 64 years of age. Since the risk of cerebrovascular disease increases with age, there is also an increase in seizures and epilepsy after 65 years of age (Annegers, 1997).

Clinical Manifestations at Time of Diagnosis

A diagnosis of seizures or epilepsy is based on obtaining an accurate history of the event, a physical and neurologic examination, and ancillary tests and consultations as necessary. The most important information is obtained through a thorough and accurate history obtained from the individual and/or family. Information should include details of the events before, during, and after the episode (Browne, 2000). Box 25-3 lists the key elements when taking a history of a suspected seizure. It is important to determine when the event occurred, if there was a warning, what signs and symptoms were present, and what part or parts of the body were involved and how. In addition, the duration of the event, whether consciousness was intact or not, and the frequency of the episodes are important. Precipitating factors should be evaluated (Box 25-4). The history should also

BOX 25-3

Key Elements in the History of a Suspected Seizure

BEFORE THE EVENT

Unusual stress (e.g., severe emotional trauma)
Sleep deprivation
Recent illness
Unusual stimuli (e.g., flickering lights)
Use of medication and drugs
Activity immediately before event (e.g., change in posture, exercise)

DURING THE EVENT

Symptoms at onset (e.g., aura)
Temporal mode of onset: gradual vs. sudden
Duration: brief (ictal phase <5 minutes) vs. prolonged
Stereotypy: duration and features of episodes nearly identical vs. frequently changing
Time of day: related to sleep or occurring on awakening
Ability to talk and respond appropriately
Ability to comprehend
Ability to recall events during the seizure
Abnormal movements of the eyes, mouth, face, head, arms, and legs
Bowel or bladder incontinence

AFTER THE EVENT

Confusion
Lethargy
Abnormal speech
Focal weakness or sensory loss (i.e., Todd's paralysis)
Headache, muscle soreness, or physical injury

From Prego-Lopez, M. & Devinsky, O. (2002). Evaluation of a first seizure: Is it epilepsy? *Postgrad Med, 111*(1), 34-48. Reprinted with permission.

BOX 25-4

Precipitating Factors for Seizures

Sleep deprivation
Stimulant use
Alcohol or sedative drug withdrawal
Substance abuse
High fever
Hypoglycemia
Electrolyte imbalance
Hypoxia
Flickering lights
Antiepileptic drug (AED) noncompliance
Menstrual cycle
Dehydration
Hyperventilation
Improper diet
Specific "reflex" triggers
Intense exercise

Data from Leppick, I. (2001). *Contemporary diagnosis and management of the patient with epilepsy* (5th ed.). Newtown, Pa.: Handbooks in Health Care; Brodie, M. & Schachter, S. (2001). *Epilepsy* (2nd ed.). Oxford: Health Press.

BOX 25-5

Evaluation of a Neonatal Seizure

With a history that suggests a probable cause (intrauterine insult, hypoxia, etc.):
Serum chemistries: glucose, calcium, magnesium, electrolytes, blood urea nitrogen, or creatinine
Serum pH, PO_2 (arterial or capillary)
Urine screen for toxic substances
Lumbar puncture: CSF protein, glucose, cells, smear, and culture
A cranial ultrasound or noncontrast CT scan of the brain
EEG
Without a probable cause also include:
TORCH titers
Quantitative urine and amino acids
Serum and urine organic acids
AIDS testing
Drug screen

From Prensky, A. (2001). An approach to the child with paroxysmal phenomenon with emphasis on nonepileptic disorders. In J. Pellock, W. Dodson, & B. Bourgeois (Eds.). *Pediatric epilepsy: Diagnosis and therapy* (2nd ed.). New York: Demos, pp. 97-116. Reprinted with permission.
CSF, Cerebrospinal fluid; *CT,* computed tomography; *EEG,* electroencephalogram; *TORCH,* toxoplasmosis, other (congenital syphilis and viruses), rubella, cytomegalovirus, and herpes simplex virus; *AIDS,* acquired immunodeficiency virus.

ancillary tests are performed as necessary (Box 25-5 and Table 25-2).

Classification of Seizures

The first and most important step in the treatment of epilepsy is the correct diagnosis, thereby correctly classifying the seizure or the epilepsy syndrome (Nordli, 2002; Shields, 1999). The classification of epileptic seizures and epileptic syndromes that is widely used today is the classification developed by the ILAE (Table 25-1 and Box 25-1). This classification system groups seizures that have similar clinical presentations.

There are numerous important reasons for classifying seizures and epileptic syndromes. One of the most important is for communication purposes. In order to communicate effectively, there needs to be a common understanding of terms. With common terminology, professionals can communicate information in order to improve the treatment of epilepsy (Dreifuss & Nordli, 2001; Nordli, 2002). Classification can help with information regarding seizure control and long-term outcomes. Classification can also assist in identifying patient populations for investigational trials and genetic research. Finally, co-morbid conditions often accompany many epileptic syndromes, and therefore health care providers can be alerted to screen for subtle disorders that may accompany a particular syndrome (Nordli, 2002).

Partial Seizures. Partial (focal or localization-related) seizures are characterized by seizure activity that begins in specific loci in the cortex of the brain in one hemisphere (Dreifuss & Nordli, 2001; Wyllie & Luders, 1997). Partial seizures are then divided into simple partial seizures, complex partial seizures, and partial seizures with secondary generalization (Wyllie & Luders, 1997). *Simple partial seizures* arise from the isocortex (Dreifuss & Nordli, 2001). A simple partial seizure refers to seizure activity where consciousness has been

include questions about febrile seizures, birth complications, development, serious infections, head trauma, drug or alcohol abuse, and family history of epilepsy (Browne, 2000). A complete physical and neurologic examination should be performed, looking for any abnormalities. Once this is completed,

TABLE 25-2

The Basis for Laboratory Studies

History and Physical Examination	Seizure Types	Type of Evaluation
1. Normal	Generalized	Routine EEG; serum glucose, calcium, magnesium
2. Normal	Partial (focal)	Routine or sleep-deprived EEG; brain scan (CT or MRI); serum glucose, calcium, magnesium
3. Suggests a chronic neurologic insult not previously evaluated with focal physical findings	Generalized or partial	Routine or sleep-deprived EEG; brain scan (CT or MRI); serum glucose, calcium, magnesium
4. Presence of mental retardation or slow development without focal signs	Generalized or partial	Routine EEG; serum glucose; calcium; serum and urine amino acids; chromosome studies, if otherwise indicated; TORCH titers, if under age 12 mo; if seizure is partial, brain imaging is indicated
5. Normal other than for presence of fever ± vomiting or diarrhea		
Seen acutely	Generalized or partial	LP; serum glucose, calcium, electrolytes, BUN; EEG
Seen some days later when well	Generalized	Fasting glucose, calcium; EEG
6. Normal other than for a clouded sensorium	Generalized or partial	Brain imaging (CT or MRI); if scan normal, an LP, glucose, calcium, electrolytes; if these are normal, liver chemistries including a serum ammonia, urine ketones, drug screen; EEG; AIDS testing
7. Presence of increased ICP ± focal signs	Generalized or partial	Brain imaging with contrast enhancement (CT or MRI); calcium, electrolytes, urinalysis; LP if scan is normal; EEG; if no cause is found, an MRI may be indicated at a later date
8. Presence of focal signs of recent onset	Generalized or partial	Contrasted brain scan (CT or MRI); LP if scan is normal; EEG; glucose, calcium electrolytes; if CT scan is normal, cardiac evaluation; screen for hemoglobinopathies and coagulation defects, sedimentation rate, antinuclear antibodies, serum cholesterol, triglycerides; anticardiolipin antibodies if an infarct is seen on imaging

From Prensky, A. (2001). An approach to the child with paroxysmal phenomenon with emphasis on nonepileptic disorders. In J. Pellock, W. Dodson, & B. Bourgeois (Eds.). *Pediatric epilepsy: Diagnosis and therapy* (2nd ed.). New York: Demos, pp. 97-116. Reprinted with permission.
EEG, Electroencephalogram; *CT,* computed tomography; *MRI,* magnetic resonance imaging; *TORCH,* toxoplasmosis, other agents, rubella, cytomegalovirus, herpes simplex; *LP,* lipoprotein; *BUN,* blood urea nitrogen; *AIDS,* acquired immunodeficiency syndrome; *ICP,* intracranial pressure.

preserved. During a simple partial seizure, the individual remains alert, can understand what is happening in the environment, and can respond appropriately to questions or direction. Simple partial seizures can cause motor symptoms (jerking, twitching, shaking) that are usually unilateral, and they can have somatosensory symptoms (change in vision, sound, smell, or taste), autonomic symptoms (dilated pupils, altered heart or breathing rate, flushing), or psychic symptoms (fear, anger, hallucinations, déjà vu) (AES, 2000; Wyllie & Luders, 1997).

It is believed that *complex partial seizures* involve the limbic system of the brain and therefore can lead to early bilateral dysfunction, affecting the frontal or temporal lobes of the brain. A complex partial seizure refers to seizure activity where consciousness has been impaired. A complex partial seizure can follow a simple partial seizure, or it can begin as a complex partial seizure, having altered consciousness at the onset (AES, 2000; Dreifuss & Nordli, 2001). During a complex partial seizure, the individual's ability to pay attention or respond to questions or direction is impaired or lost. Complex partial seizures can have all the same symptoms of a simple partial seizure, but in addition, the individual is confused, disoriented, or unresponsive. In addition, automatisms (automatic movements) can occur, including mouth movements (lip smacking, chewing), upper extremity movements (picking at things), vocalization (grunting, repeating), or complex motor acts. The individual may be aware of the seizure or have no recollection of the seizure that occurred (AES, 2000).

Some individuals experience an aura (or warning) before a complex partial or generalized seizure. Many professionals believe that the aura (sensory, autonomic, or psychic disturbance) is actually a simple partial seizure (Wyllie & Luders, 1997). Todd's paralysis can occur after a complex partial or secondarily generalized seizure. This is a weakness (associated with the affected region of the brain) of a part or whole side of the body that can last from minutes to hours after a seizure (AES, 2000). Lastly partial seizures can begin as a simple partial seizure or a complex partial seizure and then spread to a generalized seizure.

Generalized Seizures. Generalized seizures are characterized by abnormal activity that involves large parts of the brain, usually both cerebral hemispheres, from the onset. The initial manifestations are bilateral with loss of consciousness. The individual has no memory of the seizure. There are a variety of generalized seizures, including absence, tonic, tonic-clonic, myoclonic, akinetic, atonic, and infantile spasms (Dreifuss & Nordli, 2001).

Absence seizures, previously known as petit mal seizures, are characterized by a brief (up to 20 seconds) stare that begins and ends suddenly, with a total impairment of consciousness. There is what is described as a blank facial expression. There can be slight automatisms that accompany the seizure. There is no warning, and the individual is totally attentive when the seizure ends. Hyperventilation or flashing lights can provoke absence seizures. The seizure is accompanied by an EEG pattern of 3 Hz spike-wave activity. *Atypical absence seizures* vary slightly in that they can begin and end gradually, they are generally not provoked by hyperventilation, and they can last slightly longer (up to 30 seconds). The EEG pattern is slow spike-wave (<2.5 Hz) activity (AES, 2000; Pearl & Holmes, 2001).

Tonic seizures are characterized by the individual's body becoming stiff and rigid. Individuals may have slight tremors or fine shaking. Tonic seizures are usually brief, lasting about 5 to 20 seconds. Rapid diffuse polyspikes are usually seen on the EEG. *Tonic-clonic seizures* were previously known as grand mal seizures or convulsive seizures. The body stiffens initially. There is often a short cry as the air is forced through contracted vocal cords. The body then jerks in a rhythmic pattern. Generalized tonic-clonic seizures usually last about 30 to 120 seconds. Because of lack of swallowing during the seizure there is usually drooling or foaming at the mouth. There is often bowel or bladder incontinence as well. The EEG usually shows generalized polyspikes (AES, 2000).

Myoclonic seizures are described as very brief (<1 second), very quick muscle jerks that are uncontrollable. They often involve the arms or face, but they may also involve the whole body. They look like a quick startle but are not precipitated by an event, such as a loud noise, light, or movement. Myoclonic seizures can also occur in succession. The EEG pattern can show multiple spike–and–slow-wave discharges (AES, 2000).

Akinetic seizures are also known as drop attacks. The individual suddenly and forcefully drops to the ground but immediately recovers. *Atonic seizures*, on the other hand, consist of a sudden loss of muscle tone. The individual suddenly drops (or melts) to the ground and is limp for a period of time. Slow–spike-wave or multiple spike–and–slow-wave complexes are usually seen on the EEG for these seizure types (AES, 2000; Dreifuss & Nordli, 2001; Farrell, 1997). Some professionals use the terms *akinetic* and *atonic seizures* interchangeably, but they are actually two different seizure types.

Infantile spasms are very quick seizures and usually occur in clusters. There are three varieties of infantile spasms: flexor, extensor, and mixed. Flexor spasms, often called jackknife or salaam seizures, are characterized by abrupt flexing (bending) spasms of the neck, trunk, arms, and legs. Extensor spasms, often called a cheerleading spasm, are the least common. They are characterized by extensor (straightening) spasms involving abrupt movements of the neck, trunk, and legs. Mixed infantile spasms are the most common and are characterized by flexion of the neck, trunk, and arms and extension of the legs (Wong & Trevathan, 2001). The EEG shows a characteristic pattern called hypsarrhythmia, but a modified version of this reading can also be seen (Dulac et al, 1997).

Classification of Epileptic Syndromes

The epilepsy syndromes are classified into the following categories: localization-related, generalized, undetermined, and special syndromes (Leppik, 2001). The syndromes are benign or catastrophic disorders (Shields, 1999). Benign epilepsy disorders involve mild infrequent seizures; the disorder resolves fairly quickly and is not associated with psychologic or cognitive delays that affect long-term development (Camfield & Camfield, 2002; Shields, 2002). The catastrophic disorders consist of those disorders with very frequent, intractable (difficult to control) seizures that are treatment resistant and are associated with significant cognitive and psychosocial issues that affect long-term development. If the catastrophic epilepsies begin in a young child during the developmental stages, the long-term effects are permanent (Camfield & Camfield,

2002). For those catastrophic disorders that do not have a structural or metabolic cause, the seizures are the greatest problem. If the seizures can come under control, then there can be a positive effect on development (Shields, 1999). Some of the more common epilepsy syndromes will be discussed.

Localization-Related Idiopathic Epilepsies and Syndromes. *Benign childhood epilepsy with centrotemporal spikes* (BECTS), also known as benign rolandic epilepsy, is one of the most common epilepsy syndromes in childhood, representing approximately 15% of childhood epilepsies. The age of onset of seizures typically occurs between 3 and 10 years of age. The seizures usually occur on awakening and are simple partial with twitching of the face and tongue. The seizures can secondarily generalize, but this is uncommon. The EEG is consistent with bilateral centro-temporal spikes. The etiology is an autosomal dominant genetic disorder. The prognosis is good in that BECTS usually resolves during adolescence. Treatment is optional since the seizures usually occur at night (Camfield & Camfield, 2002).

Benign occipital epilepsy is less common than BECTS, and the seizures occur during the day. It usually consists of a visual aura, followed by automatisms or a hemiclonic seizure (Dreifuss & Nordli, 2001); however, the seizure can be of any type (Camfield & Camfield, 2002). The individual can have a migraine headache after the seizure (Dreifuss & Nordli, 2001). The EEG shows spike-wave discharges in the occipital region and is blocked with eye opening. There is no clear etiology (Camfield & Camfield, 2002).

Localization-Related Symptomatic Epilepsies and Syndromes. These epilepsy syndromes are less common in children compared with adults, and they have a variety of causes (Box 25-6). The seizures are usually partial and can secondarily generalize if not treated (Leppik, 2001). An example of a syndrome in this category is *epilepsia partialis continua* (EPC). The seizures are characterized by muscular twitches that affect a particular part of the body, usually the distal limb and face, but that can also involve the trunk, diaphragm, neck, and throat muscles. The seizure lasts for a minimum of 1 hour. The duration, rhythm, amplitude, and the limb involved, as well as the extent of involvement, can change throughout the episode. The EEG usually shows continuous focal spike discharges that spread and often have a mirror focus (Deray et al, 2001). The prognosis depends on the etiology of EPC (Arunkumar et al, 2001).

Generalized Idiopathic Epilepsies and Syndromes with Age-Related Onset. *Benign neonatal familial convulsions* is a rare disorder, with generalized seizures usually occurring on the second or third day of life. The seizures are clonic or apneic and usually resolve within a few days. There is no particular EEG finding. Etiology is unclear, but it has been associated with a deletion of chromosome 20q13.3. About 14% of these infants develop epilepsy later in life (Dreifuss & Nordli, 2001; Leppik, 2001).

Benign neonatal convulsions are also known as fifth-day fits, because they usually occur on the fifth day of life. The seizures are characterized by partial clonic or apneic seizures and can be prolonged, lasting several days (Tharp, 2002). Alternating sharp theta waves are seen on the interictal EEG. Etiology is unknown. Prognosis is good with no recurrence of seizures and no developmental problems (Dreifuss & Nordli, 2001).

BOX 25-6
Some Causes of Symptomatic Localization-Related Epilepsies

VASCULAR
Stroke
Infantile hemiplegia
Arterivenous malformations subarachnoid
Sturge-Weber syndrome
Aneurysms (subarachnoid hemorrhage)
Venous thrombosis
Hypertensive encephalopathy
Blood dyscrasias (sickle cell anemia)

INFECTIOUS
Abscess
Meningitis and encephalitis
Toxoplasmosis
Rubella
Rasmussen syndrome (presumed viral)
Cysticercosis

TUMORS
Meningiomas
Gliomas
Hamartomas
Metastatic tumors

CONGENITAL
Heterotopias
Cortical dysplasias

TRAUMATIC
Prenatal injuries
Perinatal injuries
Head injuries

CRYPTOGENIC
No cause identified

Adapted from Leppik, I. (2001). *Contemporary diagnosis and management of the patient with epilepsy* (5th ed.). Newtown, Pa.: Handbooks in Health Care.

Childhood absence epilepsy (CAE) is also known as pyknolepsy (referring to crowding) because the seizures can occur many times in an hour and usually occur daily. CAE used to be known as petit mal epilepsy. Age of onset is 4 to 10 years of age, with peak manifestation at age 6 to 7 years, and it occurs more frequently in girls. These individuals can also develop generalized tonic-clonic seizures (Dreifuss & Nordli, 2001). Seizures and the EEG reading are consistent for typical absence seizures and can be activated by hyperventilation. These children are neurologically normal, and there can be a family history of idiopathic generalized epilepsy (AES, 2000; Camfield & Camfield, 2002). These seizures are usually fairly easy to control.

Juvenile absence epilepsy (JAE) is similar to CAE; however, age of onset is during puberty. The typical absence seizures occur sporadically and are seen less frequently than in CAE. Generalized tonic-clonic seizures are common, usually on awakening, and myoclonic seizures can also be seen. The EEG reading is often faster than the usual three per second spike-wave seen in CAE. Individuals usually respond well to treatment (Dreifuss & Nordli, 2001).

Juvenile myoclonic epilepsy (JME) was previously known as impulsive petit mal epilepsy (Dreifuss & Nordli, 2001). Age of onset is in adolescence, usually at 12 to 13 years of age (Shields, 1999). Single or repetitive myoclonic seizures usually occur on awakening, often because of sleep deprivation or stress. The seizure can be intense, causing the individual to suddenly fall, and there is not a noticeable change in consciousness (Dreifuss & Nordli, 2001). The individual often complains of being clumsy or jittery (Leppik, 2001). There are often generalized tonic-clonic seizures associated with JME; and less often there are rare absence seizures (AES, 2000; Dreifuss & Nordli, 2001). Individuals can have photosensitive seizures, which are diagnosed using strobe lights during an EEG (AES, 2000). Rapid, generalized, and often irregular spike waves and polyspike waves are seen on EEG. JME often responds well to appropriate treatment (Dreifuss & Nordli, 2001).

Generalized Cryptogenic or Symptomatic Epilepsies and Syndromes. *West syndrome* is the most common catastrophic epilepsy in children (Shields, 2000). West syndrome consists of infantile spasms (occurring up to hundreds of times per day), hypsarrhythmia on the EEG, and psychomotor retardation, although this may be absent (AES, 2000; Wong & Trevathan, 2001). It occurs in the first year of life, with a peak around 5 months of age. The infant usually develops normally up to this point (Shields, 2002). The etiology of West syndrome includes structural abnormalities (i.e., tuberous sclerosis), metabolic diseases (i.e., phenylketonuria, hypoxia), or cryptogenic etiologies (Shields, 2002; Wong & Trevathan, 2001). Prognosis depends on the etiology; however, mental retardation is seen in approximately 70% to 93%. Approximately 50% of those with West syndrome have epilepsy in later years, and about one half of these develop Lennox-Gastaut syndrome (Leppik, 2001; Wong & Trevathan, 2001).

Lennox-Gastaut Syndrome (LGS) is also a catastrophic epilepsy, with a prevalence of approximately 4% of all childhood epilepsies being attributable to this syndrome. LGS consists of intractable mixed seizures, cognitive impairment that deteriorates over time, and a particular EEG reading (Crumrine, 2002). Onset is usually between 1 and 8 years of age, but it primarily begins in the preschool child (Dreifuss & Nordli, 2001). The main seizure types are tonic, atonic, and atypical absence, although the individual can have other seizure types as well (Crumrine, 2002; Dreifuss & Nordli, 2001). The EEG usually shows abnormal background activity, slow spike-wave discharges of less than three per second, and multifocal abnormalities. Bursts of fast rhythms are seen during sleep (Dreifuss & Nordli, 2001). Most children with this syndrome are mentally retarded; however, a few individuals (<10%) remain intellectually normal (Camfield & Camfield, 2002). The etiology of LGS varies. Nine to thirty percent of individuals have previously had infantile spasms. Most etiologies (30% to 75%) are symptomatic, and about 33% of the cases are cryptogenic (Crumrine, 2002). Seizures are very difficult to control, and the prognosis for these individuals is poor (Dreifuss & Nordli, 2001).

Undetermined Epilepsies and Syndromes. *Landau Kleffner syndrome* (LKS) is a rare syndrome also known as acquired epileptic aphasia (Glauser & Morita, 2001). Onset is usually between 1 and 8 years of age. Typically these children are previously cognitively normal with normal speech development (Camfield & Camfield, 2002). They then develop language regression with verbal auditory agnosia (the inability to know the meaning of words) and rapid reduction of spontaneous oral expression (Camfield & Camfield, 2002; Glauser & Morita, 2001). Speech often stops altogether, and the child often develops behavioral and psychomotor problems. Approximately 50% of individuals with LKS have a severe language delay or mental handicap that continues throughout life. About 40% to 50% can lead a normal social and professional life if their speech returns before adulthood (Camfield & Camfield, 2002). Epileptic seizures, either complex partial or generalized tonic-clonic, occur in approximately two thirds of the individuals and usually remit by 15 years of age (Glauser & Morita, 2001). The EEG often shows high-frequency bilateral spikes, often over the posterior temporal regions, that can be continuous. These abnormalities on EEG often lessen during rapid-eye-movement (REM) sleep (Camfield & Camfield, 2002). Etiology is unknown. Some individuals' seizures improve with antiepileptic drugs (AEDs).They often require intensive language therapy for speech (Camfield & Camfield, 2002; Glauser & Morita, 2001).

Special Syndromes: Situation-Related Seizures. *Febrile seizures* occur in approximately 2% to 4% of children in the United States, making this type of seizure the most common seizure disorder in childhood (Shinnar & Glauser, 2002). Onset is usually between 6 months and 7 years of age and is associated with an acute febrile illness (AES, 2000; Hauser, 2001). Seizures are either simple febrile seizures or complex febrile seizures. Simple febrile seizures are generalized and last less than 15 minutes. Complex febrile seizures are longer than 15 minutes, may be focal in their onset, or may recur during the febrile illness (AES, 2000; Shinnar & Glauser, 2002). The overall risk of recurrence of febrile seizures is approximately 34%. In children who have their first febrile seizure before 12 months of age, the recurrence is higher, approximately 50% (Leppik, 2001). There are no long-term consequences of simple febrile seizures. On the other hand, those with complex febrile seizures have an increased chance of developing epilepsy (Shinnar & Glauser, 2002). Epilepsy occurs in approximately 3% of these children by 7 years of age and in 7% by 25 years of age (Leppik, 2001). Children with simple febrile seizures do not need long-term AED treatment. Their seizures can be treated at the time of the event. Once the seizure is managed, it is important to determine the etiology of the fever and to treat it (Shields, 1999).

The American Academy of Pediatrics and its Provisional Committee on Quality Improvement, in collaboration with neurologists, pediatricians, and research methodologists, developed a practice parameter for the *evaluation of a child with a first febrile seizure*. A lumbar puncture (LP) should be performed based on the circumstances. If the child is younger than 12 months of age, an LP should be strongly considered, since the symptoms associated with meningitis can be minimal or absent at this age. If the child is between 12 to 18 months of age, an LP should be considered, because the symptoms associated with meningitis can be subtle at this age. If the child is older than 18 months of age, an LP is recommended if meningeal signs are present. An EEG and medical imaging studies are not recommended for a normal healthy child with a first febrile seizure. Laboratory studies are not routinely recommended for a simple febrile seizure. Laboratory evaluation should be aimed at determining the cause of the fever. Figure 25-1 depicts the practice parameter to provide recommendations for the neurodiagnostic evaluation of the child with a first simple febrile seizure (Provisional Committee on Quality Improvement, Subcommittee on Febrile Seizures, 1996).

Status epilepticus (SE) is 30 minutes or more of either continuous seizure activity or recurrent seizures without recovery of consciousness between the seizures (Fountain, 2000). Generalized convulsive status epilepticus (GCSE) is the most common form, but nonconvulsive status epilepticus (NCSE) can also occur (Brenner, 2002; Kaplan, 2000). NCSE consists of seizures that do not have convulsive motor activity, such as absence status, complex partial status, or myoclonic status (Fountain, 2000; Kaplan, 2000). Of the approximately 50,000 to 152,000 cases of SE that occur in 1 year, the highest proportion is in children. SE is a medical emergency that must be treated immediately. Children are at a higher risk to develop SE compared with adults; however, morbidity and mortality rates are lower. Death after SE is usually due to the underlying cause of the prolonged seizure (Wheless, 1999).

Treatment (Box 25-7)
Decision to Treat

The question continues to be whether to treat an individual with seizures. There are many factors to consider when making this decision. These include kindling, the recurrence rate, the fear of brain damage and other physical injury, and the possibility of death (Camfield & Camfield, 2002).

Kindling is only documented in animal studies where seizure activity is artificially stimulated (Velisek & Moshe, 2001). The premise is that the abnormal activity that occurs in a particular part of the brain that causes the seizures will eventually spread to other areas, resulting in worsening seizures that are more difficult to control.

Recurrence rate refers to whether a seizure recurs or is a one-time event, whether it is a febrile or afebrile seizure. This will affect treatment. Recurrent seizures often require treatment, whereas one-time seizures often do not require treatment.

BOX 25-7
Treatment

PHARMACOLOGIC THERAPY (ANTIEPILEPTIC DRUGS [AEDS])
NONPHARMACOLOGIC INTERVENTIONS
Ketogenic diet
Vagus nerve stimulator (VNS)
Epilepsy surgery
Resective surgery
   Temporal lobectomy
   Extratemporal resection
   Hemispherectomy
Functional surgery
   Corpus callosotomy
   Multiple subpial transection

ALTERNATIVE THERAPIES
Herbal preparations
Supplements

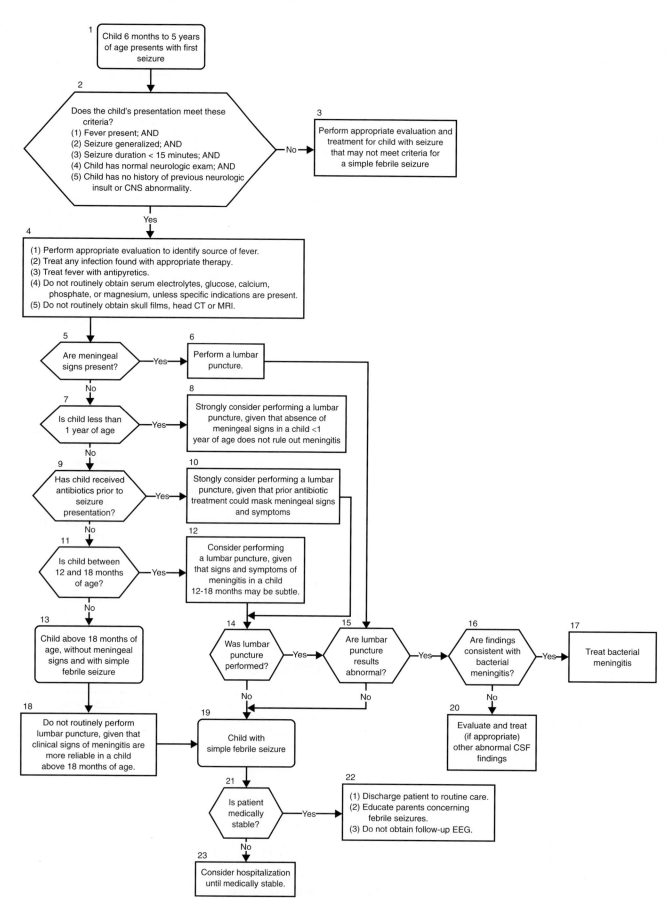

FIGURE 25-1 The neurodiagnostic evaluation of the child with a first simple febrile seizure. (From American Academy of Pediatrics, Provisional Committee on Quality Improvement, Subcommittee on Febrile Seizures. [1996]. Practice Parameter: The neurodiagnostic evaluation of the child with a first simple febrile seizure. *Pediatrics, 97,* 5. Reprinted with permission.)

The fear of injury with a seizure must take into account the seizure type, age of the child, and the activity in which the child is involved. Individuals at a continued risk for neurologic (brain) or other body injuries because of seizure activity need to be treated. Brain injury is usually caused by the loss of consciousness and the resulting fall (Shinnar & O'Dell, 2001); the seizure itself is usually not the actual cause of the brain damage.

Status epilepticus can sometimes cause brain damage, but it rarely causes brain damage in children (Camfield & Camfield, 2002). However, in rare cases status epilepticus can result in death. Sudden unexplained death in epilepsy (SUDEP) is also a concern. SUDEP refers to a sudden death in an individual with epilepsy without an identifiable cause. SUDEP is responsible for approximately 2% to 17% of deaths in individuals with epilepsy (Ficker, 2000).

Treatment Options

Once the decision to treat is made, there are various treatment options. Pharmacologic treatment consists of AEDs. Nonpharmacologic treatment consists of the ketogenic diet, vagus nerve stimulation (VNS), and brain surgery. Some individuals have elected to treat their child's epilepsy with alternative therapies, such as herbal preparations. The decision to treat should be made after considering the risks and benefits of the option chosen.

Pharmacologic Treatment. *Pharmacologic therapy* is usually the first course of action in treating epilepsy. The discussion with the family must include common side effects, including the risk of teratogenesis in future pregnancies. Other issues to discuss include fears and misconceptions about drug treatment and the importance of complete compliance with the medication regimen (Brodie & Schachter, 2001). The goal of therapy is maximum seizure control with minimum or no side effects. Approximately 60% to 70% of individuals with newly diagnosed epilepsy remain seizure free on monotherapy, leaving 30% or more who continue to have seizures and require additional medications. The localization-related epilepsies are more difficult to control. Approximately 60% of individuals can become seizure free with the first or second AED, and the response to the first AED is a good predictor of the prognosis for seizure control. When seizure control is not possible with monotherapy, then polytherapy must be considered (Brodie & Kwan, 2002).

There are a variety of established AEDs on the market for seizure control (Table 25-3). Since the 1990s, a variety of new AEDs were approved for the adjunctive treatment of intractable epilepsy (Table 25-4). Although some of these AEDs have not been approved in children, nor have they been approved as first-line treatment of seizures, many epilepsy centers use the newer AEDs in children as first-line treatment of seizures or as adjunctive therapy for seizures. The efficacy of the established and newer AEDs on common seizure types and epilepsy syndromes is presented in Table 25-5.

Nonpharmacologic Treatment.

Ketogenic diet. The ketogenic diet is another treatment for epilepsy. It is not clear why the diet works to control seizures. It is a rigid, mathematically calculated, physician-supervised diet that is high in fat and low in carbohydrate and protein.

There is usually three to five times as much fat as carbohydrate and protein combined. Calories and liquid intake are limited. The human body normally burns glucose and glycogen to meet its energy needs. If there are no new sources of glucose within 24 to 36 hours, then the body burns energy that is stored as fat. However, the body cannot do this indefinitely, because once it runs out of fat stores, it burns its own muscle protein. The ketogenic diet therefore simulates the metabolism of a person who is fasting and primarily burns the fat in the diet for energy. The diet allows the individual to maintain this state over an extended period. More than 50% of those children who have been tried on the ketogenic diet have improved seizure control, with some having their AEDs reduced and some being medication free. This diet has been shown to be effective in all seizure types and is particularly effective in controlling the absence, atonic, and myoclonic seizures associated with Lennox-Gastaut syndrome. It should not be tried without the supervision of a health care provider and dietitian, both of whom are knowledgeable in the diet (Freeman et al, 2000).

Vagus nerve stimulator. The vagus nerve stimulator (VNS) is a biomedical technique that uses the Neuro Cybernetic Prosthesis (NCP) system as a treatment option for reducing seizure frequency. It was approved in July of 1997 as adjunctive treatment for refractory partial-onset seizures in children over 12 years of age and adults. Many epilepsy centers use the VNS in children under 12 years of age as well. The mechanism of action is unknown, but it has been hypothesized that the VNS inhibits seizure activity by using projections from the nucleus solitarius to the limbic structures. The nucleus solitarius is the main afferent nucleus of the vagus nerve and has projections to a number of areas in the forebrain and brainstem that are important for epileptogenesis. The VNS affects the locus ceruleus (LC), a nucleus in the brain that is associated with seizure activity. Another hypothesis is that the intermittent stimulation of the vagus nerve alters the limbic activity in the brain and decreases epileptogenesis and therefore limits seizure activity (Kennedy & Schallert, 2001).

The VNS is effective in all seizure types and is available to those individuals who have failed or are unable to tolerate several AEDs and are not candidates for epilepsy surgery. The NCP generator is implanted usually in the left side of the chest area, with the bipolar leads threaded under the skin and wrapped around the left vagus nerve. The pulse generator is then programmed through a computer to stimulate the vagus nerve. A neurology health care provider can adjust these parameters when the individual comes into the office. A special very strong magnet is provided to the family and can be swiped across the device to prevent or stop a seizure. The pulse generator can also be turned off by taping the magnet over the device. Side effects include possible infection at the incision site after surgery. In addition, some people experience hoarseness, coughing, gagging, or tingling in the neck when the stimulus is activated (Kennedy & Schallert, 2001). The VNS device is a therapy for seizures that actually gives children and families some sense of control over the seizures.

Surgery. Children who have epilepsy with a focal origin and are refractory to other treatment methods should be evaluated for *epilepsy surgery.* An evaluation is performed to determine if there is a definable focal site for the seizures and if the

TABLE 25-3

Established Antiepilepetic Drugs

Drug	Dosage and Interval	Plasma Half-Life	Therapeutic Plasma Level	Side Effects
Adrenocorticotropic hormone (ACTH)	Varied: 20 U/m²/day to 100-150 U/m²/day for 2-8 wks			Intracranial hemorrhage Irritability Gastrointestinal disturbances/bleeding Fluid retention Electrolyte disturbance Immune system and adrenal suppression Hypertension Cushingoid facies
Bromides (Three Bromides Elixir)	300 mg to 1 g tid	12-14 days	75-125 mg/0.1 L or 10-15 mEq/L	Sedation Anorexia Rash Dementia Delirium
Carbamazepine (Tegretol, Tegretol XR, Carbatrol)	15-30 mg/kg/day bid to tid	12-17 hr	4-12 mg/L	Lethargy Ataxia Gastrointestinal upset Weight gain Pancreatitis Leukopenia Rash/Stevens-Johnson syndrome Arrhythmias in patients with conduction defects
Clonazepam (Klonopin)	0.1-0.2 mg/kg/day qd to tid	18-50 hr	20-80 mg/L	Sedation Ataxia Hyperactivity Increased salivation Rash Increased bronchial secretions
Ethosuximide (Zarontin)	15-20 mg/kg/day bid to tid	30-60 hr	40-100 mg/L	Sedation Headache Nausea/vomiting Rash/erythema multiforme/Stevens-Johnson syndrome
Phenobarbital	3-7 mg/kg/day bid Neonates: 2-5 mg/kg/day bid	24-110 hr	15-40 mg/L	Hyperactivity Drowsiness/sedation Behavioral problems Subtle cognitive changes Hepatic dysfunction Rash/Stevens-Johnson syndrome
Phenytoin (Dilantin)	4-8 mg/kg/day bid to tid	7-42 hr	10-20 mg/L Unbound: 0.5-3 mg/L (nonlinear kinetics)	Ataxia Nystagmus Lethargy Hirsutism Coarse facies Gingival hyperplasia Movement disorder Neuropathy Rash/Stevens-Johnson syndrome Bone marrow suppression Lupus

TABLE 25-3
Established Antiepilepetic Drugs—cont'd

Drug	Dosage and Interval	Plasma Half-Life	Therapeutic Plasma Level	Side Effects
Primidone (Mysoline)	10-25 mg/kg/day tid	10-21 hr	5-12 mg/L	Sedation Ataxia Hyperactivity Cognitive dysfunction Thrombocytopenia Rash/Stevens-Johnson syndrome
Valproic acid, divalproex sodium, valproate sodium (Depakene, Depakote, Depacon)	15-60 mg/kg/day bid to qid	9-12 hr	50-130 mg/L	Tremor Hyperactivity Sedation Gastrointestinal disturbances Pancreatitis Hepatotoxicity Thrombocytopenia Rash/Stevens-Johnson syndrome Polycystic ovarian syndrome

Data adapted from Crumrine, P. (2002). Lennox-Gastaut syndrome. *J Child Neurol 17*(suppl. 1), S70-S75; Deray, M., Resnick, T., & Alvarez, L. (Eds.). (2001). *Complete pocket reference for the treatment of epilepsy*. Miami: C.P.R. Educational Services; Leppik, I.E. (2001). *Contemporary diagnosis and management of the patient with epilepsy* (5th ed.). Newtown, Pa.: Handbooks in Health Care.

TABLE 25-4
Newer Antiepileptic Drugs

Drug	Dosage and Interval	Plasma Half-Life	Therapeutic Plasma level	Side Effects
Felbamate (Felbatol)	15-45 mg/kg/day tid to qid	15-23 hr	30-80 mg/L	Headache Drowsiness Insomnia Anorexia/weight loss Nausea/vomiting Rash/Stevens-Johnson syndrome Liver and renal failure Aplastic anemia
Fosphenytoin (Cerebyx)	Loading dose: 15-20 mg/kg IV or IM Maintenance: 4-8 mg/kg/day IV or IM qd to tid	12-29 hr	10-25 mg/L	Paresthesias Ataxia Nystagmus Lethargy Liver failure Hypotension Burning/itching Stevens-Johnson syndrome/toxic epidermal necrolysis
Gabapentin (Neurontin)	30-60 mg/kg/day tid to qid	4-6 hr	2-12 mg/L	Fatigue/somnolence Dizziness Ataxia Eye problems Weight gain Hypertension/hypotension
Lamotrigine (Lamictal)	With valproate: 1-5 mg/kg/day bid With monotherapy or enzyme inducer: 5-15 mg/kg/day bid	11-61 hr	4-20 mg/L	Lethargy Dizziness Nausea Pancreatitis Thrombocytopenia Rash/Stevens-Johnson syndrome/toxic epidermal necrolysis

Continued

TABLE 25-4

Newer Antiepileptic Drugs—cont'd

Drug	Dosage and Interval	Plasma Half-Life	Therapeutic Plasma level	Side Effects
Levetiracetam (Keppra)	10-80 mg/kg/day bid to tid	6-8 hr	5-40 mg/L	Sedation Asthenia Ataxia Agitation Hallucinations Emotional lability
Oxcarbazepine (Trileptal)	10-60 mg/kg/day	8-10 hr	MHD 12-30 mg/L	Headache Dizziness Tiredness/somnolence Nausea/vomiting Hyponatremia

Tiagabine (Gabatril)	20-32 mg/day bid to qid
	Increase every 2-4 days
	   by 0.1-0.2 mg/kg to maximum
	   3 mg/kg/day
		4-9 hr	0.1-0.3 mg/L	Dizziness
				Insomnia
				Somnolence
				Ataxia
				Nausea
				Increased appetite
				Concentration loss
				Rash/Stevens-Johnson syndrome

Topiramate (Topamax)	5-15 mg/kg/day bid 24 mg/kg/day in infantile spasms	19-23 hr	4-10 mg/L	Lethargy Ataxia Psychomotor slowing Paresthesias Anorexia/weight loss Rash Renal stones Pancreatitis
Zonisamide (Zonegran)	8-12 mg/kg/day qd to tid	60 hr	15-40 mg/L	Fatigue Dizziness Somnolence Ataxia Memory impairment Anorexia Rash/Stevens-Johnson syndrome Renal stones

Data adapted from Deray, M., Resnick, T., & Alvarez, L. (Eds.). (2001). Complete pocket reference for the treatment of epilepsy. Miami: C.P.R. Educational Services; Leppik, I.E. (2001). Contemporary diagnosis and management of the patient with epilepsy, (5th ed.). Newtown, Pa.: Handbooks in Health Care; Wheless, J. (2002). Using the new antiepilepsy drugs in children. *J Child Neurol, 17*(suppl. 1), S58-S64.
MHD, 10-Monohydroxyl metabolite (active metabolite).

removal of that particular area will affect function. Surgery is divided into either resective or functional surgery. Focal resection of the seizure focus is performed when the seizures are coming from an exact focus in the brain. Temporal lobectomy, removal of the temporal lobe, is the most common of these procedures. Extratemporal resection is considered in some children with the help of advances in neuroimaging techniques. Hemispherectomy is the complete or partial removal of one hemisphere of the brain (Cross, 2002).

The goal of functional procedures is to modify brain function. Corpus callosotomy and multiple subpial transection are two procedures that may be considered. In corpus callosotomy, there is either a two-thirds or complete division of the corpus callosum in order to stop the spread of the seizure from one side of the brain to the other. Multiple subpial transection is a more recent procedure being performed in children with Landau-Kleffner syndrome who have epileptic aphasia. The transverse fibers over the leading side of the Wernicke area in the brain are transected, leaving the longitudinal fibers intact. The result of this procedure is improved or normal speech in some of the children (Cross, 2002).

When considering epilepsy surgery the risks and benefits of the procedure must be discussed. Possible risks of the procedure include perioperative mortality, postoperative neurologic deficits, and failure to gain seizure control. The benefits of epilepsy surgery include improved or complete seizure control with resultant improvement in development and dysfunctional behavior (Wyllie, 1999).

Complementary and Alternative Therapies

More families are using alternative therapies, such as *herbal preparations and supplements*, to treat medical conditions. Often people are using multiple herbal preparations in conjunction with prescription drugs, and polypharmacy is becom-

TABLE 25-5

Efficacy of AEDs against Common Seizure Types and Epilepsy Syndromes

Drug	Partial	Secondarily Generalized Seizures	Atonic/Tonic	Tonic-Clonic	Absence	Myoclonic	Lennox-Gastaut	Infantile Spasms
Carbamazepine	+	+	0	+	–	–	0	0
Clonazepam	+	+	?+	+	?	+	?+	?+
Ethosuximide	0	0	0	0	+	0	0	0
Felbamate	+	+	+	+	?+	?+	+	?
Gabapentin	+	+	0	+	–	–	?	?
Lamotrigine	+	+	+	+	+	+	+	?+
Levitracetam	+	+	?	+	+	+	?	?
Oxcarbazepine	+	+	0	+	?–	?–	0	0
Phenobarbital	+	+	?	+	0	?+	?	?
Phenytoin	+	+	0	+	–	–	0	0
Primidone	+	+	?	+	0	?	?	?
Tiagabine	+	+	0	+	–	–	?	?+
Topiramate	+	+	+	+	?	+	+	?+
Sodium valproate	+	+	+	+	+	+	+	+
Zonisamide	+	+	?+	+	?+	+	?+	?+

Adapted from Brodie, M. & Kwan, P. (2002). Staged approach to epilepsy management. *Neurology, 58*(8, suppl. 5), S2-S8; Brodie M. & Schachter, S. (2001). *Epilepsy* (2nd ed.). Oxford: Health Press.
+, Proven efficacy; ?+, probable efficacy; 0, ineffective; –, worsens control; ?–, may worsen control; ?, unknown.

ing a common practice (Fugh-Berman, 2000). A number of herbs have been described as being effective or possibly effective in the treatment of seizures: American hellebore, betony, blue cohosh, kava, mistletoe, mugwort, pipsissewa, and skullcap (Blumenthal et al, 2000; Fetrow & Avila, 2001; Skidmore-Roth, 2001). However, none are recommended in the pediatric age-group (Skidmore-Roth, 2001).

All ingested substances have the potential to interact or result in some type of adverse reaction (Fugh-Berman, 2000). As a result, the herbal preparation may have a positive effect on seizures but may adversely affect another condition. Children and families must be aware of these issues when using herbal preparations.

Anticipated Advances in Diagnosis and Management

There have been significant advances in the diagnosis and subsequent management of pediatric epilepsy in the last 10 years. Advances in medical technology with EEG and neuroimaging studies have resulted in improved diagnosis and treatment of epilepsy. Newer AEDs give improved control to many individuals with previously intractable epilepsy. Surgical advances in regard to epilepsy surgery and the VNS have given hope to many who had none. In addition, the VNS has empowered many in the control of their epilepsy. However, the greatest advances have been in the molecular genetics of epilepsy, including the familial idiopathic epilepsies and the many inherited symptomatic epilepsies (Kaneko et al, 2002b). Future studies in the genetics of epilepsy can lead to new and improved treatment options, such as new types of AEDs and gene therapy. Gene therapy may lead to the need for fewer treatment modalities or an eventual cure for epilepsy (Kaneko et al, 2002a).

BOX 25-8
Associated Problems

Injuries
Cognitive dysfunction
Psychiatric complications

Associated Problems (Box 25-8)

The etiology, age of onset, seizure type, frequency of occurrence, and success of treatment influence problems related to epilepsy.

Injuries

Injury during a seizure is always possible. One must take into account the seizure type, age of the child, and the activity in which the child is involved. A child may sustain direct trauma or may fall during a seizure, but this is usually as a result of the loss of consciousness that occurs during the seizure (Shinnar & O'Dell, 2001). There is also an elevated risk of mortality in a child with seizures. The risk may be associated with the underlying cause of the epilepsy, but it is also associated in some cases with accidents that occur during a seizure (Berg & Chadwick, 2000), such as death from drowning or as a result of a motor vehicle accident. A child may also aspirate during a seizure, especially if the child has recently eaten. It is therefore vital for parents, teachers, and health care providers to be knowledgeable about the appropriate precautions (e.g., helmet for a child with uncontrolled akinetic or atonic seizures) and first aid measures to be taken in order to minimize injury during a seizure (Box 25-9).

BOX 25-9
First Aid for Seizures

GENERALIZED SEIZURES
Gently lower the child to the floor, if not already there.
Position the child to his or her side to prevent aspiration.
Support the child's head so it is in straight alignment with the body by using a small pillow, towel, jacket, or hand.
Do not put anything into the child's mouth so as not to cause injury (e.g., broken object, broken tooth, bite to the individual providing aid).
Loosen any tight clothing around the neck, chest, or abdomen of the child.
Do not restrain the child.
Move furniture away from the child.
Remain with the child.
If the seizure is prolonged, there are respiratory difficulties, or there is any concern, contact emergency medical services (EMS).

COMPLEX PARTIAL SEIZURES
Remain with the child.
Do not restrain the child.
Speak softly to the child.
If the child is walking, gently guide the child by placing hands on the child's shoulders from behind, to prevent injury.
If the seizure spreads to a generalized seizure, follow the first aid guidelines for a generalized seizure.

ABSENCE SEIZURES
Stay with the child.
Do not restrain the child.
Guide the child from behind as necessary to prevent injury.
Reorient the child to his or her surroundings after the seizure is over.

Cognitive Dysfunction

Most individuals with epilepsy have normal intelligence. However, children with epilepsy are at an increased risk for cognitive dysfunction. Numerous factors can affect cognitive function in children with epilepsy, including etiology of seizures; cerebral lesions; seizure type and age of onset; severity, frequency, and duration of the seizures; physiologic dysfunction as seen on the EEG; structural brain damage caused by prolonged or repetitive seizures; hereditary factors (e.g., the intelligence quotient [IQ] of the parent); psychosocial issues; and the result of treatment for epilepsy, including AEDs and epilepsy surgery (Meador, 2002).

Austin et al (1999) found that academic achievement in children remained stable over time. They found that children with low-severity seizure disorders had average school performance. Children with high-severity seizure disorders did not show improvement in their academic achievement, even when their seizures improved. They concluded that children with high-severity seizure disorders are at high risk for academic underachievement.

Cognitive effects can be associated with AEDs. Factors affecting cognition include polytherapy, high doses of AEDs, and higher AED blood levels (Meador, 2002). Health care providers should treat epilepsy with the lowest dose of an AED that is possible, and as few drugs as possible to limit the untoward effects.

Epilepsy surgery is not usually associated with cognitive decline since the goal of surgery is to remove dysfunctional tissue in the brain. Cognition may improve after surgery because of the reduction of seizures and the need for fewer treatment modalities. However, cognitive deficits such as memory and language deficits may occur postoperatively. The most common epilepsy surgery is the temporal lobectomy, and cognitive deficits are usually related to the language-dominant hemisphere for that individual (Meador, 2002). Improved neuropsychologic testing and medical imaging techniques result in better identification of the language-dominant hemisphere and consequently the predictive risk of these adverse effects.

Psychiatric Complications

Approximately 50% of individuals with epilepsy have been reported to have psychiatric syndromes accompanying the different stages of brain activity associated with seizures. When assessing for psychiatric disorders in individuals with epilepsy it is important to determine if the disorder is associated with the ictal, periictal, or interictal state (Marsh & Rao, 2002).

Various affective and behavior disorders occur as a result of seizure activity (ictal phase). Anxiety is the most common. However, depressed feelings, ictal psychosis phenomena, violence (extremely rare), and aggression may also be seen during this time. Adequate seizure control with AEDs and nonpharmacologic treatments (e.g., observation, education) are the recommended therapies for these disorders (Marsh & Rao, 2002).

Periictal disturbances are either preictal or postictal. Preictal disturbances include irritability, apprehension, mood swings, depression, psychosis, or aggression that can last for minutes, hours, or days before a seizure occurs. Postictal psychiatric disturbances include delirium, psychosis, mania, and violence. Postictal disturbances usually resolve quickly, but they can also last for several hours, days, or weeks. Treatment includes maintaining safety, environmental support, and behavioral redirection. Sometimes medications are necessary, such as neuroleptics (in severe cases), sedatives (for a calming effect), and diuretics (if associated with changes in gonadal hormones and fluid balance) (Marsh & Rao, 2002).

Interictal psychiatric disorders are common in epilepsy, especially in those with temporal lobe epilepsy (Marsh & Rao, 2002). Mood disorders (ranging from short-lived episodes of low or elevated mood to persistent mood disturbances) and anxiety disorders (intensity and duration of anxiety are greater than what should be expected) are the most common (Hermann et al, 2000; Marsh & Rao, 2002). Major depression, dysthymic and atypical depressive syndromes, adjustment disorders with depressed mood, bipolar disorder, generalized anxiety disorders (worrying about a number of minor matters, along with having impaired functioning), phobias, panic disorders, obsessive-compulsive disorders (OCDs), and psychotic disorders are also seen. In addition, medication-induced psychiatric disorders occur because of the positive or negative psychotropic effects of various AEDs (Marsh & Rao, 2002).

Therefore treatment consists of improved seizure control, psychiatric and psychologic therapy, and psychotherapeutic management (Hermann et al, 2000; Marsh & Rao, 2002).

Prognosis

The majority of children with epilepsy become seizure free with AEDs within a few years of diagnosis (Shinnar & Pellock,

2002), will achieve long-term remission, and continue in remission with the discontinuation of treatment (Sander & Pal, 2000; Shinnar & Pellock, 2002). Children with a single seizure have also done well without treatment (Shinnar & Pellock, 2002).

About 70% of individuals with epilepsy achieve long-term remission, leaving approximately 30% continuing to be refractory to treatment (Bebin, 2002; Shinnar & Pellock, 2002). After the first seizure onset, approximately 40% achieve remission within 5 years, either on or off medication. At 10 years, approximately 61% achieve remission, and at 20 years, approximately 70% achieve remission. Factors that influence achieving remission include etiology, epilepsy syndrome, childhood onset at less than 10 years of age, and seizure frequency or early treatment response. Those with childhood-onset epilepsy and cryptogenic epilepsy have a better prognosis (Shinnar & Pellock, 2002).

Approximately 60% to 75% of children who have remained seizure free on medication for 2 to 4 years continue to be seizure free off medication. Factors that influence recurrence risk of seizures include etiology, age of onset, and EEG findings. The rate of seizure recurrence after the withdrawal of all AEDs is approximately 15% in those who do not have any major risk factors. These include children who have cryptogenic or idiopathic seizures, have a normal EEG before discontinuation of the AEDs, and have the onset of seizures before 12 years of age. Those children with remote symptomatic epilepsy have a worse prognosis, yet approximately 50% of those children who remained seizure free on AEDs continue to remain seizure free once off medication (Shinnar & Pellock, 2002).

PRIMARY CARE MANAGEMENT

Health Care Maintenance

Growth and Development

Obtaining heights and weights regularly on children with epilepsy is particularly important. These children are at risk for significant changes in growth (i.e., loss or gain in weight), either because of the medication they are taking or because of associated problems they may have (e.g., mental retardation [MR], cerebral palsy [CP] [see Chapter 18]). In addition, medications are based on children's weight as well as their response to the AED dose.

Some children with epilepsy are at risk for developmental delays because of frequent seizures, the epilepsy syndrome, or other associated disorders. The primary care provider must monitor development in these children in regard to the child's social, cognitive, and motor development. If a delay is noted referrals should be made for appropriate screening and treatment (i.e., physical therapy, occupational therapy, speech therapy, psychoeducational testing, early intervention or infant stimulation programs, learning support in the school setting).

Diet

Feeding issues in children with epilepsy are more often related to the associated problems that children with epilepsy may have. It is therefore vital to monitor the child's growth pattern using growth charts. If there is a significant change in the child's

weight, it is important to determine if the change is associated with the medication or other factors. Once this determination is made, then appropriate measures can be taken. If the change is due to an increase or decrease in appetite because of the AED, then the primary care provider will need to discuss this with the child's specialist. The medication may need to be changed. If the change is due to other factors, then a nutritional evaluation with a referral to a dietitian may be indicated. Dietary supplements may need to be added to the child's diet if the issue is one of weight loss. A weight management program may need to be implemented if the issue is excessive weight gain. In cases of children who are compromised by other problems such as CP, a gastrostomy (G) tube may need to be considered to ensure that the child receives proper nutrition.

Weight gain is a significant issue in infants with infantile spasms when treated with adrenocorticotropic hormones (ACTH). A side effect of this drug is weight gain. The child's weight must be monitored closely while taking this medication. Children will usually return to a normal weight after the ACTH treatment is discontinued.

Children on the ketogenic diet do not usually have significant fluctuations in their weight. However, the nutritional status of these children must be carefully monitored, and a dietitian knowledgeable in the ketogenic diet must be closely involved throughout therapy.

Safety

Being aware of the many safety issues particular to infants and children with epilepsy is important. In addition, parents and families of children with epilepsy must be educated in regard to first aid for seizures (Box 25-9). Emergency medical services (EMS) should be called in situations of prolonged seizure activity or whenever there is a concern for the child's safety. Parents and child care providers of children with life-threatening seizures should be certified to perform cardiopulmonary resuscitation (CPR) in the event of a respiratory or cardiac arrest.

There is always the potential for injury during a seizure. Children and families should be educated about the appropriate type of seizure precautions necessary. In regard to *water*, the child should take showers instead of baths, if old enough, making sure the water drains well from the tub. If taking a bath, the child should be watched by an adult at all times to prevent drowning if a seizure occurs while in the water. The child should not lock the bathroom door or take a shower or bath when home alone. The child should never swim alone. The child should have one-to-one supervision while in the water so if a seizure occurs, the adult can get the child out of the water immediately. If a seizure does occur in the water, the child should be evaluated for aspiration pneumonia.

Children who have uncontrolled seizures should not be allowed to climb in *high places* (e.g., rope climbing, mountain climbing, rock climbing, tree climbing, parallel bars). If going on amusement park rides, the child should be securely strapped into the ride and not go alone. If playing on park equipment, there should be soft ground (e.g., mulch) beneath the equipment. The child should not mountain ski if seizures are uncontrolled.

The child must take precautions around *heat* (e.g., fire, electricity). When cooking on the stove, the pot and pan handles should be turned toward the center of the stove. If the child is cooking, an adult should be present at all times. The child should never use the stove when home alone; the child may use a microwave when alone. If the child is near a campfire or bonfire, the child should be standing or sitting away from the fire so if a seizure occurs the child does not fall into the fire.

If the child's seizures are uncontrolled, the child should not use *electrical/mechanical equipment* (e.g., lawn mower, power tools). When using this equipment, an adult should supervise the child at all times. Caution must be taken with *sport activities*. Children who have seizures and sustain a head injury have the potential to develop worsening seizures that are difficult to control. A helmet should be worn at all times when bike riding, horseback riding, ice skating, roller skating, and roller blading. The child should not participate in contact sports, such as ice hockey and boxing. Participation in other sports should be determined on an individual basis.

There are a few activities in which the children and adolescents with epilepsy should not participate. They cannot pilot a plane, sky dive, or scuba dive. If a seizure occurs during any of these activities, the result can be fatal. Driving laws vary by state. The health care provider can contact the Department of Motor Vehicles (DMV) for each state to determine the laws for that particular state in regard to driving restrictions for an individual with epilepsy. As in all cases, each person should be evaluated individually in regard to seizure precautions.

Immunizations

Infants and children with an underlying seizure disorder or a family history of seizures are at an increased risk of having a seizure after receiving either the DTaP (diphtheria, tetanus toxoid, acellular pertussis) or the measles vaccine (usually MMR [measles, mumps, rubella]). The risk of fever is less with the DTaP vaccine as compared with the DTP (diphtheria, tetanus toxoid, and pertussis) vaccine. The seizures that occur after immunization are usually brief, generalized, and associated with a fever (febrile seizures). No evidence suggests that these seizures cause permanent brain damage or epilepsy, worsen already present neurologic disorders, or affect the prognosis of children with underlying disorders (American Academy of Pediatrics [AAP], 2003).

Since the DTaP vaccine is given in early infancy, its side effects may be confused with the development of a neurologic disorder that is associated with seizures and may cause confusion as to the etiology of the disorder. The measles vaccine, on the other hand, is given at an older age when neurologic disorders of infancy most likely have already been established (AAP, 2003). Consequently, there is less confusion when side effects are noted.

The incidence of seizures usually occurs after the third or fourth dose of the vaccine series within 48 hours after the DTaP vaccine has been administered and usually is associated with fever. The recommendations of the AAP (2003) in regard to immunization with DTP/DTaP vaccine in infants and children with active seizures are as follows: (1) administration of the pertussis vaccine should be deferred until the exclusion of a progressive neurologic disorder has been made, (2) administration of the pertussis vaccine should be deferred in those children with a known or suspected neurologic condition that

predisposes the child to seizures (i.e., tuberous sclerosis, inherited metabolic or degenerative diseases) or unstable neurologic disorders, (3) children with well-controlled seizures or those where a recurring seizure is unlikely may be immunized, (4) administration of an antipyretic at the time of the immunization and every 4 hours for 24 hours should be considered, (5) families should be informed that there is a slight risk of seizure occurrence after the DTaP vaccine, (6) all infants and children should be evaluated on an individual basis to determine if they can be immunized, and (7) a family history of seizures is not a contraindication for the child to receive the pertussis vaccine.

Post–measles vaccine fevers usually occur within 1 to 2 weeks after the vaccine is administered. Therefore it is difficult to prevent vaccine-related febrile seizures that may occur. The recommendations of the AAP (2003) in regard to immunization with measles vaccine in infants and children with active seizures are as follows: (1) children with a history of seizures should be immunized with the measles vaccine, (2) a family history of seizures is not a contraindication for the child to receive the measles vaccine, (3) families should be informed that there is a slight risk of seizure occurrence after the measles vaccine, and (4) all infants and children should be evaluated on an individual basis to determine if they can be immunized.

If there is any question or concern in regard to providing immunizations to children with seizures, the health care provider should contact the child's specialist. All other immunizations should be given according to the routine schedule.

Screening

Vision. Routine screening is recommended.

Hearing. Routine screening is recommended.

Dental Care. Routine dental care is recommended. Those children taking phenytoin (Dilantin) should have routine dental care at least every 6 months. Gingival hyperplasia is a potential side effect of phenytoin (Greenwood, 2000); therefore children taking phenytoin require more frequent brushing and flossing with particular attention given to gums. The dentist should be informed that an individual is taking phenytoin so that frequent dental cleaning can be performed.

Blood Pressure. Routine screening is recommended. Hypertension is a potential side effect of ACTH therapy (Deray et al, 2001). Infants treated with ACTH therapy require frequent blood pressure monitoring, at least twice weekly. Children on home ACTH therapy usually have a nurse who makes home visits to monitor the child. Parents can be taught how to take and monitor the infant's blood pressure while the infant is receiving ACTH therapy.

Hematocrit. Routine screening is recommended.

Urinalysis. Routine screening is recommended.

Tuberculosis. Routine screening is recommended.

Condition-Specific Screening

Drug Toxicity Screening. Therapies used in the treatment of epilepsy have adverse effects that may affect body systems. Therefore blood tests are recommended routinely for children who are on particular AEDs or the ketogenic diet. Deray et al (2001) have made the following recommendations.

ACTH. Electrolytes and glucose are recommended at onset and end of therapy to monitor for electrolyte imbalance. Guaiac testing of all stools should be done to look for blood.

Bromides. Perform baseline complete blood count (CBC), electrolytes, and liver function tests (LFTs). Repeat monthly or as needed.

Carbamazepine (Carbatrol, Tegretol). Perform baseline complete blood count (CBC) and liver function tests (LFTs). Repeat at 6 weeks, 3 months, 6 months, and every 3 to 6 months throughout therapy.

Felbamate (Felbatol). Full hematologic evaluation should be done before therapy, frequently throughout therapy, and for a significant time after completion of therapy (*Epilepsy: Disease Management Guide*, 2000).

Ethosuximide (Zarontin). Perform CBC and LFTs monthly for the first 6 months. Repeat periodically throughout therapy.

Oxcarbazepine (Trileptal). Hyponatremia is a rare side effect. If there is a sudden increase in seizure activity in a child taking this medication, consider obtaining a serum sodium level.

Prednisone. Measure electrolytes and serum glucose at onset of therapy and on completion of therapy.

Valproic acid, divalproex sodium, and valproate sodium (Depakene, Depakote). Perform baseline CBC with platelets and LFTs. Repeat LFTs every 6 months throughout therapy.

Ketogenic Diet. At baseline, 1 month after initiation of diet, and then every 4 months thereafter, evaluate the following: CBC; liver, renal, and lipid functions; electrolytes; CO_2; calcium; and urinalysis. A baseline electrocardiogram (ECG) is recommended. Repeat the ECG 3 months after initiation of the diet, and twice yearly thereafter. If bruising occurs or there is pending surgery, it is recommended that platelet aggregation or platelet function, and prothrombin time (PT) and partial thromboplastin time (PTT) be performed.

AED Drug Levels. Serum drug levels are measured throughout therapy at varying intervals. In many of the newer AEDs, drug levels are not recommended. Efficacy is based on the individual's response to the drug.

Electroencephalogram. An EEG is performed during the diagnostic work-up for epilepsy. Only about 40% of individuals have an epileptiform EEG on the initial test. Sleep deprivation before the test to capture sleep on the EEG, activation procedures (e.g., photic stimulation, hyperventilation), and prolonging the length of the study may increase the yield on the EEG (Prego-Lopez & Devinsky, 2002). Ambulatory EEGs and inpatient video EEGs are performed at the discretion of the treating physician. Repeat EEGs should be performed at the discretion of the treating physician and before discontinuation of therapy.

Medical Imaging Studies. During the diagnostic work-up for epilepsy, medical imaging studies may be performed to determine the etiology. Computerized tomography (CT) scans can detect gross structural abnormalities or bleeding. Magnetic resonance imaging (MRI) is more sensitive and specific for evaluating brain parenchyma and structural abnormalities (Prego-Lopez & Devinsky, 2002). These studies are performed at the discretion of the treating physician and repeated throughout therapy as warranted. Other studies (e.g., SPECT [single photon emission computed tomography] scans) are performed at the discretion of the treating physician.

Common Illness Management
Common Illnesses

Various precipitating events can trigger a seizure (Box 25-4), including sleep deprivation and illness or fever. When a child is ill with a fever, the child can have an increase in seizure activity. Upper respiratory infections, viral illnesses, otitis media, and streptococcus infection of the throat are just a few of the common illnesses that can cause a fever in children. It is important to manage a fever aggressively with the use of antipyretics and increased fluids to keep the elevated temperature down. It is also important to manage bacterial infections with antibiotics. The family should be educated to treat the fever early in the course of an illness.

Vomiting and diarrhea are often seen with a viral illness. It is important for the child to continue taking the prescribed AED throughout the illness. Routine management of vomiting and diarrhea should be provided. For example, the parent or caregiver can be instructed to keep the child NPO for 4 hours after vomiting. When starting fluids, the parent or caregiver can begin with 1 teaspoon of clear fluids every 10 to 15 minutes for the first 1 to 2 hours and then increase the fluids every 1 to 2 hours by 1 teaspoon, if tolerated. The dose of AED can be divided over 1 hour and placed into the clear fluids for the child to take. If the vomiting continues, and the child cannot keep fluids or the medication down, then the parent or caregiver should be instructed to take the child to the local emergency room to get the AED or AEDs through an intravenous (IV) line.

Children on the ketogenic diet have their diet managed by a dietitian who is knowledgeable in the diet. These children are kept in ketosis and a partially dehydrated state at all times. If a child on the ketogenic diet develops vomiting and diarrhea, the family must keep in close contact with the dietitian for dietary instructions. If the vomiting and diarrhea continue despite micromanagement by the dietitian, then the child will need to go to a local emergency room for IV management. There can be no glucose added in the IV line in order to keep the child in ketosis while managing the illness.

There is no research to support that constipation causes an increase in seizure activity. However, many parents and caregivers have reported this to occur in their child with a seizure disorder. Chronic constipation is common in children with disabilities (Elawad & Sullivan, 2001) and therefore can be seen in many children with epilepsy who have associated problems, such as CP. It is important to provide adequate treatment for the child with constipation.

Head trauma can permanently alter the brain and trigger mechanisms that can eventually result in the development of epilepsy (DeLorenzo, 2001). It can lower the seizure threshold in an individual (Brodie & Schachter, 2001). In the child or adolescent who already has a seizure disorder, a head injury can result in worsening of the seizures. It is important for the person with epilepsy to follow the safety precautions necessary to prevent a head injury (e.g., wearing a helmet when riding a bike, horseback riding, roller skating, ice skating). If a child has a head injury, the child should be evaluated by his or her health care provider immediately or go to the closest emergency room to be evaluated.

Differential Diagnosis

Nonepileptic Events. Also known as nonepileptic paroxysmal disorders, are common in the pediatric population (Paolicchi, 2002). These disorders can produce behaviors that are similar to that exhibited by an individual with epilepsy (Box 25-10). Children with epilepsy can develop these disorders, and it is important to differentiate them from the child's or adolescent's seizure disorder so that the AED dosages are not increased or the AED changed unnecessarily. Most of these disorders are benign; some need no treatment and resolve on their own, and some need medication other than AEDs (Paolicchi, 2002; Prensky, 2001). Some of the more common paroxysmal disorders will be discussed.

Psychogenic Seizures. Also called *pseudoseizures,* are a common symptom of conversion disorder or dissociation disorder (AES, 2000). They are more common in the adolescent population as compared with young children and are more common in females (Paolicchi, 2002). When events are refractory to medication, psychogenic seizures should be considered (AES, 2000; Paolicchi, 2002). Often individuals who have psychogenic seizures also have true epileptic seizures (Prensky, 2001). A video EEG during the event is necessary to make the proper diagnosis (AES, 2000; Paolicchi, 2002). True psychogenic seizures should be treated as a serious psychiatric illness that requires intense treatment. These events are a learned behavior, and treatment focuses on new coping mechanisms (Gumnit, 1997). However, it is important to remember that some seizures can have symptoms that are often misdiagnosed as psychogenic seizures (Prego-Lopez & Devinsky, 2002).

Benign Neonatal Myoclonus. The most common paroxysmal event in infancy (Prensky, 2001). It usually occurs during sleep, and onset is usually in the first weeks to months of life (Paolicchi, 2002; Prensky, 2001). Quick, forceful jerks usually recur every 2 to 3 seconds and can last up to 30 minutes. They resolve only to recur again throughout the night (Prensky, 2001). They do not resolve when gently restrained, and they stop on arousal. The EEG shows no abnormal activity other than movement artifact (Paolicchi, 2002). If the infant develops the disorder early in infancy, it usually resolves within 3 to 4 months. However, some children can continue to exhibit this disorder until the second year of life (Prensky, 2001). A small dose of clonazepam (Klonopin) before bed can reduce the events if necessary (Paolicchi, 2002).

Sandifer Syndrome. This can present as tonic posturing in infants that can be mistaken for tonic seizures. The syndrome consists of abnormal posturing of the neck, trunk, and limbs usually because of gastroesophageal reflux (GER). The symptoms may also be the result of a hiatal hernia or esophageal dysmotility. The history reveals that the tonic posturing is usually associated with feedings, occurring within about 30 minutes of a feeding. In addition, there is often a history of "spitting up" or intolerance of formula. These infants need a gastrointestinal (GI) evaluation (Paolicchi, 2002).

Migraines. There is a fine line between migraines and seizures. Migraines are usually characterized by headache and accompanying focal neurologic deficits. About 20% to 30% of people with migraines develop an aura. The aura usually lasts longer than 5 minutes. The accompanying symptoms can include psychologic (e.g., euphoria, restlessness), neurologic (e.g., loss of consciousness, photophobia, phonophobia), and autonomic (e.g., flushing, diaphoresis) features. An EEG can show spike and wave. Diagnosis is based on the clinical history (Bauer, 2000).

Narcolepsy. Often confused with seizures, narcolepsy is characterized by excessive daytime sleepiness, cataplexy, hypnagogic hallucinations, and sleep paralysis (Kohrman, 1999). It is usually not seen until adolescence (Paolicchi, 2002). Children usually fall suddenly and unexpectedly asleep for brief periods during the day. They can have an abrupt and reversible loss of muscle tone in response to some type of emotion (e.g., laughter), known as cataplexy. These children have hallucinations that occur on arousal, known as hypnagogic hallucinations. They may also have sleep paralysis, which is the inability to move on awakening (Prensky, 2001). An EEG will not be positive during the events. The diagnosis is made when the child's history reveals one or more of the associated symptoms and the child has a positive multiple sleep latency test (MSLT) (Kohrman, 1999; Paolicchi, 2002).

BOX 25-10
Nonepileptic Events

MOVEMENTS
Jitteriness
Shuddering
Benign neonatal sleep myoclonus
Tics
Pseudoseizures
Masturbation
Paroxysmal torticollis
Hyperekplexia—excessive
   startle response
Self-stimulation
Eye/head movements
Dystonia
Tremors

LOSS OF TONE OR CONSCIOUSNESS
Syncope
Narcolepsy
Attention deficit
Daydreaming
Staring spells
Stereotypies
Acute hemiplegia

RESPIRATORY
Apnea
Breath-holding spells
Hyperventilation

PERCEPTUAL DISTURBANCES
Headache/pain
Dizziness
Vertigo
Hallucinations

BEHAVIOR DISORDERS
Head banging
Rage
Confusion
Fear

SLEEP DISORDERS
Sleep walking
Nightmares
Pavor nocturnus—night terrors
Somniloquy

FEATURES OF SPECIFIC DISORDERS
Tetralogy spells
Cardiac arrhythmias
Sandifer syndrome
Migraines
Cyclic vomiting
Benign paroxysmal vertigo
Recurrent abdominal pain

OTHER EVENTS
Phobias
Panic attacks
Munchausen by proxy
Drug reactions
Transient global amnesia
Withholding, constipation

Data from Paolicchi, J. (2002). The spectrum of nonepileptic events in children. *Epilepsia, 43*(suppl. 3), 60-64; Pellock, J. (1997). The differential diagnosis of epilepsy: Nonepileptic paroxysmal disorders. In E. Wyllie (Ed.). *The treatment of epilepsy: Principles and practice* (2nd ed.). Philadelphia: Williams & Wilkins, pp. 681-690.

Sleepwalking. Approximately 15% of all children have at least one episode of sleepwalking in their lifetime. It usually begins between age 5 and 10 years and can continue into the adult years. The episode usually occurs 1 to 3 hours after the child falls asleep. The child's eyes are open, and he or she walks around the house, can perform semipurposeful behaviors, mumbles, and can walk back to bed unassisted. If restrained, these children can become agitated. The child has no memory of the event in the morning. The behaviors are often confused with complex partial seizures (Prensky, 2001).

Nightmares and Night Terrors. *Nightmares* usually occur during REM sleep. The child may be restless but does not usually scream out. He or she usually remembers the dream in the morning and can develop a fear of sleeping alone. The EEG is normal during the event (Prensky, 2001). On the other hand, *night terrors* (pavor nocturnus) occur from 30 minutes to several hours after onset of sleep, during stage 3 or 4 of slow-wave sleep. Night terrors are more common between 5 and 12 years of age (Pellock, 1997). The child sits up in bed, seems terrified, and screams inconsolably. There are symptoms of increased sympathetic activity (diaphoresis, dilated pupils) during the event. Night terrors can last up to 15 minutes, and then the child falls back to sleep. There is no memory of the event in the morning, and the EEG during the event is generally normal (Prensky, 2001).

Staring Spells. These are common in children and often reflect daydreaming or inattention. Staring spells can be misdiagnosed as absence seizures or complex partial seizures. With daydreaming and inattention, the individual may not respond to verbal stimuli but usually responds immediately to noxious tactile stimulation. The EEG does not show epileptic activity during these events (Paolicchi, 2002; Prensky, 2001).

Tics. Often occurring while the individual is awake, tics resolve during sleep (Pellock, 1997) (see Chapter 40). They can involve one muscle group or many, are stereotypic and repetitive, and appear intermittently. They can be simple or complex. Simple tics are stereotypic movements involving one or two muscle groups, usually of the face and neck. The most common simple tics are eye blinking, shoulder shrugging, head turning, sniffing, and grunting. Complex tics involve a number of muscle groups and have more complex movements (Prensky, 2001). When the individual has both motor and vocal tics that wax and wane for longer than 6 months, this is considered Tourette syndrome. The EEG is normal. Tics can be treated with medication if necessary (Singer, 1999).

Breath-Holding Spells. Common in the younger child, age of onset for breath-holding spells is typically between 6 to 18 months of age. By 4 years of age, breath-holding spells resolve in approximately 50% of the children. Breath-holding spells will completely resolve in the majority of children by 7 to 8 years of age (Roddy, 1999). There are two types: cyanotic breath-holding spells and pallid breath-holding spells. *Cyanotic breath-holding spells* are usually precipitated by fear, frustration, or minor injury. The child cries vigorously, develops apnea on expiration, turns blue, and develops a loss of consciousness. Cerebral anoxia causes the child to become limp and unresponsive for 1 to 2 minutes; he or she is usually alert on arousal (Prensky, 2001). *Pallid breath-holding spells* occur as a result of a minor injury or fright. Crying is usually absent. There is no obvious apneic episode, and the child becomes pale. The child

then becomes limp and may have tonic or clonic movements. The episode lasts a few minutes, and the child is alert on arousal. Pallid spells are due to transient cardiac asystole (Roddy, 1999). Epileptic discharges are not associated with either event (Prensky, 2001).

Syncope. Either vasovagal or cardiogenic, syncope can often be confused with epilepsy, especially if tonic or tonic-clonic movements accompany the event (AES, 2000). However, prodromal symptoms are often associated with syncope such as lightheadedness, blurred vision, visual dimming, pallor, and diaphoresis. In addition, environmental factors, such as dehydration, change in position or posture, hunger, or heat exposure, also play a role in the individual with syncope. A cardiac evaluation is often valuable in distinguishing between syncope and seizures (Paolicchi, 2002).

Drug Interactions

Most AEDs are metabolized by the liver and therefore can interact with other AEDs and other commonly used drugs. The drug interactions occur because of induction or inhibition of the hepatic enzymes. It is therefore important to have an understanding of the specific cytochrome P450 (CYP450) isoenzyme that metabolizes each AED. Many newer AEDs do not induce or inhibit metabolic enzymes significantly but are affected by drugs that do alter this system. Phenytoin (Dilantin), carbamazepine (Carbatrol, Tegretol), phenobarbital, lamotrigine (Lamictal), and primidone (Mysoline) are AEDs that are hepatic enzyme inducers (Cloyd & Remmel, 2000; Faught, 2001; Patsalos et al, 2002). Felbamate, oxcarbazepine, and topiramate have shown some enzyme-inducing activity (Patsalos et al, 2002). Valproate (Depakene, Depakote) and felbamate (Felbamate) are enzyme inhibitors (Faught, 2001).

Other medications may be affected by or affect AEDs. Enzyme-inducing AEDs increase the metabolism and clearance of *oral contraceptive hormones*, therefore making contraceptive hormones ineffective (Patsalos et al, 2002). Approximately 7% of women who take both AEDs and contraceptive hormones have reported failure compared with the baseline population risk of 1% to 2% (Penovich, 2000). Increasing the estrogen to 50 μg or more in the contraceptive hormones may prevent failure (Patsalos et al, 2002; Penovich, 2000; Yerby, 2001). Depo-medroxyprogesterone acetate (Depo-Provera), which is an injectable synthetic progestin that is derived from progesterone, has no drug interactions with AEDs (Micromedex Healthcare Series, 2003).

Erythromycin and *clarithromycin* can increase the plasma concentration of carbamazepine (Carbatrol, Tegretol); therefore, when these medications are used together, carbamazepine levels must be closely monitored. Many *antiviral agents* (e.g., nevirapine, indinavir, ritonavir, saquinavir) are metabolized by CYP3A4 (subfamily of the CYP isoenzymes). When these medications are used in conjunction with enzyme-inducing AEDs, insufficient plasma concentrations of the antiviral agent will likely result. *Fluconazole* (an antifungal agent) is a CYP450 inhibitor, and co-administration of this drug and phenytoin (Dilantin) can result in increased plasma concentrations of phenytoin. *Griseofulvin* is metabolized by the liver, and concomitant use of this medication and an enzyme-inducing AED may increase the metabolism of griseofulvin, thereby reducing the antifungal efficacy of the drug. In addition, AEDs may also decrease the GI absorption of griseofulvin (Patsalos et al, 2002).

Antacids have been shown to reduce the serum concentrations of carbamazepine (Carbatrol, Tegretol), gabapentin (Neurontin), phenobarbital, and phenytoin (Dilantin). *Omeprazole* can increase the plasma concentration of phenytoin, resulting in increased phenytoin levels. When omeprazole is discontinued, the phenytoin levels can drop if there is not an adjustment made in the dose, resulting in increased seizures. *Cimetidine* is an inhibitor of the CYP450 system and can prolong the half-lives of the AEDs metabolized by the same system, such as phenytoin and carbamazepine. Since phenobarbital and primidone (Mysoline) are also metabolized by this system, they may also be affected by cimetidine (Patsalos et al, 2002).

The drug interactions that occur with concomitant use of AEDs and the psychotropic drugs have to do with the CYP450 system. Enzyme-inducing AEDs can stimulate the metabolism of the *tricyclic antidepressants* (TCAs), such as nortriptyline, imipramine, nomifensine, and trazodone. In addition, the TCAs inhibit the metabolism of some AEDs, resulting in a reduced plasma concentration of the TCA and an increase of the plasma concentration of the AED. *Fluoxetine* (a serotonin reuptake inhibitor) inhibits the CYP system and may cause an increase in the plasma concentration of carbamazepine (Carbatrol, Tegretol) and phenytoin (Dilantin). *Sertraline* (a 5HT-reuptake inhibitor) can cause lamotrigine (Lamictal) toxicity. The *anxiolytic benzodiazepines* are metabolized by the CYP450 system, and the effect on these drugs depends on whether the isoenzyme is induced or inhibited. For example, carbamazepine and phenytoin (Dilantin) decrease the plasma concentrations of medazolam, but sodium valproate (Depakene, Depakote) increases the concentration of lorazepam (Ativan) (Patsalos et al, 2002).

Enzyme-inducing AEDs may reduce the therapeutic effect of *corticosteroids* by increasing the metabolism of the corticosteroid. When an individual is taking *cyclosporine* (metabolized by CYP3A) for immunosuppression in conjunction with an enzyme-inducing AED, the result may be a reduced plasma concentration of the cyclosporine. It may be beneficial to change individuals over to a second-generation AED that is not known to induce CYP3A (e.g., tiagabine [Gabatril], levetiracetam [Keppra], lamotrigine [Lamictal], gabapentin [Neurontin]) if they must continue on cyclosporine (Patsalos et al, 2002).

CYP450 isoenzymes are important in the metabolism of *anticancer* agents. Phenobarbital and phenytoin (Dilantin) can enhance drug clearance of the anticancer drugs up to threefold. There are no data on the effect that the newer AEDs have on anticancer drugs. Theoretically, those drugs that do not undergo metabolism or affect the CYP450 system should not interact with anticancer drugs (Patsalos et al, 2002).

Promethazine, an antihistamine, can lower the seizure threshold (Micromedex Healthcare Series, 2003), resulting in seizures. If it is necessary to give this medication, the lowest dose needed should be prescribed and it should be given as infrequently as necessary. The parent should be instructed that promethazine can lower the seizure threshold.

Enzyme-inducing AEDs can increase the metabolism of *theophylline*, which is metabolized by the hepatic enzymes. In addition, enzyme-inducing AEDs can increase the metabolism of *dicumarol* and *warfarin* (anticoagulants), resulting in a reduced anticoagulant effect of the drug. The newer AEDs that do not induce the CYP450 system theoretically should not affect theophylline or the anticoagulants (Patsalos et al, 2002).

Interactions with *digoxin* are related to renal excretion, protein binding, distribution within the body, changes in gut absorption, and pharmacodynamic sensitivity to digoxin. Phenytoin (Dilantin) used with digoxin may cause a reduced plasma concentration of digoxin. Digoxin levels must therefore be closely monitored. When topiramate (Topamax) is used in conjunction with digoxin, the plasma level of the digoxin may be reduced slightly (Patsalos et al, 2002).

Developmental Issues
Sleep Patterns

Seizures that occur at night may affect the individual's sleep pattern. In addition, seizures that occur during the day followed by a prolonged postictal state characterized by sleep can affect the individual's sleep pattern at night. Sleep deprivation may also cause an increase in seizure activity. It is very important to instruct the parent or caregiver to continue with the normal bedtime routines. A two-way baby monitor or intercom can be put into the child's room so that the parent or caregiver can be alerted to nighttime seizures or sleep disturbances.

Parents or caregivers of children with seizures may get very anxious at night. They may often change their previous sleeping arrangements and bring the child into their room to sleep at night. It is important to counsel the family in regard to the pros and cons of this sleeping arrangement. Once the family begins to feel comfortable with the child's diagnosis of seizures, the family should be encouraged to resume the previous sleeping arrangements that had been established. This is important for both the child and the parent or caregiver.

Toileting

There are no particular concerns about toileting the child with seizures or epilepsy. Toilet training should be appropriate for the child's developmental age. Although there may be bowel or bladder incontinence with particular seizures (usually generalized tonic-clonic), this is not something that the individual can control. If incontinence does occur with a seizure, the child should be cleaned and clothes changed as soon as the child is stable. The child should be assured that he or she did not have control over this occurrence.

Discipline

Parents or caregivers of a child with epilepsy often treat the child as if he or she is sick. Illnesses are transient; however, epilepsy can continue for years or a lifetime. Parents and caregivers may think that they can make the epilepsy worse. They may fear disciplining their child, believing that if the child gets upset a seizure will occur. Children learn very quickly how to play on parental fears. The child learns how to manipulate a parent or caregiver and may threaten the parent or caregiver that a seizure will occur (Lechtenberg, 1999). Families should be instructed that disciplining a child will not provoke a seizure. Parents and caregivers should continue to discipline their child when warranted, in keeping with the expectations for other children.

Supervision

Parents and caregivers are often frightened by their lack of control over their child's seizures. They often compensate by trying to extend their influence and protection over various aspects of the child's life. Approximately one third of parents of children with epilepsy believe that the child needs constant supervision. The parents may try to regulate friendships, travel, activities, and play. This overprotection may affect the child's development in regard to self-esteem, self-reliance, and initiative. Often the child will also eventually rebel against the parent who is too restrictive (Lechtenberg, 1999). It is important to instruct the family to allow the child to live a normal life, taking into consideration the safety precautions necessary for those children with a seizure disorder. Encouragement of a child's developing independence should be an ongoing process.

Child Care

Finding an appropriate daycare can present a challenge for parents, especially if the child has seizures. Primary care providers can assist the family in this endeavor by helping to identify local agencies or providers familiar with the care involved with a child with epilepsy or by providing the necessary education about epilepsy to the child care agencies or providers willing to support these children's special needs. Child care providers should be educated in regard to the seizure type the particular child has, appropriate seizure precautions, and first aid procedures for the child with seizures. If medication must be administered at the child care facility, the providers should be informed of the following: (1) the rationale for the AED, (2) dosage and proper administration of the AED, and (3) potential side effects of the AED. All medications should be stored properly out of the reach of children to prevent accidental ingestion.

If the child is on the ketogenic diet, the child care provider should be instructed on the administration of the diet. Often the child care provider is invited to the hospital when the diet is initiated to learn about the diet. For those children with the VNS, the provider should be instructed on the use of the magnet to prevent or stop a seizure that occurs.

All federally funded child care programs must accept children with disabilities such as epilepsy under the Individual's with Disabilities Education Act (IDEA) (see Chapter 5) if space is available. An individualized family service program (IFSP) should be established to identify goals and services needed by the child and family. Staff from early intervention or infant stimulation programs should be consulted if the child with a seizure disorder has an associated delay. Early assessment allows appropriate interventions to begin, maximizing learning potentials.

Schooling

Children with epilepsy may have social, intellectual, and cognitive difficulties. These difficulties must be assessed and identified so that interventions for a child's particular learning needs can be individualized and addressed.

If needed, the early intervention plan (IFSP) can be carried into the formal educational program as a child ages. Core evaluations by the individual school systems are necessary and appropriate for children at risk. The individualized education plan (IEP) should be performed at intervals throughout the child's schooling. The IEP contains specific educational goals and strategies to enable the child to be successful in the school setting.

Exercise may improve epilepsy. Epileptiform discharges on EEG have been noted to decrease during exercise. Two mechanisms, compensatory hyperventilation and beta-endorphins released during exercise, may be responsible for the improved EEG. It is also believed that increased attention and awareness during exercise may have a positive antiepileptic effect, reducing seizure activity. A feeling of well-being, which may be achieved through exercise, may also help to reduce the frequency of seizures (Sirven & Varrato, 1999). It is therefore important for the child to participate in physical education class in the school setting, within the limitations of the safety precautions for the child's particular seizure type to prevent serious injury.

As in the child care setting, if the child is on the ketogenic diet or has a VNS, the school staff should be educated about the therapies. Contact people in the specialist's office should be provided to the school staff in the event there are questions or concerns about these modalities.

Establishing a supportive, well-informed environment for a child is important. School staff should be informed of a child's medical diagnosis, even if the child progresses well and does not require special educational classes. This information allows teachers to help in assessing behavioral side effects of AED therapy. A teacher who is informed of the potential for seizure occurrence and who has been instructed by the parents and the primary care provider on proper interventions is more apt to be calm and intervene appropriately if necessary.

The primary care provider must recognize the stress the diagnosis of epilepsy can place on a child and its effect on the child's self-esteem and relationships with peers, as well as on the educational system. The unpredictability and lack of control of seizure activity can add to this stress. Primary care providers should explore opportunities to educate the faculty and children in the school about epilepsy. Greater understanding of epilepsy may help to erase the social stigma that may accompany epilepsy. Health care providers should facilitate communication between themselves and the nurse or teacher at the child's school.

Sexuality

The most common endocrine problems in women with epilepsy include the effects of hormones on seizures, the changes of seizures during the changes in reproductive hormonal status, and the effects of seizures on reproductive function. The most common endocrine problem in males is altered sexuality. In both men and women, seizures can cause alterations in hormonal secretions, AEDs can cause problems with endocrine function, and hormonal therapy is sometimes used for adjunctive therapy for seizures (Klein & Herzog, 2000).

Catamenial epilepsy refers to seizures that occur related to the female menstrual cycle, usually just before or during the onset of menstruation or at the time of ovulation. There are three patterns of seizure exacerbation, including perimenstrually, at the time of ovulation, or throughout the second half of the menstrual cycle. The first two patterns are noted in females with normal menstrual cycles, and the third is associated with those who have abnormal cycles (Klein & Herzog, 2000). The patterns are as a result of fluctuations of estrogen and progesterone. Estrogen will promote seizures, and progesterone will inhibit seizures (Klein & Herzog, 2000; Sheth, 2002).

Some seizures may resolve during menarche, and some may be exacerbated. For example, BECTS and benign occipital epilepsy often resolve spontaneously. On the other hand, complex partial seizures may increase in frequency. During pregnancy, some females have seizures for the first time and they only occur during pregnancy (Klein & Herzog, 2000). About one third of women have a worsening of their seizures during pregnancy (Klein & Herzog, 2000; Penovich, 2000). This has been attributed to a greater volume of distribution and a higher clearance rate of AEDs, resulting in decreased levels. Conversely, about one sixth of women have a decrease in seizure frequency during pregnancy (Klein & Herzog, 2000). Reproductive problems (fertility problems) and endocrine disorders (anovulatory cycles) are also common among women with epilepsy (Klein & Herzog, 2000; Penovich, 2000).

Hyposexuality is seen more often in men and women with epilepsy than in those without epilepsy. It is manifested by lack of libido and difficulty in achieving an orgasm. Hyposexuality may be a result of psychosocial problems, medication, or dysfunction of the limbic system as a result of epilepsy. AEDs may also affect reproductive function in men and women. In men this is usually due to the effect of certain AEDs on testosterone. In women this may be due to the fact that sodium valproate (Depakene, Depakote) has been associated with polycystic ovarian syndrome (PCOS) (Klein & Herzog, 2000).

Hormonal therapy has been effective in reducing seizure frequency in some individuals. Some hormones used as adjunctive therapy for seizure control include progesterone, estrogen antagonists (e.g., clomiphene), and medications that suppress the activity of the hypothalamo-pituitary-adrenal axis (e.g., ACTH, prednisone) (Klein & Herzog, 2000).

Teratogenesis is a problem for women with epilepsy. Women with epilepsy have a higher incidence of birth malformations even if they are not being treated with AEDs at the time of pregnancy. The incidence of congenital malformations is increased with polytherapy. Neural tube defects have been associated with valproate (Depakene, Depakote) and carbamazepine (Carbatrol, Tegretol). The newer AEDs have not been around long enough to determine these effects. However, the utilization of monotherapy, the lowest effective AED dose, and initiation of folate have all been beneficial in reducing the incidence of fetal malformations (Penovich, 2000).

Transition into Adulthood

Adolescence is a time when young persons strive for independence on the way to adulthood. This is also a critical time in life for the development of their self-esteem. Having a chronic condition such as epilepsy can make that transition more difficult. The young adult may be fearful of peers witnessing a seizure and therefore not be willing to participate in social events. The young adult wants to "fit in" with peers, which is

an important element of socialization. He or she may believe that taking medication makes him or her different, which in turn may interfere with medication compliance. In addition, adolescents who have active social lives may forget to take their medication, which can result in uncontrolled seizures. Those individuals with uncontrolled seizures are less likely to be allowed to participate in activities outside the home. The young adult with uncontrolled seizures will also not be allowed to drive, which results in dependence on family and friends and may further restrict participation in social events. These restrictions can have a devastating effect on the young adult's ability to test limits and explore the boundaries of independence, which is critical at this stage of development. This in turn will affect the young adult's development of self-esteem (Nordli, 2001; Sheth, 2002).

As the adolescent is stepping toward adulthood, there are numerous issues to consider. Will he or she be able to drive? Can the adolescent go on for further education? Can he or she live away from home while in college? Can the adolescent live independently? Can he or she gain useful employment? Will he or she be able to enlist in the military if desired? Will the adult be able to get health insurance? For the young adult with a significant delay or other associated problems, the parent may need to find residential placement. With many, there is also the need to transfer care to an adult specialist rather than the pediatric specialist who may have been caring for the adolescent.

Children and adolescents with epilepsy are at risk for not being able to achieve their goals in regard to education, vocation, and socialization. The primary care provider can assist the adolescent during this time of transition. Psychologic health can be improved through education, counseling, and advocacy (Nordli, 2001).

Family Concerns and Resources

Family Adjustment

There are many different feelings that the child and family members will experience as they learn to adjust to the diagnosis of epilepsy. These feelings occur in various stages that may include the following: shock and disbelief, anger, depression/fear, hope/defense building, acceptance/understanding, and adjustment/effective coping. It is often difficult for family members to hear information during the stages of shock and disbelief, anger, and depression/fear. Health care providers must realize that they may need to repeat information many times to the family members during these stages of adjustment. As family members experience the various stages of adjustment, they may project their feelings onto others in either positive or negative ways. It is important for the health care provider to understand that different family members will go through different stages at different times. Family members must be educated about the stages of adjustment and be informed that this may be a difficult time for all. They must be encouraged to be understanding of each other during this stressful time.

Cultural Differences

When providing care to a child with epilepsy it is very important to determine if there are any normative cultural values, folklores, language issues, or parent/caregiver/child health beliefs that may affect care (Flores et al, 2000). These issues may have an adverse effect on treatment if the health care provider is not aware of them. For example, a family may believe that the cause of the seizures may be related to disfavor by the gods and choose increased religious activity over prescribed medication therapy. It is important to be able to communicate with families of varying cultures, respect their cultural health beliefs, and educate them in regard to the treatment of epilepsy.

Community Resources

Health care providers must be empathetic to the many needs of the children with epilepsy and their families. Health care workers provide the physical, emotional, and social care that individuals with epilepsy may need. Nevertheless, no one understands or feels the problems these children and families face in their day-to-day lives as well as another child or family with the same disorder. For this reason, parent and peer support groups are available to provide this network of support within the community. These resources not only are necessary but also have proven to be a major factor in coping and adaptation for these families. Individuals and families can get further information from the Epilepsy Foundation of America or from the Citizens United for Research in Epilepsy (CURE):

Epilepsy Foundation of America
4351 Garden City Dr
Landover, MD 20785-2267
(800) EFA-1000 (state and local associations)
(800) EFA-4050 (library for medical referrals)
www.epilepsyfoundation.org

CURE—Citizens United for Research in Epilepsy
505 North Lake Shore Dr
Suite 4605
Chicago, IL 60611
(312) 923-9117
www.cureepilepsy.org

Summary of Primary Care Needs for Children with Epilepsy

HEALTH CARE MAINTENANCE

Growth and Development

Obtain height and weight at each visit. Children are at risk for significant growth changes because of medication or associated problems.

Medications are based on the child's weight.

Monitor the child's development in regard to social, cognitive, and motor development. Provide referrals for appropriate evaluations and treatment as necessary.

Diet

Feeding issues are usually due to associated problems the child may have.

Pharmacologic and nonpharmacologic interventions may cause an increase or decrease in the child's weight.

Consider dietary supplements as necessary.

Consider nutritional evaluation with a dietitian as necessary.

Consider referral to a weight management program as necessary.

Safety

Provide instructions for first aid/emergency interventions for seizure activity.

Provide instructions for seizure precautions, including high places, water, heat, and mechanical/electrical equipment.

Use caution with sports activities.

Provide instruction on state laws in regard to driving a motor vehicle.

Immunizations

There is an increased risk of a seizure after a DTaP or measles vaccination for those children with an underlying seizure disorder or family history of seizures. Fever management is suggested.

Follow the American Academy of Pediatrics (AAP) recommendations for childhood immunizations.

Contact the child's specialist if there are any questions or concerns regarding immunizations.

Screening

Vision. Routine screening is recommended.

Hearing. Routine screening is recommended.

Dental. Routine care is recommended. For those children taking phenytoin (Dilantin), routine dental care is recommended every 6 months. Phenytoin may cause gingival hyperplasia. Children taking phenytoin require frequent cleaning by a dental hygienist and more frequent brushing and flossing.

Blood Pressure. Routine screening is recommended. Hypertension is a side effect of adrenocorticotropic hormone (ACTH) therapy.

These children need blood pressure monitoring at least twice weekly.

Hematocrit. Routine screening is recommended.

Urinalysis. Routine screening is recommended.

Tuberculosis. Routine screening is recommended.

Condition-Specific Screening

Drug Toxicity Screening. Treatment-specific blood tests are recommended routinely for children who are on particular antiepileptic drugs (AEDs) or the ketogenic diet.

AED Drug Levels. Serum drug levels are performed for particular AEDs at varying intervals.

Electroencephalogram. EEGs are often performed during the diagnostic work-up for epilepsy. EEGs are repeated at the discretion of the child's specialist.

Medical Imaging Studies. Studies may be performed during the diagnostic work-up for epilepsy and repeated throughout therapy at the discretion of the child's specialist.

Continued

Summary of Primary Care Needs for Children with Epilepsy—cont'd

COMMON ILLNESS MANAGEMENT

Differential Diagnosis

Fever can be a precipitating factor for seizures. The parent or caregiver should treat fevers early in the course of an illness with antipyretics and increased fluids space. Antibiotics should be administered as prescribed.

Vomiting and diarrhea can accompany an illness. The child or adolescent must continue to take the prescribed AEDs during this time. AEDs can be given over 1 hour in small amounts of clear liquids. If vomiting continues and the child or adolescent cannot keep the medication down, then the child or adolescent must go to the local emergency room (ER) to get the AEDs through an intravenous (IV) line.

The child on a ketogenic diet must keep in close contact with the dietitian knowledgeable in the ketogenic diet for dietary instructions. If the vomiting or diarrhea continues despite management by the dietitian and specialist, then the child must go to a local ER for IV management. There can be no glucose added to the IV line.

Parents or caregivers report an **increase in seizure activity** when their child has constipation, although there is no evidence to support this. Manage constipation appropriately.

Head trauma can cause a worsening of seizures in an individual who already has a seizure disorder. The individual should follow the seizure precautions necessary to prevent a head injury. If a head injury does occur, the individual should be evaluated by the health care provider immediately or go to the local ER for evaluation.

Nonepileptic events can produce behaviors that are similar in appearance to seizures. These events must be differentiated from epilepsy.

Drug Interactions

Most AEDs are metabolized by the liver and can interact with other AEDs and other commonly used drugs.

Carbamazepine (Carbatrol, Tegretol), lamotrigine (Lamictal), phenytoin (Dilantin), phenobarbital, and primidone (Mysoline) are hepatic enzyme-inducers.

Felbatol (Felbamate), oxcarbazepine (Trileptal), and topiramate (Topamax) have some enzyme-inducing activity.

Sodium valproate (Depakene, Depakote) and felbatol (Felbamate) are enzyme-inhibitors.

Enzyme-inducing AEDs can make *contraceptive hormones* ineffective. Increasing the estrogen to 50 μg or more in the contraceptive hormones may prevent failure.

Depo-Provera (injectable synthetic progestin) has no drug interactions with AEDs.

Erythromycin and *clarithromycin* can increase the plasma concentration of carbamazepine (Carbatrol, Tegretol).

AEDs can decrease the plasma concentration of *antiviral agents.*

Fluconazole can increase the plasma concentration of phenytoin (Dilantin).

Enzyme-inducing AEDs can increase the metabolism of *griseofulvin.*

AEDs may decrease the gastrointestinal absorption of *griseofulvin.*

Enzyme-inducing AEDs can stimulate the metabolism of *tricyclic antidepressants (TCAs).*

TCAs inhibit the metabolism of some AEDs, causing decreased plasma concentration of the TCA and increased plasma concentration of the AED.

Fluoxetine can increase the plasma concentration of carbamazepine (Carbatrol, Tegretol) and phenytoin (Dilantin).

Sertraline can cause lamotrigine (Lamictal) toxicity.

Anxiolytic benzodiazepines: carbamazepine (Caratrol, Tegretol) and phenytoin (Dilantin) decrease the plasma concentration of *medazolam; sodium valproate (Depakene, Depakote)* increases the plasma concentration of *lorazepam (Ativan).*

Enzyme-inducing AEDs may increase the metabolism of *corticosteroids.*

Enzyme-inducing AEDs can cause decreased plasma concentrations of *cyclosporine.*

Phenobarbital and phenytoin (Dilantin) increase the clearance of *anticancer drugs.*

Promethazine can lower the seizure threshold. Use the lowest dose necessary and administer as infrequently as necessary.

Enzyme-inducing AEDs increase the metabolism of *theophylline, dicumarol,* and *warfarin.*

Digoxin: phenytoin (Dilantin) decreases the plasma concentration of digoxin; topiramate (Topamax) may slightly decrease the plasma concentration of digoxin.

Antacids can decrease the plasma concentration of carbamazepine (Carbatrol, Tegretol), gabapentin (Neurontin), phenobarbital, and phenytoin (Dilantin).

Omeprazole can increase the plasma concentration of phenytoin (Dilantin).

Cimetidine can prolong the half-life of AEDs metabolized by the CYP450 system (e.g., phenytoin [Dilantin], carbamazepine [Carbatrol, Tegretol], phenobarbital, primidone [Mysoline]).

DEVELOPMENTAL ISSUES

Sleep Patterns

Sleep patterns may be affected if seizures occur at night or seizures occur during the day followed by a prolonged postictal state.

Sleep deprivation can cause an increase in seizure activity.

There is increased anxiety in family members after a child experiences a seizure, and often the parents or caregivers have the child sleep with them in their bed at night. Counseling in support of independent sleeping as the family becomes more comfortable with the child's seizures is recommended.

Toileting

Toileting is reflective of the child's developmental age. Incontinence of bowel or bladder can occur with some seizures.

Discipline

Parents or caregivers should continue to discipline their child without the fear of provoking a seizure or making the child's seizures worse.

Summary of Primary Care Needs for Children with Epilepsy—cont'd

Supervision

The family should be encouraged to allow the child to lead a normal life, with some safety precautions. Independence should be encouraged.

Child Care

Early intervention and infant stimulation programs should be provided as necessary.

Children may be eligible for individualized family service programs (IFSPs) and federally funded daycare programs as per the Individuals with Disabilities Education Act (IDEA).

Appropriate epilepsy education should be provided to the child care staff.

Schooling

Learning needs must be assessed and identified.

Continue early intervention plans into the formal education program as needed.

An individualized education plan (IEP) should be constructed to determine the need for special education or related services.

Appropriate epilepsy education should be provided to the school staff.

Establish a supportive, well-informed environment in the school setting through ongoing open communication with the school staff.

The child should participate in physical education classes within the limitations of the seizure precautions for the child's seizure type.

Sexuality

Some women develop catamenial epilepsy caused by fluctuations of hormones during the menstrual cycle.

Approximately one third of women will have a worsening of seizures during pregnancy; approximately one sixth of women have a decrease in seizure activity during pregnancy.

Reproductive and endocrine problems are common in women with epilepsy.

Some AEDs are teratogenic. It is recommended to administer folate daily to all women of child-bearing age.

Transition into Adulthood

The restrictions that are placed on a young adult with epilepsy can affect the young person's striving for independence and ultimately the development of self-esteem.

Young people with epilepsy are at risk for not being able to achieve their goals in regard to education, vocation, and socialization.

Education, counseling, and advocacy should be provided for the adolescent as needed to assist with the transition to adulthood.

FAMILY CONCERNS

Family Adjustment

All family members will experience various stages of adjustment as they learn about the diagnosis of epilepsy. Family members will experience different stages of adjustment at different times and must be understanding of this in each other.

It is difficult for family members to hear information as they are adjusting to the diagnosis of epilepsy.

Health care providers may need to repeat information several times during these times.

Cultural Differences

Cultural sensitivity is necessary when providing care to a child or adolescent with epilepsy. The individual's cultural health beliefs should be respected as they are educated in the treatment of epilepsy.

Community Resources

Epilepsy Foundation of America
Citizens United for Research in Epilepsy

REFERENCES

American Academy of Pediatrics. (2003). *2000 Red book: Report of the Committee on Infectious Diseases* (26th ed.). Elk Grove Village, Ill.: American Academy of Pediatrics.

American Epilepsy Society (AES). (2000). Medical education program—residents version;
Web site: www.aesnet.org/edu_pub/med_edu_residents.cfm.

Annegers, J.F. (1997). The epidemiology of epilepsy. In E. Wyllie (Ed.). *The treatment of epilepsy: Principles and practice.* Philadelphia: Williams & Wilkins, pp. 165-172.

Arunkumar, G., Kotagal, P., & Rothner, A. (2001). Localization-related epilepsies: Simple partial seizures, complex partial seizures, benign focal epilepsy of childhood, and epilepsia partialis continua. In J. Pellock, W. Dodson, & B. Bourgeois (Eds.). *Pediatric epilepsy: Diagnosis and therapy* (2nd ed.). New York: Demos, pp. 243-264.

Austin, J., Huberty, T., Huster, G., & Dunn, D. (1999). Does academic achievement in children with epilepsy change over time? *Dev Med Child Neurol, 41,* 473-479.

Bauer, J. (2000). Rational diagnosis of non-epileptic seizures. In D. Schmidt & S. Schachter (Eds.). *Epilepsy: Problem solving in clinical practice.* London: Martin Dunitz, pp. 29-41.

Bebin, M. (2002). Pediatric partial and generalized seizures. *J Child Neurol, 17*(suppl. 1), S4-S17.

Berg, A. & Chadwick, D. (2000). Starting antiepileptic drugs. In D. Schmidt & S. Schachter (Eds.). *Epilepsy: Problem solving in clinical practice.* London: Martin Dunitz, pp. 207-219.

Berkovic, S.F. & Ottman, R. (2000). Molecular genetics of the idiopathic epilepsies: The next steps. *Epileptic Disord, 2*(4), 179-181.

Blumenthal, M., Goldberg, A., & Brinckmann, J. (Eds.). (2000). *Herbal medicine: Expanded Commission E monographs.* Newton, Mass.: Intergative Medicine Communications.

Brenner, R. (2002). Is it status? *Epilepsia, 43*(suppl. 3), 103-113.

Brodie, M. & Kwan, P. (2002). Staged approach to epilepsy management. *Neurology, 58*(8, suppl. 5), S2-S8.

Brodie, M. & Schachter, S. (2001). *Epilepsy* (2nd ed.). Oxford: Health Press.

Browne, T. (2000). Managing epilepsy: Diagnostic and clinical strategies. In *Epilepsy: Disease management guide.* Montvale, N.J.: Medical Economics Co., pp. 101-135.

Camfield, P. & Camfield, C. (2002). Epileptic syndromes in childhood: Clinical features, outcomes, and treatment. *Epilepsia, 43*(suppl. 3), 27-32.

Clark, S. & Wilson, W. (1997). Mechanisms of epileptogenesis and the expression of epileptiform activity. In E. Wyllie (Ed.). *The treatment of epilepsy: Principles and practice* (2nd ed.). Philadelphia: Williams & Wilkins, pp. 53-81.

Cloyd, J. & Remmel, R. (2000). Antiepileptic drug pharmacokinetics and interactions: Impact on treatment of epilepsy. *Pharmacotherapy, 20*(8), 139S-151S.

Commission on Classification and Terminology of the International League Against Epilepsy. (1981). Proposal for revised clinical and electroen-cephalographic classification of epileptic seizures. *Epilepsia, 22,* 489-501.

Commission on Classification and Terminology of the International League Against Epilepsy. (1989). Proposal for revised classification of epilepsies and epileptic syndromes. *Epilepsia, 30*(4), 389-399.

Cross, J. (2002). Epilepsy surgery in childhood. *Epilepsia, 43*(suppl. 30), 65-70.

Crumrine, P. (2002). Lennox-Gastaut syndrome. *J Child Neurol, 17*(suppl. 1), S70-S75.

DeLorenzo, R. (2001). Ion channels, membranes, and molecules in epilepsy and neuronal excitability. In J. Pellock, W. Dodson, & B. Bourgeois (Eds.). *Pediatric epilepsy: Diagnosis and therapy* (2nd ed.). New York: Demos, pp. 25-36.

Deray, M., Resnick, T., & Alvarez, L. (Eds.). (2001). *Complete pocket refer-ence for the treatment of epilepsy.* Miami: C.P.R. Educational Services.

Dreifuss, F. (1992). Classification of epileptic seizures and the epilepsies. *Uni-versity Reports on Epilepsy, 1*(1), 1-7.

Dreifuss, F. & Nordli, D., Jr. (2001). Classification of epilepsies in childhood. In J. Pellock, W. Dodson, & B. Bourgeois (Eds.). *Pediatric epilepsy: Diag-nosis and therapy* (2nd ed.). New York: Demos, pp. 69-80.

Dulac, O., Plouin, P., & Schlumberger, E. (1997). Infantile spasms. In E. Wyllie (Ed.). *The treatment of epilepsy: Principles and practice* (2nd ed.). Philadelphia: Williams & Wilkins, pp. 540-572.

Elawad, M. & Sullivan, P. (2001). Management of constipation in children with disabilities. *Dev Med Child Neurol, 43,* 829-832.

Engel, J. (2001). A proposed diagnostic scheme for people with epileptic seizures and with epilepsy: Report of the ILAE task force on classification and terminology. *Epilepsia, 42*(6), 796-803.

Epilepsy: Disease management guide. (2000). Montvale, N.J.: Medical Economics Co.

Farrell, K. (1997). Generalized tonic and atonic seizures. In E. Wyllie (Ed.). *The treatment of epilepsy: Principles and practice* (2nd ed.). Philadelphia: Williams & Wilkins, pp. 522-529.

Faught, E. (2001). Pharmacokinetic considerations in prescribing antiepileptic drugs. *Epilepsia, 42*(suppl. 4), 19-23.

Fetrow, C. & Avila, J. (Eds.). (2001). *Professional's handbook of complemen-tary and alternative medicines* (2nd ed.). Springhouse, Pa.: Springhouse Corp.

Ficker, D. (2000). Sudden unexplained death and injury in epilepsy. *Epilepsia, 41*(suppl. 2), S7-S12.

Flores, G., Abreu, M., Schwartz, I., & Hill, M. (2000). The importance of lan-guage and culture in pediatric care: Case studies from the Latino commu-nity. *J Pediatr, 137*(6), 842-848.

Fountain, N. (2000). Status epilepticus: Risk factors and complications. *Epilep-sia, 41*(suppl. 2), S23-S30.

Freeman, J.M., Freeman, J.B., & Kelly, M. (2000). *The ketogenic diet: A treat-ment for epilepsy* (3rd ed.). New York: Demos.

Fugh-Berman, A. (2000). Herb-drug interactions. *Lancet, 355*(2), 134-138.

Glauser, T. & Morita, D. (2001). Encephalopathic epilepsy after infancy. In J. Pellock, W. Dodson, & B. Bourgeois (Eds.). *Pediatric epilepsy: Diagnosis and therapy* (2nd ed.). New York: Demos, pp. 201-218.

Greenwood, R. (2000). Adverse effects of antiepileptic drugs. *Epilepsia, 41*(suppl. 2), S42-S52.

Gumnit, R. (1997). Psychogenic seizures. In E. Wyllie (Ed.). *The treatment of epilepsy: Principles and practice* (2nd ed.). Philadelphia: Williams & Wilkins, pp. 677-680.

Hauser, W.A. (2001). Epidemiology of epilepsy in children. In J. Pellock, W. Dodson, & B. Bourgeois (Eds.). *Pediatric epilepsy: Diagnosis and therapy* (2nd ed.). New York: Demos, pp. 81-96.

Hermann, B., Seidenberg, M., & Bell, B. (2000). Psychiatric comorbidity in chronic epilepsy: Identification, consequences, and treatment of major depression. *Epilepsia, 41*(suppl. 2), S31-S41.

Kaneko, S., Iwasa, H., & Okada, M. (2002). Genetic identifiers of epilepsy. *Epilepsia, 43*(suppl. 9), 16-20.

Kaneko, S., Okada, M., Iwasa, H., Yamakawa, K., & Hirose, S. (2002). Genet-ics of epilepsy: Current status and prospectives. *Neurosci Res, 44,* 11-30.

Kaplan, P. (2000). Prognosis in nonconvulsive status epilepticus. *Epileptic Disord, 2,* 185-192.

Kennedy, P. & Schallert, G. (2001). Practical issues and concepts in vagus nerve stimulation: A nursing review. *J Neurosci Nurs, 33*(2), 105-112.

Klein, P. & Herzog, A. (2000). Hormones and epilepsy. In D. Schmidt & S. Schachter (Eds.). *Epilepsy: Problem solving in clinical practice.* London: Martin Dunitz, pp. 413-433.

Kohrman, M. (1999). Pediatric sleep disorders. In K. Swaiman & S. Ashwall. *Pediatric neurology: Principles and practice* (3rd ed.). St. Louis: Mosby, pp. 773-785.

Lechtenberg, R. (1999). *Epilepsy and the family—A new guide.* Cambridge, Mass.: Harvard University Press.

Leppik, I. (2001). *Contemporary diagnosis and management of the patient with epilepsy* (5th ed.). Newtown, Pa.: Handbooks in Health Care.

Marsh, L. & Rao, V. (2002). Psychiatric complications in patients with epilepsy: A review. *Epilepsy Res, 49,* 11-33.

Meador, K. (2002). Cognitive outcomes and predictive factors in epilepsy. *Neu-rology, 58*(8, suppl. 5), S21-S25.

Micromedex Healthcare Series. (March 2003). Vol. 115 (*Drug-reax interactive drug interaction*).

Nordli, D., Jr. (2001). Special needs of the adolescent with epilepsy. *Epilepsia, 42*(suppl.8), 10-17.

Nordli, D., Jr. (2002). Diagnostic difficulty in infants and children. *J Child Neurol, 17*(suppl. 1), S28-S35.

Paolicchi, J. (2002). The spectrum of nonepileptic events in children. *Epilep-sia, 43*(suppl. 3), 60-64.

Patsalos, P., Froscher, W., Pisani, F., & van Rijn, C. (2002). The importance of drug interactions in epilepsy therapy. *Epilepsia, 43*(4), 365-385.

Pearl, P. & Holmes, G. (2001). Absence seizures. In J. Pellock, W. Dodson, & B. Bourgeois (Eds.). *Pediatric epilepsy: Diagnosis and therapy* (2nd ed.). New York: Demos, pp. 219-231.

Pellock, J. (1997). The differential diagnosis of epilepsy: Nonepileptic parox-ysmal disorders. In E. Wyllie (Ed.). *The treatment of epilepsy: Principles and practice* (2nd ed.). Philadelphia: Williams & Wilkins, pp. 681-690.

Penovich, P. (2000). The effects of epilepsy and its treatment on sexual repro-ductive function. *Epilepsia, 41*(suppl. 2), S53-S61.

Prego-Lopez, M. & Devinsky, O. (2002). Evaluation of a first seizure: Is it epilepsy? *Postgrad Med, 111*(1), 34-48.

Prensky, A. (2001). An approach to the child with paroxysmal phenomenon with emphasis on nonepileptic disorders. In J. Pellock, W. Dodson, & B. Bourgeois (Eds.). *Pediatric epilepsy: Diagnosis and therapy* (2nd ed.). New York: Demos, pp. 97-116.

Provisional Committee on Quality Improvement, Subcommittee on Febrile Seizures. (1996). Practice parameter: The neurodiagnostic evaluation of the child with a first simple febrile seizure. *Pediatrics, 97*(5), 769-772.

Roddy, S. (1999). Breath-holding spells and reflex anoxic seizures. In K. Swaiman & S. Ashwall. *Pediatric neurology: Principles and practice* (3rd ed.). St. Louis: Mosby, pp. 759-762.

Sander, J. & Pal, D. (2000). Long-term prognosis of epilepsy. In D. Schmidt & S. Schachter (Eds.). *Epilepsy: Problem solving in clinical practice,* London: Martin Dunitz, pp. 367-380.

Serratosa, J.M. (1999). Idiopathic epilepsies with a complex mode of inheri-tance. *Epilepsia, 40*(suppl. 3), 12-16.

Sheth, R. (2002). Adolescent issues in epilepsy. *J Child Neurol, 17*(suppl. 2), 2S23-2S27.

Shields, W. (1999, December). Special syndromes. *Child Neurology Rounds,* 14-17.

Shields, W. (2000). Catastrophic epilepsy in childhood. *Epilepsia, 41*(suppl. 2), S2-S6.

Shields, W. (2002). West's syndrome. *J Child Neurol, 17*(suppl. 1), S76-S79.

Shinnar, S. (December 1999). Epidemiology of pediatric epilepsy. *Child Neu-rology Rounds,* 6-11.

Shinnar, S. & Glauser, T. (2002). Febrile seizures. *J Child Neurol, 17*(suppl. 1), S44-S52.

Shinnar, S. & O'Dell, C. (2001). Treatment decisions in childhood seizures. In J. Pellock, W. Dodson, & B. Bourgeois (Eds.). *Pediatric epilepsy: Diag-nosis and therapy* (2nd ed.). New York: Demos, pp. 291-300.

Shinnar, S. & Pellock, J.M. (2002). Update of the epidemiology and prognosis of pediatric epilepsy. *J Child Neurol, 17*(suppl.1), S4-S17.

Singer, H. (1999). Tourette syndrome and its associated neurobehavioral prob-lems. In K. Swaiman & S. Ashwall. *Pediatric neurology: Principles and practice* (3rd ed.). St. Louis: Mosby, pp. 598-605.

Sirven J. & Varrato, J. (1999). Physical activity and epilepsy: What are the rules? *The Physician and Sportsmedicine, 27*(3), 63-70.

Skidmore-Roth, L. (2001). *Mosby's handbook of herbs and natural supple-ments.* St. Louis: Mosby.

Steinlein, O.K. (1999). Idiopathic epilepsies with a monogenic mode of inher-itance. *Epilepsia, 40*(suppl. 3), 9-11.

Tharp, B. (2002). Neonatal seizures and syndromes. *Epilepsia, 43*(suppl. 3), 2-10.

Upadhyay, A., Aggarwal, R., Deorari, A.K., & Paul, V.K. (2001). Seizures in the newborn. *Indian J Pediatr, 68,* 967-972.

Velisek, L. & Moshe, S. (2001). Pathophysiology of seizures and epilepsy in the immature brain: Cells, synapses, and circuits. In J. Pellock, W. Dodson, & B. Bourgeois (Eds.). *Pediatric epilepsy: Diagnosis and therapy* (2nd ed.). New York: Demos, pp. 1-23.

Wheless, J. (1999, December). Treatment of acute seizures and status epilepticus in children. *Child Neurology Rounds*, 47-51.

Wheless, J. (2002). Using the new antiepilepsy drugs in children. *J Child Neurol, 17*(suppl. 1), S58-S64.

Wong, M. & Trevathan, E. (2001). Infantile spasms. *Pediatr Neurol, 24*(2), 89-98.

Wyllie, E. (1999, December). Surgery in the refractory patient. *Child Neurology Rounds*, 42-45.

Wyllie, E. & Luders, H. (1997). Classification of seizures. In E. Wyllie (Ed.). *The treatment of epilepsy: Principles and practice* (2nd ed.). Philadelphia: Williams & Wilkins, pp. 355-357.

Yerby, M. (2001). Modern management of women with epilepsy. In H. Luders (Ed.). *Epilepsy: Comprehensive review and case discussions*. London: Dunitz, pp. 307-326.

26 Fragile X Syndrome

Randi J. Hagerman

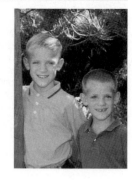

Genetic Etiology

Fragile X syndrome is a genetic disorder that causes cognitive impairment ranging from mild learning disabilities to severe mental retardation. This condition derives its name from the presence of a fragile site or break in the X chromosome at Xq27.3 (Figure 26-1), which is identifiable by chromosome analysis. Because of the phenotypic variability among children with fragile X syndrome and because this condition was only recently discovered, most individuals with fragile X syndrome remain undiagnosed.

Fragile X syndrome is caused by a mutation in the gene called the fragile X mental retardation 1 gene (FMR1), which is located at Xq27.3. The FMR1 gene was discovered and sequenced in 1991 by an international collaborative effort (Oberlé et al, 1991; Verkerk et al, 1991; Yu et al, 1991). The FMR1 gene has a unique trinucleotide expansion located within the gene. This expansion is the source of the mutation that causes fragile X syndrome. All individuals have the FMR1 gene, but when the trinucleotide repeat expansion $(CGG)_n$ increases in size dramatically, this expansion causes silencing of the gene leading to a deficiency or lack of the FMR1 protein. Normal individuals in the general population have between 6 and 53 CGG repeats within their FMR1 gene. Individuals who are carriers for fragile X syndrome have an expansion of the CGG repetitive sequence that goes beyond approximately 54 repeats up to 200. This change in the DNA is called a "premutation" and causes an increased instability of this region so that further expansion can take place when this mutation is passed on to the next generation through a female carrier. Individuals who are significantly affected by fragile X syndrome have more than 200 repeats (i.e., "full mutation"). This full mutation is usually associated with methylation, which is a process of silencing the gene so that no FMR1 protein is produced from a full mutation. The absence of protein production actually causes the physical, behavioral, and cognitive problems that comprise fragile X syndrome.

Fragile X syndrome is inherited in an X-linked fashion. Males are typically affected by any deleterious gene that they carry on the X chromosome. Females, on the other hand, are usually normal because the abnormal gene on one X chromosome is compensated for by the normal gene on the other X chromosome. Heterozygous females have a 50% chance of passing the abnormal gene to their children. Males who carry the fragile X gene, however, will pass the premutation to all of their daughters but none of their sons. Males who are carriers have the premutation, which is a CGG repeat between 54 and 200. When males pass on this premutation to all their daughters, only minimal changes occur in the CGG repeat number and it never increases to the full mutation. All sperm of affected males have only the premutation. When the premutation is passed on by a female, however, there is a high probability that the premutation will increase to a full mutation in the offspring who inherit the fragile X chromosome. The larger the size of the premutation in the carrier mother, the greater the chance that expansion will occur to a full mutation. In women with a premutation of 100 CGG repeats or larger, the expansion to the full mutation will occur 100% of the time when the fragile X chromosome is passed on to the next generation.

Incidence and Prevalence

Fragile X syndrome is the most common cause of inherited mental retardation known. Down syndrome, which rarely is inherited, has an incidence of approximately 1 per 1000. In comparison, fragile X syndrome causes mental retardation in approximately 1 per 4000 individuals in the general population (Turner et al, 1996; Sherman, 2002). Studies by Dombrowski et al (2002) have shown that approximately 1 in 250 females, and 1 in 800 males in the general population is a carrier of the premutation. Screenings of individuals with mental retardation in institutional and other residential settings have shown that 2% to 10% (Sherman, 1996; Sherman, 2002) of this high-risk population have fragile X syndrome as the cause of their mental impairment.

Population studies of such diverse groups as the Aborigines in Australia, the Zulus of Africa, and individuals screened in Sweden, Finland, New South Wales, England, and France suggest that fragile X is equally common among all racial and ethnic groups (Sherman, 1996). As mentioned, however, the majority of families affected by this syndrome are still undiagnosed and therefore remain unaware of available treatment and intervention.

Clinical Manifestations at Time of Diagnosis

When most health care providers hear the word syndrome, they think of an individual who appears phenotypically abnormal. Similarly, most syndromes have consistent cognitive and physical features that succinctly describe the clinical manifestations (Box 26-1). Although most individuals with fragile X syndrome share certain clinical findings, there is much variability. Health care providers should note that children with this syndrome may not be immediately recognizable by their phenotype.

To improve diagnosis in fragile X syndrome, primary care providers must be familiar with the characteristic gestalt that

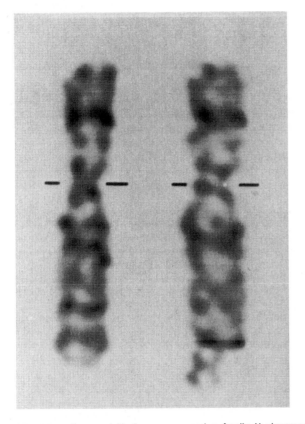

FIGURE 26-1 A normal X chromosome and a fragile X chromosome demonstrating the fragile X site at Xq27.3.

BOX 26-1

Clinical Manifestations

MALES
Severe learning disabilities or mental retardation
Delayed onset of language
Long or narrow face
Prominent or cupped ears
Enlarged testicles
Hyperextensible finger joints, pes planus
Hyperactivity or attention deficit hyperactivity disorder
Perseveration in speech

FEMALES
Mild cognitive deficits to mental retardation
Language delays
Shyness, social anxiety
Prominent ears
Long, narrow face or high palate
Hyperextensible finger joints, pes planus
Attentional problems but less prominent hyperactivity

---

defines this very common condition. None of the physical, behavioral, or psychologic characteristics looked at individually are diagnostic of fragile X syndrome. The finding of one or more of the typical features, such as prominent ears, hyperextensible finger joints, and poor eye contact in combination with developmental delay or mental retardation of unknown cause, however, should alert the clinician to order a DNA study for the FMR1 mutation.

Males

Most males with fragile X syndrome have intelligence quotients (IQs) in the mild to moderate range of mental retardation. A significantly smaller percentage is severely to profoundly retarded. Approximately 13% of males with fragile X syndrome have an IQ above 70 and are therefore not mentally retarded (Bennetto & Pennington, 2002; Hagerman, 2002c). Most of these males have a variant pattern on DNA testing, including a lack of complete methylation of the full mutation or a mosaic pattern, some cells with the premutation, and some cells with the full mutation. The cognitive profile of males with fragile X includes difficulty with abstract reasoning, math, and attention.

Delayed onset of language skills is present in approximately 85% of males with fragile X syndrome. In some children, particularly females or normal IQ males, difficulties are only evidenced by language problems related to weaknesses in abstract reasoning. Other children as young as 18 months of age have delayed speech and significant deficits in receptive and expressive language. Perseveration and echolalia (i.e., repetitive speech) are common speech characteristics of individuals with fragile X. A fast rate of speech, cluttering, mumbling, rambling, and poor topic maintenance are also frequent findings (Bennetto & Pennington, 2002; Scharfenaker et al, 2002).

The three classic physical features associated with the fragile X syndrome phenotype are a long narrow face, prominent or large ears, and, in males, enlarged testicles. Approximately 80% of males with fragile X will exhibit one or more of these features (Hagerman, 2002c). A long, narrow face is a common feature in adults and less common in young children. Large ears (i.e., >2 SD above the norm) are seen in 50% of boys with fragile X (Figure 26-2). Prominent or cupped ears are often a more useful discriminating feature among this younger group. This finding is observed in 60% to 70% of boys and is often the only obvious physical feature associated with fragile X syndrome (Hagerman, 2002c).

Enlarged testicles are often seen in the mentally retarded population; 70% to 90% of men with fragile X have a testicular volume greater than 30 ml (Hagerman, 2002c). An orchidometer (Figure 26-3) consisting of ellipsoid shapes of varying size is a useful instrument to measure testicular volume. However, most young children with fragile X syndrome do not have enlarged testicles. Macroorchidism begins to develop between 8 and 10 years with the largest size reached in late puberty with a mean volume of 50 ml (Lachiewicz & Dawson, 1994).

Other more subtle physical features noted in the fragile X population include a prominent jaw, prominent forehead, and long palpebral fissures (Butler et al, 1991; Hagerman, 2002c). A high-arched palate, mitral valve prolapse, hypotonia, hyperextensible finger joints, and flat feet suggest that these individuals may have an underlying connective tissue disorder (Hagerman, 2002c).

It is very important to recognize that the majority of males with fragile X—especially the younger boys—appear physically normal (Figure 26-4). What is often more concerning to the parents are the behavioral characteristics. Hyperactivity is observed in more than 70% of boys with fragile X syndrome but it frequently disappears after puberty. Poor attention span,

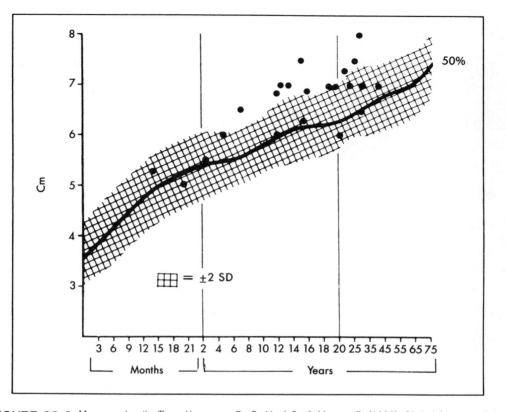

FIGURE 26-2 Mean ear length. (From Hagerman, R., Smith, A.C., & Manner, R. [1983]. Clinical features of the fragile X syndrome. *The fragile X syndrome: diagnosis, biochemistry and intervention*. Dillon, CO: Spectra. Reprinted with permission.)

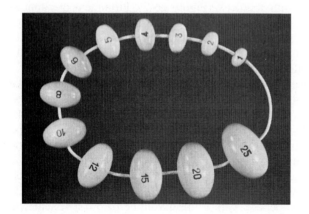

FIGURE 26-3 Prader orchidometer used to measure testicular volume.

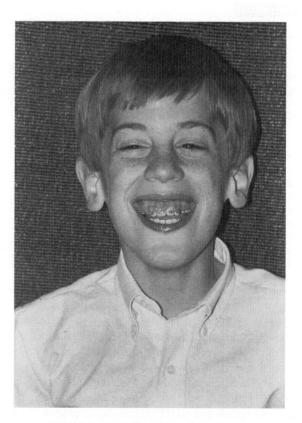

FIGURE 26-4 Prepubertal fragile X male.

often combined with impulsivity, is also problematic for all boys with fragile X—regardless of the level of cognitive functioning (Hagerman, 2002c). Approximately 90% have poor eye contact, and 60% to 70% display unusual hand mannerisms, including hand flapping and hand biting (Hagerman, 2002c).

Males with the premutation are typically unaffected intellectually, although anxiety may be seen. Recently a new tremor/ataxia syndrome has been described in a subgroup of older male carriers more than 50 years of age (Hagerman et al, 2001). The tremor is typically an action tremor, and the ataxia is often characterized by frequent falling. These symptoms are usually

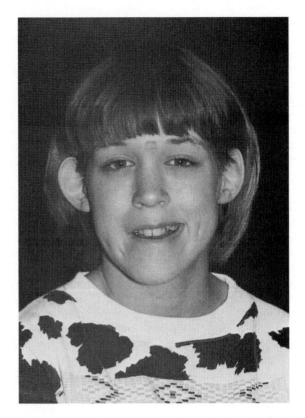

FIGURE 26-5 Young heterozygous fragile X female who is affected physically and cognitively by fragile X.

TABLE 26-1
Fragile X Checklist

	Score		
	0 **(Not Present)**	**1** **(Borderline** **or Present** **in the Past)**	**2** **(Definitely** **Present)**
Mental retardation			
Perseverative speech			
Hyperactivity			
Short attention span			
Tactile defensiveness			
Hand flapping			
Hand biting			
Poor eye contact			
Hyperextensible finger joints			
Large or prominent ears			
Large testicles			
Simian crease or Sydney line			
Family history of mental retardation			

TOTAL SCORE:

(From Hagerman, R.J. [1987]. Fragile X syndrome. *Curr Probl Pediatr, 17*, 621-674. Reprinted with permission.)

slowly progressive and may include cognitive decline in the 60s or 70s. The prevalence of this problem among older male carriers is not yet known. It has not been seen in female carriers or in those affected by fragile X syndrome.

Females
Overall, females affected by fragile X syndrome display milder phenotypic features than males, although some have been described with moderate and severe retardation (Figure 26-5).

Females who carry the premutation (i.e., CGG repeat number between 54 and 200) are usually unaffected intellectually by fragile X. Females who carry the full mutation, however, are often affected to a mild or severe degree. Approximately 70% of females with the full mutation have cognitive deficits including a borderline IQ or mild to moderate mental retardation (de Vries et al, 1996; Bennetto et al, 2001). Executive function deficits—including attention and organizational difficulties—are common in most females with the full mutation but with an overall normal IQ. In addition, math difficulties, shyness, social anxiety, and poor eye contact are also common in females with the full mutation (Braden, 2002; Hagerman, 2002c).

The physical characteristics in females are less obvious than those described for males with fragile X. Prominent ears, a long narrow face, a prominent forehead and jaw, and hyperextensible finger joints have been described (Hagerman, 2002c). Phenotypic expression is more frequently observed in the mentally impaired population, but penetrance of the fragile X gene or genes is also seen in normal functioning heterozygous females (Riddle et al, 1998).

The fragile X checklist (Table 26-1) was designed to assist primary care providers with screening children who have developmental delays or mental retardation. A child receives a zero for each feature not present, one point for those present in the past or questionably present, and two points for those definitely present. The higher the score, the greater the risk for fragile X syndrome (Hagerman 2002c).

Treatment
Few health care professionals are knowledgeable about the diagnosis and treatment of individuals with fragile X syndrome. It is not uncommon, however, for an undiagnosed child with fragile X to be seen by the primary care provider for one of several associated medical problems including repeated ear infections, strabismus, hyperactivity, delayed language, tantrums, violent outbursts, seizures, or hypotonia. Although much of the medical intervention is approached as it would be with any child, certain treatment options specific to the fragile X diagnosis can significantly improve the developmental outcome for these children.

Any signs that indicate developmental delay, sensory integration dysfunction, or language delays deserve immediate and aggressive treatment in a child with fragile X. All areas of a child's presenting signs and symptoms should be addressed, and thus a multidisciplinary approach to evaluation and therapy is essential (Box 26-2).

Medication
Management of hyperactivity and attentional problems with medication can augment learning and behavioral management at home and in school. Central nervous system (CNS) stimulant medication has proved the most reliable, with

Treatment

MEDICATIONS FOR HYPERACTIVITY
Methylphenidate (Ritalin, Concerta, Metadate), dextroamphetamine (Dexedrine), or dextroamphetamine/amphetamine (Adderall)
Catapres (clonidine) or Tenex (guanfacine)

MEDICATIONS FOR AGGRESSION OR SEVERE MOOD LABILITY
Anticonvulsants (carbamazepine) (Tegretol), or valproic acid (Depakote)
Selective serotonin reuptake inhibitors (SSRIs)

SPECIAL EDUCATION SUPPORT INCLUDING SPEECH AND/OR LANGUAGE THERAPY AND OCCUPATIONAL THERAPY

GENETIC COUNSELING FOR ALL EXTENDED FAMILY MEMBERS AT RISK

improvements in as many as two thirds of affected children (Hagerman, 2002b). No one drug is effective for all children. Children are most commonly prescribed methylphenidate (Ritalin, Concerta, Metadate), but dextroamphetamine (Dexedrine) or dextroamphetamine/amphetamine (Adderall) is also beneficial (Hagerman, 2002b) (see Chapter 28).

Clonidine (Catapres) has been beneficial in approximately 80% of children with fragile X syndrome who have significant hyperactivity. Clonidine is a high blood pressure medication that lowers plasma and CNS norepinephrine levels. This medication is particularly helpful for children with severe hyperactivity, overexcitability, and aggression, which are typical problems in fragile X, so clonidine is often used before stimulants. It has an overall calming effect on hyperactivity and can be used in conjunction with stimulants (Hagerman et al, 1995).

Individuals who suffer from significant mood lability, mood instability, or aggression may benefit greatly from the mood-stabilizing effects of anticonvulsants (e.g., carbamazepine [Tegretol] or valproic acid [Depakote] (Hagerman, 1999; Hagerman, 2002b). In our clinical experience, gabapentin has not been helpful for individuals with fragile X syndrome.

In adolescence, aggression can be a significant difficulty, and Selective serotonin reuptake inhibitors (SSRIs) (e.g., fluoxetine [Prozac], sertraline [Zoloft], or citalopram [Celexa]) have been helpful in fragile X syndrome (Hagerman et al, 1994). A survey of fluoxetine's efficacy in fragile X reported that 70% of the individuals had a beneficial response, including a decrease in aggression, improvement in anxiety, and improvement in moodiness or outburst behavior. SSRIs are widely known as antidepressant medication but may also be helpful in decreasing obsessive-compulsive behavior and anxiety. The side effects of fluoxetine can include gastrointestinal upset or nausea and an activation effect, which can sometimes exacerbate hyperactivity. A rare child may experience an increase in obsessive-compulsive behavior, aggression, or suicidal ideation while taking an SSRI. For this reason, children should be followed in therapy, preferably weekly, while taking this medication.

The use of atypical antipsychotic medication such as risperidone, olanzepine, quetiapine, or ziprazidone can also be helpful to treat aggression or mood instability (Hagerman, 2002b). The use of low doses is helpful in avoiding side effects such as tardive dyskinesias, although weight gain is often a problem particularly for risperidone and olanzepine.

Educational Intervention

Whenever possible, children should be mainstreamed into the regular classroom and receive speech and language and occupational therapy and special education support on an individual basis (see school section of this chapter for further details). Studies have indicated that IQ declines with age in children with fragile X syndrome (Wright Talamante et al, 1996; Bennetto & Pennington, 2002). Some males, however, whose IQs have remained stable over time have been followed, and an occasional individual may maintain an IQ within the normal range. This finding has been associated with a novel pattern on DNA testing: an unmethylated or partially unmethylated full mutation (i.e., CGG expansion >200). This finding is unusual because the full mutation is typically completely methylated. The lack of methylation in these high-functioning males has been associated with a limited level of FMR1 protein production, leading to a less severe degree of involvement intellectually and behaviorally than typical fragile X males (Tassone et al, 1999; Bennetto & Pennington, 2002). There is a tendency for individuals with fragile X to perform better on some academic tests than their IQ score would predict. Children with fragile X syndrome are typically better visual than auditory learners. Significant memory abilities and well-developed skills in recognizing visual gestalts make reading, spelling, and vocabulary obvious areas of strength for many (Braden, 2002; Scharfenaker et al, 2002).

Because children with fragile X are easily overstimulated, occupational therapy should be geared toward helping them reorganize, interpret, and adjust to sensory stimulation. For this reason sensory integration therapy is the method of choice when working with these children. With this form of treatment, improvements should be noticeable in motor skills, balance, coordination, movement, sequencing, and attention (Scharfenaker et al, 2002).

Genetic Counseling

Fragile X syndrome is known to affect generation after generation, and many families have two or more children affected by this condition (Figure 26-6). Early diagnosis can provide relatives with important information about fragile X inheritance, recurrence risks, carrier testing, and family planning options (Gane & Cronister, 2002).

Because fragile X syndrome is inherited, it is essential that a thorough family history or pedigree be taken. Questions about intellectual deficits, learning disabilities, emotional problems, and physical features associated with fragile X syndrome should be asked. Any relative with positive findings should be suspected as either a carrier or an affected individual.

Prenatal diagnosis is available to all families with a confirmed diagnosis of fragile X syndrome or those with a history of mental retardation. This testing includes amniocentesis (performed at 14 to 18 weeks' gestation), chorionic villus sampling (performed at $9\frac{1}{2}$ to 12 weeks' gestation), and percutaneous umbilical blood sampling (18 to 22 weeks' gestation). Each procedure has specific benefits and drawbacks that should be carefully discussed with a genetic counselor before pregnancy or testing is pursued (Gane & Cronister, 2002). The accuracy of prenatal diagnostic testing has improved significantly (i.e., >98% accurate) with DNA-FMR1 studies. All family

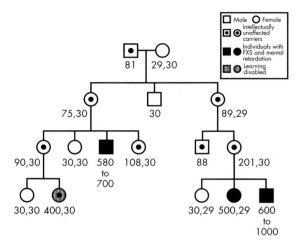

FIGURE 26-6   A family tree with individuals affected by fragile X syndrome (FXS). The numbers underneath the circles and squares represent the CGG repeat number in the FMR1.

members who are at risk to carry either the premutation or the full mutation should be studied by DNA testing, which is done on a blood sample. DNA testing is available throughout the United States and at large genetic centers internationally. For a list of laboratories that can carry out DNA testing for fragile X syndrome, contact the National Fragile X Foundation (see resources at the end of this chapter).

Complementary and Alternative Treatments

Folic acid therapy appears to be helpful for approximately 50% of prepubertal boys with fragile X although the reason for this is unknown (Hagerman, 2002b). Its use is controversial, however, and several studies have shown a lack of efficacy. Other studies have shown noticeable improvements in activity level, attention span, unusual mannerisms, and coping skills. The mechanism of action of folate is unclear, but it does not appear to be specific to fragile X syndrome. Because harmful side effects are rare, many families request that their child be given folic acid as a trial. A prepubescent child can be placed on a regimen of 10 mg/day (i.e., divided twice daily) for 3 to 6 months. Regardless of the dosage, careful follow-up is warranted to monitor vitamin B_6 and zinc serum levels, which may become deficient. If improvements are not noticeable within the trial period, the clinician should consider an alternative treatment.

Anticipated Advances in Diagnosis and Management

A significant advance is the use of antibodies to the FMR1 protein to identify individuals who have fragile X syndrome in both blood and/or hair roots (Willemsen et al, 1997; Tassone et al, 1999; Oostra & Hoogeveen, 2002). Because unaffected individuals produce a normal level of FMR1 protein, the antibody test will light up the protein within the lymphocytes or hair roots of individuals who are normal. An antibody test, however, usually detects little or no protein in males with the full mutation (Tassone et al, 1999; Oostra & Hoogeveen, 2002). Females,

on the other hand, produce some level of FMR1 protein because their other normal X chromosome is producing FMR1 protein to a level dependent on the pattern of X inactivation (the percentage of cells with the normal X as the active X). Therefore this diagnostic test does not clearly differentiate females with the full mutation compared with controls. This antibody test should be considered as a screening for individuals who may be affected by fragile X syndrome, and then the diagnosis should be confirmed by DNA testing.

Within the next 10 years the technology to either replace the FMR1 protein or add a normal FMR1 gene in individuals who are affected by this syndrome will probably be developed. This very important advance could mean a cure or significant alleviation of this disorder. Extensive animal studies will be needed over the next decade to improve methods for inserting a gene or normal FMR1 protein inside of neurons. It is unclear at this time how significant the improvements will be in children or adults who receive a new gene or normal levels of FMR1 protein (Hagerman, 2002a).

Associated Problems (Box 26-3)

Speech and Language Difficulties

Speech and language difficulties are noted in both males and females with a full mutation. Although more work is needed in this area, receptive and expressive language deficits (i.e., including difficulties with auditory processing, inappropriate and tangential speech, poor topic maintenance, and written language difficulties) have been reported (Bennetto & Pennington, 2002; Scharfenaker et al, 2002).

Otitis Media

Recurrent otitis media has been reported in 45% to 60% of all children with fragile X syndrome. Approximately 40% of these children will require myringotomy tube insertions (Hagerman, 2002c). There has been some speculation that this may be caused by an unusual angle or collapsibility of the eustachian tube. Appropriate intervention is critical to avoid conductive hearing loss and a compounding of language deficits typical for fragile X.

BOX 26-3

Associated Problems

Speech and language difficulties
Otitis media
Connective tissue problems
   Pes planus
   Scoliosis
   Mitral valve prolapse
Vision problems
   Strabismus
   Nystagmus
Seizures
Oral problems
Autistic-like features (e.g., hand flapping, hand biting)
Psychiatric manifestations
Sensory integration difficulties

Connective Tissue Problems

Of all individuals with fragile X syndrome, 50% will have pes planus, and joint laxity is seen in approximately 70% of children 10 years or younger (Hagerman, 2002c). Clubfoot has also been reported and may be related to hypotonia in utero. For reasons not clearly understood, hypotonia tends to disappear with age. Scoliosis may be present, and hernias appear to be more common in children with fragile X than in the general population. Gastroesophageal reflux is also common in infancy and is thought to be attributed to an underlying connective tissue disorder. Routine intervention is recommended.

Cardiac problems have also been noted in individuals with fragile X syndrome and may be secondary to a connective tissue disorder. Mitral valve prolapse has been diagnosed in 22% to 55% of affected adult individuals, but it is rarely seen in children (Hagerman, 2002c). Although usually benign, mitral valve prolapse can predispose a person to arrhythmias, and prophylactic antibiotics prior to surgery or dental procedures are generally recommended (see Chapter 21). Approximately 30% of heterozygous females complain of heart palpitations. Mild dilation of the base of the aorta has also been observed with ultrasound studies in as many as 50% of this population but does not appear to be progressive.

Vision Problems

Strabismus (i.e., either esotropia or exotropia) appears to be present in approximately 8% to 30% of those with fragile X syndrome (King et al, 1995; Hatton et al, 1998). Other eye problems, such as myopia, nystagmus, and ptosis, have been observed with and without strabismus (Hagerman, 2002c).

Seizures

Seizures have been documented in approximately 20% of individuals with fragile X. Generalized seizures and partial complex seizures have been reported (Musumeci et al, 1999). A careful history should be taken and if clinical seizures are present, treatment with an anticonvulsant such as carbamazepine or valproic acid is warranted (Hagerman, 2002c) (see Chapter 25).

Oral Problems

A high-arched palate is seen with greater frequency among the fragile X population and can explain the increased incidence of dental malocclusion. Several reports of Pierre Robin syndrome (micrognathia and cleft palate) have also been noted in combination with fragile X syndrome (Hagerman, 2002c) (see Chapter 19).

Autistic-like Tendencies

Much has been written to suggest an association between autism and fragile X syndrome. Studies have estimated that approximately 15% to 33% of individuals with fragile X meet the *Diagnostic and Statistical Manual of Mental Disorders (DSM-IV)* criteria for autism (Bailey et al, 1998; Rogers et al, 2001). Most individuals, however, are interested in social interactions but have autistic-like features, such as poor eye contact, unusual hand mannerisms, tactile defensiveness, and obsessive interests. What differentiates most individuals with fragile X without autism from those with autism is that those who are autistic characteristically lack an ability to relate (see Chapter 13). Although social anxiety is obvious at times, many children with fragile X can be intermittently quite sociable, demonstrating a spontaneous and natural sense of humor (Scharfenaker et al, 2002).

Psychiatric Manifestations

Researchers have only recently investigated the psychiatric manifestations of the fragile X gene in females. As with males with fragile X, social anxiety is a common complaint. Many of the affected girls appear shy, are withdrawn, and have poor eye contact (Franke et al, 1998; Hagerman, 2002c). Cognitively normal women occasionally recall that their childhood was burdened by similar types of problems. Poor self-image, schizotypal features, and depression have also been described (Franke et al, 1998; Hagerman, 2002c). The schizotypal features appear to be related to the executive function or frontal deficits that are seen in most females with the full mutation (Bennetto et al, 2001; Bennetto & Pennington, 2002).

Sensory Integration Difficulties

Other behavioral concerns include a child's inability to calm when overstimulated or overwhelmed. New stimuli or novel situations can be frightening. Many parents describe their child as being hypersensitive to touch or tactilely defensive and an enhanced sympathetic response to a variety of sensory stimuli has been documented in research studies (Miller et al, 1999; Roberts et al, 2001). Sensory integration difficulties are evidenced by an inability to screen out noises, lights, or confusion. Common responses to this overloading can include tantrums or outburst behavior, aggressive behavior, and emotional instability (Hagerman, 2002c; Scharfenaker et al, 2002).

Prognosis

Individuals with fragile X syndrome are expected to live a normal life span regardless of intellectual functioning. However, reports of sudden death have occurred and this may relate to a rare cardiac arrhythmia (Sabaratnam, 2000; Hagerman, 2002c).

Health Care Maintenance

Growth and Development

Growth parameters usually fall within the normal range, although head circumference greater than 75% has been reported (Hagerman, 2002c). Sometimes the large head circumference may lead to a misdiagnosis of Sotos' syndrome.

In addition to deficits in cognitive functioning and speech, children with fragile X may be delayed in meeting other age-appropriate developmental milestones. Hypotonia is usually obvious in infancy. Developmental delay will be evident with early developmental testing, such as the Denver II and the Bayley Scales of Infant Development (see Chapter 2). Other early warning signs are clumsiness and poor balance. Toe walking, unusual gait, lack of flow of movement, and trouble with motor planning may also occur secondary to hypotonia, joint laxity, and sensory integration difficulties (Scharfenaker et al, 2002). These children are easily overstimulated and tantrums are common particularly while shopping or visiting a mall. They usually like to watch their favorite videotapes over and over again.

Diet

Obsessive-compulsive behavior can be seen in children with fragile X syndrome and may involve food cravings. Obesity has been a problem for a small subgroup of children with fragile X, which may be secondary to perseverative eating or hypothalamic dysfunction. A subgroup of children with fragile X may have a Prader-Willi–like phenotype or general overgrowth (de Vries et al, 1995). Parents of obese children should be encouraged to place their children on appropriate diets. Exercise programs for older children may also be beneficial, as well as exercise videos, which encourage children to use their visual and mimicking abilities. Failure to thrive is not uncommon in infants with fragile X syndrome but may be the result of gastroesophageal reflux, aversion to some food textures, frequent infections, or problematic mothering skills (i.e., if the mother herself is affected by the syndrome) (Hagerman, 2002c).

Safety

Families and educators should not expect every child with fragile X to be able to learn age-appropriate safety. It will depend on each child's individual strengths and weaknesses. With strong visual and mimicking abilities and through the use of repetition, many children can be taught to follow safety tips.

Hyperactivity may lead to more accidents, so these children should be monitored closely. Home safety precautions such as safety cabinet latches and switchplate covers should be based on the child's developmental rather than chronologic age. Because children with fragile X can be overstimulated by their environment, the home setting—particularly the child's playroom and bedroom—should be a calm and uncluttered environment. The use of bean bag chairs, vibrating pillows, musical tapes, and appropriate environmental changes can be discussed with an occupational therapist (Scharfenaker et al, 2002). Tools and motorized equipment need additional precautions. Please refer to the Chapter 12 on ADHD for further impulsive/inattention safety issues.

Parents also may be concerned about the safety of their child if self-injurious behavior is displayed. Head banging is rare but can be harmful to the child; hand biting usually causes a callus and rarely scarring. Behavior management therapies to decrease the frequency of these behaviors are often helpful (Hills-Epstein et al, 2002; Scharfenaker et al, 2002). Safety issues are a concern when the parents are also affected. Recommendations include referral to a public health nurse and early infant stimulation programs to get professionals into the home to evaluate safety. Parents and professionals should also be advised of possible seizure activity and taught appropriate intervention (see Chapter 25).

Immunizations

The vaccination regimen is the same as it would be for any infant or child. Prevnar (for *Pneumococcus*) can decrease otitis media by 8% to 20%, which is important in fragile X because of the increased frequency of otitis. Because of mental retardation there is an increased risk for oral and fecal contamina-

---

> **BOX 26-4**
> ## Screening
>
> Vision
> Hearing
> Dental
> Cardiac examination
> Speech and/or language delays
> Connective tissue problems
> Seizures

tion, so immunization for hepatitis A and B is important. If a child has a seizure disorder, the American Academy of Pediatrics guidelines for administering pertussis and measles vaccinations to those with seizures should be followed (see Chapter 25) (Committee on Infectious Diseases, 1994).

Screening (Box 26-4)

Vision. An eye examination is recommended as early as possible after fragile X is diagnosed to rule out strabismus and the less frequent findings of myopia, hyperopia, astigmatism, nystagmus, and ptosis. The evaluation should include a complete case history, visual acuity evaluation, refractive error determination, oculomotor assessment, and funduscopy. Other testing may include an assessment of focusing function and visual developmental-perceptual skills. Yearly screening is sufficient unless visual difficulty is suspected. Early intervention is encouraged to avoid the development of blurred vision, amblyopia, or diplopia as a result of an uncorrected refractive error or strabismus. Treatment for many of the ophthalmologic problems includes corrective lenses or patching or both (i.e., treatment that is relatively inexpensive and noninvasive). For some cases of strabismus, however, surgery may be the treatment of choice. Corrected vision will maximize a child's learning potential.

Hearing. Because of the increased risk for recurrent ear infections, hearing evaluations are strongly recommended in newly diagnosed children. Audiometry testing is usually sufficient to assess hearing. Any child with a history of recurrent ear infections is best referred to an ear, nose, and throat (ENT) specialist to determine whether pressure-equalizing (PE) tubes are warranted.

Dental. A routine dental screening by the practitioner may reveal a high-arched palate, cleft palate, or dental malocclusion, all of which compound speech problems. Adults who need dental work should be assessed for mitral valve prolapse; if present, prophylactic antibiotic treatment to avoid subacute bacterial endocarditis is warranted (see Chapter 21). Although not always possible, families should be referred to a pedodontist experienced in working with children who are developmentally delayed or hyperactive.

Blood Pressure. Routine screening is recommended.

Hematocrit. Routine screening is recommended.

Urinalysis. Routine screening is recommended.

Tuberculosis. Routine screening is recommended.

Condition-Specific Screening

Mitral Valve Prolapse. Children with fragile X syndrome are at increased risk of mitral valve prolapse. Careful auscultation for a click or murmur is essential to detect this problem or any other cardiac involvement. Any child or adult with an abnormal cardiac examination should be referred to a cardiologist for formal evaluation.

Speech and Language. Some children will have early speech delays that may be so subtle that they go undetected by parents or teachers. An early and annual speech and language evaluation should be performed to detect any speech or language deficits that can be improved through early intervention. Because of the diversity of speech and language difficulties in children with fragile X, no one screening tool is recommended. Each child should be approached on an individual basis. Children identified with fragile X syndrome should have a formal evaluation by a licensed speech and language pathologist who is preferably experienced with fragile X syndrome. Speech evaluation should be included in each IEP evaluation in school to determine the benefit of speech therapy.

Connective Tissue Problems. Early detection of scoliosis can often prevent further sequelae. Screening should also include a careful examination for excessive joint laxity and other complications of loose connective tissue (e.g., hernias).

Seizures. When the clinical history suggests seizures, an electroencephalogram (EEG) is indicated. Unusual findings can include a slow background rhythm and spike-wave discharges that are often similar to rolandic spikes (Musumeci et al, 1999). Any child who appears to be having seizures should be treated with anticonvulsant medication and followed closely by a pediatric neurologist (Hagerman, 2002b). If a child is taking medication to control seizures, anticonvulsant serum levels should be followed (see Chapter 25).

Common Illness Management
Differential Diagnosis (Box 26-5)

Recurrent Otitis Media. These children must be vigorously monitored and treated for recurrent otitis media to avoid sequelae that could further compromise language development and learning. Parents of young children may not recognize otitis as the cause of their child's irritability. It may be helpful to inform parents of children with fragile X that recurrent otitis media is a common problem and review which signs or symptoms are indicators of infection.

To best determine a child's individualized medical management, newly diagnosed families should be referred to a health care team with expertise in fragile X syndrome for a thorough evaluation and consultation.

BOX 26-5
Differential Diagnosis
Attention deficit hyperactivity disorder (ADHD)
Autism
Pervasive developmental disorder, not otherwise specified (PDD NOS)
Sotos syndrome or cerebral gigantism
Prader-Willi syndrome
X-linked mental retardation
Fetal alcohol syndrome
Tourette syndrome

Drug Interactions

Carbamazepine is a commonly prescribed anticonvulsant that is also used to control behavior problems (e.g., violent outbursts, aggression, and self-injurious behavior). Concurrent treatment with macrolide antibiotics (Zithromax, erythromycin), cimetidine (Tagamet), propoxyphene (Darvon), and isoniazid (INH) can interfere with the breakdown of carbamazepine, causing nausea, vomiting, and lethargy. Folic acid therapy may worsen the seizure frequency in children with epilepsy.

Developmental Issues
Sleep Patterns

Frequent wakefulness in early childhood is a common problem in children with fragile X. Overstimulation can often interfere with sleeping, and calming techniques (e.g., music) are useful in quieting the child in preparation for bedtime. Melatonin also helps sleep disturbances.

Toileting

Parents of children with fragile X often need help setting realistic expectations about toilet training. Some children achieve this milestone on time, but delayed training is more common. Parents should not be discouraged if a child takes longer to learn. Establishing a predictable routine and consistent positive reinforcement are general principles that are helpful for children with fragile X (Crepeau-Hobson & O'Connor, 2002). As with parents of any child having toilet-training difficulties, parents are discouraged from being overly critical or reprimanding.

Discipline

Children with fragile X syndrome are especially noncompliant in response to an unexpected event or change in routine and therefore need a highly structured environment. Sending the child to school the same way each day, having meals on a scheduled basis, and using the same nightly routines are encouraged. Behavior problems should be anticipated if a child is faced with an unexpected event. The prevention of unpredictable events in the home or at school is obviously an unrealistic expectation and should not be overemphasized. On the other hand, change and transitions should be gradually programmed into the child's learning and home environment. Setting limits, giving the child timeouts, and being consistent are appropriate responses when disciplinary action is required.

Child Care

Issues related to child care are common concerns for parents of a child with fragile X. Because of the short attention span and hyperactivity of children with fragile X, child care providers should be knowledgeable about behavior modification techniques. The environment in which a child is placed is also important. Colors, noise level, and the amount of light can be altered to avoid overstimulation both at home and in a child care setting. Slowly but gradually new events can be programmed into a child's day. Setting a common time each week to introduce a new game, playing in a new space, or meeting a new daycare provider can help a child anticipate and deal more effectively with change. If these aspects of daycare are well managed, there is no reason why a child with fragile X cannot be placed in full-day or half-day programs. Placement with nonaffected children is very helpful for modeling appropriate behavior. Children can be mainstreamed in preschool programs as well, but child care providers should be experienced in specialized education. Children with fragile X are eligible for special education from age 3 on, so preschool programs affiliated with a school system should be able to provide special services such as speech and language therapy and occupational therapy.

Schooling

Most children with fragile X syndrome that have been identified are receiving special education. Inclusion is a potential goal as described under the treatment section in this chapter (see Chapter 2). Speech therapy, occupational therapy, learning assistance, and psychologic counseling can all be accessed through special education. A program that provides for individualized attention and a high teacher-student ratio is best. The success of any approach depends on a number of factors specific to each child, including the child's level of cognitive functioning, distractibility, impulsivity, the structure of the class, classroom environment, and appropriate role models. All children with fragile X will need a consistent routine and help with transitions in school (Braden, 2002). Sometimes their behavior problems require taking medication in school such as stimulants or clonidine. It is important for the school nurse to be familiar with these medications and their use in children with fragile X (Hagerman, 2002b).

Because few educators are knowledgeable about fragile X syndrome, the health care professional can play an active role in helping families educate the teachers and therapists about the specialized needs of their child and why an integrative approach that emphasizes a child's overall strengths and remediates the weaknesses is essential for effective learning.

Parents should be encouraged to become actively involved in their child's program. Frequent visits to the classroom and observing therapy sessions help establish open communication among parents, teachers, and support personnel.

When developing an educational program, a child's overall intellectual abilities must be considered. Inclusion is a realistic goal for some children, but others may need a more structured and specialized program. Children with fragile X will improve most significantly if they are shown appropriate role models. Educational intervention strategies should emphasize a child's strengths (e.g., imitating abilities, memory, computer skills, visual skills, and vocabulary). The curriculum should focus on areas of a child's interest (Braden, 2002; Scharfenaker et al, 2002). Logo reading is an example of a learning tool developed to capitalize on a child's strength for incidentally acquired knowledge (Braden, 2002). The idea is to use logos from popular television commercials and advertisements as the basis for a sight word vocabulary. The logos are gradually faded away so that only the word, phrase, or number remains.

Another learning tool that has proved successful is the use of computers for learning enhancement. This medium may be used to enhance language ability and academic progress in reading, spelling, and math. It can use visual matching skills and can help focus attention with colorful programs (Braden, 2002).

Speech and language and occupational therapy intervention are critical components of the education program and are recommended for all children with fragile X syndrome. Therapy is most effective when it incorporates a child's primary areas of interest. When possible, speech and language therapy sessions should include one or two other children who function at a higher level. Again, early intervention and vigorous treatment can optimize a child's speech and language abilities (Scharfenaker et al, 2002).

Sexuality

Masturbation and other forms of self-stimulatory behavior are common among individuals with mental retardation and are sometimes problematic for adolescents with fragile X. Families can be supportive by providing appropriate sex education and talking openly about sexuality issues. This need can also be met through family or individual counseling (Hills-Epstein et al, 2002). Counseling or therapy can also train new behaviors that can replace socially inappropriate behavior (e.g., masturbation in public). Most important, counseling provides adolescents a place to discuss and deal with issues of sexuality in a supportive environment.

Fertility is usually normal in men with fragile X, although reproduction is rare because of cognitive deficits (Hagerman, 2002c). Most males with fragile X are not sexually active but they may obsess on women they like and on rare occasions can become physically aggressive toward these women. All female children of males with fragile X will have the premutation because only the premutation—not the full mutation—is carried in the sperm. Ovarian problems and premature menopause have been reported in women with the premutation (Gane & Cronister, 2002; Hagerman, 2002c). Females with the full mutation are more likely to reproduce than males because they have higher cognitive abilities. However, they are at a 50% risk to have a child affected by fragile X, unlike the males. Sex education and genetic counseling should be available to them.

Transition to Adulthood

The transition to adulthood is usually difficult for adolescents with fragile X syndrome because living independently is a problem as a result of mental retardation. It is important for adolescents to have adequate vocational training. Most individuals affected by fragile X syndrome can carry out jobs in the community that are consistent with their level of mental functioning. Many individuals require a job trainer who can work with them for the first several days or first few weeks when a new job is started. If they are to be successful in living independently or semi-independently, a focus on daily living skills is also critical for young adults with fragile X syndrome. Individuals with mild or moderate mental retardation can learn how to use public transportation and carry out activities in the home, including laundry, self-care, and cooking. Most adults affected by fragile X syndrome do well with limited supervision in an apartment living situation.

Females affected with fragile X syndrome have most difficulty when trying to raise their children who are affected by fragile X syndrome. This role can be extremely stressful and may overwhelm their limited resources, particularly if the mother is mildly retarded. Additional help from family or from social services agencies is usually necessary. They should be referred to a public health nurse and parenting classes, and their children affected by fragile X should have intervention from birth on. Adults with fragile X should also have protection under the Americans for Disabilities Act for employment and housing issues (see Chapter 9).

The connective tissue problems usually improve in adulthood, and medical complications are uncommon. Hernia and mitral valve prolapse are more common in adulthood than childhood. Follow-up with a cardiologist and the use of antibiotic prophylaxis for subacute bacterial endocarditis (SBE) prevention are necessary for mitral valve prolapse.

Most adults with fragile X and cognitive deficits can receive supplemental security income and therefore can obtain health care and counseling through Medicaid and/or Medicare. This coverage is important for ongoing care and medication.

Approximately 30% of young adults—particularly males—with fragile X syndrome may have difficulty with episodic outburst behavior. This behavior should be treated with medications such as SSRIs and/or atypical antipsychotics, in addition to counseling. Counseling can help with development of calming techniques and recognition of environmental situations that can lead to outburst behavior (Hills-Epstein et al, 2002). The occupational therapist can also help with calming techniques in adults with fragile X.

Family Concerns and Resources

Perhaps the most frustrating aspect of having a child with fragile X syndrome is realizing that few professionals have a good understanding of this disorder and how it can affect a child and other family members. As a consequence many parents become the main advocate for their child in both the educational and medical settings. Health care professionals who are unfamiliar with fragile X syndrome should make every effort to listen carefully to families. It is also the parents' responsibility to educate themselves about this unique disorder so that they too appreciate the specialized needs of these children, as well as recognize their own needs if they require additional support because they may also be affected by the syndrome.

Fragile X syndrome occurs in all ethnic and racial groups that have been studied. There is no evidence of increased prevalence in any individual group. In some cultural groups, such as certain Asian populations, it is sometimes difficult to do genetic counseling in extended family members because of the negative cultural implications of knowing about a genetic disorder that affects large numbers within the family tree. When these cultural concerns exist, often permission will not be given to inform extended family members about this genetic disorder. In these cases it is helpful to write an explanatory letter about fragile X syndrome that the immediate family can pass out to other family members who may be affected or be carriers for fragile X syndrome.

The National Fragile X Foundation was established to educate parents, professionals, and the public on the diagnosis and treatment of fragile X syndrome and other forms of X-linked mental retardation. In addition, the National Fragile X Foundation promotes research pertaining to fragile X syndrome in the areas of biochemistry, genetics, and clinical applications. All parents who have a child diagnosed with fragile X syndrome and professionals interested in working with the developmentally delayed population are encouraged to write or call the foundation so that they may receive the newsletter and other services available to them.

Resources

Foundations

National Fragile X Foundation
PO Box 190488
San Francisco, CA 94119
(925) 938-9300
www.nfxf.org

FRAXA Research Foundation
PO Box 935
West Newbury, MA 01985-0935
(978) 462-1866; (978) 463-9985 (fax)
www.fraxa.org; info@fraxa.org
Fragile X syndrome listserv sponsored by FRAXA: to be added to the listserv, email "SUBSCRIBE FRAGILEX-L" to listserv@ listserv.cc.emory.edu

Fragile X Research Foundation of Canada
167 Queen Street West
Brampton, ON
Canada L6Y 1M5
(905) 453-9366
FXRFC@ibm.net;
www.fragile-x.ca

The Fragile X Society (England)
53 Winchelsea Lane
Hastings, East Sussex
TN35 4LG
011-424-813147

The International Fragile X Alliance (Australia)
263 Glen Elra Road
Nth Caulfield 3161
Melbourne, Australia
(03) 9528-1910; (03) 9532-9555 (fax)
jcohen@netspace.net.au

Fragile X Association of Australia, Inc.
15 Bowen Close
Cherrybrook, NSW
Australia
(019) 987012
fragilex@ozemail.com.au

Newsletters

National Fragile X Foundation Newsletter—Call the National Fragile X Foundation at (800) 688-8765.

FRAXA Research Foundation Newsletter—Subscriptions through FRAXA, PO Box 935, West Newbury, MA 01985

Reading for Children

O'Connor, R. (1995). *Boys with Fragile X Syndrome*. Can be obtained from the National Fragile X Foundation: (800) 688-8765
Steiger, C. (1998). *My Brother Has Fragile X Syndrome*. Chapel Hill: Avanta Publishing. (800) 434-0322

Summary of Primary Care Needs for the Child with Fragile X Syndrome

HEALTH CARE MAINTENANCE
Growth and development

Physical growth is usually within normal limits.
Some children are reported to have large heads for body size.
Deficits in cognitive function and speech are common.
Developmental delays in gross motor skills are common.

Diet

Obsessive eating may result in obesity in older children.
Infants may have failure to thrive.

Safety

Cognitive dysfunction may limit these children's awareness of safety issues.
Hyperactivity may make these children more accident prone.
Self-injurious behavior may occur, and parents can be taught behavior management therapies.
If seizures are present, seizure precautions are necessary.
Home safety may be further compromised if the parents also have fragile X.

Immunizations

Routine immunizations are recommended.
AAP guidelines for immunizations in children with seizures should be followed where indicated.

Screening

Vision. Eye examination for strabismus, refractive errors, and visual perceptual skills is recommended at the time of diagnosis. If no problems are found, annual vision screening is recommended.

Hearing. An increased risk of otitis media warrants audiometric testing. A child may need referral to an ENT specialist for PE tubes.

Dental. Screening for palate and dental abnormalities is recommended. If mitral valve prolapse is present, prophylactic antibiotics will be needed for dental work.

Blood Pressure. Routine screening is recommended.
Hematocrit. Routine screening is recommended.
Urinalysis. Routine screening is recommended.
Tuberculosis. Routine screening is recommended.

Condition-specific screening

Mitral Valve Prolapse. In the presence of an abnormal cardiac examination, mitral valve prolapse must be evaluated by a cardiologist.

Speech and Language. Speech and language evaluation should be done annually, with early intervention if a problem is detected.

Connective Tissue Problems. Children should be screened for flat feet, scoliosis, and excessive joint laxity.

Seizures. A clinical history suggestive of seizures should be evaluated by electroencephalography. If a child is taking anticonvulsants, blood levels must be monitored.

COMMON ILLNESS MANAGEMENT
Differential Diagnosis

Recurrent otitis media is common.

Drug Interactions

Carbamazepine is altered by macrolide antibiotics, cimetidine, propoxyphene, and isoniazid.
See Chapter 25 for drug interactions with seizure medications.

DEVELOPMENTAL ISSUES
Sleep Patterns

Frequent wakefulness in early childhood is not uncommon.
Overstimulation should be avoided.

Toileting

Delayed continence is not uncommon.

Discipline

Children behave better in highly structured environments.
Consistent limit setting is beneficial.
Positive reinforcement is essential.

Child Care

Short attention span and hyperactivity may be modified by subdued environments.
New activities must be introduced slowly.

Schooling

Most children receive special education services. The provider can help educate the school system personnel on condition and treatment.

Sexuality

Self-stimulatory behaviors are common. Counseling may help decrease inappropriate behavior.
Fertility is normal in men; but reproduction is rare due to cognitive delay.
Carrier females may experience premature menopause.
Sex education, birth control, and genetic counseling are necessary.

Transition to Adulthood

Living independently is difficult; individuals will likely need support from others. Housing and employment opportunities are protected under ADA.
Connective tissue problems will improve.
Outburst behavior may be a problem and should be treated with medication and counseling.

FAMILY CONCERNS

Families may have difficulty adjusting to the diagnosis; parents may also be affected.
Genetic counseling is warranted.
Because the condition is not well known, care may be nonspecific.

REFERENCES

Bailey, A., Palferman, S., Heavey, L., & Le Couteur, A. (1998). Autism: the phenotype in relatives. *J Autism Dev Disord, 28*, 369-392.

Bennetto, L. & Pennington, B.F. (2002). Neuropsychology. In: R.J. Hagerman & P.J. Hagerman (Eds.), *Fragile X Syndrome: Diagnosis, Treatment, and Research*, (3rd ed., pp. 206-248). Baltimore: The Johns Hopkins University Press.

Bennetto, L., Pennington, B.F., Taylor, A., & Hagerman, R.J. (2001). Profile of cognitive functioning in women with the fragile X mutation. *Neuropsychology, 15*(2), 290-299.

Braden, M. (2002). Academic interventions in fragile X. In: R.J. Hagerman, & P.J. Hagerman (Eds.), *Fragile X Syndrome: Diagnosis, Treatment and Research* (3rd ed., pp. 428-464). Baltimore: The Johns Hopkins University Press.

Butler, M.G., et al. (1991). Anthropometric comparison of mentally retarded males with and without the fragile X syndrome. *Am J Med Genet, 38*, 260-268.

Committee on Infectious Diseases. (2000). *2000 red book: Report of the committee on infectious diseases* (25th ed.), Elk Grove Village, IL: American Academy of Pediatrics.

Crepeau-Hobson, F. & O'Connor, R. (2002). Appendix 4. Toilet Training the Child with Fragile X Syndrome. In: R.J. Hagerman & P.J. Hagerman (Eds.), *Fragile X Syndrome: Diagnosis, Treatment, and Research* (3rd ed., pp. 527-529). Baltimore: The Johns Hopkins University Press.

de Vries, B.B., et al. (1995). General overgrowth in the fragile X syndrome: variability in the phenotypic expression of the FMR1 gene mutation. *J Med Genet, 32*, 764-769.

de Vries, B.B., et al. (1996). Mental status of females with an FMR1 gene full mutation. *Am J Med Genet, 58*, 1025-1032.

Dombrowski, C., et al. (2002). Premutation and intermediate-size FMR1 alleles in 10,572 males from the general population: loss of an AGG interruption is a late event in the generation of fragile X syndrome alleles. *Hum Mol Genetics, 11*, 371-378.

Franke, P., et al. (1998). Genotype-phenotype relationship in female carriers of the premutation and full mutation of FMR-1. *Psychiatry Res, 80*, 113-127.

Gane, L. & Cronister, A. (2002). Genetic Counseling. In: R.J. Hagerman & P.J. Hagerman (Eds.), *The Fragile X Syndrome: Diagnosis, Treatment, and Research* (3rd ed., pp. 251-286). Baltimore: The Johns Hopkins University Press.

Hagerman, P.J. (2002a). FMR1 Gene Expression and Prospects for Gene Therapy. In: R.J. Hagerman & P.J. Hagerman (Eds.), *Fragile X Syndrome: Diagnosis, Treatment and Research*, (3rd ed., pp. 465-494). Baltimore: The Johns Hopkins University Press.

Hagerman, R.J. (1999). Psychopharmacological Interventions in Fragile X Syndrome, Fetal Alcohol Syndrome, Prader-Willi Syndrome, Angelman Syndrome, Smith-Magenis Syndrome, and Velocardiofacial Syndrome. *Ment Retard Dev Disabil Res Rev, 5*, 305-313.

Hagerman, R.J. (2002b). Medical follow-up and pharmacotherapy. In: R.J. Hagerman & P.J. Hagerman (Eds.), *Fragile X Syndrome: Diagnosis, Treatment and Research*, (3rd ed., pp. 287-338). Baltimore: The Johns Hopkins University Press.

Hagerman, R.J. (2002c). Physical and Behavioral Phenotype. In: R.J. Hagerman & P.J. Hagerman (Eds.), *Fragile X Syndrome: Diagnosis, Treatment and Research* (3rd ed., pp. 3-109). Baltimore: The Johns Hopkins University Press.

Hagerman, R.J., et al. (1994). Fluoxetine therapy in fragile X syndrome. *Dev Brain Dys, 7*, 155-164.

Hagerman, R.J., et al. (2001). Intention tremor, parkinsonism, and generalized brain atrophy in male carriers of fragile X. *Neurology, 57*, 127-130.

Hagerman, R.J., Riddle, J.E., Roberts, L.S., Brease, K., & Fulton, M. (1995). A survey of the efficacy of clonidine in fragile X syndrome. *Dev Brain Dys, 8*, 336-344.

Hatton, D.D., Buckley, E.G., Lachiewicz, A., & Roberts, J. (1998). Ocular status of young boys with fragile X syndrome: A prospective study. *J AAPOS, 2*, 298-301.

Hills-Epstein, J., Riley, K., & Sobesky, W. (2002). The Treatment of Emotional and Behavioral Problems. In: R.J. Hagerman & P.J. Hagerman (Eds.), *Fragile X Syndrome: Diagnosis, Treatment, and Research* (3rd ed., pp. 339-362). Baltimore: The Johns Hopkins University Press.

King, R.A., Hagerman, R.J., & Houghton, M. (1995). Ocular findings in fragile X syndrome. *Dev Brain Dys 8*, 223-229.

Lachiewicz, A.M. & Dawson, D.V. (1994). Do young boys with fragile X syndrome have macroorchidism? *Pediatrics, 93*, 992-995.

Miller, L.J., et al. (1999). Electrodermal responses to sensory stimuli in individuals with fragile X syndrome: a preliminary report. *Am J Med Genet, 83*, 268-279.

Musumeci, S.A., et al. (1999). Epilepsy and EEG findings in males with fragile X syndrome. *Epilepsia, 40*, 1092-1099.

Oberlé, I., et al. (1991). Instability of a 550-base pair DNA segment and abnormal methylation in fragile X syndrome. *Science, 252*, 1097-1102.

Oostra, B.A. & Hoogeveen, A.T. (2002). FMR1 Protein Studies and Animal Model for Fragile X Syndrome. In: R.J. Hagerman & P.J. Hagerman (Eds.), *Fragile X Syndrome: Diagnosis, Treatment, and Research* (3rd ed., pp. 169-190). Baltimore: The Johns Hopkins University Press.

Riddle, J.E., et al. (1998). Phenotypic involvement in females with the FMR1 gene mutation. *Am J Ment Retard, 102*, 590-601.

Roberts, J., Mirrett, P., & Burchinal, M. (2001). Receptive and expressive communication development of young males with fragile X syndrome. *Am J Ment Retard, 106*, 216-230.

Rogers, S.J., Wehner, E.A., & Hagerman, R.J. (2001). The behavioral phenotype in fragile X: symptoms of autism in very young children with fragile X syndrome, idiopathic autism, and other developmental disorders. *J Dev Behav Pediatr, 22*, 409-417.

Sabaratnam, M. (2000). Pathological and neuropathological findings in two males with fragile X syndrome. *J Intel Disabil Res, 44*, 81-85.

Scharfenaker, S., O'Connor, R., Stackhouse, T., & Noble, L. (2002). An integrated approach to intervention. In: R.J. Hagerman & P.J. Hagerman (Eds.), *Fragile X Syndrome: Diagnosis, Treatment and Research* (3rd ed., pp 363-427). Baltimore: The Johns Hopkins University Press.

Sherman, S. (1996). Epidemiology. In: R.J. Hagerman & A. Cronister (Eds.), *Fragile X Syndrome: Diagnosis, Treatment, and Research* (2nd ed., pp. 165-192). Baltimore: The Johns Hopkins University Press.

Sherman, S. (2002). Epidemiology. In: R.J. Hagerman & P.J. Hagerman (Eds.) *Fragile X Syndrome: Diagnosis, Treatment and Research* (3rd ed., pp. 136-168). Baltimore: The Johns Hopkins University Press.

Tassone, F., et al. (1999). FMRP expression as a potential prognostic indicator in fragile X syndrome. *Am J Med Genet, 84*, 250-261.

Turner, G., Webb, T., Wake, S., & Robinson, H. (1996). Prevalence of fragile X syndrome. *Am J Med Genet, 64*, 196-197.

Verkerk, A.J., et al. (1991). Identification of a gene (FMR-1) containing a CGG repeat coincident with a breakpoint cluster region exhibiting length variation in fragile X syndrome. *Cell, 65*, 905-914.

Willemsen, R., et al. (1997). Rapid antibody test for prenatal diagnosis of fragile X syndrome on amniotic fluid cells: a new appraisal. *J Med Genet, 34*, 250-251.

Wright Talamante, C., et al. (1996). A controlled study of longitudinal IQ changes in females and males with fragile X syndrome. *Am J Med Genet, 64*, 350-355.

Yu, S., et al. (1991). Fragile X genotype characterized by an unstable region of DNA. *Science, 252*, 1179-1181.

27 Head Injury

Rhonda Burton and Kimberly Moffatt

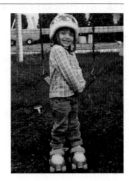

Etiology

Traumatic brain injury (TBI) is defined as a brain insult caused by an external force, which may produce a reduced or altered state of consciousness (Murdoch & Theodoros, 2001). Traumatic brain injury can cause primary and/or secondary injuries. Skull fractures, epidural hematomas, subdural hematomas, intracerebral hematomas, and diffuse axonal injuries are examples of primary injuries. Primary injury to the brain occurs from a direct traumatic force at the moment of impact and is classified as either focal or diffuse. Focal injuries are most commonly associated with a blow to the head, whereas diffuse axonal injuries are the result of inertial forces (violent motion inside the skull) such as those experienced in a motor vehicle accident. Brain damage that occurs as a result of a primary injury is irreversible (Marik et al, 2002).

The primary injury elicits a secondary response from the brain, which includes a cascade of biochemical and physiologic events that can cause neuronal damage and secondary brain injury (Marik et al, 2002). Secondary injuries include the development of intracranial hypertension, cerebral edema, cerebral hemorrhage, seizures, systemic hypotension, hypercapnia, infection, or hypoxemia and significantly increase the morbidity and mortality in children with TBI. Unlike the primary injury, secondary responses and the resulting injury to the brain are amenable to medical and pharmacologic intervention. Although the damage from secondary complications is more diffuse in children than adults, it is more likely to resolve during recovery and rehabilitation (Cronin, 2001).

Mechanisms of Injury

The mechanisms of TBI are a result of forces of deceleration, acceleration, coup-contrecoup, or rotational trauma (Figure 27-1). Deceleration occurs when the head strikes an immovable object, whereas acceleration forces occur when a moving object strikes the head. A coup injury occurs when the brain strikes the cranium on the side of impact, whereas a contrecoup injury occurs when the brain rebounds and strikes the cranium on the contralateral side. Contrecoup injuries are considered more severe, and the size of the impact area affects the injury severity; the smaller the area of impact, the greater the severity of the injury as a result of the concentration of force in the smaller area (Walleck & Mooney, 1994).

Rotational trauma is characterized by a twisting of the brain during deceleration or acceleration, which frequently occurs in combination with coup-contrecoup injuries, resulting in shearing of the tissues (Woestman et al, 1998).

Head Injury Classification

Mild or Severe Head Injury. Head injuries are classified by severity of response (mild, moderate, severe) during the immediate postinjury period. The Glasgow Coma Scale (GCS) has been the most reliable indicator of injury severity and deterioration or improvement (Table 27-1). In 1999 the American Academy of Pediatrics (AAP) and the American Academy of Family Practitioners (AAFP) defined children with minor closed head injury as "those who have normal mental status at the initial examinations, who have no abnormal or focal findings on neurologic exam, and no physical evidence of skull fracture" (AAP and AAFP, 1999, page 1407). Mild head injuries are typically associated with GCS scores of 13 to 15 and moderate head injuries are typically associated with GCS scores of 9 to 12 (Table 27-2). More than 90% of children with TBI injury fall within the mild to moderate range of severity (Cronin, 2001). Severe head injuries are associated with GCS scores of 8 or less and have potential long-term morbidity or mortality (Franzen, 2000; Weiner et al, 2000).

Open or Closed Head Injuries. Open head injuries are the result of penetrating wounds to the skull such as falling onto sharp

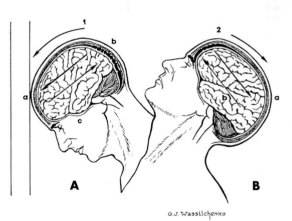

G.J. Wassilchenko

FIGURE 27-1 Coup and contrecoup head injury following blunt trauma. **A,** Coup injury: impact against object. Site of impact and direct trauma to brain (a). Shearing of subdural veins (b). Trauma to base of brain (c). **B,** Contrecoup injury: impact within skull. Site of impact from brain hitting opposite side of skull (a). Shearing forces through brain (b). These injuries occur in one continuous motion—the head strikes the wall (coup), then rebounds (contrecoup). (From Rudy, E. [1984]. *Advanced neurological and neurosurgical nursing.* St. Louis: Mosby. Reprinted with permission.)

TABLE 27-1
Glasgow Coma Scale

	Child >2 Years Old or Adult		Child < 2 Years Old or Developmentally Delayed	
Best eye-opening response	Spontaneously	4	Spontaneously	4
	To verbal command	3	To verbal command	3
	To pain	2	To pain	2
	No response	1	No response	1
Best verbal response	Oriented, converses	5	Coos, babbles	5
	Disoriented, converses	4	Irritable cry	4
	Inappropriate words	3	Cries to pain	3
	Incomprehensible sounds	2	Moans to pain	2
	No response	1	None	1
Best motor response				
To verbal command	Obeys	6	Spontaneous	6
To painful stimulus	Localizes pain	5	Withdraws to touch	5
	Flexion-withdrawal	4	Withdraws to pain	4
	Flexion-decorticate	3	Abnormal flexion	3
	Extension-decerebrate	2	Abnormal extension	2
	No response	1	None	1
Total		(3-15)		(3-15)

From Chipps, E.M., Clanin, N.J., & Campbell, V.G. (1992). *Neurologic disorders*. St. Louis: Mosby; Hazinski, M.F. (1992). Neurologic disorders. In Hazinski, M.F. (Ed.), *Nursing care of the critically ill child*, St. Louis: Mosby. Adapted with permission.

objects or gunshot wounds. In penetrating brain injuries, skull fragments tear the dura mater. Open wounds are most commonly associated with focal brain pathology (Murdoch & Theodoros, 2001). Closed head injuries are the result of nonpenetrating wounds and can result in cerebral concussion, contusion, or hematoma.

Focal or Diffuse Injuries. Focal vascular lacerations or contusions occur when brain damage is localized to one area due to an expanding mass. Diffuse injuries occur when brain damage is widespread due to generalized brain edema or ischemia, systemic hypoxia, or hypotension. Brain injuries in children are most commonly diffuse closed head injuries.

Intracranial Injury

Skull Fracture. Skull fractures occur when external forces exceed the skull's tolerance (Roth & Farls, 2000). Skull fractures may or may not show bony displacement or swelling. The incidence of skull fracture is higher in children when compared with adults, especially in children younger than 2 because infants have thinner cranial bones (Weiner & Weinberg, 2000). Skull fractures are a predictor for intracranial injury. When fractures do occur, about 60% to 70% involve the parietal bone and are most often linear (Evans & Wilberger, 1999; Schutzman & Greenes, 2001). Though most linear fractures are associated with overlying hematomas of soft tissue swelling, they typically heal without complications. Linear fractures can result from low velocity and blunt or compression trauma (Roth & Farls, 2000). They don't play a significant role with severe head injury; however, with mild head injury, the presence of a fracture increases the risk of intracranial injury fourfold (Evans & Wilberger, 1999). Other less common skull fractures include depressed and basilar fractures (Schutzman et al, 2001; Marik et al, 2002). Depressed skull fractures occur in the presence of greater force velocity and blunt or compression trauma and can cause tissue damage or hemorrhage. Because of this, depressed

TABLE 27-2
Severity of Head Injury

Mild	Moderate	Severe
Asymptomatic or Minimal loss of consciousness with rapid clearing of mental status or Headache or Vomiting or Irritability GCS 13-15	>10 min posttraumatic unconsciousness or Posttraumatic seizures or Focal neurologic deficits or Retrograde amnesia lasting >30 min or Evidence of depressed skull fracture, basilar skull fracture, or CSF leak or Severe headache or Persistent vomiting or Irritability GCS 9-12	Respiratory distress or Circulatory instability or Altered mental status (unresponsiveness, coma) or Marked irritability or Signs of increased intracranial pressure GCS ≤ 8

GCS, Glasgow Coma Score.
From Fox, J. (1997). *Primary healthcare of children*. St. Louis: Mosby; Berman, S. (1997). *Pediatric decision making*. St. Louis: Mosby. Adapted with permissions.

skull fractures are neurosurgical emergencies (Roth & Farls, 2000). Basilar fractures should be monitored more closely than linear fractures secondary to cerebrospinal fluid leakage, infection and/or cranial nerve palsies (Evans & Wilberger, 1999).

Concussion. The least serious type of TBI is a concussion, which is a transient alteration in mental status post head trauma (Schutzman & Greenes, 2001). Rapid acceleration/deceleration injuries or sudden blows to the head cause concussions. The

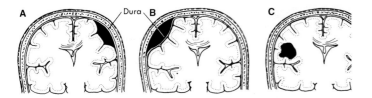

FIGURE 27-2 Different types of hematomas. **A,** Subdural. **B,** Epidural. **C,** Intracerebral. (From Thelan, L.A., et al [1994]. *Critical care nursing: diagnosis and management* [2nd ed.]. St. Louis: Mosby. Reprinted with permission.)

typical concussion presentation is loss of consciousness (LOC) for less than 6 hours and retrograde posttraumatic amnesia. The symptoms are usually reversible, but in some instances there may be subtle residual neurological impairment. Several weeks postinjury, children should be observed for the presence of symptoms suggestive of postconcussion syndrome. These symptoms include dizziness, headache, irritability, poor concentration, emotional lability and poor judgment, which can last up to 1 year postinjury (Roth & Farls, 2000).

Contusion and Laceration. Cerebral contusions are the result of the brain moving within the skull causing bruises along the surface of the brain. Cerebral contusions can occur at the site of impact (coup) and/or opposite the side of impact (contrecoup). Contusions are the most frequently seen lesions in older children after a head injury. Common locations for contusions include the frontal, occipital, and parietal areas. Lacerations may also occur with contusions and are due to a penetrating head injury or depressed skull fracture. Lacerations involve tearing of the cortical surface with damage to the surrounding tissues (Roth & Farls, 2000).

Diffuse Axonal Injury. Diffuse axonal injury (DAI) is a term used to describe diffuse degeneration of white matter, global neurologic dysfunction, and diffuse cerebral swelling at the time of impact. This damage results from axonal shearing, which causes swelling, degeneration, and disconnection of axons (Roth & Farls, 2000; Marik et al, 2002). The symptoms of DAI include prolonged unconsciousness, increased intracranial pressure, hypertension, and decerebrate posture. The severity of injury corresponds with the amount of shearing force applied. The resulting injury to the brain tissue leads to widespread cerebral edema and neuronal dysfunction. Children with DAI have a high mortality rate. Those who survive typically do so in a persistent vegetative state (Evans & Wilberger, 1999; Marik et al, 2002).

Cerebral Hemorrhage. Cerebral hemorrhage, or hematoma, results in a mass lesion effect that causes elevated intracranial pressure (Figure 27-2). Of individuals with skull fractures, 25% develop significant hematoma. Epidural hematomas are relatively uncommon and present in less than 1% of those with head injury. These rare hematomas occur between the dura and the skull and are often arterial. Subdural hematomas occur in 30% of children with severe head injury (Evans & Wilberger, 1999; Marik et al, 2002). Blood collects between the dura and arachnoid meninges layer. They are classified as acute (occurred in the past 48 hours), subacute (occurred in the past 2-14 days), and chronic (occurred >14 days ago). Intracerebral hemorrhage produces mass lesions primarily in the frontal and temporal lobes. These hemorrhages occur mainly in the presence of

moderate and severe head injuries such as significant blows to the head or depressed skull fractures (Roth & Farls, 2000; Marik et al, 2002). Surgical evacuation of an intracerebral hemorrhage occurs only when medical therapies to decrease intracranial pressure fail.

Cerebral Edema. Cerebral edema, either focal or generalized, is the result of an increase in tissue fluid from intracellular or extracellular sources. It may be caused by either the initial injury to the neuronal tissue or secondarily in response to hypoxia, hypercapnia, or cerebral ischemia. Cerebral edema can cause increased intracranial pressure (ICP). Signs and symptoms of increased intracranial pressure include irritability, lethargy, nausea and vomiting, headache, photophobia, pupillary changes, abnormal reflexes, seizures, widening pulse pressure, bradycardia, and apnea.

Peak response for cerebral edema usually occurs up to 72 hours after the neurologic insult, and gradually resolves over a 2- to 3-week period (Walleck & Mooney, 1994). If left untreated or poorly controlled, cerebral edema can have a devastating effect, resulting in intracranial hypertension and altered cerebral perfusion. These results can lead to neuronal tissue hypoxia, ischemia, cerebral herniation, and death.

Known Genetic Etiology

There is no known genetic predisposition to head injury.

Incidence and Prevalence

Injuries represent the leading cause of death and disability among children in the United States, with a majority of death and disability resulting from head trauma (Youngblut et al, 2000; Tilford et al, 2001). Head trauma in children accounts for an estimated 600,000 emergency department visits, 95,000 hospital admissions, and 550,000 hospital days annually (Schutzman & Greenes, 2001; Schutzman et al, 2001). Approximately 180 children per 100,000 sustain closed head injuries annually (Ponsford et al, 2001). It is estimated that children between 1 and 15 years of age have fatal head trauma injuries at a rate of 10 per 100,000 annually (Reece & Sege, 2000). Head trauma is the third leading cause of death in children younger than the age of 1 and the most common cause of death and new disabilities in childhood. Whereas the majority of head injuries are considered minor, requiring no intervention, it is estimated that at least 29,000 children experience permanent neurologic symptoms and another 7,000 are fatally injured from head injuries (Schutzman & Greenes, 2001). In the United States more than $1 billion is spent providing hospital care to children with head injuries annually (Weiner & Weinberg, 2000; Schutzman et al, 2001; Tilford et al, 2001).

Head injuries in children commonly result from falls, child abuse, and bicycle and motor vehicle accidents. In children less than 2 years of age, child abuse is the main cause of head injury. In children 2 to 4 years of age, falls are the main cause of head injury. In older children, bicycle, vehicle, and recreational accidents are the main cause of head injury (Weiner & Weinberg, 2000). Of traumatic head injuries in children, 82% are considered mild, 14% are moderate or severe, and 5% are fatal. An estimated 2.5 million to 6.5 million individuals (both children and adults) are living with lasting effects of TBI (NIH, 1999).

BOX 27-1
Clinical Manifestations at Time of Diagnosis
Physical findings determined by severity and type of injury
Assessment tools for TBI
Glasgow Coma Scale (GCS)
Children's Coma Scale (CCS)

Factors influencing traumatic head injury in children include gender (i.e., males are affected more often than females at a ratio as high as 2:1 during adolescence), socioeconomic factors (i.e., increased incidence in low socioeconomic classes), and time of year (i.e., increased incidence in spring and summer) (Adelson & Kochanek, 1998; Alexander & Moore, 2001). Peak occurrence is evenings, nights, weekends, and holidays when children are outside playing, swimming, riding bicycles, traveling in cars, or victims of gunshot wounds.

Clinical Manifestations at the Time of Diagnosis

The clinical manifestations at the time of diagnosis vary depending on the primary brain injury and the extent and involvement of secondary responses (Box 27-1). Children with head injuries can present with varying degrees of alertness and responsiveness, depending on the degree of increased intracranial pressure. Children who have sustained a mild TBI can experience headache, dizziness, and fatigue up to 1 week postinjury (Ponsford et al, 2001). If the child sustains an epidural hematoma, clinical manifestations include immediate loss of consciousness, followed by a lucid period of wakefulness, followed by rapid deterioration in neurologic status. Other symptoms may include headache, seizure, vomiting, hemiparesis, and fixed and dilated pupils. Prompt surgical removal of the hematoma results in a favorable outcome. Clinical manifestations of a subdural hematoma range from headache and fatigue to seizure, papilledema, and hemiparesis. Clinical manifestations of intracranial hemorrhage (ICH) are headache, deteriorating LOC, dilated pupil on the side of the hemorrhage, and hemiplegia on the opposite side of the hemorrhage. It takes at least 24 hours after the insult to see ICH on a computed tomography (CT) scan (Roth & Farls, 2000; Marik et al, 2002).

As cerebral edema and increased intracranial pressure rise, herniation ensues (Schutzman & Greenes, 2001). Clinical manifestations of herniation are changes in level of consciousness, abnormal respiratory patterns, loss of protective reflexes (e.g., gag or corneal), changes in blood pressure and pulse pressure with bradycardia, pupillary dysfunction, papilledema, changes in motor function or posturing, nausea and projectile vomiting, positive Babinski sign, and visual disturbances (Adelson & Kochanek, 1998).

The GCS has become the standard tool to measure a child's level of consciousness and severity of head injury (Alexander & Moore, 2001). The GCS objectively scores the child's best responses to motor, verbal, and eye-opening stimulation (see Table 27-1). The highest combined score is 15 and the lowest is 3. Any score less than 15 is considered an alteration in the level of consciousness. The GCS, along with the clinician's

BOX 27-2
Children's Coma Scale
Maximum score = 11
Minimum score = 3
Motor response: maximum score = 4
4   flexes and extends
3   withdraws from painful stimulus
2   hypertonic
1   flaccid
Verbal response: maximum score = 3
3   cries
2   spontaneous respirations
1   apneic
Ocular response: maximum score = 4
4   pursuit
3   extraocular muscles (EOM) intact, reactive pupils
2   fixed pupils of EOM impaired
1   fixed pupil and EOM paralyzed

From Ghajar, J. & Hariri, R. (1992). Management of pediatric head injury. *Pediatr Clin North Am, 39*, 1093-1125.

physical assessment, should be used in evaluating children with a head injury during the acute care period.

Despite its limitations for use in infants and preverbal children, individuals with a preinjury deficit (i.e., hemiparesis, cognitive deficit), or individuals that are intubated, a Children's Coma Scale (CCS) was developed (Box 27-2) (Gharjar & Hariri, 1992). However, it is not used as commonly as the GCS.

Treatment
Mild Traumatic Brain Injury

The goal of treatment in children with minor traumatic brain injury is to maximize the ability to function independently while minimizing any disability (Goka, 2000). Children younger than 2, who have sustained minor head trauma, provide a challenge to providers because their assessment is more difficult. They may be asymptomatic postinjury despite having an intracranial injury. Children considered at high risk of developing intracranial injury are those who are difficult to arouse, have an abnormal neurologic exam, signs or symptoms of a skull fracture, irritability, progressively worsening vomiting, or a bulging fontanelle. Children with any of these signs or symptoms should receive a CT scan.

Children considered at moderate risk of developing intracranial injury are those with four or fewer episodes of vomiting, LOC less than 1 minute, reports of lethargy or irritability, skull fracture present more than 24 hours, behavior reportedly not at baseline, a fall onto a hard surface, a scalp hematoma, or unwitnessed trauma. They should receive a CT scan at the discretion of the provider. Children in the moderate risk group who do not receive a CT scan should be observed for up to 6 hours for the development of neurologic symptoms.

Children considered at low risk of developing intracranial injury are those who fell less than 3 feet and have a normal neurologic exam at least 2 hours' postinjury. In children considered low risk a CT scan is typically not warranted (Schutzman et al, 2001). However, children younger than 2 years of age have a

BOX 27-3
Pediatric Brain Injury Sign/Symptom Checklist

Please take a few minutes to check off any of the following concerns for yourself and/or your child since the brain injury occurred:

— decrease in smell
— ringing in ears
— sudden changes in emotion
— irritability
— change in personality
— trouble naming things
— problems swallowing
— attention difficulties
— change in appetite
— neck or back pain
— bowel problems
— bladder problems
— nausea or vomiting
— memory problems
— school problems
— anxiety

— change in food tastes
— vision changes
— impulsivity
— depression
— trouble speaking
— problems chewing
— choking on food
— easy distractibility
— headaches
— seizures
— sleep problems
— dizziness
— confusion
— bizarre statements
— tics
— violent behavior

From Alexander, J. & Moore, D. (2001). Primary care for children with brain injury. *NC Med J, 62*(6), 344-348.

BOX 27-4
Treatment of Severe Head Trauma

Prehospital stabilization
Early treatment determined by severity of TBI
Need to control hypoxia, increased cerebral CO_2 and brain edema
Surgical intervention for bleeding, trauma, or cerebral edema may be necessary
Recovery from coma follows predictable patterns but with varied time sequence
Rehabilitation program key to long-term recovery

higher risk of intracranial injury even with minor mechanisms of injury (Schutzman & Greenes, 2001).

The AAP and AAFP (1999) devised parameters to manage minor closed head injury in children older than 2, within the first 24 hours of the injury (Figure 27-3). Children with minor closed head trauma are defined as those with normal mental status at initial examination with no abnormal or focal findings on neurologic examination and have no physical evidence of a skull fracture. The parameter also considers those children who may have experienced temporary loss of consciousness (<1 minute), had a seizure or vomited and/or exhibited headache or lethargy postinjury.

For a child with *mild closed head injury with no loss of consciousness*, an initial evaluation should include a thorough history, physical, and neurologic exam. Observation is sufficient with the goal of recognizing worsening symptoms and subsequently seeking appropriate medical assistance. Fewer than 1 in 5,000 people with mild closed head injury with no loss of consciousness have intracranial injuries that require medical or neurosurgical interventions (AAP & AAFP, 1999). CT and magnetic resonance imaging (MRI) scans are not necessary because they provide only marginal benefits of early detection of intracranial injury. However, a cranial CT is the preferred imaging technique if desired.

For a child *with mild closed head injury with loss of consciousness (<1 minute)*, an initial evaluation should include a thorough history, physical, and neurologic exam. Although observation is sufficient, a cranial CT scan may be ordered at the discretion of the provider. Because children with signs and symptoms such as headache, vomiting, or lethargy are more likely to have intracranial injury, a cranial CT or MRI is the preferred brain imaging study.

Because most brain injuries are minor and observation is the most common treatment, instructions should be given to guardians/parents/caretakers describing postinjury signs and symptoms that require medical attention (Box 27-3).

Severe Traumatic Brain Injury (Box 27-4)

Medical management in the prehospital setting is an important predictor of outcome following TBI. The goal of treatment is to stabilize the effects of the primary injury and prevent secondary injuries due to hypoxia, hypercarbia, cerebral edema, seizures, infection, and aspiration, and to surgically treat correctable intracranial lesions. Initial treatment begins with cervical stabilization and support of the airway, breathing, and circulation (Schutzman & Greenes, 2001; Marik et al, 2002).

Children who have sustained a severe TBI are best managed at a trauma center with neurologic and neurosurgical services. To prevent secondary injuries, treatment includes intubation, ventilation, fluid resuscitation, diuretics, and blood pressure monitoring (Evans & Wilberger, 1999; Marik et al, 2002).

Recovery from Coma

Most children who lapse into a coma as a result of a traumatic brain injury eventually regain consciousness (Adelson & Kochanek, 1998). Ninety percent of children younger than 15 years of age who have survived a severe head injury will recover to a moderately disabled state or better over a 3-year period postinjury. The duration of a coma is the length of time from its onset until the display of meaningful response to external stimuli (Alexander & Moore, 2001). Its length is directly proportional to neurologic sequelae. A coma less than 6 hours is rarely associated with severe neuropsychologic problems. A coma lasting more than 7 days is associated with a decline in IQ. About 90% of children in a coma lasting less than 6 weeks will return to independent function (Weiner & Weinberg, 2000).

Long-Term Management and Rehabilitation

Rehabilitation can hasten and maximize restoration of lost functions, promote adaptation to disabilities, and aid in age-appropriate independence and reintegration into family and school life. Rehabilitation can enhance the quality of life of children with TBI and reduce future health care expenditures. Most post-brain injury undergoes spontaneous recovery in the first 6 months postinjury. Deficits remaining after this period typically are permanent (Goka, 2000). The GCS helps predict rehabilitation outcomes on the basis of four categories: mild, moderate, severe, and vegetative state (Table 27-3).

The broad range of symptoms present after TBI include movement disorders, seizures, visual deficits, and sleep disorders. Management of these symptoms requires an

Evaluation and Triage of Children and Adolescents with Minor Head Trauma

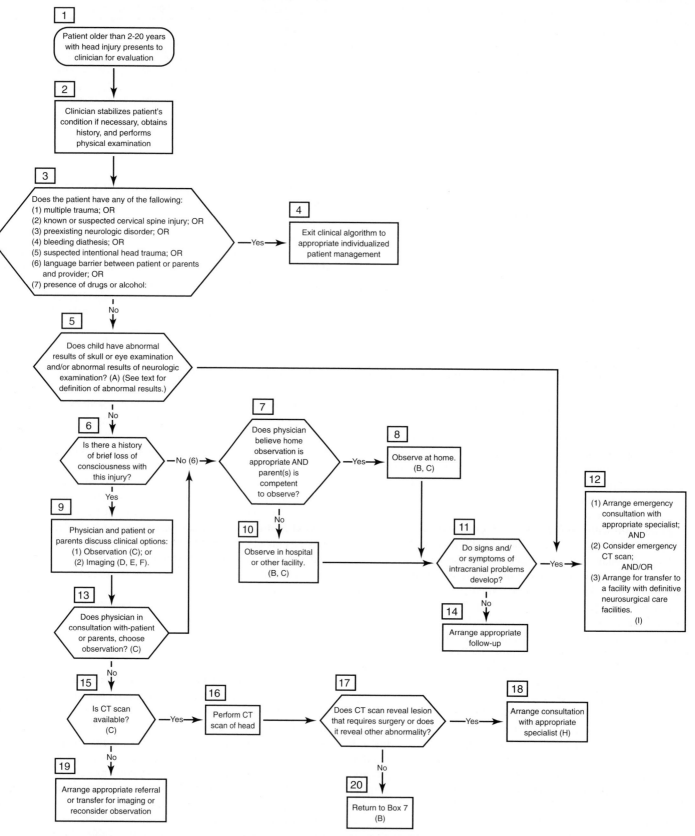

FIGURE 27-3 Treatment of mild head trauma. (From Committee on Quality Improvement, American Academy of Pediatrics and Commission on Clinical Policies and Research, American Academy of Family Physicians. [1999]. The management of minor closed head injury in children, *Pediatrics, 106*(6)1407-1415.)

TABLE 27-3
Glasgow Coma Scale: Outcomes

Category and Score	Description
Vegetative state (<5)	A persistent state of impaired consciousness.
Severe (5-8)	Child is conscious but requires 24-hour care and supervision because of cognitive, behavioral, or physical disabilities. Slow response time and difficulties with short-term memory predominate.
Moderate (9-12)	Child is expected to achieve eventual independence in activities of daily living and home and community activities with persistent disability. Children in this group may have memory impairments, hemiparesis, dysphagia, ataxia, and other neuromotor problems.
Mild (13-15)	Good recovery is expected. Child is able to reintegrate into normal social life. There may be mild persisting sequelae.

From Winkler, P. (1995). Head injury. In Umphred, D. (Ed.), *Neurological rehabilitation* (3rd ed.). St. Louis: Mosby. Adapted with permission.

BOX 27-5
Associated Problems

Neurologic dysfunction
  Posttraumatic hydrocephalus
  Posttraumatic seizures
  Postconcussion syndrome
Abnormal motor and sensory function
Feeding problems
Endocrine dysfunction
Altered cognitive and neuropsychologic functions
Speech/communication deficits
Psychosocial and psychiatric deficits
Additional physiologic problems (see Box 27-5)

interdisciplinary or multidisciplinary approach to develop an individualized treatment plan (NIH, 1999). The team of specialists is generally directed by a pediatric physiatrist (a physician of physical medicine rehabilitation). Within the team of experts, physical and occupational therapists attend to physical limitations by passive range-of-motion exercises, limb splinting, and proper support and positioning, which prevent physical deformities (e.g., extremity contractures) that result from prolonged immobilization and increased tone. Rehabilitation reestablishes learning through repetitive stimulation. Daily repetition permanently programs or reprograms the brain (Goka, 2000).

The team's psychologists, psychiatrists, social workers, and recreational life therapists guide emotional, social, and behavioral aspects of a child's recovery. The team's speech and language pathologists and special education teachers direct school reentry (Goka, 2000).

The role of the primary care provider is often incorporated into the final stages of inpatient rehabilitation. The provider is updated on the child's medical conditions and functional limitations, the team of subspecialists providing services, and the types of therapy and equipment necessary after discharge. Together the primary care provider and the rehabilitation staff evaluate the community resources and services and implement the support that will be necessary to the child and family upon returning home.

The process of recovery does not stop when a child is discharged from the inpatient unit. Continued emotional, physical, medical, nursing, and cognitive support for the child and family is needed until the quality of life is acceptable to the child, family, and care providers. In addition, respite opportunities for the family and other providers are important and should be arranged. The decision to discharge the child from a rehabilitation program should be considered when reasonable treatment goals have been achieved or no further progress is demonstrated.

Complementary and Alternative Treatments
Interventions such as music and art therapy, therapeutic recreation, acupuncture, and other alternative approaches are com-

monly used; however, their efficacy has not been substantiated (NIH, 1999). One study showed homeopathic medication may actually have a role in treating persistent mild TBI (Chapman et al, 1999).

Anticipated Advances in Diagnoses and Management

Current advances in the management and treatment of children with head injuries center around monitoring and preventing or treating secondary responses and injuries. Maintaining adequate cerebral perfusion pressure at a minimum of 70 mm Hg is recommended to avoid cerebral ischemia. Intracranial pressure monitoring is recommended in those with GCS less than or equal to 8. Intraventricular catheters have become the standard when treating severe head injuries and have been attributed to improved outcomes (Marik et al, 2002).

There have been attempts to decrease brain damage after TBI with free radical scavengers, aminosteroids, calcium antagonists, glutamate antagonists, ion channel blockers, and adenosine agonists; however, these have not yet been shown to be efficacious (Marik et al, 2002).

Associated Problems (Box 27-5)
Neurologic Dysfunction

Posttraumatic Hydrocephalus. Posttraumatic hydrocephalus occurs in a small number of individuals after head trauma, most commonly in those who have suffered a subarachnoid hemorrhage. Cerebral ventriculomegaly may arise weeks or months after head injury. In children with severe head injury, the ventriculomegaly may be due to cerebral atrophy. If a diagnosis of hydrocephalus is made, treatment consists of placement of a valve-regulating shunt. Surgical management via a shunt relieves the acute symptoms (see Chapter 29).

Posttraumatic Seizures. The incidence of posttraumatic seizures in children is about 10% (Pellock et al, 2001). Posttraumatic seizures are classified as early (i.e., occurring within 7 days of injury) or late (i.e., occurring 7 days after injury). Studies have indicated that prophylactic administration of anticonvulsants during the first week reduces the incidence of early seizures. Extended use of anticonvulsants, however, does not reduce the incidence of late seizures. Anticonvulsants should therefore only be given prophylactically for 1 week and then discontinued unless chronic seizures develop. Chronic seizures are usually well controlled with anticonvulsant medications. The onset of these seizures varies greatly, from soon after the initial injury to 2 years following the injury (Evans & Wilberger, 1999) (see Chapter 25).

Postconcussion Syndrome. Postconcussion syndrome can occur after a mild head injury. The most common symptoms include headaches, irritability, anxiety, behavioral disturbances, dizziness, fatigue, impaired concentration, forgetfulness, blurred vision, nausea, sleep disturbances, and noise sensitivity. This syndrome usually appears days to weeks after the initial injury and can persist up to a year postinjury (Evans & Wilberger, 1999; Roth & Farls, 2000). Management is symptomatic.

Abnormal Motor and Sensory Function

Common motor disabilities for children following a head injury include muscle stiffness (i.e., spasticity), movement problems (i.e., ataxia), changes in muscle elasticity (i.e., contractures), paralysis and speech impairments. The incidence and severity increase with coma following injury. Although 5% to 30% of children with traumatic brain injury manifest some motor control problems, many show improvements for up to 7 years postinjury. In addition, audiologic problems and visual deficits may develop. Occupational and physical therapies are provided at regular intervals to maximize balance, coordination, and strength, as well as to retrain individuals in assisted, and ultimately independent, ambulation and other functional activities leading to developmentally appropriate self-care. Adaptive equipment (crutches, walkers, wheelchairs, lifts, and mechanical seats) may be used as needed. Surgical and pharmacologic interventions are available to address motor problems (Cronin, 2001).

Feeding Problems

Many children with severe TBI cannot eat on their own because of physical limitations or inability to coordinate chewing and swallowing (Alexander & Moore, 2001). Children often have nasogastric or gastrostomy tubes to facilitate nutrition. A child's ability to feed is often an area of focus for a family due to the emotional, social, and cultural beliefs surrounding feeding and nutrition. Use of a registered dietitian to maintain fluid balance, appropriate caloric intake, and nutrition status for growth is highly recommended.

Endocrine Dysfunction

Children post–severe head injury may experience hyperphasia, hypothyroidism, precocious puberty, amenorrhea, growth failure, and leg length discrepancy from fractures and an enlarging skull defect (Alexander & Moore, 2001). After a severe head injury, children may initially show signs of antidiuretic dysfunction such as (1) diabetes insipidus, which presents as hypernatremia, polydipsia, and polyuria, or (2) syndrome of inappropriate secretion of antidiuretic hormone (SIADH), which consists of hyponatremia and decreased urinary output. Either dysfunction resolves in most children but is a lifelong issue for some. Children who have any sign of endocrine dysfunction should be evaluated and followed by an endocrinologist.

Altered Cognitive and Neuropsychologic Function

Deficits may be noted in the areas of memory, word retrieval, naming, verbal organization, comprehension of verbal information, comprehension of verbal abstractions, efficient verbal learning, and effective conversation and discourse. Difficulties in attention and concentration, poor judgment, and impulsivity may persist. There may also be perceptual impairment, poor motor planning, tactile sensory dysfunction, and spatial disorientation (Cronin, 2001). Neuropsychologic testing can identify deficits.

Speech/Communication Deficits

Impairments in expressive and receptive language are common in children with traumatic brain injury with mild to moderate injury being more impaired in expressive language, notably deficits of memory, word retrieval, labeling, and verbal organization. Improvement of speech is consistent with gains in motor function. Improvement in language ability (predominantly a cognitive function) may lag in severe cases despite aggressive therapy by speech and language specialists (Cronin, 2001).

Psychosocial and Psychiatric Deficits

There is an increased risk for persistent and transient psychological sequelae following significant pediatric traumatic brain injury (Bloom et al, 2001). Emotional or behavioral difficulties that predate the brain injury are likely to be exacerbated (Alexander & Moore, 2001; Vasa et al, 2002).

Organic personality syndrome is the most common psychiatric disorder among children who have sustained a severe TBI. Organic personality syndrome includes affective instability, aggression, markedly impaired social judgment and occasionally apathy or paranoia (Max et al, 1998). The most frequent anxiety symptoms seen post–severe TBI are being overanxious, obsessive-compulsive disorders, separation anxiety, and phobia symptoms (Vasa et al, 2002).

Additional Problems Associated with Traumatic Brain Injury

A variety of other associated problems or complications can occur after traumatic brain injury and are listed in Box 27-6. Primary care providers must recognize these as potential complications when providing care to children with a history of significant head injury.

Prognosis

The key factor associated with overall outcome is the severity and type of traumatic brain injury. Of the children who sustain traumatic brain injury, 95% survive; however, of the children who sustain a severe head injury, only 65% survive (Michaud et al, 1993; Jennett, 1998). Children with diffuse injury have better outcomes than children with focal lesions in addition to a diffuse injury (Weiner & Weinberg, 2000). Significant extracranial injuries and related problems of hypoxia and hypotension are associated with a poorer survival rate and

BOX 27-6
Additional Problems Associated with Traumatic Brain Injury

Focal neurologic deficits
Neurogenic pulmonary edema
Pneumonia
Gastrointestinal hemorrhage
Cardiac dysrhythmias
Disseminated intravascular coagulation
Pulmonary emboli
Heterotopic ossifications
Increased muscle tone
Contractures
Aspiration
Hypertension
Disturbances of respiratory control
Hypopituitarism
Impaired nutritional status
Bladder incontinence
Bowel incontinence
Hyperphagia

Adapted from Chipps, E.M., Clanin, N.J., & Campbell, V.G. (1992). *Neurologic disorders.* St. Louis: Mosby.

TABLE 27-4
Glasgow Coma Scale Scores vs. Glasgow Outcomes Scale

GCS at 24 Hrs	Good Recovery or Moderate Disability %	Vegetative or Dead %
11-15	91	6
8-10	59	27
5-7	28	54
3-4	13	80

From Chipps, E.M., Clanin, N.J., and Campbell, V.G. (1992). St. Louis: Mosby. Reprinted with permission.

outcome (Weiner & Weinberg, 2000; Marik et al, 2002). Length of coma, changes in GCS scores in the first 24 hours, age, postresuscitation GCS scores, neurological reflex, posttraumatic seizures, CT scan findings, and availability of rehabilitation services also are considered prognostic indicators. However, there is debate whether rehabilitation optimizes functional outcomes or quickens the time to reach the functional plateau (Cronin, 2001) (Table 27-4).

Despite improvements in imaging techniques and aggressive management for infants, toddlers, and young children with traumatic brain injuries, the clinical examination is the strongest predictor of outcome (Yoon & Narayan, in press). Potential outcomes range from coma and permanent neurologic damage to a brief loss of consciousness followed by the resumption of full neurologic functioning. Of survivors with mild traumatic brain injury, 20% will have a residual disability (Hawley et al, 2002).

Long-term prognosis is more difficult to evaluate. The reasons for higher percentages of good neurologic outcome in the pediatric population are unclear but could be attributed to the resilient properties of the immature brain (Beaulieu, 2002).

PRIMARY CARE MANAGEMENT

Health Care Maintenance
Growth and Development

Because of the risk of hydrocephalus and altered nutritional intake, weight, height, and head circumference should be measured and plotted on a growth chart at each clinic visit.

Precocious puberty may occur in association with head trauma as a result of potential disruption of the normal hypothalamus and pituitary function. Premature sexual characteristics can include isolated breast, axillary, or pubic hair development. Referral to a pediatric endocrinologist is recommended for more in-depth management.

Severe head injury may affect major milestone attainment or cause milestone regression, and therefore developmental progress should be monitored and community services obtained for physical therapy, occupational therapy, and speech therapy as needed and available.

Diet

Children with severe TBI may experience swallowing difficulties due to oral-motor incoordination and problems chewing. In turn, this can lead to dysphagia, aspiration, or poor weight gain (Alexander & Moore, 2001). Placement of a gastrostomy tube and fundoplication may be considered for long-term management. Potential aspiration or gastroesophageal reflux concerns may be addressed by placing the child in a side-lying position during and after meals. Difficulty with immobility may lead to increased bone calcium loss as a result of inadequate weight bearing (Boss, 1994). Because these problems can lead to poor nutritional status, referrals to a gastroenterologist, nutritionist, and/or occupational therapist may be necessary.

Safety

As with all pediatric visits, counseling about safety practices and injury prevention at a child's age and developmental level is appropriate. Although it is impossible to prevent all minor head injury, efforts to minimize head trauma should be discussed. Use of appropriate motor vehicle passenger seat restraints, helmets, and home childproofing should be reinforced. Adolescents with severe post-TBI may have increased safety risks as a result of neuropsychiatric sequelae impairing judgment, and motor coordination. Parents may need help determining appropriate adolescent responsibilities and activities, including driving.

Children with severe traumatic brain injury are at an increased risk for future injury due to neuropsychologic and neurobehavioral deficits resulting in overactivity, poor judgment, impulsivity, and perceptual deficits similar to children with attention deficit hyperactivty disorder (Michaud et al, 1993) (see Chapter 12). Assistive devices if used (e.g., wheelchairs and walkers) should be assessed for safety. Family members and care providers should also be knowledgeable of seizure precautions and seizure first aid if seizures are a complication of the head injury (see Chapter 25).

Minor head injury is rarely associated with significant long-term sequelae with the exception of sports-related head injuries. *Second impact syndrome* refers to cerebral edema from a relatively mild head trauma after a concussion. The syndrome is believed to be caused by impaired cerebral autoregulation. This swelling can be irreversible and fatal if one minor head injury is followed by another injury in close succession, while still symptomatic from the first injury. The American Academy of Neurology defined three grades of concussion and recommendations for return to sports activities (Box 27-7) (Evans & Wilberger, 1999; Schutzman & Greenes, 2001). The primary care provider must educate families, children, and school personnel regarding this potential serious complication.

Immunization

Routine immunizations are recommended. In general, immunizations can be given when the child's neurologic situation is stabilized. The risk of contracting these preventable diseases versus the risk of the immunization side effects should be discussed with the family. Postimmunization fever management with antipyretics is recommended. Children with known seizure history may be more susceptible to febrile seizures following the administration of diphtheria, tetanus, and acellular pertussis (DTaP) (CDC, 2000).

Screening

Vision. Vision can be adversely affected in children after a TBI. People with TBI may experience symptoms of double vision, movement of fixed objects such as walls, eyestrain, visual fatigue, and loss of peripheral vision (Padula & Argyris, 2001-02; Fisk et al, 2002). In the presence of visual deficits, a referral to a pediatric ophthalmologist is recommended.

Routine periodic screening for vision is recommended if deficits are not determined in the immediate postinjury period.

Hearing. Hearing can be adversely affected after TBI, and the most common sequelae reported are tinnitus, vestibular dysfunction, intolerance to loud/sudden noises, and sensorineural hearing impairment (Jury & Flynn, 2001). An audiologist referral is recommended in the presence of hearing deficits. Routine periodic screening for hearing is recommended if deficits are not determined in the immediate postinjury period.

Dental. Routine dental care is recommended. Children with head injuries may have fractured or missing teeth secondary to facial trauma and a pediatric orthodontist referral is necessary.

Blood Pressure. Routine screening and evaluation are recommended. Persistently elevated blood pressure should be evaluated, particularly in the presence of an intracranial shunt (see Chapter 29).

Hematocrit. Routine screening is recommended. Intracranial bleeding, especially in the newborn and young infant, may result in anemia.

Urinalysis. Routine screening is recommended to rule out indications of trauma and low urine specific gravity (a possible indicator of diabetes insipidus).

Tuberculosis. Routine screening is recommended. If prophylactic medications are needed, evaluate potential drug interactions in children taking other medications.

Condition-Specific Screening

Posttraumatic Seizure Therapy. For those children on anticonvulsant medication for seizures, periodic blood testing will be necessary to determine medication blood levels and test for hematologic effects and liver dysfunction. These tests should be ordered in consultation with the child's neurologist (see Chapter 25).

Common Illness Management

Differential Diagnosis (Box 27-8)

Children with traumatic brain injury are susceptible to common childhood illnesses, just like any other child; however, the management of these illnesses may differ depending upon the sequelae.

Alterations in Cognition or Level of Consciousness. Knowledge of the child's baseline neurologic status and behavior is the key to accurate assessment. A significant change in cognitive function should be viewed as pathologic, and assessed. Trauma, infections, tumors, and metabolic imbalances may cause alterations in arousal or cognition. The onset may be sudden, subacute over

---

BOX 27-7

Summary of Recommendations for Return to Sports Activity after Concussion

GRADE 1 CONCUSSION

Definition. Transient confusion, no loss of consciousness, and duration of mental status abnormalities <15 minutes.

Management. Return to sports activity same day only if all symptoms resolve within 15 minutes: if a second grade 1 concussion occurs, no sports activity until asymptomatic for 1 week.

GRADE 2 CONCUSSION

Definition. Transient confusion, no loss of consciousness, and a duration of mental status abnormalities ≥15 minutes.

Management. No sports activity until asymptomatic for 1 full week, if a grade 2 concussion occurs on the same day as a grade 1 concussion, no sports activity until asymptomatic for 2 weeks.

GRADE 3 CONCUSSION

Definition. Concussion involving loss of consciousness (LOC).

Management. No sports activity until asymptomatic for 1 week if loss of consciousness is brief (seconds); no sports activity until asymptomatic for 2 weeks if loss of consciousness is prolonged (minutes or longer).

FOR A SECOND GRADE 3 CONCUSSION, NO SPORTS ACTIVITY UNTIL ASYMPTOMATIC FOR 1 MONTH

If an intracranial pathology is detected on CT or MRI, no sports activity for remainder of season and the athlete should be discouraged from future return to contact sports.

Data from Schutzman, S. & Greens, D. (2001). Pediatric minor head trauma. *Ann Emerg Med, 37*(1), 65-74. Centers for Disease Control and Prevention. (1997). Sports related recurrent brain injuries—United States. *MMWR Morb Mortal Wkly Rep, 46,* 224-227.

BOX 27-8

Differential Diagnosis

Need to know child's current baseline neurologic status.

Fever may increase potential for seizure in children with TBI seizures.

Nausea and vomiting may be indicative of shunt malfunction in children with posttraumatic hydrocephalus. Prolonged or severe vomiting may require aggressive rehydration in children with poor nutritional intake.

Headaches post-TBI often associated with frequent headaches. Headache diaries may help determine frequency, intensity, and effectiveness of mild analgesics.

a period of several days, or progressive over several weeks to months.

Fevers. Fevers are a common occurrence in the presence of viral and bacterial illnesses. Routine fever management is appropriate. In children with a history of seizures, the risk of seizures may increase during a febrile illness (see Chapter 25).

Nausea and Vomiting. Routine management of nausea and vomiting is advised. However, persistent vomiting or development of lethargy should be evaluated urgently in the child with an intracranial shunt (see Chapter 29).

Headaches. Posttraumatic headaches can be concerning to the family. Use of a headache diary can be valuable in recording onset, frequency, and associated symptoms. Symptom management with mild analgesics is usually adequate. If the headaches persist in frequency, further evaluation is recommended and a preventive medication may be warranted.

Drug Interactions

Children post-TBI may receive a variety of medications including antiepileptics, stimulants for behavior, headache prophylaxis, and muscle relaxants for spasticity. In the event that additional medications such as antibiotics are necessary, it is helpful to consult the Physicians Desk Reference or pharmacist to prevent potential drug interactions.

Developmental Issues

Sleep Patterns

Alterations in sleep patterns may be present after TBI. Transient insomnia is treated symptomatically with short-term use of antihistamines (for their sedative effect), antidepressants, or intermediate-acting hypnotics (e.g., chloral hydrate). Long-acting hypnotics are contraindicated because of impairment in daytime functioning. Regular sleep patterns are recommended and are generally managed with behavioral therapy. A regular bedtime that allows a sleep period of at least 8 hours is recommended. Activities that can enhance sleep patterns include regular daily exercise, a soothing evening bath or shower to increase relaxation, and adjusting the timing of medication doses to promote sleep. Caffeine, especially in the evening, late evening exercise, and napping during the day should be avoided to encourage nighttime sleeping.

Toileting

Bowel and bladder continence may be disrupted postinjury and generally can be managed in conjunction with the rehabilitation team. Frequent toileting can help obtain bowel and bladder control. The goal should be to obtain bowel and bladder control during the waking hours and then progress to nighttime hours. Fluid intake should be limited 2 hours prior to bedtime. The child who is immobile is prone to constipation and can benefit from anticipatory guidance regarding its prevention and management. These children may require the use of natural or medicated stool softeners, glycerin suppositories, or additional fluid intake for assisted elimination.

Discipline

Alterations in behavior and personality should be anticipated following brain injury. Although it may be difficult to determine how TBI contributes to a child's behavior, the effects from brain injury should always be included in the differential diagnosis. Behavioral changes commonly seen after brain injury are anger, apathy, anxiety, depression, disinhibition, emotional lability, impaired judgment, and impulsivity (Alexander and Moore, 2001).

Parents and primary care providers must be encouraged to be consistent with discipline and reinforce normal household rules as much as possible (Diamond, 1994). Persistent behavior difficulties at home, altered family and peer relationships, disruption in the school setting, or issues in the use of leisure time can lead to interruption in learning situations.

Difficulties with behavior and discipline are generally managed with behavioral therapy. Clear, simple expectations should be established and explained at an appropriate cognitive level for the child. Consistency in the style of discipline and behavior management of care providers is important to avoid giving mixed messages of appropriate and acceptable behavior. The parents, care providers, and other family members should do role modeling of acceptable behavior.

Pharmacologic management with the use of stimulants or other psychotropic medications may be considered (see Chapter 12). These medications should be used in conjunction with behavioral therapy.

Child Care

Mildly disabled children may be appropriately cared for in a daycare or home care setting. For children in a daycare or preschool setting, an individualized health program (IHP) can be useful in communicating medical information with early childhood educators and individual curriculum goals. Children who experience a TBI prior to the age of 3 are eligible for early intervention services. Occupational therapists and early intervention programs are helpful in determining age-appropriate activities. Other interventions include parent support, education, and training to create an environment that fosters the child's ability to work independently. The Individuals with Disabilities Education Act (IDEA) of 1997, mandates preschool services, which include occupational therapy for children with TBI, if the resulting impairments affect the child's ability to benefit from special education. Occupational therapists help to plan the child's transition to elementary school. Severely disabled children often require assisted nursing care in the home. Federal funds from Title XX of the Social Security Act are available for respite services, homemaker services, and foster home care.

Schooling

A critical phase in recovery for children with a head injury is the return to school. Successful school reentry is determined by intellect and cognitive ability, social skills, and peer relationships. Homeschooling, tutoring, or part time attendance may initially be appropriate on return to a school program, especially if limited endurance or fatigue problems are present.

The child with TBI must be supported in the transition to school. Recommended transition services are (1) establishing communication among all persons caring for the child, (2) initiating an evaluation process, (3) integrating information in an interdisciplinary forum, (4) adapting education programs to meet the child's needs, (5) preparing the child for transitions, and (6) providing ongoing monitoring for possible late-developing problems (Cronin, 2001).

Depending on the depth of persistent deficits, children with TBI can receive services in regular classes or special education classes. They are also eligible for speech-language therapy, occupational or physical therapies, special services for hearing or visual impairments, behavior management, and counseling as components of an individualized education program (IEP) (see Chapter 5).

There are documented academic difficulties in children with TBI. As a result, there may be a poor fit between their needs and school education programs (NIH, 1999). Children who did not qualify for special education in the preschool period may qualify later, as late emerging problems may surface. In the school age child, the occupational therapist assesses for learning disabilities and works in conjunction with the educational team and primary care provider to ensure that these problems are addressed (Cronin, 2001).

Sexuality

Individuals who have sustained a head injury may have altered inhibitions or may make socially inappropriate sexual comments and gestures. Impairment in motor and sensory function or impaired communication may alter sexual functioning. Concerns about sexuality expressed by the child or adolescent, family, and significant others should be addressed early. For adolescents, educational programs or counseling sessions should include the topics of sexuality, substance abuse, and other risk-taking behaviors. Caution should be used when prescribing medication to female adolescents, i.e., seizure medications, because of possible teratogenic effects.

Transition to Adulthood

Traumatic brain injury may have a major effect on the subsequent education, vocational development, independent living skills, and future productivity of affected individuals. Supported living programs, supervised housing, shared services, or foster care should be evaluated with respect to the level of assistance provided for the activities of daily living (Jackson, 1994). Supervised work experiences may be necessary to develop appropriate skills and work habits in order to succeed in gainful employment and contribute to the community. Health care insurance coverage and financial assistance programs should also be addressed as adolescents enter adulthood (see Chapter 9).

Family Concerns and Resources

TBI can be stressful for the child and the family. This stress can have negative effects on the parent's mental health and can potentially deteriorate the parent-child and family relationships. Parents are suddenly faced with fears about survival, current condition, and uncertainty about the future. While caring for the child with TBI, parents may even feel guilty about neglecting the child's siblings (Youngblut et al, 2000). Siblings may experience emotional disturbances, school problems, and aggression. They may also demonstrate guilty feelings after initially experiencing a sense of relief that the injury happened to their brother or sister and not to them. Parents, family members, and primary care providers should be encouraged to become actively involved in the day-to-day care of the child because this

will reduce their sense of helplessness and result in confidence building (Appleton, 1994).

Significant financial issues, change in employment due to care responsibilities, the loss of a job, and the conflict related to the parents' return to work may arise, adding to the family's stress. Long-term family support and counseling should be advocated. Families that seek support and try to accept the situation may experience less stress and family dysfunction over time (Wade et al, 2001).

Primary health care providers are in a key position to help provide comprehensive care services that are congruent with and respectful toward the child's and family's cultural background. Primary health care providers can facilitate the family's acceptance of the injury and help them set attainable goals (Wade et al, 2001). Anticipatory guidance should focus on the length of time that symptoms may occur and the importance of routine follow-up during the first 12 months postinjury (Youngblut et al, 2000).

Caring for a child with a head injury is a complex task because of the physical, cognitive, and psychosocial concerns that must be addressed. The following is a list of additional resources.

Resources

General Organizations

American Speech, Language, Hearing Association
10801 Rockville Pike
Rockville, MD 20852
(800) 638-8255
www.asha.org

Brain Injury Association
105 N. Alfred Street
Alexandria, VA 22314
(800) 444-6443 (Family Helpline)
www.biausa.org

Brain Injury Society
1890 E. 4th Street Corner Kings Highway,
Suite 2S
Brooklyn, NY 11230
(718) 645-4401
www.bisociety.org

Family Caregiver Alliance
690 Market Street, Suite 600
San Francisco, CA 94104
(415) 434-3388
www.caregiver.org

Head Injury Hotline
212 Pioneer Building.
Seattle, WA 98104-2221
(206) 621-8558
www.headinjury.com

San Diego Head Injury Foundation, Inc.
PO Box 84601
San Diego, CA 92138
(619) 294-6541 (helpline)

Organizations for Professionals

American Congress of Rehabilitative Medicine
6801 Lake Plaza Drive, Suite B-205
Indianapolis, IN 46220
(317) 915-2250
www.acrm.org

Association of Rehabilitation Nurses
4700 W. Lake Avenue
Glenview, IL 60025-1485
(800) 299-7530; (847) 375-4710
www.rehabnurse.org

National Stroke Association
9707 E. Easter Lane
Englewood, CO 80112
(303) 649-9299; (800)-STROKES
www.stroke.org

Summary of Primary Care Needs for the Child with a Head Injury

HEALTH CARE MAINTENANCE

Growth and Development

Height, weight, and head circumference should be assessed to monitor growth. Medications are based on current accurate weight measurements for therapeutic effectiveness.

Delayed development may be present. Cognitive and motor skills should be regularly screened and assessed. Interventional therapy programs are recommended.

Signs of precocious puberty and short stature should be monitored.

Diet

Eating and feeding problems can contribute to poor growth patterns. Decreased physical activity and immobility may lead to excessive weight gain. Dietary intake should be tailored to meet the child's caloric needs.

Protective reflexes should be regularly monitored to prevent potential of aspiration.

Occupational therapy can assist with optimal feeding programs.

Safety

Increased risk of injury is present as a result of instability, incoordination, potential seizures, and delays in motor skill acquisition.

Ongoing anticipatory guidance on general safety precautions should be provided.

Emergency seizure procedures should be reviewed.

Caution should be taken with risk-taking sports and activities.

Immunization

Routine immunizations should be avoided in the acute postinjury recovery stage.

Children with posttraumatic seizures may be at increased risk for having a seizure after a DTP/DTaP.

Fever prophylaxis with acetaminophen or ibuprophen is recommended, not aspirin.

Screening

Vision. A complete evaluation is recommended postinjury during the recovery period, with correction of minor deficits.

Hearing. A complete evaluation is recommended postinjury during the recovery period, with correction of minor deficits.

Dental. Routine screening is recommended.

Possible dental trauma should be evaluated after a head injury.

More frequent evaluations may be necessary for children on phenytoin.

Blood Pressure. Monitor blood pressure with each visit.

Hematocrit. Routine screening is recommended.

Urinalysis. Routine screening is recommended.

Tuberculosis. Routine screening is recommended. If prophylactic medications are needed, potential drug interactions should be evaluated in children receiving other medications.

Condition-Specific Screening

Posttraumatic Seizure Therapy. Monitor CBC counts and chemistry panels along with anticonvulsant levels for the first 6 months postinjury and periodically thereafter.

COMMON ILLNESS MANAGEMENT

Differential Diagnosis

A thorough knowledge of the baseline neurologic status and behavior is key in assessing significant pathologic deviations.

Risk of seizures is increased with acute illness and fever.

The potential for increased intracranial pressure should be monitored in the presence of an intracranial shunt with signs of nausea and vomiting.

Evaluation of headaches will require careful history and symptom management.

Drug Interactions

Potential drug interactions can occur if the child post-TBI is taking epileptic drugs, stimulants for behavior, headache prophylaxis, and/or muscle relaxants for spasticity. Careful monitoring required.

DEVELOPMENTAL ISSUES

Sleep Patterns

Disruption in sleep patterns may be evident. A structured behavioral program is recommended.

Toileting

Bowel and bladder continence may be delayed in younger children or disrupted in older children who previously had voluntary control. Establishment of a progressive training program with positive reinforcement as cognition increases will help them regain control.

Discipline

Alterations in behavior and personality should be anticipated with early guidance counseling instituted. Standard developmentally appropriate discipline is recommended with reinforcement of normal household rules.

Persistent difficulties with behavior and discipline are managed with behavioral therapy. Referral and evaluation by a behavior specialist may be warranted.

Continued

Summary of Primary Care Needs for the Child with a Head Injury—cont'd

Child care

Child care and respite care have been identified as priority needs by the primary caretakers. Assistance in this area is priority.

Schooling

Cognitive changes continue to occur from weeks to months following the recovery from head trauma.

Assessment of learning needs must be fully individualized and addressed as soon as feasible postinjury. Public Law 99-457 and 101-476 outline mandated educational programs.

Families may require assistance with IEP process.

Toddlers and preschoolers need close monitoring because of increasing cognitive demands with age.

Formal neuropsychologic and school performance testing may be necessary.

Sexuality

Impairment in the motor and sensory function or impaired communication may alter sexual functioning. Anticipatory guidance in counseling is advised.

Transition to Adulthood

Traumatic brain injury can have a major effect on the future education, vocational development, and independent living skills of the affected adolescent. School guidance and vocational counseling are recommended.

FAMILY CONCERNS

Severe stresses on the family unit arise following the sudden occurrence of a head injury. Support groups or family counseling for parents and siblings may be helpful.

Cultural differences can be considered a barrier to adequate services despite the benefits of family-centered care. Comprehensive care that is congruent with and respectful toward the child's and family's cultural background is a key element.

REFERENCES

Adelson, P.D. & Kochanek, P.M. (2001). Head injury in children. *J Child Neurol, 13*(1), 2-15.

Alexander, J. & Moore, D. (2001). Primary care for children with brain injury. *NCMJ, 62,* 344-348.

American Academy of Pediatrics, American Academy of Family Physicians. (1999). The Management of Minor Closed Head Injury in Children. *Pediatrics, 104*(6), 1407-1415.

Appleton, R. (1994). Head injury rehabilitation for children. *Nurs Times, 90,* 29-31.

Bagnato, S.J. et al. (1988). An interdisciplinary neurodevelopmental assessment model for brain-injured infants and preschool children. *J Head Trauma Rehabil, 3,* 75-86.

Beaulieu, C.L. (2002). Rehabilitation and outcome following pediatric traumatic brain injury. *Surg Clin North Am, 82*(2), 393-408.

Bloom, R. et al. (2001). Lifetime and novel psychiatric disorders after pediatric traumatic brain injury. *J Am Acad Child Adolesc Psychiatry, 40*(5), 572-579.

Boss, B.J. (1994). Coma and Cognitive Deficits. In E. Barker (Ed.). *Neuroscience Nursing.* St. Louis: Mosby.

Centers for Disease Control. (2000). Contradictions for Childhood Immunization.

Chapman, E.H., Weintraub, R.J., Milburn, M.A., Pirozzi, T.O., & Woo, E. (1999). Homeopathic treatment of mild traumatic brain injury. *J Head Trauma Rehabil, 14*(6), 521-542.

Chipps, E.M., Clanin, N.J., & Campbell, V.G. (1992). *Neurological Disorders.* St. Louis: Mosby.

Coffman, S.P. (1992). Home care of the child and family after near drowning. *J Pediatr Health Care, 6,* 18-24.

Cronin, A.F. (2001). Traumatic brain injury in children: issues in community function. *Am J Occup Ther, 55*(4), 377-384.

Diamond, J. (1994). Family-centered care for children with chronic illness. *J Pediatr Health Care, 8,* 196-197.

Evans, R. & Wilberger, J.E. (1999). Traumatic disorders. In C. Goetz & E. Pappert (Eds.). *Textbook of Clinical Neurology* (pp. 1035-1058). Philadelphia, PA: W.B. Saunders Company.

Folden, S.L. & Coffman, S. (1993). Respite care for families of children with disabilities. *J Pediatr Health Care, 7,* 103-110.

Franzen, M.D. (2000). Neuropsychological assessment in traumatic brain injury. *Crit Care Nurs Q, 23*(3), 58-64.

Ghajar, J. & Hariri, R. (1992). Management of pediatric head injury. *Pediatr Clin North Am, 39,* 1093-1125.

Goka, R.S. (2000). Mild traumatic brain injury: treatment paradigms. In G. Jay (Ed) *Minor Traumatic Brain Injury Handbook.* Boca Raton: CRC Press LLC.

Hawley, C.A., Ward, A.B., Magnay, A.R., & Long, J. (2002). Children's brain injury: a postal follow-up of 535 children from one health region in the UK. *Brain Inj, 19*(11), 969-985.

Humphrey, R.P. (1991). Complications of pediatric head injury. *Pediatr Neurosurg, 17,* 274-278.

Jackson, J.D. (1994). After rehabilitation: meeting the long-term needs of persons with traumatic brain injury. *Am J Occup Ther, 48,* 251-255.

Jennett, B. (1998). Epidemiology of head injury. *Arch Dis Child, 78*(5), 403-413.

Jury, M.A. & Flynn, M.C. (2001). Auditory and vestibular sequelae to traumatic brain injury: a pilot study. *N Z Med J, 114*(1134), 286-288.

Marik, P.E., Varon, J., & Trask, T. (2002). Management of head trauma. *Chest, 122*(2), 122, 699-711.

Max, J.B., et al. (1998). Psychiatric disorders in children and adolescents after severe traumatic brain injury: a controlled study. *J Am Acad Child Adolesc Psychiatry, 37*(8), 832-840.

Michaud, L.J., Duhaime, A.C., & Batshaw, M.L. (1993). Traumatic Brain Injury in Children. *Pediatr Clin North Am, 40,* 553-565.

Miller, L. (1991). Significant others: treating brain injury in the family context. *J Cognit Rehabil, 9,* 16-25.

Murdoch, B.E. & Theodoros, D.G. (2001). *Introduction: epidemiology, neuropathophysiology, and medical aspects of traumatic brain injury. Traumatic brain injury.* Canada: Delmar.

Murdoch, B.E. & Theodoros, D.G. (2001). Traumatic brain injury: Associated speech, language and swallowing disorders. Traumatic brain injury. Canada: Delmar.

NIH Consensus Development Panel on Rehabilitation of Persons with Traumatic Brain Injury. (1999). Rehabiliation of persons with traumatic brain injury. *JAMA, 282*(10), 974-983.

Padula, W.V. & Argyris, S. (2001-2002). *Post-traumatic vision syndrome: Part 1.* Neuro-optometric Rehabilitation Association International, Inc.

Pellock, J.M., Dodson, W.E., & Bourgeois, B.F. (Eds.). (2001). *Pediatric Epilepsy Diagnosis and Therapy*. New York: Demos.

Ponsford, J., et al. (2001). Impact of early intervention on outcome after mild traumatic brain injury in children. *Pediatrics, 108*(6), 1297-1303.

Reece, R.M. & Sege, R. (2000). Childhood head injuries: accidental or inflicted? *Arch Pediatr Adolesc Med, 154,* 11-15.

Roth, P. & Farls, K. (2000). Pathophysiology of traumatic brain injury. *Crit Care Nurs Q, 23*(3), 14-25.

Schutzman, S.A. & Greenes, D.S. (2001). Evaluation and management of children younger than two years of with apparently minor head trauma: proposed guidelines. *Pediatrics, 107*(5), 983-993.

Schutzman, S.A. & Greenes, D.S. (2001). Pediatric minor head trauma. *Ann Emerg Med, 37*(1), 65-74.

Tilford, J.M., et al. (2001). Variation in therapy and outcome for pediatric head trauma patients. *Crit Care Med, 29*(5), 1056-1061.

Vasa, R.A., et al. (2002). Anxiety after severe pediatric closed head injury. *J Am Acad Child Adolesc Psychiatry, 41*(2), 148-157.

Wade, S.L., et al. (2001). The relationship of caregiver coping to family outcomes during the initial year following pediatric traumatic injury. *J Consult Clin Psychol, 69*(3), 406-415.

Walleck, C.A. & Mooney, K.F. (1994). Neurotrauma: Head Injury. In E. Barker (Ed.). *Neuroscience Nursing*. St. Louis: Mosby.

Weiner, H.L. & Weinberg, J.S. (2000). Head injury in the pediatric age group. In P.R. Cooper & J. Golfinos (Eds.). *Head Injury*. New York: McGraw-Hill.

Woestman, R., Perkin, R., Serna, T., Van Stralen, D., & Knierim, D. (1998). Mild head injury in children: Identified clinical evaluating, neuroimaging and disposition. *J Pediatr Health Care, 12,* 288-298.

Yoon, M.S. & Narayan, R.K. (in press). Treatment of severe closed head injury. *Pediatr Radiol, 27,* 790-793.

Youngblut, J.M., et al. (2000). Effects of pediatric head trauma for children, parents, and families. *Crit Care Nurs Clin North Am, 12*(2), 227-235.

28 HIV Infection and AIDS

Rita Fahrner and Sostena Romano

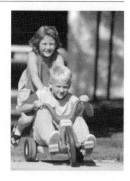

Etiology

The human immunodeficiency virus (HIV) causes a continuum of infection to occur, the end stage of which is acquired immune deficiency syndrome (AIDS). HIV type 1 (HIV-1) is a member of the lentivirus genus of the Retroviridae family, which means that its viral RNA is copied into DNA using reverse transcriptase. This virus selectively infects the T-helper (i.e., T4 or CD4) subset of T-cell lymphocytes. Other cells that express CD4 (e.g., monocytes, macrophages, and glial cells) and some cells without detectable cell surface CD4 can become infected. Through a process of replication, HIV perpetuates and integrates itself into the genetic material of the organism it infects. Full intracellular viral life cycling requires the generation of a DNA copy of the HIV-1 RNA genome; integration of this proviral DNA into the host genomic DNA permits viral persistence and impedes the eradication of virus from infected individuals (Luzuriaga & Sullivan, 1998). The primary pathologic condition of HIV causes specific immunodeficiency that destroys the host's ability to withstand infection. In addition, the HIV directly invades other major organ systems, including the peripheral and central nervous system (CNS), lungs, heart, kidneys, and gastrointestinal (GI) tract.

Although HIV infection in children and adults has common pathologic conditions, infants with perinatally acquired HIV infections represent a distinctive immunologic host with a developing, immature immune system (Kamani & Douglas, 1991). The fetus and neonate have a well-developed T cell, or cell-mediated, immune system, whereas their B cell, or humoral, immune system, is physiologically immature. Although the function of both B and T cells is altered in HIV-infected children, the consequences of B-cell dysfunction, including hypergammaglobulinemia and failure to form functional antibodies, are often problematic early in the course of disease. For this reason, children with HIV are more susceptible to bacterial infections than their adult counterparts. T-cell defects, allowing for opportunistic infections (OIs), such as *Pneumocystis carinii* pneumonia (PCP), are also often seen in young infants. In addition, the degree of lymphopenia, percentage of T4 (CD4) cells, absolute T4 (CD4) count, and degree of reversal of the helper-suppressor (T4-T8) ratio are more variable in infants. Depletion of T-cell numbers and inversion of the helper-suppressor ratio generally occurs at a later stage of disease in children than in adults. Another major difference between adults and children with HIV is that the time period from infection to development of signs and symptoms seems to be shorter in children.

HIV is transmitted to children by a variety of modes (Layton, 2000) (Table 28-1). Perinatal transmission is the most common (91%) mode of transmission and may occur transplacentally in utero (vertically from mother to fetus), during delivery by exposure to infected maternal blood and vaginal secretions, and by postpartum ingestion of infected breast milk (Centers for Disease Control and Prevention [CDC], 1994). Many factors (i.e., maternal, fetal, viral, placental, obstetrical, and neonatal) seem to influence mother-to-infant transmission of the virus. The success of the Pediatric AIDS Clinical Trials Group (PACTG) 076 study demonstrated that when zidovudine (AZT) was administered during pregnancy and labor, as well as to the newborn, the risk for perinatal HIV transmission was reduced by two thirds; infection rates were 25% in the placebo group compared with 8% in the treatment group (Stiehm et al, 1999) (Boxes 28-1 and 28-2).

Children have become infected with HIV from contaminated blood and blood products, tissues, and factor concentrates received between 1978 and 1985. The risk for infection, however, was extremely high during these years, with infection estimated to occur in up to 95% of those receiving contaminated products. Because of the safeguards instituted in blood and tissue collection and heat treatment of factor concentrates during the mid-1980s, few new cases of infection from blood and blood products, tissues, and factor concentrates have been reported.

A small number of children have become infected with HIV as a result of sexual abuse. Practitioners caring for children who have experienced abuse must include HIV infection in their differential diagnosis of sexually transmitted diseases. HIV has also rarely been transmitted through blood exposure within household settings, but no cases of transmission within daycare or school settings have been reported (Courville et al, 1998).

Adolescents and young adults aged 13 through 24 years comprise approximately 4% of the AIDS cases in the United States (CDC, 2002c). Of the HIV infection cases reported by the states who track HIV infection, however, adolescents and young adults aged 13 through 24 years comprise 16%, a percentage that has been rising of late (CDC, 2002c). The average time from HIV infection to the development of AIDS is about 11 years, so most young adults with AIDS were infected as teenagers. Teenagers are especially at risk for HIV because many of the behaviors that put a person at risk for HIV begin during adolescence (i.e., unprotected sexual activity, drug use, etc.). In addition, as the management and therapeutic treatments for children with perinatally acquired HIV infection improve, more of these children are reaching adolescence before receiving a formal AIDS diagnosis.

TABLE 28-1

U.S. Pediatric AIDS Cases by Route of Transmission*

Mode of transmission	%
Mother has or is at risk for HIV infection	91
Recipient of blood, blood product, or tissue	4
Hemophilia or coagulation disorder	3
Undetermined	2
TOTAL	100

*N = 9074
From Centers for Disease Control and Prevention. (2002). *HIV/AIDS surveillance report, year-end 2001.*

BOX 28-1

AZT to Reduce Vertical Transmission (from ACTG 076 Protocol)

MATERNAL
Antepartum
Begin after 14 weeks' gestation
Zidovudine 100 mg PO 5 times daily

Intrapartum
Zidovudine loading dose 2 mg/kg IV over 1 hr then 1 mg/kg/hr continuous IV infusion until delivery
Zidovudine 1000 mg should be diluted with 250 mg D_5W to prepare a final concentration of 4 mg zidovudine/ml D_5W.

INFANT
Begin as soon as possible within the first 12 hours of life

FOR PO INFANT
Zidovudine 2 mg/kg PO q6h 3 to 6 weeks plus extra week supply

FOR NPO INFANT
Zidovudine 1.5 mg/kg IV q6h infuse over 30 to 60 minutes
Zidovudine should be diluted with D_5W to prepare a final concentration of 0.5 mg zidovudine/ml D_5W.

BOX 28-2

Results of ACTG 076

A randomized, double-blind, placebo-controlled clinical trial of the efficacy and safety of zidovudine (AZT) in reducing the risk of maternal-infant HIV transmission:
The mothers and infants who took zidovudine had an 8.3% risk of transmission.
The mothers and infants who took the placebo had a 25.5% risk of transmission.

Data from Connor, E.M. (1994). Reduction of maternal-infant transmission of human immunodeficiency virus type I with zidovudine treatment. *N Engl J Med, 331,* 1173-1180.

Known Genetic Etiology

There is no evidence of any genetic predisposition to HIV/AIDS. Because it is an infectious disease, one must be infected with the virus in order to develop the disease. There is nothing specific known about genetic susceptibility, nor are there any data to suggest genetic defense against developing the

TABLE 28-2

Pediatric AIDS Cases (N 8284) by Maternal Exposure Category and Race*

Maternal Exposure Category	White (%)	Black (%)	Asian/ Latino (%)	Am Ind/ Pac Is (%)	Alaskan (%)	Total (%)
Injection drug use (IDU)	41	31	40	17	48	39
Sex with IDU	20	15	26	17	21	18
Sex with another at-risk person	21	19	17	31	14	19
Recipient of blood, blood products, or tissue	4	1	2	3	3	2
Risk unspecified	14	27	15	32	14	22

*Pac Is, Pacific Islander; Am Ind, American Indian; IDU, injection-drug user.
From Centers for Disease Control and Prevention. (2002). *HIV/AIDS surveillance report, year-end 2001.*

infection. There may be host factors at play because there have been cases of discordant twins, in which one twin is infected and the other is not. Another theory regarding discordant twins born to HIV-infected mothers is that birth order may be relevant; the first born seems more likely to be infected.

Incidence and Prevalence

Although pediatric and adolescent AIDS is a reportable condition, the actual incidence and/or prevalence is unknown because AIDS cases are significantly underreported in the United States and worldwide. The actual incidence and/or prevalence of HIV infection in children, however, is becoming increasingly known as national confidential HIV infection reporting continues to increase; it now occurs in 35 states as well as 4 US dependencies, possessions, and associated nations. The occurrence of AIDS in children was established as early as 1982; 20 children younger than 13 years of age were diagnosed by the end of 1981 (CDC, 1994). By the end of 2001, more than 9,074 cases of AIDS in children (i.e., 1.1% of the total number of reported AIDS cases in the United States) were reported to the CDC (CDC, 2002c). Estimates from the CDC suggest that there are 18,000 to 23,000 infants and children infected with HIV in the United States. The incidence of pediatric HIV is increasing as HIV infection increases in the injection drug-using and heterosexual communities. All states in the United States have reported at least one case of pediatric AIDS (CDC, 2002c).

Because most children with AIDS have been perinatally infected, the demographics of this group closely parallel that of women with AIDS (Table 28-2). In this population, HIV is a disease primarily associated with poverty and drug use and is clustered in inner cities and ethnic minority communities. On the other hand, parenteral cases have a broader geographic distribution and a wider ethnic apportionment.

Clinical Manifestations at Time of Diagnosis

Developing a clinical definition of HIV infection and AIDS in children is a complex task (Box 28-3). The initial pediatric

AIDS definition directed surveillance but did not describe the spectrum of infection. Therefore in 1987 the CDC developed a classification system for HIV infection in children; as more information about pediatric HIV became available, however, the 1987 classification system was inadequate. In 1994 the CDC again revised the classification system for children younger than 13 years of age. The current classification system places perinatally exposed and infected children into mutually exclusive categories according to infection and clinical and immunologic status (Box 28-4). Although HIV infection is most accurately identified by viral culture from blood or tissue, it is generally diagnosed in adults by the presence of specific antibodies to the virus. The presence of passively acquired maternal antibodies, however, limits the use of HIV antibody testing in infants up to 18 months of age suspected of perinatal infection. For this reason, two definitions of infection in children are necessary: one for infants up to 18 months of age and one for older children (see Box 28-4).

Children who meet the definition of HIV exposure or infection may be further grouped into one of six mutually exclusive classes based on clinical signs, symptoms, and immunologic status (Table 28-3). This classification system is helpful for health care planning and for epidemiologic purposes.

Pediatric HIV/AIDS centers can use more specific laboratory tests to determine infection in perinatally exposed infants. HIV blood culturing is considered the gold standard in virologic testing of infants. Blood culturing is very expensive and labor intensive, however, and results are not usually available for 4 to 6 weeks after specimen processing. The p24 antigen assay is another virologic test that is rather inexpensive and has been available for many years. In the presence of HIV

antibodies, however, an immune complex is formed with the p24 antigen, making detection of the antigen itself impossible. This test becomes more accurate in children at 6 months of age, when maternal antibody titers in infants begin to drop. A third test, the polymerase chain reaction (PCR), has proved to be superior to viral culture and p24 antigen assay. PCR is a method

---

BOX 28-4
Diagnosis of HIV Infection in Children*

DIAGNOSIS: HIV INFECTED

A. A child <18 months of age who is known to be HIV seropositive or born to an HIV-infected mother and:
  Has positive results on two separate specimens (excluding cord blood) from any of the following HIV detection tests:
    HIV culture
    HIV polymerase chain reaction
    HIV antigen (p24)
      or
  Meets criteria for AIDS diagnosis based on the 1987 AIDS surveillance case definition

B. A child >18 months of age born to an HIV-infected mother or any child infected by blood, blood products, or other known modes of transmission (e.g., sexual contact) who:
  Is HIV antibody positive by confirming Western blot or immunofluorescence assay (IFA)
      or
  Meets any of the criteria in A

DIAGNOSIS: PERINATALLY EXPOSED (PREFIX E)

  A child who does not meet the previously listed criteria who:
  Is HIV seropositive by ELISA and confirming Western blot or IFA and is ≤18 months of age at the time of test
      or
  Has unknown antibody status but was born to a mother known to be infected with HIV

DIAGNOSIS: SEROREVERTER (SR)

  A child who is born to an HIV-infected mother and who:
  Has been documented as HIV antibody negative (i.e., two or more negative ELISA tests performed at 6 to 18 months of age or one negative ELISA test after 18 months of age)
      and
  Has had no other laboratory evidence of infection (i.e., has not had two positive viral detection tests, if performed)
      and
  Has not had an AIDS-defining condition

From Centers for Disease Control and Prevention. (1994). *MMWR Morb Mortal Wkly Rep, 43,* 2-3.

BOX 28-3
Clinical Manifestations at Time of Diagnosis

Failure to thrive
Chronic or recurrent diarrhea
Fever of unknown origin
Atopic dermatitis
Persistent or recurrent fungal infections (e.g., thrush or diaper dermatitis)
Thrombocytopenia
Hepatosplenomegaly
Parotitis
Frequent infections
Developmental delay; loss of milestones

TABLE 28-3
Pediatric HIV Classification*

Immunologic Categories	Clinical Categories			
	N: No Signs/Symptoms	A: Mild Signs/Symptoms	B: Moderate Signs/Symptoms	C: Severe Signs/Symptoms
1: No evidence of immune suppression	N1	A1	B1	C1
2: Evidence of moderate immune suppression	N2	A2	B2	C2
3: Severe immune suppression	N3	A3	B3	C3

*Children whose HIV infection status is not confirmed are classified by using the above grid with a letter E (for perinatally exposed) placed before the appropriate classification code (e.g., EN2).
From Centers for Disease Control and Prevention (1994). *MMWR Morb Mortal Wkly Rep, 43,* 2-3.

of gene amplification that directly detects proviral sequences of HIV within DNA using small amounts of blood. PCR is less expensive than viral culture and more sensitive than p24 antigen assays. In addition, PCR results are usually available within 1 week of processing the specimen.

By using HIV culture, PCR, or both, an infant's infection status can be determined with 90% to 100% certainty by 3 to 6 months of age (Khoury & Kovacs, 2001). Although these tests are becoming more widely available, many community clinicians caring for these children may not have direct access to them but will need to refer children to the closest pediatric HIV specialty center or contact the National Institute of Allergy and Infectious Diseases or the Maternal-Child Health Bureau for the nearest participating research group.

Because HIV infection is clearly a multisystem disease process, infected infants and children may have a wide range of signs and symptoms. The clinical manifestations that occur early in infection are often nonspecific and may be seen in healthy children and children with other conditions. Children with HIV infection, however, generally experience more chronic and severe signs and symptoms and often fail to respond to appropriate therapy. Some children have acute opportunistic infections (OIs) with the same protozoal, viral, fungal, and bacterial pathogens as adults, which are indicator diseases for an AIDS diagnosis. Others may have nephropathy, hepatitis, cardiomyopathy, and hematologic abnormalities (Pizzo & Wilfert, 1998).

Most children are diagnosed with HIV infection before they exhibit any signs or symptoms of illness. Infants and children born to mothers who are infected with HIV or known to be at risk should be tested to determine if they are also infected. Retrospective transfusion programs have identified many children who are infected. Children with hemophilia or other hematologic conditions who received factor concentrates or other blood products before 1985 should be counseled about HIV testing (see Chapter 14).

Treatment

HIV infection has become a chronic, treatable, life-threatening disease (Forsyth, 2000). The most significant treatments are those aimed at interfering with the replicative process of HIV in an attempt to reduce the body's burden of HIV and thereby reduce the destruction of the individual's immune system (Palumbo, 2000) (Box 28-5). Combination antiretroviral therapy using a variety of agents has become standard therapy (Pizzo & Wilfert, 1998).

Although the pathogenesis of HIV infection and the general virologic and immunologic principles for the use of antiretroviral therapy are similar for all individuals with HIV, there are unique considerations for their use in infants, children, and adolescents. These considerations include the following: (1) perinatal transmission; (2) in utero exposure to antiretrovirals; (3) differences in diagnostic evaluations in perinatal infection; (4) differences in immunologic markers in young children; (5) changes in pharmacokinetics with age caused by the continuing development and maturation of organ systems involved in drug metabolism and clearance; (6) differences in the clinical and virologic manifestations of perinatal HIV infection in relation to the occurrence of primary infection in growing, immunologically immature bodies; and (7) special issues associated with treatment adherence for children and adolescents (Working Group, 2000).

Many questions about the use of antiretrovirals in children are now being answered because there are a growing number of investigational treatment protocols for children that address issues such as the optimal time to start treatment, when and how to modify dosage, and how to determine disease progression. Rather than having to prove their efficacy in adults before children are allowed access to them, new drugs are now simultaneously tested in adults and children. This process parallels the approval process for new chemotherapeutic agents used in cancer therapy. Combination therapy has proved to be superior to monotherapy and is the hallmark of HIV treatment (McKinney et al, 1998). A variety of agents including nucleoside reverse transcriptase inhibitors (i.e., zidovudine [AZT], lamivudine [Epivir], stavudine [Zerit], didanosine [Videx], abacavir [Ziagen]), nonnucleoside reverse transcriptase inhibitors (i.e., nevirapine [Viramune], delavirdine [Rescripton], efavirenz [Sustiva]), and protease inhibitors (i.e., ritonavir [Norvir], nelfinavir [Viracept], indinavir [Crixivan], amprenavir [Agenerase], saquinavir [Invirase or Fortovase], lopinavir/ritonavir [Kaletra]) are currently used (CDC, 2001c).

Intravenous immune globulin (IVIG) is still used in some centers in an attempt to reconstitute the immune systems of children with HIV infection. IVIG has been shown to reduce serious bacterial infections in children with HIV but has not increased survival time (Wood, 1998). This benefit, however, did not hold true in children receiving zidovudine in addition to trimethoprim-sulfamethoxazole (TMP-SMX) as *Pneumocystis carinii* pneumonia (PCP) prophylaxis (Spector, 1994).

Without a definitive cure, children with HIV infection are treated with comprehensive, multidisciplinary care with prompt diagnosis and aggressive therapy of concurrent infections and other clinical manifestations of disease. Recurrent and severe systemic bacterial infection, which can progress to pneumonia, meningitis, and sepsis, is one of the most frequent problems in children with HIV disease. Although this type of infection contributes greatly to morbidity, it is potentially preventable and treatable. The major bacterial pathogens encountered are those seen in pediatric practice with children who are immunocompetent. Reducing the frequency and intensity of bacterial infection may potentially modify HIV replication and primary disease progression (Krasinski, 1994).

Most children with HIV infection, even those with symptomatic disease, are active, playful, functional children who see themselves as healthy. They may take medications and spend time in the hospital and in outpatient clinics, but also attend daycare and engage in many after-school activities. It is

---

BOX 28-5

Treatment

Antiretroviral drugs
Intravenous immune globulin
Therapies for concurrent infectious and other clinical manifestations

important for primary care providers to remember that these children will develop common childhood illnesses and that all symptoms are not related to their underlying immunodeficiency. Children with HIV, however, must be quickly assessed and aggressively managed when the possibility of intercurrent illness occurs (Luzuriaga et al, 1997). A wait-and-see attitude is rarely appropriate. These children and their families must develop strong partnerships with both their primary care provider as well as their HIV specialists to ensure prompt evaluation and treatment. Children infected with HIV must be linked with a comprehensive pediatric HIV/AIDS treatment center whenever possible (Palumbo, 2000). Centers ensure access to clinical trials and the most up-to-date information and expertise, as well as to other children and families living with this condition. Clear lines of access to and responsibility of the primary care provider and the center team must be developed for each family.

Complementary and Alternative Therapies

Complementary or alternative treatments are frequently used in chronic conditions, and adults with HIV/AIDS have been at the forefront of this movement. These therapies may be used alone but are more frequently used in combination with traditional treatments. Forms of therapy include massage, exercise, dietary supplements, vitamins, and acupuncture (MacIntyre et al, 1997; Standish et al, 2001). Although no studies have been completed in the pediatric populations, those that involved adolescents have shown an improved sense of well-being when used in conjunction with traditional medicine (Duggan, 2001). In some individuals using complementary therapies, enhanced immune function was seen after 12 weeks (Diego & Field, 2001). No recommendations can be made, but future research may shed more light on the subject.

Anticipated Advances in Diagnosis and Management

In 2002 the CDC published an update to the 1994 Public Health Service guidelines for the use of antiretroviral drugs—both for maternal health and for reducing perinatal transmission of HIV—in pregnant women with HIV (CDC, 2002d). These guidelines are based on the ACTG (AIDS Clinical Trials Group) 076 protocol and confirmation of the efficacy of AZT for reducing perinatal transmission. Along with the substantial advances in the understanding of the pathogenesis of HIV infection and in the treatment and monitoring of HIV disease, standard antiretroviral therapy for adults with HIV now comprises more aggressive combination drug regimens that maximally suppress viral replication. Pregnancy is not a reason to defer standard therapy; therefore, offering antiretroviral therapy to infected pregnant women—whether to primarily treat the disease or to reduce the risk of perinatal transmission, or both, is recommended. Treatment discussions should include the known and unknown short- and long-term benefits and risks of such therapy for infected women and their infants (CDC, 2002d).

Advances in the early diagnosis of infants at risk for HIV have been dramatic. One of the reasons that the ACTG 076 efficacy results were available earlier than anticipated is because when the study was first drafted in 1990, it was thought that

infection could only be ruled out when maternal antibody levels in the infant dissipate (i.e., at 15 to 18 months of age). More recently, the use of repeated PCR testing has made diagnosis of HIV possible by 3 to 6 months of age.

The advances in combination antiretroviral therapy have provided substantial clinical benefit to children with HIV with immunologic and/or clinical symptoms of disease (Sullivan & Luzuriaga, 2001). Studies have shown concrete improvements in neurodevelopment, growth, and immunologic and/or virologic status with initiation of monotherapy. Recent trials have shown that combination therapy is clinically, immunologically, and virologically superior to monotherapy in previously untreated symptomatic children, as well as that combination therapy including a protease inhibitor is superior to dual nucleoside combination therapy in children who were previously treated (CDC, 2001c).

Recently HIV drug resistance assays, which may include genotyping and/or phenotyping of an individual's HIV, have become available. These tests may be useful in guiding antiretroviral regimen changes by identifying specific viral mutations. These assays help determine which medications might be successful in reducing the amount of HIV replication. However, these methods may be less effective in predicting children's response to treatment when compared with usage in adults with HIV (Cohen, 2002).

Adult treatment guidelines are appropriate for postpubertal adolescents who have been infected by sexual activity or needle-sharing behaviors because their clinical course is more similar to that of adults than to that of perinatally infected children (CDC, 2002b). Adolescents who are long-term survivors of perinatal HIV infection or transfusion-related infection as young children, however, may have a unique clinical course. Dosages of medications for HIV infection and opportunistic infection should be based on Tanner staging of puberty rather than age; adolescents in early puberty should be given dosages based on pediatric schedules, and those in late puberty should follow adult dosing schedules (CDC, 2002b).

Associated Problems (Box 28-6)

Failure to Thrive

Nutrition can be a significant problem for children with HIV, particularly for those with chronic diarrhea and *Candida* esophagitis. Many infants and children with symptomatic disease demonstrate poor weight gain and often fall below the fifth percentile on the National Center for Health Statistics growth curves for weight (Arpadi, 2000). Because most children with HIV/AIDS also experience nutritional deficits, malnutrition is thought to be a cofactor of immune dysfunction (Miller & Garg, 1998).

Specific causes of chronic diarrhea (e.g., *Cryptosporidium* spp., *Giardia* spp., and *Mycobacterium avium-intracellulare* [MAI] spp.) are rarely found, even after exhaustive gastrointestinal (GI) and stool examinations. Some children thrive better on lactose-free diets, whereas others experience cyclical diarrhea unresponsive to dietary manipulations. The GI tract is a major target for HIV because it constitutes 60% of all the lymphocytes in the body. Therefore these problems are thought to be caused by changes in the GI tract secondary to direct invasion by HIV (Miller & Garg, 1998). HIV-associated

BOX 28-6
Associated Problems

FAILURE TO THRIVE
Chronic diarrhea
Candida sp. esophagitis
Malnutrition

NEUROLOGIC MANIFESTATIONS
HIV encephalopathy
Developmental delay
Deterioration of motor skills and/or cognitive functions

Acquired microcephaly
Impaired brain growth
Cortical atrophy
Calcifications

Gait disturbances
Deficits in expressive language

OPPORTUNISTIC INFECTIONS (OI)
Major cause of death
PCP most common OI

PULMONARY DISEASE
Noninfections
PLH/LIP
Nonspecific pulmonary fibrosis
Pulmonary hypertension
Aspiration pneumonia

Infections
PCP
CMV
RSV
MTB
Rubeola
Varicella

PANCYTOPENIA
Thrombocytopenia
Anemias
Leukopenia
Neutropenia
Lymphopenia

FUNGAL INFECTIONS
Candidiasis

DRUG EXPOSURE
Delayed development
Learning/behavioral difficulties

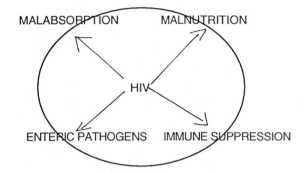

FIGURE 28-1 Link between malabsorption, malnutrition, and HIV infection. From Winter, H.S. & Miller, T.L. (1995). Gastrointestinal and nutritional problems in HIV disease. In Pizzo, P.A. & Wilfert, C.M. (Eds.). *Pediatric AIDS: the challenge of HIV infection in infants, children, and adolescents* (2nd ed.). Baltimore: Williams & Wilkins. Reprinted with permission.

Neurologic Manifestations

The brain is a target site for HIV infection in infants and children, and a variety of clinical patterns of neurodevelopmental involvement emerge (Pearson et al, 2000). In most children the neurologic dysfunction appears to be a result of direct infection of the CNS by HIV (Browers et al, 1998). HIV encephalopathy may result in developmental delay, deterioration of motor skills and cognitive functioning, and behavioral abnormalities. This course may be static, progressive, or episodic with plateaus of relative stability that last months alternating with intervals of marked deterioration that last weeks. The degree of neurologic deficit is variable and related to an individual's age at first symptom, stage of disease, rate of disease progression, and the current age (Brewers et al, 1998; Khoury & Kovacs, 2001). Some degree of neurologic impairment is usually found in all symptomatic children, but CNS involvement may be the first and only sign of HIV disease in a child.

Acquired microcephaly is often observed in infants and young children with HIV disease. Computed tomography (CT) scanning and magnetic resonance imaging (MRI) often show impaired brain growth with diffuse cortical atrophy and basal ganglia calcifications in severely affected infants. Cerebrospinal fluid (CSF)—even if positive for HIV culture—usually shows normal glucose, protein levels, and cell count.

Children with acquired microcephaly may demonstrate gradual apathy, progressive motor deficits resulting in generalized weakness and gait disturbances, and difficulties with expressive language. It is often perplexing to differentiate the effect of HIV infection from the effects of prenatal and perinatal drug exposure, prematurity, chronic disease, and chaotic social environments.

Opportunistic Infections

Opportunistic infections (OIs), including bacterial, mycobacterial, fungal, protozoal, and viral infections, are the major cause of death for children with HIV infection (Hines, 2000; Dankner et al, 2001). Serious bacterial infections often occur in children with HIV, and the risk of infection continues throughout childhood (Wilfert, 1998). *Pneumocystis carinii* sp. pneumonia (PCP) is the most frequent AIDS-defining illness in children with HIV, and most cases occur between the third and sixth

malnutrition is no different from malnutrition of other causes. Children with chronic conditions who are experiencing malabsorption may also have malnutrition-induced immunodeficiency, which creates an atmosphere in which enteric pathogens are likely to thrive. Therefore malabsorption, malnutrition, immunodeficiency, and enteric infections appear to be interrelated (Miller & Garg, 1998). Figure 28-1 shows the obvious necessity of good nutrition in supporting the immune system of children with HIV infection (Butensky 2001; Guarino et al, 2002).

months of life. The initial episode of PCP is most often fatal, even with appropriate treatment (Pizzo & Wilfert, 1998). The high rate of recurrence makes prophylaxis imperative.

Pulmonary Disease

Pulmonary disease and resultant respiratory failure profoundly contribute to the morbidity and mortality of pediatric HIV infection. Despite successful trends in the treatment of HIV disease, pulmonary disease remains a common clinical manifestation of pediatric HIV disease (Perez Mato & Van Dyke, 2002). More than 80% of HIV-infected children develop lung disease during the course of their illness (Andiman & Shearer, 1998). Pulmonary complications of pediatric HIV infection may be divided by noninfectious and infectious etiologies. The lymphoid infiltrates represent a continuum from focal lymphocytic hyperplasia in lung parenchyma (PLH) to more diffuse infiltration of alveolar septa and interstitial tissue (LIP) and then to neoplastic lymphoproliferative disease (Andiman & Shearer, 1998). Symptoms may be subtle and include tachypnea, dyspnea, cough, and exercise intolerance. Treatment is generally symptomatic and supportive but also depends upon antiretroviral therapy aimed at the underlying HIV infection, as well as corticosteroids. PLH/LIP may be complicated by superinfection with viral, bacterial, or other pathogens.

PCP, which is a diffuse, desquamative alveolopathy that results in hypoxia, is the OI seen most often in pediatric AIDS. The clinical manifestations of children with PCP are age and immune status dependent. Symptoms are likely to be acute with fever, dyspnea, dry cough, cyanosis, and hypoxemia. Treatment of acute infection usually begins with TMP-SMX (Bactrim, Septra) and corticosteroids. Prophylaxis, both primary and secondary, with oral Bactrim or Septra is extremely effective.

Other pathogens causing pulmonary infection include cytomegalovirus (CMV); respiratory syncytial virus (RSV); *Mycobacterium tuberculosis* spp.; MAI; rubeola; varicella; and other viral, fungal, and bacterial sources. Reactive airway disease is common and considered to be chronic airway inflammation associated with frequent and persistent infection.

Pancytopenia

Hematologic abnormalities, occurring as a result of HIV infection or as an adverse effect of treatment, are common in children with HIV. Some children have thrombocytopenia, which is usually an immune response to circulating platelets, because their bone marrow produces megakaryocytes, which break down into platelets in the peripheral blood. Intravenous immunoglobulin (IVIG) is sometimes effective in raising the platelet count. An alternative treatment is administering pulses of high-dose corticosteroids. Platelet transfusions are rarely required. Anemias of chronic disease, drug-induced bone marrow suppression and iron deficiency, are common in this population and often require iron supplementation. Red blood cell (RBC) transfusions are sometimes indicated—especially in AZT-induced anemia. Cytomegalovirus-negative, washed, and irradiated RBCs and platelets are used to avoid introducing new infection and to protect against graft-versus-host disease. Abnormalities of the white blood cell (WBC) line (i.e., neutropenia, lymphopenia, and leukopenia) are also often seen.

The newer drugs that increase red blood cell production (erythropoietin) and white blood production are being used more routinely in pediatric HIV disease.

Fungal Infections

Candidiasis occurs frequently and may be manifested as either oral thrush or diaper dermatitis. Mucosal *Candida* sp. is the most prevalent opportunistic infection in all individuals with HIV (Walsh et al, 1998). First-line treatments for oral thrush usually include topical nystatin (Mycostatin) and clotrimazole (Mycelex) oral troches. Clotrimazole vaginal suppositories (100 mg) used orally are often more effective because they are 10 times more potent than oral suspensions or troches. Infants can be treated either by placing the suppository into the nipple of a bottle, allowing the infant to suck formula through it, or by dissolving the suppository in warm water and swabbing the mouth. Older children can suck the suppositories. Both nystatin and clotrimazole creams are available for skin infections. Refractory cases of mucous membrane and dermatologic infections may be treated systemically with oral ketoconazole (Nizoral) or fluconazole (Diflucan); IV amphotericin B may be necessary for refractory cases of mucosal candidiasis.

Prenatal and Perinatal Drug Exposure

Children with HIV who were born to mothers who have HIV and have had drugs and/or alcohol abuse are often premature and small for gestational age and have very immature immune systems. Their development is often delayed, and learning and behavioral difficulties are common (see Chapters 12, 36, and 37).

Prognosis

HIV infection is now the seventh leading cause of death in US children 1 to 14 years of age and is the leading cause of death in children 2 to 5 years old in many US cities (CDC, 2001c). More than 50% of the children diagnosed with AIDS have died, but the actual mortality rates appear to be changing along with treatment advances. Two distinct courses of disease of perinatally infected children seem to exist. Infants who have a shorter median survival time seem to develop symptoms by 4 to 6 months of age, qualify for an AIDS diagnosis by 1 year of age, and often die by 2 years of age; and infants with a longer median survival time usually develop mild symptoms during the first year that resolve over the second and third years, may not have an AIDS diagnosis for many years, and may live into adolescence and adulthood.

Data now exist to support the well-accepted hypothesis that prenatally infected children who have a rapidly progressive HIV course were infected early in gestation and those with a more indolent course were infected late in gestation or during the delivery process (Pizzo & Wilfert, 1998).

HEALTH CARE MAINTENANCE

Health Care Maintenance

All children followed by HIV centers must also have a primary care provider. The HIV specialty provider and primary care provider work together, partnering with the family, to provide the highest level of care.

Growth and Development

The poor growth of children with symptomatic HIV disease appears to be more related to the general failure to thrive associated with the underlying HIV infection than to specific problems with caloric intake or GI losses. A practitioner or a skilled assistant should carefully measure height and weight at least monthly and plot the findings on the child's individual National Center for Health Statistics growth chart. Tracking the child's BMI also should be done. The same scale should be used at each visit if possible.

As previously noted, cortical atrophy and acquired microcephaly are common findings in severely affected infants. All children up to 3 years of age require serial head circumference measurements at least every 3 months, with results plotted on their growth charts and carefully evaluated.

Standard developmental screening tests used by primary care providers (e.g., the Denver Developmental Screening Test II) are of little value in assessing children with HIV disease. Developmental delay is a hallmark of pediatric HIV infection, and early intervention seems to produce significant results; therefore, children must be regularly assessed by a skilled clinical psychologist as part of the comprehensive team approach. It is important for the primary care provider and the psychologist to discuss their developmental assessments and formulate a plan of action together.

Intervention strategies must begin as early as possible in an attempt to maximize a child's capabilities. Infant stimulation programs that focus on motor and language skills and additional specialties (e.g., physical, occupational, and speech therapy) can be provided at home, in the hospital, or in clinic or group settings. Preschool and school-aged children with the necessary physical stamina can best be mainstreamed into regular programs with special services added (Abramowitz et al, 1998).

Diet

Children with HIV need a well-balanced diet with emphasis on adequate calories to maintain and increase their weight with growth. Nutritionists must be part of the multidisciplinary primary care team, taking dietary histories and performing nutritional assessments to guide clinical decisions. There are no special dietary recommendations or restrictions based on HIV infection. Because failure to thrive is common in these individuals, however, early nutritional intervention before wasting occurs is important (Deatrick, 1998). Dietary supplementation and special formulas (e.g., Scandi-shakes [Scandipharm] and Instant Breakfast [Carnation] for those who can tolerate dairy products; Pediasure [Ross] for infants and younger children; Ensure/Ensure Plus [Ross], Boost/Boost Plus and Advera for older children and adolescents who are lactose intolerant) are often beneficial for weight stabilization and potential gain. Enteral feedings and IV alimentation may be used acutely, intermittently, or chronically for children with severe anorexia, vomiting, diarrhea, and other GI problems. Families should regularly consult the primary care provider regarding the child's particular needs. Oral megestrol (Megace) has proved to increase appetite in some children.

Safety

Primary care providers must teach the families safety precautions for children with neutropenia and thrombocytopenia, as well as how to evaluate a child with neutropenia for signs and symptoms of infection (see Chapter 17).

Caretakers may benefit from education on infectious disease transmission and control (e.g., the need for frequent handwashing and avoiding people with known contagious infections). Children with HIV and their household contacts must learn universal/standard blood and body substance precautions; daycare and school personnel must also be knowledgeable. Because there is such concern about casual contagion in the community, families must be well educated and able to withstand the apprehension of others if they choose to disclose. Several prospective studies of family and school contacts have found no evidence of the spread of HIV within these settings (Courville et al, 1998). Although HIV has been isolated in a variety of body fluids (including blood, CSF, pleural fluid, breast milk, semen, cervical secretions, saliva, and urine), only blood, semen, cervical secretions, and human milk have been implicated in its transmission.

It is important to counsel the child's caretaker about the safe storage of medications and equipment in the home (Maloney et al, 1998). Families may have many potentially hazardous medications at home. Children with HIV may be developmentally delayed or exhibit neurologic regression as the infection progresses, and safety precautions must be adjusted accordingly. If an HIV-infected parent cares for the child, the parent's ability to provide safe care must be frequently assessed because of the dementia often associated with HIV infection in adults.

Immunizations

Controversy continues about immunization practices in children with HIV. Live-virus vaccines have not been recommended for children with congenital or drug-induced immunodeficiencies because of the concern that live, attenuated vaccine viruses can produce infection in an immunocompromised host. Prospective studies, however, failed to reveal such problems in HIV-infected children (Committee on Infectious Diseases, 1999).

In addition, the dysfunction of the B-cell system typical of infants with HIV disease, which includes markedly elevated immunoglobulins, reflects nonspecific stimulation that is suggestive of a poor immune response to antigens and therefore to vaccines. Because of this immunologic dysfunction, immunogenicity and efficacy of vaccines may be lower in these children than in children who are immunocompetent. In general, children with symptomatic HIV infections have poor immunologic responses to vaccines and therefore should be considered susceptible regardless of history of vaccination, as well as receive passive immunoprophylaxis if indicated, when exposed to a vaccine-preventable disease such as measles or tetanus (CDC, 2002c).

Because live-virus, attenuated immunizations may be ineffective in children who have received IVIG within the past 3 months, the general practice is to administer these vaccinations at the midpoint between monthly IVIG infusions.

Hepatitis B Virus (HBV). Hepatitis B vaccine is recommended as part of the regular schedule of immunizations for all children, including those who are symptomatic with HIV infection.

Hepatitis A Virus (HAV). Hepatitis A vaccine is recommended in some states as part of the regular schedule of childhood immunizations, including those who are symptomatic with HIV infection.

Tetanus. Children with HIV should receive human tetanus immune globulin (TIG) regardless of vaccine status following an injury that places them at risk for tetanus infection (CDC, 2002a).

Polio. Currently inactivated poliomyelitis vaccine (EIPV) is recommended for all children (CDC, 2002a).

Measles, Mumps, and Rubella. The measles, mumps, and rubella (MMR) vaccination should be administered at the standard age of 12 to 15 months with a second dose at 4 to 6 years of age unless the risk for measles or rubeola exposure is increased. Monovalent measles vaccine can be used for infants 6 to 11 months old, with MMR revaccination at 12 months of age or older (CDC, 2001a). Regardless of vaccination status, children with both asymptomatic and symptomatic HIV infection should receive prophylaxis with immune globulin (IG) after exposure to measles (CDC, 2002a). Immune globulin may help prevent or minimize measles if administered within 6 days of exposure and is indicated for household contacts of children with HIV disease who are measles susceptible, especially for infants younger than 12 months of age. IG may be unnecessary if a child is receiving regular IVIG infusions and the last dose was within 3 weeks of exposure (CDC, 2002a).

***Haemophilus influenzae* Type B (HIB).** Conjugated polysaccharide-diphtheria HIB vaccine is recommended for all children at 2 months of age (CDC, 2002a). As previously noted, *H. influenzae* organisms are a common and serious pathogen in children with HIV, increasing the importance of immunization. Even children who have had one or more episodes of documented infection with *H. influenzae* before 2 years of age may not produce enough antibody to prevent subsequent infections, making vaccination imperative. Prophylaxis with rifampin (Rifadin) is required even after vaccination if there is a known contact with HIB (CDC, 2002a).

Pneumococcus. Pneumococci are a prevalent pathogen in children with HIV. The heptavalent pneumococcal conjugate vaccine (Prevnar) and polyvalent pneumococcal vaccine are recommended for all children ages 2 through 59 months in a series of two to four vaccinations depending on age (Committee on Infectious Diseases, 2000). Infants at risk for HIV should receive this vaccine as early as possible to provide some possible protection against pneumococci infections.

Influenza. Yearly influenza vaccination with the subvirion (i.e., split virus) bivalent vaccine is recommended for children older than 6 months of age with HIV exposure or infection and their household contacts (CDC, 2001b).

Varicella. Varicella (VZV) poses significant risks for dissemination, encephalitis, and pneumonia in children who are immunosuppressed. Limited data on the use of varicella vaccine in HIV positive children have shown it to be safe and effective for asymptomatic or mildly symptomatic HIV-infected children with age-specific CD4+ percentages of 25% or greater. A study of the use of varicella vaccine in HIV-infected children

with greater immune suppression is in progress (CDC, 1999). Children with HIV who are susceptible to varicella need to receive varicella-zoster immune globulin (VZIG) intramuscularly within 72 hours of exposure if they have not received IVIG within the past 3 weeks (CDC, 2001a).

Screening

Vision. Because of the incidence of CMV retinitis in adults with HIV disease and therefore the theoretical risk of a similar process affecting children, primary care providers must elicit a thorough visual history and provide a careful visual and funduscopic examination. Comprehensive pediatric HIV centers may recommend that all children with HIV be referred to a knowledgeable pediatric ophthalmologist for baseline screening and annual follow-up. If the findings are normal, the primary care provider can then continue to provide regular follow-up.

Hearing. Because of the frequent acute suppurative otitis media (OM) in children with HIV infection and the possibility of hearing loss, periodic audiometry and tympanometry should be performed. Children who require myringotomy tube placement require special precautions for swimming and showers (e.g., regular use of well-fitting earplugs).

Children with severe neurologic disease, some children with chronic OM, and those on maintenance aminoglycoside therapy need baseline brainstem, auditory-evoked response hearing testing if routine acuity testing cannot be done or is abnormal.

Dental. Early screening (i.e., starting at 2 to 3 years of age) is strongly recommended because dental caries can create a focus of infection. Fluoride treatments are recommended if the community water supply does not contain adequate amounts to protect enamel. Severe dental caries and gingivitis, as well as dental abscesses, are reported in some infected children (Ramos-Gomez, 1997). Clinicians must educate families on appropriate oral hygiene and encourage regular dental care. Liquid medications contain sweeteners to increase drug palatability, which also increases the risk of caries.

Blood Pressure. Blood pressure measurements should be taken every 3 to 6 months unless changes warrant more frequent measurements. Increased blood pressure can indicate renal disease.

Hematocrit. Screening is deferred because of the need for frequent assessment of CBCs.

Urinalysis. Children with HIV require urinalysis with microscopic examination at least every 3 months because urine abnormalities can be the first sign of illness. Findings can include hematuria and proteinuria and can result in azotemia and nephrotic syndrome. Children taking the protease inhibitor indinavir (Crixivan) need frequent (i.e., at least monthly) urinalysis with microscopic examination for blood and crystals because this drug is known to cause renal stones.

Tuberculosis. Yearly screening is strongly advised. As tuberculosis is being diagnosed more often in adults with HIV, more children in infected households are at risk. Because many individuals infected with HIV demonstrate anergy to skin testing, close surveillance of families may include regular chest radiographic studies. MAI is a common bacterium of the same family as *Mycobacterium tuberculosis,* which is prevalent in individuals with HIV. Unlike *M. tuberculosis,* MAI is not contagious by the respiratory route but may be transmitted through infected GI secretions. Because it can invade many organ systems, including the bone marrow and the GI system, MAI may be responsible for much morbidity.

Condition-Specific Screening

Vital Signs. Vital signs should be assessed and documented at each visit. Children can be asymptomatic yet febrile, needing a work-up. Elevations in heart and respiratory rates can indicate pulmonary or cardiac dysfunction.

Complete Blood Count. Because of bone marrow suppression caused by HIV and some OIs, as well as by many of the drugs used in treatment, children with HIV require that CBCs—with differential and platelet counts—be regularly determined. Asymptomatic children should have a CBC done every 3 to 6 months; symptomatic children usually need them done at least monthly. This bloodwork can be performed by the primary care provider or at the pediatric HIV center.

If anemia is present, its cause should be investigated because children with iron deficiency anemia usually benefit from oral iron supplementation. A specific cause, however, is not often discovered. Children taking antiretrovirals need their CBCs and reticulocyte counts assessed frequently because anemia is a common adverse effect. CBCs are usually completed every 2 weeks for the first 2 months and then done monthly as long as they are stable. Some children taking antiretrovirals require RBC transfusions. Neutropenia and thrombocytopenia are also common side effects of antiretroviral treatment. Dosages of antiretrovirals may be modified based on the degree of bone marrow suppression. Bone marrow–stimulating drugs such as filgrastim (Neupogen) and granulocyte colony–stimulating factor (G-CSF) may be used.

Immunologic Markers. Baseline T- and B-cell counts and quantitative immunoglobulin (QUIG) determinations are necessary to assess immunologic status. T-cell subset values and T4/T8 ratios are usually checked every 3 to 6 months. T4 counts below 350 mm^3 generally indicate that antiretrovirals should be prescribed. Children receiving monthly IVIG infusions do not have serial QUIG assessments because the infused—rather than endogenous—immunoglobulins would be represented.

Clinicians interpreting immunologic markers for children must consider age as a variable. These markers are used in conjunction with other markers to guide antiretroviral treatment decisions and primary prophylaxis for PCP after 1 year of age.

HIV Markers. Viral burden can be determined by using quantitative HIV RNA viral load assays of peripheral blood. During primary infection in adults and adolescents, the HIV RNA viral load rises to high peak levels and then—coinciding with the body's humoral and cell-mediated immune response—declines by 2 to 3 logs to a stable lower level some 6 to 12 months later. This leveling off reflects the balance, or steady state, between ongoing viral production and immune elimination (CDC, 2001c). This pattern differs in perinatally infected infants in that high HIV RNA levels usually persist during the first year of life and then gradually decline over the next few years. This pattern may reflect an immature but developing immune system's lower efficiency in containing viral replication and more HIV-susceptible cells.

Trends in HIV RNA levels can be helpful in determining antiretroviral therapy and when the agents should be changed. Because of the complexities of testing and the age-related changes in values, interpretation of HIV RNA levels for clinical decision making should be done by or in consultation with pediatric HIV experts.

Chemistry Panel. Routine serum chemistry panels should be obtained every 3 to 6 months and more often for symptomatic children or those taking medications (i.e., AZT, didanosine [ddI]) that might affect liver or kidney function. Children taking ddI, d4T, and/or 3TC must also be monitored for pancreatitis by having their amylase and lipase levels regularly checked. Children taking protease inhibitors need regular lipid panels (including lipase, cholesterol, triglyceride, and glucose levels). Many children with HIV have elevated baseline liver function test results, often with both aspartate aminotransferase (AST) and alanine aminotransferase (ALT) enzyme levels two to three times that of normal.

Pulmonary Function. Children with chronic lung disease need baseline pulmonary function testing with oxygen saturation and regular serial testing based on disease severity. When available, pulse oximetry—a noninvasive technique—is used in place of arterial blood gas sampling. A baseline radiograph is useful as a comparison study for pulmonary complaints. Children with either acute infection or chronic pneumonitis often have no adventitious sounds. Pulmonary consultation is a useful adjunct for the primary care provider in following these children.

Common Illness Management
Differential Diagnosis (Box 28-7)

Fever. Fever is often a sign in children with HIV disease and can be caused by the HIV itself or can indicate a separate infectious process. Practitioners must ensure that families have a thermometer that they can use accurately, as well as clear guidelines about when to contact their primary care provider. Whenever a child's temperature measures at least 38.5° C (101° F), the child generally needs to be examined and a treatment plan initiated based on the objective and subjective findings.

BOX 28-7
Differential Diagnosis

Fever
   HIV infection vs. other infectious process

Respiratory distress
   LIP vs. PCP
   Cardiomyopathy
   Reactive airway disease

Otitis media
   ENT referral for tube placement

Sinusitis
   Untreated infection can lead to meningitis

Varicella
   Risk of dissemination high

A thorough interval history and complete physical examination are the most important part of the work-up of a febrile child with HIV. Some of these children will have otitis media, sinusitis, pneumonia, or sepsis; others will have common colds and other viral infections that can be traced to school or household contacts.

In consultation with the infectious disease specialist or the HIV center, the primary care provider can order cultures of blood and other body fluids as indicated for aerobic, anaerobic, and fungal organisms. Cultures are essential to identifying the infectious process. Cultures are often negative—even in seriously ill children, but positive cultures will determine specific antibiotic therapy. Chest radiographic studies may be an important part of the work-up of a febrile child with HIV.

Respiratory Distress. A variety of respiratory complaints may plague children with HIV. History and physical examination are paramount to the differential diagnosis. A dry, hacking cough is a common complaint of children with LIP but can also be a sign of PCP. Children with acute onset of respiratory distress require quick evaluation because the condition can progress extremely rapidly—sometimes within hours. Pulmonary consultation is often necessary. Children with cardiac disease occasionally have respiratory complaints and need cardiologic consultation and diagnosis.

Children with known reactive airway disease may benefit from having equipment and medications for aerosol delivery at home. The primary care provider must evaluate the family's ability to provide such sophisticated assessment and treatment; if parents are capable, they can be taught the necessary skills.

Otitis Media. Otitis media (OM) is one of the most common infectious diseases in children with HIV and is often diagnosed on routine physical examination when no pain or fever is present, even when the tympanic membrane may be ruptured with pus filling the external canal. Follow-up must be done after treatment is completed because the OM may not resolve and complications may occur. Children who have persistent and refractory OM should be referred to an ear, nose, and throat (ENT) specialist for evaluation for placement of myringotomy tubes.

Sinusitis. Although sinusitis is uncommon in children, it is seen commonly in children with HIV disease and often occurs after a viral respiratory tract infection. Primary care providers can teach families to report changes in nasal mucus from clear or white to yellow or green, which may indicate infection. If not appropriately treated, sinusitis can lead to mastoiditis and directly extend into the brain, causing meningitis.

Varicella. Because of the risk of dissemination as a result of immunocompromise, varicella is potentially life threatening in children with HIV. Because these children may not respond adequately to vaccines and the general herd immunity to varicella will not be high until the vaccine has been widely distributed for many years, herpes zoster virus (HZV) will continue to cause chickenpox as a primary manifestation and zoster as a secondary manifestation of infection in most children with HIV. If primary prevention with VZIG fails or if a child was not known to be exposed until the rash occurs, the usual practice at most centers is to quickly evaluate these children. Most will start oral treatment with acyclovir right away regardless of their immune status. Some will require hospitalization for treatment with IV acyclovir. With this treatment, few children progress to disseminated disease, and most go home within 5 days of starting therapy, continuing with oral therapy to complete a 7- to 10-day course.

Drug Interactions

Antiretrovirals. The following three groups of agents are used to treat HIV infection: (1) nucleoside reverse transcriptase inhibitors (e.g., AZT, 3TC, ddI, zalcitabine [ddC], d4T, abacavir); (2) nonnucleoside reverse transcriptase inhibitors (e.g., nevirapine, delavirdine, sustiva); and (3) protease inhibitors (e.g., saquinavir, ritonavir, indinavir, nelfinavir, lopinavir/ritonavir) (CDC, 2001c). There are variations in whether each drug may be given on an empty or full stomach, and some must be given separately from other drugs. Many of these drugs have significant drug interactions. It is best to identify the specific considerations of each and every drug that a child with HIV is taking.

TMP-SMX. Two of the major toxicities of this sulfa combination are hematologic: neutropenia and thrombocytopenia. Children on PCP prophylaxis or treatment regimens who develop persistent neutropenia secondary to TMP-SMX either alone or with AZT must often discontinue TMP-SMX. Dapsone, atovaquone, and intravenous or aerosolized pentamidine can be used as alternatives in older children. Allergic reactions to sulfa are not uncommon, and primary care providers must teach families how to recognize the symptoms of skin rash and hives as part of the reaction complex. Several studies have shown successful treatment using TMP-SMX with a history of previous adverse reactions (Simonds & Orejas, 1998).

IVIG. There are no specific drug interactions noted with IVIG. Allergic reactions have been documented but appear to be rare.

Developmental Issues

Sleep Patterns

Children taking AZT or other medications that interrupt normal sleeping hours may experience difficulty in returning to sleep. Findings from a study on sleep disturbances in children with HIV suggest that sleep disturbances occur frequently (Franck et al, 1998). Therefore parents may need to try a variety of schedules to find one that works best for them and their child to minimize interruptions in their child's sleeping hours.

Toileting

Children with HIV who are in diapers may experience diaper dermatitis, which is often associated with candidiasis, as well as with chronic and cyclic diarrhea. Impeccable perineal care—including frequent diaper changes, exposure of the perineum to air, and the use of topical medications—can significantly reduce morbidity. When the perineum is bloody or the child has hematuria or diarrhea, caretakers should wear gloves to protect themselves during diapering. Neurologic deterioration can lead to incontinence in children who have previously been out of diapers.

Discipline

Discipline is often difficult for the family of a child with a life-threatening illness. Some parents are unable to set developmentally appropriate and necessary limits and need guidance and information from their primary care provider. Discipline needs and appropriate expectations will vary as the illness progresses and neurologic and motor deterioration occurs, so caretakers must be given anticipatory guidance in these areas. Other factors (e.g., homelessness, chaotic lifestyle, and parental illness) can make consistent discipline difficult. Practitioners may need to help families and caregivers understand the child's needs for safety and limits.

Child Care

Child care, respite care, and preschool placement are difficult issues for families of children with HIV. Primary care providers must advise parents that children in group settings are at increased risk for exposure to infectious diseases and common childhood illnesses compared with children who stay at home (Takala et al, 1995). The particular setting must be individualized for each child based on the child and family's needs and resources. Practitioners can provide education on universal infection control and infectious disease guidelines for these agencies.

Child care and respite care are important resources for families caring for children with chronic conditions. Some foster families have access to respite hours through their social services division, but others do not. In some areas there are few, if any, child care or respite workers willing to care for infants and children with HIV, which is an enormous problem for families who need time to care for their own HIV, as well as for their infected and uninfected children. The regular availability of respite care and other support services may allow many infected mothers to continue to care for their children. It is important to note that uninfected parents and caregivers also need respite care.

Public Laws 101-476 and 99-457, as well at the IDEA, ADA, and Lanterman Act, may offer valuable services for children with HIV (see Chapter 5). Head Start, a federal preschool program that provides preschool for economically deprived children, is specifically mandated to enroll children with HIV.

Because daycare and preschool are not a legal requirement for children, individual daycare providers may develop their own policies in accordance with local, state, and federal regulations. Many private daycare centers and preschools do not accept children with HIV, probably because of their fears of casual contagion, litigation, and disenrollment if other families discover the diagnosis. Some areas of the country with a high prevalence of pediatric HIV have developed daycare programs specifically for these children. Such services are directed toward children who are too ill to attend regular daycare programs.

Daycare and preschool personnel and families should be educated before a child with HIV is enrolled. It may be useful for the primary care provider to call the preschool, stating that a family is interested in enrolling their child with HIV. The school is notified that there is no "duty to inform" and that the child will not be identified. Feelings about children with HIV infection are explored, and an offer is made to provide in-service training about pediatric HIV and control of general infection.

Some families choose to conceal the HIV in their family, but other families openly discuss it (Wiener et al, 1998). As more

children take antiviral medications such as AZT that must be administered frequently, it is becoming harder to conceal HIV infection from daycare providers. Many families schedule dosing around school hours and create unusual stories about why they need to immediately know about chickenpox or other contagious illnesses in the classroom. Clinicians have an important role to play in helping families decide how, when, and to whom information about HIV disease should be disclosed (Committee on Pediatric AIDS, 1999a). Nondisclosure may be an appropriate consideration in some cases when there is no duty to disclose.

Schooling

The major school issues faced by young children with HIV have little to do with their educational needs and much to do with concerns about confidentiality, information sharing, and infection control. These issues have created strife in many communities nationwide. As children with HIV age, however, their needs for special education programs will undoubtedly increase. Primary care providers can help the families secure the appropriate services (see Chapter 5).

Because AIDS is recognized as a handicap, Public Law 101-476 supports attendance in public schools. In some areas of the country, committees of educators and public health officials, along with the child's primary care provider if the child's HIV status is disclosed, decide public school attendance. If the decision to ban the child from attending school is made, the school district must provide home teaching. Children benefit greatly from attending school, so this option should be strongly discouraged. When children are too ill to attend, home teaching is a viable alternative for that time period only. As a child's condition progresses, particularly with neurologic deterioration, frequent meetings of school resource personnel, health care providers, and family members will be needed to ensure that appropriate services are provided.

The legal duty to inform school officials about a child's HIV diagnosis varies from state to state (Cohen, 1997). As more children become aware of their own HIV infection, there will be more discussion among these children, which will make more of the school and larger community aware that a child with HIV is in attendance. Providers should be available to the school (i.e., students, faculty, and parents) for educational discussion sessions.

Teenagers with HIV often have difficulty in school. Rumors that circulate about HIV infection and the students thought to be infected can cause tremendous anxiety for an infected adolescent—regardless of the route of infection (Chabon & Futterman, 1999). Primary care providers can support their teenaged clients, helping them gain more knowledge and determine whom they might trust with this sensitive information. Referral to the school nurse or counselor may be appropriate.

Disclosure. Many children are not told their diagnosis because of the family's concerns that the child will become depressed, angry or may tell others and expose the family to discrimination or stigmatization (Hines, 2000). Now that these children are surviving into adolescence and adulthood, disclosure is becoming a common clinical issue. Recommendations and guidelines for disclosure are available (AAP, 1999). Nondisclosure can result in anxiety and depression. The process of disclosure should take the child's age, psychologic maturity, and family dynamics into account (Gerson et al, 2001).

Sexuality

Children and adolescents with HIV need to learn about all modes of transmission of this condition, with an emphasis on sexual, injection-drug use, and perinatal transmission. Adolescence is the time for sexual experimentation and the emergence of sexual identity, and sexual activity increases steadily throughout these years. Teens with HIV face much difficulty in attaining a healthy, integrated sexual identity because of the risks of oral and genital sexual transmission (Ledlie, 2002). Some teens deny the reality of their HIV, refusing to practice safe sex. Some teens suffer from cognitive delays stemming from neurologic effects of HIV. Primary care providers must be comfortable discussing transmission and sexual risk reduction strategies, as well as demonstrating the proper use of condoms and dental dams in developmentally appropriate and cognitively limited teens.

Transition to Adulthood

The advent of new and more effective HIV therapies has transformed HIV infection from a terminal illness to a chronic but manageable condition. Survival times have continued to increase; there are now long-term survivors among children who were perinatally infected (Forsyth, 2000). These individuals will continue to need a vast array of medical and psychosocial services throughout their childhood and transition to adulthood (Ledlie, 2002). Because these children were born to mothers with HIV, many infected family members are often at risk for death from HIV while these children are young. As they reach sexual maturity, these children must be educated about and helped to deal with the fact that they can transmit HIV to their sexual or drug partners. Of course, all children need to be taught about STD prevention in general.

Children and teenagers who have been infected as a result of nonperinatal transmission (i.e., sexual activity, injection-drug use, transfusion, or transplantation) have many other concerns to face. Some of these issues include the risk for sexual transmission, intimacy, and stigma. As HIV infection becomes a more chronic, life-threatening disease integrated into the mainstream of health care, these special issues may gradually decline.

Family Concerns and Resources

HIV infection is a family disease, and when a child is diagnosed, a family crisis results. Many children with HIV have infected mothers who are ill, dying, or deceased and may have an infected father and siblings in the family, as well. Most mothers who transmit HIV to their children experience tremendous guilt. The physical and emotional burden of caring for a child who requires frequent medical and supportive treatments, may have developmental delay, and will probably die as a result of the illness is enormous for all parents and caregivers, regardless of whether the adults are infected.

The most significant psychosocial issue facing children with HIV and their families is the social stigmatization associated with the disease. Many families initially feel isolated and unable to call on their normal support systems for fear of rejection and retaliation. Infected families may also lack other resources; they are primarily poor, of minority heritage, undereducated, and burdened by the social ills of inner-city life. With support, these families may reach out to extended family, friends, and community agencies. Noninfected parents and caregivers also need support in caring for their children and in getting the community support that is available.

The majority of children who were perinatally infected with HIV are of African-American and Latino descent. Some children are placed in foster or adoptive care after birth if their mother is unable to care for them. Others are placed out of the home later when resources cannot support their parents' ability to care for them. Foster and adoptive parents need considerable support (i.e., ongoing education, financial support, respite care, emotional support and counseling, and social and legal counseling) to provide optimal care for these children. Because children in foster care are wards of the juvenile court, decisions about consent for investigational drugs and experimental protocols, as well as do-not-resuscitate orders, must be court ordered. Working relationships between the primary care provider, HIV center, and social services must be developed to ensure that children with HIV receive optimal care in the child welfare system.

Helping children and families face a chronic life-threatening illness that may ultimately lead to death is a pivotal role for primary care providers. Counseling about the physical and emotional issues of death and the dying process, options for hospital or home death, hospice services, funeral plans, and bereavement are an integral part of the clinician's role. Support groups are invaluable resources for networking, keeping current, and decreasing social isolation. Most pediatric HIV/AIDS comprehensive treatment centers offer such groups on an ongoing basis. Primary care providers should become familiar with the local, national, and international organizations (see the list of organizations that follows).

Resources

Camps

Camp Heartland
www.campheartland.org

Camp Pacific Heartland
3663 Wilshire Boulevard
Los Angeles, CA 90010-2798
(213) 464-1235
www.campheartland.org/camping/campingprograms

Camp Sunburst National AIDS Project
5350 Commerce Boulevard, Suite I
Rohnert Park, CA 94928
(707) 588-9477
www.sunburstprojects.org

National Organizations

CDC National AIDS Clearinghouse
PO Box 6003
Rockville, MD 20849-6003
(800) 458-5231
www.cdcnpin.org

HIV and AIDS Malignancy Branch (HAMB), National Cancer Institute
(301) 496-0328
http://ccr.cancer.gov/Labs/Labs.asp?LabID=63

National AIDS Hotline
(800) 342-AIDS
www.ashastd.org/nah

National Center for Youth Law
114 Sansome Street, Suite 900
San Francisco, CA 94104-3820
(415) 543-3307
www.youthlaw.org

National Foundation for Children with AIDS
3505 South Ocean Drive
Hollywood, FL 33019
www.childrenwithaids.org

National Pediatric and Family HIV Resource Center
15 S. 9th Street
Newark, NJ 07107
(800) 362-0071
www.pedhivaids.org

NIAID Intramural Trials for HIV Infection and AIDS
(800) AIDS-NIH or (800) 243-7644

Safe Haven
PO Box 24
Vineyard Haven, MA 02568
(508) 693-1767

Sunshine for HIV Kids, Inc
C/o Richard Merck
PO Box 3537
Kingston, NY 12402
(888) SUN-4-KIDS
www.songshine.com

The Elizabeth Glaser Pediatric AIDS Foundation
1311 Colorado Avenue
Santa Monica, CA 90404
(310) 395-9051
www.pedaids.org

Local and State Resources
County health department
State health department
AIDS task forces
AIDS hotlines

Summary of Primary Care Needs for the Child with HIV

HEALTH CARE MAINTENANCE
Growth and development

Growth in both weight and height may be poor and should be measured and plotted monthly.

Cortical atrophy and acquired microcephaly are common in severely affected infants.

Measure and plot head circumference every 3 months until a child is 3 years of age.

Standard developmental screening tests are not useful; if available, serial screening by a psychologist is recommended.

Early intervention programs are recommended.

Diet
A balanced high-calorie diet should be emphasized.
Nutritional supplements are often beneficial.

Safety
The risk of infection because of immunocompromise is increased. Frequent hand washing and avoiding people with known infections is recommended.

The risk of bleeding because of thrombocytopenia is increased.

Universal/standard blood and body substance precautions should be taught to the family and community.

Safe storage of medication in the home is important.

Developmental delay or regression may alter safety requirements.

Parents with HIV must be evaluated for safe care practices because of symptoms of dementia.

Uninfected parents may also benefit from home evaluation especially as medications/treatments become more complex.

Immunizations
General poor immune response to vaccines. Passive immunoprophylaxis may be indicated when exposure occurs.

Hepatitis B vaccine should be given to all children with HIV.

Hepatitis A vaccine should be given according to state recommendations.

Tetanus immunoglobulin (TIG) should be given to children at risk for infection due to injury.

EIPV is recommended.

Give immune globulin within 6 days of measles exposure to prevent or modify course unless a child received IVIG in the previous 3 weeks.

Haemophilus influenzae type b is recommended. Known exposure to HIB requires prophylaxis with rifampin.

Pneumococcal vaccine series are recommended starting at 2 months of age.

Yearly influenza vaccine is recommended.

Varicella-zoster immune globulin is recommended within 72 hours of varicella exposure.

Screening
Vision. An ophthalmologist should do a baseline funduscopic examination with practitioner follow-up every 3 to 6 months; consider ophthalmologist follow-up every 1 to 2 years.

Hearing. Periodic audiometry and tympanometry screenings are recommended. Frequent acute otitis media and treatment with aminoglycosides may affect hearing.

A brain stem evoked-response (BSER) hearing test should be given to children with chronic OM or abnormal screening.

Dental. Early screening is recommended to prevent dental infections and should be followed up regularly to prevent and/or treat dental caries.

Blood Pressure. Measurements should be taken every 3 to 6 months. Increased BP may indicate renal disease.

Hematocrit. Routine screening is deferred because of the need for frequent CBC tests.

Continued

Summary of Primary Care Needs for the Child with HIV—cont'd

Urinalysis. Urinalysis with microscopic examination should be done at least every 3 months to rule out renal disease and monthly for children taking indinavir (Crixivan).

Tuberculosis. Yearly screening is recommended. Chest radiographic studies may be needed if a child is anergic. MAI infections are responsible for significant morbidity.

Condition-Specific Screening

Vital Signs. Temperature, heart rate, and respiratory rate should be checked at each visit.

Complete Blood Count. A CBC should be assessed every 3 to 6 months if a child is asymptomatic and every 2 to 4 weeks if a child is taking antiretrovirals or other myelosuppressive agents; those who are stabilized on antiretroviral therapy may require only quarterly blood counts. Anemia, neutropenia, and thrombocytopenia are common side effects of antivirals.

Immunologic Markers. Baseline T- and B-cell counts, QUIG values, repeat T-cell subset levels, and T4/T8 ratios should be checked every 3 to 6 months.

HIV Markers. HIV RNA viral load assays are taken periodically to determine disease progression and antiviral therapy.

Chemistry Panel. Serum chemistry panels should be obtained every 3 to 6 months if a child is asymptomatic and more often if a child is symptomatic or taking liver or kidney toxic agents. Serum amylase and lipase should be obtained for children taking d4T/3TC/ddI. Lipid panel and glucose should be obtained for children taking protease inhibitors.

Pulmonary Function. Baseline pulmonary function testing, including pulse oximetry if available, is recommended for children with lung disease.

COMMON ILLNESS MANAGEMENT

Differential diagnosis

Fever. Rule out bacterial infection and OI.

Respiratory Distress. Rule out LIP, PCP, and cardiac disease.

Otitis Media. Rule out tympanic membrane perforation.

Sinusitis. Rule out bacterial sinusitis, mastoiditis, and meningitis.

Varicella. Use VZIG as primary prevention and acyclovir as secondary prevention.

Drug interactions

Zidovudine. Bone marrow suppression may occur.

Didanosine (ddI), Stavudine (d4T), Epivir (lamivudine). Check amylase, lipase for pancreatitis.

Protease Inhibitors. Hyperglycemia, hypercholesterolemia, hypertriglyceridemia, and hyperbilirubinemia may occur. Many drug interactions occur with protease inhibitors. The provider needs to consult the *PDR*.

Nonnucleoside Analogs (NNRTIs). Allergic reactions may occur, including severe allergic rash.

TMP-SMX. Bone marrow suppression (neutropenia, thrombocytopenia) and allergic reactions may occur.

IVIG. No specific drug interactions and allergic reactions are rare.

DEVELOPMENTAL ISSUES

Sleep Patterns

Sleep patterns may be disturbed because of medications needed around the clock, as well as prenatal drug exposure issues.

Toileting

Impeccable perineal care is necessary to reduce morbidity of diaper dermatitis. Caretakers should use gloves for blood or diarrhea. Neurologic deterioration can lead to incontinence.

Discipline

Discipline is often difficult for the family; lifestyle issues can exacerbate problems.

Child Care

Participation in child care and preschool increases the risk of infections. The child care program should be individualized to meet the child and family's needs.

Public Laws 99-457 and 101-476, Lanterman Act cover early intervention services; all babies born to infected mothers are potentially at risk and qualify for services until the age of 3.

Head Start is mandated to enroll children with HIV. Child care personnel need education on condition, infection control, and medications.

Schooling

Public Law 101-476 aids public school attendance.

There is no duty to inform school officials of a child's HIV status.

The school community may benefit from education.

Teens may need extra support from the school nurse or counselor.

Sexuality

Sexual and perinatal transmission should be discussed.

Safer sex techniques and the use of condoms and dental dams should be demonstrated.

Transition to Adulthood

With improved treatment, HIV disease has become a chronic condition.

Parents may have died from condition years before.

Individuals must be educated about the possible transmission of HIV to others.

FAMILY CONCERNS

HIV is a family disease.

Many families lack resources.

HIV is an enormous physical and emotional burden.

Stigmatization is a major issue.

Many children with HIV are placed in foster or adoptive homes.

Counseling on death and dying and during bereavement is helpful.

Many children with HIV are of African-American and Latino descent. Primary care providers must be sensitive to specific cultural issues.

REFERENCES

Abramowitz, S., Obten, N., & Cohen, H. (1998). Measuring case management for families with HIV. *Soc Work Health Care, 27,* 29-41.

Andiman, W.A. & Shearer, W.T. (1998). Lymphoid interstitial pneumonitis. In P.A. Pizzo & C.M. Wilfert (Eds.), *Pediatric AIDS: the challenge of HIV infection in infants, children and adolescents* (3rd ed.). Baltimore: Williams & Wilkins.

Arpadi, S.M. (2000). Growth failure in children with HIV infection. *J Acquir Immune Defic Syndr Hum Retrovirol, 15*(Suppl. 1), S37-S42, 2000.

Browers, P., Wolters, P., & Civitello, L. (1998). Central nervous system manifestations and assessment. In P.A. Pizzo & C.M. Wilfert (Eds.), *Pediatric AIDS: the challenge of HIV infection in infants, children and adolescents* (3rd ed.). Baltimore: Williams & Wilkins.

Butensky, E.A. (2001). The role of nutrition in pediatric HIV/AIDS: a review of micronutrient research. *J Pediatr Nurs, 16*(6), 402-411.

Butz, A.M., Joyner, M., Friedman, D.G., & Hutton, N. (1998). Primary care for children with human immunodeficiency virus infection. *J Pediatr Health Care, 12,* 10-19.

Centers for Disease Control and Prevention. (1994). 1994 revised classification system for human immunodeficiency virus infection in children less than 13 years of age. *MMWR Morb Mortal Wkly Rep, 43*(RR-12), 1-10.

Centers for Disease Control and Prevention. (1999). Rotavirus vaccine for the prevention of rotavirus gastroenteritis among children: recommendations of the advisory committee on immunization practices (ACIP). *MMWR Morb Mortal Wkly Rep, 48*(RR-2), 1-23.

Centers for Disease Control and Prevention. (1999). Prevention of varicella update recommendations of the advisory committee on immunization practices (ACIP). *MMWR Morb Mortal Wkly Rep, 48*(RR-6), 1-5.

Centers for Disease Control and Prevention. (2001a). Recommended childhood immunization schedule—United States. *MMWR Morb Mortal Wkly Rep, 50,* 7-10.

Centers for Disease Control and Prevention. (2001b). Prevention and control of influenza: recommendations of the advisory committee on immunization practice (ACIP). *MMWR Morb Mortal Wkly Rep, 50*(RR-4).

Centers for Disease Control and Prevention. (2001c). Guidelines for the use of antiretroviral agents in pediatric HIV-infection [online]. Available: www.hivatis.org.

Centers for Disease Control and Prevention. (2002a). Notice to reader: recommended childhood immunization schedule—United States. *MMWR Morb Mortal Wkly Rep, 50*(02), 31-33.

Centers for Disease Control and Prevention. (2002b). Guidelines for the use of antiretroviral agents in HIV-infected adults and adolescents. *MMWR Morb Mortal Wkly Rep, 51*(NORR-7), 1-64.

Centers for Disease Control and Prevention. (2002c). HIV/AIDS surveillance report: U.S. HIV and AIDS cases reported through December 2001 Year-end edition. Vol.13, No.2,10.

Centers for Disease Control and Prevention. (2002d). Public Health Task Force recommendations: use of antiretroviral drugs in pregnant HIV-1 infected women for maternal health and interventions to reduce perinatal HIV-1 transmission in the United States [online]. Available: www.hivatis.org.

Chabon, B. & Futterman, D. (1999). Adolescents and HIV. *AIDS Clin Care, 11,* 1.

Cohen, J., et al. (1997). School-related issues among HIV-infected children. *Pediatrics, 100,* E8.

Cohen, N.J., Oram, R., Elsen, C., & Englund, J.A. (2002). Response to changes in antiretroviral therapy after genotyping in human immunodeficiency virus-infected children. *Pediatr Infect Dis J, 21*(7), 647-653.

Committee on Infectious Diseases. (1997). *Report of the Committee on Infectious Disease* (24th ed.). Elk Grove Village, IL: The American Academy of Pediatrics.

Committee on Infectious Diseases. (1999). Poliomyelitis prevention: revised recommendations for use of inactivated and live oral poliovirus vaccines, American Academy of Pediatrics. *Pediatrics, 103,* 171-172.

Committee on Infectious Diseases. (2000). Policy statement: recommendations for the prevention of pneumococcal infections, including the use of pneumococcal conjugate vaccine (Prevnar), pneumococcal polysaccharide vaccine and antibiotic prophylaxis (RE9960), American Academy of Pediatrics. *Pediatrics, 106*(2), 362-366.

Committee on Pediatric AIDS. (1999a). Disclosure of illness status to children and adolescents with HIV infection, American Academy of Pediatrics. *Pediatrics, 103,* 164-166.

Committee on Pediatric AIDS. (1999b). Planning for children whose parents are dying of HIV/AIDS, American Academy of Pediatrics. *Pediatrics, 103,* 509-511.

Courville, T.M., Caldwell, B., & Brunell, P.A. (1998). Lack of evidence of transmission of HIV-1 to family contacts of HIV-1 infected children. *Clin Pediatr, 37,* 175-178.

Dankner, W.M., Lindsey, J.C., & Levin, M.J. (2001). The Pediatric AIDS Clinical Trials Group Protocol Teams 051, 128, 138, 144, 152, 179, 190, 220, 240, 245, 254, 300 and 327. *Pediatr Infect Dis J, 20*(1): 40-48, 2001.

Deatrick, J.A., et al. (1998). Nutritional assessment for children who are HIV-infected. *Pediatr Nurs, 24,* 137-141.

Diego, M. & Field, T. (2001). HIV adolescents show improved immune function following massage therapy. *Int J Neurosci, 106*(1/2), 35-44.

Duggan, J., Peterson, W., Schutz, M., Khuder, S., & Charkraborty, J. (2001). Use of complementary and alternative therapies in HIV-infected patients. *AIDS Patient Care STDS, 15*(3), 159-167.

Forsyth, B. (2000). HIV infection in children, a new hope. *Child Adolesc Psychiatr Clin N Am, 9*(2), 279-294.

Franck, L.S., et al. (1999). Sleep disturbances in children with HIV infection. *Pediatrics, 104*(5): e62.

Gerson, A.C., et al. (2001). Disclosure of HIV diagnosis to children: when, where, why and how. *J Pediatr Health Care, 15*(4), 161-167.

Guarino, A., et al. (2002). Effects of nutritional rehabilitation on intestinal function and on CD4 cell number in children with HIV. *J Pediatr Gastroenterol Nutr, 34*(4), 366-371.

Hines, S. (2000). Primary care for HIV-exposed and infected children: translating progress into practice. *Lippincotts Prim Care Pract, 4*(1), 43-65.

Kamani, N.R. & Douglas, S.D. (1991). Structure and development of the immune system. In D.P. Sites & A.F. Terr (Eds.), *Basic and clinical immunology* (7th ed.). Norfolk, CN: Appleton & Lange.

Khoury, M. & Kovacs, A. (2001). Pediatric HIV infection. *Clin Obstet Gynecol, 44*(2), 243-275.

Krasinski, K. (1994). Bacterial infections. In P.A. Pizzo & C.M. Wilfert (Eds.), *Pediatric AIDS: the challenge of HIV infection in infants, children, and adolescents* (2nd ed.). Baltimore: Williams & Wilkins.

Layton, T.L. & Davis-McFarland, E. (2000). Pediatric human immunodeficiency virus and acquired immunodeficiency syndrome: an overview. *Semin Speech Lang, 21*(1), 7-17.

Ledlie, S. (2002). The psychological issues of children with perinatally acquired HIV disease becoming adolescents: a growing challenge for providers. *AIDS Patient Care STDs, 12*(5), 231-236.

Luzuriaga, K. & Sullivan, J.L. (2002). Pediatric HIV-1 infection: advances and remaining challenges. *AIDS Rev, 4*(1), 21-26.

Luzuriaga, K. & Sullivan, J.L. (1998). Prevention and treatment of pediatric HIV infection. *JAMA, 280,* 17-18.

Luzuriaga, K. & Sullivan, J.L. (1998). Viral and immunopathogenesis of vertical HIV-1 infection. In P.A. Pizzo & C.M. Wilfert (Eds.), Pediatric AIDS: the challenge of HIV infection in infants, children and adolescents (3rd ed.). Baltimore: Williams & Wilkins.

Luzuriaga, K., et al. (1997). Combination treatment with zidovudine, didanosine, and nevirapine in infants with human immunodeficiency virus type 1 infection. *N Engl J Med, 336,* 1343-1349.

MacIntyre, R.C., Holzemer, W.L., & Philippek, M. (1997). Complementary and alternative medicine and HIV-AIDS. Part I: issues and context. *J Assoc Nurses AIDS Care, 8,* 23-31.

Maloney, C., Damon, B., & Regan, A.M. (1998). Pediatric compliance in combination HIV therapy: getting it right the first time. *Adv Nurse Pract, 6,* 35-38.

McKinney, R.E. Jr., et al. (1998). A randomized study of combined zidovudine-lamivudine versus didanosine monotherapy in children with symptomatic therapy-naïve HIV-1 infection: the pediatric AIDS clinical trials group protocol 300 study team. *J Pediatr, 133,* 500-508.

Miller, T.L. & Garg, S. (1998). Gastrointestinal and nutritional problems in pediatric HIV disease. In P.A. Pizzo & C.M. Wilfert (Eds.), *Pediatric AIDS: the challenge of HIV infection in infants, children and adolescents* (3rd ed.). Baltimore: Williams & Wilkins.

Palumbo, P.E. (2000). Antiretroviral therapy of HIV infection in children. *Pediatr Clin North Am, 47*(1), 155-169.

Pearson, D.A., et al. (2000). Predicting HIV disease progression in children using measures of neuropsychological and neurological functioning. Pediatric AIDS clinical trials 152-study team. *Pediatrics, 106*(6), E76.

Perez Mato, S. & Van Dyke, R.B. (2002). Pulmonary infections in children with HIV infection. *Semin Respir Infect, 17*(1), 33-46.

Pizzo, P.A. & Wilfert, C.M. (Eds.), *Pediatric AIDS: the challenge of HIV infection in infants, children and adolescents.* (3rd ed.). Baltimore: Williams & Wilkins.

Ramos-Gomez, F.J. (1997). Oral aspects of HIV infection in children. *Oral Dis,* (Suppl 1), S31-S35.

Simonds, R.J. & Orejas, G. (1998). *Pneumocystis carinii* pneumonia and toxo-plasmosis. In P.A. Pizzo & C.M. Wilfert (Eds.), *Pediatric AIDS: the challenge of HIV infection in infants, children and adolescents* (3rd ed.). Baltimore: Williams & Wilkins.

Spector, S.A., et al. (1994). A controlled trial of intravenous immune globulin for the prevention of serious bacterial infections in children receiving zidovudine for advanced human immunodeficiency virus infection. *N Engl J Med, 331*, 1181-1187.

Stiehm, E.R., et al. (1999). Efficacy of zidovudine and human immunodefi-ciency virus (HIV) hyperimmune immunoglobulin for reducing perinatal HIV transmission from HIV-infected women with advanced disease: results of pediatric AIDS clinical trials group protocol 185. *J Infect Dis, 179*, 567-575.

Standish, L., et al. (2001). Alternative medicine use in HIV-positive men and women: demographics, utilization patterns and health status. *AIDS Care, 13*(92), 197-208.

Sullivan, J. & Luzuriaga, K. (2001). The changing face of pediatric HIV-1 infec-tion. *N Engl J Med, 345*(21): 1568-1569.

Takala, A.K., et al. (1995). Risk factors for primary invasive pneumococcal disease among children in Finland. *JAMA, 273*(11), 859-864.

Walsh, T.J., et al. (1998). Fungal infections in children with HIV. In P.A. Pizzo & C.M. Wilfert (Eds.), *Pediatric AIDS: the challenge of HIV infection in infants, children and adolescents* (3rd ed.). Baltimore: Williams & Wilkins.

Wiener, L.S., Battles, H.B., & Heilman, N.E. (1998). Factors associated with parents' decision to disclose their HIV diagnosis to their children. *Child Welfare, 77*, 115-135.

Wilfert, C.M. (1998). Invasive bacterial infections in children with HIV infec-tion. In P.A. Pizzo & C.M. Wilfert (Eds.), *Pediatric AIDS: the challenge of HIV infection in infants, children and adolescents* (3rd ed.). Baltimore: Williams & Wilkins.

Wood, L.V. (1998). Immunomodulation and immune reconstitution. In P.A. Pizzo & C.M. Wilfert (Eds.), *Pediatric AIDS: the challenge of HIV infec-tion in infants, children and adolescents* (3rd ed.). Baltimore: Williams & Wilkins.

Working Group on Antiretroviral Therapy and Medical Management of HIV-Infected Children. (2000). *HIV Clinical Trials, 1*(3), 58-99.

29 Hydrocephalus

Sue Ditmyer

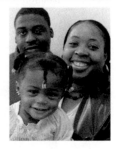

Etiology

Hydrocephalus is a condition that results from an imbalance between the production and absorption of cerebrospinal fluid (CSF), leading to an increase in the volume of intracranial CSF, enlargement of the ventricular system, and possible increased intracranial pressure (ICP). Hydrocephalus is most commonly caused by an obstruction in the normal circulation and absorption of CSF. The rare tumor, choroid plexus papilloma, has been shown to produce excessive volumes of CSF. Whether this overproduction is sufficient to produce hydrocephalus is controversial and seems unlikely (Albright et al, 1999).

CSF is continuously produced by the choroid plexus within the lateral, third, and fourth ventricles and as a by-product of cerebral and spinal cord metabolism. Clinical and experimental studies have reported that CSF forms at a rate of approximately 20 ml/hour or 500 ml/day in adults as well as children (Choux et al, 1999). The rate of CSF production has been shown to be relatively constant among individuals and within the same individual over time. Premature and small infants do produce less CSF than adults, but these differences are negligible after about 1 year of age (Albright et al, 1999). Under normal circumstances, an equal amount of CSF is absorbed from the subarachnoid space into the venous system by projections called arachnoid villi. To reach the subarachnoid space and villi, CSF passes through a series of channels and pathways (see Figure 29-1). Pulsations of the choroid plexus propel CSF through the ventricular system. From the lateral ventricles, CSF flows into the third ventricle via the foramen of Monro. It then passes from the third ventricle into the fourth ventricle through the aqueduct of Sylvius and out of the fourth ventricle through either the lateral foramina of Luschka or the foramen of Magendie. CSF exits the ventricular system and travels around the brainstem and spinal cord and over the surface of the brain, where it is absorbed by the arachnoid villi. Alternate pathways for CSF absorption may come into play when ICP is increased. CSF may travel into the paranasal sinuses, conjunctiva of the eye, and lymphatics, as well as along the cranial or spinal nerves to be absorbed into the systemic circulation.

Hydrocephalus is classified as either noncommunicating or communicating (Box 29-1). Noncommunicating hydrocephalus is characterized by failure of CSF to flow through its normal pathways from one ventricle to another or from the ventricles to the subarachnoid cisterns, resulting in an enlargement of the ventricles proximal to the site of the obstruction. An example of noncommunicating hydrocephalus would be an obstruction of the aqueduct of Sylvius in which the lateral and third ventricles are enlarged but the fourth ventricle's size is normal.

Noncommunicating hydrocephalus can be further classified as congenital or acquired. Conditions, which occur congenitally, include Chiari malformation, aqueductal stenosis, aqueductal gliosis or obstruction from lesions such as neoplasms or vascular malformations. Aqueductal stenosis, obstruction of flow through the aqueduct of Sylvius, is the most common form of noncommunicating hydrocephalus. Noncommunicating hydrocephalus can be acquired through an infectious ventriculitis, a neoplasm, chemical ventriculitis, or a ventricular hemorrhage.

Communicating hydrocephalus occurs when CSF flows freely through the normal pathways but cannot be absorbed through the subarachnoid spaces, the basal cisterns or the arachnoid villi. Common causes of communicating hydrocephalus are meningitis, intraventricular hemorrhage, trauma, or congenital malformation of the subarachnoid spaces.

Known Genetic Etiology

Isolated hydrocephalus due to congenital stenosis of the aqueduct of Sylvius is almost always an X-linked recessive inherited condition (Hamada et al, 1999). Most cases of X-linked hydrocephalus with associated stenosis of the aqueduct of Sylvius are caused by mutations in the gene for neural cell adhesion molecule (Chalmers et al, 1999). Couples who have had one previous child with hydrocephalus have a recurrence risk of 4%. Primary care practitioners should recommend genetic counseling to couples with one child with hydrocephalus prior to attempting to conceive a second child. Those couples that have conceived should be offered prenatal diagnosis in the second trimester for all subsequent pregnancies.

Incidence and Prevalance

Hydrocephalus is the most frequent neurosurgical problem encountered in the pediatric age group. With an incidence rate of 1 in 2,000 births, it occurs in nearly one third of all congenital malformations of the nervous system. Hydrocephalus is often associated with neural tube defects, which have an incidence in the United States of approximately 0.7 to 1 for every 1,000 live births each year. It is also a common complication of virtually any insult to the child's nervous system, including intraventricular hemorrhage, brain tumors, infections, and head injury. CSF shunting procedures comprise roughly half of most modern pediatric neurosurgical practices (McLone, 2001).

According to Emily Fudge, executive director of the San Francisco–based Hydrocephalus Association, it is difficult if not impossible to get accurate prevalence rates for hydrocephalus.

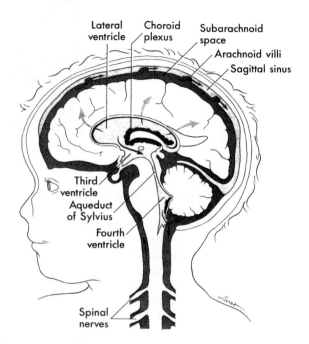

FIGURE 29-1 CSF circulatory pathway showing a view of the center of the brain. Solid arrows show the major pathway of CSF flow; broken arrows show additional pathways. Illustration © Lynne Larson. Reprinted with permission.)

BOX 29-1

Classification of Hydrocephalus

NONCOMMUNICATING

Congenital
Chiari malformation (usually associated with myelomeningocele)
Aqueductal stenosis
Aqueductal gliosis (postperinatal hemorrhage or infection)
Obstruction from congenital lesions (neoplasms, vascular malformation, vein of Galen)
Arachnoid cyst, benign intracranial cyst

Acquired
Infectious ventriculitis
Obstruction from lesions (neoplasms, vascular malformation)
Chemical ventriculitis
Intraventricular hemorrhage

COMMUNICATING

Congenital
Arachnoid cyst
Encephalocele
Associated with congenital malformation: craniofacial syndromes, achondroplasia
Dandy-Walker malformation

Acquired
Chemical arachnoiditis
Infections (postmeningitis)
Posthemorrhagic (postsubarachnoid hemorrhage, intraventricular hemorrhage)
Associated with spinal tumors and seeding from CNS tumors

Data from Carey, C.M., Tullous, M.W., & Walker, M.L. (1994). Hydrocephalus: etiology, pathologic effects, diagnosis, and natural history. In Cheek, W.R. (Ed.). *Pediatric neurosurgery: surgery of the developing nervous system* (3rd ed.). Philadelphia: W.B. Saunders; Barkovich, A.J. (1995). Hydrocephalus. In Barkovich, A.J. *Pediatric neuroimaging*, New York: Raven Press.

This is because reporting is done based on ICD-9 and CPT codes, most of which are an overall diagnosis, which may not be hydrocephalus. An example would be brain tumor in which there may be hydrocephalus that may or may not need shunting (personal communication). The Hydrocephalus Foundation, Inc. reports on its Web site (www.hydrocephalus.org) that there are 25,000 shunt operations performed each year in the United States. Of those, some 18,000 are initial shunt placements.

Clinical Manifestations at Time of Diagnosis

Clinical Manifestations in Infancy

Due to incomplete myelination in the infant brain, ventricular size can increase significantly before the skull circumference increases. Macrocrania in the premature or full-term infant should strongly suggest the diagnosis of hydrocephalus. Normal head circumference at birth is 33 to 36 cm. An increase in head circumference of 0.5-1 cm in the newborn infact is considered normal. An increase of more that 2 cm/week in an infant with a head circumference more than two standard deviations above normal should be attributed to hydrocephalus until proven otherwise. Other associated findings include bulging of the anterior fontanelle and splitting of the cranial sutures. The skin over the skull can appear shiny with distention of the scalp veins. The setting-sun phenomenon, coupled with an inability to look up, is attributed to dysfunction of the tectal plate. Papilledema, poor feeding, and vomiting are rare findings (Box 29-2) (Choux et al, 1999). If the accumulation of excessive CSF occurs slowly, an infant or young child may be asymptomatic until the hydrocephalus is advanced. Infants are less likely to be acutely ill because their skull and sutures can expand to accommodate increasing ventricular size, thereby minimizing an elevation in ICP (Dias & Li, 1998).

Clinical Manifestations in Children

Hydrocephalus in children, beyond infancy, is usually associated with a neoplasm or mass secondary to obstruction of flow of CSF. The ability of the brain to compensate for intracranial hypertension is limited if the sutures are closed. Macrocrania is not necessarily a component of the presentation in older children. For this reason the presentation of hydrocephalus in older children is typically acute. The classic history involves rapid onset of headache that is most pronounced in the morning, vomiting, and alterations of consciousness. Apnea and bradycardia are far less prevalent than in the infant population. Double vision attributable to palsies of the third, fourth, and sixth cranial nerves is common, with sixth nerve palsy being the most frequent (Choux et al, 1999).

In children with a chronic course of hydrocephalus, such as that which is caused by a slow-growing tumor of the brainstem, the history is usually significant for headache, abdominal pain, nausea, vomiting, behavioral change, memory loss, worsening of school performance, and impaired mentation (Choux et al, 1999).

Treatment

The ultimate goal of the treatment of hydrocephalus is to prevent or to reverse the neurologic damage caused by the

---

BOX 29-2
Clinical Manifestations at Time of Diagnosis

> Manifestations are determined by degree of hydrocephalus, degree of increased ICP, and etiology.

ASSOCIATED SYMPTOMS
Associated symptoms in infants:
Rapid skull growth
Macrocrania
Bulging fontanelle
Split cranial sutures
Apnea
Bradycardia
Distention of scalp veins
Setting-sun phenomenon
Ophthalmoplegia
Papilledema
Poor feeding
Vomiting
Drowsiness
Frontal bossing
Head bobbing

Associated symptoms in children >18 months:
Headache
Vomiting
Alteration in level of consciousness
Ophthalmoplegia
Macrocephaly
Abdominal pain
Behavioral changes
Memory loss
Worsening school performance
Impaired mentation
Papilledema
Irritability

From Choux, M., Rocco, C.D., Hockley, A.D., & Walker, M.L. (1999). *Pediatric neurosurgery.* London: Churchill Livingstone. Modified with permission.

---

distortion of the brain from increased intracranial pressure and accumulation of CSF. Intermediate goals include allowing the actual brain tissue volume to increase and reconstitution of the mantle. Secondary goals of treatment include the prevention of complications and the avoidance of shunt dependency if at all possible (Albright et al, 1999).

Pharmacologic Treatment

Drugs that reduce CSF formation have been used in an attempt to delay or avoid shunting. Furosemide interferes with chloride transport in the apical cells of the choroid plexus and can decrease CSF production by as much as 50%. Acetazolamide inhibits carbonic anhydrase and can decrease CSF formation by approximately 50%. The combination of these two drugs can decrease production by as much as three quarters of its original volume. These two modalities have been useful as temporizing measures but have been abandoned in the treatment of chronic hydrocephalus. Physiologically the production of CSF is not sufficiently reduced to decrease intracranial pressure enough to be efficacious (Choux et al, 1999).

BOX 29-3
Treatment

> Treatment is determined by the cause. The goal is to restore CSF flow by removing the obstruction or creating a new pathway.

Drug therapy
Surgical treatment
Shunting pathways
    Ventriculoperitoneal
    Ventriculoatrial
    Ventriculopleural
Management of shunt malfunction
    Shunt infection
    Shunt malfunction
Neuroendoscopy
Spontaneously resolving hydrocephalus
Neuroimaging

Surgical Treatment

Surgical treatment for hydrocephalus is directed at restoring CSF flow by either removing the obstruction to CSF flow or creating a new CSF pathway (Box 29-3). In most cases of hydrocephalus, the obstruction to CSF flow cannot be effectively or safely removed; therefore, surgical shunting is required. Shunting involves placement of a ventricular catheter or shunt to divert CSF flow to another body cavity, where it can be absorbed. The peritoneal cavity is the preferred location and most commonly utilized. If the peritoneal cavity is not appropriate for placement of the distal tubing—either due to abdominal malformation, postsurgical adhesions, infection, or inadequate absorption—the shunt may be placed in the atrium of the heart (i.e., ventriculoatrial [VA] shunt) or the pleural space (i.e., ventriculopleural shunt). The distal portion is tunneled under the child's skin to the designated location, where a small incision is made and the shunt is inserted either through the peritoneum into the peritoneal cavity (i.e., VP shunt) or through the neck into the superior vena cava and into the right atrium (i.e., VA shunt) (Figure 29-2). The distal end of the ventriculopleural shunt is guided subcutaneously to an area just below the nipple, where an incision is made, and the tube is inserted into the pleural space.

CSF shunts regulate flow by means of a one-way valve. The "standard" valves that have been in use for decades simply open or close depending on the pressure across them. They can be grouped into four general design categories: silicone rubber slit valves, silicone rubber diaphragm valves, silicone rubber miter valves, and metallic spring-and-ball valves. The pressure at which they open is termed the opening pressure. Typically there are low, medium, and high designations that generally correspond to 5, 10, and 15 cm of H_2O pressure (McLone, 2001). No one type of shunt is superior in function over another type. The choice of which type of shunt to be placed is the personal preference of the neurosurgeon based on training and personal experience. No data exist to support a recommendation of one particular shunt design over another.

The reservoir and tubing are palpable from the burr hole in the skull to the tube's insertion at either the abdomen or chest. Identification of and access to the shunt reservoir are important in evaluating shunt infection and/or malfunction. The reservoir

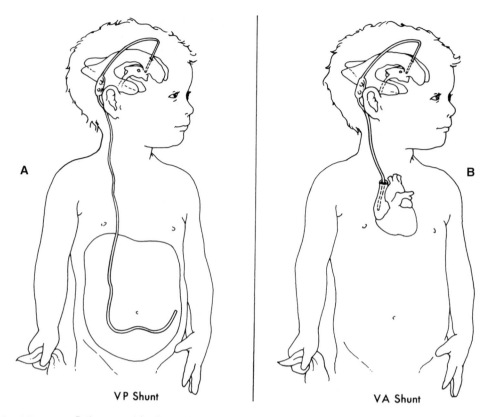

A

B

VP Shunt

VA Shunt

FIGURE 29-2 Pathway used for **A,** ventriculoperitoneal shunt and, **B,** ventriculoatrial shunt. Illustration © Lynne Larson. Reprinted with permission.)

should be easy to depress and should rebound readily when released. A small 25-gauge needle can be inserted into the reservoir to collect CSF for culture, obtain ICP readings, or inject radioisotopes for shunt-flow studies.

Complications of Surgical Treatment. Although CSF shunting has dramatically improved the prognosis for children with hydrocephalus, shunts still have inherent problems. Shunt mechanical complications may occur at any time from immediately after the shunt placement to years later. The most common time for a shunt to fail is in the first 6 months after insertion (McLone, 2001). The incidence of mechanical shunt malfunction is approximately 30% over 1 year. Shunt occlusion is the most common shunt complication in the pediatric population and constitutes approximately 50% of all shunt complications (Choux et al, 1999). Shunt revisions are necessary at some time in almost all children who have shunted hydrocephalus. The average number of shunt revisions a child undergoes in a lifetime is five to seven. Shunt obstruction may occur as a result of chronic or acute inflammation, overgrowth of the choroid plexus, accumulation of cellular debris or blood, or occlusion of either the distal or proximal end of the shunt as a result of the child's growth. Repeated shunt failure requiring multiple revisions is a problem for some children. One study found that the interval between revisions became progressively shorter as the number of surgeries increased. So it seems that the primary pathology that resulted in hydrocephalus in these children elicits a reactive inflammatory process that is perpetuated by repeat shunt procedures.

The incidence of shunt infections has decreased significantly over the past decade but continues to be a major source of shunt malfunction and potential morbidity. Previously, shunt infection was the most common cause of morbidity with an occurrence rate of 10%. Almost 90% of shunt infections are diagnosed within 6 months after surgery, supporting a basic premise of direct contamination at the time of surgery (Camboulives et al, 2002). As a foreign body, the implanted shunt creates a medium in the host where normal phagocytosis is impaired, allowing a child to be susceptible to infection of the shunt and cerebrospinal fluid. There seems to be consensus that very young children have a higher incidence of shunt infection than older individuals. However, the exact age at which this increased liability to infection diminishes is unclear, ranging in various reports from 6 months to 4 years. The most common risk factors for infection include concurrent infection, previous shunt infections, and postoperative disruption of the wound exposing the shunt (Albright et al, 1999). Irregularities in the wall of the shunt and the glycoproteinaceous film that forms along the shunt tubing increase the risk of infection by providing a niche for adherence and growth of bacteria (Madikians & Conway, 1997). A shunt infection is identified when a bacterial pathogen or pathogens are isolated from ventricular CSF. Although shunt infections have been as high as 40% in the past three decades, most recent studies have reported operative infection rates less than 4% (McLone, 2001).

More than two thirds of all shunt infections are caused by staphylococcal species, with *Staphylococcus epidermidis* isolated in 47% to 64% of all infections, and *S. aureus* the next most common organism occurring in 12% to 29%. Gram-negative enteric organisms, usually *Escherichia coli* and *Klebsiella* spp., are responsible for 6% to 20% of infections. *Proteus* and *Pseudomonas* spp. also are not infrequently isolated, and streptococcal species are found in 8% to 10% of infections. Other less common organisms, such as fungi and other commensal microbes, make up the remainder of the infections (McLone, 2001). Although shunt malfunction has not been associated with cognitive deficits, shunt infections—especially resulting from gram-negative organisms—can have significant detrimental effects on cognition in the host.

The treatment of shunt infections varies among neurosurgeons. In one study (Whitehead & Kestle, 2001) pediatric neurosurgeons were surveyed about their practices with regard to the treatment of infected shunts. The most popular treatment strategies for the management of shunt infections involve surgical removal of the infected shunt followed by a period of external drainage until CSF cultures are sterile, and finally surgical replacement of a new shunt. Other methods of treatment that involve antibiotic therapy only or the immediate removal and replacement of the shunt during the same surgery are seldom used.

Prevention of shunt infections is the key to improving outcomes in children with shunted hydrocephalus and decreasing the cost of the care of these individuals. The one approach to the prevention of postoperative shunt infections that has been sufficiently studied and proven to reduce shunt infections is the use of prophylactic systemic antibiotics (Albright et al, 1999).

Neuroendoscopy

A significant development in pediatric neurosurgery during the past decade has been the evolution of neuroendoscopy and its application to the management of childhood hydrocephalus. Before this evolution, the standard treatment for all types of hydrocephalus was the implantation of ventriculoextracranial shunts. Although many children were spared the devastating effects of uncontrolled hydrocephalus with these shunt systems, a variety of problems emerged that prompted continued refinement of shunt systems or alternative therapies with similar if not superior results (McLone, 2001).

A decade ago few pediatric neurosurgical centers in the world offered third ventriculostomy as an alternative to shunting for obstructive hydrocephalus. Today, however, few major centers in the United States do not have a neurosurgeon skilled in this procedure. The procedure was first described by Dandy in 1922 but was not widely practiced because of the many complications and unacceptable failure rates. The renewed enthusiasm for this surgical procedure arises from the expectation that approximately half or more of appropriately selected individuals may remain or become shunt free. Furthermore, the safety of the procedure compared with approaches used in the past has greatly increased related to the availability of high-quality endoscopes, light sources, camera equipment, and instrumentation. The capability through MRI to visualize the oscillatory flow of CSF, as well as obstruction in the ventricular system, has improved selection as well as preoperative and postoperative monitoring of children. It is also clear, however, that this "rediscovered" procedure is not yet well characterized for its potential complications and long-term success rates. Clearly, late failures after prolonged effective control of hydrocephalus are now emerging (McLone, 2001).

One group has reported a 48% success rate over a period of 18 months in infants with newly diagnosed hydrocephalus. In their study, children with newly diagnosed hydrocephalus secondary to aqueductal stenosis were treated with third ventriculostomy regardless of age. Their data suggest that etiology, not age of the infant or child is the most important factor in determining the success rate of the procedure (Javadpour et al, 2001).

Spontaneously Resolving Hydrocephalus

Children with communicating hydrocephalus occasionally outgrow the need for a shunt. Alternative pathways for absorption are thought to be established as a result of persistent increased ICP, therefore compensating for the diminished absorption from the arachnoid villi. This compensated or resolved hydrocephalus usually occurs during the first year of life, although it may not be identified until later when lengthening of the shunt appears necessary as a result of growth. Compensated hydrocephalus is accompanied by stable ventricular size despite documented shunt obstruction. Shunt failure may be verified by the absence of flow after injection of a radioisotope into the shunt reservoir (i.e., shunt function study) or by radiologic confirmation of shunt disconnection (i.e., radiographic shunt series) or, where available, MRI CSF flow study. When it is determined that the child is no longer shunt dependent, the shunt is left in place unless the risk of infection is high. The child is monitored by periodic brain scans and neuropsychologic examinations. Annual neuropsychologic testing is recommended because intellectual deterioration has been associated with arrested hydrocephalus.

Neuroimaging

Neuroimaging of the brain is essential for the diagnosis and management of hydrocephalus. The three major imaging modalities include ultrasonography, computed tomography (CT) scan, and magnetic resonance imaging (MRI). Ultrasound is only possible in infants while the anterior fontanelle is open. CT scans are most commonly obtained if acute hydrocephalus or shunt malfunction is suspected. Although all techniques are reasonable for follow-up of ventricular size and shunt placement, MRI is superior in defining the cause of hydrocephalus. MRI scans illustrate the central nervous system anatomy in multiple planes and allow for detailed imaging of the cerebrum and posterior fossa. Advances in MRI technology can also be used to study the flow dynamics of CSF. MRI is also useful in determining the success of third ventriculostomy in restoring CSF circulation.

CT and MRI studies are used to evaluate shunt failure and the need for shunt revision. These scans must be compared with prior imaging studies and reviewed in conjunction with clinical findings of probable shunt failure, as assessed by an experienced clinician. In one study, initial radiologic reports did not support the diagnosis of shunt malfunction in as many as one third of children presenting with shunt failure (Iskandar et al, 1998). In some cases, ventricular size did not change despite shunt malfunction. In other cases, ventricular enlargement was only noted when compared with previous scans. Primary care providers must remember that a negative or stable CT scan does not rule out shunt malfunction.

Other diagnostic tools to evaluate shunt function include radionuclide CSF shunt studies, a shunt series (i.e., a lateral radiograph of the skull, neck, chest, and abdomen to ascertain the location and continuity of the shunt apparatus), shunt tap for CSF for culture, and ICP monitoring. A measurement of ICP can be obtained either intermittently via the shunt reservoir or by placement of an ICP monitor. Keeping in mind the morbidity associated with a delay in the diagnosis of a shunt malfunction, primary care providers must have a low threshold for ordering a brain scan or referring a child to the neurosurgeon when symptoms of increased ICP or shunt infection are apparent.

Complementary and Alternative Treatments

No evidence is available in the current literature regarding complementary or alternative treatment of hydrocephalus.

Anticipated Advances in Diagnosis and Management

Fetal shunting was first performed in the early 1980s with the hope that early intervention would improve the outcome for children diagnosed with fetal hydrocephalus. Unfortunately, knowledge about the natural history and outcome of the fetus with hydrocephalus was limited. Imaging as compared with today's techniques was suboptimal and other brain anomalies were missed at the time of diagnosis and fetal shunting. Therefore, a moratorium on fetal surgery was initiated. Due to improved diagnostics and surgical techniques of the present, there may now be a place for fetal shunting. The key to positive outcomes will depend upon careful selection of the appropriate fetus (Harrison et al, 2001).

Advances in obstetric and neonatal intensive care have decreased the incidence of hydrocephalus as a result of intraventricular hemorrhage and meningitis. In addition, nutritional guidelines recommending supplementation of folic acid in women of childbearing age have lowered the incidence of hydrocephalus by decreasing the number of children born with myelomeningocele and other neural tube defects.

Prenatal evaluation (i.e., including high-resolution ultrasound and measures of maternal alpha-fetoprotein [AFP]) has increased the number of fetal anomalies identified. Neural tube defects may be identified by fetal ultrasound and elevated levels of maternal AFP. Assessment for other congenital anomalies and follow-up ultrasounds to detect progressive ventricular enlargement are essential when counseling families. If severe brain dysfunction or other congenital anomalies are suspected, parents may decide to terminate the pregnancy; otherwise pregnancy can be continued as close to term as possible and a shunt or ventricular access device placed soon after birth.

Over the years, medical equipment manufacturers have developed new and improved shunt designs with the claim that their shunt will dramatically change the treatment of hydrocephalus. However, there are no data published to validate the performance of one shunt over another. Neuroendoscopic treatment of children with hydrocephalus is an established surgical

modality. Open magnetic resonance imaging (MRI) technology introduces new imaging features that, in combination with endoscopy, seem particularly valuable for performing these operations. "Near" real-time production of MR images in three dimensions during the procedure allows real-time neuronavigation, thus facilitating guidance of an endoscope. Additionally, intraoperative changes such as brain shift, effects of perforation, and drainage of cysts are shown during an ongoing procedure (Balmer et al, 2002).

The use of programmable shunts has increased over the past decade. The programmable shunt system was designed by Dr. Hakim to relieve under and over drainage problems in hydrocephalus. The system allows for noninvasive postimplantation adjustment of the opening pressure of the valve through a range of 30 to 200 mm H_2O in 10 mm differentials according to the individual needs of the child. (Tsuji & Sato, 1998). Slit ventricle syndrome and nonhemorrhagic postshunting subdural collections are examples of over drainage problems for which the programmable shunt is now being used successfully. The programmable shunt has been found to be useful for reducing the need for shunt revision for headache (Kay et al, 2002). And the programmable shunt system is beginning to be used to wean children with shunted hydrocephalus from their shunts through careful control of the valve pressure (Takahashi, 2001). Programmable shunts are sensitive to magnets. Therefore the primary care practitioner should notify the child's primary neurosurgeon when ordering a diagnostic magnetic resonance imaging study.

It is hoped that the current advances in computer technology will be applied to shunts for hydrocephalus. A computer chip will likely be developed for shunts, which can anticipate the changing requirement for pressure settings based on the child's personal needs (Sun, personal communication, 2002).

Associated Problems (Box 29-4)
Intellectual Problems

Intellectual function is difficult to predict early after diagnosis. Some infants with extreme hydrocephalus and virtually no cortical mantle visible on the initial imaging studies have grown up to be remarkably normal adults. Serial imaging studies of infants with hydrocephalus often show dramatic reconstitution of the brain over time, and the mechanism of this process remains a topic of active investigation (Harrison et al, 2001). Although the precise nature of the neuropsychologic deficits in hydrocephalus are not completely known, several factors such as etiology, raised intracranial pressure, ventricular size, and changes in gray and white matter tissue composition, as well as shunt treatment complications, have been shown to influence

---

BOX 29-4
Associated Problems

Intellectual deficits
Ocular abnormalities
Motor disabilities
Seizures

cognition (Mataro, 2001). In long-term studies, approximately 30% of the children with hydrocephalus had intelligence quotients (IQs) in the normal range above 90; 30% to 60% had mild to moderate mental retardation; and 7% to 20% had severe retardation. Integration into the normal school system was possible for 60% of these children, although many required some special education services (Hoppe-Hirsch et al, 1998). The younger the individual is when hydrocephalus is diagnosed the greater the risk for intellectual impairment. Those children diagnosed in utero have the poorest outcome intellectually as compared with those diagnosed during the first year of life (Futagi et al, 2002). Regardless of the etiology, children with hydrocephalus compared with nonaffected children exhibited a pattern of performance suggestive of encoding and retrieval deficits on both verbal and nonverbal tasks, showing a pervasive disturbance of memory processes (Scott et al, 1998). Children with hydrocephalus are able to decode words when reading but exhibit poor comprehension of what is decoded (Barnes, 2002).

Children and young adults with spina bifida and hydrocephalus are at an even greater risk for cognitive deficits than those who have hydrocephalus without spina bifida. This combination of problems causes significant dysmorphology of the cerebellum. As a result, these children and young adults have been found to have more motor speech deficits than those individuals without spina bifida and hydrocephalus (Huber-Okrainec et al, 2002). Of interest is a difference in the cognitive ability of children with spina bifida with hydrocephalus who are walking as compared with those who are wheelchair-bound (Rendeli, 2002).

As with most developmental measures, social risk factors also affect cognitive outcomes. One study found that socioeconomic status was the factor most strongly associated with verbal scores in children with hydrocephalus (Bier et al, 1997). The importance of both social and biologic factors in developmental outcomes must be remembered in counseling families and planning intervention strategies. Preschool and school counseling with neuropsychologic evaluations must be completed early to identify areas of learning disability and resources for intervention.

Ocular Problems

Ocular abnormalities are often found at the time of diagnosis or during episodes of shunt malfunction. Increased ICP results in optic nerve pressure, limited upward gaze, extraocular muscle paresis, and papilledema. Without prompt treatment for acute hydrocephalus or shunt malfunction, permanent visual damage is a definite risk. Before the era of successful CSF shunting, optic atrophy secondary to hydrocephalus was the leading cause of blindness from congenital malformations. Even with a functioning shunt and controlled hydrocephalus, however, visual problems are common. Gaze and movement problems such as strabismus, astigmatism, nystagmus, and amblyopia are found in approximately 25% to 33% of children with hydrocephalus (Rosen, 1998). Refractive and accommodative errors are found in about the same percentage of children but not necessarily in the same children. The optic disk is often found to be abnormally light or pale, but papilledema is not normally found. These children may require the use of large print and increased contrast in work materials, as well as placement of work items within their visual field. Abnormalities in vision are associated with lower intelligence scores and may help identify children at risk for developmental delay. Close follow-up and referral to infant stimulation programs for the visually impaired may be necessary (Rosen, 1998). Correctable visual problems should be attended to as soon as possible so that poor vision does not interfere with learning potential. Children with slit ventricle syndrome are at an increased risk for significant visual loss. Therefore these children require special attention and prompt treatment when increased intracranial pressure is discovered (Nguyen et al, 2002).

Motor Disabilities

Unfortunately as many as 60% of the children with hydrocephalus will have some form of motor disability (Hoppe-Hirsch et al, 1998). These disabilities vary from severe paraplegia to mild imbalance or weakness. The severity of the motor deficit is most often related to the diagnosis, with conditions such as porencephaly, Dandy-Walker malformation, and myelomeningocele having more serious motor defects than simple congenital hydrocephalus. Hydrocephalus also affects fine motor control. The kinesthetic-proprioceptive abilities of the hands are often negatively affected and—coupled with the impaired bimanual manipulation and frequent visual deficits—make it difficult for children with hydrocephalus to perform well on time-limited, nonverbal intelligence tests.

Seizures

Since the introduction of ventriculoatrial and/or ventriculoperitoneal shunting for individuals with hydrocephalus, controversies have arisen regarding the likelihood of epileptic seizures developing as a result of the shunting itself and/or its complications. Hydrocephalus is not commonly recognized as a cause of seizures in general, although epilepsy is reported to be frequently associated with shunt-treated hydrocephalus, especially in children. Several authors have reported an increased risk of epileptic seizures after shunt placement, but the underlying mechanisms are still controversial. The insult to the brain at the time of ventricular catheter insertion, the presence of the shunt tube itself as a foreign body, the burr hole location, the number of shunt revisions after malfunction, associated infection, the etiology of hydrocephalus, and associated developmental delay are thought to be related to the risk of epilepsy. Age at the time of initial shunt placement also seems to be an important factor. Early shunting is a well-known determinant of risk in shunt obstruction, and children younger than 2 years old are consequently at a higher risk of developing epilepsy than older children. It is reported that antiepileptic drug treatment is not as efficacious as might be expected. Routine electroencephalogram (EEG) recordings in children being treated with antiepileptic medications may be beneficial during follow-up. The incidence of seizures in shunted children is reported to be quite high, ranging from 20% to approximately 50% (Sato et al, 2001). Although ventriculoextracranial shunts have been the standard treatment for hydrocephalus for decades, the long-term morbidity, including postshunt epileptic seizures, has to be taken seriously. The use of neuroendoscopic techniques when indicated may ameliorate this problem significantly in the future (Sato et al, 2001). (See Chapter 25 for further discussion on seizure disorders.)

Prognosis

Hydrocephalus is the result of some event on the nervous system, and a child's prognosis is not so much based on the hydrocephalus as the cause of the hydrocephalus. The prognosis for successful management of hydrocephalus is excellent. It is, however, the underlying cause that will ultimately determine a child's outcome (Columbia University Department of Neurological Surgery Web site). Shunt dependency may carry with it a mortality rate as high as 1% per year, with most of the mortality due to delays in accessing a responsive system in time to prevent death. Primary care providers should remember that children with hydrocephalus are still at risk for increased morbidity and early mortality after years of excellent progress and shunt function. Early detection and treatment of shunt malfunction and complications can reduce morbidity and mortality significantly.

Research and experience show that children with hydrocephalus have excellent opportunities to attain their full potential through comprehensive integrated medical care and programs that stimulate their development (Fudge, 2000).

PRIMARY CARE MANAGEMENT

Shunt dependency will always be a "preexisting condition," making it difficult for the individual with hydrocephalus to maintain health insurance. A disproportionate number of these individuals, particularly young adults, are living either at or below the poverty line and dependent on governmental programs for their health care, or are unable to obtain insurance at all until they have difficulties with their shunts, become bankrupt because of the experience, and then become indigent. Guaranteed access to a responsive system is not just a good idea for these people; it is literally a matter of life and death and as caregivers we must always attempt to be mindful of the economics of health care delivery and be good stewards of our resources. However, we must above all be advocates for the care of the children whose lives we touch. We must be involved in the creation of and constant fine-tuning of a responsive system to ensure access for all individuals with hydrocephalus (Albright et al, 1999).

Health Care Maintenance

Growth and Development

Measurements of children seen in a primary care practice are typically done by minimally trained office or clinic personnel. If a child is suspected of having hydrocephalus or known to have hydrocephalus, the primary care provider should measure the head circumference and plot it on a head circumference chart appropriate for age (Figures 29-3 and 29-4). Until the cranial sutures are completely fused, which is often delayed in these children, head circumference is a major diagnostic tool in evaluating a child's condition. Normal head circumference at birth is 33 to 36 cm. During the first year, head circumference increases 2 cm/month during the first 3 months, 1 cm/month

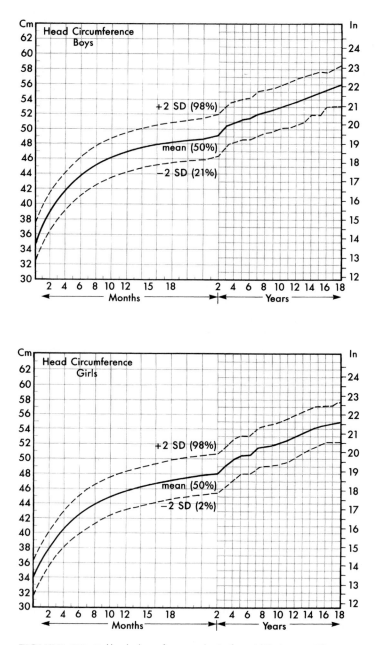

FIGURE 29-3 Head circumference charts from birth to age 18 years. (From Neilhaus, G. [1968]. Head circumference from birth to eighteen years. *Pediatrics, 41,* 106-114.)

from 4 to 6 months, and 0.5 cm/month from 7 to 12 months. A diagnosis of hydrocephalus is indicated more by increases across growth percentiles than by a normal rate of growth paralleling the 95th percentile. Increasing head circumference from hydrocephalus is usually associated with a full fontanelle, splayed sutures, and frontal bossing.

Once the diagnosis of hydrocephalus has been made and a shunt inserted, head circumference may decrease 1 to 2 cm as the pressure is relieved. The sutures may become overriding, and the fontanelle sunken. After this initial decrease, the head should only grow in proportion to the child's body. Therefore a newborn whose weight and height are in the 50th percentile for age and who has a head size of 40 cm when a shunt is placed shortly after birth may not resume head growth for 2 to 4

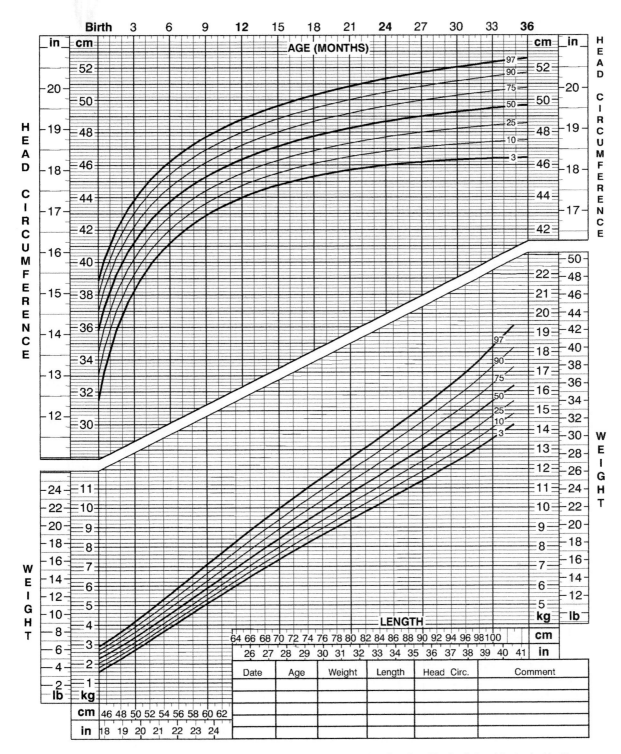

FIGURE 29-4 Boys head circumference chart from birth to 36 months. (Developed by the National Center for Health Statistics in collaboration with the National Center for Chronic Disease Prevention and Health Promotion, 2000, available at www.cdc.gov/growthcharts, modified May 30, 2000.)

months (see Figure 29-3). Resumption of growth before that time might indicate shunt malfunction. The significance of head size measurements in a child with a shunt cannot be overestimated, and daily measurements may be necessary during evaluation of shunt-dependent infants for possible shunt malfunction. Weight gain must be assessed carefully because

the increasing weight of the head of the infant with hydrocephalus may mask failure to thrive.

Hydrocephalus may cause disorders of growth and puberty. However, short stature is frequently due to meningomyelocele and rarely to growth hormone deficiency. Central early puberty is the most frequent endocrine disorder. Treatment is available

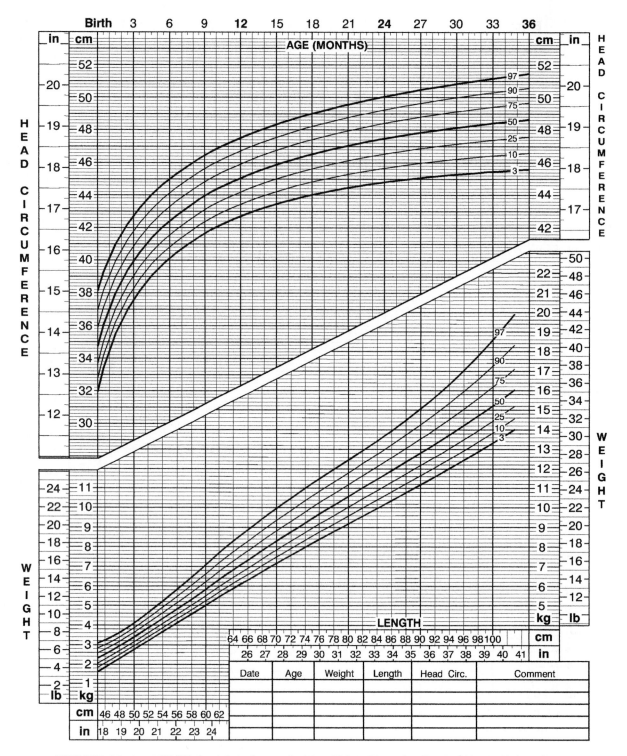

FIGURE 29-4, cont'd Girls head circumference chart from birth to 36 months. (Developed by the National Center for Health Statistics in collaboration with the National Center for Chronic Disease Prevention and Health Promotion, 2000, available at www.cdc.gov/growthcharts, modified May 30, 2000.)

and the primary care practitioner should refer the child to a pediatric endocrinologist should a question arise.

The standard early infant developmental assessment tools used in primary care practice (e.g., Denver Developmental Screening Test II) are of little help in assessing infants with hydrocephalus. Tasks that require head control (e.g., elevating the head while in the prone position, rolling over, pulling to a sitting position without head lag, and even sitting unassisted) will be delayed in infants with macrocrania. It is important for primary care providers to interpret developmental findings in light of other clinical observations to help parents set reasonable expectations for their infant.

Other motor delays can be expected during infancy and childhood given that approximately 60% of children with hydrocephalus have some form of motor disability. Primary care providers must carefully document motor skill acquisition (i.e., even in infants and older school-aged children) because a loss of skill may indicate shunt malfunction or progression of the primary cause. Ataxia, slurred speech, lack of progression in school, incontinence, or other regression in developmental ability may indicate a deterioration in neurologic status and need for further evaluation.

In surgically treated hydrocephalus, survival rate is at least 90%, and the IQ is normal or nearly normal in approximately two thirds of affected individuals. As a rule, verbal IQ is higher than performance IQ, and the classic cocktail chatter of a child with hydrocephalus is a common occurrence. Verbal skills are usually commensurate with intellectual abilities, and these children will perform better on verbal tests than on fine motor-visual perception tests. Neither site of obstruction nor number of shunt revisions has an adverse effect on IQ. No evidence exists that prompt shunting enhances the ultimate IQ. Rather, IQ is a function of the etiology of the hydrocephalus, in particular, the presence or absence of concurrent cerebral malformations (Menkes & Sarnat, 2000). Primary care providers must assess speech carefully with each health care visit. These children often benefit from infant stimulation programs or speech therapy. Primary care providers should become familiar with the program offerings in the family's community to help them identify services that would be most beneficial for their child.

Diet

There are no special dietary requirements for children with hydrocephalus. Many parents become overly concerned about the episodes of regurgitation or vomiting that are common in all infants, and clarification as to what is normal and what is pathologic vomiting should be made soon after the diagnosis of hydrocephalus. Parents may be hesitant to burp their infant because of poor head control or concern over dislodging the shunt. Alternate positions for burping can be demonstrated. If repeated regurgitation does occur, parents should be advised on how to use an infant seat for postfeeding positioning and introduction of solids (if age-appropriate). The primary care provider can be supportive of the parents of a child with newly diagnosed hydrocephalus by reassuring them that their concerns are valid. Neurosurgical practitioners reassure these same parents that it is better to notify too often regarding a symptom of possible shunt malfunction even if there is no malfunction rather than to miss something and cause the child harm. Eventually the majority of parents of children with shunted hydrocephalus become expert at knowing when there is a real problem with the shunt.

Safety

Primary care providers play a major role in educating parents and children about safety. Families may be so overwhelmed with the task of parenting a child with a chronic condition that routine safety measures are overlooked. The prolonged lack of head control predisposes children with hydrocephalus to head injury. Care seat use must be altered accordingly. Children

with hydrocephalus and physical disabilities may require special devices and individualized fitting to ensure safety while being transported in a vehicle. A referral to a pediatric physical therapist may be helpful in determining the appropriate equipment.

For infants up to 20 pounds and 1 year of age, car safety seats must face the rear of the vehicle. The safest location for the safety seat is the middle of the backseat. Infants should never be placed in the front passenger seat of a car with an airbag. If the family only has a truck with an airbag, the airbag must be disengaged. The child may be upgraded to a booster/toddler seat when the weight reaches 20 pounds. The child should continue to be restrained in a booster seat in a vehicle until age 8 years. For additional assistance with car seat safety, the parents may be referred to the Auto Safety Hotline at 800-434-9393 (The Cleveland Clinic Web site, 2002).

As a child grows, activities should be limited as little as possible to encourage normal development and peer relationships. Many parents of children with shunted hydrocephalus become overly concerned about head injuries. Parents may ask about the child wearing a helmet at all times to protect the shunt in the event of a fall or head injury. Children with shunts need only wear helmets for the same reasons all children should wear helmets, i.e., while riding, scooters, bicycles, skateboards, etc. unless they are having difficulty with head control or seizures. It is important for the primary care provider to encourage parents not to be overly protective of their child with shunted hydrocephalus. A child's neurologic disabilities and visual perceptual integration may make competitive sports difficult and operation of motor vehicles hazardous. Few sports are absolutely contraindicated in children with hydrocephalus. Violent contact sports such as wrestling, tackle football, and hockey might increase the risk of shunt damage or head trauma, so participation in these sports may need to be restricted. Each individual's ability must be regularly assessed so that the risks and benefits of activities can be determined.

Immunizations

Diphtheria and Tetanus Toxoids and Acellular Pertussis Vaccine. Whether and when to administer DTP or DTaP to children with proven or suspected underlying neurologic disorders should be decided individually. Generally infants and children with stable neurologic conditions, including well-controlled seizures, may be vaccinated (Committee on Infectious Diseases, 2002). As stated, seizures at the time of diagnosis during the newborn period may be present in infants with hydrocephalus, but it is difficult to determine which of these infants will continue to have recurrent seizures. An infant's neurologic status should be evaluated at each primary care visit to determine if the pertussis vaccine is contraindicated. Use of acellular pertussis is associated with fewer neurologic side effects and is recommended for children with hydrocephalus. Because outbreaks of pertussis still occur in the United States, deferral of the vaccine must be weighed against the potential for disease and disease-related complications. Children in daycare, attending special developmental programs, or receiving care in residential centers are exposed to other children who also may not be immunized and are therefore at increased risk for developing pertussis. In such difficult situations consultation with the child's neurosurgeon or neurologist may help in assessing the child's seizure potential. If the primary care provider, with parental consent, decides early in infancy that the pertussis immunization will be withheld, diphtheria and tetanus vaccines should be given on schedule.

Measles. Measles vaccine had been contraindicated for children with seizures or with the potential for seizures due to the possibility of postvaccine seizures. However, seizures are no longer a contraindication for giving the measles vaccine (Committee on Infectious Diseases, 2002).

***Haemophilus influenzae* Type B (HIB).** Because of the increased risk of CNS infections in children with shunts, children with shunted hydrocephalus should be vaccinated for *H. influenzae* type B (Committee on Infectious Diseases, 2002).

Other Immunizations. Vaccination for polio, hepatitis B, pneumococcal varicella, mumps, and rubella should be given as routinely scheduled. Pneumococcal polysaccharide vaccine (PPV) is recommended in addition to pneumococcal conjugated vaccine (PCV) for certain high-risk groups. Influenza vaccine is recommended annually for children age older than 6 months with disabling conditions that make them more susceptible to acute respiratory infections (Committee on Infectious Diseases, 2002).

Screening

Vision. Because of the high incidence of visual defects in children with hydrocephalus, practitioners must pay particular attention to visual screening. The Hirschberg light reflex, cover test, tracking, and funduscopic examinations should be performed at each office visit and the results carefully documented in the record. At approximately 6 months of age, the child should be referred to a pediatric ophthalmologist for a thorough examination. Yearly examinations should be scheduled thereafter. Children with hydrocephalus often need surgery on their eye muscles to correct esotropia or exotropia. Practitioners can be instrumental in completing preoperative examinations and preparing the families for surgery. The primary care provider must remember that alterations in the funduscopic examination, eye muscle control, or visual ability may be associated with shunt malfunction and must be evaluated carefully when shunt malfunction or infection is part of the differential diagnosis. Referral to an ophthalmologist for evaluation of an infant or young child for papilledema or evidence of increased pressure may help to differentiate benign headaches from those due to shunt malfunction.

Hearing. In addition to routine office screening for hearing acuity, an auditory evoked–response test should be ordered if an infant has a history of CNS infection or antibiotic treatment with aminoglycosides. Subsequent shunt malfunctions or CNS infections require reassessment of hearing. Periodic evaluation by an audiologist is recommended.

Dental. Routine dental care is recommended. If a child is taking phenytoin (Dilantin) for seizure control, dental care may need to be more frequent because of hyperplasia of the gums. Poor dental hygiene and periodontal infections may produce bacteremia—even without dental procedures (Helpin et al, 1998). Because intravascular foreign bodies are susceptible to bacterial colonization, any episode of transient bacteremia places a child with a ventriculoatrial shunt at risk for infection

(Helpin et al, 1998). Antibiotic prophylaxis is recommended for children with VA shunts undergoing dental work likely to cause gingival bleeding (including routine cleaning of teeth). The spontaneous shedding of primary teeth or simple adjustment of orthodontic appliances does not require prophylaxis to prevent bacterial endocarditis. The recommended prophylaxis is the same for prevention of bacterial endocarditis in children with congenital heart disease (see Chapter 25). Children with ventriculoperitoneal shunts do not require prophylaxis for routine dental procedures.

Blood Pressure. Blood pressure readings should be recorded on each clinic or office visit. Elevations in blood pressure with a widening pulse pressure are a late sign of increased ICP. Having an established baseline reading can help the practitioner assess a child for possible shunt malfunctions or progression of disease process.

Hematocrit. Routine screening is recommended.

Urinalysis. Routine screening is recommended.

Tuberculosis. Routine screening is recommended.

Condition-Specific Screening

Head Circumference. Head circumference measurements should be taken at every clinic or office visit until a child's sutures are completely fused (see the discussion of growth and development in this chapter).

Common Illness Management
Differential Diagnosis

Unfortunately, many of the symptoms of shunt malfunction or infection are the same symptoms commonly found with routine childhood illness (Box 29-5). It is important to remember that children with hydrocephalus will develop otitis media, gastrointestinal (GI) illnesses, headaches, and viral infections with fever just like their unaffected peers. Primary care providers must approach these children as they would children without hydrocephalus. A calm manner and a thorough history and examination are reassuring to parents and productive for the primary care provider. The most frequent symptoms of shunt malfunction include irritability, headache, nausea, vomiting, lethargy, and delays or loss of developmental milestones. Other symptoms include personality changes, diplopia, new seizures or a change in seizure pattern, and worsening school performance, as well as—in infants—decreased level of conscious-

---

BOX 29-5
Differential Diagnosis

Fever—concern about shunt malfunction
Gastrointestinal symptoms—concern about/that:
  Peritoneal shunt placement and malfunction
  Abdominal infection may seed shunt
  Brain tumors may metastasize to abdomen via shunt
  Constipation may result in peritoneal shunt malfunction
Headaches—concern about increased ICP
Scalp infections—concern about spread of infection to shunt reservoir
Alterations in behavior—concern about shunt malfunction

ness, loss of upward gaze, nuchal rigidity, sixth nerve palsy, papilledema, and hemiparesis or loss of coordination and balance. With a shunt malfunction, the shunt reservoir may not pump and refill as expected, although the sensitivity and predictive value of a shunt pumping are questionable. If the shunt is infected, additional signs and symptoms may include fever, redness and swelling along the shunt tract, abdominal pain, skin breakdown or drainage along incision sites, leakage of CSF from a recent surgical wound, nuchal rigidity, neck or back pain, headache, and photophobia (Madikians & Conway, 1997).

Fever. There is no characteristic combination of signs and symptoms of shunt infections. Perhaps the most important clinical aspect of identifying a shunt infection is to understand that the presentation is highly variable and the diagnosis of shunt infection must be sought rather than simply found. Systemic signs and symptoms of infection such as fever, swelling, erythema, warmth, pain, and tenderness are frequently not present (Albright et al, 1999). Early in an infant's first year when shunt infections are most common, parents should be encouraged to consult the primary care provider whenever the infant has a temperature above 38.5° C. The practitioner, with the consulting physician, can then evaluate the child early in the course of illness and note progression of symptoms. If a focus of infection other than the shunt is identified, it should be treated appropriately. No studies indicate that frequent antibacterial therapy for illnesses of questionable origin reduces the incidence of shunt malfunction. Children being treated for bacterial infections (e.g., otitis media, pneumonia, or streptococcal sore throat) should be carefully reassessed in the office or clinic 24 to 48 hours after treatment is initiated. Continued or worsening symptoms may indicate progression of the infection into bacteremia or a CNS infection caused by the increased susceptibility resulting from the shunt. The child with an indwelling CSF shunt who presents with the signs and symptoms of infection involving the intracranial space, the shunt tract, or the abdomen must be presumed to have a shunt infection until proven otherwise (Albright et al, 1999). The primary care provider should obtain a CBC, urinalysis, and blood cultures and then immediately consult a neurosurgeon.

If a child has a mild or moderate fever of unknown origin with other symptoms compatible with a common childhood illness and no obvious signs of shunt malfunction, the primary care provider can assume a wait-and-see attitude. Arrangements for telephone follow-up or a return appointment in 24 hours should be made. The parents must be instructed to report symptoms such as lethargy, confusion, or recurrent vomiting (more than three times/24 hours), immediately if they occur.

Children who have very high temperatures (i.e., 40° C) and symptoms of moderate to severe illness must be assumed to have a shunt infection until proven otherwise. Consultation with a neurosurgeon is advised. Blood cultures for both aerobic and anaerobic organisms should be drawn, although they are often not initially positive. A CBC is also indicated, but minimal leukocytosis does not rule out shunt infection. CSF should be obtained by the neurosurgeon for culture through the shunt reservoir. Although CSF leukocytosis (i.e., 50 to 200 cells/cm³) is common with shunt infection, an infection can be present despite normal CSF cell count, protein, and glucose. CSF

eosinophilia (i.e., more than 7% of the total CSF white blood cell count) is also indicative of shunt infection (Madikians & Conway, 1997). Shunt aspiration should be done with meticulous aseptic technique so as not to contaminate a sterile shunt system or introduce a second organism into an already infected shunt. An LP is not advised in a child with a shunt due to the possibility of downward brain herniation and death if there is ventriculomegaly with increased ICP.

A chest radiograph and urine culture are recommended to rule out pneumonia or urinary tract infection. However, if the history and physical findings strongly suggest shunt involvement, these may be omitted. The neurosurgeon may prefer that all tests be done at the hospital because hospitalization is often required to complete the evaluation and treatment process. Throughout the work-up for the source of fever, the primary care practitioner should be in close communication with the primary neurosurgeon.

GI Symptoms. Nausea and vomiting are common clinical symptoms during childhood, often accompanying such diverse conditions as influenza, otitis media, and urinary tract infections. Diarrhea and abdominal pain are also frequent complaints in childhood. Children with hydrocephalus can be expected to have these common complaints as often as other children. When a child has mild GI symptoms, the practitioner must consider the presence or absence of other symptoms and the history of exposure to GI illness. The diagnostic work-up should include an evaluation for shunt infection and GI disease. The primary care provider must recognize that abdominal symptoms may be the presenting symptom of peritoneal shunt malfunction or an acute condition in the abdomen in children with shunts (Pumberger et al, 1998).

Children with a peritoneal shunt infection may have mild to moderate fever, abdominal pain, anorexia, nausea, vomiting, and diarrhea. They may guard their abdomen and be unwilling to ambulate. Swelling, redness, or inflammation along the catheter tract or at the incision site is highly suggestive of shunt involvement. Abdominal ultrasound and CSF cultures should help differentiate between an acute condition in the abdomen and a shunt infection. Specific signs of appendicitis can be demonstrated by a CT scan of the abdomen, but identification of an abdominal pseudocyst is more characteristic of a distal shunt infection (Pumberger et al, 1998). Abdominal pseudocysts may develop around the peritoneal end of the VP shunt and usually result from past or current shunt infection. A history of recent or recurrent shunt revisions also substantially increases the risk for infection. The primary care practitioner may be able to differentiate the symptoms of an acute condition in the abdomen from peritoneal shunt malfunction. Consultation with and referral to the attending neurosurgeon are advised.

Many children with hydrocephalus have other neurologic problems that may increase the incidence of constipation. Stool trapped in the colon may put pressure on the peritoneal shunt, resulting in a malfunction. Maintenance of regular stool patterns may prevent unnecessary hospitalization and need for shunt revision.

Another abdominal concern for infants with inguinal or umbilical hernias is the potential for CSF or shunt tubing to migrate into the hernia. The hernia becomes enlarged with a collection of CSF; treatment includes repair of the hernia and possible shunt revision.

Metastasis of brain tumor cells from the ventricular cavities into the abdominal cavity is a possible side effect of ventriculoperitoneal shunts (Rickert, 1998). This side effect must be considered when a differential diagnosis is made in children with chronic or recurring abdominal complaints if these children also have a history of a brain tumor. Appropriate referral is required to rule out this possibility after more common reasons for the complaint have proven negative.

Headaches. Children often complain of headaches, which can also occur in children with a shunt and may have the same origin as in children without hydrocephalus. Children with hydrocephalus are reported to have migrainous headaches twice as often (i.e., 8.5% vs. 4%) and nonmigrainous headaches almost three times as often as children without hydrocephalus (Stellman-Ward et al, 1997). The incidence of headaches in these children did not decrease with shunt revision and was not associated with seizures or the underlying condition causing the hydrocephalus. These headaches have been called shunt migraines and occur more often in individuals who have very small ventricles after shunting and are thought to be due to poor brain compliance in response to physiologic variations in ICP. If routine treatment with mild analgesics and rest does not relieve the symptom or if the headaches become frequent, affect school attendance, or are associated with lethargy or irritability, then evaluation by the neurologist and/or neurosurgeon is required. Repetitive and vigorous investigation of shunt malfunction may not be necessary in the absence of other symptoms. Shunt malfunction can be partial or variable, depending on cerebral blood flow, CSF production, and a child's activity, and may result in periodic episodes of increased ICP. Children with shunts occasionally experience headaches and vomiting in the early morning after sleeping all night. These symptoms may be caused by temporary partial blockage of the shunt from cellular debris, inactivity, and the horizontal sleeping position, which negates the beneficial effect of gravity for ventricular drainage. These symptoms usually subside after children have been up for a few hours. If these episodes are infrequent and self-limited, they do not require treatment other than acetaminophen or ibuprofen for pain. Parents should be instructed to call the primary care provider if these symptoms continue for more than 6 hours or are associated with a decrease in the level of consciousness or loss of motor ability.

Scalp Infections. A thin layer of skin covers the shunt reservoir on the scalp. If the skin around the shunt reservoir becomes infected, the integrity of the skin barrier may be broken and infection of the shunt is possible. The primary care provider should manage scalp infections aggressively in collaboration with the neurosurgeon.

Alterations in Behavior. All children experience mood swings and temporary behavior changes. Parents of children with hydrocephalus may comment on them not being themselves; school performance may falter, normal interest in activities may dwindle; and lethargy or irritability may develop. If these changes persist beyond a few days, a child should be seen by the neurosurgeon for an evaluation. Subtle changes in behavior, cognition, or motor ability may be symptoms of shunt malfunction.

Drug Interactions

No routine medications are prescribed for children with hydrocephalus. (See Chapter 25 for drug interactions with anticonvulsant therapy.)

Developmental Issues

Sleep Patterns

Parents may be concerned about their infant or child sleeping in a position that might adversely affect the shunt. During the immediate period after shunt placement, these children should be positioned off the reservoir site to avoid skin breakdown. With the exception of this brief period of time after shunt placement or revision, parents and caretakers must be reassured that their child can sleep in any comfortable position without fear of affecting the shunt. Infants and young children should be encouraged to assume a normal sleeping pattern at night.

Toileting

Children with neurologic deficits associated with hydrocephalus may have a delayed ability to develop bowel and bladder control. Parents need to be counseled on the possibility of this difficulty, and the methods of toilet training should be reviewed. The neurologist, neurosurgeon, and physiatrist (if applicable) following a child's development should be consulted about the child's neurologic capability to attain satisfactory toilet training. If necessary, special bowel training and clean intermittent catheterization education should be provided and can usually be obtained through referral to a pediatric urologist or physiatrist (see Chapter 33).

Discipline

Discipline for children with hydrocephalus should be managed as for other children, recognizing the limitations of cognitive and motor development of the individual child. Some parents may have difficulty understanding the discrepancy between their child's verbal and performance skills and may have expectations that are too high for the child to attain, which may lead to inappropriate discipline. On the other hand, parents may be afraid to discipline their child and must be encouraged to set appropriate limits.

Practitioners must always be concerned with the increased possibility of child abuse in children with chronic conditions. Head injuries and abdominal injuries are common in child abuse and may result in further brain injury or shunt malfunction.

Child Care

Most mothers work outside the home. Child care and preschool placement are major issues for all working parents but are even more so when a child has a chronic condition. Fortunately, the current shunt systems are self-maintained and do not require special care (e.g., pumping periodically) throughout the day. There are no special care needs for children with hydrocephalus unless other disabilities (e.g., cerebral palsy with spasticity or dystonia, seizures, or developmental delay) are present. If a child has significant disabilities, child care arrangements must be evaluated for their ability to meet the child's needs. Public Law 101-476, the Individuals with Disabilities Education Act

(1997), extended services to children with disabilities from birth to school entry, so federally funded programs are accessible to children with disabilities (see Chapter 5). Parents of children with disabilities such as spina bifida and hydrocephalus may visit the Web site www.ideapractices.org/law/index.php to obtain more information about the law and current amendments.

Children with hydrocephalus, however, are at greater risk for CNS infections than their peers because of their shunt. Parents must understand that children who attend daycare or preschool are exposed to childhood infections and have illnesses (i.e., usually respiratory or gastrointestinal) more often than those who stay at home. Children up to 2 years of age should receive child care at home or in a small daycare program to minimize exposure to common pediatric pathogens.

Schooling

In general, 60% of children with hydrocephalus attend regular school, but many function below their expected grade level (Casey et al, 1997; Hoppe-Hirsch et al, 1998). Primary care providers can help families plan their child's individualized educational program (IEP) to ensure appropriate interventions for the child. Although Public Law 101-476 requires the school district to assess a child's needs, financial constraints of the school district may limit neuropsychologic testing. Therefore any testing done before school may be beneficial and should be forwarded to the school district. Parents may need help obtaining medical records to facilitate formulation of their child's IEP. The primary care practitioner can be of assistance to the family during this process.

Because of physical or intellectual limitations, some children with hydrocephalus qualify for separate special education classes. Other children can be mainstreamed into regular classrooms and receive special services (e.g., adaptive physical education to help with motor control and balance, occupational therapy to assist with kinesthetic-proprioceptive deficits, speech therapy, or psychologic counseling to address emotional issues). As these children reach junior high school and high school, some limitations may be made on competitive, high-impact violent sports. Tackle football, boxing, wrestling, and ice hockey have a much higher risk of head and abdominal injury than track, swimming, tennis, or golf. If a child has mild to moderate neuromotor deficits, an evaluation by a sports medicine professional may help identify sports activities that the child can successfully perform. Being involved in sports activities is often beneficial to a child's self-esteem and encourages peer relationships, both of which may be problematic areas for children with hydrocephalus.

Children with less severe disabilities may experience psychosocial difficulty because they may have a difficult time fitting in with nondisabled peers but also do not fit in with more disabled children. Their disabilities may not be recognized by teachers and peers unable to understand why these individuals have difficulty in school or sports. Adolescents who are trying not to be different may not disclose their learning or motor deficit but will not be able to successfully compete with unaffected peers. The resulting incongruity between expectations and ability can lead to a sense of failure and lowered self-esteem.

Primary care providers should routinely ask parents and children about school progress. If academic difficulties develop, these children should be referred for repeat neuropsychologic testing to rule out medical reasons for these problems. Shunt malfunction may result in gradual changes in cognition, fine motor abilities, or personality and must be ruled out as a contributing factor. If difficulties are assessed to be more emotional, which often happens during adolescence when children struggle with their body image and identity, children should be referred for counseling. This referral should be made to a professional experienced in working with children with disabilities.

Sexuality

As previously mentioned, delayed or precocious puberty may occur in children with hydrocephalus. Their progression through puberty must be assessed and monitored, and counseling may be indicated to support them during this period. Research indicates that children with precocious puberty may have lowered self-esteem, poor peer relationships, and a higher incidence of sexual abuse than normally developing children. Sexuality and reproductive issues should be managed the same as with other children. Female adolescents receiving anticonvulsive therapy should be informed of the possible teratogenic effects of the medications they are taking (see Chapter 25). Adolescents with associated motor disabilities may have additional needs (see Chapter 18).

Transition to Adulthood

Each health care provider, including neurosurgeons, manages the ongoing care of the child with hydrocephalus differently. Changes in the way this care is given are being mandated as the economics of medical care changes in response to market forces.

Since the 1970s, improvements in shunt techniques and management of shunt complications have resulted in a dramatic increase in the survival of individuals with hydrocephalus. Researchers have been following these young people as they make their transition into adulthood. They have identified concerns about how these individuals deal with vocational training, career placement, sexuality, and family roles. Their social outcomes are highly influenced by their associated disabilities, especially developmental delay and motor handicaps. Many adults who were shunted during childhood have achieved full-time employment and successful personal relationships because either their disabilities were minor or they were able to overcome them. Results of studies assessing the employment rate of young adults with hydrocephalus associated with spina bifida have been less promising, with as many as 70% to 80% failing to maintain employment. Some of these individuals have been described as lacking drive or initiative, but more accurately they lack an environment that fosters independence. Parents are often overcautious and overprotective and do not discipline appropriately, inadvertently causing children to be socially inappropriate and dependent.

A supportive climate that encourages independence, maturity, and responsibility is essential if young adults with hydrocephalus are to complete school, maintain employment, and function as adults. Professional guidance is often necessary to create this environment. Health professionals should emphasize a positive prognosis for young adults with hydrocephalus. Parents must be prepared to face the normal problems of adolescence and let their young children develop independence. The National Information Center for Children and Youth with Disabilities (NICHCY) can provide information and referrals for social skills programs that may be useful to parents, teachers, and others. (See listing and Web site under "Resources.") At the college level, vocational training and special education resources can help young adults prepare for job placement. Young adults dependent on a shunt should be cautious about living alone because they could become acutely ill, confused, or even comatose during a shunt malfunction. These individuals should form a buddy system to ensure their well-being, thereby minimizing their risk of permanent brain injury from an unrecognized shunt malfunction.

Hydrocephalus alone should not interfere with a woman's ability to conceive, but reports suggest that shunt function can be affected by pregnancy (Bradley et al, 1998). Neurologic complications that have been known to occur during pregnancy include seizures, headaches, nausea, vomiting, lethargy, ataxia, and gaze paresis. In most cases symptoms of increased ICP resolve during the postpartum period. Therefore prenatal counseling and assessment should include an evaluation of medications—especially anticonvulsants, genetic counseling, and a review of family history for neural tube defects. A complete assessment of shunt function should be obtained if pregnancy is being considered. In addition, maternal supplementation with folic acid significantly diminishes the number of infants born with neural tube defects (Manning et al, 2000). Therefore women of childbearing age must be strongly encouraged to supplement their intake of folic acid before conception.

Family Concerns and Resources

Parents of children with hydrocephalus constantly worry about continued shunt function. With every malfunction there is the need for surgery and the perceived threat of further brain damage. This constant worry and the daily responsibility and stress of caring for a child who may have multiple medical problems are hard on families. The financial strain from numerous medical visits or surgical procedures may deplete a family's financial reserves. Private insurance may not be obtainable unless offered through a large group employment policy. Concern about a child's ability to be self-supporting and independent in the future is also an issue for parents as their child grows into adolescence.

Parent-to-parent support groups can offer support by publishing newsletters and even hosting major medical conferences for both health professionals and parents. These organizations also provide a network for children with hydrocephalus, offering them the opportunity to make new friends, develop peer support, and exchange knowledge. Support groups are now readily available on the Internet to both the adolescent with

hydrocephalus and his/her parents. (See Web sites listed below.) Primary care providers should become familiar with the organizations in the community and Web connections so that appropriate referrals can be made. It is better to make such referrals soon after a child's diagnosis than to wait to see how the parents cope. All parents need support above and beyond what is reasonable for a physician or nurse to provide.

Resources

Organizations and Web Sites

The Cleveland Clinic
www.clevelandclinic.org

Hydrocephalus Foundation, Inc.
910 Rear Broadway, Rt. 1
Saugus, MA 01906
(781) 942-1161
www.hydrocephalus.org

HOPE (Hydrocephalus Opens People Eyes)
104-47 120th Street
Richmond Hill, NY 11419

Hydrocephalus Association
870 Market Street, Suite 705
San Francisco, CA 94102
(415) 732-7040; (888) 598-3789
www.hydroassoc.org

Individuals with Disabilities Education Act
www.ideapractices.org/law/index.php

National Hydrocephalus Foundation
12413 Centralia Road
Lakewood, CA 90715-1623
(562) 402-3532 or (888) 857-3434
http://nhfonline.org

National Information Center for Children
and Youth with Disabilities (NICHCY)
PO Box 1492
Washington, DC 20013
(202) 884-8441; (800) 695-0285
www.nichcy.org

National Organization for Rare Disorders (NORD)
PO Box 8923
New Fairfield, CT 06812
(203) 746-6518
www.rarediseases.org

Columbia-Presbyterian Department of Neurological Surgery
http://cpmcnet.columbia.edu/dept/nsg

Spina Bifida Association of America
4590 MacArthur Boulevard NW, Suite 250
Washington, DC 20007-4226
(202) 944-3285: (800) 621-3141
www.sbaa.org; sbaa@sbaa.org

United Cerebral Palsy Association, Inc
1660 L Street, Suite 700
Washington, DC 20036
www.uscpa.org

Summary of Primary Care Needs for the Child with Hydrocephalus

HEALTH CARE MAINTENANCE

Growth and Development

Height and weight are usually within normal range unless a child is severely handicapped.

If enlarged head size is diagnosed in infancy and a shunt is placed, head size should follow the normal growth curve.

The head should be measured at each visit until the sutures are fused.

Both precocious puberty and short stature are reported.

Standard infant development tests may indicate delay because of poor head control.

Of all children with hydrocephalus, 75% will have some motor disability.

Verbal skills must be assessed and compared with intellectual ability.

Diet

A normal diet is indicated.

There are concerns about and difficulty in assessing infant vomiting as normal or as a sign of increased ICP.

Safety

The risk of head injury is increased because of poor head control.

A rear-facing car seat should be recommended until a child can sit unsupported.

A helmet should be used for bike and skateboard riding.

Neurologic deficits may make competitive sports difficult and operation of motor vehicles hazardous.

Immunization

Pertussis vaccine may be deferred in infants with seizures.

Measles vaccine may cause seizures in children with seizure disorders but is recommended because of the prevalence of measles.

H. influenzae type B conjugated vaccine is strongly recommended.

Pneumococcal vaccine and influenza vaccine should be considered for children with multiple shunt infections or significant disabilities.

Screening

Vision. Hirschberg examination, cover test, ability to track, and funduscopic examination should be done at each visit. Children should be examined by an ophthalmologist at 6 months of age and then yearly thereafter.

Alterations in eye examination may be associated with shunt malfunction.

Hearing. A routine office screening is recommended. An auditory-evoked response test should be given to children with a history of CNS infection or who have been treated with aminoglycosides.

Dental. Routine dental care is recommended.

Children on phenytoin therapy require more frequent dental care.

Prophylactic antibiotics are recommended for dental procedures likely to cause bleeding.

Blood Pressure. Blood pressure should be recorded at each visit.

Blood pressure increases with increased ICP.

Hematocrit. Routine screening is recommended.
Urinalysis. Routine screening is recommended.
Tuberculosis. Routine screening is recommended.

Condition-Specific Screening

Head Circumference. Head circumference should be measured at each visit until the sutures are completely fused.

COMMON ILLNESS MANAGEMENT

Differential Diagnosis

Fever. Shunt or CNS infection should be ruled out.

Gastrointestinal Symptoms. Increased ICP with nausea and vomiting should be ruled out.

Peritonitis with abdominal pain or acute diarrhea should be ruled out.

Shunt infection caused by abdominal infection should be ruled out.

Constipation should be ruled out as cause of shunt malfunction.

Metastatic abdominal tumor should be ruled out in children with primary brain tumors and ventriculoperitoneal shunts.

Headaches. Shunt malfunction should be ruled out as the cause of acute or chronic headaches.

Scalp Infections. Possible infection spread to shunt reservoir should be ruled out.

Alterations in Behavior. Alterations in behavior should be ruled out as a symptom of shunt malfunction.

Drug Interactions

No routine medications are prescribed.

DEVELOPMENTAL ISSUES

Sleep Patterns

Standard developmental counseling is advised.

Toileting

Delayed bowel and bladder training may occur because of neurologic deficit.

Constipation may cause peritoneal shunt malfunction.

Discipline

Expectations are normal with recognition of the possible discrepancy between verbal and motor abilities. Physical punishment is a hazard because it may cause head or abdominal injury.

Child Care

No special care needs are required except when a child has a severe motor disability or seizures.

Home care or small daycare programs are recommended during a child's first 2 years of life to reduce infections.

Schooling

Associated problems are often covered by Public Law 101-476.

Families should be assisted in IEP hearings.

Children may have possible adjustment problems during adolescence.

Continued

Summary of Primary Care Needs for the Child with Hydrocephalus—cont'd

Children may need psychometric testing for poor school performance.

Low-impact sports should be selected to prevent head trauma and abdominal injury.

Minor, unseen disabilities should not be overlooked.

Sexuality

Children should be evaluated for delayed or precocious puberty.

Standard developmental counseling is advised unless associated problems warrant additional care.

Transition to Adulthood

Research has identified difficulty with vocational training, career, sexuality, and family roles associated with hydrocephalus and mental retardation and motor handicaps.

Independence must be fostered from an early age to prepare young adults for independence.

Shunt-dependent individuals should develop a buddy system to ensure that shunt malfunction leading to acute illness, confusion, or coma does not go unrecognized.

Pregnancy may interfere with peritoneal shunt drainage. Securing independent health and life insurance may be difficult for individuals with hydrocephalus.

FAMILY CONCERNS

Families are concerned about continued shunt function and the possibility of brain damage caused by shunt failure or infection.

REFERENCES

Albright, A., Leland, Pollack, Ian, F., Adelson, P., & David. (1999). *Principles and practice of pediatric neurosurgery.* New York: Thieme.

Balmer, B., Bernays, R.L., Kollias, S.S., & Yonekawa, Y. (2002). Interventional MR-guided neuroendoscopy: a new therapeutic option for children. *J Pediatr Surg, 37*(4), 668-672.

Barnes, M.A., Faulkner, H.J., & Dennis, M. (2002). Poor reading comprehension despite fast word decoding in children with hydrocephalus. *Brain Lang, 80*(2), 253-259.

Bier, J.A., Morales, Y., Liebling, J., Geddes, L., & Kim, E. (1997). Medical and social factors associated with cognitive outcome in individuals with myelomeningocele. *Dev Med Child Neurol, 39*(4), 263-266.

Camboulives, J., Meyrieux, V., & Lena, G. (2002). Infections of cerebrospinal fluid shunts in the child: prevention and treatment. *Ann Fr Anesth Reanim, 21*(2), 84-89.

Casey, A.T., et al. (1997). The long-term outlook for hydrocephalus in childhood. *Pediatr Neurosurg, 27*, 63-70.

Chalmers, R.M., et al. (1999). Familial hydrocephalus. *J Neurol Neurosurg Psychiatry, 67*, 410-417.

Choux, M., DiRocco, C., Hockley, A.D., & Walker, M.L. (1999). *Pediatr Neurosurg.* London: Churchill Livingstone.

Committee on Infectious Diseases. (2000). *Report of the committee on infectious diseases* (25th ed.) Elk Grove Village, IL: The American Academy of Pediatrics.

Dias, M.S. & Li, V. (1998). Pediatric neurosurgical disease. *Pediatr Clin North Am, 45*(6), 1539-1545.

Frim, D.M., Scott, R.M., & Madsen, J.R. (1998). Surgical management of neonatal hydrocephalus. *Neurosurg Clin North Am, 9*(1), 105-110.

Fudge, R.A. (2000). About hydrocephalus—a book for parents. San Francisco: Hydrocephalus Association.

Futagi, Y., Suzuki, Y., Toribe, Y., & Morimoto, K. (2002). Neurodevelopmental outcome in children with fetal hydrocephalus. *Pediatr Neurol, 27*(2), 111-116.

Hamada, H., et al. (1999). Autosomal recessive hydrocephalus due to congenital stenosis of the aqueduct of Sylvius. *Prenat Diagn, 19*(11), 1067-1069.

Harrison, M.R., Evans, M.I., Adzick, N.S., & Holzgreve, W. (2001). *The unborn patient. The art and science of fetal therapy* (3rd ed.). Philadelphia: W.B. Saunders.

Helpin, M.L., Rosenberg, H.M., Sayany, Z., & Sanford, R.A. (1998). Antibiotic prophylaxis in dental patients with ventriculo-peritoneal shunts: a pilot study. *J Dent Child, 65*(4), 244-247.

Hoppe-Hirsch, E., et al. (1998). Late outcome of the surgical treatment of hydrocephalus. *Childs Nerv Syst, 14*, 97-99.

Huber-Okrainec, J., Dennis, M., Brettschneider, J., & Spiegler, B.J. (2002). Neuromotor speech deficits in children and adults with spina bifida and hydrocephalus. *Brain Lang, 80*(3), 592-602.

Iskander, B.J., McLaughlin, C., Mapstone, T.B., Grabb, P.A., & Oakes, W.J. (1998). Pitfalls in the diagnosis of ventricular shunt dysfunction: radiology reports and ventricular size. *Pediatrics, 101*(6), 1031-1036.

Javadpour, M., Mallucci, C., Brodbelt, A., Golash, A., & May, P. (2001). The impact of endoscopic third ventriculostomy on the management of newly diagnosed hydrocephalus in infants. *Pediatr Neurosurg, 35*, 131-135.

Kay, A.D., Fisher, A.J., O'Kane, C., Richards, H.K., Pickard, J.D. (2002). United Kingdom and Ireland Medos Shunt Audit Group. A clinical audit of the hakim programmable valve in patients with complex hydrocephalus. *Br J Neurosurg, 14*(6), 535-542.

Madikians, A. & Conway, E.E. (1997). Cerebrospinal fluid shunt problems in pediatric patients. *Pediatr Ann, 26*, 613-620.

Manning, S.M., Jennings, R., & Madsen, J.R. (2000). Pathophysiology, prevention, and potential treatment of neural tube defects. *Ment Retard Dev Disabil Res Rev, 6*(1), 6-14.

Mataro, M., Junque, C., Poca, M.A., & Sahuquillo, J. (2001). Neuropsychological findings in congenital and acquired childhood hydrocephalus. *Neuropsychol Rev, 11*(4), 169-178.

McLone, D.G. (2001). *Pediatric neurosurgery: surgery of the developing nervous system* (4th ed.). Philadelphia: W.B. Saunders.

Menkes, J.H. & Sarnat, H.B. (2000). *Child neurology* (6th ed.). Philadelphia: Lippincott Williams & Wilkins.

Nguyen, T.N., Polomeno, R.C., Farmer, J.P., & Montes, J.L. (2002). Ophthalmic complications of slit-ventricle syndrome in children. *Ophthalmology, 109*(3), 520-524.

Pumberger, W., Lobl, M., & Geissler, W. (1998). Appendicitis in children with a ventriculoperitoneal shunt. *Pediatr Neurosurg, 28*, 21-26.

Rendeli, C., et al. (2002). Does locomotion improve the cognitive profile of children with meningomyelocele? *Childs Nerv Syst, 18*(5), 231-234.

Rickert, C.H. (1998). Abdominal metastases of pediatric brain tumors via ventriculo-peritoneal shunts. *Childs Nerv Syst, 14*, 10-14.

Rosen, S. (1998). Educating students who have visual impairments with neurological disabilities. In S.Z. Sacks & R.K. Silberman (Eds.). *Educating students who have visual impairments with other disabilities.* Baltimore: Paul H. Brookes.

Sato, O., Yamguchi, T., Kitaaka, M., Toyama. (2001). Hydrocephalus and epilepsy. *Childs Nerv Syst, 17*(1-2), 76-86.

Scott, M.A., et al. (1998). Memory functions in children with early hydrocephalus. *Neuropsychology, 12*(4), 578-589.

Stellman-Ward, G.R., Bannister, C.M., Lewis, M.A., & Shaw, J. (1997). The incidence of chronic headache in children with shunted hydrocephalus. *Eur J Pediatr Surg, 7*(Suppl 1),12-14.

Takahashi, Y. (2001). Withdrawal of shunt systems—clinical use of the programmable shunt system and its effect on hydrocephalus in children. *Childs Nerv Syst, 17*, 472-477.

Tsuji, O. & Sato, K. (1998). CSF dynamics in a patient with a programmable shunt. *Acta Neurochir Suppl (Wien), 71*, 364-367.

U.S. Department of Health and Human Services, Public Health Service. (2000, October). *Guide to contraindications to childhood vaccinations.* Washington, DC: CDC.

Whitehead, W. & Kestle, J. (2001). The treatment of cerebrospinal fluid shunt infections. *Pediatr Neurosurg, 35*, 205-210.

30 Inflammatory Bowel Disease

Betsy Haas-Beckert and Melvin B. Heyman

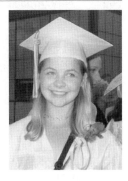

Etiology

The term inflammatory bowel disease (IBD) encompasses the diagnoses of Crohn's disease (CD) and ulcerative colitis (UC). These two forms of IBD are commonly discussed together in the literature because they share many of the same presenting signs, symptoms, approaches to diagnosis, and management.

Crohn's disease is a chronic inflammatory disease of the bowel that may involve any portion of the gastrointestinal (GI) tract—from mouth to anus. CD is characterized by inflammation that is transmural (extending through the entire wall of the intestine). It may begin as mild superficial disease and subsequently slowly extend from the intestinal mucosal lining through the serosal layer. In this condition diseased segments of the bowel may border on segments of healthy tissue, giving it a segmental or uneven appearance. CD most commonly affects the terminal ileum (30%-70% of cases), involves the ileum and colon in 60%, and is limited to the colon in 10% to 20% of cases (Baldassano & Piccoli, 1999; Hyams, 2000). Ten percent to 15% of children have diffuse small bowel disease involving the more proximal ileum or jejunum. Isolated gastroduodenal involvement has been previously thought to be less common, but has recently been reported in 30% to 40% of all individuals with CD when these areas are examined for endoscopic or histologic evidence of disease (Baldassano & Piccoli, 1999). Perianal disease in children with CD ranges from 25% to 30% (Hyams, 1999). Affected children may have skin tags, fissures, and fistulas.

Ulcerative colitis is an inflammatory disease limited to the colon, including the rectal mucosa. The inflammatory process starts in the rectum and progresses proximal in an uninterrupted pattern to involve parts or all of the large intestine. Inflammation limited to the rectum is found in 10% of cases (termed ulcerative proctitis), 30% is found in the sigmoid and descending colon, distal to the splenic flexure ("left-sided colitis"), and in 40% to 50% the entire colon from rectum to cecum (termed pancolitis) is involved (Hyams, 2000).

A subgroup of children with disease limited to the colon but whose condition cannot be clearly categorized as CD or UC is termed "indeterminate colitis" and may comprise 10% to 15% of cases. Usually after 1 to 2 years, many (approximately 50%) can be reclassified as UC or CD (Present, 2002).

A thorough history is extremely important, with emphasis on recent antibiotic intake, family history, and length of time of symptoms. The diagnostic tools for IBD include radiographic examination of the GI tract, endoscopy and biopsy, physical examination, including growth and nutrition parameters, and assessment of laboratory values (including stool cultures). Common laboratory findings associated with IBD include increased acute-phase reactants (e.g., erythrocyte sedimentation rate [ESR] and C-reactive protein [CRP]), thrombocytosis, low serum iron, low hematocrit value, and low hemoglobin level. Hypoalbuminemia and a decreased total protein serum value may also be noted, particularly in CD that affects the small bowel and in moderate to severe UC.

Radiologic studies and upper and lower endoscopy are useful to define the nature and extent of intestinal inflammation and to help differentiate UC from CD. Colonoscopy and upper endoscopy are the preferred methods to evaluate the intestinal tract; they can identify mucosal inflammation and permit mucosal biopsies to obtain histologic assessment. Colonoscopy to the terminal ileum is the preferred method to assess disease involving the large intestine (colon). Upper endoscopy, in conjunction with an upper gastrointestinal radiograph, including a small-bowel follow-through are the preferred methods to evaluate the small bowel, stomach, and esophagus. The small bowel follow-through radiograph allows for evaluation of the entire small intestine to the terminal ileum, the most common site for disease involvement in CD. Computed tomography (CT) scan may be useful to delineate small intestinal wall thickening, extramural extension of inflammation by fistulization to adjacent structures, and the presence of abscesses (Hyams, 1999).

Advances in the immunologic and genetic factors that are associated with CD and UC suggest that these inflammatory bowel diseases are not simply two disorders that share similar clinical manifestations, but more likely are composed of a group of diseases triggered and sustained by a variety of diverse genetic, environmental, and immunologic factors (Oliva-Hemker et al, 2002). Recent studies, however, have discovered specific genotypes that might provide subgroups of each of these diseases (Ahmed et al, 2002). Despite the research progress over the past two decades, the etiology and pathogenesis of IBD still remain to be clearly defined. Several investigators now hypothesize that IBD results from an unregulated immune response to environmental and bacterial triggers, probably in a genetically susceptible host. Investigations into genes associated with and/or predisposing to IBD are being studied in many research centers throughout the world.

Known Genetic Etiology

Some investigators hypothesize that a complex immunogenetic model for IBD is in part responsible, whereby genetically susceptible individuals harbor an aberrant response to yet unidentified environmental factors (Cuthbert et al, 2002).

Many researchers have worked to identify and localize IBD-susceptible genes. Recently groups of researchers have found an area of apparent linkage on chromosome 16 (Ogura et al, 2000; Cuthbert et al, 2002; Podolsky, 2002). Detailed mapping of chromosome 16 has resulted in the identification of a gene, NOD2, that correlates strongly and is responsible in part for CD, particularly fibrostenosing Crohn's disease of the ileum and proximal colon, but not UC (Hampe et al, 2002). To date no combination of genes appears sufficient alone for the development of CD or UC, but additional factors, such as the use of nonsteroidal antiinflammatory drugs (NSAIDs), altered intestinal flora, or other environmental factors, may be associated with an unregulated immune system leading to the evolution of IBD in an individual.

Incidence and Prevalence

The incidence of CD increased considerably during the middle of this century. The overall increase began to level off in the early 1980s, although controversy prevails over this point. The incidence and prevalence of IBD in the pediatric population is less than in adults. However, over the past several decades the prevalence appears to have increased among children and adolescents (Oliva-Hemker et al, 2002). Twenty-five percent to 30% of individuals with CD and 20% of those with UC are now presenting before 20 years of age (Baldassano & Piccoli, 1999). This increase may be due to earlier diagnoses rather than a true increase in the occurrence of CD and UC in children (Hyams, 1996; Logan, 1998). An incidence rate for CD reported in a US study was 5.8 per every 100,000 individuals per year (Loftus et al, 1997). The incidence of UC in children range from 1 to 10 cases per 100,000 individuals is thought to be relatively stable (Calkins & Mendeloff, 1995; Kirschner, 1996; Logan, 1998).

The incidence and frequency of IBD vary greatly depending upon geographic location and racial or ethnic background. The highest rates are found in the Scandinavian countries and Scotland, then England and North America, and followed by central and southern Europe (Oliva-Hemker et al, 2000). The risk of having IBD is greater in urban compared with rural areas, in higher versus lower socioeconomic classes, and in developed versus less developed countries (Oliva-Hemker et al, 2002). However, probably the single greatest risk factor for developing IBD is a first-degree relative with the disease (Hyams, 2000; Oliva-Hemker et al, 2002; Podolsky, 2002). Children diagnosed with IBD show a 30% greater family history. The family risk pattern appears to be greater for CD compared with UC. Additionally, high rates of Crohn's disease have been observed in monozygotic twins compared with dizygotic twins (Podolsky, 2002). Although monozygotic twins share identical genomic material, they may be disconcordant for CD, leading researchers to believe that multiple gene products contribute to a person's risk of IBD (Podolsky, 2002)

The risk for UC and CD is greater for Jewish people of middle European origin living in the United States than for those living in Israel. Blacks are less commonly affected with CD than whites. Men and women appear to be equally affected (Hyams, 1996).

Clinical Manifestations at Time of Diagnosis

Presentation of symptoms and signs of CD is determined primarily by the location and extent of disease involvement. The diagnosis of IBD is often difficult or delayed because of the subtle manner in which it may present and symptoms that can be associated with many other disease entities. Infectious conditions of the gastrointestinal tract, such as *Salmonella, Shigella, Campylobacter, Yersinia, Aeromonas* and *Clostridium difficile,* and the parasite *Entamoeba histolytica,* can mimic IBD and need to be ruled out. Fortunately most laboratories can culture for these organisms. Recurrent abdominal pain is a common complaint in the pediatric population, with 10% of the population complaining of nonspecific periumbilical pain at some time during childhood and it can be secondary to many different causes (Baldassano & Piccoli, 1999). Common causes of abdominal pain in the pediatric population can include constipation, gastroesophageal reflux, urinary tract infection, giardiasis, lactose intolerance, and functional abdominal pain. If the abdominal pain is also associated with other symptoms such as growth failure, anorexia, diarrhea, or other extraintestinal manifestations as described below, then a more extensive evaluation for IBD should be performed.

Nearly 80% of IBD in the pediatric population present with abdominal pain, diarrhea, anorexia, and/or weight loss (Griffiths & Buller, 2000). Periumbilical or right lower quadrant abdominal pain is the most common single symptom related to disease in the region of the distal ileum and proximal colon. It tends to be persistent and severe, frequently awakening the child from sleep. Diarrhea, which is common, may not be present, especially if the disease is located in the small bowel. However, malabsorption, diarrhea, abdominal pain, growth failure, fever, weight loss, and anorexia are typical symptoms of small intestine involvement. Blood is usually occult, although stools in about 20% may be grossly bloody in CD of the colon. Crohn's colitis may be clinically difficult to distinguish from ulcerative colitis (UC), with symptoms of bloody diarrhea, cramping abdominal pain, and urgency to defecate (tenesmus). Perianal disease may be an isolated presenting feature of CD (see Table 30-1).

Growth failure in stature and concomitant delay in sexual maturation may precede the development of overt intestinal manifestations by years in children with CD.

Protein-energy malnutrition (PEM) is a common finding and may occur in 85% of children hospitalized with an acute exacerbation of IBD. At the time of initial diagnosis, 85% of children with CD and 65% of children with UC have lost weight. Children with IBD, particularly with CD, are at significant risk for growth failure (Graham et al, 2002). The cause of growth failure is thought to be multifactorial, including increased energy expenditure, increased nutrient losses, and catabolic effects of medications, especially corticosteroids. However, the consensus is that inadequate caloric intake is the fundamental cause. Children may ingest too few calories because of anorexia associated with the symptoms of disease activity. They may also consciously skip meals to minimize embarrassing symptoms such as diarrhea. Nutritional intervention directed toward achieving adequate caloric intake for growth and development is a crucial goal for treatment of IBD.

TABLE 30-1

Comparison of Crohn's Disease and Ulcerative Colitis: Presenting Symptoms

	Crohn's Disease	Ulcerative Colitis
Alteration in bowel pattern	Diarrhea is common; constipation, alternating with diarrhea, may also be seen.	Diarrhea is a hallmark; an increase in frequency of bowel movements with urgency is often a component. Constipation may be seen if the disease is obstructive.
Blood in stool	Grossly bloody stools are occasionally seen, most often when colonic disease is present. Occult blood is not uncommon in Crohn's disease.	It is common to see grossly bloody diarrhea; pus or mucus may also be seen.
Abdominal pain	Abdominal pain is often present in association with meals; pain is often periumbilical.	Abdominal cramping is often present in association with passage of stool. Pain is often noted in the lower part of the abdomen.
Fever	It is not uncommon to have intermittent, usually low-grade fever.	Fever is sometimes seen.
Onset of disease	Classically the signs of Crohn's disease are more subtle than those of ulcerative colitis, though in a smaller percentage onset may be abrupt.	Onset may be insidious or abrupt.
Weight loss/growth failure	Weight loss is a common feature of Crohn's disease; it may have occurred for many months to years before diagnosis.	Weight loss is not uncommon and is typically more abrupt than in Crohn's disease.
Perianal disease	Perianal disease is common.	Perianal disease is rarely seen.

The most common presenting symptoms of UC are diarrhea, abdominal pain, and rectal bleeding with blood and mucus. Children with UC may present with one of several patterns. Mild disease, characterized by insidious diarrhea progressing to hematochezia, is seen in 50% to 60% of the pediatric population (Baldassano & Piccoli, 1999; Hyams, 1999). In mild disease the inflammation is usually confined to the distal colon and usually readily responds to treatment. Thirty percent of children, however, present with moderate disease, characterized by bloody diarrhea, cramping pain, tenesmus, and abdominal tenderness (Baldassano & Piccoli, 1999; Hyams, 1999). Other systemic symptoms are seen, such as anorexia, weight loss, fever, and mild anemia. Severe colitis with an acute, fulminant presentation is seen in only 10% of children (Baldassano & Piccoli, 1999; Hyams, 1999). These children appear moderately to severely toxic, have more than six bloody stools per day, cramping abdominal pain, fever, anemia, leukocytosis, and hypoalbuminemia. Serious complications such as toxic megacolon, life-threatening hemorrhage, and perforation are rare in the pediatric population.

An unusual but relevant issue to pediatric practitioners is the observation that children's presenting symptoms can sometimes be limited to abnormalities of the anogenital region. Children with CD have presented with histories of chronic constipation, even encopresis; often a thorough perianal examination will provide clues to the correct diagnosis. Published cases document children with CD being initially referred for evaluation of suspected sexual abuse (Sellman & Hupertz, 1996). Although physical findings consistent with sexual abuse must be appropriately investigated, organic causes of anogenital disease must also be properly evaluated. The course of the signs and symptoms of illness observed at diagnosis (e.g., the extraintestinal manifestations previously noted) may remain with a child, disappear with treatment, only to reappear with exacerbations of the disease, or may never return. New symptoms (i.e., GI or extraintestinal) may also appear with exacerbations.

Serologic markers, a somewhat controversial test, may occasionally be useful to help diagnose people with IBD and to distinguish individuals with CD from UC. The serologic markers are inappropriate antibody responses to self or foreign antigens. The two best-studied antibodies are perinuclear antineutrophil cytoplasmic antibodies (pANCAs) and anti-*Saccharomyces cerevisiae* antibodies (ASCA). Specificities of ASCA-positive and pANCA-negative results for CD are 97% to 100%, and ASCA negative and pANCA positive for UC are 92% to 97%. Although initially thought to be helpful in the diagnosis of IBD, studies have shown that when combined, these tests have only 49% to 57% sensitivity. The pANCA result is positive in only 60% to 70% of people with UC, and is positive in 5% to 15% of individuals with CD, and 5% to 10% of people without IBD. Likewise, ASCA is positive in 60% to 70% of people with Crohn's, but is also found to be positive in 10% to 15% of people with UC and 0% to 5% of controls (Present, 2002).

Results of these tests can vary when performed in different laboratories. The serologic markers may be helpful in distinguishing UC from CD in a small percentage of the population who have been diagnosed with indeterminate colitis.

IBD may manifest with symptoms other than those attributed to the GI tract (Figure 30-1). Extraintestinal symptoms or signs of an underlying IBD may be clinically significant in about 25% to 35% of children with IBD (Baldassano & Piccoli, 1999; Hyams, 1999; Griffiths & Buller, 2000). The most common target organs are the skin, joints, liver, eyes, and bone. Skin manifestations of IBD are erythema nodosum (raised, red tender nodules that appear primarily on the anterior surfaces of the leg), affecting 3% of children with CD and pyoderma gangrenosum (chronic ulcer), affecting 1% of children with UC and even fewer with CD (Baldassano & Piccoli, 1999). Aphthous ulceration in the mouth is the most common oral manifestation in CD. These lesions may appear before any gastrointestinal symptom. Arthritis is the most common extraintestinal manifestation, occurring in 7% to 25% of children with IBD. It usually involves the large joints of the lower extremities and can appear in children many years before any gastrointestinal symptoms develop (Baldassano & Piccoli, 1999). Hepatobiliary disease, both intrahepatic and extrahepatic, is a relatively common extraintestinal manifestation of IBD. Liver disorders may be present before the onset of IBD

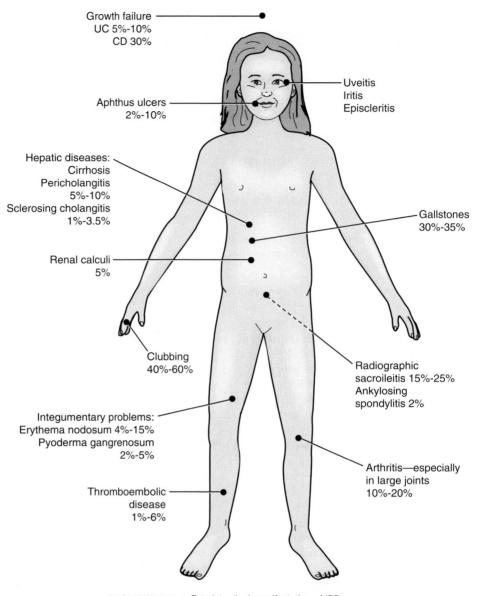

Growth failure
UC 5%-10%
CD 30%

Aphthus ulcers
2%-10%

Hepatic diseases:
Cirrhosis
Pericholangitis
5%-10%
Sclerosing cholangitis
1%-3.5%

Renal calculi
5%

Clubbing
40%-60%

Integumentary problems:
Erythema nodosum 4%-15%
Pyoderma gangrenosum
2%-5%

Thromboembolic
disease
1%-6%

Uveitis
Iritis
Episcleritis

Gallstones
30%-35%

Radiographic
sacroileitis 15%-25%
Ankylosing
spondylitis 2%

Arthritis—especially
in large joints
10%-20%

FIGURE 30-1 Extraintestinal manifestation of IBD.

and during active disease, or develop after surgical resection of diseased bowel. Sclerosing cholangitis is reported in 3.5% of children with UC and less than 1% of children with CD (Baldassano & Piccoli, 1999). Of note is that up to 90% of people with primary sclerosing cholangitis are eventually diagnosed with IBD, most commonly UC.

Ophthalomologic findings for both UC and CD usually appear when the condition is active. The most common ocular findings are episcleritis and anterior uveitis; glaucoma has been reported in some teenagers, independent of corticosteroid usage.

An exacerbation of CD or UC may sometimes be preceded by an intercurrent illness or emotional stress or may occur for no apparent reason. Intercurrent GI infections may also trigger an exacerbation of disease activity, with *Clostridium difficile* and viral infections (e.g., rotavirus and adenovirus) being implicated (Gryboski, 1991; Kirschner, 1996). Exacerbations of symptoms may be seen after dietary indiscretions, but such

indiscretions are not considered to be a cause of genuine flare-ups of disease activity because they are not accompanied by changes in histologic, radiographic, or laboratory parameters. Children with IBD often become adept at anticipating which activities are likely to trigger a flare-up of their disease. For example, adolescents with IBD may find that their symptoms worsen during school examinations or near important social events.

Treatment

Treatment of IBD includes medical, pharmacologic (Table 30-2), nutritional, and surgical therapies. The goals of treatment for IBD include clinical and laboratory control of inflammation, alleviation of symptoms with the fewest possible side effects from medications, optimal growth and development through nutrition, facilitation of normal social development with a good quality of life, and avoidance of long-term

TABLE 30-2

Drugs Used for Treatment of Inflammatory Bowel Disease

Drug / Dosage	Uses in IBD	Side Effects	Special Considerations
SULFASALAZINE (Azulfidine) 50-60 mg/kg/day	Treatment of UC and Crohn's colitis	*Common:* headache, malaise, GI upset, decreased sperm production *Less common:* skin eruption, hepatitis, pancreatitis, pneumonia, hemolysis, allergic reaction 5-ASA side effects (see below)	Fewer adverse reactions may be noted if the dosage is gradually increased to reach the planned therapeutic dosage. Enteric coated tablets may alleviate GI upset. Monitor WBC count over first 3 months of treatment. Impairs folic acid absorption; give folic acid 1 mg/day
OLSALAZINE (Dipentum) 30-50 mg/kg/day	Treatment of UC and Crohn's colitis (not used often in pediatrics because of diarrhea)	For all 5-ASAs: *Common:* GI upset, abdominal pain, dizziness, headache, diarrhea, rash, hair loss *Less common:* pancreatitis, pericarditis, aplastic anemia, allergic reaction	For all 5-ASAs: Fewer adverse reactions than sulfasalazine; useful for individuals unable to tolerate sulfasalazine Dipentum, Pentasa, and Colazal capsules may be opened and mixed in food for younger children.
BALSALAZIDE (Colazal) 40-60 mg/kg/day	Treatment of UC and Crohn's colitis	5-ASA side effects	5-ASA special considerations
MESALAMINE (Asacol) 40-60 mg/kg/day (Pentasa) 40-60 mg/kg/day	Treatment of UC and ileocolonic CD	5-ASA side effects	5-ASA special considerations
	Treatment of small intestinal and colonic CD Can be used to treat UC	5-ASA side effects	5-ASA special considerations
(Rowasa enema) 60 ml/4 g nightly (Canasa suppository) 500 mg one QD or BID	Topical therapy for proctitis and distal colitis	5-ASA side effects *Common:* perianal irritation, pruritus *Less common:* pancreatitis, pericarditis	5-ASA considerations Child should be instructed to try to retain the suppository or enema overnight
CORTICOSTEROIDS (Prednisone, Prednisolone) 1-2 mg/kg/day up to 60-80 mg/day	Useful in children who do not respond adequately to 5-ASAs Useful in moderate to severe disease Also available as foam (Cortifoam) and retention enemas (Cortenema) for rectal disease	*Common:* adrenal suppression, growth retardation, cushingoid facies, weight gain, striae, mood swings, acne, impaired calcium absorption, osteoporosis, hypertension, hyperglycemia *Less common:* cataracts, aseptic necrosis of the femoral head	Alternate-day therapy at lowest possible dose is often used to minimize adverse effects once in remission. Child should be warned to not discontinue corticosteroid use suddenly; this could result in an adrenal crisis and a flare-up of symptoms. Ophthalmic examination, urine dipstick, and blood pressure monitoring should be done at each visit. Child should see an ophthalmologist once or twice a year if on corticosteroids.
BUDESONIDE (Entocort) 9 mg/day	Mild to moderate CD	*Common: (much less than corticosteroids)* headache, respiratory infection, nausea, cushingoid facies, acne, and bruising	90% of drug does not go into the bloodstream; it is a nonsystemic corticosteroid Avoid eating grapefruit during administration. Recommended duration of therapy is 8 weeks.
METRONIDAZOLE (Flagyl) 10-15 mg/kg/day	Effective adjunct treatment for CD Useful in the management of perianal disease, fistulas, abscesses	*Common:* GI upset, metallic taste in mouth, paresthesias	Assess for paresthesias at each office visit; these are usually reversible after discontinuation of the medication. Disulfiram-like effect (i.e., vomiting) occurs if taken with alcohol or products containing alcohol.
CIPROFLOXACIN (Cipro) 10-20 mg/kg/day	Effective adjunct treatment for CD Useful in the management of perianal disease, fistulas, and abscesses	*Common:* headache; rash; GI upset; anemia	Ciprofloxacin has caused damage to growing bone in some laboratory animals, but to date no such adverse reactions have been observed in children.
6-MERCAPTOPURINE (6-MP, purinethol) 1.5-2.0 mg/kg/day	Used as a primary therapy in CD and UC, when 5-ASA therapy and corticosteroids have failed, or when child cannot be weaned from corticosteroids	*Common:* leukopenia, pancreatitis, hepatitis, allergic reactions, increased risk of infection	If fever develops, drug should be discontinued until illness resolves. It may take 3 to 4 months to see response
AZATHIOPRINE (Imuran) 2.0-2.5 mg/kg/day	Same as 6-mercaptopurine	*Common:* GI upset, leukopenia, hepatitis, pancreatitis, allergy, risk of infection	CBC, transaminases, amylase, and lipase should be monitored during therapy.

Continued

TABLE 30-2
Drugs Used for Treatment of Inflammatory Bowel Disease—cont'd

Drug / Dosage	Uses in IBD	Side Effects	Special Considerations
METHOTREXATE 15 mg/wk IM 25 mg/wk SC	Steroid-dependent CD	*Common:* malaise, fatigue, headache, rash, GI upset, stomatitis, myelosuppression. *Less common serious:* toxic reactions: death, encephalopathy, cortical blindness	Folate may decrease drug response.
INFLIXIMAB (Remicade) 5/mg/kg/dose at 0, 2, and 6 weeks then every 8-12 weeks IV	Used with moderate to severe active CD in children or adolescents who have inadequate response to conventional therapy. Active fistulas in CD. Refractory UC	*Common:* headache, itching, fatigue, nausea, dizziness, fever, upper respiratory infection, autoimmune antibody formation conventional therapy. *Less common:* tuberculosis, sepsis, malignancies, and formation of human antichimeric antibody (HACA)	The concomitant treatment with azathioprine, 6-MP, methotrexate, or corticosteroid (or pretreatment) appears to reduce the frequency of formation of HACA antibodies. HACA is associated with loss of clinical response to infliximab or increased infusion reactions.
CYCLOSPORINE (Sandimmune, Neoral) 1-2 mg/kg/day IV 4-8 mg/kg/day PO	Used in steroid refractory UC, difficult to treat CD and indeterminate colitis when colectomy is suggested and family is not ready	*Common:* immunosuppression, increased risk for malignancy (lymphomas, lymphoproliferative disorder, and squamous cell tumor), nephrotoxicity, hypertension, seizure, hirsutism, acne, GI upset, gingival hyperplasia, and headache. *Less common:* encephalopathy, convulsions, vision and movement disturbances, and impaired consciousness	Trough levels (before AM dose) should be drawn periodically. Grapefruit juice will increase absorption.
TACROLIMUS (Prograf, FK506) 0.1 mg/kg/day	Same as cyclosporine. Available in topical ointment	Same as cyclosporine	Same as cyclosporine. Many drugs can increase or decrease serum levels. Topical ointment should not be used in occlusive dressing.

BOX 30-1
Treatment

DRUG THERAPY
See Table 30-2

NUTRITIONAL THERAPY
An elemental diet is less effective in achieving remission than corticosteroids but can improve nutritional status.
Total parenteral nutrition is generally reserved for individuals with severe disease who cannot tolerate enteral feedings.

SURGICAL INTERVENTION
Surgical intervention is indicated when disease activity or complications do not respond to medical management.
Ulcerative colitis: Colectomy is the procedure of choice. For many individuals the option exists for reanastomosis and surgical construction of a "rectum" or pouch to maintain continence.
Crohn's disease: Procedures are limited resection of diseased bowel segment or colectomy with permanent ileostomy.

EMOTIONAL SUPPORT
Stress is a factor in exacerbations. Stress management techniques can be helpful.

disease-related complications. The specific treatment plan depends on the location and severity of the disease, the effect of the disease on growth and development, and the degree of debilitation experienced by the child. When medical therapies do not adequately control symptoms or complications (e.g., toxic megacolon, severe hemorrhage, obstruction, fistulas, or abscesses) or symptoms do not respond to medical management, surgical intervention is indicated. Children with severe disease who are experiencing debilitating symptoms accompanied by abnormal laboratory values require aggressive medical intervention. These children may require hospitalization; restricted diets, intravenous corticosteroid therapy, or total parenteral nutrition may then be initiated (Box 30-1).

Pharmacologic Therapy
Pharmacologic therapy is the mainstay of treatment of disease and maintenance of remission of IBD (see Table 30-2). The medications are often classified as antiinflammatory, immunosuppressive, and biologic immunotherapeutic agents. The 5-aminosalicylic acid (5-ASA) preparations, corticosteroids, and antibiotics usually are considered antiinflammatory, whereas 6-mercaptopurine, azathioprine, cyclosporine A, FK-506 (tacrolimus) and methotrexate are classified as immunosuppressive therapies (see Table 30-2). The newer biologic agents are therapies that can target specific immune-related actions

to block precise immune pathways. Biologic agents include antibody-based therapies, recombinant proteins, and nucleic acid-base therapies. Most clinicians use a stepwise approach to therapy employing increasingly more potent agents to the regimen if less active drugs fail to achieve remission. A combination of drugs from the different categories may be necessary for treatment depending upon the child or adolescent's response. Treatment plans vary by individual clinician; each physician/nurse practitioner relies upon his or her experience, clinical knowledge, and the observed clinical response of the child. In addition, nutritional therapies are used as a primary therapy for Crohn's disease and as adjunctive therapy for either UC or CD; these are discussed below.

Antiinflammatory Therapy. The 5-aminosalicylate preparations include the oral agents sulfasalazine (Azulfidine), olsalazine (Dipentum), balsalazide (Colazal), and mesalamine (Asacol, Pentasa); enema and suppository forms of mesalamine (Rowasa and Canasa) are available as the first step in treatment of distal colonic IBD. For many years, sulfasalazine was the primary drug used to treat colonic disease. Sulfasalazine is a combination of 5-aminosalicylic acid and sulfapyridine. Sulfapyridine is primarily used as a delivery agent that—when bound to 5-ASA—inhibits its absorption in the proximal GI tract. Unfortunately 20% to 25% of individuals who take sulfasalazine experience significant allergic or other adverse side effects, mostly related to the sulfapyridine component (Griffiths & Buller, 2000). Although generally well tolerated, 5-ASA medications are reported to cause occasional headache, malaise, nausea, vomiting, anorexia, heartburn, and/or diarrhea. Less common but more severe reactions include skin eruptions, hepatitis, pancreatitis, pneumonia, hemolysis or bone marrow suppression, and allergic reactions (PDR, 2001). Sulfasalazine (due to the sulfapyridine) may also interfere with folate absorption, which can lead to megaloblastic anemia; this problem may be prevented by coadministering 1 mg of folic acid per day (Griffiths & Buller, 2000; PDR, 2001).

Sulfasalazine, or one of the other 5-ASA medications, may be used as primary therapy in mild to moderate UC. Sulfasalazine is the only 5-ASA preparation that can be formulated into a suspension at this time for children who cannot take pills or capsules. When initiating therapy, a child's dose is gradually increased in an effort to alleviate or avoid the dose-dependent side effects of sulfasalazine, to the therapeutic range (i.e., 50 to 60 mg/kg/day) (PDR, 2001). During the initiation of therapy, leukopenia and hemolytic anemia should be monitored at least monthly by a complete blood count (CBC). If either of these becomes apparent, the dosage should be decreased or stopped until the blood values return to normal. The dosage may then be slowly returned to therapeutic range. If this approach is unsuccessful, the drug should be discontinued and therapy with another 5-ASA preparation attempted. Eighty percent to 90% of people who did not tolerate or are allergic to sulfasalazine will tolerate another oral 5-ASA preparation (Griffiths & Buller, 2000).

The 5-ASA drugs have the advantage of being more site-specific and having a lower incidence of side effects and are as effective compared with sulfasalazine in prolonging remission in UC (Hyams, 1999; Griffiths et al, 2000; Katz, 2002). Adverse effects with the newer 5-ASA preparations occur less frequently than those of sulfasalazine but include nausea, vomiting, dizziness, headache, abdominal pain, worsening of diarrhea and rectal bleeding, rash, and hair loss. Pancreatitis, pericarditis, aplastic anemia, and hypersensitivity reactions are rare but more worrisome (Stein et al, 1999; Griffiths & Buller, 2000). Although pediatric doses of mesalamine have not been fully established, it has been recommended to start at 40 to 60 mg/kg/day (Baldassano & Piccoli, 1999). Recommended monitoring of toxicity includes monthly complete blood cell (CBC) counts, liver function tests, blood urea nitrogen and creatinine levels, and urinalysis for 3 months, then every 3 to 6 months (Stein & Hanauer, 1999). Asacol only comes in an enteric coated tablet form, which is difficult for children who cannot swallow pills; Dipentum, Colazal, and Pentasa capsules may be opened and mixed in food to ease administration.

Mesalamine enemas (Rowasa) and suppositories (Canasa) can be effective to treat distal colonic ("left-sided disease") and rectal disease. Rectal therapy has been found to enhance the efficacy and rapidity of oral therapy in achieving remission when given concomitantly (Katz, 2002). Enemas are typically instilled at bedtime with the goal of retaining the fluid overnight. Suppositories are useful to treat proctitis and are inserted twice a day. Treatment may be provided for a few weeks or longer. Adverse effects of these topical preparations include perianal irritation, pruritus and, rarely, pancreatitis, and pericarditis (PDR, 2001).

In moderate to severe disease, as well as during exacerbations, corticosteroids are often used to induce remission. For many decades corticosteroids have been the mainstay of treatment of inflammatory bowel disease. However, recently many pediatric IBD centers have been steering away from the use of corticosteroids due to recognition of serious and long-term side effects, the availability and increased experience with the use of immunosuppressive medications, and the introduction of new biologic agents. Corticosteroids are still used in step one or two of treatment depending upon the child or adolescent's symptoms.

Corticosteroids are prescribed as prednisone, prednisolone, methylprednisolone, hydrocortisone, and the newest form, budesonide. They differ in duration of action, strength of glucocorticoid, and relative mineralocorticoid activity. Children are started with a dosage ranging from 1 to 2 mg/kg/day, usually with a maximum dose of up to 60 to 80 mg/day. Intravenous therapy is used for severe disease and disease refractive to oral therapy. Treatment with daily prednisone at high doses should continue for 2 to 3 weeks, usually when remission is achieved. A tapering regimen is then carefully prescribed, decreasing the dose gradually in 5- to 7-day intervals. Occasionally if children have difficulty tapering, the prednisone can be tapered to an alternating day cycle and then gradually discontinued (Griffiths & Buller, 2000). The dose is then gradually tapered while a child's symptoms and laboratory values—especially ESR, CBC, and albumin—are monitored.

Side effects of prednisone are related to the amount administered and duration of therapy or the total dosage to which the child is exposed. The major side effects include acute reactions: moon facies, weight gain, fluid retention with hypertension, hyperglycemia, acne, striae, hirsutism, and mood swings.

Long-term effects include calcium depletion (and osteoporosis), immunosuppression, cataract formation, glaucoma, and aseptic necrosis of the hip or knees (Griffiths & Buller, 2000). Growth inhibition is a major problem in children and adolescents with daily therapy due to direct suppression of IGF-1 and consequent inhibition of linear growth (Griffiths & Buller, 2000). Alternate-day steroid dosing will allow IGF-1 to normalize and preserve normal growth rates. Corticosteroid-induced bone disease results from decreased calcium absorption, increased urinary calcium excretion, increased bone resorption, and diminished bone formation. Trials are under way to test the efficacy of biphosphonates to prevent bone demineralization in children exposed to large doses of corticosteroids. Adequate calcium and physical activity may reduce the rate of bone disease.

Budesonide is a synthetic steroid that has decreased adverse systemic effects compared with the other group of corticosteroids. Budesonide, which has been widely tested in Europe and Canada, exerts a strong topical antiinflammatory effect in the distal small intestine and proximal colon, but when absorbed, it is rapidly metabolized by the liver and in low doses has minimal effect on adrenal suppression (Hyams, 1999; Griffiths et al, 2000; Katz, 2002). Because of its low bioavailability, the incidence of prednisone-like side effects is much lower. Rapid metabolism in the liver to compounds with vastly lower affinity for the glucocorticosteroid receptors results in only 10% bioavailability, in contrast with prednisolone, which is 80% available (Griffiths & Buller, 2000). Some recent studies have suggested that to achieve efficacy, the higher dose needed causes systemic reactions similar to prednisone. More studies need to be done to determine if budesonide will be an effective therapy in children with IBD.

Long-term corticosteroid use also leads to adrenal suppression, which persists for 6 to 12 months after prednisone therapy has been completed. Rapid cessation (often inadvertently) of prednisone during therapy or stressful incident (e.g., an accident, serious infection, or surgery) in the year following treatment with prednisone may precipitate acute adrenal insufficiency. Symptoms of acute adrenal insufficiency include fever, hypotension, dehydration, vomiting, electrolyte abnormalities, hypoglycemia, severe abdominal pain, and lethargy (see Chapter 20). Treatment consists of intravenous hydrocortisone administration until oral therapy can be resumed and, if needed, fluid replacement to treat dehydration. Children should also be given stress doses of corticosteroids during episodes of significant illness or for scheduled surgical procedures (Spahn & Kamada, 1995).

Antibiotic therapy has been used as a primary treatment, as an adjunct to other treatments, or to specifically treat complications of Crohn's disease, and is used less frequently in individuals with UC. Although their mechanism of action is unclear, antibiotics are hypothesized to affect the enteric bacterial flora that has been implicated in the pathophysiology of intestinal inflammation in CD. Metronidazole is the most frequently studied and used antibiotic in children with IBD, but recently ciprofloxacin has been added to the armamentarium.

Metronidazole is effective in the treatment of perianal disease, fistulas, and abscesses, but when its dose is lowered or it is discontinued, perianal disease commonly relapses (Grand et al, 1995; Cohen et al, 1998). The effects of long-term use of metronidazole are not known, but concern has been raised that it may potentially be carcinogenic or mutagenic, a concern supported by studies conducted in mice and rats. However, no cases have been reported in which either cancer or chromosomal aberrations have been proven to be attributable to metronidazole in humans (PDR, 2001). The recommended pediatric dosage ranges from 10 to 15 mg/kg/day (Markowitz et al, 1991; Kirschner, 1995a). Side effects of metronidazole include GI upset and a metallic taste. A more worrisome side effect is peripheral neuropathy, which appears to be related to dose and duration of therapy (Grand et al, 1995, Griffiths & Buller, 2000). Adolescents should be warned of the disulfiram-like effect if they ingest alcohol while taking metronidazole.

Ciprofloxacin at a dose of 10 to 20 mg/kg/day has been used alone or in combination with metronidazole to treat perirectal disease. Ciprofloxacin has caused damage to growing bone in some laboratory animals, but to date such adverse effects have not been observed in children despite substantial use in a host of pediatric conditions, particularly in children with cystic fibrosis (Griffiths & Buller, 2000) (see Chapter 22).

Immunsuppressive Therapy. Immunomodulators, 6-mercaptopurine (6-MP) and azathioprine (Imuran) are widely used to treat IBD in children. Initially 6-MP was used as a steroid-sparing agent and was prescribed as a third-line therapy in children for whom more conservative medical management had failed or who could not be weaned from steroids. Because of the increased experience using these medications over the past 20-plus years, immunomodulators are being prescribed much earlier in the course of treatment, even in some cases upon initial presentation. They improve control of symptoms, reduce corticosteroid requirements in 60% to 70% of children, and prevent relapses (Hyams, 1999; Griffiths & Buller, 2000; Katz, 2002). The recommended doses are 1.5 to 2 mg/kg/day for 6-MP and 2.0-2.5 mg/kg/day for azathioprine. Response to these agents is not immediate, averaging 3 to 4 months. A relatively new assay that tests for metabolism of 6-MP (by the enzyme thiopurine methyltransferase, or TPMP) may be useful to identify children in whom the drug will not be effective or may be severely toxic (Cuffari et al, 1996). Individuals with normal enzyme activity can have the dosage increased more rapidly and thus achieve medication effect within 4 to 6 weeks (rather than 3-4 months).

The most commonly cited complications of 6-MP and azathioprine are GI irritation manifested by vomiting and abdominal pain, leukopenia, fever, hepatitis, and pancreatitis. All immunomodulators predispose individuals to an increased risk of infection due to bone marrow suppression or toxicity. Concern about the possible increased risk of lymphoma for individuals treated with these agents has been allayed by multiple clinical studies showing their safety for long-term use (Hanauer, 1996; Kirschner, 1998; Markowitz, 2000). During the first 1-2 months of therapy a CBC with differential (to monitor for leukopenia and lymphopenia), liver enzyme levels, and amylase and lipase levels should be checked every 2 weeks to assess for adverse reactions. These parameters should then be checked monthly for several months and then every 3 months thereafter (Kirschner, 1996, 1998; Markowitz, 2000). The dose is reduced or therapy discontinued if the total WBC count falls below 2,500 or the transaminases rise (>2 times normal). Levels of the active metabolites (6-TG or 6-thioguanine) may prove to be useful to monitor for compliance and possibly efficacy and safety. Hepatotoxicity appears to correlate with elevated levels of another metabolite (6-methylmercaptopurine [6-MMP] levels), although the clinical relevance and usefulness of this test is controversial. Therapy may be reattempted after the liver enzymes return to normal. Elevation of amylase and/or lipase levels may signify pancreatitis, but this laboratory finding may also be transient, so the significance of this observation must be taken cautiously and in the context of the clinical setting (Griffiths & Buller, 2000; Markowitz, 2000). The primary care provider, family, and child must be aware that any febrile illness during therapy with 6-MP or azathioprine is an indication for concern and must be evaluated. Temporary discontinuation of the drug may be necessary until the illness resolves. Exposure to varicella infection in those who have not been vaccinated or had prior varicella infection and who are taking 6-MP or azathioprine warrants administration of varicella zoster immune globulin (VZIG) within 48 hours of exposure; the 6-MP, or azathioprine (Imuran), should then be temporarily discontinued.

Cyclosporine (Sandimmune) and FK506 (Tacrolimus) are potent inhibitors of cell-mediated immunity and are sometimes administered to selected individuals with refractory UC or CD, and are occasionally employed in cases of severe indeterminate colitis (in which the health care provider is trying to avoid colectomy until the disease "declares itself"). Response to cyclosporine therapy is inconsistent. Treated individuals have had a significant incidence of relapse while receiving therapy and recurrence when discontinuing the drug (Kirschner, 1994, 1996; Ramakrishna et al, 1996). Cyclosporine and Tacrolimus have been used to induce remission in children and adolescents with severe UC who are hospitalized, failed standard medical management, and otherwise are in need of urgent proctocolectomy but are psychologically or emotionally unprepared to accept the surgical option (Podolosky, 2002). If remission can be achieved, then other therapies such as 6-MP or azathioprine are used to sustain the remission and cyclosporine or tacrolimus are weaned (Grand et al, 1995; Hanauer, 1996; Ramakrishna et al, 1996).

Cyclosporine is usually first administered intravenously at 1 to 2 mg/kg/day. If clinical improvement is achieved, children are then changed to the oral form at 4 to 8 mg/kg/day. Because absorption of cyclosporine can be erratic, trough blood levels frequently need to be checked and the dosage adjusted to maintain a blood level between 100 and 200 mg/ml (Jani & Regueiro, 2002). Many of the individuals who respond initially to cyclosporine still eventually require colectomy.

Tacrolimus seems to be more potent than cyclosporine, and the advantage of reliable oral absorption reduces the need for intravenous therapy (Bousvaros et al, 1996; Bousvaros et al, 1997). Ongoing studies of Tacrolimus in children with fulminant colitis show efficacy of this agent to induce remission while permitting individuals to be weaned from steroids and make a transition to other immunosuppressant medications. The side effects of Tacrolimus appear to be the same or less than those of cyclosporine. A pediatric trial using oral tacrolimus showed improvement in 9 out of 14 subjects with steroid-

refractory severe colitis given a dose of 0.1 mg/kg every 12 hours, aiming for whole blood trough levels of 10 to 15 mg/ml (Bousvaros et al, 1997).

Side effects of cyclosporine and tacrolimus include hypertension, tremor, paresthesias, hirsutism, seizures, nausea and vomiting, and the potential for renal insufficiency. Careful monitoring of children and adolescents for serious infections, especially those who are taking corticosteroids and 6-MP is essential. Prophylaxis with oral trimethoprim-sulfamethoxazole (TMP-SMX) is suggested for those taking cyclosporine or tacrolimus. Frequent monitoring of vital signs, serum laboratory studies (including blood urea nitrogen and creatinine), and drug levels is mandatory during treatment (Jani & Regueiro, 2002). Toxicity of these agents, especially cyclosporine, limits their use, particularly in UC, which is "curable" with surgery.

Use of methotrexate to treat Crohn's disease has been reported in both children and adults who have been steroid dependent (Podolsky, 2002). Methotrexate is administered as a weekly injection by the intramuscular route (15 mg/wk) or subcutaneously (25 mg/wk). Response may take several weeks. In a study of 14 children who were steroid dependent and had failed treatment with 6-MP or azathioprine (Mack et al, 1998), 64% showed improvement after administration of methotrexate. Methotrexate has also been shown to have a faster onset of action compared with 6-MP or azathioprine.

Biologic Immunotherapy. The biologic agents, the newest family of medications to be developed for treatment of IBD, are becoming more common therapy in children with CD. These new therapies are directed toward specific targets of the inflammatory reaction, rather than the broad-based approach by the commonly used immunosuppressive and immunomodulatory medications.

The first genetically engineered product to be approved by the FDA for treatment of IBD is an antibody against tumor necrosis factor (TNF)-alpha, infliximab (Remicade). First approved for use in CD with active fistulas, infliximab is now also being used in individuals with medically resistant, moderate to severe CD and for some people with refractory UC. Infliximab is administered as a series of intravenous infusions at a dose of 5 mg/kg/dose at 0, 2, and 6 weeks then every 8 to 12 weeks if needed. Infliximab therapy is quite costly, and concern remains regarding potential side effects when altering the immune response. The side effects of infliximab therapy include infections (tuberculosis and sepsis with opportunistic and unusual infections), infusion reactions, autoantibody formation, and malignancies. The US Food and Drug Administration (FDA) approved the use of infliximab in the United States in 1998 for two indications: single-dose therapy for the treatment of individuals with moderate to severe inflammatory CD refractory to conventional therapy and three-dose infusion therapy for individuals with actively draining external fistulas (Mamula et al., 2002). The use of infliximab in UC remains uncertain, but studies are ongoing to evaluate its potential.

Numerous other biologic agents are under development. In preliminary studies, etanercept (Enbrel), a TNF-alpha receptor antagonist, has been used successfully for treatment of rheumatoid arthritis but has not proved to be effective therapy for Crohn's disease.

Nutritional Therapy

Nutritional therapy has been used for primary management of disease activity and as adjunctive therapy to correct or avoid malnutrition and to facilitate growth in children and adolescents with IBD.

The role of nutritional therapy as a primary method of treating IBD is controversial. Elemental formulas were first proposed and successfully employed as an acceptable and equivalent alternative to corticosteroid therapy for treating intractable small bowel CD. A recent Canadian multicenter study in children with CD showed a semielemental diet induced a higher (83%) remission in newly diagnosed children compared with remission rates with individuals with relapsing disease (50%) (Ruemmele et al, 2000). Although aggregate studies suggest that enteral therapy with elemental formula is less effective than corticosteroids in achieving remission in active CD with distal or colonic involvement or in those who have severe anorectal involvement, small bowel disease appears to be amenable to enteral therapy almost equally to corticosteroids, thus avoiding potential adverse effects of the corticosteroid medications. Enteral nutrition with an oligopeptide formula had fewer relapses when used over 4 weeks of a 20-week cycle, when compared with children receiving alternate-day prednisone (0.33 mg/kg every other day) (Baldassano & Piccoli, 1999). The newer oligopeptide formulas are more palatable compared with earlier formulas, and many children are able to drink them without having to use a nasogastric tube. Many insurance carriers refuse to cover these costly formulas, and the burden of this expense must be shouldered by the families alone. Some studies and meta-analyses have supported the position that the composition of the formula used for nutritional replenishment may not be critical (Graham & Kandil, 2002). The therapeutic benefit to individuals may result from improvement in nutritional status rather than as a direct result of a benefit from the elemental preparation (Tolia, 1997). Thus less expensive, more palatable preparations may be used when necessary.

Enteral nutrition offers important benefits for children experiencing growth failure—particularly when disease affects the small intestine. The "ideal" child for enteral nutrition would be a newly diagnosed adolescent with CD limited to the ileum but complicated by growth failure and delayed maturation (Ruemmele et al, 2000). Another suitable management strategy for these children may be to combine use of steroids and nutritional therapy for faster induction. In this situation the nutritional therapy is useful to maintain remission by permitting rapid tapering of the corticosteroids to a lower dose (Tolia, 1997). Enteral nutrition can also be used in children who refuse corticosteroids or who refuse repeat courses because of their concerns about adverse effects.

Total parenteral nutrition (TPN) can also be instituted as a primary therapy and is used to provide "bowel rest," theoretically reducing intestinal inflammation and thereby decreasing disease activity. TPN has been documented to diminish disease activity and reverse growth failure (Hyams, 1999; Griffiths & Buller, 2000; Graham & Kandil, 2002). TPN is used to provide nutrition support in individuals with fulminant IBD who cannot tolerate enteral feedings and is necessary in individuals with short bowel syndrome due to multiple surgical resections. Graham and Kandil (2002) report a review of pooled data from studies assessing the effects of TPN on closure of intestinal fistulas in CD revealed a 44% initial closure rate of 154 fistulas in 127 people. Forty-seven (38%) fistulas remained closed after follow-up intervals of 3 to 120 months.

Risks of TPN include sepsis, mechanical complications of central lines (right atrial catheters), and thrombosis, particularly in children and adolescents with IBD who have an underlying risk for a hypercoagulable state. The implementation of TPN in any child must be done taking into consideration the risks versus benefits of the therapy.

Probiotics have been gaining increasing popularity over the past several years. Probiotics are "healthy" bacteria that may prevent an overgrowth of pathogenic bacteria and maintain the integrity of the mucosal barrier. They are nonpathogenic food-grade organisms that are usually of the genera *Bifidobacterium* and *Lactobacillus* or may include nonbacterial organisms, such as *Saccharomyces boulaardi*. Individuals with pouchitis have had the best response to the treatment; recent studies show a dramatic decline in pouchitis in postsurgical subjects maintained on probiotic therapy (Gionchetti et al, 2000).

Surgical Intervention

Ulcerative Colitis. Indications for surgical intervention for children with UC include intractable disease, refractory growth failure, toxic megacolon, hemorrhage, perforation, and cancer prophylaxis (Griffiths & Buller, 2002). The most commonly performed surgery is the ileal pouch anal anastomosis. This curative procedure can be performed either as a primary operation or in a two-stage approach. If surgery is urgent, a total colectomy with preservation of a rectal stump and creation of a diverting ileostomy is the procedure of choice. The ileoanal pull-through procedure takes advantage of UC as a mucosal disease. The rectal mucosa is dissected and removed to the dentate line of the anus. This preserves an intact rectal muscular cuff and anal sphincter apparatus, thus allowing for greater fecal continence. A two-stage procedure is typically performed. The first stage consists of colectomy, mucosal proctectomy, endorectal ileal pouch-anal anastomosis, and diverting loop ileostomy. At the second surgery the loop ileostomy is closed (Becker, 1999). Benefits of the pouch procedure are resumption of rectal continence and avoidance of a permanent ostomy, which makes it much easier for children and their parents to accept. One-stage surgery is now commonly performed when the colectomy is elective. The colon is removed and ileum is brought down into the pelvis and sutured to the anus in an end-to-end fashion. An ileal pouch or reservoir is constructed proximally to the ileoanal anastomosis (Becker, 1999). This eliminates the loop ileostomy. Many surgeons are performing both the one- and two-stage colectomy laparoscopically. Bowel movements initially occur frequently with fecal soiling at night, but in time decrease to four to six times a day. Pouchitis, an inflammatory process in the ileal pouch, is the most common single long-term complication occurring in 19% of the time in children and adolescents (Hyams, 1999; Griffiths & Buller, 2000). It can lead to increased diarrhea, tenesmus, and bleeding. Episodes respond well to antibiotics (metronidazole and ciprofloxacin), and maintenance may be achieved using a probiotic agent. Long-term follow-up is still needed with regular endoscopic surveillance of the pouch and especially if there is residual rectal mucosa, which can still put them at risk for dysplastic changes (Griffiths & Buller, 2000).

Crohn's disease. Indications for surgery in CD include intractable disease, hemorrhage, toxic megacolon, bowel perforation, stricture with obstruction, and abscesses and fistulas unresponsive to medical management (Hyams, 1996; Cohen et al, 1998). Surgery may also be indicated for prepubertal children or early adolescents who have growth failure and relatively localized disease, including stenotic segments of bowel (Cohen et al, 1998). Surgery will not cure Crohn's disease as it does UC. The most common indication for surgery of the small bowel is intestinal obstruction caused by fibrosis and stricture (Becker, 1999). Recurrence of disease is common in CD after surgery; 50% of children have a recurrence within 5 years of their first surgery. Prophylactic postoperative treatment with 6-MP or azathioprine (Imuran) may help to delay recurrence of disease. Because a child with CD may have multiple surgical resections over a lifetime, the goal of surgery should be to relieve symptoms while preserving as much bowel as possible. An isolated nonprogressive area of bowel may be removed. Alternatively, strictureplasty, aimed at opening a stenotic area while avoiding resection of bowel, may be performed. It is accomplished by incising the strictured area of intestine longitudinally, applying traction sutures perpendicular to the bowel, and closing the incision transversely (Becker, 1999). A greater percentage of children have surgery for intractability, fulminant disease, or anorectal disease. In cases of fulminant colitis, a total proctocolectomy with a loop ileostomy may suffice or a permanent ileostomy may be necessary. Children with CD are not good candidates for pouch procedures because of the high rate of disease recurrence (Griffiths & Buller, 2002). Despite the risk of recurrent disease after resection, surgery is still an attractive option for children because of the potential of a significant asymptomatic interval during which normal growth and development can occur. In one pediatric study it was found that children undergoing intestinal resection within 1 year of onset of symptoms have a delayed recurrence of active disease, compared with children whose preoperative duration of symptomatic disease was greater than 1 year (Hyams, 1999). Skin tags are rarely excised during surgery.

Complementary and Alternative Therapies

The use of complementary medicine has been dramatically increasing over the past 10 years worldwide and especially in the United States (Heuschkel et al, 2002). Complementary and alternative medicine (CAM) can incorporate chiropractic, homeopathy, naturopathy, acupuncture, aromatherapy, massage, biofeedback, probiotics, herbal medicines, and dietary supplements. It has been postulated that people use CAM because they find these therapies more "natural and because they may allow more choice and autonomy (Heuschkel et al, 2002). In 2000, a multicenter international study was conducted in Boston, Detroit, and London to examine the use of CAM in children and young adults with IBD. The researcher found that the frequency of CAM was 41%. The most common CAMs were megavitamin therapy (19%), dietary supplements (17%), and herbal medicine (14%). The most common reasons cited for using CAM were side effects from prescribed medicines,

prescribed medicines not working as they hoped, and wish for a cure (Heuschkel et al, 2002). Because stress has been identified as a factor that may contribute to the exacerbation of IBD symptoms, some children find it helpful to master relaxation and stress management techniques for controlling or preventing flare-ups of their disease, as well as for managing daily stressors. Primary care providers may help families find programs that promote the development of stress management and problem-solving skills.

Anticipated Advances in Management

Many new therapies for the treatment of IBD have been developed and are undergoing further clinical trials. Almost all data on their effectiveness are from research done with adults; clinical trials are just beginning with children. Over the past several years advances in immunology have led to discovery of novel therapeutic modalities. Biologic therapies have begun to assume a prominent role and include recombinant cytokines, chimeric, and humanized monoclonal antibodies, surface proteins and adhesion molecules, antisense oligonucleotides, vaccines, and gene therapies (Sands, 1999; Mamula et al, 2002). Many agents are under investigation, including CDP571, etanercept (discussed above), ISIS2302, anti-alpha 4 integrin antibody, IL-10, IL-11, anti-IL-12, and parasites (Mamula et al, 2002). Nonbiologic agents are also being investigated. The potent teratogen, thalidomide, has resurfaced for treatment of IBD because of its TNF-blocking action. However, because of its history as a teratogen, its use is limited at this time and requires rigorous supervision. The antiinflammatory effects of heparin are being studied as a potential treatment, especially in UC. Growth hormone therapy has been used in the treatment of growth failure in CD. It has also been found to correct the abnormally increased levels of TNF-alpha in children with growth hormone deficiency, thus decreasing the catabolic process associated with mucosal inflammation (Mamula et al, 2002).

Specific nutritional therapies offer another alternative treatment. Omega-3 fatty acids (fish oil) reduce the production of leukotriene B_4 and thromboxane A_2, inhibit synthesis of cytokines, and act as free radical scavengers in CD (Baldassano & Piccoli, 1999). Studies suggest that fish oil in high dosages (up to 3 g/day) may help sustain remission in CD (Belluzzi, 1996).

Associated Problems (Box 30-2)
Growth Failure and Delayed Sexual Development

Growth failure and delayed sexual development associated with IBD in childhood affect children with CD more than those with UC. Activity of disease is the major determinant of adequacy of growth (Griffiths & Buller, 2000). The proposed etiology for growth failure includes chronic malnutrition, corticosteroid administration, and the growth-retarding effects of chronic inflammation (Hyams, 1996). Inadequate calorie intake resulting from disease-related symptoms and anorexia most likely accounts for the malnutrition in children with IBD, rather than increased losses or requirements.

Associated Problems

GROWTH FAILURE
Musculoskeletal problems
Osteoporosis
Peripheral arthritis
Ankylosing spondylitis
Sacroiliitis
Bone demineralization and osteoporosis

DERMATOLOGIC MANIFESTATIONS
Erythema nodosum
Pyoderma gangrenosum

VISUAL CHANGES
Iritis
Episcleritis
Uveitis
Conjunctivitis
Cataracts

HEPATOBILIARY COMPLICATIONS
Primary sclerosing cholangitis
Pericholangitis
Gallstones

RENAL CHANGES
Renal calculi

PERIANAL DISEASE
Fistulas, abscesses
Fissures, skin tags

FULMINANT COLITIS OR TOXIC MEGACOLON
Intestinal malignancy

LACTOSE INTOLERANCE
ANEMIA
Vitamin B_{12} deficiency
Iron deficiency due to chronic blood loss

Musculoskeletal Problems

Musculoskeletal problems associated with IBD include peripheral arthritis, ankylosing spondylitis (see Chapter 31), and sacroiliitis. Peripheral arthritis is seen in approximately 20% of individuals with IBD, usually in association with active intestinal disease (Kirschner, 1995a). Arthritis is the most likely of the extraintestinal manifestations to precede the gastrointestinal manifestations of CD. Inflammation and discomfort are noted in the large joints, especially those of the hip, knee, and ankle. Inflammation does not occur symmetrically. Unlike the other musculoskeletal manifestations of IBD, the arthritic symptoms often fluctuate with the activity of the bowel disease and respond to treatment of the disease. NSAIDs may be used to treat refractory joint complaints, but due to the possibility of causing a disease exacerbation, their duration is limited (Kirschner, 1996). Ankylosing spondylitis may be seen in up to 11% of individuals with IBD and is more common in individuals with CD. Sacroiliitis may be noted on radiographs in 4% to 18% of individuals with IBD, with far fewer individuals noting symptoms such as low back pain.

Although not manifestations of IBD, osteoporosis and decreased bone mineral density (BMD) can be seen in children with IBD. Reported causes of decreased BMD include malabsorption of calcium and vitamin D, macro- and micronutrient deficiencies, decreased level of physical activity, estrogen deficiency in females, and—importantly—corticosteroid use (Pigot et al, 1992; Semeao et al, 1997). A report by Semeao and associates (1997) described five children with CD, all of whom had received significant amounts of corticosteroids, who developed vertebral compression fractures. In CD a major factor to decrease bone density is the inhibition of bone formation by cytokines (Griffiths & Buller, 2000). In UC, decreased bone density is more often associated with chronic corticosteroid use. Examination of BMD by dual-energy radiographic absorptiometry (DEXA) has revealed BMD more than two standard deviations below the mean. Semeao and associates recommend that all children with CD receive routine DEXA scanning in addition to careful evaluation of back pain complaints. Calcium and vitamin D supplementation should also be considered, especially if milk intake is limited.

Dermatologic Manifestations

Dermatologic manifestations occur in up to 5% to 15% of individuals with IBD (Hyams, 1999; Griffiths & Buller, 2002). Erythema nodosum is a tender, reddened nodule that commonly appears on the anterior aspect of the lower leg, although it may be seen on the foot, back of the leg, or arm. Erythema nodosum is seen more often with CD (8%-15%) than with UC (4%). It usually occurs when the intestinal disease is active, but does not indicate severity (Griffiths & Buller, 2000). Therapy involves treating the underlying bowel disease.

Pyoderma gangrenosum is a more serious dermatologic condition that may be found in 1% to 5% of individuals with UC and 1% to 2% of those with CD and is usually seen in those with active pancolitis, but can occur even when the disease is in remission. The lesions typically appear on the anterior of the lower leg and have dark red or purple borders surrounding deep skin ulcerations with necrotic centers (Powell & O'Kane, 2002). Control of the intestinal disease can result in healing of these lesions, but topical or systemic therapy directed at the lesions themselves may also be necessary. Recurrence of the pyoderma gangrenosum is common (Powell & O'Kane, 2002).

Visual Changes

Ocular manifestations of IBD include iritis, episcleritis, uveitis, and conjunctivitis and correlate with disease activity. Uveitis is usually symptomatic, causing pain or possibly decreased vision. Children treated with corticosteroids are also at increased risk for cataracts and elevated intraocular pressure, although glaucoma has been reported in children and adolescents without corticosteroid exposure (Hyams, 1999).

Hepatobiliary Complications

A particularly troublesome extraintestinal manifestation of IBD involves the hepatobiliary system. Hepatobiliary complications in pediatrics, such as pericholangitis, cirrhosis, and primary sclerosing cholangitis, may precede the onset of IBD, or may occur during active disease or develop even after surgical resection (Baldassano & Piccoli, 1999). Transient elevation of liver enzymes is common in IBD and appears to be related to medications or disease activity. Physical examinations should be closely monitored for hepatic enlargement or signs of portal hypertension. Primary sclerosing cholangitis (PSC) can present before diagnosis or during the illness (Hyams, 1999). Sclerosing cholangitis develops in 3.5% of children with UC and 1% of children with CD (Baldassano & Piccoli, 1999). Gallstones are seen more often with CD than with UC and occur in 13% to 34% of individuals with IBD, particularly in those with extensive ileal disease or ileal resection. The occurrence of gallstones seems to be related to the malabsorption of bile salts with concomitant cholesterol precipitation and calculus formation (Hyams, 1999).

Renal Changes

Renal calculi may also be seen in individuals with IBD. They have been noted in 8% to 19% of individuals with IBD—the highest incidence occurring in people with CD after small bowel resection or ileostomy. Children with severe ileal disease or resection of the ileum are at risk for formation of calcium oxalate stones (Retsky & Kraft, 1995).

Perianal Disease

Reports of perianal disease in children with CD vary from 14% to 62%. These lesions include fissures, skin tags, fistulas, and abscesses (Cohen et al, 1998). Because of the transmural nature of the inflammation in CD, fistulas and abscesses may form between the bowel and surface of the skin or between the bowel and other orifices. Clinicians should question children and/or parents about the passage of air or stool through the vagina or the urethra, because this may indicate a rectovaginal or rectourethral fistula. Complaints of pain, fullness, or drainage from the perianal area may alert clinicians to active perianal disease or abscess. Metronidazole has been most useful in treating perianal disease, but other therapies (e.g., corticosteroids, 6-MP, or cyclosporine) may also be used. In cases of refractory perianal disease, surgery may be necessary (Cohen et al, 1998).

Fulminant Colitis or Toxic Megacolon

Fulminant colitis presents with grossly bloody diarrhea, fever, tachycardia, abdominal pain, and abnormal laboratory findings. When these symptoms occur accompanied by a markedly distended colon on radiographs, toxic megacolon is present (Cohen et al, 1998). Although fulminant colitis and toxic megacolon may be managed medically, most individuals eventually receive a colectomy. Both conditions can occur with UC or Crohn's colitis. Toxic megacolon has been found in up to 5% of children and adolescents with UC (Hyams, 1999). It is a medical and potential surgical emergency. The incidence of toxic megacolon has decreased over the years due in part to the decreased use of opiates and antispasmodics, as well as the avoidance of tests such as barium enema or colonoscopy during periods of severe colitis—all of which have been known to precipitate toxic megacolon.

Lactose Intolerance

During periods of active disease, some children with IBD may experience symptoms of lactose intolerance including bloating, abdominal cramping, and diarrhea related to the intake of dairy products (Grand et al, 1995). For this reason, some health care providers recommend that children eliminate lactose from their diet during the initial period of diagnosis and recovery to minimize confusion about a child's response to therapy. A breath hydrogen test may be performed to definitively diagnose lactose intolerance if such a clarification is desired. Ultimately a significant proportion of children with IBD will eventually be able to tolerate some amount of lactose in their diet.

Anemia

As a result of chronic malnutrition, malabsorption, the interference of sulfasalazine in the absorption of folates, and chronic blood loss, children with IBD are at increased risk for vitamin B_{12} deficiency and hypochromic microcytic or iron deficiency anemia. Daily supplementation with folic acid is recommended for children receiving sulfasalazine, and monitoring of the CBC is recommended for all children with IBD. Iron supplementation is recommended for children with iron deficiency anemia.

Hypercoagulability

Both UC and CD are associated with hypercoagulable states (about 1%-2% of cases), manifested by thrombocytosis, low prothrombin time, and low partial thromboplastin time, and clinically by thromboses. Peripheral vein thromboses and even pulmonary emboli have been reported as complications of IBD. Postoperative thromboembolic events must be considered when following these children and adolescents after surgical procedures.

Carcinoma

Adenocarcinomas are the colorectal tumors associated with IBD. A significantly greater risk for intestinal malignancies exists among children with IBD than among those who do not have IBD, especially in individuals with pancolitis beginning in childhood. The risk of malignancy in UC increases with the extent and duration of the disease, as well as with a younger age at the time of diagnosis (Hyams, 1999; Griffiths & Buller, 2000). The risk of cancer begins to increase 10 to 15 years after diagnosis (Baldassano & Piccoli, 1999). According to Baldassano and Piccoli (1999), children who develop UC before 14 years of age have a cumulative colorectal cancer incidence rate of 5% at 20 years and 40% at 35 years. Children who develop the disease between 15 and 39 years of age have a cumulative incidence rate of 5% at 20 years and 30% at 35 years. This gives an estimate of an 8% risk of dying of colon cancer 10 to 25 years after diagnosis of UC if colectomy is not performed to cure the disease. The risk of malignancy in CD is not as high as in UC. Adenocarcinoma of the colon with CD is 4 to 20 times that of the general population. Factors increasing the risk are early age of disease onset, male sex, location and extent of the disease, and presence of strictures or fistulas.

Most authors agree that surveillance colonoscopy should be performed on children with UC, but disagree on when this should start and how often it should occur. Annual or biannual colonoscopies are recommended when biopsy findings are negative for dysplasia; colonoscopies are recommended every 6 months when biopsies show indeterminate dysplasia, and a colectomy is recommended when a biopsy shows any signs of dysplasia (Cohen et al, 1998). Cohen and associates (1998) also point out that dysplastic lesions and carcinomas may be difficult to detect in early stages, and although frequent biopsy during colonoscopy is recommended, lesions may be missed. Some gastroenterologists recommend prophylactic colectomy for individuals with long-standing UC—especially when diagnosed in childhood (Cohen et al, 1998; Baldassano & Piccoli, 1999). Finally, carcinoma has been detected in ileoanal pouches, which must also be screened for malignancy (Cohen et al, 1998). Recommendations for cancer surveillance are the same as for UC.

Psychosocial Issues

Chronic disease, by itself, places children and adolescents at risk for secondary psychiatric disorders. Engstrom and Lindquist (1982) reported that psychiatric disorders were four times as frequent in children with IBD than in healthy cohorts. Dealing with the uncertainty of the symptoms and their effect on the child or adolescent's lifestyle contributes to the psychosocial issues commonly found with IBD. This reinforces the need to address the psychologic and psychosocial impact of IBD in the pediatric population as well as on their families.

Research has increased over the past few years in the area of health-related quality-of-life issues in chronic disease. Two validated tools have been developed that examine disease-related quality of life in the adult IBD population (Dudley-Brown, 2001). One tool assesses four aspects of adults' lives: symptoms directly related to the primary bowel disturbance, systemic symptoms, and emotional and social function. The other assessed four broad categories of daily living: functional/economic, social/recreational, affect/life, and medical/symptoms. Individuals with IBD had significantly lower quality-of-life scores (Dudley-Brown, 2001).

Prognosis

The severity of presenting symptoms of IBD may not be indicative of the course that the condition will follow for a child. One of the most frustrating aspects of IBD for children and their parents is the inability to learn the "anticipated course" of the condition. In one retrospective study of children with UC, 70% were in clinical remission within 3 months of diagnosis. Remission was achieved within 6 months in 80% to 90% of the children studied. The course of the disease beyond 1 year from diagnosis was similar for all of the children, regardless of the initial degree of severity of their disease. The percentage of children with inactive (absence of GI or extraintestinal symptoms) disease was 55% to 57%. The percentage of children whose disease was moderate to severe ranged from 37% to 39%. The percentage of those who had continuous symptoms (i.e., absence of symptom-free intervals or daily corticosteroid therapy with recurrence of symptoms when corticosteroids were discontinued) ranged from 4% to 8% (Hyams, 1999).

PRIMARY CARE MANAGEMENT

Health Care Maintenance

Growth and Development

Children with IBD should have growth parameters measured and graphed on a National Center for Health Statistics chart at each primary care visit. For recently diagnosed children it is helpful to go back through previous visit records to assess growth in the years before the diagnosis was made. This review will help primary care providers to assess for any deceleration in growth rate. School health or athletic offices may often be of assistance in reconstructing the growth curve. Height and weight for age, Tanner stage for pubertal development, and arm anthropometry are growth parameters of particular importance. Once growth retardation is identified as an actual or potential problem, bone age should be obtained to identify the child's remaining growth potential. Continued careful measurement and graphing of growth parameters are essential. Catch-up growth is considered to be adequate if children return to their pre-illness growth percentiles.

Cognitive abilities are unimpaired in children with IBD, and development usually progresses normally.

Diet

No specific dietary restrictions have been documented as helpful in controlling symptoms for individuals with IBD. Some individuals may feel more comfortable when they avoid certain foods; however, the child and family can be helped to identify such foods. Practitioners must be aware that concerned parents, who feel able to attribute symptoms to multiple foods, may overly restrict the diet. Such overrestriction may result in a diet that is unappealing to the child and too restrictive to provide enough calories for growth and development.

Many centers consider a referral for nutritional consultation to be a standard of care for children and adolescents who have been recently diagnosed with IBD. The dietitian may assess a child's intake and nutritional status and, if necessary, counsel the child and family regarding augmentation of caloric intake.

If growth retardation associated with IBD is identified, nutritional supplementation with high-caloric formulas or an enriched diet is necessary. Consultation with a clinical nutritionist is beneficial for the family to help with ways to increase calories that are palatable for the child or adolescent. It is generally agreed that given adequate calories, children or adolescents (i.e., before epiphyseal closure) may recover lost growth. As nutritional replenishment begins, children or adolescents with IBD may have greater caloric requirements than their unaffected peers. Recommendations for caloric intake range from 75 to 95 kcal/kg/day. It is not routinely necessary for children with IBD to receive more calories than those without IBD (Kirschner, 1995a).

During periods of active disease, many children may feel more comfortable on a low-roughage diet. Children with CD of the small bowel are also more likely to experience some degree of lactose intolerance, which may even persist during periods of remission. During periods of inactive disease, these children may drink LactAid (Merck) milk or use lactase capsules and tablets, which are readily available. For children who feel especially deprived or set apart from their peers because of their dietary restrictions, such products may be of value. Experience has shown, however, that these products are not helpful for all lactose-intolerant individuals. Children on milk-restricted diets and those taking corticosteroids should receive calcium supplementation (amount should be based on RDA for age) because they are at risk for osteoporosis.

Safety

Children with IBD require no special restriction of activities. They should be encouraged to participate in all sports they can enjoy. Vigorous activities (e.g., lacrosse or tackle football) should pose no problem for children in remission. Children with osteoporosis, however, should refrain from such sports. Because—as in many populations with special needs—anxious families may tend to shelter their child from uncomfortable or tense situations, primary care providers can play an integral role in advocating for a normal lifestyle for these children.

Children and adolescents with IBD who plan to travel may need to make some special modifications. Referral or consultation with a tropical medicine or travel clinic may be beneficial when travel abroad is planned. General considerations include the purity of the water supply, ova, parasites, and proper immunization. Children and adolescents who are immunosuppressed should not receive live virus immunizations.

Alcohol consumption by adolescents with IBD who are in remission is of the same concern as alcohol consumption by their unaffected peers. Alcohol ingestion may cause discomfort for some individuals with IBD. If so, these individuals should limit intake. Individuals taking metronidazole should be informed that alcohol intake will induce a disulfiram (Antabuse) type of reaction.

Children who are immunosuppressed should wear a Medic-Alert bracelet or use other easily identifiable methods of communicating this fact to emergency medical personnel. Children who have received steroids in the past year may need a stress dose of corticosteroids at times of serious illness, accident, or surgery (Spahn & Kamada, 1995) (see Chapter 20).

Immunizations

No change from the normal immunization schedule is necessary unless a child receives maintenance therapy of corticosteroids or other immunosuppressive agents (e.g., 6-MP or cyclosporine). These children should not receive live virus immunizations until they have been tapered from these drugs. If this is not feasible or if exposure is of particular concern, a killed virus vaccine or condition-specific immunoglobulin may be given. Exposure to varicella infection in those who have not been vaccinated or had prior varicella infection and who are taking 6-MP or azathioprine warrants administration of VZIG within 48 hours of exposure; the 6-MP or azathioprine (Imuran) should then be temporarily discontinued. Children who are immunosuppressed should receive a yearly flu shot, as well (Committee on Infectious Diseases, 2000).

Screening

Vision. Ophthalmic examinations are necessary at each well-child visit because children with IBD are at risk for ocular manifestations of the disease. In the case of iritis, examiners may note redness of the eye, eye pain, photophobia, or blurred vision. In uveitis, abnormal pupillary reaction may also be assessed. A reddened eye may be noted in episcleritis or conjunctivitis. If the child is receiving prolonged corticosteroid therapy, ophthalmologic referral for assessment for cataracts is recommended twice a year (Kirschner, 1996). Any child with an abnormal ophthalmoscopic examination or complaints of the previously mentioned symptoms should be referred to an ophthalmologist, as well as to the gastroenterology team.

Hearing. Routine screening is recommended.

Dental. Children who are being treated with cyclosporine are at risk for gingival hyperplasia. Proper dental hygiene and the need for dental visits twice a year should be reinforced at each well-child visit.

Blood Pressure. Children who are taking cyclosporine or corticosteroids are at increased risk for hypertension. Their blood pressures should be measured and graphed at every visit. Evidence of hypertension should be reported to the gastroenterology team.

Hematocrit. Hemoglobin and hematocrit values should be measured yearly for children who are asymptomatic and have no history of anemia. A CBC count should be checked every 6 months or as needed for children with a history of anemia or those experiencing increased symptoms of their disease.

Urinalysis. No change in the usual protocol for screening is necessary unless the history indicates renal involvement or the child is experiencing symptoms indicative of any of the previously mentioned conditions.

Tuberculosis. Children who are receiving immunosuppressive therapy may not respond to testing. Screening may be withheld until immunosuppressive drugs are discontinued. If exposure is suspected, a control may be placed along with the purified protein derivative of the tuberculosis to assess for anergy. Chest radiography may be necessary to screen for active disease (Committee on Infectious Diseases, 2000). TB screening and a chest radiograph must be done before treatment with infliximab (Remicade) because of the risk of reported disseminated tuberculosis.

Condition-Specific Screening

It is customary for even asymptomatic children and adolescents to be seen on a regular basis by the gastroenterology team. The following condition-specific screening studies are typically obtained at the time of these visits. Primary care practitioners must be aware that these studies should be routinely evaluated. In some circumstances the primary care setting may be the most convenient or appropriate place to monitor these values.

Erythrocyte Sedimentation Rate (ESR). An ESR should be measured yearly for asymptomatic children. The ESR may be used for some children with IBD as an index of disease activity, which is seen in up to 90% of individuals with CD and more than 50% of those with UC (Calenda and Grand, 1995). The ESR should be normal in children with inactive disease. A variation from baseline should be followed with close questioning about current disease activity and onset of new symptoms.

Fecal Occult Blood Test. For asymptomatic children, stool should be monitored yearly with a fecal-occult blood reagent (e.g., Hemoccult) for the presence of occult blood. The results should usually be negative in children with inactive disease. Some children with IBD always carry a trace of blood in their stool. Children whose stools are routinely normal but have a positive occult blood result should be assessed more carefully for indications of increased disease activity and anemia.

Chemistries. Children taking cyclosporine, azathioprine, or 6-MP should have renal (i.e., blood urea nitrogen and creatinine levels) and liver function studies (i.e., fractionated bilirubin, aspartate aminotransferase, alanine aminotransferase, and alkaline phosphatase values) monitored at least every 4 months throughout therapy. Liver function studies should be assessed every year in otherwise asymptomatic children with IBD. Children with CD should also have albumin levels checked yearly.

Lactose Intolerance. The diagnosis of lactose intolerance may be made empirically by eliminating lactose-containing products from the diet and monitoring for changes in symptoms such as cramping, distention, and diarrhea. The diagnosis may also be made by the breath hydrogen test. Clinicians may also do a cursory screen for lactose intolerance by testing stool for reducing substances or testing the pH of the stool. An acidic pH (i.e., 6.0 or less) could be indicative of lactose intolerance.

Neurologic Examination. Children who are being treated with metronidazole should be assessed for peripheral neuropathy at each visit.

Radiologic Studies. Children with CD or those treated with long-term corticosteroids should have their bone mineral density assessed by means of DEXA scanning.

Endoscopy. Endoscopy may be performed during times of disease exacerbation, and routine colonoscopy should be performed in children with UC starting 10 years after diagnosis.

Common Illness Management

Differential Diagnosis (Box 30-3)

The symptoms of IBD and its associated problems vary. Symptoms of common childhood illnesses may be difficult to differentiate from exacerbations of a child's underlying disease process. GI symptoms will most likely concern or alarm the child, family, and primary care provider. An index of disease activity for some—but not all children—is the ESR, which may sometimes help to clarify a child's symptoms. Because this value is a nonspecific indicator of systemic inflammation, however, it is not a specific indicator of IBD activity. Some primary care providers use the CRP (C-reactive protein) as an alternative indicator for disease activity.

Intercurrent illnesses, such as a viral or bacterial gastroenteritis or another illness that must be treated with antibiotics, may contribute to flare-ups of a child's IBD. These flare ups may result from the alteration of the normal flora of the bowel (i.e., usually a predominance of *Clostridium difficile*) after antibiotic therapy.

Diarrhea. Children with IBD have bouts of gastroenteritis similar to those of their peers and family members. A child's

---

physical examination and history should include an evaluation of any IBD-like symptoms, including the presence of any blood, pus, or mucus in the stool; cramping pain or urgency associated with bowel movements; weight loss or anorexia; and any symptoms that might be extraintestinal manifestations of the disease. A child's abdomen should be closely examined for any change. Stool cultures should always be obtained, because infections with *Yersinia*, *Campylobacter*, *Shigella*, and *C. difficile* may mimic IBD. Children should be treated for any identified pathogen. A child with prolonged symptoms, including bloody diarrhea (with no identified pathogen), or weight loss should be referred to the gastroenterology team.

Abdominal Pain. Children with abdominal pain should be examined for any changes that might indicate a progression of the disease, fulminant colitis, or an obstruction. These children should be questioned about the similarity of their current pain to the pain experienced as a part of the IBD. Similarity to previous episodes, location of known disease, and history of accompanying symptoms that would indicate IBD rather than influenza or other acute conditions of the abdomen should guide practitioners. Many of the medications used to treat IBD may cause gastritis. Children will often present with epigastric pain or refluxlike symptoms. A child who appears ill with acute pain should be immediately referred to the gastroenterology team; less acute symptoms should be watched carefully, with referral if the symptoms do not abate within 24 to 48 hours.

Vomiting. Vomiting in children with IBD, especially CD, could indicate an obstruction. The history and physical examination should elicit information about distention, associated pain and its relation to meals and the nature of the emesis, and accompanying abdominal pain. As always, information about the child's bowel pattern and the nature of the stools should be gathered.

Skeletal Complaints. Children who are receiving corticosteroid therapy are at increased risk for osteoporosis, aseptic necrosis of the hip or knee joints, and spinal fractures. In addition, children with IBD are more likely to have peripheral arthritis, sacroiliitis, and ankylosing spondylitis. Children with IBD who complain of back or hip pain require radiologic examination to adequately assess these symptoms. When children with IBD complain of joint pain, they should be questioned about the presence of erythema or swelling. If joint involvement is a concern, these children should also be assessed for any increased disease activity.

Drug Interactions

Sulfasalazine potentiates the action of both oral-form hypoglycemia agents (metformin, see Chapter 23) and may result in blood glucose values that are lower than anticipated. Sulfasalazine potentiates the action of phenytoin (Dilantin), resulting in higher than expected blood values of this drug and inhibits absorption of digoxin (Lanoxin), resulting in decreased blood levels of this drug. Metronidazole and corticosteroids potentiate the action of warfarin (Coumadin), but azathioprine (Imuran) may inhibit its effect. Increased prothrombin time has also been reported in children taking warfarin and olsalazine (Dipentum) simultaneously. Metronidazole has a disulfiram (Antabuse) type of reaction when an individual ingests alcohol or alcohol-containing elixirs during drug therapy. Phenytoin

---

BOX 30-3
Differential Diagnosis

DIARRHEA
Rule out flare-up of disease; obtain cultures

ABDOMINAL PAIN
Rule out flare-up of disease, gastritis, fulminant colitis, and obstruction

VOMITING
Rule out flare-up of disease, gastritis; assess for obstruction

SKELETAL COMPLAINTS
Rule out arthritic manifestations of the disease (i.e., sacroiliitis, ankylosing spondylitis, peripheral arthritis), aseptic necrosis of the femoral head, vertebral compression fractures, and osteoporosis

and phenobarbital increase the elimination of metronidazole, but cimetidine decreases its clearance. Individuals taking lithium may experience elevations in lithium levels if they start taking metronidazole. Their lithium levels should be checked carefully to avoid toxicity. Increased bone marrow suppression has been noted in some individuals taking TMP-SMX while on 6-MP therapy (PDR, 2001). Corticosteroids also diminish the efficacy of oral hypoglycemic agents, resulting in blood glucose levels that are higher than desired (PDR, 2001). NSAIDs should be avoided by most individuals with IBD because of the potential of bleeding.

Developmental Issues

Sleep Patterns

Children who are taking corticosteroids twice daily may feel agitated or euphoric at bedtime and may have difficulty sleeping. Dosage times may be shifted to alleviate this problem. Once the dosage is decreased, a single dose may be given in the morning. Children experiencing a flare-up of disease or whose disease is under poor control may be troubled by the need to frequently use the bathroom during the night, which may make it difficult for them to feel well rested and refreshed in the morning.

Toileting

Because most children are diagnosed with IBD after they have accomplished toilet training, families of children with IBD do not typically face this issue. For children who are not toilet trained, however, it is preferable to wait to start toilet training until the disease is quiescent and the character of bowel movements is as close to normal as possible.

Incontinence is experienced by many individuals with IBD. Children who have frequent bowel movements accompanied by urgency often fear recurrence of this problem. Children and families should be assisted in planning to prevent or handle such eventualities in a low-key way. In the context of an overview of a child's condition and its implications, the possibility of incontinence occurring should be shared with the school nurse and classroom teachers, who can make plans to ensure that incidents will be handled with sensitivity and that the child may retain as much control and dignity as possible. Classroom teachers should be encouraged to move the child's seat closer to the door and to liberalize bathroom privileges so that he or she may leave the room unobtrusively. Primary care providers may suggest that an extra change of clothing be kept in the child's locker or the nurse's office. Reminders to use the bathroom before leaving home and at regular intervals may also help to reduce the occurrence of potentially embarrassing episodes.

Management styles vary among practitioners with respect to the use of antispasmodic agents for the relief of chronic diarrhea in children with mild IBD. Drugs such as loperamide (Imodium) or diphenoxylate with atropine (Di-Atro) may be used cautiously in controlling symptoms during daytime activities (Kirschner, 1996)

Discipline

Behavioral expectations for children with IBD are similar to those for their unaffected peers. One area of concern may be the issue of compliance for children who are responsible or are assuming responsibility for their treatment regimen. Children in whom IBD remains in remission may not perceive the need for their medications because they may essentially be asymptomatic and feeling well. The concept of remission and disease being present but not discernible is difficult for school-aged children or early adolescents to master. Because a large percentage of children diagnosed with IBD are in early to middle adolescence, rebellion and testing are normal developmental issues. For adolescents with IBD, medications and treatment regimens can become a battleground for testing their independence. Primary care providers can help families identify ownership of responsibility for disease management. A particular risk facing children and adolescents with IBD is the hazard of abrupt discontinuation of steroid medications. In addition to a recurrence of IBD-related symptoms, children are at risk for adrenal crisis. Adolescents who are responsible for their own medication regimens, as well as their parents, should be educated about the significant risks associated with abruptly stopping their steroids.

Child Care

Parents of children with IBD should be encouraged to use the same guidelines for choosing child care arrangements as for their well children. Because the onset of IBD commonly occurs later in childhood, the increased risk of diarrheal illness secondary to diaper-changing areas and daycare providers handling food does not often need to be addressed by these families. If a child becomes infected, the illness should be promptly treated and the child monitored for signs of exacerbation of the disease. The overriding philosophy, however, is not to unduly isolate a child from the normal activities of daily living.

Schooling

Children with CD and UC are as able to achieve in the classroom as their unaffected peers. Similar to many children with chronic conditions, children with IBD must juggle treatment schedules and cope with stigma, pain, fatigue, and occasionally frequent or prolonged school absences. Academic performance may ultimately reflect a child's struggle to overcome these hurdles.

The nature of the disease processes and treatment regimens often set children with IBD apart from their peers in significant ways, including the cushingoid faces of children receiving corticosteroid therapy, the need for embarrassing treatments such as the instillation of rectal medications, and the use of nocturnal nasogastric feedings or restrictive diets. The isolation felt by children experiencing these treatments may cause them to limit participation in activities that enrich the school experience. Alternatively these children may choose not to comply with treatment regimens in an effort to "fit in." This behavior may set up a cycle of disease exacerbation and escalation of therapy that may concomitantly affect a child's academic achievement, reinforcing the child's sense of isolation. Sensitivity to these issues, creative problem solving, and anticipatory guidance by the primary care provider support the child and family in achieving as normal a lifestyle as possible. An issue often faced by individuals with IBD is the common misunderstanding by laypeople and some of those in the medical community that IBD is a psychologic disease. A primary role of health care providers is to educate school personnel and other significant adults in the child's life (e.g., club leaders, coaches, and daycare providers).

Sexuality

Adolescence is a time when concerns about body image, interpersonal relationships, and plans for the future are paramount. Therefore it is not unusual that adolescents or young adults with IBD are concerned about the effect this diagnosis might have on their appeal as a sexual partner, their ability to perform sexually, and their fertility. The significant changes in appearance that adolescents with IBD must withstand often include the late onset of puberty, weight gain, and acne—all of which contribute to their feelings of self-consciousness and stigmatization. Individuals with CD frequently have stomas or perianal involvement, which can be disfiguring and may affect their feelings of sexual attractiveness or acceptability to another person. Positive feelings of self-worth and a sense of acceptance must be conveyed to adolescents with IBD. The option of joining a network of other adolescents with common concerns should be offered whenever possible. Formal organizations or casual social gatherings may provide opportunities for teens and families to obtain support and acceptance.

Sulfasalazine has been shown to cause infertility in men, due to a decrease in sperm count and dysmotility and sperm malformation. These effects have been shown to be reversible, however, when men stop taking sulfasalazine for 3 months. No infertility is reported in men receiving the newer, oral 5-ASA preparations (PDR, 2001). Neither UC nor CD increases infertility in women with inactive disease. Some studies have indicated that women with CD have higher rates of infertility than control populations. It is believed that the most common cause of infertility in women with CD is the activity of the disease. Other factors include poor nutritional status, rectovaginal fistulas, and fear of becoming pregnant. Pelvic scarring is thought to be the cause of infertility in only a small percentage of individuals (Burakoff, 1995). A recent report suggests women who are postcolectomy have more difficulty having children compared with people without surgical treatment (Ording et al, 2002).

The outcome of pregnancy in women with IBD approximates that of the general population, but some researchers have found a somewhat higher incidence of prematurity in infants born to mothers with IBD than in the general population (Burakoff, 1995).

Pregnancy does not increase the likelihood of a relapse of either UC or of CD. In two thirds of all women with active IBD at conception, the disease remains active or worsens during pregnancy.

Surgical resection for CD or UC appears to not affect fertility in men. Men who have undergone colectomy with ileostomy or one of the other continent ileostomy procedures have a low risk of impotence as a complication of the surgical procedure (Burakoff, 1995).

Transition to Adulthood

Individuals with IBD do not typically require a specialized environment or assistance with activities of daily living. The embarrassing nature of many of the required medical therapies and symptoms of active disease make private living facilities most desirable for many individuals with IBD. Practitioners may help individuals to secure such accommodations.

Specialized programs to transition adolescents with IBD to adult care are not readily available. Many primary care providers have an informal policy of caring for their adolescent clients with IBD until they have weathered most of the anticipated developmental crises of late adolescence. It is best to wait to make this transition until a time when the individual's disease is quiescent.

Family Concerns and Resources

Families of children with IBD, similar to families of children with other chronic conditions, may focus on the child's symptoms and treatment regimen. In the case of the families dealing with IBD, however, this often means disclosing such private and potentially embarrassing issues as toileting and personal hygiene. The invasion of privacy felt by the child may become a source of stress for the entire family. Common concerns shared by children with IBD include personal appearance, physical endurance, diet, and their ability to fit in when sharing a meal or snacks with friends and family. These issues are magnified as these children enter adolescence and seek increased independence from their families and become increasingly self-conscious and concerned about body image and function. Poor communication and distrust between parent and child about disease activity and compliance with treatment regimens may result. If these children can become relatively independent in disease management before this difficult time, they and their families may develop confidence and trust in one another, perhaps alleviating or avoiding some of these conflicts.

IBD may affect children of many ethnic and religious backgrounds at a wide range of ages and with varied clinical presentations and severity. When cultural or religious practices focus on food and special dietary practices, these children may feel conflicted if disease activity makes some foods difficult to tolerate. Other than during times of disease activity, it is not typically recommended that children limit their diet. Children should be encouraged to maintain a diet as unrestricted and palatable as possible to encourage adequate caloric intake to promote optimal growth and development. Health care team members' sensitivity about dietary issues relating to both everyday life and special celebrations or religious observances is important. Practitioners should work in partnership with the family and child to develop a flexible plan of care that incorporates individual cultural concerns, such as religious feasts or times of fasting.

Resources

Organizations

Crohn's and Colitis Foundation of America, Inc.
386 Park Avenue S, 17th Floor
New York, NY 10016-8804
(800) 932-2423; (212) 685-3440
www.CCFA.org; info@ccfa.org

The Crohn's and Colitis Foundation of America (CCFA) is an organization with many chapters across the country that supports research and provides education and support for its members and for members of the community. Individuals with IBD and their families are encouraged to join and attend meet-ings and educational offerings. Many chapters have subcommittees that specifically deal with issues related to the needs of children with IBD and their families. The CCFA also publishes educational books, pamphlets, and newsletters written for the lay public. Professional memberships are available.

Summary of Primary Care Needs for the Child with Inflammatory Bowel Disease

HEALTH CARE MAINTENANCE

Growth and Development

Growth failure is a common problem for children with IBD but is more commonly seen in CD than UC.

Growth parameters are important to measure and graph at each primary care visit.

Cognitive abilities are unimpaired by IBD.

Diet

No special diet is recommended. Referral to a nutritionist at time of diagnosis is recommended. Some children may be lactose intolerant, particularly when disease is active. Some children during active disease may have less pain on a diet low in roughage. Adequate caloric intake is essential for growth.

If growth retardation has occurred, supplemental diet preparations may be beneficial.

Safety

No special safety recommendations are necessary for a child with inactive disease.

Children with osteoporosis should not participate in contact sports.

Individuals on metronidazole should be cautioned about an Antabuse type of reaction to alcohol.

Children on immunosuppressive therapy should wear Medic-Alert bracelets.

Take caution with travel, especially to tropical areas. Ova, parasites, and purity of water should be concerns.

Immunizations

No change in the normal immunization protocol is indicated unless a child is taking maintenance doses of immunosuppressive agents; in this case, no live vaccines should be administered, but immune globulin may be used with exposures.

Yearly influenza vaccine is recommended for children receiving immunosuppressants.

Screening

Vision. Ophthalmic examination is necessary at each visit. Twice-yearly ophthalmologist visits are recommended for a child taking maintenance doses of corticosteroids.

Hearing. Routine screening is recommended.

Dental. Routine care is adequate, but children taking cyclosporine are at increased risk for gingival hyperplasia.

Blood Pressure. Routine screening is recommended; if a child is taking cyclosporine or corticosteroids, blood pressure should be measured at every visit.

Hematocrit. Hematocrit and hemoglobin values should be obtained yearly if a child is asymptomatic and has no history of anemia; otherwise a CBC should be obtained every 6 months or as necessary.

Urinalysis. Routine screening is recommended unless a child has a history of fistulas or abscesses.

Tuberculosis. Routine screening is recommended. TB screening and chest x-ray must be done before treatment with infliximab.

Condition-Specific Screening

Erythrocyte Sedimentation Rate. Check annually or as needed if a flare-up of disease is suspected.

Fecal occult Blood Test. Check stool yearly and with potential disease flare-ups.

Chemistries. Liver function studies should be monitored every year for an otherwise asymptomatic child with IBD. A child taking Dipentum, Asacol, or Pentasa should have renal functions studies monitored at least every 4 months. In a child receiving cyclosporine, 6-MP, or azathioprine renal and liver function studies should be monitored every 4 months. A child taking 6-MP should have amylase and lipase levels tested every 4 months.

Lactose Intolerance. Check as indicated.

Neurologic Examination. Children receiving metronidazole should be assessed for paresthesias at each routine visit.

Bone Mineral Density. Screening in children with CD is recommended.

Surveillance Endoscopy. There are new recommendations for annual or biannual colonoscopies.

COMMON ILLNESS MANAGEMENT

Differential Diagnosis

Diarrhea. Rule out flare-up of disease, obtain cultures.

Abdominal Pain. Rule out flare-up of disease, gastritis, fulminant colitis, and obstruction.

Vomiting. Rule out flare-up of disease and gastritis; assess for obstruction.

Skeletal Complaints. Rule out arthritic manifestations of the disease (i.e., sacroiliitis, ankylosing spondylitis, peripheral arthritis), aseptic necrosis of the femoral head, vertebral compression fractures, and osteoporosis.

DEVELOPMENTAL ISSUES

Sleep Patterns

Children with IBD generally have no special needs; children receiving an evening dose of corticosteroids may have some difficulty sleeping. Children may have some nighttime stooling, interrupting sleep.

Continued

Summary of Primary Care Needs for the Child with Inflammatory Bowel Disease—cont'd

Toileting

Most children with IBD are diagnosed after toilet training has been accomplished. When toilet training is a concern, it may be suggested that toilet training be instituted when the disease activity is quiescent.

For older children with active disease, occasional incontinence may be an issue.

Antispasmodics may be used cautiously for daytime incontinence.

Discipline

Standard developmental counseling is advised; monitor adherence to treatment regimen.

Children and families should be educated on the hazards of discontinuing treatment.

Child Care

Standard developmental counseling is advised.

Schooling

Children with IBD are as able to achieve in the classroom as their unaffected peers.

Frequent or prolonged absences may interfere with school performance.

School personnel must be educated about special issues related to IBD; any misunderstandings about a psychologic cause of IBD should be alleviated.

Sexuality

Self-esteem and body image issues are important to adolescents with IBD.

Adolescents may have late onset of puberty due to growth retardation.

Sulfasalazine may cause infertility in men while they are taking the drug.

Pregnancy outcomes are similar to those of the general population.

Transition to Adulthood

Self-care responsibilities may be gradually taken on by adolescents. Specialized environments and assistance with activities of daily living are not typically required by young adults with IBD.

The transition to a provider specializing in care of adults is best done during periods of quiescent disease.

FAMILY CONCERNS

Privacy issues regarding toileting are often difficult for children and families. Because IBD affects individuals of disparate backgrounds and varies in its clinical presentation and severity, care of a child with IBD should be individualized. The practitioner should be sensitive to the needs of children and families whose cultural or religious practices focus on food if dietary restrictions are indicated during periods of active disease.

REFERENCES

Ahmed, T., et al. (1999). Inflammatory bowel disease in pediatric and adolescent patients. *Gastroenterol Clinic North Am, 28*, 445-458.

American Academy of Pediatrics. (2000). In L.K. Pickering (Ed.), *2000 Red book: report of Committee on Infectious Diseases* (25th ed.). Elk Grove Village, IL.

Becker, J.M (1999). Surgical therapy for ulcerative colitis and Crohn's disease. *Gastroenterol Clinic North Am, 28*, 371-390.

Belluzzi, A., et al. (1996). Effect of an enteric-coated fish-oil preparation on relapses in Crohn's disease. *N Engl J Med, 334*, 1557-1560.

Bousvaros, A., et al. (2000). Oral tacrolimus treatment of severe colitis in children. *Gastroenterology, 112*, PA941.

Bousvaros, A., Wang, A., & Leichtner, A. (1996). Tacrolimus (FK-506) treatment of fulminant colitis in a child. *J Pediatr Gastroenterol Nutr, 23*, 329-333.

Burakoff, R. (1995). Fertility and pregnancy in inflammatory bowel disease. In J.B. Kirsner & R.C. Shorter (Eds.), *Inflammatory bowel disease*. Baltimore: Williams & Wilkins.

Calkins, B.M. & Mendeloff, A.I. (1995). The epidemiology of idiopathic inflammatory bowel disease. In J.B. Kirsner & R.C. Shorter (Eds.), *Inflammatory bowel disease*. Baltimore: Williams & Wilkins.

Cohen, M.B., et al. (1998). Controversies in pediatric inflammatory bowel disease. *Inflamm Bowel Dis, 4*, 203-227.

Colenda, K. & Grand, R. (1995). Clinical manifestations of pediatric inflammatory bowel disease. In J.B. Kirsner & R.C. Shorter (Eds.), *Inflammatory bowel disease*. Baltimore: Williams & Wilkins.

Committee on Infectious Diseases. (2000). *Report of the committee on infectious disease* (25th ed.). ELK Grove Village, Il: the American Academy of Pediatrics.

Cuffari, C., Theoret, Y., Latour, S., & Seidman, G. (1996). 6-Mercaptopurine metabolism in Crohn's disease: correlation with efficacy and toxicity. *Gut, 39*, 401-406.

Cuthbert, A.P., et al. (2002). The contribution of NOD2 gene mutations to the risk and site of disease in inflammatory bowel disease. *Gastroenterology, 122*, 867-874.

Dudley-Brown, S. (1992). Psychosocial issues in IBD. *Nurse/Patient Link (Centocor)2*, 1-10.

Engstromm, I. & Lindquist, B.L. (1992). Inflammatory bowel disease in children and adolescents: a somatic and psychiatric investigation. *Acta Paediatr Scand, 80*, 640-647.

Gionchetti, P., et al. (2000). Oral bacteriotherapy as maintenance treatment in patients with chronic pouchitis: a double-blind, placebo-controlled trial. *Gastroenterology, 119*, 305-309.

Graham, T.O. & Kandil, H.M. (2002). Nutritional factors in inflammatory bowel disease. *Gastroenterology Clinics, 31*, 203-219.

Grand, R.J., Ramakrishna, J., & Calenda, K.A. (1995). Inflammatory bowel disease in the pediatric patient. *Gastroenterol Clin North Am, 24*, 613-632.

Griffiths, A.M. & Buller, H.B. (2000). Inflammatory bowel disease. In W.A.Walker, P.R. Durie, J.R. Hamilton, J.A. Walker-Smith & J.B. Watkins (Eds.), *Pediatric Gastrointestinal Disease*. Canada: B.C. Decker.

Gryboski, J.D. (1991). *Clostridium difficile* in inflammatory bowel disease relapse. *J Pediatr Gastroenterol Nutr, 13*, 39.

Hampe, J., et al. (2002). Association of NOD2 (CARD 15) genotype with clinical course of Crohn's disease: a cohort study. *Lancet, 359*, 1661-1665.

Hanauer, S.B. (1996). Inflammatory bowel disease. *New Engl J Med, 334*, 841-848.

Harrison, J. & Hanauer, S.B. (2002). Medical treatment for Crohn's disease. *Gastroenterol Clin North Am, 31*, 167-185.

Heuschkel, R., et al. (2002). Complementary medicine use in children and young adults with inflammatory bowel disease. *Am J Gastroenterol, 97,* 382-388.

Hyams, J.S. (1999). Crohn's disease. In R. Wyllie & J.S. Hyams (Eds.), *Pediatric Gastrointestinal Disease.* Philadelphia: W.B. Saunders.

Hyams, J.S., Markowitz, J., & Wyllie, R. (2000). Use of infliximab in the treatment of Crohn's disease in children and adolescents. *J Pediatr, 137,* 192-196.

Hyams, J.S. (1996). Crohn's disease in children. *Pediatr Clin North Am, 43,* 255-277.

Hyams, J.S., et al. (1996). Clinical outcome of ulcerative colitis in children. *J Pediatr, 129,* 81-88.

Hoffenberg, E.J., Fidanza, S., & Sauaia, A. (1999). Serologic testing for inflammatory bowel disease. *J Pediatr, 134,* 447-452.

Jani, N. & Regueiro, M.D. (2002). Medical therapy for ulcerative colitis. *Gastroenterol Clin North Am, 31,* 147-167.

Katz, S. (2002). Update in medical therapy of ulcerative colitis: a practical approach. *J Clin Gastroenterol, 34,* 397-407.

Kirschner, B.S. (1995). Medical management of inflammatory bowel disease in children. In J.B. Kirsner & R.C. Shorter (Eds.), *Inflammatory bowel disease.* Baltimore: Williams & Wilkins.

Kirschner, B.S. (1996). Ulcerative colitis in children. *Pediatr Clin North Am, 43,* 235-254.

Kirschner, B.S. (1998). Safety of azathioprine and 6-mercaptopurine in pediatric patients with inflammatory bowel disease. *Gastroenterology, 115,* 813-821.

Levine, A., et al. (2002). Evaluation of oral budesonide for treatment of mild and moderate exacerbations of Crohn's disease in children. *J Pediatr, 140,* 2002.

Loftus, E.V., et al. (1997). (abstract). Incidence and prevalence of Crohn's disease in Olmsted County Minnesota, 1970-1993. *Gastroenterology, 112,* A1027.

Logan, R.F. (1998). Inflammatory bowel disease incidence: up, down, or unchanged? *Gut, 42,* 309-311.

Mamula, P., Mascarenhas, M.R., & Baldassano, R.N. (2002). Biological and novel therapies for inflammatory bowel disease in children. *Ped Clinics of N Amer, 49,* 125.

Markowitz, J.F., Grancher, B.S., Kohn, N., & Daum, F. (2002). Immunomodulatory therapy for pediatric inflammatory bowel disease: changing patterns of use, 1990-2000. *Am J Gastroenterol, 97,* 928-932.

Markowitz, J., Grancher, K., Kohn, N., Lesser, M., & Daum, F. The pediatric 6MP collaborative group. (2000). A multicenter trial of 6-mercaptopurine and prednisone in children with newly diagnosed Crohn's disease. *Gastroenterology, 119,* 895-902.

Markowitz, J. (1999). Ulcerative colitis. In R. Wyllie & J.S. Hyams (Eds.), *Pediatric Gastrointestinal Disease.* Philadelphia: W.B. Saunders.

Markowitz, J. & Bengmark, S. (2002). Probiotics in health and disease in the pediatric population. *Pediatr Clin North Am, 49,* 127-141.

Markowitz, J., et al. (1995). Highly destructive perianal disease in children with Crohn's disease. *J Pediatr Gastroenterol Nutr, 21,* 149-153.

Markowitz, J., et al. (1991). Immunology of inflammatory bowel disease: summary of the proceedings of the subcommittee on immunosuppressive use in IBD. *J Pediatr Gastroenterol Nutr, 12,* 411-423.

Markowitz, J., et al. (2000). A multicenter trial of 6-mercaptopurine and prednisone in children with newly diagnosed Crohn's disease. *Gastroenterology, 110,* 895-902.

Ogura, Y., et al. (2000). A frameshift mutation in NOD2 associated with susceptibility to Crohn's disease. *Nature, 31*(411), 603-606.

Oliva-Hemker, M. & Fiocchi, C. (2002). Etiopathogenesis of inflammatory bowel disease: the importance of the pediatric perspective. *Inflamm Bowel Dis, 8,* 112-128.

Ording, O.K., Juul, S., Berndtsson, I., Oresland, T., & Laurberg, S. (2002). Ulcerative colitis: female fecundity before diagnosis, during disease and after surgery compared with a population sample. *Gastroenterology, 122,* 15-19.

Physicians' Desk Reference. (2001). Montvale, NJ: Medical Economics Data Production Company.

Pigot, F., et al. (1992). Low bone mineral density in patients with inflammatory bowel disease. *Dig Dis Sci, 37,* 1396-1403.

Podolsky, D.K. (2002). Inflammatory bowel disease. *New Engl J Med, 347,* 417-429.

Powell, F.C. & O'Kane, M. (2002). Management of pyoderma gangrenosum. *Dermatol Clin, 20,* 29-38.

Present, D.H. (2002). Serological tests are not helpful in managing inflammatory bowel disease. *Inflamm Bowel Dis, 3,* 227-228.

Ramakrishna J., et al. (1996). Combined use of cyclosporine and azathioprine or 6-mercaptopurine in pediatric inflammatory bowel disease. *J Pediatr Gastroenterol Nutr, 23*(39), 296-302.

Retsky, J.D. & Kraft, S.C. (1995). The extraintestinal manifestations of inflammatory bowel disease. In J.B. Kirsner & R.C. Shorter (Eds.), *Inflammatory bowel disease.* Baltimore: Williams & Wilkins.

Ruemmele, F.M., Roy, C.C., Levy, E., & Seidman, E.G. (2000). Nutrition as primary therapy in pediatric Crohn's disease: fact or fancy? *J Pediatr, 136,* 285-291.

Sanborn, W.J. & Targan, S.R. (2002). Biologic therapy of inflammatory bowel disease. *Gastroenterology, 122,* 1592-1608.

Sands, B.E. (1999). Novel therapies for inflammatory bowel disease. *Gastroenterol Clinic North Am, 28,* 323-352.

Sellman, S.P., Hupertz, V.F., & Reece, R.M. (1996). Crohn's disease presenting as suspected abuse. *Pediatrics, 97,* 272-274.

Semeao, E.J., Stallings, V.A., Peck, S.N., & Piccoli, D.A. (1997). Vertebral compression fractures in pediatric patients with Crohn's disease. *Gastroenterology, 112,* 1710-1713.

Spahn, J.D. & Kamada, A.K. (1995). Special considerations in the use of glucocorticoids in children. *Pediatr Rev, 16,* 266-272.

Stein, R.B. & Hanauer, S.B. (1999). Medical therapy for inflammatory bowel disease. *Gastroenterol Clin North Am, 28,* 297-321.

Swidsinski, A., et al. (2002). Mucosal flora in inflammatory bowel disease. *Gastroenterology, 122,* 44-54.

Tolia, V. (1997). Crohn's disease: to feed or not to feed at night is the question. *J Pediatr Gastroenterol Nutr, 25,* 246-247.

31 Juvenile Rheumatoid Arthritis and Juvenile Spondyloarthropathy

Patricia A. Rettig, Stephanie L. Merhar, and Randy Q. Cron

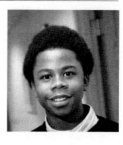

Etiology

Chronic arthritis in childhood represents a heterogeneous group of diseases, of which the two most common forms are juvenile rheumatoid arthritis (JRA) and juvenile spondyloarthropathy (JSpA). Chronic arthritis is defined as swelling within a joint or limitation in the range of movement with joint pain and tenderness that persist for at least 6 weeks and for which all other causes are excluded (Petty & Cassidy, 2001b).

Over the past 3 decades, international leaders in the field of pediatric rheumatology have debated the criteria for classification of childhood arthritis (Foeldvari & Biddle, 2000; Petty, 2001). In 1997, pediatric rheumatologists in the International League of Association for Rheumatology (ILAR) proposed the term "juvenile idiopathic arthritis" (JIA) rather than the more common "JRA" classification and terminology (Kulas & Schanberg, 2001; Petty et al, 1998). ILAR criteria attempt to combine the current American College of Rheumatology (ACR) criteria for JRA and the European League Against Rheumatism (EULAR) criteria for juvenile chronic arthritis (JCA) along with JSpA (Table 31-1). The ultimate goal of the JIA classification is to promote a greater understanding of persistent arthritis that begins in childhood. However, until JIA is universally accepted, published, and scientifically validated, the specific conditions of JRA and JSpA will be either referred to individually or in general as chronic arthritis for the purposes of clarity in this chapter. Moreover, the importance of recognizing JSpAs in any discussion of chronic arthritis in children is emphasized, since the incidence of these conditions may be similar to JRA, and JSpA is frequently underdiagnosed or misdiagnosed (Bauman et al, 1996; Garcia-Consuegra Molina et al, 1998).

The etiology of chronic arthritis in childhood is unknown. This condition is not a single disease entity but represents a heterogeneity of phenotypes with several modes of onset (Cassidy & Petty, 2001). Differences in onset and clinical course need to be considered when researching causes. Current hypotheses focus on the roles of autoimmunity, abnormal immunologic regulation, infection, psychologic stress, trauma, and hormonal factors as potential triggers in a child with a genetic predisposition. Substantial evidence points to an autoimmune process, including synovial pathology, presence of autoantibodies, and T-cell abnormalities (Cassidy & Petty, 2001; Glass & Giannini, 1999; Grom & Hirsch, 2000). There is also increasing evidence of excess cytokine production and abnormal immunoregulatory processes as contributors to chronic arthritis. In a recent comparison study of individuals with JRA and JSpA, proinflammatory cytokines were detected in both disease groups at a similar rate (Murray et al, 1998). Epidemiologic studies have shown familial, seasonal, geographic, and ethnic differences among the subtypes of chronic childhood arthritis, suggesting environmental and genetic factors (Gare, 1999).

Known Genetic Etiology

JRA is thought to be a complex genetic (polygenic) trait. One abnormal gene or one mutation is not sufficient to result in the disease, and one or more genetic factors must interact. This explains why there is a low probability of disease occurring in more than one family member (Glass & Giannini, 1999). Concurrence of chronic arthritis in siblings is uncommon. There are an estimated total of only 300 sibling pairs with JRA in the United States among the total population of 30,000 to 50,000 with JRA (Glass & Giannini, 1999). Certain human leukocyte antigen (HLA) alleles are associated with disease susceptibility and with the different types of chronic arthritis in childhood. For example, HLA-DR4 is associated with polyarticular rheumatoid factor (RF)–positive JRA. HLA-A2, HLA-DR8, and HLA-DR5 are strongly associated with early susceptibility to pauciarticular JRA (Murray et al, 1997). A recent study of 80 sibling pairs with JRA demonstrated the genetic linkage between JRA and more than one chromosomal region (Prahalad et al, 2000a). Again, these results lend support to the hypothesis that JRA is a complex genetic trait in which more than one chromosomal region is likely to influence disease phenotype (Prahalad et al, 2000b).

In contrast to JRA, there is a high familial occurrence of JSpA among children, parents, and first-degree relatives. The association of the genetic marker HLA-B27 in JSpA is well described. In one study, the association of juvenile ankylosing spondylitis (JAS), a form of JSpA, and HLA-B27 was as high as 91%, but this is probably an overestimate (Cabral et al, 1992).

Incidence and Prevalence

The estimated incidence and prevalence of childhood chronic arthritis differ markedly across a range of studies, in part because of the discrepancies in classification criteria as described above (Manners & Bower, 2002). Results from 34 epidemiology studies reported a prevalence range of 0.07 to 4.01 per 1000 children and an incidence range of 0.0008 to 0.226 per 1000 children per year for chronic arthritis (Grom et al, 1994). The specific incidence of JRA based on ACR criteria has varied from 2 to 20 per 100,000 (Cassidy & Petty, 2001). Prevalence of JRA based on ACR criteria ranges from

TABLE 31-1

Comparison of Classifications of Childhood Arthritis

ACR	EULAR	ILAR
Juvenile rheumatoid arthritis	Juvenile chronic arthritis (JCA)	Juvenile idiopathic arthritis
Systemic	Systemic JCA	Systemic
Polyarticular	Polyarticular JCA	Polyarticular, RF positive
	Juvenile rheumatoid arthritis	Polyarticular, RF negative
Pauciarticular	Pauciarticular JCA	Oligoarticular Persistent Extended
	Juvenile psoriatic arthritis	Psoriatic arthritis
	Juvenile ankylosing spondylitis	Enthesitis-related arthritis Other arthritis

From Cassidy, J.T. & Petty, P.E. (2001). *Textbook of pediatric rheumatology* (4th ed.). Philadelphia: W.B. Saunders. Reprinted with permission.
ACR, American College of Rheumatology; *EULAR,* European League Against Rheumatism; *ILAR,* International League of Associations for Rheumatology; *RF,* rheumatoid factor.

BOX 31-1

Criteria for the Classification of Juvenile Rheumatoid Arthritis

1. Age at onset <16 yr
2. Arthritis (i.e., swelling or effusion or presence of two or more of the following signs: limitation of range of motion, tenderness or pain on motion, increased heat) in one or more joints
3. Duration of disease >6 wks
4. Type of onset defined by type of disease in first 6 mo:
    a. Polyarthritis: ≥5 inflamed joints
    b. Oligoarthritis: <5 inflamed joints
    c. Systemic: arthritis with characteristic fever
5. Exclusion of other forms of juvenile arthritis

From Cassidy, J.T. & Petty, P.E. (2001). *Textbook of pediatric rheumatology* (4th ed.). Philadelphia: W.B. Saunders. Reprinted with permission.

BOX 31-2

Reasons to Refer to Pediatric Rheumatology

Child with:
    Joint pain, swelling, stiffness, decreased mobility
    Limp, refusal to walk, or hip pain
    Unexplained rash or fever
    Prolonged or cyclic fevers
    Muscle weakness associated with rash
    Multisystemic disease

16 to 150 per 100,000 (Cassidy & Petty, 2001). Incidence and prevalence studies are believed to represent low estimates; clearly, chronic arthritis in childhood is not an uncommon condition (Cassidy & Petty, 2001).

It is notable that the incidence and prevalence of JSpAs may reach or even exceed that of JRA in some geographic areas (Cassidy & Petty, 2001). Previous reports on these statistics have failed to differentiate between early JSpA and JRA. Moreover, increasing awareness of the occurrence of JSpAs and their clinical and diagnostic differentiation from JRA will result in an increased proportion of children with chronic arthritis in the JSpA category.

Clinical Manifestations at Time of Diagnosis

The diagnostic criteria for JRA have been developed and are listed in Box 31-1. Misdiagnosis of JRA results when four key points are missed: (1) Arthralgia, or joint pain, alone is not sufficient to make the diagnosis; arthritis must be present. (2) The arthritis must persist for *at least* 6 weeks. (3) All other causes of chronic arthritis in children must be excluded. These causes include, but are not limited to, other pediatric rheumatic diseases such as JSpAs, lupus, dermatomyositis, vasculitis, sarcoidosis, scleroderma, and periodic fever syndromes. In addition, other nonrheumatic causes of arthritis must be ruled out, including metabolic, infectious (Lyme arthritis being the most common), neoplastic, congenital, traumatic, degenerative, and psychogenic causes. (4) There are no signs, symptoms, or laboratory investigations pathognomonic for JRA or JSpA. Children should be referred to a pediatric rheumatology center (Box 31-2) when the clinician is suspicious of an underlying rheumatic, inflammatory, or autoimmune disorder.

A joint with arthritis exhibits one or more of the following signs of inflammation: swelling, heat, pain, or reduced range of motion. Swelling results from an intraarticular effusion or hypertrophy (thickening) of the synovial membrane (Figure 31-1). Synovitis may develop insidiously and exist for months or years without causing joint destruction; or it may damage cartilage, subchondral bone, or other joint structures in a relatively short time (Baeten et al, 2002; Laxer & Schneider, 1998; Prieur, 1998; Sherry et al, 1998). Clinical features range from mild synovitis in one joint with no systemic symptoms to moderate or severe disease in many joints.

Common clinical manifestations in addition to synovial inflammation include morning stiffness and "gelling." Stiffness is defined as discomfort when the person attempts to move joints after a period of inactivity. Children may also experience stiffness after prolonged sitting (gelling), such as during classes or after a long car ride. At every rheumatology visit, children are asked about the duration of stiffness. The length of time is a good indicator of disease activity (Cron & Finkel, 2002). Mild stiffness will resolve within a few minutes of walking; however, severe stiffness may take several hours to dissipate. The child or parents will report that the child has stiffness or a limp that is worse in the morning and improves as the day progresses.

Children with arthritis may not complain of pain, and the manner in which they do so depends on their age, disease status, and psychosocial measures, such as social support, stress, and locus of control (Varni & Bernstein, 1991). Many children present with pain-free large joint effusions (Sherry et al, 1990), and some may have joint contractures. However, because these children are able to maintain normal activity levels and keep up with their peers without discomfort, the diagnosis is often delayed. Unfortunately, delay in diagnosis and treatment can have serious consequences for the child, including permanent leg length discrepancy (Sherry et al, 1999) and permanent vision loss (Oren et al, 2000).

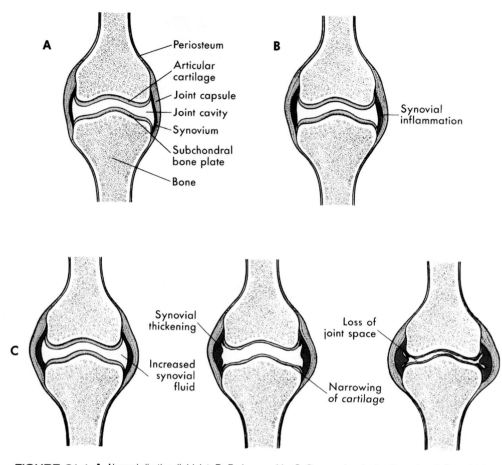

FIGURE 31-1 **A,** Normal diarthrodial joint. **B,** Early synovitis. **C,** Progressive destruction of an inflamed joint.

Children who present with a chief complaint of musculoskeletal pain are highly unlikely to have chronic inflammatory arthritis. In a recent study of 414 children referred to a pediatric rheumatology service over a 2-year period, 226 children were referred for pain. Of these 226 children, only 12 were diagnosed with JRA and only 4 had JspA (McGhee et al, 2002). These results suggest that primary care providers should not order antinuclear antibody (ANA) or rheumatoid factor (RF) studies on children with musculoskeletal pain and an otherwise normal physical examination. The likelihood of these children having a chronic inflammatory condition is extremely low (McGhee et al, 2002). At least 10% of the general population carries a positive ANA with no evidence of disease, and the percentage is higher if they have a relative with an autoimmune illness. The rheumatoid factor is even less significant in pediatrics and is only ordered after the diagnosis of polyarticular JRA is established (Table 31-2). The primary care provider must remember that childhood arthritis is a totally different disease entity with different clinical and diagnostic parameters than the adult form of rheumatoid arthritis (RA).

Types of Onset

Manifestations at the time of onset and throughout the first 6 months of the disease determine classification into one of three major subtypes: pauciarticular, polyarticular, or systemic JRA. These subtypes are characterized by several factors, including the number of joints, variations in patterns and severity of joint disease, extraarticular manifestations, immunogenetic characteristics, age at onset, and gender of the child (Cassidy & Petty, 2001; Jarvis, 2002; Sherry et al, 1998)(Table 31-2). JRA is a disease characterized by exacerbations ("flares") and remissions. Exacerbations may occur during episodes of acute illness or stress. The frequency and duration of flares are unpredictable, but they are easily recognized and rapidly treated. Children, especially those with systemic JRA, may also experience constitutional symptoms, such as fever, anorexia, weight loss, growth failure, and anemia.

Pauciarticular Juvenile Rheumatoid Arthritis. Close to 60% of children with JRA have the mildest form, pauciarticular JRA, which involves four or fewer joints during the first 6 months of the disease. In this type, the peak age of onset is between 1 and 3 years of age, and the female/male ratio is 5:1. Often there is only one joint, typically the knee, involved. A classic presentation of pauciarticular disease is the toddler with a limp, no complaints of pain, and a large knee effusion with a flexion contracture on examination. Physical findings may also include thigh and calf atrophy of the involved side and a leg length discrepancy, with the involved leg being longer. Uveitis is a major complication in this group, especially in those who are ANA positive, and it is imperative that the child see a pediatric ophthalmologist at onset and at designated periodic intervals (see Associated Problems).

Polyarticular Juvenile Rheumatoid Arthritis. Approximately 30% of children with JRA have five or more affected joints

Characteristics of JRA by Type of Onset

	Polyarthritis	Oligoarthritis (Pauciarticular Disease)	Systemic Disease
Frequency of cases	30%	60%	10%
Number of joints involved	≥5	≤4	Variable
Age at onset	Throughout childhood; peak at 1-3 yr	Early childhood; peak at 1-2 yr	Throughout childhood; no peak
Gender ratio (F/M)	3:1	5:1	1:1
Systemic involvement	Moderate involvement	Not present	Prominent
Occurrence of chronic uveitis	5%	20%	Rare
Frequency of seropositivity			
Rheumatoid factors	10% (increases with age)	Rare	Rare
Antinuclear antibodies	40%-50%	75%-85%*	10%
Prognosis	Guarded to moderately good	Excellent except for eyesight and those who develop polyarticular course	Moderate to poor

From Cassidy, J.T. & Petty, P.E. (2001). *Textbook of pediatric rheumatology* (4th ed.). Philadelphia: W.B. Saunders. Reprinted with permission.
*In girls with uveitis.

(polyarticular onset) during the first 6 months of the disease. Rheumatoid factor is rarely positive in JRA in general and is present in only 10% of the children with this type. The small subgroup with polyarticular JRA and RF positivity may develop a more severe form of arthritis with early onset of erosive arthritis, rheumatoid nodules, and a chronic course persisting into adulthood (Cassidy & Petty, 2001; Jarvis, 2002). Extraarticular manifestations include fatigue, low-grade fevers, anemia, osteopenia, mild lymphadenopathy, and rheumatoid nodules. Greatest disability occurs with unremitting neck, jaw, and hip arthritis. Conversely, children with RF-negative arthritis, which is much more common, exhibit less aggressive joint destruction but have widespread large and small joint involvement (Prieur, 1998). Laboratory findings include elevated or normal sedimentation rate, leukocyte count, and platelet count. A possible presentation for polyarticular JRA is a girl with mild fatigue and anemia who has bilateral wrist, finger, knee, and ankle arthritis; joint contractures; and a limp.

Systemic Juvenile Rheumatoid Arthritis. Systemic JRA (10% of all children with JRA) presents with severe systemic involvement that may precede the arthritis by weeks or months. The diagnostic hallmark of this type of arthritis is the fever pattern. The fevers are characterized by daily or twice-daily spiking temperatures over 102° F, with a rapid return to normal or below baseline. The fever usually occurs in the late afternoon or evening in conjunction with the classic systemic JRA rash. The rash consists of discrete, small, macular, pink- or salmon-colored lesions that are blanching, transient, and nonpruritic in most cases. This rash is commonly seen on the trunk, and it may be present on the extremities (Cassidy & Petty, 2001). Arthritis may be absent at onset, but arthralgias or myalgias are usually present. Other systemic clinical features include diffuse lymphadenopathy, hepatosplenomegaly, leukocytosis, thrombocytosis, progressive anemia, and elevated acute-phase reactants, such as an elevated sedimentation rate (often greater than 80 mm/hr by Westergren method [Jarvis, 2002]), C-reactive protein, and serum ferritin. Normochromic, normocytic anemia of chronic disease may also be present (Cassidy & Petty, 2001; Laxer & Schneider, 1998). Other laboratory abnormalities may include elevated D-dimers, hypoalbuminemia, elevated liver function studies, elevated aldolase levels, and hypergamma-

Criteria for the Classification of Spondyloarthropathy

Inflammatory spinal pain
  or
Synovitis
  Asymmetric or
  Predominantly in the lower limbs and one or more of the following:
    Positive family history
    Psoriasis
    Inflammatory bowel disease
    Urethritis, cervicitis, or acute diarrhea within 1 mo before arthritis
    Buttock pain alternating between right and left gluteal areas
    Enthesopathy
    Sacroiliitis

From Dougados, M. et al. (1991). The European Spondyloarthropathy Study Group preliminary criteria for the classification of spondyloarthropathy. *Arthritis Rheum, 34,* 1218-1227. Reprinted with permission.

globulinemia (Bloom et al, 1998; Laxer & Schneider, 1998). In addition, joint involvement is often polyarticular, involving the wrists, carpal bones, knees, ankles, tarsal bones, neck, and any or all other joints. Children with systemic JRA can develop macrophage activation syndrome (MAS), which is an uncommon but acute complication associated with morbidity and sometimes death (Grom & Passo, 1996).

Juvenile Spondyloarthropathies. Four discrete entities make up the chronic JSpAs (Box 31-3): SEA (seronegative enthesopathy and arthropathy) syndrome, juvenile ankylosing spondylitis, psoriatic arthritis, and arthritis associated with inflammatory bowel disease (IBD) (see Chapter 30). These diseases all have noted associations with the HLA-B27 gene product. HLA-B27 is present in about 8% of the general white population but is present in around 50% to 90% of children with the JSpAs. The JSpAs occur predominantly in males, except for psoriatic arthritis, which has a slightly higher percentage of females. Certain ethnic groups have higher incidences of SpAs, particularly native North Americans in and around Alaska (Peschken & Esdaile, 1999). The JSpAs also are known for a more chronic waxing and waning disease course than JRA, but some children have a more debilitating illness not unlike those with severe

RF-positive JRA. A significant distinguishing feature of the JSpAs is the presence of enthesitis, which is absent in children with JRA. Enthesitis is inflammation at tendon and ligament insertion sites into bone. Most commonly these sites are found around the knees and feet (Petty & Cassidy, 2001a). The mechanism for enthesitis is thought to be similar to arthritis except that the inflammation does not occur within a defined joint capsule. Certain forms of reactive arthritis and Reiter syndrome are also considered in the category of SpAs, but they are not usually chronic and will not be discussed in this chapter.

SEA syndrome. SEA (seronegative enthesopathy and arthropathy) syndrome is probably the most common form of JSpA. Seronegative refers to ANA negative and RF negative, and arthropathy refers to the fact that joint pain, not frank arthritis, is all that is required to make the initial diagnosis (Cabral et al, 1992). SEA syndrome typically affects boys who are usually HLA-B27 positive, and there is often a family history of chronic lower back pain, psoriasis, or known SpAs. Enthesitis on examination and the pattern of involved joints are often clues to the diagnosis (Faustino et al, 2001). SEA syndrome is sometimes the precursor for other forms of JSpAs, such as juvenile ankylosing spondylitis (JAS).

Juvenile ankylosing spondylitis. Because the criteria are so strict, true JAS is uncommon in childhood but does afflict some older adolescent boys (Burgos-Vargas et al, 1996; Garcia-Consuegra Molina et al, 1998). Ultimately, boys with JAS will go on to develop axial skeleton involvement with sacroiliitis and lumbosacral spine arthritis. This can be quite debilitating and is often best assessed clinically by the modified Schober examination, which measures lower back movement, and radiologically by magnetic resonance imaging (MRI) (Luong & Salonen, 2000). True JAS often requires aggressive pharmacotherapy and physical therapy to maintain good range of motion and function of the pelvis, lower back, and lower extremities.

Psoriatic arthritis. Children with psoriasis and arthritis are said to have psoriatic arthritis. The diagnosis of psoriatic arthritis or probable psoriatic arthritis can be made even in the absence of psoriasis by the presence of nail pits, dactylitis, or a strong family history for psoriasis. Girls slightly outnumber boys, and the HLA-B27 association may be 50% or lower. An aggressive form of psoriatic arthritis, arthritis mutilans, is uncommon in childhood (Ansell, 1994).

Arthritis associated with inflammatory bowel disease. Up to 30% of children with IBD, either Crohn disease or ulcerative colitis (see Chapter 30), will develop chronic arthritis at some point during their illness. The onset of arthritis may occur before, concurrent with, or subsequent to the diagnosis of IBD. A recent prospective analysis, however, puts the prevalence of peripheral arthritis in individuals with IBD closer to 12% (Palm et al, 2001). There is certainly an association with the inflammation of the bowels and inflammation of joints in the SpAs, and several immune-based hypotheses connecting the gut and the joints have been proposed (Baeten et al, 2002). The arthritis of IBD often begins peripherally but may end up affecting the axial skeleton. Moreover, the bowel disease may eventually become quiescent, but the child may go on to develop an aggressive form of axial arthritis not unlike that of JAS or ankylosing spondylitis.

BOX 31-4
Treatment

GOAL OF TREATMENTS
Induce disease remission
Decrease systemic and joint inflammation
Prevent disease complications and disability
Promote maximal growth and development
Promote psychosocial well-being of child and family

TREATMENT PLAN
Pharmacotherapy: PO, SC, or IV administration
Aerobic, range of motion, and stretching exercise program
PT, OT, splints, orthotics, and supportive footwear
Nutritional counseling
Heat and cold application: moist heating pad, warm bath/shower, sometimes ice
Social support
Surgery

PO, By mouth; *SC,* subcutaneous; *IV,* intravenous; *PT,* physical therapy; *OT,* occupational therapy.

Treatment

Management of chronic arthritis in childhood is most successful when there is early diagnosis and institution of early aggressive treatment with targeted interventions (Box 31-4) (Wallace, 2000).

The cornerstone of treatment is antiinflammatory and disease-modifying medication, with newer, more effective treatments available now than even 3 years ago. Interdisciplinary, family-centered treatment interventions incorporate the team approach and include the family and child, pediatric rheumatologist, advanced practice nurse, clinic nurse, primary care provider, physical therapist, occupational therapist, and social worker. Consultations with the ophthalmologist, orthopedist, psychologist, dietitian, orthodontist, interventional radiologist, and other pediatric specialists are sought as indicated.

Pharmacotherapy for Childhood Chronic Arthritis

Treatment of chronic arthritis in childhood has come a long way in the last one-half century. New therapies are becoming available for use at a quick pace. The days are long gone when pediatric rheumatologists inched up the aspirin dose based on increased weight of the child. Equally rare are JRA-associated blindness and use of wheelchairs.

In general, JRA and the JSpAs are treated similarly. Specific pharmacologic agents used to treat JRA and the JSpAs are identified in Table 31-3. Nonsteroidal antiinflammatory drugs (NSAIDs) remain one of the cornerstones of treatment for the childhood chronic arthritides (Brunner et al, 2001; Cron et al, 1999; Minden et al, 2002). Recently, the use of preferential cyclooxygenase-2 inhibitors (NSAIDs with less gastrointestinal toxicity) has begun to filter into pediatric practice (Foeldvari et al, 2002). However, the trend of universal NSAID use in treating childhood chronic arthritis is slowly being

TABLE 31-3

Medications Commonly Used in Treatment of Juvenile Rheumatoid Arthritis

Drug	Trade Name	Dosing	Side Effects	Laboratory Monitors
NONSTEROIDAL ANTIINFLAMMATORY DRUGS (NSAIDs)*				
Naproxen[†]	Anaprox Naprosyn Aleve (OTC)	15-20 mg/kg/day bid	For all NSAIDs: abdominal pain, dizziness, drowsiness, fluid retention, gastric ulcers and bleeding, greater susceptibility to bruising or bleeding, heartburn, indigestion, lightheadedness, nausea, rash, reduction in kidney function, anemia, increase in liver enzymes For naproxen and some others: pseudoporphyria with sun exposure	ALL NSAIDs: CBC with differential, UA, BUN, creatinine, and LFTs initially at 6 wk, then every 3-6 mo
Ibuprofen[†]	Advil (OTC) Motrin IB (OTC) Nuprin (OTC) Motrin (Rx)	30-40 mg/kg/day tid		
Indomethacin[†]	Indocin Indocin SR	1-3 mg/kg/day tid or qid 75 mg qd or bid	For indomethacin only: depression, severe headaches, "spaced out" feeling	
Nabumetone[‡] Tolectin sodium	Relafen Tolectin	500 or 750 mg PO bid 30-40 mg/kg/day tid; max 1800 mg/day		
Sulindac[‡]	Clinoril	3-4 mg/kg/day bid		
COX-2 INHIBITORS				
Celecoxib[‡]	Celebrex	100 or 200 mg PO qd or bid	Same as traditional NSAIDs, but less likely to cause gastric ulcers, bleeding, and bruising	
Rofecoxib[†]	Vioxx	12.5, 25, or 50 mg qd	Cautions: sensitivity to sulfonamides or allergies to aspirin or other NSAIDs	
DISEASE-MODIFYING ANTIRHEUMATIC DRUGS (DMARDs)				
Methotrexate (MTX)	Rheumatrex Trexall	1 mg/kg/dose weekly up to 40 mg subcutaneously PO only	Nausea, vomiting, mouth sores, increased liver enzymes, myelosuppression, hair loss Cautions: abnormal blood count, liver or lung disease, active infection or fever; NO alcohol; causes birth defects if taken during pregnancy	CBC with differential and LFTs every month ×2, then every 2 mo
Sulfasalazine	Azulfidine Azulfidine EN-tabs	30-50 mg/kg tid; maximum 3 g/day	Stomach upset, diarrhea, dizziness, headache, light sensitivity, itching, rash, loss of appetite, nausea, vomiting, increased liver enzymes, lowered blood count Cautions: allergy to sulfa or aspirin; kidney, liver, or blood disease; avoid prolonged sun exposure; take with food; do not take with Maalox or Mylanta type of antacids	Same as for methotrexate
CORTICOSTEROIDS				
Prednisolone*[‡]	Prelone[†] Pediapred[†] Orapred[†]	0.5-2 mg/kg/day qd or bid Varies with disease Used mostly for sJRA	Indigestion, weight gain, increased appetite, mood changes, insomnia With long-term therapy: cushingoid features, weight gain, striae, osteoporosis, cataracts, glaucoma, elevated blood glucose, immunosuppression	CBC with differential, BP every month, yearly ocular exams
Prednisone*[‡]	Deltasone Orasone		Cautions: active infection, hypertension, osteoporosis Same as Prednisolone	

Continued

TABLE 31-3

Medications Commonly Used in Treatment of Juvenile Rheumatoid Arthritis—cont'd

Drug	Trade Name	Dosing	Side Effects	Laboratory Monitors
BIOLOGIC RESPONSE MODIFIERS				
Etanercept	Enbrel	0.4 mg/kg per dose 2 doses SC injections weekly	Possible redness, itching, or swelling at injection site Cautions: hold drug if active infection, no live vaccines; keep refrigerated	Obtain baseline chest x-ray to rule out tuberculosis, no laboratory tests; assess for signs of infection, fever when ill
Infliximab (usually given in conjunction with MTX)	Remicade	IV infusion weeks 1, 3, 7; then every 4-8 wk depending on response	Upper respiratory infection, headache, chest pain, infusion reaction	

CBC, Complete blood count; *UA*, urinalysis; *BUN*, blood urea nitrogen; *LFTs*, liver function tests; *OTC*, over the counter; *Rx*, prescription; *BP*, blood pressure.
*Do not take NSAIDs with other OTC NSAIDs. Always take NSAIDs with food. Remind parents that NSAIDs are mainly to treat chronic inflammation and are to be continued as prescribed even if child does not complain of pain.
†Available as suspension.
‡Drugs not listed as mg/kg are actual adult doses; pediatric doses are estimated based on a 70-kg adult.

reversed by the increased use of intraarticular corticosteroids and by early aggressive therapy (Cron et al, 1999).

Intraarticular corticosteroids are now the second most common form of treatment for pauciarticular JRA (Cron et al, 1999). Long-lasting corticosteroids, such as triamcinolone hexacetonide, are safe and highly effective (Breit et al, 2000; Padeh & Passwell, 1998). The use of intraarticular corticosteroids can substantially decrease the use of systemic therapy and the associated side effects.

In addition to NSAIDs, there are a growing variety of medicines used to treat chronic childhood arthritis, referred to as slow-acting antirheumatic drugs (SAARDs) or disease-modifying antirheumatic drugs (DMARDs). The most commonly used DMARD for SEA syndrome is sulfasalazine, whereas methotrexate is the most common DMARD for all forms of JRA (Cron et al, 1999). DMARDs such as gold and D-penicillamine are rarely, if ever, used anymore to treat chronic childhood arthritis (Brunner et al, 2001; Cron et al, 1999). In the last 2 decades, methotrexate has largely replaced most DMARDs as the treatment of choice for arthritis and treatment-resistant uveitis based on its high efficacy–to–side effect profile in children (Hashkes et al, 1997). It is also well tolerated at doses up to 1 mg/kg/wk, with a maximum of 40 mg per dose, particularly if given in a subcutaneous route (Wallace, 1998). Methotrexate is also commonly used in combination with other agents.

When the combination of NSAIDs, methotrexate, and intraarticular injections is not enough to get the arthritis into remission, a variety of other agents are available for use. Recently, biologic agents, particularly tumor necrosis factor (TNF) inhibitors, are finding widespread use among pediatric rheumatologists caring for children with chronic arthritis. These include etanercept (Enbrel) twice weekly subcutaneous injections and infliximab (Remicade) intravenous administration at regular intervals. The TNF inhibitors are typically used in conjunction with methotrexate and have been helpful for difficult to treat individuals with polyarticular disease (Lovell et al, 2000). Newer biologics are being studied in adults, including

interleukin-1 blockers and inhibitors of lymphocyte activation by co-stimulatory blockade (Arkachasisri & Lehman, 2000). It will not be long before these become available for use in pediatrics.

For the sickest children, particularly those with systemic-onset JRA, systemic glucocorticoids are often necessary to control disease activity. The steroids are usually given as daily oral doses and as weekly or monthly intravenous boluses. Unfortunately, systemic corticosteroids are associated with a large list of adverse side effects (e.g., striae, cushingoid features, hirsutism, weight gain, reduced growth velocity, diabetes, glaucoma, cataracts, osteopenia) (Cassidy, 1999). In order to limit steroid usage to the shortest possible duration, more aggressive therapy is necessary. Both immunosuppressive medications such as cyclosporine (Gerloni et al, 2001) and cytotoxic agents such as cyclophosphamide (Wallace & Sherry, 1997) have proven effective. However, these medicines are associated with significant short-term and long-term complications, such as opportunistic infections, infertility, mutagenesis, and oncogenesis; therefore, their use is clinically limited (Laxer & Schneider, 1998; Singsen & Rose, 1995).

Exercise and Therapy

Numerous research studies of adults with rheumatoid arthritis demonstrate the benefits of a regular exercise program (van den Dende et al, 1998). However, there are few studies on children with chronic arthritis concerning the effects of exercise and physical therapy. Existing evidence does demonstrate that individualized conditioning programs, such as aerobic exercise and aquatic training, have both physical and psychologic benefits. These programs have the potential to increase aerobic capacity, muscular strength, endurance, and stamina for daily activities without aggravating joint disease (Klepper, 1999; Scull, 2000; Takken et al, 2001).

Physical and occupational therapy goals include the following: (1) to increase range of motion, endurance, strength, and conditioning; (2) to teach principles of joint protection and energy conservation; (3) to utilize appropriate splints; (4) to recommend modalities and assistive devices; (5) to assess and treat limitations in current function; and (6) and to reinforce a home exercise program, appropriate sports, and play activities (Klepper, 1999; Scull, 2000). Today, with early, advanced, aggressive pharmacotherapy, many children with arthritis may not require physical therapy or splints. For example, the child with pauciarticular disease who presents with a joint contracture in an inflamed knee will be treated with an intraarticular corticosteroid injection and/or an NSAID. This treatment will decrease inflammation and the contracture and may produce a full remission. Unfortunately, if treatment is delayed for a child with persistently swollen joints, the child may hold the joints in a position of comfort, usually flexion. This position contributes to a flexion contracture with decreased joint mobility and causes joint malalignment. This child may require therapy and splinting to reduce residual limitations after the institution of medications.

Occupational therapists usually evaluate and fabricate splints for the upper extremities, and physical therapists construct splints for the lower extremities, including foot orthotics. Splints can be useful adjuncts to therapy to regain motion in an involved joint or to rest a joint experiencing a disease flare. Three categories of splints are used: resting splints, corrective splints, and functional splints (Lindsley, 1999). Resting splints are used during active disease. Night resting splints place the wrist in a cock-up position (i.e., 20 degrees of wrist extension) and are the most common. Corrective splints include both serial casting and dynamic splints. Functional splints include supportive wrist splints that can be worn during the day, ankle-foot orthoses, molded shoe inserts, and heel cups (Lindsley, 1999).

Nutrition

Nutritional counseling is particularly recommended for children who are underweight, overweight, systemically ill, or taking long-term steroids (Henderson et al, 2000). Nutritional education and dietary changes are necessary to minimize weight gain associated with long-term corticosteroid treatment (see Primary Care Management).

Social Support

The chronicity and unpredictability of childhood arthritis and the necessary lifestyle changes lead to many situations in which psychologic support is helpful. Counseling, support groups, and peer activities such as camps for children with chronic diseases are helpful adjuncts to care (see Resources).

Surgery

Orthopedic surgery plays a very limited but important role in correcting joint deformities or replacing joints entirely (Cassidy & Petty, 2001; Drew, Cohen, & Witt, 1999). Arthroscopy is rarely performed for synovial biopsy or synovectomy. Prophylactic synovectomies are controversial, and their long-term benefits are limited, but they can be effective in selected cases (Sherry et al, 1998). For a child with functional impairment or secondary mechanical problems, soft tissue releases, osteotomies, posterior capsulotomy, and tendon lengthening may be performed (Cassidy & Petty, 2001; Prieur, 1998). Children with micrognathia (small, receded jaw) may profit

---

BOX 31-5
Children with Chronic Arthritis: Presurgical Considerations

Stop NSAID therapy 4-7 days before surgery to prevent excessive bleeding.
With long-term steroid use, give stress dose of corticosteroids PO/IV to prevent adrenal insufficiency.
Consult pediatric anesthesiologist for airway considerations. With neck or TMJ disease, obtain cervical and TMJ imaging studies.
Give prophylactic antibiotics for total joint replacements or if child is immunosuppressed.
Monitor child's preoperative complete blood count and platelet count.

NSAID, Nonsteroidal antiinflammatory drug; *PO,* by mouth; *IV,* intravenously; *TMJ,* temporomandibular joint.

---

from a combined orthodontic and surgical approach to temporomandibular disease.

Total joint replacements are beneficial to those with marked disability and pain secondary to joint destruction (Cassidy & Petty, 2001; Drew et al, 1999). Total hip and knee replacements usually result in major improvements in functional ability (Drew et al, 1999). As a child approaches adulthood and reaches bone maturity, reconstructive surgery plays a more vital role. Preoperative considerations for joint surgery and other surgical procedures are listed in Box 31-5.

Complementary and Alternative Therapies

The unpredictable, chronic, and sometimes progressive nature of childhood arthritis compels many parents to consider using treatments outside of standard medical practice for their children (Ernst, 1999). Approximately 68% of parents with a child with JRA have used an unconventional therapy or unproven remedy, such as wearing copper bracelets or using herbal or nutritional supplements (Tucker et al, 1996). Because parents are often reluctant to divulge their use of complementary and alternative treatments to the primary care provider, it is important to create an accepting environment where frustrations with conventional treatment can be aired and unproven remedies openly discussed. Primary care providers can help families differentiate between harmless and potentially harmful interventions and help them evaluate the claimed efficacy of unconventional remedies (Tucker et al, 1996). For example, many parents ask about the popular dietary supplements glucosamine and chondroitin sulfate. They should be informed that these substances have improved symptoms in osteoarthritis *only,* not inflammatory arthritis such as JRA and JSpAs (Reginster et al, 2001). Almost no controlled clinical trials for alternative therapies have been done on children, and therefore the risks and benefits are unknown (Henderson, 2002; Henderson & Panush, 1999). Potential risks include interaction with prescribed medications, financial considerations, and the perceived strain on the provider-client relationship (Tucker et al, 1996).

Cognitive behavioral therapy may be used to reduce stress, pain, and psychologic disability (Simon et al, 2002). Anecdotal reports from families reveal that some children do benefit from massage, relaxation techniques, visual imagery, and exercise such as Tai Chi or yoga. A study of 13 children with JRA showed significant pain reduction after an 8-week program of cognitive behavioral therapy. The investigators taught the children how to do progressive relaxation, meditative breathing, and guided imagery (Walco & Ilowite, 1992). Benefits include improved coping, pain control, and self-confidence. Moreover, the results were sustained 12 months after the intervention.

In general, parents are advised to be wary of any product that is labeled as a "cure" and to discuss any additional treatments with the rheumatology team. Parents can be reassured that when a significant medical advance is made, and reported in a reputable scientific journal, the rheumatology specialists will know about it (Arthritis Foundation, 1998).

Anticipated Advances in Diagnosis and Management

JRA and the JSpAs are considered complex genetic diseases. A current model of a pathogenetic mechanism for chronic arthritis in childhood involves a *tri*molecular complex. The complex is composed of an *HLA* (human leukocyte antigen/major histocompatibility [MHC]) gene product on antigen-presenting cells (macrophages, dendritic cells, B cells), which presents a peptide *antigen* to a T-lymphocyte via its *T-cell receptor* (TCR), which in turn specifically recognizes the antigen in the context of the HLA protein (Grom et al, 1994).

A molecular mimicry model has been proposed for the spondyloarthropathies and for Lyme disease, another cause of chronic arthritis in childhood. In this model, a foreign (infectious) peptide in the context of self-MHC triggers genetically susceptible hosts to mount an autoimmune response against self-antigens present in the joint space that appear similar to the foreign antigen (Marker-Hermann & Schwab, 2000; Trollmo et al, 2001). However, recent theories dispute even the requirement for immunologic recognition of HLA-B27 in the JSpAs (Turner & Colbert, 2002). Nevertheless, the interplay of certain genetically determined elements of the trimolecular complex is thought to trigger the inflammatory process through local release of proinflammatory cytokines (e.g., tumor necrosis factor [TNF]). Interesting insights into the pathology of different subgroups in JRA have been attained by the measurement of serum and synovial fluid cytokines and their agonists and antagonists (Murray et al, 1997; Woo, 1997). Ultimately, the classification schemes for the different forms of chronic childhood arthritis should incorporate criteria based on genetic susceptibility loci.

Thalidomide has been explored as a new therapy for steroid-dependent JRA with some success (Lehman et al, 2002). In addition, bone marrow transplantation has been reserved for the sickest of the children with polyarticular JRA. To date, the long-term effects and rates of remission following bone marrow transplantation for JRA are unknown. There has also been a significant percentage of deaths in these early attempts at autologous bone marrow transplantation for JRA (Barron et al, 2001). Time will tell whether thalidomide and/or bone marrow transplantation will become viable options for larger numbers of children with JRA. As newer biologics are made available, this may not even be an issue.

Associated Problems (Box 31-6)

Uveitis

Uveitis (i.e., iridocyclitis) is one of the most devastating complications associated with JRA (Cassidy & Petty, 2001) and remains one of the major causes of visual impairment in children (Reiff et al, 2001). Uveitis of JRA is a chronic, nongranulomatous inflammation that primarily affects the anterior uveal tract (iris, ciliary body) (Sherry et al, 1998). Persistent uveitis leads to multiple ocular complications, such as glaucoma, cataracts, band keratopathy, posterior synechiae, and loss of vision (Jarvis, 2002). Risk factors associated with developing uveitis include female gender, young age, ANA positivity, and pauciarticular onset. Uveitis is generally *asymptomatic*; therefore regular screening with a slit-lamp examination by a pediatric ophthalmologist is required for early detection (Box 31-7). When uveitis is symptomatic, the child may experience ocular pain and redness, change in vision, photophobia, headache, and eye pain. The pattern of remissions and exacerbations of uveitis does not parallel articular disease (Sherry et al, 1998).

Recently, several studies reported a decrease in prevalence of uveitis from greater than 21% to approximately 13% of children with JRA, possibly because more methotrexate and other systemic medications are used now to treat arthritis, thus preventing uveitis (Oren et al, 2000). Early and aggressive treatment of the uveitis with topical corticosteroid drops with or without a mydriatic drug has been effective in preserving the vision of children without advanced disease (Cassidy & Petty, 2001). Low-dose weekly methotrexate is considered the drug of choice for treating uveitis resistant to topical corticosteroids

Ophthalmologic Screening Schedule

High risk: every 3-4 mo
    Pauciarticular—ANA+, onset ≤7 yr
    Polyarticular—ANA+, onset ≤7 yr
Medium risk: every 6 mo
    Pauciarticular—ANA+, onset ≥7 yr
    Pauciarticular—ANA–, any age onset
    Polyarticular—ANA+, onset ≥7 yr
    Polyarticular—ANA–, any age onset
Low risk: yearly
    Systemic—any age onset

From American Academy of Pediatrics. (1993). Guidelines for ophthalmic examinations in children with juvenile rheumatoid arthritis. *Pediatrics, 92,* 295-296. Reprinted with permission.

(Reiff et al, 2001). Cataracts and glaucoma are associated with topical corticosteroid drops, and therefore methotrexate and other DMARDs are beginning to be used more frequently and earlier in the course of uveitis therapy (Cron, 2001). More recently, cyclosporine and etanercept have been used for treatment-resistant uveitis (Reiff et al, 2001).

Children with JSpA may develop a *symptomatic* iritis manifested by acute onset of eye pain, redness, and photophobia. The iritis is typically unilateral, recurrent, and frequently without residua (Petty & Cassidy, 2001a). With acute iritis, ophthalmology evaluation and treatment are required only when the eye symptoms are present. Therefore the child with JSpA does not need more than routine eye screening.

Skeletal and Growth Abnormalities

In childhood chronic arthritis, the growing skeleton undergoes unique deformities because of systemic and local growth disturbances. Up to 30% of children will develop generalized or local growth disturbances (Cassidy & Petty, 2001; Ostrov & Levine, 1999). Disease severity is a crucial factor in the association of skeletal abnormalities, bone mineralization, and low bone formation (Pepmueller et al, 1996). Each subgroup of JRA affects growth differently. Children with systemic onset and those requiring long-term steroids experience growth failure more than the other types (Ostrov & Levine, 1999). Factors contributing to short stature and growth abnormalities are largely a result of poor disease control, including undertreatment, side effects of corticosteroids, poor nutritional status, temporomandibular joint (TMJ) disease, vertebral fractures, and hip and knee contractures (Cron, 2001; Prahalad & Passo, 1998).

Chronic hyperemia of inflammation in a joint may accelerate maturation of the epiphyseal plates, resulting in skeletal overgrowth of the affected extremity (Ostrov & Levine, 1999; Prieur, 1998). This process is characteristically seen in children with early-onset pauciarticular disease who have unilateral knee involvement, bony enlargement of the medial femoral condyle, and valgus deformity (Lovell & Woo, 1998; Sherry et al, 1998). Eventually, limb shortening may result in chronic arthritis when there is premature fusion of the epiphyseal growth plates in the affected extremity (Cassidy & Petty, 2001).

TMJ involvement may lead to growth aberrations of the mandible and destruction of the condyle of the mandible, causing micrognathia, which has dental, nutritional, hygienic, speech, and cosmetic consequences. With destructive TMJ disease, combined orthodontic and reconstructive surgery may improve function, decrease pain, and improve appearance (Cassidy & Petty, 2001). Thus early treatment with adequate therapy, including the use of intraarticular injections for TMJ and peripheral joints, is imperative to prevent complications (Sherry et al, 1999; Wallace et al, 1994).

Characteristic abnormalities of the cervical spine in systemic or polyarticular disease include apophyseal joint space narrowing, irregularity and undergrowth of the vertebral bodies, fusion (especially at C2-C3), and atlantoaxial subluxation or instability leading to impingement on the spinal cord and brainstem (Cassidy & Petty, 2001; Lovell & Woo, 1998; Prieur, 1998). Stiffness and pain of the cervical spine with rapid loss of extension and rotation are common early findings in polyarticular JRA (Laxer & Schneider, 1998). Children with chronic arthritis have structural scoliosis more often than nonaffected children because of postural curves associated with asymmetric involvement of the lower limb joints causing pelvic tilting (Swann, 1998).

Hip pathology occurs in up to 50% of children with chronic arthritis. It is almost always bilateral and is usually associated with polyarticular arthritis. These children experience limitation of full flexion, abduction, and rotation as a result of iliopsoas and adductor muscle spasm (Laxer & Schneider, 1998). In time, anatomic changes in the hip from persistent inflammation may include femoral head overgrowth, decreased development of the femoral neck, and acetabular modifications with erosions or protrusions (Prieur, 1998). A compensatory lumbar lordosis can occur with a hip contracture. Flexion contractures of the knees are common. Children with arthritis of the knee joint can develop valgus of the knee with compensatory valgus deformity of the hindfoot and varus of the forefoot (Prieur, 1998). Subtalar joint involvement often results in a valgus deformity or, rarely, in a varus deformity. Disturbances of gait and balance can occur as a result of retarded growth and development of the feet with active persistent inflammatory disease (Lindsley, 1999).

Anemia and Systemic Disease

The anemia most often seen in JRA is a result of chronic disease and is more severe in systemic JRA. Its pathogenesis is unclear, but its severity correlates with underlying disease activity and inflammation. This anemia usually presents with low iron and transferrin, as well as with an elevated serum ferritin that does not typically respond to iron supplementation (Richardson et al, 1998). The anemia of chronic disease is normocytic and may be related to abnormal levels of hepcidin (Fleming & Sly, 2001). Children with poor nutrition or NSAID-induced gastrointestinal blood loss, however, may also develop iron deficiency anemia, resulting in microcytosis and hypochromia (Laxer & Schneider, 1998; Mulberg & Verhave, 1993).

Systemic JRA can involve significant extraarticular manifestations, including hepatosplenomegaly, lymphadenopathy, pericarditis, pleuritis, or other evidence of serositis (Cabral et al, 1992). Nutritional problems, especially protein energy malnutrition, are common in systemic JRA.

Prognosis

The prognosis for children with chronic arthritis depends on the disease type and course, severity during the first 6 months, degree of joint destruction, and complications (Prieur & Chedeville, 2001). A recent study suggests that children with JSpA and JRA have a favorable prognosis, with only one half requiring rheumatology care in adulthood (Minden et al, 2002). Different criteria for classification and remission, in addition to a lack of uniform methods to assess outcome, make a comparison of studies difficult (Cassidy & Petty, 2001; Tucker, 2000). In a Norwegian study (Flato et al, 1998) of 72 children with JRA and juvenile spondyloarthropathy over 10 years, remission occurred in 60%. This study demonstrated that (1) 60% of children had no disability on the Childhood or Adult Health Assessment Questionnaire; (2) 25% of children with JRA had joint erosions; (3) DMARDs were used in 68% of children after a disease duration of 0.8 years; and (4) having active disease 5 years after onset was a predictor of disability (Flato et al, 1998). Future studies are expected to show a more favorable prognosis because of the current trend toward early, aggressive treatment and because of the availability of newer targeted biologic agents.

Children with pauciarticular arthritis have a good prognosis for articular disease. In fact, 80% of these children have no musculoskeletal disability after 15 years of follow-up (Sherry et al, 1998). A recent study on long-term outcome and prognosis of children with pauciarticular disease identified two to four affected joints, upper limb involvement, and high ESR as predictors for poor outcome (Guillaume et al, 2000).

The prognosis in regard to uveitis is less favorable, however, ranging from remission without sequelae to severe visual loss. Children with a polyarticular course have a fair to poor prognosis for articular disease. Adolescent females presenting with a positive RF follow a course similar to those with adult-onset RA, developing persistent erosive joint disease (Cassidy & Petty, 2001). Children with systemic disease can have a monocyclic course with remission, a polycyclic course with exacerbations of systemic disease activity, or a course of persistent polyarticular arthritis without systemic features. Long-term studies show that 15% to 37% of children with chronic articular disease in this subset develop chronic destructive arthritis and have the poorest outcomes (Spiegal et al, 2000). The prognosis for the JSpAs is just as variable, depending on onset type, course, and complications. Children with SEA syndrome who have HLA-B27 positivity, arthritis at onset, and progressive occurrence of sacroiliac and back pain were found to be more likely to progress to ankylosing spondylitis in several studies (Prieur & Chedeville, 2001).

Primary Care Management

Health Care Maintenance

Growth and Development

Linear growth may be retarded or delayed during periods of active disease. Therefore monitoring height and weight via the growth chart is important. Some children have growth abnormalities that persist into adulthood. Osteopenia is a frequent finding in children with chronic arthritis. One study demonstrated that osteopenia was associated with decreased weight, decreased stature, decreased body mass index (BMI), protein energy malnutrition, decreased physical activity, and active chronic arthritis in postpubertal females, none of whom had received corticosteroid treatment (Henderson et al, 2000). Moreover, the current body of scientific knowledge demonstrates that children with a history of chronic arthritis are at an increased risk for the premature development of osteoporosis when studied as adults (Zak et al, 1999). Therefore assessment and recommendation of adequate calcium and vitamin D intake by foods, milk, or supplementation are crucial. Children with arthritis have higher calcium needs than normal children, and children receiving long-term steroid treatment have an even higher requirement (up to 2200 mg of calcium per day). The variety of forms of calcium supplementation includes chewable tablets, flavored chews, and regular tablets of varying dosages.

Children with chronic arthritis generally do not have any cognitive or language delay; however, they may have a delay in fine and gross motor skills. Fine motor skills are less likely to be delayed if the child is provided with toys and activities that encourage hand manipulation. Limited mobility and decreased opportunities to actively interact with the peer group place the child at a risk for both motor and social delays. In these areas, the child's rheumatology team, occupational therapist, and physical therapist can be valuable resources for primary care providers (Arthritis Foundation, 1998).

The acquisition of independence and self-care skills may be delayed in children with JRA. Certain skills, such as transition from a bottle to a cup or toilet training, should be postponed during periods of diagnosis or of active disease. Children with severe JRA often fall behind in acquiring hygiene, toileting, dressing, feeding, and handwriting skills. Regression in performance of these skills is common during acute illness and may be sustained during remissions as a result of lowered parental expectations and continued reinforcement of a child's dependent behaviors. Adaptive clothing (e.g., shoes with Velcro closures) and dressing aids can facilitate activities of daily living (ADLs). Every office visit can be an opportunity for discussion about and promotion of independence in a child with arthritis. Educational materials are available for parents of children with arthritis regarding growth and development (see Family Concerns and Resources). Moreover, developmentally appropriate functional assessment tools for children with arthritis exist. These include the following standard and validated tools: the Childhood Health Assessment Questionnaire (CHAQ), the Juvenile Arthritis Functional Assessment Report (JAFAR), and the Juvenile Arthritis Self-Report Index (JASI) (Tucker, 2000).

Diet

Nutritional problems are common in JRA. Factors contributing to the occurrence of these problems include increased inflammatory activity (i.e., hypercatabolism in the systemic subgroup), anorexia, gastrointestinal side effects of medication, physical limitations, depression, poor food choices, and limited movement of the TMJs. In addition, increased weight gain can occur with corticosteroid use because of increased appetite and fluid retention.

Alternative diets and dietary supplements have long been popular with people with rheumatic disease. The most common unconventional dietary remedies for arthritis are avoiding nightshade vegetables (e.g., potatoes, eggplant) and acidic foods (e.g., tomatoes), increasing dietary omega-3 fatty acids (found in fish), fasting, herbal remedies, and megavitamin therapy (Henderson, 2002). Although omega-3 fatty acids have been shown to cause improvement in adult rheumatoid arthritis (Harrison & Harrison, 2001; Grom & Passo, 1996), neither they nor any other specific dietary intervention has been proven to ameliorate the symptoms of arthritis in children. Given the current knowledge of childhood arthritis and diet, educating families about proper nutrition for a growing child with a chronic condition and evaluating potentially harmful dietary manipulations, especially those involving nutrient restrictions, are important responsibilities of the primary care provider. Nutritional education and referral to a dietitian may be indicated.

Safety

Education about medication safety is an important responsibility of the primary care provider. All medications must be kept in childproof containers out of reach of young children, which is especially important when older children assume responsibility for self-care (because of their limited grip strength, special grippers may be used to open containers). Children taking long-term immunosuppressant drugs are encouraged to wear Medic-Alert bracelets or necklaces. Photosensitive skin reactions may occur with several JRA medications, including naproxen and other NSAIDs, methotrexate, sulfasalazine (Azulfidine), and hydroxychloroquine (Plaquenil). Therefore hypoallergenic sun block lotion with a minimum sun protection factor (SPF) of 45 should be used on exposed skin.

Orthotic appliances are often recommended to prevent or correct deformities. Important safety issues related to splint wearing include care of the splint to maintain integrity, proper skin care, signs and symptoms of a poorly fitted splint (e.g., potential pressure points), and proper splint application. The splint should be adjusted to maintain correct function and ensure that the child has not outgrown it. Superficial heat and cold modalities are often recommended to relieve pain and stiffness. Determining the type of applications used by the family and reviewing safety precautions specific to each type of application are important.

Some children with JRA use adaptive equipment (e.g., elevated toilet seats) to minimize joint stress and increase independence. Adaptive equipment should be evaluated for the safety of all family members. Bath safety can be improved by the use of safety strips, rubber mats, wall grab bars, and tub chairs. As with all family members, a home fire safety plan should include a specific plan for the child with JRA.

Immunizations

Children with chronic arthritis in disease remission who are not taking immunosuppressive medications can receive all routine immunizations. If possible, children with arthritis should be immunized on schedule. Children whose immunocompetence is altered by antimetabolites such as methotrexate or by large doses of corticosteroids (2 mg/kg/day or more, a dose usually reserved for the sickest children with systemic JRA) should not receive live vaccines for at least 3 months after cessation of these medications (Committee on Infectious Disease, 2000). Fortunately, the polio vaccine is now administered as an inactivated virus (IPV). Live vaccinations (varicella, measles mumps rubella [MMR]) may be administered to children with JRA whose only exposure to steroids is topically applied ophthalmic medication or intraarticular injections or low-dose maintenance and/or physiologic doses (Committee on Infectious Disease, 2000). It is unknown if the newer biologic agents pose a significant risk for receiving live vaccines. At this time, one should avoid live vaccines when receiving these agents. All children with chronic arthritis should receive the current recommended influenza vaccine each year. Early concerns that influenza immunization may cause a disease flare seem to be unjustified (Cassidy & Petty, 2001). Overall, there has been a widespread concern about the possibility of immunizations causing a flare of the underlying disease or immunologic disorder in chronic arthritis. Anecdotal experience views this as a potential problem, but scientific data to support this theory do not exist. These concerns should not discourage primary care providers from immunizing children with chronic arthritis with inactivated vaccines.

Screening

Vision. A thorough funduscopic examination and visual acuity screening should be performed at each routine office visit. At the time of diagnosis, every child must be examined for uveitis by an ophthalmologist. Frequent ophthalmologic examinations are recommended for children at risk for uveitis, glaucoma, and cataracts. Eye examinations are scheduled every 3 to 6 months for children with pauciarticular and polyarticular disease. Young children with ANA-positive arthritis are at greatest risk for development of ocular inflammation. The rheumatology section of the American Academy of Pediatrics (1993) has developed an ophthalmologic screening schedule (Box 31-7). More frequent follow-up is needed for children with active uveitis. Medications such as corticosteroids can cause glaucoma or cataracts. Children taking hydroxychloroquine (Plaquenil) should have a baseline and biyearly ophthalmologic examination that includes visual field determinations.

Hearing. Routine office screening is recommended.

Dental. Dental visits should occur at least every 6 months and more frequently if malocclusions, crowded teeth, and dental caries occur as a result of TMJ disease. Orthodontic referrals are made as needed. Increased incidence of dental caries can potentially occur in children with JRA, possibly because of poor oral hygiene secondary to TMJ or upper extremity limitations. Malocclusions and crowded teeth occur as a result of micrognathia (Cassidy & Petty, 2001). Children with JRA should be checked for bleeding gums and poor dental hygiene. In these situations, consultation with the pediatric rheumatology team and the dentist is necessary. Routine dental visits are recommended, and orthodontic referrals are made as needed. Dental work for children who develop thrombocytopenia or leukopenia should be postponed until blood counts have returned to normal. Individuals with joint replacements should have prophylactic antibiotics before dental work (see Chapter 21).

Blood Pressure. Routine screening is recommended. Mild hypertension may occur in children taking NSAIDs. Steroid-induced hypertension can occur, although it is less frequent when lower doses are prescribed (Singsen & Rose, 1995).

Anemia. Hematologic testing is frequently ordered by the rheumatologist to screen for disease activity and medication toxicity. Therefore routine screening may not be required in the pediatric office.

Tuberculosis. Routine screening is recommended, especially before the initiation of TNF inhibitors.

Common Illness Management

Children with an established diagnosis of chronic arthritis will seek care for common childhood illnesses from the primary care provider. There are several signs and symptoms of common illnesses that need to be differentiated from a potential arthritis flare or from arthritis treatment, side effects, or toxicity.

Differential Diagnosis (Box 31-8)

Fever. The fever of systemic JRA is easily differentiated from the fever of an infectious process because of the characteristic pattern with normal or below normal temperature most of the day with once or twice daily high spikes. In addition, children with systemic JRA often appear ill and have a pronounced classic rash during the febrile spikes, but they are relatively well when afebrile. A careful history and complete physical examination usually determine the source of the fever.

Dermatologic Symptoms. The classic systemic JRA fever is usually accompanied by a rash of 2 to 6 mm evanescent (fleeting), salmon pink, generally circumscribed macular lesions. This rash may become confluent, with larger lesions developing pale centers and pale peripheries, and it is most commonly seen on the trunk, on the extremities, and over pressure areas, but the face, palms, and soles may also be involved. The rash is most prominent during fever spikes and may be visible only after the skin is rubbed or scratched. Stress or a hot bath may also induce the rash (Cassidy & Petty, 2001). Other types of rashes are rarely seen as part of the JRA condition and should be assessed and treated as are routinely done for children without JRA.

BOX 31-8

Differential Diagnosis of Chronic Arthritis vs. Treatment Side Effects vs. Other Illnesses

Fever: Rule out systemic JRA fever vs. infectious process.
Dermatologic: Rule out systemic JRA rash vs. infectious process vs. photosensitive skin reaction.
Otologic: Rule out referred TMJ pain vs. infectious process.
Respiratory: Rule out pleuritis vs. cricoarytenoid arthritis vs. infectious process.
Cardiac: Rule out pericarditis.
Gastrointestinal: Rule out NSAID gastropathy vs. drug-induced GI bleeding vs. inflammatory bowel disease associated with JSpA.
Renal: Rule out urinary tract infection vs. medication toxicity.

Photosensitive skin reactions may occur with several of the medications used to treat JRA, including naproxen, methotrexate, sulfasalazine, and hydroxychloroquine, with the most common rash being pseudoporphyria associated with naproxen (Naprosyn, Anaprox) and other NSAIDs (Cron & Finkel, 2000).

Otologic Symptoms. TMJ arthritis may cause referred pain to the ear, which should be considered when evaluating children for otitis media.

Respiratory Symptoms. Cricoarytenoid arthritis (i.e., laryngeal arthritis) can cause stridor, dyspnea, and cyanosis in JRA. Pleuritis and pericarditis can occur in systemic JRA. Rarely, methotrexate therapy may lead to hypersensitivity pneumonitis (Cron et al, 1998).

Gastrointestinal Symptoms. Gastrointestinal tract disease is rarely described in children with JRA. However, gastrointestinal symptoms may be difficult to evaluate because the medications can cause some degree of nausea, dyspepsia, abdominal pain, and diarrhea. Drug-induced gastrointestinal bleeding also must be considered in children receiving NSAIDs or steroids, particularly in those complaining of abdominal pain at night (Keenan et al, 1995). Peptic ulcers are rare in children on NSAID treatment, and they may present as chronic anemia secondary to occult blood loss. The classic peptic ulcer symptom of epigastric pain that improves with eating and worsens with an empty stomach is more common in adolescents and is virtually absent in young children. IBD should be ruled out in children experiencing major gastrointestinal problems. A careful history and physical examination, as well as consultation with the pediatric rheumatologist as needed, will help the primary care provider to evaluate the differential diagnoses.

Renal. Urinary tract infection vs. renal toxicity from medications must be considered with abnormal urinalyses.

Drug Interactions

Potential interactions exist among medications commonly used to treat JRA and over-the-counter or prescription drugs used to manage common pediatric conditions. Major drug interactions of concern to primary care providers are identified in Box 31-9. Generally, providers should not discontinue a child's condition-specific medications without consulting the pediatric rheumatologist. Conditions warranting temporary cessation of arthritis medications include the following: (1) exposure to chickenpox in unimmunized children; (2) significant bleeding of the nose, gums, or gastrointestinal tract; or (3) significant emesis and dehydration as a result of infectious illness. Communication with the rheumatology team would be essential in these circumstances.

Developmental Issues
Sleep Patterns

A child fatigues more readily during flares, especially with systemic JRA. The child may require periods of rest during the day. Teaching a child to recognize body signals, set limits and priorities, pace activities, and plan ahead will help conserve energy (Arthritis Foundation, 1998). The severity and duration of morning stiffness increase with increased disease activity. Recommendations to alleviate morning stiffness include

BOX 31-9
Potential Drug Interactions

Concurrent use of **NSAIDs** and **glucocorticoids** may increase risk of gastrointestinal side effects.

Antacids may alter the absorption rate of **NSAIDs** and **glucocorticoids**, resulting in subtherapeutic serum levels.

Methotrexate concentrations are increased by **NSAIDs**, which is generally not a concern in weekly low-dose methotrexate therapy.

Concomitant use of **methotrexate** and **alcohol** may increase the risk of gastrointestinal and hepatic side effects.

Sulfonamides may displace or be displaced by other highly protein-bound drugs (e.g., **NSAIDs**, **methotrexate**). Monitor children for increased effects (i.e., increased hepatotoxicity) of highly bound drugs when sulfonamides (e.g., **trimethoprim/sulfamethoxazole [Bactrim]**) are added.

Estrogen-based oral contraceptives may alter metabolism or protein binding, leading to decreased clearance and increased elimination, half-life, and therapeutic or toxic effects of **glucocorticosteroids**.

NSAIDs plus **acetaminophen** increase the risk of adverse hepatic side effects.

NSAIDs displace **anticoagulants** from protein binding sites.

NSAID, Nonsteroidal antiinflammatory drug.

TABLE 31-4
Common School Problems for Students with Chronic Arthritis

Problem	Intervention Strategies
Difficulty climbing stairs or walking long distance	Obtain elevator permit.
	Schedule classes to decrease walking and climbing.
	Have two sets of books: keep one in appropriate class, other at home.
	Use wheelchair if needed.
	Wear proper footwear—supportive sneakers.
Inactivity, stiffness from prolonged sitting	Move! Change position every 20 min.
	Sit to the side or back of the room to allow for standing or walking without disturbing the class.
	Ask to be assigned jobs that permit walking (pass out or collect papers).
Difficulty carrying books or cafeteria tray	Sit in an accessible desk.
	Use backpack for books.
	Have two sets of books.
	Determine cafeteria assistance plan (helper, reserved seat, wheeled cart) or pack lunch.
Handwriting problems (slow, messy, painful)	Use fat pen or pencil, crayons.
	Use a felt-tip pen.
	Use Dr. Grip pens and pencils.
	Stretch hands about every 10 min.
	Use a tape recorder for note taking.
	Use a computer for reports.
	Consider alternatives for timed tests (oral test, extra time, computer).
	Educate teacher; messy writing may be unavoidable at times.
Difficulty with shoulder movement, dressing, putting on coat, boots, tying shoes	Wear loose-fitting clothing without buttons or zippers.
	Use Velcro closures.
	Obtain adaptive equipment from an occupational therapist.
	Assistance may be needed for some things, especially on stiff days.
Reaching locker, opening locker	Modify locker, or use alternative place for storage.
	Have two lockers.
	Use key for locker instead of combination.
Raising hand	Devise alternative signaling method.

administration of medications 30 to 60 minutes before arising and stretching in a warm bath or shower before starting daily activities. In addition, flannel sheets, thermal underwear, warmed clothing, and a sleeping bag may decrease morning stiffness. An electric blanket with a timer set to warm the blanket 1 hour before a child is scheduled to wake is another option.

Toileting

The acquisition of self-care skills may be delayed in children with JRA. Toilet training should be postponed during periods of active disease because a child may lack the motivation and physical capability to perform tasks necessary for successful toileting. Limitations in the upper and lower extremities make it difficult for children to transfer on and off the toilet, manage toilet paper, and undress. Safety bars and elevated toilet seats are reliable assistive devices for children with lower extremity involvement. For children with upper extremity limitations, effective aids for wiping after toileting can be obtained from occupational therapists. Adaptive clothing and dressing aids can facilitate toileting. In severely affected children, bedpans, urinals, and commodes may also be required at night if pain and stiffness limit mobility.

Discipline

Parents of children with arthritis may have difficulty dealing with their guilt and concern over their child's condition. They may become overprotective and not handle behavioral issues as firmly as they would if the child was not "sick." In addition, overindulgence during periods of active disease alternating with normalization of discipline practices during remissions fosters inconsistent limit setting. The primary care provider can reinforce normalcy in childhood expectations, responsibilities, and chores, as well as appropriate behavioral expectations and discipline.

Child Care

Parents of children receiving medications may have difficulty locating child care providers who are willing to administer medications. For caregivers who accept this responsibility, parents can prepare a list that includes the name, dose, time, and method of administration, as well as the side effects of each medication. The parents should list the name and telephone number of the person to contact for questions or problems. Caregivers need to understand that chronic arthritis is characterized by fluctuations in disease activity and symptoms. Therefore a child's functional capacity, energy level, and developmental progress may change on different days. Education about the child's abilities, limitations, disease, and treatments is likely to decrease anxiety among caregivers and promote appropriate interactions among caregivers, children, and families. Infants and young children with chronic arthritis may be eligible for special education services and related services under Public Law (PL) 99-457 and PL 101-476 (see Chapter 5).

Schooling

Children with chronic arthritis can participate fully in school, physical education, and extracurricular activities with certain interventions and adaptations listed in Table 31-4. Many children have special needs that must be communicated to the school by verbal and written communication and addressed in an individualized educational plan (IEP; see Chapter 5). Most pediatric rheumatology centers have a standard letter for the school nurse and personnel that describes the condition and recommended adjustments. Educating school personnel about morning stiffness and variability of clinical manifestations is very important. Severe disease flare-ups or surgery may necessitate temporary home instruction and should be planned for in a child's IEP.

Primary care providers can periodically question children and parents about school-related problems, such as fatigue, distractibility, limited mobility, absences, and medications. The provider may interface with the family, school staff, and pediatric rheumatology team to identify and remedy problems before, or when, they occur. The student can participate in school athletic programs with modifications as necessary. Swimming as a sport is strongly encouraged since it strengthens muscle groups around joints, provides good range of motion therapy, is less stressful on joints than weight-bearing activities of contact sports, and promotes aerobic fitness.

Sexuality

Sexual maturation may be delayed in adolescents with chronic arthritis, especially in those with systemic disease. Menarche has been shown to occur later in girls with JRA (mean age 13.2 years) than in unaffected controls (mean age 12.5 years) because of active inflammatory disease (Ostrov & Levine, 1999; Petty, 1998). Contraceptive advice should include discussion of interactions among arthritis medications and various oral contraceptives, as well as any effects of arthritis medications on fertility and fetal development (Siegel & Baum, 1999). This is particularly important for young women taking methotrexate, which can act as a teratogen to the fetus (Buckley et al, 1997).

Obstetric management of women with JRA who are pregnant is best managed with a team effort between an obstetrician and rheumatologist (Ostrov & Levine, 1999). In a retrospective study of 76 pregnancies in 51 women with JRA, the following two conclusions were reached: (1) pregnancy had no adverse effects on the signs and symptoms of JRA, and (2) maternal and fetal outcomes of pregnancy were generally good (Ostensen, 1991).

Transition into Adulthood

Thoughtful planning for transition into adulthood is necessary and useful. The optimal goal of health care transition planning for the teenager with arthritis is to provide coordinated, uninterrupted care that addresses the developmental topics of this age period (Rettig & Athreya, 1999), including vocational, career, sexuality, independence, and financial issues. Successful health care transition is influenced by a number of variables. These include: the serious shortage of internist-rheumatologists in the United States, the limited number of pediatric rheumatology programs associated with adult tertiary centers, delayed emotional maturity and learned dependency of some adolescents, fear of "moving on" to adult care, overprotectiveness of parents, health insurance restrictions, and/or lack of health insurance (Rettig & Athreya, 1999). The primary care provider can promote the transition process for the teenager in many ways. The provider can help the family identify a local rheumatologist, encourage independence in self-care, address adolescent developmental issues, counsel parents and teens, and refer to community programs as needed. In the future, the primary care provider will have an increasing role as a family advocate, family counselor, and care coordinator and will be expected to work with schools and community agencies to promote successful transition of teenagers with chronic disease (Kelly, 1995).

Family Concerns and Resources

Raising a child with chronic arthritis can be difficult. There are many misconceptions about arthritis. Families must repeatedly explain and educate others that arthritis is not just a problem to be quickly remedied by the multitudes of treatment offered on television advertisements and in magazines. Others often believe that arthritis is a condition affecting only older people and express disbelief when children discuss their arthritis. After hearing about the diagnosis, well-meaning family and friends sometimes tend to overwhelm the family with information about the diagnosis and "cures" of which they have heard or read. Children with arthritis often appear healthy, which makes it difficult to explain their need for modifications at school and work. They have appropriate concerns about school attendance, sports participation, growth, and any limitations that make them feel different. Parents have concerns about long-term side effects of medications (e.g., fertility), whereas children are more concerned about the short-term effects (e.g., cushingoid facies with corticosteroids).

Children are asked to engage in several treatment regimens, such as medications, exercise, lifestyle changes, splint wear, and added appointments to the primary care provider, rheumatologist, ophthalmologist, and other specialists. The child, adolescent, or parent may decide not to comply with the recommendations. Families and older children need to be made aware of the risk/benefit ratios of treatments and the consequences of poor adherence to treatment regimens. The primary care provider has the longest relationship with the family and can therefore encourage and support adherence, refer to social services (e.g., when finances or transportation interferes with treatment), and promote parental supervision and organization when necessary (Rapoff, 2002). Teaching problem-solving and decision-making skills and utilizing contracts are helpful strategies to use with the adolescent.

Even with all these issues, however, children with arthritis have been found to be remarkably similar to controls on measures of social functioning, emotional well-being, and behavior, suggesting considerable psychologic hardiness among children with chronic arthritis (Noll et al, 2000). Key family resources and programs are available through several organizations. Families of children with chronic arthritis are strongly encouraged to utilize these educational and support services.

RESOURCES

American Juvenile Arthritis Organization (AJAO)
Arthritis Foundation National Office
1330 West Peachtree Street NW
Atlanta, GA 30309
(404) 872-7100 (ext. 6277); (800) 283-7800
www.arthritis.org

The AJAO is a national membership association of the Arthritis Foundation that serves the special needs of young people with rheumatic diseases and their families. The AJAO provides local, regional, and national family conferences, quarterly newsletters, and printed educational materials for children, parents, and health professionals. In addition, local chapters of the Arthritis Foundation may offer summer camps, pen pal clubs, and family support groups. Educational literature and information about these programs are available on the Arthritis Foundation's Web site. AJAO offers the following materials:

"Arthritis in Children," "When Your Student Has Arthritis," "Decision Making for Teenagers with Arthritis" (pamphlets)
Arthritis Today (magazine)
Educational Rights for Children with Arthritis: A Manual for Parents (manual)
Kids Get Arthritis Too (newsletter)
Raising a Child with Arthritis—A Parents' Guide (book)

Other Resources

National Institute of Arthritis and Musculoskeletal and Skin Diseases Information Clearinghouse
NIAMS/National Institutes of Health
www.nih.gov/niams/healthinfo

Tucker, L.B. et al. (1996). *Your child with arthritis—a family guide for caregiving*, Baltimore: Johns Hopkins University Press.

Transition Resources

National Center for Youth with Disabilities
University of Minnesota, Box 721-UMHC
420 Delaware Street SE
Minneapolis, MN 55455
(612) 626-2825
www.peds.umn.edu/peds-adol/NCYD.html

Post-secondary Education for Individuals with Disabilities
HEATH Resource Center
2121 K Street, NW, Suite 220
Washington, DC 20037
(202) 973-0904; (800) 544-3284
www.heath.gwu.edu

Acknowledgment   The authors would like to acknowledge the work done by Gail R. McIlvain-Simpson and Patricia M. Reilly on previous editions of this chapter.

Summary of Primary Care Needs for the Child with Juvenile Rheumatoid Arthritis and Juvenile Spondyloarthropathy

HEALTH CARE MAINTENANCE

Growth and Development

Linear growth may be delayed during active systemic disease.

Catch-up growth occurs with disease control or during remission.

Corticosteroids may suppress growth at doses >0.15 mg/kg/day.

Poor weight gain may be a result of systemic disease.

Excessive weight gain may occur as a result of decreased activity, depression, poor nutrition, or corticosteroid usage.

Gross motor delays and temporary regressions are not uncommon during periods of flares/ active disease.

Fine motor skills are less likely to be affected.

Standard infant development screening tools are of questionable value with severely affected children.

Age-appropriate physical activities are important and should be based on a child's capabilities, energy level, and activity tolerance.

Diet

The risk of protein-calorie malnutrition is increased.

Increased inflammatory activity, anorexia, gastrointestinal side effects of medication, physical limitations, depression, corticosteroid usage, poor food choices, and limited movement of the temporomandibular joint (TMJ) may contribute to nutritional problems.

Calcium intake in the diet should be assessed and supplementation provided if necessary.

A daily vitamin should be added.

"Arthritis diets" should be evaluated for nutritional adequacy, and families should be educated about proper nutrition for a growing child with a chronic disease.

Safety

Childproof containers should be used for medications.

Children taking immunosuppressive agents should wear a Medic-Alert bracelet or necklace.

Safety issues related to splint wear, heat and cold applications, and adaptive equipment should be reviewed.

Sun block should be used on exposed skin because of photosensitive skin reactions occurring with some medications.

Immunizations

Children who are not taking immunosuppressive drugs or experiencing systemic disease symptoms should be routinely immunized.

In the absence of neurologic symptoms, a child with classic, intermittent JRA fever can be immunized during febrile episodes.

No live virus vaccines (varicella, measles mumps rubella [MMR]) should be given to children receiving antimetabolites, large doses of corticosteroids, or biologic agents.

All children with chronic arthritis should receive the current recommended influenza vaccine each year.

Screening

Vision. A funduscopic examination and acuity screening should be performed at each visit. Children should be examined by an

Continued

Summary of Primary Care Needs for the Child with Juvenile Rheumatoid Arthritis and Juvenile Spondyloarthropathy—cont'd

ophthalmologist for uveitis (Box 31-7). Children taking topical or systemic steroids require close ophthalmologic follow-up.

Hearing. Routine visits are recommended.

Dental. Children with TMJ involvement and micrognathia should have frequent dental visits (at least every 6 months). Prophylactic antibiotics should be used for dental work in children with total joint replacements or those taking steroids.

Blood Pressure. Routine screening is recommended.

Laboratory Monitoring. Complete blood count (CBC), differential, erythrocyte sedimentation rate (ESR), C-reactive protein (CRP), platelet count, urinalysis, and liver function tests are routinely ordered by the rheumatologist to monitor disease activity, response to therapy, and drug toxicity and to assess for anemia of chronic disease.

Tuberculosis. Routine screening is recommended.

COMMON ILLNESS MANAGEMENT

Differential Diagnosis

Fever. Classic, intermittent JRA fever should be differentiated from infectious processes.

Dermatologic. Rheumatoid rash should be ruled out in systemic JRA. Drug-related photosensitivity skin reactions should be ruled out.

Otologic. TMJ arthritis with referred ear pain should be differentiated from otitis media.

Respiratory. Colds and flu may cause arthritis flare-ups. Infectious processes must be differentiated from pleuritis or cricoarytenoid arthritis.

Gastrointestinal. Drug-related gastrointestinal symptoms should be differentiated from a gastroenteritis infection. Drug-related gastropathy should also be differentiated from inflammatory bowel disease associated with JSpA.

Renal. Urinary tract infection should be distinguished from medication toxicity.

DEVELOPMENTAL ISSUES

Sleep Patterns

Fatigue associated with disease flares may necessitate rest periods during the day.

Recommendations to promote comfort and sleep and to alleviate morning stiffness (e.g., use of electric blanket with timer) should be discussed with the family.

Toileting

Training should be postponed during periods of active disease.

Assistive devices may be needed with individuals with severe disease, joint deformities, and limited mobility.

Discipline

Overprotection, overindulgence, and inconsistent limit setting should be identified. Reinforce the need for consistent expectations (e.g., daily chores). Discuss impact of chronic arthritis on age-specific developmental tasks so parents have a framework for decision making about discipline.

Child Care

Caregivers will need to be knowledgeable of medications, use of assistive devices, and applying splints.

Parents should provide caregivers with information about child's medications.

Caregivers should be educated on the effect of JRA on a child's functional capacity, energy level, and developmental progress.

A home-based, single-provider daycare setting rather than group child care is recommended for children taking steroids or immunosuppressants.

Most infants and young children with JRA are eligible for Public Law (PL) 99-457 and PL 101-476 educational programs.

Schooling

PL 101-476 entitles most students with JRA to occupational therapy, physical therapy, adaptive physical education, and transportation to and from school, home, and facilities where services are provided (Table 31-4).

Most students with JRA can participate in modified school athletic programs "to their own tolerance level."

Disease flare-ups or surgery may necessitate home instructions for a brief period.

Teaching families about their educational rights and how to advocate for their child in school is important.

Sexuality

Puberty may be delayed in children with JRA.

Discussion of puberty, sexual activity, appropriate contraception, and pregnancy is imperative with all adolescents.

Medication modifications (i.e., methotrexate is an abortifacient and is teratogenic) must be made before planning a pregnancy.

Transition into Adulthood

Adolescents can be referred to the state office of vocational rehabilitation for assistance with postsecondary educational opportunities.

Primary care providers can assist the family with decisions regarding health care, psychosocial, vocational, financial, and family issues.

Teenagers are advised to avoid drinking any alcohol. Alcohol significantly increases the risk of liver toxicity when taking methotrexate.

FAMILY CONCERNS

Family frustration and concern over the lack of a cure and the unpredictability of the illness should be acknowledged.

The impact of the illness on the child's ability to fully participate in school, sports, and social activities raises concerns for parents.

Multiple treatment regimens and concern about side effects may lead to nonadherence.

Referral for psychosocial and family issues may be necessary.

Encouragement to participate in educational and support programs (see Resources) is helpful to families.

REFERENCES

American Academy of Pediatrics. (1993). Guidelines for ophthalmic examinations in children with juvenile rheumatoid arthritis. *Pediatrics, 92,* 295-296.

Ansell, B. (1994). Juvenile psoriatic arthritis. *Baillieres Clin Rheumatol, 8*(2), 317-332.

Arkachasisri, T. & Lehman, T. (2000). Use of biologics in the treatment of childhood rheumatic diseases. *Curr Rheumatol Rep, 2*(4), 330-336.

Arthritis Foundation. (1998). *Raising a child with arthritis: A parents guide.* Atlanta: Author.

Baeten, D., De Keyser, F., Mielants, H., & Veys, E.M. (2002). Immune linkages between inflammatory bowel disease and spondyloarthropathies. *Curr Opin Rheumatol, 14*(4), 342-347.

Barron, K.S., Wallace, C., Woolfrey, C.E., Laxer, R.M., Hirsch, R., et al. (2001). Autologous stem cell transplantation for pediatric rheumatic diseases. *J Rheumatol, 28*(10), 2337-2358.

Bauman, C., Cron, R.Q., Sherry, D.D., & Francis, J.S. (1996). Reiter syndrome initially misdiagnosed as Kawasaki disease. *J Pediatr, 128*(3), 366-369.

Bloom, B.J., Tucker, L.B., Miller, L.C., & Schaller, J.G. (1998). Fibrin D-dimer as a marker of disease activity in systemic onset juvenile rheumatoid arthritis. *J Rheumatol, 25*(8), 1620-1625.

Breit, W., Frosch, M., Meyer, U., Heinecke, A., & Ganser, G. (2000). A subgroup-specific evaluation of the efficacy of intraarticular triamcinolone hexacetonide in juvenile chronic arthritis. *J Rheumatol, 27*(11), 2696-2702.

Brunner, H. et al. (2001). Current medication choices in juvenile rheumatoid arthritis II—Update of a survey performed in 1993. *J Clin Rheum, 7,* 295-300.

Buckley, L.M., Bullaboy, C.A., Leichtman, L., & Marquez, M. (1997). Multiple congenital anomalies associated with weekly low-dose methotrexate treatment of the mother. *Arthritis Rheum, 40*(5), 971-973.

Burgos-Vargas, R., Vazquez-Mellado, J., Cassis, N., Duarte, C., Casarin, J., et al. (1996). Genuine ankylosing spondylitis in children: A case-control study of patients with early definite disease according to adult onset criteria. *J Rheumatol, 23*(12), 2140-2147.

Cabral, D., Oen, K., & Petty, R. (1992). SEA syndrome revisited: A long-term follow-up of children with a syndrome of seronegative enthesopathy and arthropathy. *J Rheumatol, 19*(8), 1282-1285.

Cassidy, J. (1999). Medical management of children with juvenile rheumatoid arthritis. *Drugs, 58*(5), 831-850.

Cassidy, J. & Petty, R. (2001). Juvenile rheumatoid arthritis. In J. Cassidy & R. Petty (Eds.). *Textbook of pediatric rheumatology* (4th ed.). Philadelphia: W.B. Saunders.

Committee on Infectious Diseases. (2000). *2000 Red book: Report of the Committee on Infectious Diseases* (24th ed.). Elk Grove Village, Ill.: American Academy of Pediatrics.

Cron, R.Q. (2001). Treatment for JRA in the new millenium. *J Clin Rheum, 7*(5), 1-3.

Cron, R.Q. & Finkel, T.H. (2000). Nabumetone induced pseudoporphyria in childhood. *J Rheumatol, 27*(7), 1817-1818.

Cron, R.Q. & Finkel, T.H. (2002). Approach to the child with joint pain. In S. West (Ed.). *Rheumatology secrets* (2nd ed.). Philadelphia: Hanley & Belfus Inc, pp. 483-490.

Cron, R.Q., Sharma, S., & Sherry, D.D. (1999). Current treatment by United States and Canadian pediatric rheumatologists. *J Rheumatol, 26*(9), 2036-2038.

Cron, R.Q., Sherry, D.D., & Wallace, C.A. (1998). Methotrexate-induced hypersensitivity pneumonitis in a child with juvenile rheumatoid arthritis. *J Pediatr, 132*(5), 901-902.

Drew, S., Cohen, B., & Witt, J. (1999). Surgical management of adolescents with rheumatic diseases. In D. Isenberg & J. Miller (Eds.). *Adolescent rheumatology.* Malden, Mass.: Blackwell Science Inc.

Ernst, E. (1999). Prevalence of complementary/alternative medicine for children: A systematic review. *Eur J Pediatr, 158,* 7-11.

Faustino, P.C., Terreri, M.T., Andrade, C.T., Len, C., & Hilario, M.O. (2001). Clinical features of spondyloarthropathies in childhood: Analysis of 26 patients. *Rev Assoc Med Bras 47*(3), 216-220.

Flato, B., Aasland, A., Vinje, O., & Forre, O. (1998). Outcome and predictive factors in juvenile rheumatoid arthritis and juvenile spondyloarthropathy. *J Rheumatol, 25*(2), 366-375.

Fleming, R. & Sly, W. (2001). Hepcidin: A putative iron-regulatory hormone relevant to hereditary hemochromatosis and the anemia of chronic disease. *Proc Natl Acad Sci USA, 98*(15), 8160-8162.

Foeldvari, I. & Bidde, M. (2000). Validation of the proposed ILAR classification criteria for juvenile idiopathic arthritis. *J Rheumatol, 27*(4), 1069-1072.

Foeldvari, I., Burgos-Vargas, R., Thon, A., & Tuerck, D. (2002). High response rate in the phase I/II study of meloxicam in juvenile rheumatoid arthritis. *J Rheumatol, 29*(5), 1079-1083.

Garcia-Consuegra Molina, J., Merino Munoz, R., Fernandez Revuelta, S., & Soler Balda, C. (1998). Juvenile spondyloarthropathies: Descriptive study of 40 patients. *An Esp Pediatr, 48*(5), 489-494.

Gare, B. (1999). Juvenile arthritis—Who gets it, where, and when? A review of current data on incidence and prevalence. *Clin Exp Rheumatol, 17*(3), 367-374.

Gerloni, V., Cimaz, R., Gattinara, M., Arnoldi, C., Pontikaki, I., et al. (2001). Efficacy and safety profile of cyclosporin A in the treatment of juvenile chronic (idiopathic) arthritis: Results of a 10-year prospective study. *Rheumatology, 40*(8), 907-913.

Glass, D. & Giannini, E. (1999). Juvenile rheumatoid arthritis as a complex genetic trait. *Arthritis Rheum, 42*(11), 2261-2268.

Grom, A., Giannini, E., & Glass, D. (1994). Juvenile rheumatoid arthritis and the trimolecular complex (HLA, T-cell receptor, and antigen). *Arthritis Rheum, 37,* 601-607.

Grom, A. & Hirsch, R. (2000). T-cell and T-cell receptor abnormalities in the immunopathogenesis of juvenile rheumatoid arthritis. *Curr Opin Rheumatol, 12,* 420-424.

Grom, A. & Passo, M. (1996). Macrophage activation syndrome in systemic juvenile rheumatoid arthritis. *J Pediatr, 129*(5), 630-632.

Guillaume, S., Prieur, A.M., Coste, J., & Job-Deslandre, C. (2000). Long-term outcome and prognosis in oligoarticular-onset juvenile idiopathic arthritis. *Arthritis Rheum, 43*(8), 1858-1865.

Harrison, R. & Harrison, B. (2001). Fish oils are beneficial to patients with established rheumatoid arthritis. *J Rheumatol, 28*(11), 2563-2565.

Hashkes, P.J., Balistreri, W.F., Bove, K.E., Ballard, E.T., & Passo, M.H. (1997). The long-term effect of methotrexate therapy on the liver in patients with juvenile rheumatoid arthritis. *Arthritis Rheum, 40*(12), 2226-2234.

Henderson, C. (2002). The use of dietary supplements in rheumatic diseases: What evidence exists? *Biomechanics, 4*(9), 1-10.

Henderson, C. & Panush, R. (1999). Diets, dietary supplements, and nutritional therapies in rheumatic diseases. *Rheum Dis Clin North Am, 25*(4), 937-968.

Henderson, C.J., Specker, B.L., Sierra, R.I., Campaigne, B.N., & Lovell, D.J. (2000). Total-body bone mineral content in non-corticosteroid-treated postpubertal females with juvenile rheumatoid arthritis: Frequency of osteopenia and contributing factors. *Arthritis Rheum, 43*(3), 531-540.

Jarvis, J. (2002). Juvenile rheumatoid arthritis: A guide for pediatricians. *Pediatr Ann, 31*(7), 437-446.

Keenan, G., Giannini, E., & Athreya, B. (1995). Clinically significant gastropathy associated with nonsteroidal anti-inflammatory drug use in children with juvenile rheumatoid arthritis. *J Rheumatol, 22,* 1149-1151.

Kelly, A. (1995). The primary care provider's role in caring for young people with chronic illness. *J Adolesc Health Care, 4,* 261-265.

Klepper, S. (1999). Effects of an eight-week physical conditioning program on disease signs and symptoms in children with chronic arthritis. *Arthritis Care Res, 12*(1), 52-60.

Kulas, D. & Schanberg, L. (2001). Juvenile idiopathic arthritis. *Curr Opin Rheumatol, 13*(5), 392-398.

Laxer, R. & Schneider, R. (1998). Systemic-onset juvenile chronic arthritis. In P.J. Maddison, et al. (Eds.). *Oxford textbook of rheumatology* (2nd ed.). Oxford, England: Oxford University Press.

Lehman, T., Striegel, K., & Onel, K. (2002). Thalidomide therapy for recalcitrant systemic onset juvenile rheumatoid arthritis. *J Pediatr, 140*(1), 125-127.

Lindsley, C. (1999). Rehabilitation and recreation. In D. Isenberg & J. Miller (Eds.). *Adolescent rheumatology.* Malden, Mass.: Blackwell Science Inc.

Lovell, D.J., Giannini, E.H., Reiff, A., Cawkwell, G.D., Silverman, E.D., et al. (2000). Etanercept in children with polyarticular juvenile rheumatoid arthritis: Pediatric Rheumatology Collaborative Study Group. *N Engl J Med, 342*(11), 763-769.

Lovell, D. & Woo, P. (1998). Growth and skeletal maturation. In P.J. Maddison et al. (Eds.). *Oxford textbook of rheumatology* (2nd ed.). Oxford, England: Oxford University Press.

Luong, A. & Salonen, D. (2000). Imaging of the seronegative spondyloarthropathies. *Curr Rheumatol Rep, 2*(4), 288-296.

Manners, P. & Bower, C. (2002). Worldwide prevalence of juvenile arthritis—Why does it vary so much? *J Rheumatol, 29,* 1520-1530.

Marker-Hermann, E. & Schwab, P. (2000). T-cell studies in the spondyloarthropathies. *Curr Rheumatol Rep, 2*(4), 297-305.

McGhee, J.L., Burks, F.N., Sheckels, J.L., & Jarvis, J.N. (2002). Identifying children with chronic arthritis based on chief complaints: Absence of predictive value for musculoskeletal pain as an indicator of rheumatic disease in children. *Pediatrics, 110*(2), 354-359.

Minden, K., Niewerth, M., Listing, J., & Zink, A.; German Study Group of Pediatric Rheumatologists. (2002). Health care provision in pediatric rheumatology in Germany—National rheumatologic database. *J Rheumatol, 29*(3), 622-628.

Mulberg, A.E. & Verhave, M. (1993). Identification and treatment of nonsteroidal anti-inflammatory drug-induced gastroduodenal injury in children. *J Pediatr, 122*(4), 647-649.

Murray, K., Thompson, S., & Glass, D. (1997). Pathogenesis of juvenile chronic arthritis: genetic and environmental factors. *Arch Dis Child, 77*(6), 530-534.

Murray, K.J., Grom, A.A., Thompson, S.D., Lieuwen, D., Passo, M.H., et al. (1998). Contrasting cytokine profiles in the synovium of different forms of juvenile rheumatoid arthritis and juvenile spondyloarthropathy: Prominence of interleukin 4 in restricted disease. *J Rheumatol, 25*(7), 1388-1398.

Noll, R.B., Kozlowski, K., Gerhardt, C., Vannatta, K., Taylor, J., et al. (2000). Social, emotional, and behavioral functioning of children with juvenile rheumatoid arthritis. *Arthritis Rheum, 43*(6), 1387-1396.

Oren, B., Sehgal, A., Simon, J.W., Lee, J., Blocker, R.J., et al. (2000). The prevalence of uveitis in juvenile rheumatoid arthritis. *J Aapos, 5*(1), 2-4.

Ostensen, M. (1991). Pregnancy in parents with a history of juvenile rheumatoid arthritis. *Arthritis Rheum, 34*, 881-887.

Ostrov, B. & Levine, R. (1999). Interactions of puberty with rheumatic diseases, contraception and gynecological issues. In D. Isenberg & J. Miller (Eds.). *Adolescent rheumatology.* Malden, Mass.: Blackwell Science Inc.

Padeh, S. & Passwell, J. (1998). Intraarticular corticosteroid injection in the management of children with chronic arthritis. *Arthritis Rheum, 41*(7), 1210-1214.

Palm, O., Moum, B., Jahnsen, J., & Gran, J.T. (2001). The prevalence and incidence of peripheral arthritis in patients with inflammatory bowel disease, a prospective population-based study (the IBSEN study). *Rheumatology, 40*(11), 1256-1261.

Pepmueller, P.H., Cassidy, J.T., Allen, S.H., & Hillman, L.S. (1996). Bone mineralization and bone mineral metabolism in children with juvenile rheumatoid arthritis. *Arthritis Rheum, 39*(5), 746-757.

Peschken, C. & Esdaile, J. (1999). Rheumatic diseases in North America's indigenous peoples. *Semin Arthritis Rheum, 28*(6), 368-391.

Petty, R. (1998). Clinical presentation in different age groups. In P.J. Maddison, et al. (Eds.). *Oxford textbook of rheumatology* (2nd ed.). New York: Oxford University Press.

Petty, R. (2001). Growing pains: The ILAR classification of juvenile idiopathic arthritis. *J Rheumatol, 28*(5), 927-928.

Petty, R. & Cassidy, J. (2001a). Juvenile ankylosing spondylitis. In J. Cassidy & R. Petty (Eds.). *Textbook of pediatric rheumatology* (4th ed.). Philadelphia: W.B. Saunders.

Petty, R. & Cassidy, J. (2001b). The juvenile idiopathic arthritides. In J. Cassidy & R. Petty (Eds.). *Textbook of pediatric rheumatology* (4th ed.). Philadelphia: W.B. Saunders.

Petty, R.E., Southwood, T.R., Baum, J., Bhettay, E., Glass, D.N., et al. (1998). Revision of the proposed classification criteria for juvenile idiopathic arthritis: Durban, 1997. *J Rheumatol, 25*(10), 1991-1994.

Prahalad, S. & Passo, M. (1998). Long-term outcome among patients with juvenile rheumatoid arthritis. *Front Biosci, 3*, e13-e22.

Prahalad, S., Ryan, M.H., Shear, E.S., Thompson, S.D., Giannini, E.H., et al. (2000a). Juvenile rheumatoid arthritis: Linkage to HLA demonstrated by allele sharing in affected sib pairs. *Arthritis Rheum, 43*(10), 2335-2338.

Prahalad, S., Ryan, M.H., Shear, E.S., Thompson, S.D., Glass, D.N., et al. (2000b). Twins concordant for juvenile rheumatoid arthritis. *Arthritis Rheum, 43*(11), 2611-2612.

Prieur, A. (1998). Rheumatoid factor negative polyarthritis in children (seronegative polyarthritis). In P.J. Maddison, et al. (Eds.). *Oxford textbook of rheumatology* (2nd ed.). Oxford, England: Oxford University Press.

Prieur, A. & Chedeville, G. (2001). Prognostic factors in juvenile idiopathic arthritis. *Curr Rheumatol Rep, 3*(5), 371-378.

Rapoff, M. (2002). Assessing and enhancing adherence to medical regimens for juvenile rheumatoid arthritis. *Pediatr Ann, 31*(6), 373-379.

Reginster, J.Y., Deroisy, R., Rovati, L.C., Lee, R.L., Lejeune, E., et al. (2001). Long-term effects of glucosamine sulphate on osteoarthritis progression: A randomised, placebo-controlled clinical trial. *Lancet, 357*(9252), 251-256.

Reiff, A., Takei, S., Sadeghi, S., Stout, A., Shaham, B., et al. (2001). Etanercept therapy in children with treatment-resistant uveitis. *Arthritis Rheum, 44*(6), 1411-1415.

Rettig, P.A. & Athreya, B.H. (1999). Leaving home—Preparing the adolescent with arthritis for coping with independence in the adult rheumatology world. In D. Isenberg & J. Miller (Eds.). *Adolescent rheumatology.* Malden, Mass.: Blackwell Science Inc.

Richardson et al. (1998). Haematology. In P.J. Maddison et al. (Eds.). *Oxford textbook of rheumatology* (2nd ed.). Oxford, England: Oxford University Press.

Scull, S. (2000). Physical therapy for the child and adolescent with juvenile rheumatoid arthritis. In J. Melvin & F. Wright (Eds.). *Rheumatologic rehabilitation series,* vol. 3. *Pediatric rheumatic diseases.* Bethesda, Md.: American Occupational Therapy Association Incorporated, pp. 199-222.

Sherry, D.D., Bohnsack, J., Salmonson, K., Wallace, C.A., & Mellins, E. (1990). Painless juvenile rheumatoid arthritis. *J Pediatr, 116*(6), 921-923.

Sherry, D.D., Stein, L.D., Reed, A.M., Schanberg, L.E., & Kredich, D.W. (1999). Prevention of leg length discrepancy in young children with pauciarticular juvenile rheumatoid arthritis by treatment with intraarticular steroids. *Arthritis Rheum, 42*(11), 2330-2334.

Sherry, D.D. et al. (1998). Pauciarticular-onset juvenile chronic arthritis. In P.J. Maddison et al. (Eds.). *Oxford textbook of rheumatology* (2nd ed.). Oxford, England: Oxford University Press.

Siegel, D. & Baum, J. (1999). Adolescent rheumatic disease and sexuality. In D. Isenberg & J. Miller (Eds.). *Adolescent rheumatology.* Malden, Mass.: Blackwell Science Inc.

Simon, L. et al. (2002). *Guideline for the management of arthritis pain in osteoarthritis, rheumatoid arthritis, and juvenile chronic arthritis.* Glenview, Ill.: Clinical Pain Society.

Singsen, B. & Rose, C. (1995). Juvenile rheumatoid arthritis and the pediatric spondyloarthropathies. In M. Weissan & M. Weinblatt (Eds.). *Treatment of the rheumatic diseases: Companion to the textbook of rheumatology.* Philadelphia: W.B. Saunders.

Spiegel, L.R., Schneider, R., Lang, B.A., Birdi, N., Silverman, E.D., et al. (2000). Early predictors of poor functional outcome in systemic-onset juvenile rheumatoid arthritis: A multicenter cohort study. *Arthritis Rheum, 43*(11), 2402-2409.

Swann, M. (1998). Surgery in children. In Maddison, P.J. et al. (Eds.). *Oxford textbook of rheumatology.* New York: Oxford University Press.

Takken, T., van der Net, J., & Helders, P. (2001). Do juvenile idiopathic arthritis patients benefit from an exercise program? A pilot study. *Arthritis Care Res, 45*(1), 81-85.

Trollmo, C., Meyer, A.L., Steere, A.C., Hafler, D.A., & Huber, B.T. (2001). Molecular mimicry in Lyme arthritis demonstrated at the single cell level: LFA-1 alpha L is a partial agonist for outer surface protein A-reactive T cells. *J Immunol, 166*(8), 5286-5291.

Tucker, L. (2000). Outcome measures in childhood rheumatic diseases. *Curr Rheumatol Rep, 2*(4), 349-354.

Tucker, L. et al. (1996). *Your child with arthritis—A family guide for caregiving.* Baltimore: Johns Hopkins University Press.

Turner, M.J. & Colbert, R.A. (2002). HLA-B27 and pathogenesis of spondyloarthropathies. *Curr Opin Rheumatol, 14*(4), 367-372.

Van den Dende, C.H., Vliet Vlieland, T.P., Munneke, M., & Hazes, J.M. (1998). Dynamic exercise therapy in rheumatoid arthritis: A systematic review. *Br J Rheumatol, 37*(6), 677-687.

Varni, J. & Bernstein, B. (1991). Evaluation and management of pain in children with rheumatic diseases. *Rheum Dis Clin North Am, 17*, 985-1000.

Walco, G.A. & Ilowite, N.T. (1992). Cognitive-behavioral pain management in children with juvenile rheumatoid arthritis. *Pediatrics, 89*, 1075-1089.

Wallace, C.A. (2000). Methotrexate: More questions than answers. *J Rheumatol, 27*(8), 1834-1835.

Wallace, C.A. (1998). The use of methotrexate in childhood rheumatic diseases. *Arthritis Rheum, 41*(3), 381-391.

Wallace, C.C., Farrow, D., & Sherry, D.D. (1994). Increased risk of facial scars in children taking nonsteroidal antiinflammatory drugs. *J Pediatr, 125*(5, pt. 1), 819-822.

Wallace, C.C. & Sherry, D.D. (1997). Trial of intravenous pulse cyclophosphamide and methylprednisolone in the treatment of severe systemic-onset juvenile rheumatoid arthritis. *Arthritis Rheum, 40*(10), 1852-1855.

Walton, A.G., Welbury, R.R., Foster, H.E., & Thomason, J.M. (1999). Juvenile chronic arthritis: A dental review. *Oral Diseases, 5*(1), 68-75.

Woo, P. (1997). The cytokine network in juvenile rheumatoid arthritis. *Rheum Dis Clin North Am, 23*(3), 491-498.

Zak, M., Hassager, C., Lovell, D.J., Nielsen, S., Henderson, C.J., et al. (1999). Assessment of bone mineral density in adults with a history of juvenile chronic arthritis: A cross-sectional long-term follow-up study. *Arthritis Rheum, 42*(4), 790-798.

32 Mood Disorders

June Andrews Horowitz and Carol Marchetti

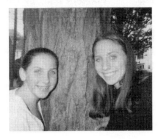

MOOD disorders in children and adolescents are not a single clinical entity with clearly determined etiology or predictable lifetime course. Rather, mood disorders include a range of mental health difficulties that feature depressed mood with or without mania and loss of pleasure or interest, and disorders characterized by mania in varying degrees with or without depression. All mood disorders in children and adolescents commonly manifest age-specific associated features. Even when diagnostic criteria for a mood disorder are met, a myriad of paths can lead to its development, continuation, and recurrence (Kaslow et al, 2000). Moreover, research outcomes have indicated that most children who experience depression also manifest a co-morbid problem, most commonly an anxiety disorder. Determination of a mood disorder in children necessitates consideration of the combination, severity, and duration of symptoms (Stark et al, 2000).

According to the *Diagnostic and Statistical Manual of Mental Disorders* (ed. 4), text revision *(DSM-IV-TR)* (American Psychiatric Association [APA], 2000), mood disorders encompass several diagnoses and their subtypes. Mood disorders are organized as depressive disorders (unipolar depression), bipolar disorders, and two etiologically based disorders: mood disorder caused by a general medical condition and substance-induced mood disorder. The diagnoses falling under depressive disorders are distinguished from bipolar disorders by a lack of any type of manic episode or features in the history. Conversely, bipolar disorders do involve current or past manic episodes or manic features in the presentation. Table 32-1 summarizes the diagnostic categories that make up the mood disorders according to *DSM-IV-TR*.

Etiology

Etiology of childhood mood disorders is multifaceted without a single, clear causal pathway (Stark et al, 2000). Considerable evidence has accumulated to indicate that mood disorders are the same fundamental disorders experienced by children, adolescents, and adults (Kaplan & Sadock, 1998); nevertheless, developmental factors in onset, course, and prognosis may be discerned. Etiologic variables identified in the research literature indicate that a variety of psychosocial and biologic factors contribute to development of a depressive disorder; even less is known about the etiology of bipolar disorders. Further, although a group of causal variables may emerge from research, etiologic factors for a given child may well differ from those of another child, and variables are likely to interact with each other and with stress to produce and maintain a disorder (Stark et al, 2000).

Psychosocial Factors

Models of depression have been developed from psychodynamic, interpersonal, cognitive, behavioral, and sociologic theoretic perspectives. No single model is adequate to explain the variations across personal history, family and peer relationships, social environment, or other factors among youth who experience depression or to explicate how some children with psychosocial risk factors for depression escape a mood disorder. However, several important psychosocial risks with empiric support are negative thinking, inadequate self-regulation, poor interpersonal relations, and family factors (Birmaher et al, 1996).

Negative Thinking. Cognitive theories of depression, developed in relation to adults (Beck, 1967; Seligman, 1975), focus on negative thinking as a cause of depressed mood. The *learned helplessness* model of depression first evolved from animal studies that demonstrated that lack of control over aversive events led to a state of helplessness (Seligman, 1975). In the revised model, cognitive attribution is the operative process. A negative attributional style in which a person takes responsibility for bad events and outcomes characterizes individuals prone to depression. Blaming oneself is an *internal attribution*; seeing the cause as unchanging is a *stable attribution*; and generalizing the cause to most situations is a *global attribution*. Such attributions create learned helplessness that can lead to hopelessness and ongoing depression (Abramson et al, 1978).

According to Beck's cognitive theory of depression (1967), biased and negative beliefs lead to faulty interpretations of life events. Problematic cognitive processing involves automatic thoughts about events based on selective attention to negative information, assumption of blame about events, exaggeration of negative outcomes, and minimization of positive aspects of events. Distortions in thinking, characterized as the *depressive cognitive triad* of thoughts about the self, the world, and the future, are thought to generate feelings of worthlessness and hopelessness that characterize depression. Rigid and enduring cognitive schemata guide information processing and do not yield to new information that could contradict negative self-perceptions.

Cognitive models of depressive disorders are useful templates for evaluation of distorted thinking and undergird cognitive therapy approaches to treatment. Clinicians who work with depressed youth validate the presence of negative interpretations of events, self-blame, and poor self-esteem. However, cognitive development among children and adolescents progresses through stages that are not comparable to adult cognitive processing that formed the foundation for this model (Mash & Wolfe, 1999). Therefore clinicians are cautioned to

TABLE 32-1

Diagnostic DSM-IV-TR Categories for Mood Disorders

Diagnosis	Summary of Key Characteristics
Major depressive disorder	Presence of one or more major depressive episodes
Dysthymic disorder	Chronically depressed mood most days for at least 1 yr for children and adolescents; criteria not met for major depressive episode
Bipolar I disorder	Presence of one or more manic episodes or mixed episodes (i.e., manic *and* major depressive)
Bipolar II disorder	Presence of one or more major depressive episodes and one or more hypomanic episodes
Cyclothymic disorder	Chronic mood disturbance with alternating periods of hypomanic and depressive symptoms; criteria not met for major depressive episode or manic episode
Depressive disorder not otherwise specified	Disorders with depressive features that do not meet criteria for other disorders
Bipolar disorder not otherwise specified	Disorders with bipolar features that do not meet criteria for other disorders
Mood disorder caused by a general medical condition	Mood disturbance caused by direct psychologic effects of a medical condition
Substance-induced mood disorder	Mood disturbance caused by direct physiologic effects of a substance

Data from American Psychiatric Association. (2000). *Diagnostic and statistical manual of mental disorders* (4th ed.). Washington, D.C.: Author.

evaluate cognitive distortions in relation to any child's developing sense of self and to weigh whether these cognitions reflect depression.

Inadequate Self-Regulation. According to self-control theory (Rehm, 1977), problems in self-monitoring, self-evaluation, and self-reinforcement contribute to development of depression. Children with inadequate self-regulation are likely to attend to negative events, establish excessively high standards for self-performance, furnish inadequate personal rewards, and use excessive self-punishment (Mash & Wolfe, 1999; Schwartz et al, 1998). Children with depression have shown self-regulation problems (Kaslowet et al, 1988; Rehm & Sharp, 1996); however, ongoing research is needed to provide more substantive empiric support.

Poor Interpersonal Relations and Family Factors. Problematic peer relations have been associated with depression in children and adolescents. Ongoing teasing and bullying, negative interactive patterns that affect 9% to 15% of children, involve social exclusion, physical violence, threats, sexual and racial harassment, and public humiliation (Nansel et al, 2001). Youth who experience long-term teasing and bullying are at increased risk for detrimental psychologic effects, including depression, anxiety, low self-esteem, social withdrawal, violent retaliation, and suicide (Forero et al, 1999; Muscari, 2002). Depressed youth also tend to exhibit aversive behaviors that produce annoyance and frustration in others (Mash & Wolfe, 1999; Schwartz et al, 1998)—exacerbating a cycle of rejection, withdrawal, social isolation, and ongoing depression.

The function of problematic family relations in development and continuation of childhood depressive disorders is yet to be explicated fully; however, direct and indirect family influences

have been described. Stark et al (2000) synthesized the literature in this area to propose a possible pathway for family influences. The route may begin with parental transmission of a genetic predisposition to a depressive disorder. When present, parental psychopathology has a negative effect on interactions within the family and interferes with the parent's ability to nurture, show affection, and support the child. Other family environmental factors, such as conflict, instability, substance abuse, and child maltreatment, may converge to increase the child's risk for development of a depressive disorder. Stress reaction models also have been proposed to explain how stressful life events, such as parental death, put children at risk for depression. In diathesis-stress models, individual vulnerability and the nature of the stressor interact to determine if depression will result (Mash & Wolfe, 1999).

Biologic Factors

Contributions of psychophysiologic factors to childhood depressive disorders are being explored and are thought to lie beneath the expression of depressive symptoms. The ability of various antidepressant medications to alleviate depressive symptoms indicates that neurotransmitter systems contribute to development and maintenance of depression. In particular, deficits in the monoamine transmitters (norepinephrine, serotonin, dopamine) and an excessive number of binding sites for these neurotransmitters are likely to be present in depressed individuals (Stark et al, 2000). The monoamine hypothesis of depression is evolving to include the possibility that depression results from a deficiency in signal transmission from the monoamine neurotransmitter to its postsynaptic neuron in the presence of normal levels of neurotransmitter and receptors rather than from a deficiency in amounts of the neurotransmitter or receptors (Stahl, 2000). Monoaminergic mechanisms play a role in regulating sleep, arousal, and response to stimuli (Stark et al, 2000).

Monoamine neurotransmitters and the neuroendocrine systems are related. Serotonin and norepinephrine are involved in limbic system functioning that regulates drives, emotions, and instincts. The hypothalamic-pituitary-thyroid (HPT) axis and the hypothalamic-pituitary-adrenal (HPA) axis are associated with depression. Dysregulations in the HPT and HPA axes modulate reactions to stress (Stark et al, 2000). Overactivation of the HPA axis is the most common biologic dysfunction in major depression. Cortisol, a stress hormone, increases in response to stress and has been related to depression. Hypercortisolemia may be linked to more severe depressive symptoms (Wolkowitz & Reus, 2001). Chronic stress may produce changes in monoamines in people who are prone to depression (Dinan, 1994). Results of research concerning neurobiologic factors in depression among children and adolescents indicate that young people who experience depression may have increased sensitivity to stress rather than a chronic dysregulation (Mash & Wolfe, 1999). A cycle may be fueled by continued neuroendocrine activation related to stress that raises risk for depression; chronic depression symptoms may lead in turn to continued activation and repeated psychosocial stresses (Birmaher et al, 1996).

Hormonal alterations also may contribute to depression risk in children and adolescents. For girls, the presence of estrogen has been associated with depression and estrogen may be related to differences in growth hormone (GH) secretion, including increased secretion among girls (Stark et al, 2000). However, contrasting evidence has indicated that estrogen is likely to mitigate depression in women. Through various mechanisms, estrogen increases the concentration and availability of serotonin in the brain (Sherman, 2001). Birmaher et al (2000) found decreased GH response to pharmacologic stimulation among children and adolescents during a major depressive episode and after recovery. When considered together with previous evidence, these results indicated that decreased GH response may be a trait marker for at-risk children and adolescents. Thyroid hormones also have been implicated in depression, but prevalence of abnormalities and pathophysiologic importance remain controversial (Wolkowitz & Reus, 2001). A relationship between hypothyroidism and depression in children suggests that the HPT axis is involved, but inconsistent responses to thyroid replacement therapy indicate that age may mediate this connection (Stark et al, 2000).

Causal pathways and interactions among neuroendocrine and neurotransmitter systems are only partially understood. "The complex relation between hormones and the HPA and HPT axes, which are mutually regulated with the monoamine neurotransmitters, contribute to the complexity of biological explanations for depression" (Stark et al, 2000, p. 308). Evidence to support biologic etiology of depressive disorders among adults is evolving, although no single model is fully explanatory. Less is known about developmental factors. Further research is needed to uncover psychobiologic mechanisms and interactions among processes that contribute to development and persistence of depression among children and adults.

Biologic rhythms involving mutual influences of sleep-wake cycles, neuroendocrine activity, and body temperature that respond to the cyclic light-dark patterns of day and night are implicated in mood disorders (Stark et al, 2000). Depressive sleep is shallow, fragmented, and shortened. During mania, sleep is fragmented and shortened, and people experience a decreased need for sleep. Unlike their depressed counterparts, people experiencing a manic episode do not feel a need for more sleep and may be energized after only 3 or 4 hours of sleep. In individuals vulnerable to bipolar disorders, sleep disruption may trigger hypomania or mania, leading to a self-reinforcing cycle of insomnia and sleep disturbance causing reduced sleep that instigates mania; in turn, mania creates need for less sleep, and thus the cycle may be perpetuated (Szuba et al, 2001). The processes involved in mutual interaction among development, sleep disturbance, and mood disorders in children and adolescents remain to be uncovered through future research.

Known Genetic Etiology

Evidence to support genetic etiology for childhood- and adolescent-onset mood disorders is extensive. No single gene abnormality has been linked to depression, and such a discovery is unlikely. Current thinking posits that multiple sites in deoxyribonucleic acid (DNA) within the genome interact independently, additively, or synergistically in combination with multiple environmental inputs to produce most depressions (Stahl, 2000).

New theories that integrate both genetic and environmental risk factors for depression propose that stress, possibly acting through monoaminergic neurotransmission, can cause depression by down-regulating critical genes, so that their key gene products are not produced (Stahl, 2000, p. 77).

Outcomes from family studies have indicated that a genetic link exists. Results of twin studies have demonstrated that monozygotic twins are at higher risk for depressive disorders than are dizygotic twins. Further, researchers who studied monozygotic twins raised separately reported a 67% concordance rate for depressive disorders, confirming that genetics make an important contribution (Stark et al, 2000). Family studies have produced complementary data. Major depressive disorder is 1.5 to 3 times more common among first-degree biologic relatives of people with this disorder (APA, 2000). First-degree relatives of adolescents with major depressive disorder have an increased lifetime incidence of depression and other psychiatric diagnoses (Williamson et al, 1995). Early onset also has been associated with depression in first-degree relatives (Harrington et al, 1996).

Empiric support from family, twin, and adoption studies has established a genetic contribution to the etiology of bipolar disorders. Having one parent with a bipolar disorder creates a 10% to 30% risk for the disorder. Odds increase to 75% when both parents have bipolar disorder. Among affected individuals, 90% have one or more biologic relatives with the disorder (Laraia, 2002).

Inheritance of bipolar disorders is likely to be multifactorial, and as many as 10 chromosomes may be involved (Laraia, 2002). In order for the disorder to manifest, additive or subtractive effects of multiple genes may be required (Philibert et al, 1997). However, researchers have not identified a specific genetic biochemical abnormality, and practitioners continue to base their diagnoses on clinical history, presentation, and evaluation (National Institute of Mental Health [NIMH] Genetics Initiative Bipolar Group, 1997). Moreover, genetic and environmental factors are likely to interact, and multiple genes may have a modifying, causative, or protective role in development of bipolar disorders. "We submit that for an individual to develop bipolar affective disorder, both a particular complement of susceptibility genes and their interactions with environmental risk factors are undoubtedly required" (Philibert et al, 1997, p. 2).

Incidence and Prevalence

Among adults, mood disorders have been widely studied and incidence rates have been determined for each of the diagnostic categories. For children and adolescents, prevalence estimates are less robust; however, evidence is accumulating that these disorders are serious problems for a significant number of youth and that they tend to persist and recur. Overall prevalence for mood disorders in children and adolescents is estimated to range from 2% to 5% in community samples and from 10% to as high as 50% in psychiatric samples (Schwartz et al, 1998).

Mood disorders in youth increase with increasing age. Preschool children rarely exhibit criteria for major depressive disorder. Estimates of prevalence for preschoolers are 0.03% in the community and 0.09% in psychiatric clinic settings.

School-aged children have an estimated incidence of 2%. Among adolescents, incidence rises to approximately 5% in the community, and 33% to 48% of adolescents have self-reported symptoms (Pullen et al, 2000). Among youth hospitalized for psychiatric reasons, approximately 20% of school-aged children and 40% of adolescents have major depressive disorder (Kaplan & Sadock, 1998).

Childhood-onset dysthymic disorder (i.e., a disorder characterized by unremitting low level depression) (Table 32-1), is less common than major depressive disorder with rates from 0.6% to 1.7% (Mash & Wolfe, 1999) but may be as high as 5% to 8% among young adolescents (Kaplan & Sadock, 1998). Because dysthymic disorder does not present with symptoms that meet criteria for major depressive disorder and may be more insidious or long-standing, many cases may remain unrecognized. More important, many children and adolescents go on to experience a major depressive disorder within 1 year of onset of dysthymic disorder (Kaplan & Sadock, 1998).

Bipolar disorder is less common than either major depressive disorder or dysthymic disorder. In pediatric populations, estimates have ranged from 0 .04% to 1.2% (Kaplan & Sadock, 1998; Lewinsohn et al, 1995). Rapid cycling of mood symptoms among children and adolescents may mask presence of bipolar I disorder (i.e., mood disorder characterized by presence of mania with or without depression). Rapid mood cycling also may lead to higher estimates for the less severe diagnoses of bipolar II (i.e., depression with hypomania) and cyclothymic disorder (i.e., a disorder characterized by numerous periods of hypomanic symptoms) (Table 32-1; Lewinsohn et al, 1995; Mash & Wolfe, 1999); moreover, as many as 10% of adolescents may exhibit some variant of mania (Kaplan & Sadock, 1998).

Increasing recognition of bipolar disorder in youth is a developing trend in psychiatric practice. Estimates of childhood disorders are rising, and average age of onset is falling from the early 30s to late teens over the course of a single generation (Laraia, 2002). Wozniak and colleagues (2001) have challenged the predominant view that pediatric-onset bipolar disorder is a rare condition. They reported that childhood mania constituted 16% of referrals to their clinic. Although this high rate in part may be a by-product of the authors' expert status and the widespread regard that clinicians have for their clinic at Massachusetts General Hospital, the percentage of children identified is likely to represent a growing recognition of childhood-onset mania as an underidentified and significant clinical problem.

Clinical Manifestations at Time of Diagnosis (Box 32-1)

Early detection of mood disorders in pediatric primary care practice is essential. Without adequate assessment, referral to specialists in pediatric mental health psychiatric evaluation and treatment, and ongoing monitoring and management by primary care providers, youth with mood disorders are more likely to experience more severe symptoms, greater chronicity, and more serious functional impairment. A primary care clinician (PCP) may be the only health care professional who observes the child, and therefore the clinician must seize the opportunity to perform a mental status evaluation, initiate treatment, and make a referral when indicated. The PCP is reminded to be mindful that the signs and symptoms of psychiatric illness are often more subtle than other common physical childhood ailments, yet the devastating effects of psychiatric illness can be pervasive and destructive.

BOX 32-1

Clinical Manifestations of Mood Disorders

Mood	Somatic	Behavior	Loss of Pleasure or Interest	Cognitive
Irritable	Vague complaints without specific illness or injury	Drop in grades	Going through the motions	Poor concentration
Sad		Poor social, academic, or occupational functioning	Bored or apathetic attitude	Indecisiveness
Gloomy	Body or facial expressions of depressed mood		Not feeling satisfaction	
Hopeless	Weight loss	Withdrawal or dropping out of activities or play	Lack of enjoyment in usual activities or play	Thoughts of death or suicide
Down	Decrease or increase in appetite	Isolation from peers		Play themes of worthlessness, guilt, death, suicide, self-destruction
Blue		Frequent angry outbursts		
Moody	Failure to meet expected weight gains for age	Temper tantrums (older child or adolescent)		Self-reproach
Grouchy				Poor or exaggerated self-esteem
Depressed	Insomnia or excessive sleeping	Excessive goal-driven or pleasure-oriented activities		
Anxious				Grandiosity
Apathetic	Diminished need for sleep			Slowed thoughts
Angry	Fatigue	Pressured speech or excessive talkativeness		Flight of ideas or racing thoughts
Cranky	Low energy			
Feeling worthless	Psychomotor retardation			Distractibility
Guilty	Psychomotor agitation			
Abnormally expansive or elated				
Euphoric				

Depressive Disorders

Major Depressive Disorder. Children and adolescents do experience depression. Unfortunately, until recently not all clinicians appreciated this. Until the 1980s researchers conducted few studies to explore depression among children and adolescents, and many clinicians even debated its existence (Scahill 2001a; Stark et al, 2000). Others considered depression to be part of normal development or a rare or transitory occurrence (Schwartz et al, 1998). Childhood depressive disorders were not even included in the psychiatric diagnostic classification until publication of *DSM-III* (APA, 1980).

Major depressive disorder, also referred to as unipolar depression, requires the presence of one or more major depressive episodes. According to the current *DSM-IV-TR* (APA, 2000), a depressive episode has common characteristics for adults as well as for children and adolescents. The essential feature of a major depressive episode is a 2-week or longer period during which a person experiences depressed mood or loss of interest or pleasure (anhedonia) in most activities. Descriptions such as feeling sad, gloomy, hopeless, down, blue, moody, grouchy, or depressed characterize mood. Children and adolescents often present with irritable mood rather than sadness. Therefore modification in symptom presentation regarding children and adolescents includes presence of *irritable* rather than only depressed or sad mood (Kaplan & Sadock, 1998). Apathetic or anxious mood may obscure the presence of an underlying depressed mood. Somatic complaints sometimes are the vehicle of expression for depression. To ascertain if the child or adolescent is feeling depressed, the clinician can question carefully and comment on nonverbal cues, for example, "You look like you might start to cry as you talk." Facial expression and body language also may infer depres-sion. Angry outbursts over rather minor events and frustrations suggest depression. Thus irritability and "cranky" mood are common features of a depressive episode for children and adolescents (APA, 2000; March & Wolfe, 1999) (Box 32-2).

Decreased interest or loss of pleasure also typifies a depressive episode. Family members may note reduced participation in activities and lack of enjoyment of formerly pleasurable activities. For children and adolescents, withdrawal from activities and friends is cause for concern. Finding excuses to avoid activities such as sports practice or school events can signal depression. Changes from previous behavior also characterize depression, including a drop in academic performance or conduct disturbances (APA, 2002a; March & Wolfe, 1999; Stark et al, 2000).

In addition to having one of the hallmarks of depressed mood or loss of interest or pleasure, four or more out of nine additional diagnostic criteria for a major depressive episode must be met, or an additional three if both depressed mood and loss of interest are present (for a total of at least five criteria). These criteria are found in Box 32-2. The presenting symptoms must cause distress and functional impairment, do not meet criteria for a mixed episode (i.e., episode with mania), are not caused by effects of a substance or medical condition, or are not better accounted for by the bereavement diagnosis (APA, 2000).

Although research to validate clinical presentation of major

BOX 32-2

Diagnostic Criteria for a Major Depressive Episode

Five or more symptoms either (a) depressed mood or (b) loss of interest or pleasure.
  (a) Depressed mood most of the day, most days, and/or diminished interest or
  (b) Pleasure in all/most activities most of the day, most days.
Additional symptoms:
  Significant loss of weight when not dieting, or increase or decrease in appetite nearly every day (For children, failure to achieve expected weight gains is considered.)
  Insomnia or excessive sleeping almost every day
  Observable psychomotor agitation or retardation
  Fatigue or reduced energy almost every day
  Feeling worthless or excessively guilty (even if delusional) almost every day
  Reduced ability to concentrate or think, or indecisiveness almost every day
  Continuing thoughts of death or suicide without a plan, a plan to commit suicide, or a suicide attempt

Data from American Psychiatric Association. (2000). *Diagnostic and statistical manual of mental disorders* (4th ed.). Washington, D.C.: Author.

---

depressive disorder for children and adolescents is limited, available data confirm that diagnostic criteria developed for adults apply within the context of a child's development. Luby et al (2002) investigated the validity of developmentally modified *DSM-IV* criteria for preschool major depressive disorder. Preschool children with major depressive disorder displayed expected age-adjusted symptoms of depression based on diagnostic criteria, as well as vegetative signs. Major depressive disorder symptoms differentiated these children from nonsymptomatic controls and controls with another psychiatric diagnosis. Anhedonia, or lack of pleasure in activities and play, could serve as a marker for major depressive disorder because only the depressed group exhibited this diagnostic marker. Death-related or suicidal themes in play also were present for 61% of the depressed group. These data provide new evidence that preschool children manifest major depressive disorder with typical age-adjusted symptoms, including vegetative signs (Box 32-3).

To investigate adolescent-onset depression symptoms, Patton et al (2000) assessed 1947 Australian adolescents. Over the 30-month study, 69 participants met criteria for depressive episodes. Diminished pleasure and interest, lessened energy and increased fatigue, disturbed sleep, decreased concentration, and thoughts of suicide differentiated depressed adolescents from controls. As depression severity increased, guilt and self-reproach, psychomotor retardation and/or agitation, and appetite and weight changes increased the most in frequency. In addition, depressed mood was endorsed by 94% of depressed adolescents but also by 20% of controls.

Dysthymic Disorder. Dysthymic disorder, also considered a unipolar depressive disorder, is characterized by a chronically depressed mood experienced most of the day on more days than not for at least 1 year for children and adolescents and for 2 years for adults (APA, 2000). The specifier "early onset" indicates occurrence before age 21 years. As in major depressive disorder, mood may be more irritable or "cranky" than sad or

Proposed Adjustments to DSM-IV-TR Criteria for Depression for Preschoolers

Five (or more) of the following symptoms have been present *but not necessarily persistently** over a 2-week period and represent a change from previous functioning; at least one of the symptoms is either (1) depressed mood or (2) loss of interest or pleasure *in activities or play. If both (1) and (2) are present a total of only 4 symptoms is needed.*

1. "Depressed mood *for a portion of the day for several days,* as observed (or reported) in behavior. Note: may be irritable mood."
2. "Markedly diminished interest or pleasure in all, or almost all, activities *or play for a portion of the day for several days* (as indicated by either subjective account or observation made by others)."
3. "Feelings of worthlessness or excessive guilt (even if delusional) *that may be evident in play themes.*"
4. "Diminished ability to think or concentrate, or indecisiveness, *for several days* (either by subjective account or as observed by others)."
5. "Recurrent thoughts of death (not just fear of dying), recurrent suicidal ideation without specific plan, or a suicide attempt or specific plan for committing suicide. *Suicidal or self-destructive themes are persistently evident in play only*" (p. 931).

Data from Luby, J.L., Heffelfinger, A.K., Mrakotsky, C., Hessler, et al. (2002). Preschool major depressive disorder: Preliminary validation for developmentally modified *DSM-IV* criteria. *J Am Acad Child Adolesc Psychiatry, 41,* 928-937.

*Suggested changes in *DSM-IV-TR* diagnostic criteria are indicated in italics.

"down." Two or more of the following symptoms are needed in addition to presence of depressed mood for a diagnosis of dysthymic disorder: "poor appetite or overeating, insomnia or hypersomnia, low energy or fatigue, low self-esteem, poor concentration or difficulty making decisions, and feelings of hopelessness" (APA, 2000, p. 377). Additional APA criteria specify conditions for diagnosis and factors for consideration in differential diagnosis by psychiatric clinicians.

When compared with youth with major depressive disorder, children and adolescents with dysthymic disorder typically have fewer neurovegetative symptoms, such as sleep disturbance, agitation, or restless behavior; seldom exhibit anhedonia (lack of pleasure) or social withdrawal; and are less likely to have thoughts of dying or somatic complaints (Kovacs et al, 1994; Mash & Wolfe, 1999). Moodiness, irritability, anger, sadness, poor self-esteem, and temper outbursts occur more prominently in dysthymic disorder than in major depressive disorder (Renouf & Kovacs, 1995). Youth with dysthymic disorder may experience "double depression" (Hersen & Ammerman, 2000, p. 295) when major depressive disorder develops. Clinicians may miss the presence of underlying dysthymia because of the more florid presentation of an acute major depressive episode indicative of major depressive disorder. However, such "double depression" negatively affects long-term prognosis and therefore merits careful evaluation (Hersen & Ammerman, 2000).

Bipolar Disorders

In 2000, the National Institute of Mental Health (NIMH) convened a roundtable meeting to discuss controversial issues about bipolar disorders in children (NIMH Roundtable, 2001). The participants reached consensus that clinicians could diagnose prepubertal children with bipolar disorder using *DSM* criteria. These experts identified two categories: (1) children who clearly meet *DSM-IV* criteria for a bipolar disorder and (2) children who do not meet criteria but who may have bipolar disorder (i.e., although full diagnostic criteria are not met, these children experience severe impairment from symptoms of mood instability). For this latter group, the diagnosis of bipolar disorder, not otherwise specified may be used. Wozniak et al (2001) also reported empiric support for bipolar diagnosis in children based on structured interview data from prepubertal children who underwent extensive clinical evaluation.

Mania, an abnormally and persistently expansive, elated, or irritable mood, is the hallmark of the bipolar disorders (APA, 2000). Manic, mixed, and hypomanic episodes with and without depressive symptomatology characterize and differentiate the various bipolar disorders. To meet criteria for a manic episode, mania (i.e., abnormally and persistently expansive, elated, or irritable mood) must be present for at least 1 week. During the mood disturbance, three or more persistent and significant symptoms are required (four or more are required if mood is only irritable) from the following list: grandiosity or exaggerated self-esteem, diminished need for sleep, excessive talkativeness or pressured speaking, racing thoughts or flight of ideas (i.e., rapid flow of thoughts), distractibility, psychomotor agitation or increased goal-driven behavior, excessive activity involving pleasurable pursuits that are likely to result in problems, and the mood disturbance causing serious impairment in functioning (social, occupational, or academic), requiring hospitalization to prevent harm to self or to other people, or including psychotic symptoms. Last, manic symptoms are not attributable to substance use or a medical condition.

A mixed episode consists of a period of at least 1 week during which criteria for both manic and major depressive episodes are met almost every day. Moods alternate rapidly across the spectrum of depression, irritability, and euphoria along with other symptoms of both types of episodes. A hypomanic episode consists of a period of 4 days or more during which elevated, expansive, or irritable mood is present. Other criteria for manic episode also are met except that changes in functioning are less severe, hospitalization is not needed, and psychotic features are not present (APA, 2000).

According to APA criteria (2000), bipolar disorders fall into two major categories: bipolar I disorder is characterized by one or more manic episodes with or without depression; bipolar II disorder is characterized by one or more major depressive episodes along with one or more hypomanic episodes (APA, 2000). Although PCPs do not diagnose precise variants among the many mood disorders, PCPs do need to recognize that any evidence of mania indicates presence of a bipolar disorder rather than a depressive disorder. Failure to identify manic or hypomanic symptoms in a child or adolescent being medicated for depression can contribute to escalation of mania. When any degree of mania is identified, a referral to an experienced child psychiatric-mental health (PMH) clinician who is authorized to prescribe is needed to ensure accurate diagnosis and appropriate treatment. Follow-up care by the PCP involves ongoing evaluation of symptoms and response to medication.

Cyclothymic Disorder. A chronic mood disturbance with

alternating periods of hypomanic and depressive symptoms characterizes cyclothymic disorder. Cyclothymic disorder is analogous to dysthymic disorder in depression. Hypomanic and depressive symptoms do not meet the threshold for severity, pervasiveness, or duration needed to meet criteria for a manic or major depressive episode, and hypomanic symptoms do not need to fulfill criteria for a full hypomanic episode. A diagnosis of cyclothymic disorder requires that children and adolescents exhibit symptoms for at least 1 year (timeframe for adults is 2 years' duration) and that no more than 2 months during this time are symptom free. Clinically significant distress and social or functional impairment also are required for a diagnosis. In addition, symptoms are not due to direct physiologic effects of a substance or general medical condition and cannot be better accounted for by schizoaffective disorder, or are not superimposed on schizophrenia, schizophreniform disorder, delusional disorder, or psychotic disorder not otherwise specified (APA, 2000).

Treatment (Box 32-4)

Psychotherapy for Depressive Disorders

Most children and adolescents respond well to psychotherapy for the treatment of depression provided by clinicians with expertise in child psychiatric practice and specialized psychotherapy training. Interventions that include parents and other family members are critical, particularly when a child is experiencing a crisis or loss, or when another family member is depressed (Waldinger, 1997). Psychodynamic therapy and cognitive-behavioral therapy are the most commonly used psychotherapeutic approaches for the treatment of depression in children. In addition, family, parent training (Russ & Ollendick,

---

BOX 32-4
Treatment

DEPRESSIVE DISORDERS
Psychotherapy
    Psychodynamic
    Cognitive-behavioral therapy (CBT)
    Adjunctive therapies
        Child centered
        Family
        Psychoeducational
Psychopharmacologic therapy
Electroconvulsant therapy (ECT) (for severe depression only)

BIPOLAR DISORDERS
Adjunctive psychoeducational therapy
Psychopharmacologic therapy
    Mood stabilizers
        Lithium
        Alternative mood stabilizers/anticonvulsants
    Antipsychotics
    Benzodiazepines
    Antihypertensives
    Anxiolytic agent
ECT (for acute mania only)

1999), and psychoeducational therapies (American Academy of Child and Adolescent Psychiatry [AACAP], 1997) may be helpful. Psychotherapeutic approaches are classified according to their underlying theoretic concepts (i.e., psychodynamic or behavioral therapy), the various settings (i.e., inpatient or outpatient), and the approach to treatment (i.e., individual therapy, family therapy, or combination of psychotherapy and medication). Practice parameters are published in the *Journal of the American Academy of Child and Adolescent Psychiatry* and are available online (http:///www.aacap.org) (Remschmidt, 2001).

Psychodynamic Psychotherapy. Psychodynamic theorists assume that a real or imagined loss leads to the development of depression in children. Many theorists maintain that depressed children harbor aggressive impulses secondary to losses that the children have experienced. The children direct these impulses toward themselves, which results in depression. Thus the goal of psychotherapy for the treatment of depression is to help the child to recognize the source of the aggressive impulses and work at integrating these impulses and thereby improve self-esteem in the therapeutic relationship. In older children and adolescents, this can often be achieved through conversation or "talk therapy." For younger children, or in those with cognitive and developmental deficits, play therapy is usually the appropriate choice of treatment (Remschmidt, 2001).

Many techniques of psychodynamic therapy that work with adults are not developmentally appropriate in treatment with children. Modifications of therapeutic strategies apply to free association, the establishment of therapeutic rapport, and transference—all central tenets of psychoanalytically oriented approaches. For example, teenagers typically have a restricted ability to free associate and children almost entirely lack this ability. As a result, techniques such as play therapy, activities, games, and outings have replaced free association in pediatric psychoanalytic therapy. Modifications also are needed because children have less capacity for introspection than do adults. In pediatric psychiatry, some of the current psychotherapy approaches derived from psychoanalytic theory include crisis intervention, and group and family therapy (Remschmidt, 2001).

Cognitive-Behavioral Therapy (CBT). The literature provides substantive support for use of CBT as an effective treatment of depression in children and adolescents (Harrington et al, 1996; Remschmidt, 2001). Kendall & Panichelli-Mendal (1995) reviewed studies in which CBT was the primary intervention to treat depression in children and adolescents, and found that the average child who had been treated for depression with CBT scored better on outcome measures than 71% of the children in the nontreatment control group.

CBT is a combination of behavioral and cognitive therapeutic approaches that emphasize how children and adolescents may use thinking processes to reframe, restructure, and solve problems (Sadock & Sadock, 2000). The underlying principle of CBT is that emotional and behavioral difficulties stem from maladaptive thinking patterns, feelings, and behavioral responses. Cognitive-behavioral theorists maintain that a change in one's thoughts will lead to a change in both behavior and emotions (Geffken, 1998). CBT is a problem-oriented therapy that targets cognitive distortions and also focuses on faulty attributions, poor self-esteem, and their behavioral manifestations. Thus the goals of CBT are to change or reconstruct maladaptive cognitions (e.g., personalization, minimization, overgeneralization), diminish negative and self-recriminating attitudes, and emphasize positive attitudes and improved social competence (Sadock & Sadock, 2000).

The following CBT techniques frequently are used to treat depression in children and adolescents (Herpertz-Dahlmann, 2001):

1. Emotional training: exploring children's or adolescents' own emotional worlds and emotional communication with others by identifying feelings and expressions or gestures indicative of others' feelings.
2. Self-control methods: changing depressive cognitions by means of self-observation, self-reinforcement, and self-appraisal.
3. Activating the individual: developing a timetable to keep the child busy. A healthy level of activity will reduce the tendency to withdraw, encourage a less passive attitude, and increase motivation. Eventually, the child will associate positive experience with improved mood.
4. Social skills training: coaching both verbal and nonverbal skills to improve accurate perception and expression of a range of emotions. Tools include instruction, modeling, and practice of appropriate social behavior and feedback from the therapist.

Psychopharmacologic Treatment for Depression

Effective treatment of mood disorders in children and adolescents frequently requires use of medication (Barnes, 1996; Scahill, 2001a, 2001b; Tarascon Publishing, 2000). Children who do not respond to psychotherapy alone tend to present with major dysfunction and vegetative symptoms and have a positive family history for depression (Waldinger, 1997). Careful assessment and accurate diagnosis of youth with a mood disorder are critical before developing a medication plan for at least two reasons. First, distinguishing between the different subtypes of mood disorders can be difficult because many symptoms overlap (i.e., depressive features of unipolar depression vs. bipolar disorder). Also, bipolar disorder in young children is underdiagnosed. Second, many antidepressants and psychostimulants are contraindicated in individuals with bipolar disorder and can induce mania (Papolos & Papolos, 1999). The American Academy of Child and Adolescent Psychiatry (AACAP, 1997) recommended the following procedures when initiating pharmacotherapy: informed consent, physical examination, including laboratory data; identification of the phase of the illness; discussion of the expected length of treatment; and discussion of medication choice.

The research literature regarding pharmacologic treatment of childhood mood disorders is limited so many treatment recommendations are based on evidence from adult studies (AACAP, 1997). Approved use of most antidepressant medications is for individuals over 12 years of age (Keltner

& Folks, 2001; Skidmore-Roth, 2002; Scahill, 2001a, 2001b), yet clinicians frequently turn to medications to reduce distressing symptoms and to prevent escalation of related functional and social problems. Psychopharmacologic treatment of children and adolescents involves consultation, referral, cautious use of available guidelines, and continued monitoring of effectiveness, side effects, and adverse effects (Table 32-2).

Psychopharmacologic Management. Psychopharmacologic management of the majority of psychiatric childhood disorders necessitates the practice called "off-label" prescribing (Laughren, 1996, p. 1276). Off-label use means that clinicians prescribe drugs for disorders other than those indicated in Food and Drug Administration (FDA)—approved labeling for those products. Off-label prescribing is *not* a violation of federal law, and the FDA does not regulate such professional practice decisions, although clinicians are cautioned that they are prescribing medications with inadequate data concerning safe and effective use for the circumstance. Without research involving pediatric populations, labeling and marketing of medications require a disclaimer to indicate that safety and effectiveness have not been established for children (McLeer & Wills, 2000). However, psychopharmacologic treatment for children and adolescents is widespread and often needed to ameliorate distressing and debilitating symptoms. Nonetheless, at least a perception of increased liability risk exists concerning such practices (Laughren, 1996).

For PCPs, potential liability risk associated with off-label prescribing of psychopharmacologic agents to children and adolescents merits serious consideration. Such risk is likely to be even greater for PCPs than risk experienced by PMH clinicians authorized to prescribe. Particularly when initiating psychopharmacologic treatment of children and adolescents with a moderate to severe major psychiatric disorder without a psychiatric referral, PCPs are practicing outside their area of specialization. PCPs are encouraged to consult and make referrals to PMH clinicians with prescriptive authority who have extensive training and experience with pediatric psychopharmacology. Further, any time that a PCP detects moderate to severe mood disorder symptoms, suspects bipolar disorder, or identifies suicidal ideation, intent, or plan, a psychiatric referral is a necessity. Subsequent medication management by PCPs is appropriate collaborative practice with PMH colleagues. Such collaboration is likely to reduce liability risk and to produce the safest, most efficacious outcomes for treatment of mood disorders among children and adolescents (Table 32-2).

Antidepressant Medications. Antidepressant medications work by inhibiting or potentiating the actions of neurotransmitters in the brain, particularly norepinephrine, serotonin, dopamine, and gamma-aminobutyric acid (GABA). The major classes of antidepressant medications include selective serotonin reuptake inhibitors (SSRIs) (e.g., fluoxetine [Prozac], sertraline [Zoloft], paroxetine [Paxil]), tricyclic antidepressants (TCAs) (e.g., imipramine, amitriptyline), and monoamine oxidase inhibitors (MAOIs) (e.g., phenelzine [Nardil], tranylcypromine [Parnate]). Trazodone and bupropion are examples of atypical antidepressants (Waldinger, 1997).

Text continued on p. 615.

TABLE 32-2
Psychotropic Medications Used to Treat Childhood and Adolescent Mood Disorders

Medication	Typical Starting Dosage*	Typical Daily Dosage*	Side Effects	Use Guidelines and Efficacy (when data available)
SELECTIVE SEROTONIN REUPTAKE INHIBITORS (SSRIs)			Gastrointestinal (GI): nausea, diarrhea, cramping, heartburn Central nervous system (CNS): insomnia, agitation, restlessness, headache, tremor, insomnia, irritability Genitourinary (GU): decreased libido	Antidepressant medications approved for use in individuals over 12 yr; fluoxetine received FDA approval for treatment of depression and obsessive-compulsive disorder in children (Jan. 2003)
Citalopram (Celexa)	5 mg	5-40 mg	Similar to other SSRIs	
Fluoxetine (Prozac)	5-10 mg	5-40 mg: children 10-60 mg: adolescents	Most common: behavioral activation (e.g., motor restlessness, insomnia, disinhibition) Also reports of suicidal ideation and self-injurious behavior	Studied for treatment of depression in children and adolescents; support as first-line medication choice; strong evidence to date of efficacy as treatment of depression in children and adolescents. FDA approved use (11/2003) for children age 8 and older
Fluvoxamine (Luvox)	12.5-25 mg	50-200 mg	Similar to other SSRIs	Approved to treat obsessive-compulsive disorder in children
Paroxetine (Paxil)	5-10 mg	10-40 mg	Similar to other SSRIs Increased suicide risk	Limited clinical experience indicates that the drug is well tolerated; Strong evidence of efficacy as treatment for depression. However, following action by UK regulations, FDA recommended (6/2003) *against* use with children and adolescents for treatment of depression.
Sertraline (Zoloft)	12.5-25 mg	25-150 mg: children	Similar to other SSRIs	Studied for treatment of depression in children and adolescents; more evidence of efficacy needed for children but adequate support as first-line medication choice; modest evidence to date of efficacy as treatment of depression in adolescents; approved to treat obsessive-compulsive disorder in children
		50-200 mg: adolescents	One study of 33 children and adolescents demonstrated evidence of 2 cases of sertraline-induced mania	Evidence from adult studies shows that some individuals respond to low doses; hence clinicians should evaluate response before increasing dose

Data from American Psychiatric Association. (2002). *Quick reference to the American Psychiatric Association practice guidelines for the treatment of psychiatric disorders: Compendium 2002.* Washington, D.C.: Author; Barnes, M.A. (1996). *The Harriet Lane handbook: A manual for pediatric house officers* (14th ed.). St. Louis: Mosby–Year Book.; Kaplan, H.I. & Sadock, B.J. (1998). *Kaplan and Sadock's synopsis of psychiatry: Behavioral sciences/clinical psychiatry.* Baltimore: Williams & Wilkins; Keltner, N.L. & Folks, D.G. (2001). *Psychotropic drugs* (3rd ed.). St. Louis: Mosby; Popolos, D. & Popolos, J. (1999). *The bipolar child: The definitive and reassuring guide to childhood's most misunderstood disorder.* New York: Broadway Books; Rankin, E.A. (2000). *Quick reference for psychopharmacology.* Albany, N.Y.: Delmar Thomson Learning; Scahill, L. (2001a). *Psychopharmacology for adolescents.* In N.L. Keltner & D.G. Folks (Eds.). *Psychotropic drugs* (3rd ed.). St. Louis: Mosby, pp. 496-514; Scahill, L. (2001b). Psychopharmacology for children. In N.L. Keltner & D.G. Folks (Eds.). *Psychotropic drugs* (3rd ed.). St. Louis: Mosby, pp. 468-495; Schatzberg, A.F. & Nemeroff, C.B. (1998). *The American Psychiatric Press textbook of psychopharmacology* (2nd ed.). Washington, D.C.: American Psychiatric Press; Skidmore-Roth, L. (2002). *Mosby's nursing drug reference:* 2002. St. Louis: Mosby; Tarascon Publishing. (2000). *The Tarascon pocket pharmacopoeia 2000* (deluxe ed.). Loma Linda, Calif.: Author.

*Dosages are indicated for children and adolescents when recommendations for each age-group are available. When not specified as child, adolescent, or adult dose, the dosages indicated are guidelines for use with children and adolescents. If child or adolescent dosage recommendations are not generally available, adult dosages are given. **Please note: Caution is recommended when prescribing and monitoring psychotropic medication use with children and adolescents**; many drugs require off-label use, demonstration of efficacy may be minimal, and dosages may not be clearly evidence based. Clinicians are advised to monitor changes in FDA approvals, warnings, and new medications and uses.

Continued

TABLE 32-2

Psychotropic Medications Used to Treat Childhood and Adolescent Mood Disorders—cont'd

Medication	Typical Starting Dosage	Typical Daily Dosage	Side Effects	Use Guidelines and Efficacy (when data available)
ATYPICAL/NOVEL ANTIDEPRESSANTS			GI: nausea, vomiting, constipation CNS: agitation, insomnia Neurologic: tremors Dermatologic: skin rashes	
Bupropion (Wellbutrin)		50-200 mg: children 100-250 mg: adolescents	Low risk of seizures	Limited evidence of efficacy for treatment of attention deficit hyperactivity disorder (ADHD), in children and adolescents; more evidence needed
Trazodone (Desyrel)	150 mg: adults	150-600 mg: adults	Specific to Desyrel: GI: nausea, dyspepsia CNS: orthostasis, sedation, restlessness Cardiovascular: effects such as risk for atrial arrhythmia GU: priapism	Not well studied in children and adolescents
Mirtazapine (Remeron)	15-45 mg: adults	15-45 mg: adults	Specific to mirtazapine: GI: increased appetite, weight gain CNS: somnolence, dizziness	Not well studied in children and adolescents
Nefazodone (Serzone)	200 mg: adults	150-600 mg: adults	Hepatic: abnormal liver function tests (LFTs), "black box" risk warning GI: nausea, dyspepsia, constipation, and varied symptoms	Not well studied in children and adolescents; *not recommended at this time for use with children and adolescents* because of risk of liver damage
Venlafaxine (Effexor)		75-150 mg in 2-3 divided doses with food: adults up to 375 mg	GI: dysphagia, eructation (belching), gastritis, stomach and mouth ulcerations, rectal hemorrhage, weight gain or loss	One study found drug to be no better than placebo in relieving depression in children
TRICYCLIC ANTIDEPRESSANTS (TCAs)			GI: weight gain CNS: tremor, agitation Cardiovascular: orthostatic hypotension, palpitations, hypertension, dizziness Anticholinergic: dry mouth, sweating, urinary retention and hesitance	Over 30 yr of use in children and adolescents; approved for use in individuals over 12 yr with depression; evidence for efficacy in treating children's depression is unconvincing Children can show tremendous variation in serum level at the same dose of these drugs Before initiating treatment with TCA, an electrocardiogram (ECG) should be performed; ECG should be repeated with dosage adjustments, when maintenance dose is achieved, and semiannually during treatment Baseline assessment should include blood pressure, pulse, and a review of medical and family history (e.g., syncope, sudden death); children thought to be more sensitive to overdoses of TCAs than adults
Amitriptyline (Elavil)	25 mg	25-150 mg: children 50-200 mg: adolescents		
Clomipramine (Anafranil) (also referred to as a serotonin reuptake inhibitor because of potential action)	25 mg	50-100 mg: children 50-150 mg: adolescents		Approved to treat obsessive-compulsive disorder in children

TABLE 32-2

Psychotropic Medications Used to Treat Childhood and Adolescent Mood Disorders—cont'd

Medication	Typical Starting Dosage	Typical Daily Dosage	Side Effects	Use Guidelines and Efficacy (when data available)
TRICYCLIC ANTIDEPRESSANTS (TCAs)—cont'd				
Desipramine (Norpramin, Pertofrane)	10-25 mg	25-125 mg: children 50-150 mg: adolescents	TCA most likely to alter electrical conduction through the heart; can also prolong the QT interval, which can increase risk of fatal ventricular tachycardia in susceptible individuals	
Imipramine (Tofranil)	25 mg	25-150 mg: children 50-200 mg: adolescents		Approved to treat enuresis in children
Nortriptyline (Aventyl, Pamelor)	10-25 mg	20-100 mg: children 50-125 mg: adolescents		Modest evidence of efficacy in treating depression for adolescents
MONOAMINE OXIDASE INHIBITORS (MAOIs)			GI: constipation, weight gain Cardiovascular: decreased heart rate, decreased vasoconstriction, hypotension, hypertensive crisis Anticholinergic: dry mouth, blurred vision, urinary hesitancy CNS: agitation, anxiety, restlessness, insomnia GU: anorgasmia or impotence Mood: euphoria, hypomania	Tyramine-containing foods (e.g., wine, aged cheese) should not be ingested by the person taking MAOIs
Phenelzine (Nardil)		30-90 mg: adults		
Tranylcypromine (Parnate)		20-60 mg: adults		
MOOD STABILIZER				
Lithium	30 mg/kg body weight/day	300-600 mg increasing over 4-5 days to 1500-1800 mg	GI: weight gain, bloated feeling, diarrhea CNS: tremor, ataxia, cognitive slowing, sedation, sleeplessness, headaches, dyspepsia, dry mouth Cardiovascular: arrhythmia, conduction disturbances, hypotension GU: polyuria, polydypsia Dermatologic: hair loss, acne, rash	Several studies for prepubertal children to treat severe aggression; not approved for use in children <12 yr, although limited use reported; evidence to support safe and effective use in adolescents During first month, check serum level every week and then monthly; thyroid every 4-6 mo, renal function every 6-12 mo; baseline ECG needed and repeated yearly Serum levels: therapeutic or normal level: 0.6-1.2 mEq/L; adverse reactions at 1.5 mEq/L and toxic reaction at 2.0-3.0 mEq/L and lethal reactions at greater than 4 mEq/L; draw blood in morning 8-12 hr after last dose and before morning dose Maintenance of adequate hydration essential
ALTERNATIVE MOOD STABILIZER/ ANTICONVULSANTS			Multiple side effects reported Specific side effects as noted by medication	
Carbamazapine (Tegretol)	100-200 mg in 2 divided doses	Increase to total of 200-600 mg in 3 divided doses (10-20 mg/kg/day): children	GI: nausea and vomiting, weight gain, GI upset CNS: sedation, poor coordination, dizziness, irritability, diplopia, tremors	Minimally studied in children, may be useful for aggression; laboratory work weekly to monitor plasma levels; after stabilization, monitor monthly; baseline ECG, hemoglobin, hematocrit,

Continued

TABLE 32-2

Psychotropic Medications Used to Treat Childhood and Adolescent Mood Disorders—cont'd

Medication	Typical Starting Dosage	Typical Daily Dosage	Side Effects	Use Guidelines and Efficacy (when data available)
ALTERNATIVE MOOD STABILIZER/ANTICONVULSANTS—cont'd				
Carbamazapine (Tegretol)—cont'd		Increase by 200 mg/day: adolescents Dose to reach serum level of 4-12 μg/ml	Dermatologic: skin reactions and rashes, transient hair loss, acne Hematologic: blood dyscrasias including agranulocytosis (most serious), leukopenia, aplastic anemia (rare), agranulocytosis, thrombocytopenia (dose related) Eyes, ears, nose, and throat (EENT): blurred vision Renal: hyponatremia Hepatic and pancreatic: hepatotoxicity and pancreatitis (rare)	complete blood count (CBC) with differential, white blood count (WBC), platelet count, LFTs; after stabilization, CBC and LFTs weekly for 1 mo, monthly for 4 mo, every 3 mo thereafter; evaluate CBC for blood dyscrasias
Gabapentin (Neurontin)		900-1800 mg in divided doses: adults and children >12 yr of age	Specific to gabapentin: GI: increased appetite, weight gain CNS: sedation, tremor, ataxia, incoordination	Open trials and case reports with adults indicate effectiveness for rapid cycling; may be more effective to treat bipolar II and in combination with another mood stabilizer; not used for children <12 yr
Lamotrigine (Lamictal)	12.5-25 mg/day with slow increase by 12.5 mg every 7-10 days: adolescents 25-50 mg/day: adults	75-100 mg/day may be effective but up to 225 mg required: adolescents 100-500 mg: adults	Specific to lamotrigine: CNS: cognitive blunting ("spacing out") Cardiac: restlessness, dizziness, conduction changes Dermatologic: rash (particularly in combination with valproate, higher dosages, during first 8 wk of treatment, and in children), Stevens-Johnson syndrome in 1%-2% of children and 0.1% of adults (severe allergic and sometimes fatal reaction; stop use immediately and treat with corticosteroids)	Used only for children >16 yr; valproate doubles plasma levels of lamotrigine; sertraline increases plasma levels of lamotrigine; carbamazapine and phenobarbital lower plasma levels of lamotrigine; alcohol increases severity of lamotrigine's side effects
Tiagabine (Gabatril)	Start low and increase weekly until good response or until max dose reached	32 mg max dose per day	CNS: dizziness, fatigue, unstable gait	FDA approved for treatment of convulsant disorders in adolescents; more evidence needed to show efficacy for bipolar treatment over other agents; may be helpful after other agents tried with limited effect
Topiramate (Topamax)	1-3 mg/kg/day or 25 mg/day (whichever is less) at bedtime	Increase by 1-3 mg/kg/day every 1-2 wk up to 5-9 mg/kg/day in 2 divided doses 200-600 mg/day: adults	GI: weight loss, anorexia CNS: sedation, fatigue, dizziness GU: dysmenorrhea and menstrual disorder EENT: diplopia, vision abnormality Respiratory: upper respiratory infection (URI), pharyngitis, sinusitis Miscellaneous: leukopenia	Decreased levels of contraceptives
Valproate/valproic acid (Depakote)		15 mg/kg/day divided in 2 or 3 doses; may increase by 5-10 mg/kg/day every week; not to exceed	GI: nausea, vomiting, constipation, weight gain, toxic hepatitis, hepatic failure, pancreatitis CNS: sedation, drowsiness, dizziness, incoordination, tremors, headache, depression	Approved for treatment of epilepsy in children and adults Minimal studies with adolescents conducted to date During first 1-2 mo, serum levels checked every 1-2 wk and liver function tests (LFTs) and

`TABLE 32-2`
Psychotropic Medications Used to Treat Childhood and Adolescent Mood Disorders—cont'd

Medication	Typical Starting Dosage	Typical Daily Dosage	Side Effects	Use Guidelines and Efficacy (when data available)
ALTERNATIVE MOOD STABILIZER/ANTICONVULSANTS—cont'd				
Valproate/valproic acid (Depakote)—cont'd		60 mg/kg/day in 2 or 3 divided doses Dose to reach serum level of 50-100 µg/ml: children and adults	GU: polycystic ovaries (more likely when treatment started in teen years) Hematologic: thrombocytopenia, leukopenia, lymphocytosis Dermatologic: transitory hair loss, skin eruptions Hepatic: hepatotoxicity (rare in children under 10 yr) Pancreatic: pancreatitis (potentially fatal and rare, usually associated with use of multiple anticonvulsants)	CBC monthly and then every 6-12 mo; potential for development of polycystic ovaries raises question about risk/benefit ratio for use in adolescent girls
ANTIPSYCHOTIC MEDICATIONS			Traditional neuroleptics/antipsychotics (e.g., chlorpromazine, haloperidol, thioridazine, thiothixene) have significant side effects including: CNS: sedation Cardiovascular: hypotension Anticholinergic: dry mouth, constipation, blurred vision Extrapyramidal side effects: dystonia, rigidity, akathisia; long-term use associated with tardive dyskinesia Neuroleptic malignant syndrome (NMS; severe muscular rigidity, autonomic system instability, changing levels of consciousness) can be fatal; associated with high-potency drugs prescribed in high doses and with rapid increase in dosing; if NMS is suspected, treat symptoms and stop the drug	With traditional neuroleptics, consider risk and monitor signs of abnormal movements that may indicate tardive dyskinesia Use lowest possible dose, and withdraw slowly, evaluate changes in symptom severity Newer atypical antipsychotic drugs (e.g., risperidone, loanzapine, quetiapine, loxapine) generally better tolerated
Chlorpromazine (Thorazine)	10-25 mg	50-300 mg: children 50-400 mg: adolescents	Same as above	Plasma levels found to be lower in children than in adults after the same weight-adjusted dose Evidence of modest effectiveness but used less because of availability of newer agents; studied in adolescents
Clozapine (Clozaril)	25-50 mg: adolescents	700 mg maximum: adolescents	Weight gain may be substantial; life-threatening agranulocytosis can occur	Not approved for use in children under 16 yr; because of risk profile, not recommended unless standard medications fail; studied in adolescents
Haloperidol (Haldol)	0.25-0.5 mg	0.5-6 mg: children 2-10 mg: adolescents	Causes more extrapyramidal side effects than chlorpromazine or thioridazine but is less sedating	Most studied neuroleptic with children; effective for treatment of autism, schizophrenia, severe aggression, tics; studied in adolescents
Loxapine (Loxitane)	10 mg bid: adolescents	60-100 mg: adolescents		Studied in adolescents
Olanzapine (Zyprexa)		2.5 mg: adolescents	GI: increased appetite, weight gain	Limited data for use with children and adolescents

Continued

TABLE 32-2

Psychotropic Medications Used to Treat Childhood and Adolescent Mood Disorders—cont'd

Medication	Typical Starting Dosage	Typical Daily Dosage	Side Effects	Use Guidelines and Efficacy (when data available)
ANTIPSYCHOTIC MEDICATIONS—cont'd				
Quetiapine (Seroquel)		100-400 mg: adolescents		Limited data for use with children and adolescents
Risperidone (Risperdal)	0.5 mg	1-3.5 mg: children 2-8 mg: adolescents	Cardiovascular: higher incidence of cerebrovascular adverse events in elderly with dementia-related psychosis	Limited data to support use in children yet several studies to support use for behavioral dyscontrol; extensive evidence for use in adults; studied in adolescents
Thioridazine (Mellaril)	25-50 mg: adolescents	0.5-3.0 mg/kg/day or 10-50 mg 2-3 times per day: children 50-400 mg: adolescents		Studied in adolescents
Thiothixene (Navane)	1-2 mg	5-40 mg: children 8-40 mg: adolescent		Approved to treat psychosis in children >12 yr; studied in adolescents; meager evidence for children <12 yr suggests less sedation than low-potency neuroleptics and fewer side effects than high-potency neuroleptics
BENZODIAZEPINES				Use only as needed for acute anxiety or adjunctively with antidepressant as brief treatment; not recommended as monotherapy for anxiety symptoms; tolerance easily develops; withdrawal and symptoms commonly occur with only 6-8 wk of treatment; slow taper over 2-4 mo at 10% dose reduction to discontinue
Diazepam (Valium)		1-2.5 mg in 3 or 4 divided doses 2-10 mg in 2-4 divided doses		
Lorazepam (Ativan)		0.05 mg./kg./day every 4-8 hr: child dose 2-6 mg/day divided doses (max 10 mg/day): adolescent and adult dosing		
Clonazepam (Klonopin)		2-16 mg: adults	CNS: drowsiness	Recommend serum bilirubun, renal function tests, CBC
ANTIHYPERTENSIVES			CNS: drowsiness, sedation, headache, fatigue, nightmares, insomnia, mental changes, anxiety, depression, hallucinations, delirium GI: nausea, vomiting, dry mouth Cardiovascular: orthostatic hypotension, palpitations, congestive heart failure (CHF), electrocardiogram (ECG) abnormalities Dermatologic: rash	Contraindicated if bleeding disorder; baseline testing for renal function, LFTs, electrolytes, ECG

TABLE 32-2

Psychotropic Medications Used to Treat Childhood and Adolescent Mood Disorders—cont'd

Medication	Typical Starting Dosage	Typical Daily Dosage	Side Effects	Use Guidelines and Efficacy (when data available)
ANTIHYPERTENSIVES—cont'd				
Clonidine (Catapres)	0.05 mg: adolescents	0.15-0.2 mg: adolescents		Minimally studied in children; modest evidence for efficacy in ADHD; approved only for treatment of hypertension for adults
Guanfacine (Tenex)	0.5 mg	1.5-3 mg		Minimally studied in children; modest evidence for efficacy in ADHD and tics; approved only for treatment of hypertension for adults
ANXIOLYTIC AGENT				
Buspirone (BuSpar)	2.5-5 mg	10-20 mg: children 60 mg max dose for adolescents in 3 divided doses	CNS: fatigue, sleep disturbance, headache, restlessness, agitation, depression, anxiety, confusion GI: abdominal discomfort, nausea	Minimally studied in children; improvement in anxiety and aggression If there is no evidence of improvement after 6 wk, buspirone should be discontinued

SSRIs act by potentiating the central nervous system (CNS) action of serotonin and norepinephrine. SSRIs are the newest class of antidepressants and the most widely used medications for treatment of depression in children and adolescents. SSRIs are the medication of choice primarily because of their favorable side effect profile. SSRIs do not cause orthostatic hypotension or anticholinergic side effects. Some of the side effects of SSRIs include restlessness, irritability, and insomnia. However, a rare and potentially fatal adverse reaction to SSRIs, serotonin syndrome, presents with heightened restlessness, confusion, and lethargy and may progress to myoclonus, hyperthermia, rigor, and increased tone. Serotonin syndrome is likely to result from overstimulation of the serotonergic centers. Risk for occurrence is greatest when a clinician changes medication from an SSRI to an MAOI. In cases of serotonin syndrome, immediately stopping use of the medication and seeking emergency medical attention are indicated actions (Waldinger, 1997).

The action of TCAs appears to be similar to that of the SSRIs, but TCAs are not the first choice of antidepressant medication for the treatment of depression in children because of their more troublesome side effect profile. Prepubescent children are more sensitive to the cardiovascular side effects of tricyclics than are adults, and therefore some experts have recommended that these medications should be prescribed with caution only by experienced child psychiatrists (Waldinger, 1997). However, imipramine (Tofranil) is an approved and frequently used treatment for enuresis, and clomipramine (Anafranil) is approved to treat childhood obsessive-compulsive disorder. Most common side effects include anticholinergic reactions (e.g., dry mouth, dizziness), weight gain, and insomnia.

MAOIs appear to work by blocking the metabolism of norepinephrine and serotonin in the CNS. MAOIs are considered less effective than the SSRIs and the TCAs, and they are asso-

ciated with more adverse side effects. MAOIs are often the medication of choice in individuals who have not responded to the SSRIs or TCAs, and for those who present with high levels of anxiety, phobias, or obsessive-compulsive symptoms (Waldinger, 1997). Overdose risk also is important to note: TCAs and MAOIs are lethal in relatively small dosages as compared with the SSRIs. This risk should be considered when treating a suicidal child.

The treatment of bipolar disorder in the pediatric population is evolving. In fact, much work remains to develop optimal treatment strategies. Because research in this area is scant, improvisation in developing a treatment plan is necessary (Mondimore, 1999). Given evidence of a biologic cause of the disorder, and the related functional and psychosocial problems, a sensible treatment strategy for moderate to severe cases combines psychopharmacology and psychotherapy. Electroconvulsant therapy (ECT) also may be indicated for partial responders and nonresponders to other treatments.

Psychotherapy for Bipolar Disorders

Although there is no evidence that psychotherapy can help to treat the core symptoms of bipolar disorders in children, adjunctive psychosocial therapies can address the functional impairments of affected individuals and families (AACAP, 1997). Supportive therapy helps families to cope with the devastating social and emotional effects of the disorder and promotes compliance with medication regimens (Waldinger, 1997). The AACAP (1997) has affirmed that appropriate psychotherapeutic interventions with this population focus on psychoeducation, relapse prevention, and reduction of morbidity.

Psychopharmacologic Treatment for Bipolar Disorders

Medication is a widely used treatment for bipolar disorders to eliminate manic (or mixed) and depressive symptoms, and to prevent recurrence (AACAP, 1997) (see Table 32-2 and Psychopharmacologic Management section above). Mood stabilizers, such as lithium, are the mainstays of treatment for bipolar disorders. Frequently, prescription of a combination of drugs within different classes is necessary to treat the complex and varied symptoms of the disorders. For example, a child may take a mood stabilizer to achieve some balance in mood, an antipsychotic medication to treat manic symptoms and severe behavioral disturbances, and an antidepressant to relieve depressive features of the illness. In treating bipolar disorder, an antidepressant should be given only if the child has been placed on a mood stabilizer. Antidepressants, and in many cases stimulants, given without the protection of a mood stabilizer, can lead to increased anxiety, aggression, temper tantrums, cycling of mood, and induction of mania (Papolos & Papolos, 1999).

Electroconvulsive Therapy

Older children and adolescents who have been resistant to alternate forms of treatment sometimes receive ECT for treatment of severe depression and acute mania. When rapid relief is required because of suicidal intent, risk for self-harm, or exhaustion, ECT may be effective (Waldinger, 1997). Although ECT is safe and effective when administered correctly, many people expect that the treatment is painful and view it as barbaric and archaic. Because of these common misperceptions about ECT, extensive education is essential when this treatment option is proposed.

Complementary and Alternative Therapies

Complementary and alternative therapies for the treatment of many childhood disorders and ailments have been a topic of intense research in the United States during the past decade. Snyder (2002, p. 4) summarized outcomes of two national surveys: "More than 33% of those surveyed in 1991 used complementary therapies with that number increasing to 42% in 1997." A central tenet underpinning these treatment approaches is that people heal themselves and physicians, nurses, and others assist in the process. Cost containment and relative noninvasiveness also are attractive features of many of these therapies.

St. John's Wort. Many people use St. John's wort *(Hypericum perforatum)*, a whole plant product with antidepressant properties, to self-medicate their depression. St. John's wort is licensed in Germany and used extensively throughout Europe for treatment of insomnia, anxiety, and depression, and surpasses sales of fluoxetine (Prozac) by a wide margin. Action involves inhibition of uptake of serotonin, norepinephrine, and dopamine, and inhibition of binding to GABA receptors. St. John's wort reduces serum levels of theophylline, digoxin, cyclosporine, and indinavir. Use is associated with increased photosensitivity and poses a theoretic risk for serotonergic crisis when taken with other agents that have similar action (Plotnikoff, 2002). Although this agent may reduce mild depression, St. John's wort is neither regulated nor approved as a depression treatment in the United States so dosage and composition are unstandardized, and efficacy is unknown: However, St. John's wort may help to reduce mild depression (APA,

2002a; Keltner & Folks, 2001). Ongoing placebo-controlled clinical trials and comparative studies with SSRIs are likely to yield data about efficacy for different types of depression, comparison with other antidepressants, and long-term maintenance (Keltner & Folks, 2001).

Light Therapy. Light therapy (phototherapy) is a complementary or alternative treatment for seasonal affective disorder, a depressive disorder associated with reduced sunlight exposure during autumn and winter. Treatment involves daily exposure to full-spectrum wavelengths (like sunlight) from a high-intensity lamp. The pineal gland receives information about light exposure through nerve pathways. This gland secretes melatonin, a sleep-inducing hormone associated with depression of mood and mental agility. Melatonin secretion is highest during winter under conditions of reduced sunlight. Thus light therapy may help to reduce melatonin production and resultant effects on mood and associated features of depression (Papolos & Papolos, 1999).

Exercise. Considerable evidence supports the positive effects of exercise on depression (Byrne & Byrne, 1993). Exercise produces physiologic and psychologic benefits that include a reduced stress response and increased well-being (Treat-Jacobson & Mark, 2002). Athletes and others who regularly engage in physical activity attest to positive feelings (e.g., "runner's high") associated with release of endorphins triggered by exercise. Positive effects of exercise have long been recognized and encouraged as complementary treatment for depression.

Anticipated Advances in Diagnosis and Management

Without early and accurate diagnosis of childhood- and adolescent-onset mood disorders, affected youth are likely to experience unabated distressing symptoms and an exacerbation of related functional, academic, social, and family problems. Clinicians recognize that children are distinctive developing persons rather than being merely "little adults"; nevertheless, practitioners persist in using nomenclature and a diagnostic system based on observations and studies from adult populations. As a result, providers must adapt information for application to children and adolescents, and they may lack relevant data. For example, although clinicians generally are familiar with signs of depression in adults, such as flat affect and increased requirement for sleep, many may not be aware that depressed children can present with irritability and aggressive outbursts.

Pediatric-based research holds promise of improved treatment options. Researchers are investigating medications expected to improve the symptoms of mood disorders while minimizing unfavorable side effects. Clinical investigators also are exploring treatment options that are less invasive. Examples of such methods for the treatment of bipolar disorder include light therapy and repeated transcranial magnetic stimulation (r-TMS) (Papolos & Papolos, 1999). However, faulty research designs have contributed to knowledge gaps about the nature, course, and best treatments of pediatric mood disorders. Developing evidence-based practice recommendations requires that investigators correct existing methodologic deficiencies, including small sample sizes, lack of comparison groups, retrospective designs, and lack of standardized measures (AACAP, 1997). Developing a research agenda for childhood and adolescent mental health remains a significant challenge: If such a research program is realized, a commitment to it holds promise for improving the quality of life and reducing future disability of affected youth.

Knowledge of genetic causation in psychiatric disorders is expanding rapidly yet many unknowns remain. Mood disorders exist in clusters within families, and genetic transmission is likely in many instances. Researchers are hopeful that developments in the field of genetics will lead to a better understanding of the complex etiology of mood disorders and expect that new knowledge will lead to better diagnosis and treatment of the disorders. Indeed, clinicians have become more skilled in the diagnosis of mood disorders, and biochemical methods available to locate and identify genes on the human chromosome have become quite sophisticated (Mondimore, 1999). The future of the genetic revolution presents unknown challenges for researchers and clinicians, yet few health care professionals are prepared to address potential effects of new discoveries on family relationships (Feetham, 1999). In relation to mood disorders, affected youth, as well as their parents, relatives, and future partners, need information about genetic etiology from clinicians in order to make informed decisions and to manage the disorder.

Associated Problems (Box 32-5)

Although research-based evidence about the interface between mood disorders and other illnesses is limited to date, expecting that youth with mood disorders are more prone to stress-related illnesses and accidents is logical. Children who experience stress tend to have higher levels of circulating cortisol. Thus they experience stress reactions much more frequently than children without a mood disorder. Children with mood disorders often exhibit hyperactivity and impulsivity that put them at higher risk for falls and accidents that are associated with aggressive behaviors that often lead to self-injury and injury of others. Social, academic, and occupational problems commonly accompany mood disorders.

BOX 32-5
Associated Problems

Social, academic, and occupational difficulties
Stress-related somatic complaints and problems
Accidents
Hyperactivity and impulsivity
Injury to self or others
Suicide
Co-morbidity with:
    Anxiety disorders (highest)
    Attention deficit and disruptive behavior disorders
    Substance use disorders
    Tourette's syndrome

Stress-Related Somatic Complaints and Problems

Children and adolescents commonly come for primary care visits because of somatic complaints, such as headaches, sleep disturbances, fatigue, and stomachaches. When a physical illness cannot fully explain somatic symptoms, emotional distress might be contributing to the problem. After ruling out possible illnesses or when such illnesses do not explain symptoms completely, exploring another source of the problem is warranted. In addition, when physical symptoms persist or occur in relation to stressful situations, a mental health problem might be present. Children sometimes express emotional distress and depressed feelings as physical symptoms. Depressive disorders in particular may present with fatigue and sleep disturbance.

Accidents

Impulsive behavior associated with bipolar disorders sometimes results in accidents. When children present with frequent accidents associated with making poor judgments or feeling frustrated, a covert bipolar disorder might be present. Further, a child, adolescent, or parent might describe a suicidal gesture as an accident because of denial or shame. When PCPs observe a pattern of injuries from accidents, assessing the child or adolescent for signs of depression, mania, or hypomania and suicidal ideation is appropriate; if one of these problems is suspected, referral for a mental health evaluation is needed. Children diagnosed with a mood disorder also require ongoing monitoring of self-injurious behavior during primary care visits.

Suicide

In the United States, suicide among adolescents has reached epidemic status, rising to one of the three leading causes of death among this population. A dramatic rise in suicide incidence has occurred among younger children between the ages of 5 and 12 years; suicide rates among these youngsters have more than doubled in the last 2 decades. Moreover, incidence statistics tend to underreport suicide because many suicidal deaths are recorded as "accidents." Although numerous factors, such as divorce or death of a parent, can prompt young people to attempt to take their own lives, depression and psychotic thinking clearly put youth at higher risk for suicide. Depression often leads to feelings of hopelessness and helplessness, and psychosis can result in a suicidal attempt as a response to a hallucination (Waldinger, 1997). Suicidal thoughts, threats, or gestures always must be taken very seriously, and children with mood disorders are considered to be high risk for self-harm. Evaluation of suicide risk includes the following considerations (that all increase risk):

- Evidence of suicidal or homicidal thoughts, intent, or plan
- Availability of means for suicide and lethality of method
- Evidence of psychotic symptoms, particularly command hallucinations, or severe anxiety
- Previous attempts and seriousness of attempts
- Family history of suicide or exposure to suicide attempts (APA, 2002b)

Co-morbid Conditions

Co-morbidity with other psychiatric disorders is high. Among youth with major depressive disorder, 40% to 70% present with one or more other psychiatric disorders (Mash & Wolfe, 1999; Siminoff et al, 1997). Among clinically referred youth, anxiety disorders are the most frequently co-occurring disorders followed by attention deficit and disruptive behavior disorders and substance-related disorders (Birmaher et al, 1996; Mash & Wolfe, 1999; Siminoff et al, 1997).Prevalence of co-morbid anxiety and depression ranges from 15% to 60% (Daleiden et al, 1999). Co-morbidity percentages of major depression and specific anxiety disorders are estimated as 55% for generalized anxiety disorder, 45% for phobias, and 9% for separation disorder (Birmaher et al, 1996; Mash & Wolfe, 1999; Siminoff et al, 1997). Youth who are co-morbid for anxiety and depression tend to have more disturbed and severe symptoms and to be older (Daleiden, 1999).

Bipolar disorder in children rarely occurs as a single diagnosis. Typically, a cluster of symptoms that suggest other disorders, such as attention deficit hyperactivity disorder, oppositional defiant and conduct disorders, substance abuse, or Tourette syndrome (see Chapter 40), accompanies bipolar disorders. As many as 90% of children and 30% of adolescents seen for evaluation of possible bipolar disorder have attention deficit hyperactivity disorder (Mash & Wolfe, 1999).

Prognosis

Depressive disorders typically have a long-term course with periods of remission that vary across diagnoses and individuals. Major depressive disorder has a high rate of recurrence. At least 60% of individuals with a single episode experience another episode, and 5% to 10% subsequently develop a manic episode. Partial remission rather than complete remission also increases the likelihood of additional episodes (APA, 2000). Most children and adolescents with a depressive disorder experience recovery. However, although recovery occurs, the cumulative chance of recurrence is about 25% by 1 year, 40% by 2 years, and 70% by 5 years (Birmaher et al, 1996). Dysthymic disorder is likely to have an insidious onset during childhood, adolescence, or early adulthood, with a chronic course. Major depressive disorder may be superimposed over a dysthymia. The spontaneous remission rate for dysthymic disorder may be as low as 10%; however, active treatment significantly improves outcomes (APA, 2000).

Bipolar disorders tend to have a chronic course. Bipolar disorder recurs in 90% of individuals who have a single manic episode. The majority of affected persons experience remission of symptoms between episodes, 20% to 30% continue to experience mood instability and other ongoing mood symptoms, and up to 60% have interpersonal and occupational or school difficulties between acute episodes. The course of bipolar disorder characterized by hypomania rather than mania tends to be less severe, and most individuals return to a good functional level between episodes; however, about 15% of affected individuals continue to have interpersonal and occupational or school difficulties. Dysthymic disorder and cyclothymic disorder tend to have an early and insidious onset and follow a chronic course. When cyclothymic disorder is present, risk for development of a more serious bipolar disorder is 15% to 50% (APA, 2000). Thus mood disorders have a high risk of recurrence of episodes, and many of these conditions have a chronic lifetime course.

When individuals experience recurrence of depression or mania, they also are at risk for self-harm. Repeated major depressive episodes contribute to hopelessness that can prompt suicidal ideation and actions. The cyclic nature of manic episodes, with or without alternating periods of depression, impairs judgment and therefore increases risk for self-harm through unintentional accidents, dangerous behaviors, and suicide attempts. Thus, to evaluate prognosis for any child or adolescent with a mood disorder, long-term risk for self-harm merits ongoing consideration.

Primary Care Management

Health Care Maintenance
Growth and Development

Mood disorders are not associated with specific alterations in normal physical growth and development, and therefore regular age-appropriate screening is recommended. However, failure to achieve expected weight gains for children, weight loss without dieting, and increases or decreases in appetite constitute a criterion for a major depressive episode requiring additional evaluation when detected during any primary health care encounter. If undetected and untreated, an underlying depression could thwart a child's normal growth over time. In addition, psychopharmacologic treatment may cause appetite and weight changes. TCAs, MAOIs, mood stabilizers, some antipsychotics, and possibly atypical/novel antidepressants (notably mirtazapine [Remeron]), frequently cause weight gain that may be distressing to children and adolescents and that requires monitoring.

Very often interruptions in social development result from or even contribute to the development and chronic course of mood disorders. Failure to reach academic standards for grades in school and poor social integration may threaten psychosocial development of affected youth. Thus evaluating information about functioning at home, in school, and in social settings is an important component of regular developmental monitoring.

Diet

Changes in eating patterns may occur with mood disorders. Decreased or increased appetite and changes in food preferences often develop as early signs of mood disorders. Hoarding and binge eating can be seen across these disorders. Excessive eating may be an attempt to fill a sense of emptiness or to self-soothe in depressive disorders. During mania, children and adolescents may become "too busy" to stop for a meal. Poor nutrition results from binge eating, filling up on junk food and sweets, or inadequate intake of calories and nutrients during mania. Nutritional planning and, in severe cases, a nutritional consultation are needed to ensure that affected children and adolescents maintain adequate dietary intake. Increased risk for development of a co-morbid eating disorder requires careful monitoring throughout treatment and recovery phases. In addition, because psychotropic medications can cause changes in appetite and weight, dietary and weight monitoring and education about side effects of medications are important clinical actions during primary care encounters. Use of MAOIs requires a special diet that excludes foods high in tyramine and foods and drug interactions that may cause hypertension, anticholinergic effects, or sympathomimetic effects (Keltner & Folks, 2001; Skidmore-Roth, 2002) (Boxes 32-6 and Box 32-7).

Safety

Assessment of potential for self-injury because of poor judgment and risky behavior also is needed when depression or a

---

BOX 32-6

Tyramine-Rich Foods

ALCOHOLIC BEVERAGES
Beer and ale
Chianti and sherry wine

DAIRY PRODUCTS
Cheese: cheddar, bleu, brie, and mozzarella
Sour cream
Yogurt

FRUITS AND VEGETABLES
Avocados
Bananas
Fava beans
Canned figs

MEATS
Bologna
Chicken liver
Fish, dried
Liver
Meat tenderizer
Pickled herring
Salami
Sausage

OTHER FOODS
Caffeinated coffee, colas, and tea (large amounts)
Chocolate
Licorice
Soy sauce
Yeast

From Keltner, N.L. & Folks, D.G. (2001). *Psychotropic drugs* (3rd ed.). St. Louis: Mosby. Reprinted with permission.

BOX 32-7

Drugs to Avoid While Taking MAOIs

Drugs	Interaction
Anticholinergic drugs	Compound anticholinergic response
Anesthetics (general)	Deepen CNS depression
Antihypertensives (diuretics, beta-blockers, hydralazine)	Compound hypotensive effect
CNS depressants	Intensify CNS depression
Meperidine	CNS depression; deaths have occurred
Guanethidine, methyldopa, reserpine	
Sympathomimetics (mixed- and indirect-acting)	Produce severe hypertension
Amphetamines, methylphenidate, dopamine, phenylpropanolamine (in many OTC medications)	Precipitate hypertensive crisis, cardiac stimulation, arrhythmias, cerebrovascular hemorrhage
Sympathomimetics (direct-acting)	Same as for mixed- and indirect-acting sympathomimetics, but theoretically should not produce as severe a reaction
Epinephrine, norepinephrine, isoproterenol	
Cyclic and newer antidepressants	Same as for epinephrine, norepinephrine, isoproterenol; possibly serotonin syndrome

From Keltner, N.L. & Folks, D.G. (2001). *Psychotropic drugs* (3rd ed.). St. Louis: Mosby. Reprinted with permission.
MAOIs, Monoamine oxidase inhibitors; *CNS*, central nervous system.

---

hypomanic or manic episode is suspected or evident. For example, adolescents who have driving violations, especially from speeding, are at risk for self-injury and harming others. Risk behaviors necessitate careful monitoring and may require parental limitations on privileges and even hospitalization in extreme situations to ensure safety.

Safety considerations also accompany psychotropic medication use. Referral to psychiatric practitioners to initiate medication use and to provide periodic evaluation over the course of treatment is recommended as appropriate and safe primary care practice when treating mood disorders in children and adolescents. Risk of overdose, particularly with TCAs, and potential for serious adverse reactions necessitate intensive education of affected youth and their parents at initiation of treatment and follow-up education at every health care visit. Medication interactions with MAOI use pose special risks (APA, 2002a; Keltner & Folks, 2001) (Boxes 32-6 and 32-7).

Youth with mood disorders may attempt to self-medicate by using substances, including alcohol and street drugs. Substance use can mask mood disorder symptoms and places youth at risk for overdose, accidents, impulsive sexual activity, date rape, and fighting. Although assessment of substance use among older children and adolescents is an important component of primary care, ongoing evaluation is essential whenever a youth has a mood disorder.

Educating parents and affected youth about psychotropic drugs is an essential component of primary care. Clinicians share medication management with children and adolescents being treated and their families. Educational goals include understanding the medication's purpose, desired effects, dosage, and administration; related tests and monitoring; potential side effects and adverse effects; risk for overdose; possible interactions and dietary requirements; and anticipated time frame for treatment (Box 32-8).

Immunizations
Routine immunizations are recommended.

Screening (Box 32-9)
Vision. Routine screening for vision is recommended. To ensure that symptoms of withdrawal, low self-esteem, distractibility, irritability, and impaired attention are not partially caused by impaired sight, conducting vision screening when assessing for a mood disorder is recommended.

Hearing. Routine screening for hearing is recommended. To ensure that symptoms of withdrawal, low self-esteem, distractibility, irritability, and impaired attention are not partially caused by impaired hearing, conducting hearing screening when assessing for a mood disorder is recommended.

Dental. Routine screening is recommended.

Speech and Language. Routine screening is recommended. If psychomotor retardation is present when a depressive disorder is suspected, or if rapid speech flow is noted when a manic episode is suspected, additional speech and language evaluation may be indicated. However, if other symptoms of a mood disorder are present and meet diagnostic criteria, treatment for the appropriate mood disorder is implemented first. If speech and language do not normalize in relation to improvement of other

BOX 32-8
Parent Education for Specific Psychotropic Drugs

ANTIDEPRESSANTS
Tricyclics can be fatal in overdose. Drug administration should be supervised, and the drug should be securely stored.

Other medications, including antibiotics and OTC agents, may interact with antidepressants. Hence all medications should be reviewed with the primary clinician.

The selective serotonin reuptake inhibitors (SSRIs) can cause motor restlessness, insomnia, and irritability.

In OCD and depression, there may be a lag between initiation of treatment and clinical response.

ANTIPSYCHOTIC AGENTS
Antipsychotic drugs are part of a comprehensive program to treat psychosis.

Traditional antipsychotic medications can cause dystonic reactions, especially early in treatment.

Watch for muscle rigidity, inability to remain still, and new abnormal movements.

Review the risk of tardive dyskinesia and withdrawal dyskinesia before treatment.

MOOD STABILIZERS/ANTICONVULSANTS
Some medications require monitoring of serum levels (involves drawing blood).

Lithium can cause serious and even fatal reactions if serum level is too high.

With lithium, keep child well hydrated with adequate liquids (10-12 glasses of water per day) and extra care during exercise and hot weather.

Topiramate (Topamax) can reduce effectiveness of oral contraceptives.

Valproate (Depakote) can cause polycystic ovaries when given to girls: use with caution.

Many side effects can occur with these medications: report changes to primary care practitioner (PCP) to evaluate.

Some side effects may decrease over time.

Contact PCP if serious side effects occur: vomiting, severe tremor, severe sedation, muscle weakness, and dizziness.

Gastrointestinal effects and weight gain occur with many of the drugs: give with food, encourage healthy diet (decrease high-calorie foods and drinks) and moderate exercise.

Sedation, blood changes, and skin problems occur with some drugs.

Learn side effects for particular medication from PCP and follow instructions for follow-up health care visits, observe changes, know changes that are serious and require immediate action, and use measures to reduce effects as suggested by PCP.

From Scahill, L. (2001). Psychopharmacology for children. In N.L. Keltner & D.G. Folks (Eds.). *Psychotropic drugs* (3rd ed.). St. Louis: Mosby, pp. 468-495. Modified with permission.

BOX 32-9
Screening

VISION AND HEARING
Determine if symptoms are related to vision or hearing deficits

SPEECH AND LANGUAGE
Additional evaluation if treatment does not correct any abnormalities

BLOOD PRESSURE
Baseline readings before starting medication treatment
Monitor throughout treatment
Alter dose or change medication if persistent elevation
Stop medication immediately if extreme increase and seek emergency intervention

CARDIAC
Baseline blood pressure, complete blood count (CBC), and electrocardiogram (ECG) before starting tricyclic antidepressants (TCAs)
Repeat if dosage is changed or if PR interval ≥0.22 seconds, QRS $\geq130\%$ of baseline, pulse $>140/90$

DRUG TOXICITY SCREENING
Monitor for safety-specific recommendations for each drug class

screening or monitoring is ineffective in such instances because onset is rapid and requires immediate emergency treatment. Thus education about risks associated with diet and medications is essential.

Hematocrit. Routine screening is recommended.

Urinalysis. Routine screening is recommended.

Tuberculosis. Routine screening is recommended.

Condition-Specific Screening

Cardiac Function. Children taking TCAs are at risk for cardiac effects, including tachycardia and orthostatic hypotension (APA, 2002a). Obtaining baseline blood pressure, complete blood count (CBC), and electrocardiogram (ECG) is recommended. If a dose is changed, blood pressure, CBC, and ECG should be repeated. Lowering the dose is warranted when the PR interval reaches 0.22 seconds or QRS reaches 130% of baseline on ECG, heart rate is greater than 140 beats/min, or blood pressure is over 140/90 (Barone, 1996).

Drug Toxicity Screening. Medications used to treat mood disorders have various adverse effects. Therefore tests for safety monitoring are recommended. Screening recommendations are provided for the most commonly prescribed medications, and for selected drugs in practice with specific recommendations (APA, 2002a; Keltner & Folks, 2001; McLeer & Wills, 2000; Scahill, 2001a, 2001b; Schatzberg & Nemeroff, 1998, 2001). (See Table 32-2 for additional medication information.)

TCAs. An ECG should be done at baseline, and regular blood pressure and pulse checks should be done; evaluate family history for cardiac disease. Repeat ECGs if dosage is changed or if dosage exceeds 3 mg/kg./day (dosing range is similar within this class).

MAOIs. Monitor diet and avoid contraindicated foods, medications, and substances (Boxes 32-6 and 32-7).

symptoms, then additional evaluation of speech and language is needed.

Blood Pressure. Routine screening is recommended. Blood pressure should be monitored regularly during the first several weeks of medication treatment if TCAs or MAOIs are prescribed, and it should be monitored every few months thereafter. If MAOIs are in use, risk of hypertensive crisis is serious if the required diet is not followed carefully or if drug interactions occur (APA, 2002a; Keltner & Folks; Skidmore-Roth, 2002) (Boxes 32-6 and 32-7). However, blood pressure

Lithium. Laboratory work should be done weekly to monitor plasma levels; after stabilization, monitor monthly. Baseline ECG should be recorded. Because lithium can cause alterations in kidney function, blood urea nitrogen (BUN) and creatinine should be checked every 4 to 6 months; because lithium can cause goiter or hypothyroidism, a thyroid-stimulating test should be done every 4 to 6 months.

Carbamazepine (Tegretol). Laboratory work should be done weekly to monitor plasma levels; after stabilization, monitor monthly. Baseline ECG should be recorded. Baseline hemoglobin, hematocrit, CBC with differential, white blood count (WBC), platelet count, and liver function tests (LFTs) should be done. Monitoring recommendations vary, but a conservative plan is as follows: CBC and LFTs weekly for 1 month, monthly for 4 months, and every 3 months thereafter. Evaluate CBC for blood dyscrasias, especially agranulocytosis and leukopenia (rare). Order tests if rash, lethargy, fever, weakness, malaise, vomiting, anorexia, increased urinary frequency, jaundice, easy bruising, bleeding, or mouth ulcers occur. Stop the drug if neutrophil count drops below 1000 or if hepatitis occurs.

Valproate/valproic acid (Depakote). Baseline and periodic CBC and LFTs should be done. Suggest scheduling lab tests as for carbamazepine (Tegretol).

Antipsychotic agents: chlorpromazine (Thorazine). Baseline and periodic (e.g., every 3 to 6 months) CBC and LFTs should be done.

Antipsychotic agents: clonazepam (Klonopin). Baseline and periodic (e.g., every 3 to 6 months) LFTs, serum bilirubin, renal function tests, and CBC should be done.

Common Illness Management
Differential Diagnosis (Box 32-10)

Differential diagnosis is an important issue in relation to all mood disorders for children and adolescents. Considerable overlap in symptoms with several other psychiatric disorders requires evaluation of diagnostic *DSM-IV-TR* criteria across conditions. Several other disorders require evaluation including, but not limited to, anxiety disorders, attention deficit hyperactivity disorder (ADHD), substance use disorders, and eating disorders. Common problems seen by PCPs that include weight loss, somatic complaints, fatigue, recurrent injuries, and school failure have overlapping presentations with mood disorders.

Anxiety often accompanies other symptoms of depressive disorders among children and adolescents yet also tends to emerge as a co-morbid condition as age and severity increase (Gurley et al, 1996). Distractibility and inattention, characteristics of ADHD, overlap with symptoms of depressive and bipolar disorders. All other diagnostic criteria merit careful evaluation to differentiate these diagnoses.

Youth who experience depression or mania often use alcohol and drugs in an attempt to manage symptoms or because of their poor judgment. If criteria for any substance use disorder are met, co-morbid conditions exist and both disorders require active treatment. Moreover, safety risks result from illegal use of substances, interactions of substances with prescribed medications, and increased incidence of accidents. Therefore, even if diagnostic criteria for a substance use disorder are unmet, the reasons, pattern, and effects necessitate exploration, and strategies to promote and monitor abstinence are important components of care.

Weight loss and reduced appetite that can occur in depressive disorders might appear like signs of anorexia nervosa; however, anorexics typically retain their desire for food even when restricting intake and mood changes can emerge as a secondary problem to the eating disorder. Binge eating, a component of bulimia nervosa, can occur with mania. Obtaining a detailed report for food intake from a single day, exploring perceptions of food and body characteristics, and evaluating other impulsive behaviors will assist the clinician to differentiate eating disorders from mood disorders (APA, 2002a). Weight loss also can be a symptom of many physical illnesses. Weight loss among children and adolescents with mood disorders requires careful investigation to detect a possible underlying illness.

Somatic complaints may be expressions of emotional distress but also may indicate another illness or problem. Fatigue is a common symptom of depression but is also associated with many physical illnesses. PCPs can evaluate such symptoms by asking the child about other signs related to the diagnosed mood disorder and about signs of other suspected illnesses. For example, a stomachache might indicate emotional upset or a gastrointestinal disorder. Before attributing a somatic complaint to a mood disorder, investigation of a possible physical cause is needed. Recurrent injuries require thorough evaluation in addition to safety education, and assessment of judgment and functioning. For example, frequent falling from athletic equipment in a playground might indicate self-injurious motivation, impulsiveness, or a physical problem such as a neurologic disorder. Poor school performance or failure could be caused by exacerbation of a mood disorder or by another problem, such as a learning or developmental disorder.

Drug Interactions

Drug interactions can occur with concurrent use of two or more psychotropic agents, or when a psychopharmacologic drug interacts with a medication used to treat a different problem. Youth being medicated for mood disorders are at risk for both types of drug interactions. Ordering plasma levels is indicated when interactions have potential to raise or lower levels to an extent that safety or efficacy is affected, and when careful monitoring is indicated to judge safety and efficacy of dosage, such as with lithium use.

BOX 32-10
Differential Diagnosis

Adjustment disorders
Anxiety disorders
Attention deficit hyperactivity disorder
Somatic complaints
Recurrent injuries
Eating disorders
Substance use disorders

Combination therapy (i.e., the use of two or more psychopharmacologic agents together) is used when a single drug has failed to produce the desired therapeutic effect. Although combination drug treatment is indicated at times to ameliorate the debilitating symptoms of mood disorders, the risk for drug interactions increases. Further, changing from one class of drugs to another can produce interactions.

Although a few interactions exist, SSRIs have a more benign profile than earlier TCA and MAOI antidepressants, including less risk from cumulative effects with concomitant CNS depressants such as alcohol, antihistamines, or anticholinergic drugs (Schatzberg & Nemeroff, 1998, 2001). Greatest risk occurs when SSRIs are administered with other antidepressants and when a change is made from one antidepressant class to another. SSRIs in combination with MAOIs can produce a potentially lethal interaction: serotonin syndrome, as discussed previously in this chapter. Changing from an SSRI to an MAOI requires that at least five half-lives elapse; the long half-life of fluoxetine (Prozac) necessitates a 5-week washout period. To change from an MAOI to an SSRI, a 2-week waiting period is recommended. SSRIs and antipsychotic medications may reduce metabolism and clearance of TCAs, causing a rise in TCA blood levels (APA, 2002a; McLeer & Wills, 2000; Scahill, 2001a, 2001b).

TCAs and MAOIs interact with a variety of other drugs. TCAs can alter the pharmacokinetics or pharmacodynamics of other medications, including lowering valproate (Depakote) levels and activity of clonidine, necessitating alteration of dosages. When taken with alcohol, TCA clearance is decreased with single or episodic alcohol ingestion, but clearance is increased with regular alcohol use in the absence of liver damage from cirrhosis (Schatzberg & Nemeroff, 1998, 2001). Potentially dangerous interactions such as hypertensive crisis can result from joint administration of TCAs and MAOIs, epinephrine, and norepinephrine. Further, because of albuterol's effect on the vascular system, albuterol inhalers should be administered with extreme caution in combination with either TCAs or MOAIs; caution should be maintained within 2 weeks of TCA or MAOI discontinuation (Warrick Pharmaceuticals Corporation, 1999). Combination therapy involving TCAs and MAOIs should be considered only after all other options have been exhausted, and this approach requires careful monitoring by an expert psychopharmacologist (APA, 2002a; McLeer & Wills, 2000; Scahill, 2001a, 2001b). (For interactions with MAOIs, see Box 32-7.)

Other notable drug interactions associated with TCAs are warfarin (increased anticoagulant activity), phenothiazines (additive anticholinergic effects), phenytoin (increased concentrations of this antiepileptic agent may become toxic), and haloperidol (Haldol) (blocked TCA metabolism potential to raise TCA plasma levels to toxic range); also possible are alterations in metabolism or effects of agents when used with barbiturates, cimetidine, clonidine, guanethidine, and methylphenidate. Other notable interactions associated with MAOIs are over-the-counter medications with sympathomimetic agents such as some cough syrups, narcotics (most notably with meperidine resulting in hypertension, hyperpyrexia, and coma), amphetamines, anticonvulsants, antihyper-

tensives, buspirone (BuSpar), and clomipramine (Anafranil) (Rankin, 2000; Schatzberg & Nemeroff, 1998, 2001).

Drug treatment of mania also poses risks for adverse effects and interactions. Lithium has remarkably few clinically significant drug interactions. Lithium is cleared by the kidneys with an approximate half-life of 14 to 30 hours. Young people tend to have a faster lithium clearance rate than older adults. To treat children safely, lithium serum levels require regular monitoring. Most individuals will experience some toxic effects with levels over 1.5 mEq/L, and levels over 2.0 mEq/L are associated with life-threatening side effects. Therefore changes in hydration, renal function, and sodium levels will alter lithium serum levels; any medication, such as a diuretic, will increase lithium levels by 30% to 50%. Agents that may produce interactions with lithium are diuretics, nonsteroidal antiinflammatory agents (e.g., ibuprofen, naproxen), neuroleptics, potassium, and antiarrhythmics (APA, 2002a; Schatzberg & Nemeroff, 1998).

Interactions of anticonvulsants and other drugs merit consideration when prescribing and monitoring medication use. Valproate (Depakote) is extensively metabolized by the liver and is highly protein bound; therefore interactions, including valproate toxicity, may occur with other metabolized or protein-bound medications, most notably aspirin. Valproate also weakly inhibits drug oxidation, resulting in increased serum concentrations of drugs, such as TCAs, phenobarbital, and phenytoin, that undergo oxidative metabolism. Co-administration of microsomal enzyme-inducing drugs, such as carbamazepine (Tegretol), can decrease serum concentrations of valproate, and drugs that inhibit metabolism, such as fluoxetine (Prozac), can increase levels (APA, 2002a; Rankin, 2000; Schatzberg & Nemeroff, 1998, 2001).

Carbamazepine (Tegretol), another mood stabilizer, induces metabolism of other drugs by the liver and is highly protein bound. Thus this medication decreases plasma levels of many other medications, including TCAs, antipsychotics (particularly haloperidol [Haldol]), thyroid hormones, hormonal contraceptives, antiasthmatics (e.g., prednisone, methylprednisone, theophylline), warfarin, valproate, benzodiazepines, and neuroleptics. Drugs that inhibit carbamazepine metabolism, including erythromycin, calcium channel blockers diltiazem and verapamil, danazol, dextropropoxyphene, propoxyphene, isoniazid, valproate, and SSRIs, will increase serum levels. Other anticonvulsants, notably gabapentin (Neurontin) and lamotrigine (Lamictal), can interact with other drugs: gabapentin may interact with antacids and cimetidine; and lamotrigine may interact with carbamazepine, phenobarbital, phenytoin, primidone, and valproate (APA, 2002a; Rankin, 2000; Schatzberg & Nemeroff, 1998, 2001).

Developmental Issues
Sleep Patterns

Sleep disturbances characterize mood disorders. Although sleep patterns among children and adolescents who experience mood disorders may not mirror the sleep of adults with depressive or bipolar disorders (Mash & Wolfe, 1999), sleeping difficulties are common symptoms. Excessive sleeping, too little sleep, disrupted sleep, and poor quality of sleep all contribute to irritability, poor school performance, and fatigue or agitation. The depressed child may sleep more or have insomnia that may be related to a co-morbid anxiety disorder or may be due to anxiety associated with the depression. The child with bipolar disorder may cycle from periods of very little sleep and hyperactivity to periods of utter exhaustion during which the child may want to sleep all day. Of course, a co-morbid hyperactivity disorder could also profoundly affect sleep cycles. As previously mentioned, the sedating effects of many psychoactive medications must also be considered.

Changes in sleep patterns may be one of the early signs of an incipient mood episode. Eliciting an account of recent sleep patterns, including any changes from usual patterns, from parents and pediatric clients will assist primary care providers to identify signs that might signify a mood disorder. Keeping a sleep diary can assist youth and their parents to track patterns and monitor response to treatment. Improvement is expected with treatment; in addition, implementing good sleep habits, including a regular bedtime, avoidance of caffeine in the evening, and relaxing routines before sleep, can assist in normalizing sleep patterns.

Toileting

Mood disorders generally are not associated with significant difficulties in toileting. In some instances, however, problems with bedwetting and soiling have been seen in children with bipolar disorder (Papolos & Papolos, 1999).

Discipline

Mood disorders can create tremendous interactive problems for children and adolescents in various environments, including the home, the classroom, and the playground. Parents and teachers may perceive depressed children who are frequently quiet and withdrawn as being uncooperative. Children with bipolar disorder are prone to aggressive behavior and outbursts that are disruptive, and that might alienate them from the other children who fear for their own safety. All children and adolescents with mood disorders are prone to irritability that often translates into lack of cooperation and lack of respect. If adults treat symptoms as discipline problems without treating the underlying disorder, discipline will be ineffective and likely exacerbate the undesired behaviors. Consistent limits and clear explanations of behavioral contingencies are appropriate discipline strategies. Enforcing rules regarding safety also is essential for purposes of protection.

Child Care

Although no specific problems concerning child care are associated with mood disorders, children with these disorders can present a challenge to child care providers. These children frequently have trouble relating to peers. Irritability makes them difficult to be around and tends to push others away. Bipolar children typically have periods of disruptive behavior that can cause safety problems and interfere with group activities. In addition, a lack of pleasure (anhedonia), a cardinal symptom of depressive disorders, limits engagement in usual social activities and even casual peer pastimes. Regular schedules and placement in small family settings or centers with high staff/child ratios and stable personnel are ideal. Once a diagnosis has been made, child care personnel should be educated about the condition and management in the setting. These issues necessitate careful placement with consistent caring caregivers for child care to be successful—not always an easy goal.

Schooling

Not surprisingly, children with mood disorders, particularly bipolar disorders, frequently experience a great deal of difficulty in school. Successful school performance requires concentration, alertness, proper behavior, individual performance, teamwork, and an ability to consolidate information quickly. A downward slide in grades, difficulty managing school-related activities, and behavior problems in the classroom are indicators that students might be experiencing a mood disorder. Although such behavioral signs are associated with many health-related problems among youth, too often they fail to trigger evaluation for a mood disorder. Poor concentration, irritability, disorganization, lack of self-confidence, or grandiosity interferes with academic work. In addition, the factors discussed above in relation to social problems also lead to difficulties in school, most notably withdrawal, bullying, and fighting.

Without timely evaluation and treatment, school-related problems can escalate and may lead to academic failure and even dropping out of school among adolescents. In severe cases, hospitalization and residential placement may be needed. In such instances, removal from school becomes necessary, and academic tutoring or schooling in a residential treatment setting must substitute for usual school attendance. Children with mood disorders often have trouble making transitions and may have co-morbid conditions that make them easily distracted and inattentive. In addition, medications may have a sedating effect that makes it difficult for these children to stay awake (Papolos & Papolos, 1999).

Clearly, these children often require special accommodations in school that are guaranteed by federal law (see Chapter 5). PCPs may help the child and family obtain educational services, negotiate modification of the educational program, or collaborate with the therapist. An individualized educational plan (IEP) may assist the student to function in the classroom. For example, a student may require adjustments in assignments, setting, or teaching modality to learn effectively. To create a viable plan, consultation is needed among learning specialists in the school system, teachers, the guidance counselor or school psychologist, and the PCP and psychiatric clinician involved in the student's care. The PCP appropriately provides information to involved school personnel, with parental consent and student assent, and monitors progress.

Sexuality

Depressive disorders may affect sexuality by reducing interest and performance ability among adolescents (APA, 2000). More importantly for young people, difficulty establishing close relationships may interfere with the development of healthy sexuality. In addition, bipolar disorders are associated with poor judg-ment during manic episodes that could lead to promiscuous behavior and related risks for unwanted pregnancy and sexually transmitted diseases (STDs). PCPs are encouraged to discuss dating and sexual behavior and to provide early contraceptive education, and pregnancy and STD testing. Because medications to manage bipolar disorders (i.e., carbamazepine [Tegretol], topiramate [Topamax]) can reduce the effectiveness of hormonal contraceptives, alternative or dual birth control methods (e.g., use of condoms with birth control pills) are recommended. Condoms also provide some protection against STDs. Exploring risks associated with sexual behavior may assist older children and adolescents to make responsible choices. In addition, genetic counseling may be indicated, given available knowledge about genetic factors in etiology of mood disorders, particularly for bipolar disorders.

If pregnancy occurs, continuation of psychotropic medications requires careful evaluation by involved providers. Because all psychotropic drugs diffuse across the placenta, the US Food and Drug Administration (FDA) has not approved any psychotropic medication for use during pregnancy. Psychotropics vary in teratogenic potential. SSRIs and typical neuroleptics have low risks; lithium has a moderate risk; older anticonvulsants have higher risks; and newer anticonvulsants and atypical antipsychotics have virtually unknown risks (Viguera et al, 2002). Treatment during pregnancy involves providing the best known information about risks associated with continuing and withdrawing medication; obtaining informed consent for any plan is essential. Determining a plan involves evaluation of severity of mood disorder symptoms and risk of relapse vs. risks of medication use. Relapse is a serious concern for pregnant adolescents with bipolar disorders. Recommendations for management of bipolar disorders during pregnancy are as follows: tapering and discontinuation during the first trimester and longer if signs of relapse do not appear for mild to moderate bipolar disorder; and consideration of treatment with a mood stabilizer throughout pregnancy for severe bipolar disorder (Viguera et al, 2002). Clearly, these complex issues necessitate collaboration among PCPs, psychiatric providers, parents/guardians, and affected adolescents.

Transition into Adulthood

Symptoms associated with mood disorders typically interfere with the ability of affected children and adolescents to relate to peers, develop intimate relationships, and manage responsibilities—important goals in preparation for transition to adulthood. Although hypomanic symptoms initially may help affected youth to be popular and to engage in a whirlwind of activities, as irritability and disorganization increase with mania, social engagement and functional ability decrease. Poor social relationships and impaired performance in school or work are hallmarks of mood disorders that directly interfere with a successful transition to adulthood. Separation from family is particularly difficult because a consistent and supportive home environment promotes recovery and helps to prevent relapse. Moreover, being sensitive to cultural practices and values is essential because the meaning of transition to adulthood varies. Effective transitions to college or work and moving away from home involve planning for continuation of treatment, including crisis management, and development of ways to maintain connection with family members, such as visits and contact by phone and E-mail.

BOX 32-11

The Rapid-Cycling Bipolar Child: A Day of Mood Swings

Mornings: Difficult to arouse; resists getting up, dressed, and off to school; irritable with a tendency to snap and gripe or sullen and withdrawn.

Midday: The darkness lifts, and the bipolar child enjoys a few clear hours, enabling the child to focus and take part in school.

Late afternoon: The child becomes increasingly wild, wired, euphoric in a giddy and strained way; laughs too loudly and too long; play has a flailing and aggressive quality; temper tantrums when needs are not met.

Late evening: Behavior can continue well into the night, accounting for the difficulty getting up in the morning.

TREATMENT

Conventional psychopharmacology recommended for adults

Stable schedules; no caffeine, drugs, or alcohol

Individual therapy to help learn to balance the day and resolve crises that can trigger a mood change

Family therapy so that parents and siblings can learn how to help

---

From Laraia, M.T. (2002). Bipolar disorder: Bipolar depression, rapid cycling, children, & pharmacology. *APNA News, 14*, 13. Reprinted with permission.

Adolescents with mood disorders may face trouble managing future responsibilities. If substance abuse also is present, difficulties multiply. Obtaining occupational preparation and holding a consistent job are challenging tasks. Functioning in the work world is necessary to receive health insurance, to obtain housing, and to manage other financial obligations. Failure to do so leads to ongoing dependency on family or government programs with increased risk for homelessness and a chronic mental illness course. PCPs can play an important role in encouraging affected adolescents and their families to plan appropriately for education and occupational preparation and to anticipate the need for ongoing or episodic treatment suitable to the child's diagnosis and its severity.

Family Concerns and Resources

Family Concerns

Mood disorders can also take a toll on the family as a whole. The "well" siblings may harbor feelings of resentment as the "ill" child gets special accommodations based on the disorder. The child with bipolar disorder also may embarrass family members with angry public outbursts of rage (Papolos & Papolos, 1999). Coping with the vicissitudes of mood and behavior, especially for children with rapid-cycling bipolar disorders, is a daily challenge for families (Box 32-11).

Families also face other worries. Stigma associated with mental illness may lead to shame and isolation. Concerns about possible genetic transmission can create feelings of guilt and anger, as well as anxiety about future generations. Parents often worry that symptoms will worsen over time and that their child will be unable to live independently or to fulfill their hopes for a productive and happy life.

Financial concerns often worry parents. Difficulty obtaining adequate health care coverage for psychiatric disorders, particularly when a long-term course develops, creates real financial burden and stress for families. Efforts at state and federal levels to pass and enforce legislation for mental health parity have improved coverage for pediatric care; however, adequacy of services, especially for pediatric chronic conditions, varies widely and remains a long-term concern.

RESOURCES

Organizations, support groups, and informational Web sites are available resources for families. The following is a list of resources and organizations presented by Demitri and Janice Papolos in *The Bipolar Child: The Definitive and Reassuring Guide to Childhood's Most Misunderstood Disorder* (1999):

Family Voices
PO Box 769
Algodones, NM 87001
(505) 867-2368
http://www.familyvoices.org

Federation of Families
1021 Prince St, Alexandria, VA 22314
(703) 684-7710
http://www.ffcmh.org

Lithium Information Center
c/o Madison Institute of Medicine
PO Box 628365
Middleton, WI 53562-8365
(608) 827-2470; fax: (608) 827-2479

Internet Resources

The Bipolar Child (Web site for Demitri and Janice Papolos)
http://www.bipolarchild.com

Dr. Bob's Psychopharmacology Tips
www.dr-bob.org/tips

Dr. Ivan Goldberg's site
http://www.psycom.net/depression.central.html

Moodswing.org
http://www.moodswings.org

Pendulum Resources
http://www.pendulum.org

Organizations

Child and Adolescent Bipolar Foundation (CABF)
1187 Wilmette Ave, # PMB 331
Wilmette, IL 60091
(847) 256-8525
http://www.bpkids.org

NAMI (The National Alliance for the Mentally Ill)
200 N Glebe Rd, Suite 1015
Arlington, VA 22203-3754
(703) 524-7600; fax: (703) 524-9094
(800) 950-NMAI
http://www.nami.org

NARSAD (National Alliance for Research on Schizophrenia and Depression)
60 Cutter Mill Rd, Suite 404
Great Neck, NY 11021
(516) 829-0091
http://www.mhsource.com

The National Mental Health Association
1021 Prince St
Alexandria, VA 22314
(800) 969-NMHA
http://www.nmha.org

NDMDA (National Depressive and Manic-Depressive Association)
730 N Franklin St, Suite 501
Chicago, IL 60610
(800) 82-NDMDA
http://www.ndmda.org

The Stanley Foundation Bipolar Network
5430 Grosvenor Lane, Suite 200
Bethesda, MD 20814
(800) 518-7326
http://www.bipolarnetwork.org

Summary of Primary Care Needs for the Child or Adolescent with a Mood Disorder

HEALTH CARE MAINTENANCE

Growth and Development

Failure to achieve expected weight gains, weight loss without dieting, and increases or decreases in appetite require additional evaluation.

Psychopharmacologic treatment may cause appetite and weight changes.

Failure to reach academic standards and poor social integration may threaten psychosocial development of affected youth. Evaluate information about functioning at home, in school, and in social settings.

Diet

Decreased or increased appetite, hoarding, bingeing, and changes in food preferences can occur.

During mania, children and adolescents may become "too busy" to stop for a meal.

Poor nutrition results from binge eating, filling up on junk food and sweets, or inadequate intake of calories and nutrients during mania.

Increased risk for development of a co-morbid eating disorder requires careful monitoring throughout treatment and recovery phases.

Psychotropic medications can cause changes in appetite and weight. Monitor diet and weight, and educate about side effects of medications.

Use of monoamine oxidase inhibitors (MAOIs) requires a special diet that excludes foods high in tyramine and avoidance of foods and drug interactions that may cause hypertension, anticholinergic effects, or sympathomimetic effects.

Continued

Summary of Primary Care Needs for the Child or Adolescent with a Mood Disorder—cont'd

Safety

Suicidal thoughts, threats, or gestures always must be taken seriously, and children and adolescents with mood disorders are considered to be at high risk for self-harm.

When a hypomanic or manic episode is suspected or evident, assess potential for self-injury because of poor judgment and risk-taking behavior.

Risk of overdose, particularly with tricyclic antidepressants (TCAs), and potential for serious adverse reactions necessitate intensive education of affected youth and their parents at initiation of treatment and follow-up education at every health care visit.

Medication and dietary interactions with MAOIs use pose special risks.

Immunizations

No changes in the routine schedule of immunizations are needed.

Screening

Vision. Routine age-related screening for vision is recommended.

Ensure that symptoms of withdrawal, low self-esteem, distractibility, irritability, and impaired attention are not caused in part by impaired sight by conducting vision screening when assessing for a mood disorder.

Hearing. Routine age-related screening for hearing is recommended.

Ensure that symptoms of withdrawal, low self-esteem, distractibility, irritability, and impaired attention are not caused in part by impaired hearing by conducting hearing screening when assessing for a mood disorder.

Dental. Routine screening is recommended.

Speech and Language. Routine screening is recommended.

If speech and language do not normalize after treatment is implemented, additional evaluation of speech and language is needed.

Blood Pressure. Routine screening is recommended.

Baseline blood pressure assessment and regular monitoring during the first several weeks of medication treatment if TCAs or MAOIs are prescribed should be done; monitoring should be every few months thereafter.

If MAOIs are in use, risk of hypertensive crisis is serious if the required diet is not followed carefully or if drug interactions occur. Education is essential to prevent this.

Hematocrit. Routine screening is recommended.

Urinalysis. Routine screening is recommended.

Tuberculosis. Routine screening is recommended.

Condition-Specific Screening

Cardiac Function. Children taking TCAs are at risk for cardiac effects, including tachycardia and orthostatic hypotension.

Obtaining baseline blood pressure, complete blood count (CBC), and electrocardiogram (ECG) is recommended.

If a dose is changed, blood pressure, CBC, and ECG should be repeated.

Lowering the dose is warranted when the PR interval reaches 0.22 seconds or QRS reaches 130% of baseline, heart rate is >140 beats/min, or blood pressure is >140/90.

Drug Toxicity. Monitor for safety and follow specific recommendations for each class of drugs.

COMMON ILLNESS MANAGEMENT

Differential Diagnosis

Overlap in symptoms with several other psychiatric disorders and common childhood illnesses requires evaluation of diagnostic *DSM-IV-TR* criteria and an assessment of physical symptoms.

The clinician must determine which symptoms are occurring in isolation and which appear to be associated with or caused by another physical or psychologic ailment.

A detailed and thorough history is often the best strategy to help the clinician create an accurate timeline of the onset of symptoms. Youngsters often are poor historians and lack an accurate recollection of dates. The parent or another important person in the child's life may be of great assistance in providing these critical data.

The most common psychiatric disorders to be considered as differential diagnoses include the following: adjustment disorder, post-traumatic stress disorder (PTSD), anxiety disorders, attention deficit hyperactivity disorder (ADHD), eating disorders, and substance use disorders. Consider other common childhood illnesses that may precipitate or result from a mood disorder.

Discerning between a symptom of a known mood disorder and a symptom that may represent another problem is difficult at times. To arrive at the most accurate diagnosis, careful observations are required, sometimes over an extended period.

Drug Interactions

Combination therapy increases the risk for drug interactions.

Changing from one class of drugs to another can produce interactions.

Selective serotonin reuptake inhibitors (SSRIs) in combination with MAOIs can produce a potentially lethal interaction: serotonin syndrome. Changing from an SSRI to an MAOI requires that at least five half-lives elapse; the long half-life of fluoxetine necessitates a 5-week washout period. Changing from an MAOI to an SSRI requires a 2-week waiting period.

Lithium is cleared by the kidneys with an approximate half-life of 14 to 30 hours.

Young people tend to have a faster lithium clearance rate than older adults.

Safe treatment requires regular monitoring of lithium serum levels.

Toxic effects from lithium typically occur with serum levels >1.5 mEq/L, and levels >2.0 mEq/L are associated with life-threatening side effects.

Changes in hydration, renal function, and sodium levels will alter lithium serum levels.

Valproate is metabolized by the liver and is highly protein bound; therefore interactions may occur with other metabolized or protein-bound medications. Valproate weakly inhibits drug oxidation,

Summary of Primary Care Needs for the Child or Adolescent with a Mood Disorder—cont'd

resulting in increased serum concentrations of drugs that undergo oxidative metabolism.

Co-administration of many other medications can decrease or increase serum concentrations of valproate, requiring careful evaluation of all medications administered. Valproate toxicity can result from co-administration with other protein-bound medications, such as aspirin.

Carbamazepine decreases plasma levels of many other medications, including TCAs, thyroid hormones, hormonal contraceptives, and neuroleptics.

Drugs that inhibit carbamazepine metabolism, including erythromycin, calcium channel blockers diltiazem and verapamil, and SSRIs, will increase serum levels.

DEVELOPMENTAL ISSUES

Sleep Patterns

Change in sleep patterns may be an early sign of a mood disorder. Excessive sleeping, too little sleep, disrupted sleep, and poor quality of sleep are common symptoms.

Abnormal sleep contributes to irritability, poor school performance, and fatigue or agitation.

In bipolar disorder, the affected youth may alternate between periods of very little sleep and hyperactivity to periods of utter exhaustion during which the child may want to sleep all day.

Sedating effects of many medications must be considered when evaluating sleep.

Eliciting an account of recent sleep patterns helps identify signs of a mood disorder.

Keeping a sleep diary helps track patterns and monitor response to treatment.

Implementing good sleep habits, including a regular bedtime, avoidance of caffeine in the evening, and relaxing routines before sleep, helps normalize sleep patterns.

Toileting

Mood disorders generally are not associated with significant difficulties in toileting. Problems with bedwetting and soiling sometimes occur with bipolar disorder.

Discipline

Parents and teachers may interpret withdrawal or irritability as a lack of cooperation or respect. Children with bipolar disorder are prone to aggressive behavior and disruptive and alienating outbursts.

Consistent limits and clear explanations of behavioral contingencies are appropriate discipline strategies. Enforcing rules regarding safety also is essential for purposes of protection.

Child Care

Children frequently have trouble relating to peers. Irritability makes them difficult to be around and tends to push others away.

Bipolar children typically have periods of disruptive behavior that can cause safety problems and interfere with group activities.

A lack of pleasure or interest limits engagement in social activities.

Regular schedules and placement in small family settings or centers with high staff/child ratios and stable personnel are ideal.

Schooling

A downward slide in grades, difficulty managing school-related activities, and behavior problems in the classroom can indicate a mood disorder.

Poor concentration, irritability, disorganization, lack of self-confidence or grandiosity, and withdrawal or fighting interfere with academic work.

School-related problems can escalate and lead to academic failure and dropping out.

In severe cases, hospitalization and residential placement may need to substitute for usual school attendance.

Children often require special accommodations, and an individualized educational plan (IEP) may assist affected students to function in the classroom.

Sexuality

Interest and performance ability may lessen among adolescents.

Difficulty establishing close relationships may interfere with development of healthy sexuality.

Bipolar disorders are associated with poor judgment during manic episodes that could lead to promiscuous behavior and related risks for unwanted pregnancy and sexually transmitted diseases (STDs).

Transition into Adulthood

Mood disorders interfere with being able to relate to peers, develop intimate relationships, and manage responsibilities.

Appropriate adjunctive therapeutic approaches include social skills training, academic and occupational counseling, and education in life skills.

FAMILY CONCERNS AND RESOURCES

Mood disorders take a toll on the family. "Well" siblings may harbor feelings of resentment as the "ill" child gets special accommodations based on the disorder.

The bipolar child also may embarrass family members with an angry public outburst of rage.

Concerns about possible genetic transmission can create feelings of guilt and anger, and anxiety about future generations.

Difficulty obtaining adequate health care coverage for long-term psychiatric disorders creates real financial burden and stress for families.

National organizations, local support groups, and informational Web sites are available resources for families.

REFERENCES

Abramson, L.Y., Seligman, M.E., & Teasdale, J.D. (1978). Learned helplessness in humans: Critique and reformulation. *J Abnorm Psychol, 37,* 49-74.

American Academy of Child and Adolescent Psychiatry. (1997). Practice parameters for the assessment and treatment of children and adolescents with bipolar disorder. *J Am Acad Child Adolesc Psychiatry, 36*(suppl. 176), 157.

American Psychiatric Association. (1980). *Diagnostic and statistical manual of mental disorders* (3rd ed.). Washington, D.C.: Author.

American Psychiatric Association. (2000). *Diagnostic and statistical manual of mental disorders: DSM-IV-TR* (4th ed., text revision). Washington, D.C.: Author.

American Psychiatric Association. (2002a). *American Psychiatric Association practice guidelines for the treatment of psychiatric disorders: Compendium 2002.* Washington, D.C.: Author.

American Psychiatric Association. (2002b). *Quick reference to the American Psychiatric Association practice guidelines for the treatment of psychiatric disorders: Compendium 2002.* Washington, D.C.: Author.

Barnes, M.A. (1996). *The Harriet Lane handbook: A manual for pediatric house officers* (14th ed.). St. Louis: Mosby–Year Book.

Beck, A.T. (1967). *Depression: Clinical, experimental, and theoretical aspects.* Philadelphia: University of Pennsylvania Press.

Birmaher, B., Dahl, R.E., Williamson, D.E., Perel, J.M., Brent, D.A., et al. (2000). Growth hormone secretion in children and adolescents at high risk for major depressive disorder. *Arch Gen Psychiatry, 57,* 867-872.

Birmaher, B., Ryan, N.D., Williamson, D.E., Brent, D.A., Kaufman, J., et al. (1996). Childhood and adolescent depression: A review of the past 10 years. I. *J Am Acad Child Adolesc Psychiatry, 35,* 1427-1439.

Byrne, A. & Byrne, D.G. (1993). The effect of exercise on depression, anxiety and other mood states: A review. *J Psychosom Res, 37,* 565-574.

Daleiden, E.L., Vasey, M.W., & Brown, L.M. (1999). Internalizing disorders. In W.K. Silverman & T.H. Ollendick (Eds.). *Developmental issues in the clinical treatment of children* Needham Heights, Mass.: Allyn & Bacon, pp. 261-278.

Dinan, T.G. (1994). Glucocorticosteroids and the genesis of depressive illness: A psychobiological model. *Br J Psychiatry, 164,* 365-371.

Feetham, S.L. (1999). Families and the genetic revolution: Implications for primary healthcare, education, and research. *Fam Syst Health, 17,* 27-43.

Forero, R., McLellan, L., Rissel, C., & Bauman, A. (1999). Bullying behaviour and psychosocial health among school students in New South Wales, Australia: Cross sectional survey. *BMJ, 319,* 344-348.

Geffken, G. (1998). Assessment and treatment of children and adolescents. In S. Cullari (Ed.). *Foundations of clinical psychology.* Needham Heights, Mass.: Allyn & Bacon, pp. 216-248.

Gurley, D., Cohen, P., Pine, D.S., & Brook, J. (1996). Discriminating depression and anxiety in youth: A role for diagnostic criteria. *J Affect Disord, 39,* 191-200.

Harrington, R.C., Rutter, M., & Fombonne, E. (1996). Developmental pathways in depression: Multiple meanings, antecedents, and endpoints. *Dev Psychopathol, 8,* 601-616.

Herpertz-Dahlmann, B. (2001). Depressive syndromes and suicide. In H. Remschmidt (Ed.). *Psychotherapy with children and adolescents.* New York: Cambridge University Press, pp. 291-305.

Hersen, M. & Ammerman, R.T. (2000.). *Advanced abnormal child psychology* (2nd ed.). Mahwah, N.J.: Lawrence Erlbaum Associates, Publishers.

Kaplan, H.I. & Sadock, B.J. (1998). *Kaplan and Sadock's synopsis of psychiatry: Behavioral sciences/clinical psychiatry.* Baltimore: Williams & Wilkins.

Kaslow, N.J., Adamson, L.B., & Collins, M.H. (2000). A developmental psychopathology perspective on the cognitive components of child and adolescent depression. In A.J. Sameroff, M. Lewis, & S.M. Miller (Eds). *Handbook of developmental psychology.* New York: Kluwer Academic/Plenum Publishers, pp. 491-510.

Kaslow, N.J., Rehm, L.P., Pollack, & Siegal, A.W. (1988). Social cognitive and cognitive correlates of depression in children. *J Abnorm Psychol, 12,* 605-620.

Keltner, N.L. & Folks, D.G. (2001). *Psychotropic drugs* (3rd ed.). St. Louis: Mosby.

Kendall, P.C. & Panichelli-Mendal, S.M. (1995). Cognitive-behavioral treatments. *J Abnorm Child Psychol, 22,* 107-121.

Kovacs, M., Akiskal, H.S., Gatsonis, C., & Parrone, P.L. (1994). Childhood-onset dysthymic disorder: Clinical features and prospective naturalistic outcome. *Arch Gen Psychiatry, 51,* 365-374.

Laraia, M.T. (2002). Bipolar disorder: Bipolar depression, rapid cycling, children & pharmacology. *APNA News, 14*(6), 12-13.

Laughren, T.B. (1996). Regulating issues in pediatric psychopharmacology. *J Am Acad Child Adolesc Psychiatry, 34,* 1276-1282.

Lewinsohn, P.M., Klein, D., & Seeley, J.R. (1995). Bipolar disorders in a community sample of older adolescents: Prevalence, phenomenology, comorbidity, and course. *J Am Acad Child Adolesc Psychiatry, 34,* 454-463.

Luby, J.L., Heffelfinger, A.K., Mrakotsky, C., Hessler, M.J., Brown, K.M., et al. (2002). Preschool major depressive disorder: Preliminary validation for developmentally modified *DSM-IV* criteria. *J Am Acad Child Adolesc Psychiatry, 41,* 928-937.

Mash, E.J. & Wolfe, D.A. (1999). *Abnormal child psychiatry.* Belmont, Calif.: Brooks/Cole-Wadsworth.

McLeer, S.V. & Wills, C. (2000). Psychopharmacological treatment. In M. Hersen & R.T. Ammerman (Eds.). *Advanced abnormal child psychology* (2nd ed.). Mahwah, N.J.: Lawrence Erlbaum Associates, Publishers, pp. 219-250.

Mondimore, F.M. (1999). *Bipolar disorder: A guide for patients and families.* Baltimore: The Johns Hopkins University Press.

Muscari, M.E. (2002). Sticks and stones: The NP's role with bullies and victims. *J Pediatr Health Care, 16,* 22-28.

Nansel, T.R., Overpeck, M., Pilla, R.S., Ruan, W.J., Simmons-Morton, B., et al. (2001). Bullying behaviors among U.S. youth: Prevalence and association with psychosocial adjustment. *JAMA, 285*(16), 2094-2100.

National Institute of Mental Health (NIMH) Genetics Initiative Bipolar Group. (1997). Genomic survey of bipolar illness in the NIMH Genetics Initiative Pedigrees: A preliminary report. *Am J Med Genet (Neuropsychiatric Genetics), 74,* 227-237.

National Institute of Mental Health (NIMH) Roundtable. (2001). National Institute of Mental Health Roundtable on prepubertal bipolar disorder. *J Am Acad Child Adolesc Psychiatry, 40,* 871-878.

Papolos, D. & Papolos, J. (1999). *The bipolar child: The definitive and reassuring guide to childhood's most misunderstood disorder.* New York: Broadway Books.

Patton, G.C., Coffey, M., Posterino, J.B., & Wolfe, R. (2000). Adolescent depressive disorder: A population-based study of ICD-10 symptoms. *Aust N Z J Psychiatry, 34,* 741-747.

Philibert, R.A., Egeland, J.A., Paul, S.M., & Ginns, E.I. (1997). The inheritance of bipolar affective disorder: Abundant genes coming together. *J Affect Disord, 43,* 1-3.

Plotnikoff, G.A. (2002). Herbal medicines. In M. Snyder & R. Lindquist (Eds). *Complementary/alternative therapies in nursing* (4th ed.). New York: Springer Publishing Company, Inc., pp. 295-271.

Pullen, L.M., Modrin-McCarthy, M.A., & Graf, E.V. (2000). Adolescent depression: Important facts that matter. *J Child Adolesc Psychiatr Nurs, 13,* 69-75.

Rankin, E.A. (2000). *Quick reference for psychopharmacology.* Albany, N.Y.: Delmar Thomson Learning.

Rehm, L.P. (1977). A self-control model of depression. *Behav Ther, 8,* 787-804.

Rehm, L.P. & Sharp, R.N. (1996). Strategies for childhood depression. In M.A. Reineke, F.M. Dattilio, & A. Freeman (Eds.). *Cognitive therapy with children and adolescents: A casebook for clinical practice.* New York: Guilford Press, pp. 103-123.

Remschmidt, H. (Ed.). (2001). *Psychotherapy with children and adolescents.* New York: Cambridge University Press.

Renouf, A.G. & Kovacs, M. (1995). Dysthymic disorder during childhood and adolescence. In J.H. Kocsis & D.N. Klein (Eds). *Diagnosis and treatment of chronic depression.* New York: Guilford Press, pp. 20-40.

Russ, S.W. & Ollendick, T.H. (Eds.). (1999). *Issues in clinical psychology: Handbook of psychotherapies with children and families.* New York: Kluwer Academic/Plenum Publishers.

Sadock, B.J. & Sadock, V.A. (Eds.). (2000). *Kaplan & Sadock's comprehensive textbook of psychiatry* (7th ed). Philadelphia: Lippincott Williams & Wilkins.

Schatzberg, A.F. & Nemeroff, C.B. (1998). *The American Psychiatric Press textbook of psychopharmacology* (2nd ed.). Washington, D.C.: American Psychiatric Press.

Schatzberg, A.F. & Nemeroff, C.B. (2001). *Essentials of clinical psychopharmacology.* Washington, D.C.: American Psychiatric Press.

Schwartz, J.A., Gladstone, T.R., & Kaslow, N.J. (1998). Depressive disorders. In T.H. Ollendick & M. Hersen (Eds.). *Handbook of child psychopathology* (3rd ed.). New York: Plenum Press, pp. 269-289.

Scahill, L. (2001a). Psychopharmacology for adolescents. In N.L. Keltner and D.G. Folks (Eds.). *Psychotropic drugs* (3rd ed.). St. Louis: Mosby, pp. 496-514.

Scahill, L. (2001b). Psychopharmacology for children. In N.L. Keltner & D.G. Folks (Eds.). *Psychotropic drugs* (3rd ed.). St. Louis: Mosby, pp. 468-495.

Seligman, M.E. (1975). *Helplessness: On depression, development, and death.* San Francisco: W.H. Freeman.

Sherman, B.B. (2001). Estrogen and depressive illness in women. In J.A. Amsterdam, M. Hornig, & A.A. Nierenberg (Eds.). *Treatment-resistant mood disorders.* Cambridge, U.K.: Cambridge University Press, pp. 80-95.

Siminoff, E., Pickles, A., Meyer, J.M., Silberg, J.L., Maes, H.H., et al. (1997). The Virginia Twin Study of adolescent behavioral development: Influences of age, sex, and impairment on rates of disorder. *Arch Gen Psychiatry, 54,* 801-808.

Skidmore-Roth, L. (2002). *Mosby's nursing drug reference: 2002.* St. Louis: Mosby.

Snyder, M. (2002). An overview of complementary/alternative therapies. In M. Snyder & R. Lindquist (Eds.). *Complementary/alternative therapies in nursing* (4th ed.). New York: Springer Publishing Company, Inc., pp. 3-15.

Stahl, S.M. (2000). Blue genes and the monoamine hypothesis of depression. *J Clin Psychiatry, 61,* 77-78.

Stark, S., Bronik, M.D., Wong, S., Wells, G., & Ostrander, R. (2000). Depressive disorders. In M. Hersen & R.T. Ammerman (Eds.). *Advanced abnormal child psychology* (2nd ed.). Mahwah, N.J.: Lawrence Erlbaum Associates, Publishers, pp. 291-326.

Szuba, M.P., Fernando, A.T., & Groh-Szuba, G. (2001). Sleep abnormalities in treatment-resistant mood disorders. In J.A. Amsterdam, M. Hornig, & A.A.

Nierenberg (Eds.). *Treatment-resistant mood disorders.* Cambridge, U.K.: Cambridge University Press, pp. 96-110.

Tarascon Publishing. (2000). *The Tarascon pocket pharmacopoeia 2000* (deluxe ed.). Loma Linda, Calif.: Author.

Treat-Jacobson, D. & Mark, D.L. (2002). Exercise. In M. Snyder & R. Lindquist (Eds.). *Complementary/alternative therapies in nursing* (4th ed.). New York: Springer Publishing Company, Inc., pp. 285-295.

Viguera, A.C., Cohen, L.S., Baldessarini, R.J., & Nonacs, R. (2002). Managing bipolar disoerder during pregnancy: Weighing the risks and benefits. *Can J Psychiatry, 47,* 426-436.

Waldinger, R.J. (1997). *Psychiatry for medical students* (3rd ed). Washington, D.C.: American Psychiatric Press, Inc.

Warrick Pharmaceuticals Corporation. (1999). *Patient's instructions for use.* Reno: Author.

Williamson, D.E., Ryan, N.D., Birmaher, B., & Dahl, R.E. (1995). A case-control family history study of depression in adolescents. *J Am Acad Child Adolesc Psychiatry, 34,* 1596-1607.

Wolkowitz, O.M. & Reus, V.I. (2001). Psychoneuroendocrine aspects of treatment-resistant mood disorders. In J.A. Amsterdam, M. Hornig, & A.A. Nierenberg (Eds.). *Treatment-resistant mood disorders.* Cambridge, U.K.: Cambridge University Press, pp. 49-79.

Wozniak, J., Biederman, J., & Richards, J.A. (2001). Diagnostic and therapeutic dilemmas in management of pediatric-onset bipolar disorder. *J Clin Psychiatry, 62*(suppl. 14), 10-15.

33 Myelodysplasia

Cynthia Colen Lazzaretti and Caroline Pearson

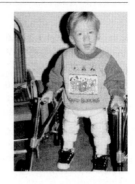

Etiology

Neural tube defects (NTDs) are malformations of the central nervous system (CNS) during embryonic development. The embryologic development of the CNS begins early in the third week of gestation with the formation of the primitive neural tube from the neural plate. The process of neurulation produces the functional nervous system (i.e., the future brain and spinal cord). Closure of the human neural tube begins in the mid-cervical region and proceeds simultaneously in the cranial and caudal directions (Hirose et al, 2001). If the neural tube fails to close the process of neurulation is interrupted, which results in the imperfect formation of the brain and spinal cord at a focal point (Elias & Hobbs, 1998). Failure of neural tube closure can occur anywhere along the length of the spinal cord. The neurologic deficits sustained by the fetus are postulated to occur in stages, as a "two-hit" hypothesis. In this theory, the first "hit" is the original defect in neurulation that creates the NTD and any associated myelodysplasia, and the second "hit" is the secondary trauma to the spinal cord as a result of its exposure to the intrauterine environment (Elias & Hobbs, 1998). Anencephaly, the incomplete development of the forebrain, occurs in 30% of NTDs (Dise & Lohr, 1998). Encephalocele, herniation of the brain and meninges through a defect in the skull, is the least common of the NTDs. Spina bifida or myelodysplasia is a collective term for malformations of the spinal cord and is the most common NTD.

Myelodysplasia is one form of an NTD that refers to the defective formation and subsequent development and function of the spinal cord. This defect can occur at any level of the spinal cord, although it more commonly affects the lumbar and sacral spine. The extent of nerve tissue and spinal cord involvement varies. The malformation results in altered body function at and below the level of the defect (Table 33-1).

The cause of neural tube defects is unknown, but there appears to be a combination of environmental and genetic factors. The genetic predisposition is through an autosomal recessive mechanism, with the risk of recurrent NTD-affected pregnancies increased to 10 times that found in the general population (Hasenau & Covington, 2002). Abnormalities are associated with trisomies 9, 13, and 18 and Meckel-Gruber syndrome and account for a small proportion of NTDs. Genetic studies have failed to identify any one gene in humans that can cause myelomenigocele (Hirose et al, 2001).

Exposure to various teratogens, including valproic acid, carbamazepine, cytochalsin, calcium antagonists, and hyperthermia, has been implicated in NTDs (Manning, Jennings, & Madsen, 2000). Further study of the mechanisms of these

tetrogens may elucidate some of the genetic programs responsible for normal neurulation (Manning et al, 2000). There is an overall increased risk of birth defects with poor prenatal care and maternal nutritional deficiencies. Maternal or fetal folate deficiency is also associated with the occurrence of NTDs, initially investigated in the early 1960s. Intervention studies in the 1980s and 1990s demonstrated a 50% to 70% reduction in NTDs with preconceptal folic acid intake (Green, 2002). Population-based research has revealed the heterogeneous frequency of defects in folic acid metabolism, although the key factors remain poorly characterized (Green, 2002). The most striking report is the 40% increase in incidence of NTDs in offspring of Hispanic descent compared with whites and blacks (Green, 2002). Variations in susceptibilities may include dietary and genetic factors (Green, 2002).

Incidence and Prevalence

NTDs occur in 1 in 2000 births, with an estimated 4000 pregnancies affected each year by an NTD, with some fetal demise through spontaneous or induced losses (Green, 2002). From 1996 to 2001, a 23% decline occurred in NTDs (spina bifida and anencephaly combined). Spina bifida declined 24% during this period, and anencephaly declined 21% (Matthews et al, 2002). The observed declines have translated into approximately 920 infants being born without these serious defects each year (Matthews et al, 2002). Reasons for the observed declining incidence include increasing utilization of prenatal screening in the form of alpha-fetoprotein assay (AFP) and ultrasonography, both of which are done early enough in the pregnancy to allow the parents the choice of terminating the pregnancy. The introduction of folic acid to women of childbearing age has also resulted in an estimated 50% reduction in neural tube defects (Green, 2002).

Clinical Manifestations at Time of Diagnosis

NTDs can vary in severity, from the congenital malformation of vertebrae alone to extensive involvement of the spinal cord and surrounding structures of nerve, bone, muscle, and skin. Myelodysplasia is classified based on the pathophysiology of the lesion or defect (Figure 33-1).

Spina bifida occulta (SBO) is the failed fusion of the vertebral arches that surround and protect the spinal cord and may involve a small portion of one vertebra or the complete absence of bone. SBO is often a benign, incidental finding, occurring in about 20% to 30% of individuals of North American descent. However, it may be associated with underlying spinal cord anomalies, such as myelomeningoceles, lipomyelomeningo-celes, diastematomyelia (split spinal cord), and a tethered cord (Greenberg, 2001). Often there are cutaneous abnormalities such as tufts of hair, dimpling, hemangiomas, and dermoid cysts located above the area of the defect. A child may be asymptomatic at birth or present with leg weakness and atrophy, bowel and bladder disturbances, or foot deformities. If left untreated, a child may develop these symptoms later in life.

A meningocele is a neural tube defect in which there is congenital absence of the vertebral arches and cystic dilation of the meninges through the defect (Greenberg, 2001). At birth the infant has a protruding sac on the back at the level of the defect. This sac is filled with cerebrospinal fluid, and the overlying skin is usually normal. In a pure meningocele, there are no abnormalities of the spinal cord, and infants remain asymptomatic before and after the repair. It is difficult to know the true incidence of meningocele because there is usually some involvement of the spinal cord or nerve roots at the area of the defect. However, it is believed to be less than one twentieth as frequent as myelomenigocele (McComb, 1999) (Table 33-1).

Myelomeningocele is the most severe form of a neural tube defect in which there is cystic dilation of meninges and the dysfunctional spinal cord through an open defect. Like meningoceles, infants present with a protruding sac at the level of the defect. However, the overlying muscle and skin are usually dysplastic. Hydrocephalus is often not apparent at birth, but it becomes present in most children within the first week of life. Approximately 85% of children born with myelomeningocele will require an internal shunt system to control the hydrocephalus (see Chapter 29). The incidence of shunting varies with the level of the spinal defect, with higher-level lesions causing more severe cases of hydrocephalus (Rintoul et al, 2002).

Treatment

Initial treatment for meningocele and myelomeningocele is early surgical closure of the defect to prevent infection and further damage of exposed neural tissue (Elias & Hobbs, 1998) (Box 33-1). Specific tissue malformation and involvement and the presence of hydrocephalus can only be determined through further diagnostic tests (e.g., ultrasonography, computerized tomography [CT] scan, magnetic resonance imaging [MRI]). Careful assessment of the infant before and during the surgical closure often aids in determination of the depth and extent of involvement. This information is important for habilitative planning and outcome.

The multisystem involvement of this diagnosis requires a comprehensive multidisciplinary team approach to treatment. This team may include nurses, neurosurgeons, urologists, orthopedists, neurologists, pediatricians, physical therapists, occupational therapists, and social workers. It is very important that the primary care provider, the multidisciplinary team, and the community resources and program work collaboratively so

---

TABLE 33-1

Functional Alterations in Myelodysplasia Related to Level of Lesion

Level of Lesion	Functional Implications
Thoracic	Flaccid paralysis of lower extremities
	Variable weakness in abdominal trunk musculature
	High thoracic level may have respiratory compromise
	Absence of bowel and bladder control
High lumbar	Voluntary hip flexion and adduction
	Flaccid paralysis of knees, ankles, feet
	May walk with extensive braces and crutches
	Absence of bowel and bladder control
Midlumbar	Strong hip flexion and adduction
	Fair knee extension
	Flaccid paralysis of ankles and feet
	Absence of bowel and bladder control
Low lumbar	Strong hip flexion, extension and adduction, knee extension
	Weak ankle and toe mobility
	Absence of bowel and bladder control
Sacral	"Normal" function of lower extremities
	May have impaired bowel and bladder function

BOX 33-1

Treatment

Assess level of involvement:
    Ultrasonography
    Computerized tomography (CT) scan
    Magnetic resonance imaging (MRI) scan
Surgical closure of deformity
Comprehensive multidisciplinary team approach to care
Rehabilitation
Prevention

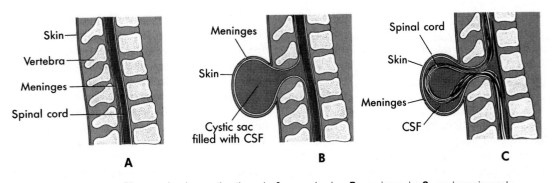

FIGURE 33-1 Diagram showing section through, **A,** normal spine; **B,** meningocele; **C,** myelomeningocele.

that the child can attain optimum function. Long-term treatment focuses on habilitation, prevention of secondary conditions, and management of associated problems.

Prevention

The purpose of prenatal diagnosis is twofold. First, it offers the parents the option to terminate the pregnancy. If the parents choose to continue the pregnancy, prenatal diagnosis provides the family and health care team the opportunity to physically and emotionally prepare for the birth of the child. Cesarean deliveries are routinely done when women are prenatally diagnosed to limit the trauma to the spine during a vaginal delivery. An elevated maternal alpha-fetoprotein (AFP) may indicate the presence of an NTD. It is important to note that a closed neural tube defect may not alter the AFP levels. When AFP levels are elevated, amniocentesis is indicated. High-resolution ultrasound is helpful in documenting the lesion, its approximate level, and the presence or absence of hydrocephalus. Genetic counseling should be offered at this time as well.

Research has demonstrated that the preconceptual and prenatal addition of folic acid can greatly reduce the incidence of NTDs. A recent published report from the Centers for Disease Control and Prevention (CDC, 2001) shows that blood serum folate levels have increased over the past few years, while the rate of neural tube defects appears to have declined by 19% (Green, 2002). In 1992 the US Public Health Service published the recommendation that all women of child-bearing age consume 0.4 mg (400 μg) of folic acid daily to prevent NTDs. Women who have had a pregnancy with an NTD should consume 0.4 mg of folic acid every day when not planning to become pregnant, and they should consult their health care provider about following the August 1991 US Public Health Service guideline for consumption of 4 mg (4000 μg) of synthetic folic acid daily beginning 1 month before they start trying to get pregnant and continuing through the first 3 months of pregnancy. Synthetic folic acid is approximately twice as absorbable as naturally occurring food folate because of the complex structure of folate (Hasenau & Covington, 2002).

Anticipated Advances in Diagnosis and Management

Fetal intervention is a relatively new and controversial treatment option:

Prenatal repair of the myelomeningocele has been performed in the United States for over 5 years with mixed results. The initial intent was to preserve distal neurological function by covering the exposed spinal cord. Although there has been relatively little effect on distal sensorimotor function, prenatal repair serendipitously led to an apparent reduction in hindbrain herniation and a possible decreased need for ventriculoperitoneal shunting. The long-term clinical consequences of these findings are not clear. What is clear, however is that further study in the form of a prospective randomized trial is mandatory (Hirose et al, 2001).

With regard to bladder function, retrospective studies have demonstrated that children treated in utero appear to have the same changes in urodynamic and anatomic abnormalities in the urinary tract as other children with spinal defects who have undergone standard postnatal care (Holmes et al, 2001).

Associated Problems (Box 33-2)
Arnold-Chiari II Malformation

Chiari II (Arnold-Chiari II) malformation is a serious, potentially life-threatening malformation that invariably occurs in 95% of children with myelodysplasia. The Chiari II malformation may be a clinically silent phenomenon or cause catastrophic events (e.g., cardiac or respiratory arrest). The malformation compresses and essentially stretches the posterior region of the cerebellum and brainstem downward through the foramen magnum into the cervical space (Figure 33-2). The exact pathogenesis of the malformation is not known. It is believed an abnormal pressure differential caused by an open spinal defect leads to a small posterior fossa and abnormal development and displacement of the brainstem and cerebellum. Approximately 95% of children with myelodysplasia have Chiari II malformations with about 33% showing symptoms. With the increased survival rate for children with myelomeningocele, adolescents and young adults appear to have a propensity to develop clinical progression attributable to this lesion (Oakes, 2001). It is very important to determine that the shunt is functioning and the intracranial pressure is normal before considering surgical intervention for the Chiari malformation.

Treatment focuses on symptomatic relief of the presenting problems (i.e., gastrostomy tube and tracheostomy may be placed for absent gag and cough). Clinical indications for surgery include severe brainstem dysfunction, cranial nerve dysfunction, and hydromyelia. Recent studies show an 80% recovery rate with early decompressive surgery (Teo et al, 1997).

Hydrocephalus and Seizures

Hydrocephalus occurs in approximately 85% of children with myelodysplasia. Hydrocephalus results from the Chiari II malformation and obstruction of the fourth ventricle. Infants with myelodysplasia and hydrocephalus can present with increased head circumference and bulging fontanel, although they may appear asymptomatic until their spinal defect is repaired. Head ultrasounds are commonly used to monitor for ventriculomegaly along with serial head circumference measurements. The decision to place a ventriculoperitoneal shunt is made based on the rate of increasing ventriculomegaly. Seizures occur in about 1 in 20 children, with the risk being greater in those

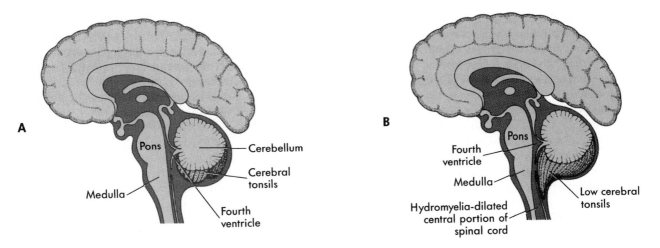

FIGURE 33-2 A, Normal brain. **B,** Brain with Chiari malformation.

who have had CNS infections, multiple shunt failures, or a history of respiratory insufficiency or arrest (Spina Bifida Association of America, 2002) (see Chapters 25 and 29).

Skin Breakdown

Newborns are at great risk for developing infection secondary to the altered skin integrity over the malformed spine, which is a possible complication until the lesion has completely healed. The risk of skin breakdown continues throughout a child's life span as a result of altered sensory function below the level of the lesion. Urinary and fecal incontinence in conjunction with altered sensation greatly increases the risk of skin breakdown.

Cognitive Deficit

Most children with myelodysplasia and hydrocephalus have IQ (intelligence quotient) scores in the average range, although this is somewhat deceptive. This is a broad range of scores on intelligence tests among this group of children and a wide range of abilities because of orthopedic and neurologic problems (Lollar, 2001a, 2001b). The precise nature of the neuropsychologic deficits in hydrocephalus is not completely known; several factors (e.g., etiology, raised intracranial pressure, ventricular size, shunt treatment complications) have been shown to influence cognition. Complications, such as infections, trauma, intraventricular hemorrhage, and other brain abnormalities, are important determinants of the ultimate cognitive status, putting the child at a higher risk of cognitive impairment. Lower intelligence and academic skills are also associated with higher-level defects and severe hydrocephalus (Mataro & Junque, 2001).

Learning Issues

Children with myelodysplasia with or without hydrocephalus have an increased incidence of learning difficulties associated with perceptual motor function, attention, impulsivity, hyperactivity, memory, sequencing, organization, and reasoning (Lollar, 2001b). These children are usually socially adept and very verbal, but because of the perceptual-motor problems, intelligence tests show higher scores on verbal abilities than nonverbal or performance abilities. In academics these children usually have higher reading and spelling skills and often much lower math skills. These children should be evaluated both psychologically and neuropsychologically so that their individual strengths and deficits can be identified and appropriate resources and strategies can be implemented. Neuropsychologic testing evaluates psychological functioning as well as evaluates the areas of memory, attention, sequencing, and reasoning (Lollar, 2001b).

Altered Motor and Sensory Function

Motor and sensory functions below the level of the lesion are invariably altered. This dysfunction may include paralysis, weakness, spasticity of lower extremities, and sensory loss. Altered motor and sensory function may also impair peristalsis, leading to constipation, impaction, and fecal incontinence. Education should start early so secondary complications of skin breakdown can be minimized. These associated problems may worsen as a child grows and the cord ascends within the vertebral canal, pulling primary scar tissue and tethering the spinal cord. As a result, tethering of the spinal cord is present in virtually all cases.

Musculoskeletal Deformities

Musculoskeletal deformities related to myelomeningocele may include clubfeet, dislocated hips, contractures, and deformities caused by decreased activity and improper musculoskeletal alignment from altered embryonic development and muscle group imbalance. Spinal deformities (e.g., scoliosis, kyphosis, gibbus) are also common as the child grows. Habilitation is essential to promoting optimum functional independence and requires close collaboration of the child's physical and occupational therapists, the family, and the myelodysplasia team. Orthotics, assistive devices such as walkers, crutches, wheelchairs, and adaptive equipment for activities of daily living are often needed and require close monitoring and adjustments. Close monitoring of muscle strength is important in assessing early signs of spinal cord tethering.

Urinary Dysfunction

Neurogenic bladder occurs in the majority of children with myelodysplasia and results in incontinence; however, all newborns with myelodysplasia have normal kidney function. The nerves that innervate the bladder are impaired, which can result in detrusor sphincter dyssynergy, incomplete emptying, high-pressure bladder, reflux, and incompetent sphincter. The goal of bladder management is to preserve kidney and bladder function and urinary continence. If continence is not attained by catheterization alone, medications such as anticholinergics and sympathomimetics may be used in conjunction with the procedure. Continence may also successfully be achieved through use of surgical interventions (e.g., artificial urinary sphincter, bladder neck reconstruction, bladder augmentation, creation of continent stomas) (McAndrew & Malone, 2002).

Bowel Dysfunction

Neurogenic bowel occurs in the majority of children with myelodysplasia and results in incontinence because of impaired sensation and impaired sphincter control. Constipation is common as a result of decreased bowel motility. Bowel management in infancy to toddler age should focus on preventing constipation. Skin integrity is at risk because of incontinence, and good skin care habits are essential.

Visual Problems

Pressure on cranial nerves that control eye movements—CN III(oculomotor), CN IV (trochlear), and CN VI (abducens)—may result in a mild disconjugate gaze or esotropia.

Latex Allergic Reactions

Research studies recently have shown that up to 73% of children and adolescents with myelodysplasia are sensitive to latex (Box 33-3) as measured by blood test or by a history of an allergic reaction (Merropol, 2001). Other research is looking at disease-associated latex sensitization in people with myelodysplasia, including genetic, antigen-mediated, early latex exposure and immunologic reasons for sensitivity (Hochleitner et al, 2001).

Careful history should be elicited regarding signs and symptoms of latex allergy. Three types of reactions may occur:
1. Irritant contact dermatitis: dry, itchy, irritated areas, usually on the hands, caused from using gloves—not a true allergy
2. Allergic contact dermatitis (Type IV): delayed hypersensitivity; may include symptoms such as watery eyes, eczematous skin eruptions, or dermatitis
3. Immediate allergic reaction (Type I) (NIOSH, 1997)

Type I reaction is an immediate hypersensitivity to exposure and may include such symptoms as rhinitis, conjunctivitis,

---

BOX 33-3
Latex Allergic Reactions

1. **Irritant contact dermatitis:** dry, itchy, irritated areas, usually on the hands, caused from using gloves—not a true allergy
2. **Allergic contact dermatitis:** delayed hypersensitivity, may include symptoms such as watery eyes, eczematous skin eruptions, or dermatitis
3. **Immediate allergic reaction:** immediate hypersensitivity to exposure, which may include symptoms of rhinitis, conjunctivitis, wheezing, bronchospasm, facial swelling, tachycardia, laryngeal edema, and hypotension (NIOSH, 1997)

---

wheezing, bronchospasm, facial swelling, tachycardia, laryngeal edema, and hypotension. Individuals with Type I reaction to latex are at extreme risk for developing anaphylaxis. Those who experience Type IV are at lower risk for developing anaphylaxis, but constant sensitization may predispose them to anaphylaxis. Avoidance of latex products is extremely important in preventing allergic reactions. Refer individuals to an allergist if latex allergy is suspected.

Prognosis

Myelodysplasia is a chronic condition. The prognosis depends on the success of prophylactic and acute treatment for potential and actual complications that affect each body system. Improved ventricular shunt systems have helped to reduce complications of malfunction and infection (see Chapter 29). Implementation of aggressive urologic management with clean intermittent catheterization starting in the newborn period and improved surgical options for bladder management have greatly reduced the incidence of renal damage and failure. Treatments and interventions will be necessary throughout the child's life span and are individualized to the child's needs and rendered when indicated by the clinical presentation, assessment, and evaluation. Life-threatening complications remain despite the vast improvement in treatment and management. If untreated or not treated quickly enough, shunt malfunction can lead to brainstem herniation and death. Those with symptomatic Chiari malformations necessitating tracheostomies and feeding tubes are at risk of aspiration and pulmonary compromise and arrest. Independent living and gainful employment are realistic goals and are directly affected by cognitive development, achievement of functional independence, good consistent medical follow-up, and continued collaboration of the family, the child, community and school resources, and the medical team.

PRIMARY CARE MANAGEMENT

Health Care Maintenance
Growth and Development

The growth and development of a child with myelodysplasia are affected by the level of the defect, the motor and sensory impairment, and the presence of hydrocephalus. As with all children, monitoring growth and development by obtaining routine heights and weights during follow-up in a spina bifida clinic as well as with their primary care provider and plotting them on a standardized growth chart are crucial. Obtaining heights may be difficult, depending on the child's ability to stand. If necessary, the primary care provider should measure the full body length with the child supine or by using arm span. Because of shortening of the spine and muscle atrophy, these children often fall below the 10th percentile in height.

Obesity is a common problem in children with myelodysplasia as a result of decreased levels of activity and can cause problems with skin breakdown and orthotic fitting. Obesity may also interfere with development of a positive self-image. Educating the family and child must begin early so that healthy eating habits can be established.

During infancy, problems related to Chiari II malformation may cause feeding problems affecting growth. Compression on CN IX (glossopharyngeal), CN X (vagus), and CN XII (hypoglossal) can affect gag and swallowing and increase the risk of aspiration, resulting in symptoms of failure to thrive, pneumonia, and respiratory compromise.

Short stature and precocious puberty are commonly seen in children with myelodysplasia and hydrocephalus and should be referred to a pediatric endocrinologist. Reasons for disturbed growth and development are the level of the spinal lesion, vertebral anomalies, and various skeletal deformities that reduce the growth of the lower limbs and spine (Trollman et al, 2000). Hydrocephalus and Chiari II malformation increase the risks of hypothalamo-pituitary dysfunctions, such as central precocious puberty and growth hormone deficiency (Trollman et al, 2000).

Head circumference should be monitored closely by the primary care provider during infancy and early childhood. If a progressive enlargement in size is noted, referral to a neurosurgeon or a spina bifida clinic should be made (see Chapter 29).

Motor development may be affected and is directly related to the level of the lesion (Table 33-1). The degree of weakness, paralysis, and decreased sensation varies. Early orthopedic and physical therapy assessment and intervention are extremely important to prevent contractures, minimize deformities, and monitor muscle strength and flexibility. Surgical intervention is often recommended and sometimes required to achieve proper muscle balance and body alignment for problems common to this population (e.g., dislocated hips, scoliosis, kyphosis, clubfeet) that would limit the child's potential. Monitoring for orthotics, adaptive equipment, and mobility needs is ongoing throughout the child's life.

The rate at which cognitive development and intellectual skills are acquired depends on a child's interaction with the environment, the severity of the defect, and the presence of hydrocephalus. Infants should be considered at risk for cognitive and developmental delays, and early intervention services should be implemented as early in infancy as possible. Language development is usually on track, although difficulties have been noted in the development of pragmatic communication and the construction of meaning (Fletcher et al, 2002). Close monitoring of hydrocephalus and the ventriculoperitoneal shunt is important.

Promoting upright positioning and independent mobility is essential for the child's overall growth and development. As the child grows and develops, other adaptive equipment (i.e., braces, wheelchairs) is used to increase mobility and independence. Each child's treatment program varies because of differences in motivation, both the child's and the family's, and access to and availability of resources.

Diet

Infancy is an excellent time to guide and educate parents on nutritional needs. It is important to teach parents early about the dangers of overfeeding, especially in children who are less mobile and therefore have fewer caloric needs. Preventing obesity and avoiding the pattern of using food as a reward are primary goals in the nutritional management of children with myelodysplasia. Children with known latex sensitivity or allergy should avoid plant products that contain the same allergy-producing proteins found in natural rubber latex because they may cause an allergic cross reaction. These include bananas, avocados, kiwis, plums, peaches, cherries, apricots, figs, papayas, tomatoes, potatoes, and chestnuts.

The child's diet should include plenty of fluids to lessen the chance of constipation and the incidence of urinary tract infections (UTIs). Dietary management is important in controlling the consistency of stools and in avoiding constipation. A diet high in fiber and low in constipating foods is usually recommended. Early nutritional assessment and guidance are essential parts of the care of children with myelodysplasia.

Difficulty in swallowing results in poor feeding and weight gain, especially in newborns and young infants, and is a common symptom of Chiari malformation (Oakes, 2001). Gagging, choking, and aspiration are other indicators of Chiari malformation. The spina bifida team or the pediatric neurosurgeon should be consulted. MRI imaging and modified barium swallow may be indicated to definitively assess and diagnose. Children and adolescents may present with increased difficulty swallowing, gagging with different textures, and choking. In children with severe symptoms, a gastrostomy tube may be needed to prevent aspiration and malnutrition.

Safety

Safety issues particular to infants and children with myelodysplasia are numerous. Because the neurologic system is the primary system involved, parents must be educated on the changes that may occur and threaten their child's safety. The congenital defect affects nerve function at and below the level of the defect on the spine, thus altering mobility and sensation of bone, muscle, and skin tissue below the level of the defect. This decreased sensation puts a child at greater risk for injuries such as burns, fractures, and skin breakdown. With proper body positioning, frequent position changes, and assurance that adaptive equipment fits properly and is used correctly, the risk of skin breakdown can be reduced. Tepid water should be used for bathing to prevent burns. The condition of the child's skin should be checked at least twice daily for redness and irritation. As soon as children are competent to assume this responsibility, they should be taught how to perform a thorough skin check.

The potential for limited cognitive ability and altered judgment exists in these children. An awareness of limitations is essential to help these children with issues such as independence, decision making, self-care, and sexuality. Instructions on the proper use of equipment for mobility (e.g., wheelchairs, braces, crutches) should be appropriate to the child's developmental and cognitive abilities.

Parents of children with seizures should be instructed on how to intervene safely and appropriately during a seizure (see Chapter 25).

Latex allergy can be life threatening; therefore the primary care provider must inform and educate the parents and individual of this potential sensitivity, observe for signs, and document the allergy. Examples of products that may contain latex are surgical gloves, balloons, catheters, and bandages. (An updated list of such products and alternatives for use is available from the Spina Bifida Association of America.) Individuals with latex sensitivity should carry an Epi-pen, a letter documenting the allergy, and nonlatex gloves, as well as wear a medic-alert bracelet indicating the allergy.

Immunizations

Routine schedule for immunizations is recommended. Alterations in the immunization schedule for children with seizures and hydrocephalus are addressed in Chapters 25 and 29.

Screening

Vision. Routine screening is recommended. Because of the high incidence of visual and perceptual deficits, ocular palsies, and astigmatism in children with myelodysplasia, practitioners should assess for these conditions during routine screening. Referral to an ophthalmologist is indicated for any positive visual findings.

Hearing. Routine screening is recommended. Children with myelodysplasia who have shunts for hydrocephalus are often hypersensitive to loud noises. Awareness of this finding may alleviate parental concern. Use of aminoglycosides may cause hearing deficits.

Dental. Routine dental screening and care are recommended. Dentists should be notified of the increased risk of latex allergy. Information should be given for safe, alternative nonlatex products. Children with hydrocephalus who have shunts do not require prophylactic antibiotics before dental procedures.

Hematocrit. Routine screening is recommended.

Tuberculosis. Routine screening is recommended.

Blood Pressure. Routine screening is recommended. Children with known renal problems such as urinary reflux or a history of hypertension should have more frequent assessment. Persistent elevated readings should be communicated to the child's urologist. In rare cases, persistent hypertension may be a sign of shunt malfunction.

Urinalysis. Baseline urinalysis and urine cultures are obtained in newborns. If a UTI is suspected, a urine culture and sensitivity should be obtained by catheterization (bag specimens have been noted to have a higher chance of contamination). A positive urine culture should be reported to the child's urologist.

Condition-Specific Screening (Box 33-4)

Complete Blood Count. If an individual is receiving long-term antibiotic therapy (e.g., sulfonamides) for prevention of UTIs, complete blood counts should be done approximately every 6 months to monitor changes.

Serum Creatinine. Serum creatinine should be checked routinely in newborns as a baseline study for renal function and should be repeated if changes on renal ultrasound are noted.

Scoliosis. Screening for scoliosis in children with myelodysplasia should begin during the first year of life and continue throughout adolescence. Spine radiographs should be obtained yearly or as indicated.

Latex Allergy. All children with myelodysplasia should be treated as latex sensitive from birth. Skin testing and blood testing or in vitro testing is available. Standardized skin testing

---

> ### BOX 33-4
> ### Condition-Specific Screening
>
> Complete blood count
> Serum creatinine
> Scoliosis
> Latex allergy

> ### BOX 33-5
> ### Differential Diagnosis
>
> Chiari II malformation
> Tethering of the spinal cord
> Hydrocephalus
> Urinary tract infections
> Fevers
> Gastrointestinal symptoms

TABLE 33-2
Implications of Cranial Nerve Dysfunction in Myelodysplasia

Cranial Nerve	Functional Implications
olfactory	Sense of smell
optic	Visual acuity, visual fields
oculomotor	Raises eyelids; constricts pupils; moves eyes up, down, and medially
trochlear	Moves eyes down
trigeminal	Sensory innervation to face, tongue; opens and closes jaw
abducens	Moves eyes laterally (out)
facial	Closes eyelids; motor and sensory for facial muscles; secretion of lacrimal and salivary glands
acoustic	Hearing; equilibrium
glossopharyngeal	Gag, swallow; taste
vagus	Muscles of larynx, pharynx, soft palate; parasympathetic innervation
spinal accessory	Shoulder shrug
hypoglossal	Moves tongue

is not available in the United States so the reliability and consistency of results vary. In vitro testing is intended for diagnosis of individuals with suspected latex allergy and not as a screening tool. These tests are very specific when the clinical symptoms are severe but less specific when symptoms are ambiguous.

Common Illness Management
Differential Diagnosis (Box 33-5)

Chiari II Malformation. Chiari II malformation compresses the brainstem. The brainstem houses the 12 cranial nerves (CNs) (Table 33-2). Pressure on this region results in altered function of these vital nerves or actual palsies. Dysfunction of the lower CNs is common. The infant's symptoms may include apnea, respiratory difficulties, stridor, and the classic barking cough of croup. Primary care providers must be cautious not to dismiss these findings as a simple upper respiratory infection but must consider the possibility that these symptoms result from pressure on CN IX (glossopharyngeal), CN X (vagus), or CN XII (hypoglossal). A depressed or absent gag may be present, leading to possible aspiration pneumonia. Feeding difficulties, poor weight gain, and symptoms of failure to thrive may also be present.

Pressure on the cranial nerves that control eye movements—CN III (oculomotor), CN IV (trochlear), CN VI (abducens)—may result in a mild disconjugate gaze or esotropia.

Subtle complaints and changes in hand function or strength, increased upper-extremity spasticity, neck pain, or behavior changes (e.g., irritability) necessitate immediate consultation with the neurosurgeon to rule out shunt malfunction or hydromyelia.

Tethering of the Spinal Cord. Myelodysplasia is not a progressive condition; thus any signs of deterioration should be evaluated closely by the primary care provider and the specialists. Virtually all children with myelodysplasia have signs of spinal cord tethering on MRI as a result of the defect and subsequent surgical closure. It is estimated that 30% to 50% of children with myelodysplasia will, at some time, require surgery to untether the spinal cord (Walker & Dias, 2001). Signs and symptoms can include changes in muscle strength, decrease in motor function, changes in bowel and bladder function, and scoliosis. The decision to intervene surgically requires careful assessment of the presenting symptoms, the impact on the child's function, and the results of diagnostic studies, such as urodynamic studies, spinal x-rays, and MRI.

Hydrocephalus. Most individuals have an internal shunt system to treat hydrocephalus. The differential diagnosis of shunt malfunction and infection must be considered in the presence of lethargy, fever, gastrointestinal distress, and headache (see Chapter 29).

Urinary Tract Infections. Urinary tract infections (UTIs) are common among children with myelodysplasia. Fever associated with UTIs may be mild or severe. Other symptoms may include abdominal pain; vomiting; cloudy, malodorous urine; and increased wetting. Frequency and burning may be masked because of decreased sensation. These symptoms should alert the primary care provider to obtain a urine specimen by catheterization for culture. A positive culture should be reported to the child's urologist, especially in cases with urinary reflux. Treatment of positive cultures may vary depending on the individual's urologist. Most children who are on clean intermittent catheterization are chronically colonized with bacteria. Treatment is usually based on the presence of urinary reflux or severe symptoms (e.g., fever, back pain, vomiting) (Elias & Hobbs, 1998). Recommendations for treatment may include a short course of appropriate antibiotics and instillation of an antibiotic solution into the bladder via catheterization. Children with urinary reflux need continuous antibiotic coverage and frequent urine cultures. Repeat cultures should be obtained once during the course of treatment and again approximately 1 week after treatment.

Fevers. Fever is a symptom found in many common childhood illnesses. Causes of fever may include shunt infection and malfunction, UTI, skin breakdown, and cellulitis. Particular consideration must be given to the presence of a fever because it may lower the seizure threshold in these children.

Fever of unknown origin may be the result of an undetected fracture of an insensate extremity. Osteoporosis associated with paralysis, decreased weight bearing, and inactivity, especially after immobilization in a cast, may contribute to the occurrence of fractures. An undetected burn of insensate areas may also result in fever. Careful examination of the area for swelling, redness, or abrasions should be undertaken by the practitioner. Obtaining a complete history from the individual and the parents may assist in determining if there has been recent trauma.

Gastrointestinal Symptoms. Nausea, vomiting, and diarrhea are all common symptoms in children. In children with myelodysplasia, however, a heightened concern and consideration to the cause should be given. Nausea and vomiting may be symptomatic of shunt malfunction. UTIs may be the cause of gastrointestinal distress. Children who have had a bladder augmentation and also have referred pain to the shoulder should seek immediate medical attention because this could indicate a urinary leak into the peritoneum. A child with a neurogenic bowel may become impacted with stool, leading to gastrointestinal distress. The presence of diarrhea may be misleading because liquid stool passes around the impacted stool. A radiograph of the kidneys, ureters, and bladder (KUB) may help differentiate diarrhea from impaction.

In children with a high lesion, practitioners should consider the possibility of appendicitis as a cause of nausea or vomiting. The classic symptom of pain may be altered as a result of the decreased sensation.

Drug Interactions

Many children with myelodysplasia are on routine medication therapy. Potential interactions among these and other medications must be carefully considered when additional medications are prescribed. Commonly used drug categories are as follows:

1. Antibiotics are given for treatment of UTIs or prophylaxis, including amoxicillin (Amoxil), trimethoprim and sulfamethoxazole (Bactrim), sulfisoxazole (Gantrisin), and nitrofurantoin (Furadantin). If a child requires other antibiotic therapy for common childhood illness, such as ear infections, the antibiotic for the UTI is discontinued during the needed course of treatment. Bladder irrigations containing antibiotics are used much less frequently.

2. Anticholinergics, most commonly oxybutynin chloride (Ditropan), are used to assist in urinary continence and reduce high bladder pressure. Oxybutynin chloride can cause heat prostration in the presence of high environmental temperatures. Extended-release oxybutynin is a fairly new form that requires administration only once per day vs. three times per day and that has fewer side effects (Youdimk & Kogan, 2002). The child must be able to swallow pills. Anticholinergics may delay absorption of other medications given concomitantly in these children (*Physicians' Desk Reference* [PDR], 2001).

3. Stool softeners, stimulants, and bulk formers aid in evacuation of stool. Many products are used for this purpose, and most are over-the-counter drugs. None of these should be administered in the presence of abdominal pain, nausea, vomiting, or diarrhea.

4. Anticonvulsants are given to control seizure activity and include phenobarbital, phenytoin sodium (Dilantin), and carbamazepine (Tegretol). Concomitant administration of carbamazepine with erythromycin may result in toxicity (PDR, 2001) (see Chapter 25).

Developmental Issues

Sleep Patterns

Individuals with Chiari II malformation may experience sleep apnea, increased stridor, and snoring with sleep. These children are at increased risk for sudden respiratory arrest. Sleep studies are helpful in determining the severity of sleep disorder and the need for bilevel positive airway pressure (BiPAP). Therefore children with such symptoms should wear a cardiac/apnea monitor during sleep. Parents must also be able to perform cardiopulmonary resuscitation in the event of an arrest.

Alteration in the child's normal sleep pattern (e.g., longer naps, increased frequency of naps) may indicate increased intracranial pressure from a shunt malfunction (see Chapter 29).

In addition, sleep may be interrupted if a child needs to be repositioned during the night to prevent pressure sores and skin breakdown from developing.

Toileting

Bowel and bladder continence is essential in the development of positive self-esteem and optimum functioning. A child's physical abilities and psychologic readiness for toileting should be assessed. Children who are unable to sit without adaptive devices or unable to master self-dressing skills need special consideration when toileting is introduced. A physical or occupational therapist should be consulted about the use of bars or adaptive seats. Special clothing or underwear may be helpful to make access to the perineum easier.

It is desirable for children to master self-care methods of toileting before entering school. Urinary and fecal incontinence can lead to difficulties socially as well as to issues with skin care. Bowel management should be monitored from birth to avoid constipation and impaction. At age 2 to 3 years the concept of toileting should be introduced to children. The goals of bowel management are to maintain soft formed stools and develop a regular schedule of evacuation on the toilet every 1 to 2 days to avoid impaction or soiling between bowel movements. These goals can be accomplished by having the child sit on the toilet at regular times, taking advantage of the gastrocolic reflex by toileting after meals, and increasing abdominal pressure by blowing bubbles, tickling the child to make him or her laugh, or placing the child's legs on a stool to increase pressure by hip flexion.

Stool consistency is crucial to developing a good bowel program. Bulking agents (e.g., Benefiber) taken with increased fluids are a key factor in avoiding constipation and eventual impaction. Children should assume responsibility for timed evacuation and good perineal care as physical and cognitive development allows. Some children will not be able to assume toileting responsibilities and will require continued assistance by parents or caretakers (Edwards-Becket & King, 1996).

The use of medicinal aids may also be necessary to control the consistency or to aid in evacuation. A number of agents are available, including stimulants, softeners, and lubricants. The antegrade continence enema (ACE) and more recently the laparoscopic ACE (LACE) are operative procedures being used frequently in those children who have failed at aggressive bowel management programs. The ACE involves surgical placement of a continent stoma to the bowel that can be catheterized for the administration of enemas for predictable bowel movements. The ACE is flushed every day or every other day with water through a catheter that is inserted into the stoma. It is a simple procedure with the goal of the child being able to manage the procedure independently.

It is important to remember that each program of management varies from child to child. A sympathetic manner in working with a child helps to avoid feelings of guilt and blame for unavoidable accidents.

Clean intermittent catheterization (CIC) is the most commonly used method to help achieve urinary continence. Ideally, CIC should be started at birth, but if not it should begin at the normal time for toilet training. If a child has been catheterized from birth, the concept of using the toilet for the procedure should be introduced at this time. The procedure is ideally taught to the parents and other individuals involved in the child's direct care. Instituting this procedure often causes varying emotions in parents related to the child's disabilities. Fear of injuring the child, difficulties with genital touching, and frustration with the mechanics of the procedure are common. Psychologic and emotional concerns are common and must be addressed before parents can be expected to understand and comply with the recommendations.

Self-catheterization is a realistic goal for most children to accomplish by early school age. An individualized approach accounting for the child's readiness is important in achieving this goal. Providing young children with an anatomically correct doll and catheter often helps them master the skill. In children with limited cognitive abilities and poor manual dexterity, adaptation, such as an abdominal continent stoma, should be considered in an effort to enable independence for the child. Noncompliance with self-catheterization may become an issue in adolescence when catheterization is used as a focus in the fight for independence.

Discipline

There can be a wide range of emotional responses to having a child with a chronic disability, from a crisis to an unfortunate event with positive implications, all of which require some degree of psychologic adjustment (Trute & Heibert-Murphy, 2002). It is very important to assess parental stress so as to assist parents with their own distress as well as guide them in seeking appropriate support and counseling that will strengthen the family's coping strategies and ultimately enhance the family's and the child's integration within society (Brinchmann, 1999; Larson, 1998). The need to overprotect a child with a disability is not uncommon and can impact a child's independence and social adjustment. Children with such a complex long-term condition are at increased risk for experiencing psychosocial adjustment problems, which may affect the parents' and family members' response to discipline. The need for discipline, direction, and encouragement of independence should be addressed early in a child's life (Lollar, 2001b).

Child Care

Primary care providers should be familiar with early intervention programs and child care placements available in the community because early intervention programs for infants vary from state to state. Preschoolers are eligible for placement in public programs that meet their physical and educational needs. It is important that the daycare or educational setting be notified in advance about a prospective student so that the staff can be educated regarding the child's abilities and medical care needs and a smooth transition can be facilitated (see Chapter 5). The child's bladder and bowel program and procedures should be taught to the care provider as well as education regarding medication and administration. The care providers should be educated regarding signs and symptoms of shunt malfunction, UTI, and latex precautions.

Many children with myelodysplasia have adaptive equipment to aid in mobilization, maintain appropriate body alignment, prevent further deformity, and increase independence. Daycare providers should be aware of proper application and fit of the equipment. It is also important to communicate the child's actual motor and sensory capacity to prevent injury.

A list of emergency telephone numbers must accompany these children. If possible, primary care providers should be available to answer questions and concerns from child care staff.

Schooling

Learning disabilities are common in children with myelodysplasia. Problems may occur in perceptual-motor skills, comprehension, attention, activity, memory, organization, sequencing, and reasoning. These areas must be assessed early in the educational process so particular needs may be met and adaptations made to minimize educational problems and frustrations for the child, family, and educators. Neuropsychologic testing is recommended (Dise & Lohr, 1998). School performance can be further compromised by frequent absences as a result of illness or medical treatment.

Federal laws protect the rights of children with disabilities to access appropriate education (see Chapter 5). Individualized education plans (IEPs) must be formulated to take care of each child's specific needs, including educational and physical requirements. The primary care provider, the child, and the family must actively collaborate with the school in this planning process. Each child's particular needs must be addressed in the IEP, including the need for catheterization; timed toileting; administration of medications; physical, occupational and speech therapy; and individual counseling. These needs may require assistance from an aide.

Adaptive equipment may be necessary and depends on a child's degree of disability. School personnel should be aware of what adaptive equipment the child has, how it functions, and what to monitor with regard to fit, skin irritation, and so on (Brown, 2001). Elevators may help a child to get to classes in a timely manner and minimize fatigue.

As children get older, they may choose to use a wheelchair for mobilization in school. This should be viewed as a means of increasing mobility and independence instead of decreasing independence. Ideally, the school should be free of structural barriers to enable the child to move freely and participate in all activities. Special provisions must be made for safe departure from the building in the event of an emergency, as well as transportation to and from home (i.e., wheelchair van or bus). Individuals with a known latex allergy will need assistance in identifying and avoiding latex in school. Common sources of latex in the school environment include art supplies, pencil erasers, and gym mats or floors. The school nurse or allergists are possible resources to assist in this process.

Both myelodysplasia and hydrocephalus affect quality of life because of the chronicity and multisystem impact of these conditions. Associated social disadvantages include decreased opportunity for peer relationships, prolonged dependency on parents, and decreased community acceptance (Kripalani, 2000). Children with myelodysplasia often have low self-concepts, low levels of general happiness, and high levels of anxiety. Awareness of these potential problems is helpful for those working with children with myelodysplasia. Emotional independence is the foundation that supports the successful development of physical independence. Appropriate referrals for further psychologic intervention and support may be advised. Primary care providers should encourage these children to be involved in extracurricular activities such as clubs, scouting, and sporting activities to enhance peer relationships, self-esteem, and independence (Lollar, 2001b).

Academic planning and career counseling must take into consideration an individual's physical as well as cognitive abilities. Education and vocational training should prepare individuals to be successful in employment, independent living, and social relationships (Johnson & Dorval, 2001).

Sexuality

The issues of sexuality and reproduction are major areas of concern for children with myelodysplasia and their parents. Information regarding sexual function, intimacy, and reproduction should be discussed early and continued throughout childhood and adolescence. The development of good self-esteem and peer relationships is important in developing satisfying intimate relationships. As with all children, sex education should begin at home with information also available through the educational system and further addressed by the spina bifida clinic team. If a primary care provider does not feel skilled in gynecologic care, the child should be referred to a sensitive specialist with experience examining individuals with disabilities.

Women with myelodysplasia are capable of normal fertility. Birth control methods must be carefully evaluated on an individual basis. The high incidence of latex allergies in this population prohibits the use of latex condoms and diaphragms. Nonlatex condoms are available, and information should be made available by the primary care provider and the spina bifida team. Because of increased risk for UTI with intercourse, women not taking routine antibiotics should take prophylactic antibiotics before and after intercourse.

Although individuals with myelodysplasia have normal sex drives, unless sensation exists in the bulbourethral, bulbocavernosus, and perineal muscles of both genders, orgasm is not likely. Women may benefit from use of additional lubricating gels when attempting intercourse because vaginal lubrication in response to sexual arousal does not occur with lower spinal cord injury.

Pregnancy in women with myelodysplasia is complicated by physical deformity, the presence of ventriculoperitoneal shunts, previous abdominal surgery for urologic and bowel management, varying degrees of impaired renal function, and hypertension. Early prenatal care is important, especially for screening the fetus for NTDs. Genetic counseling should be offered and encouraged. The American College of Obstetrics and Gynecology has guidelines on pregnancy and delivery for women with myelodysplasia.

In men with myelodysplasia, the level of spinal lesion will predict their capacity for erection and ejaculation. Because this functional ability varies among individuals, the reproductive potential is much less predictable than in women. A thorough history regarding erections and ejaculations is important in determining potential sexual function. Penile implants are available, and referral to a specialist in sexual function should be considered. Fertility will need to be evaluated as part of family planning.

Transition into Adulthood

Transition planning is a process mandated by law that must begin by age 14 years (see Chapter 9). Amendments under the Individuals with Disabilities Education Act (PL 101-476) require that goals and objectives related to employment and postsecondary education, independent living, and community participation be included in IEPs no later than age 16 years.

A successful transition is possible if there is ample preparation, motivation on the part of the young adult and family, and involvement of the school and appropriate community resources. Decision-making skills that relate to community living are necessary to a successful transition and must begin early. Development of a social support system including peers is needed to prevent social isolation, which can lead to depression and loneliness and an inability to access medical care (Johnson & Dorval, 2001).

The survival rate of individuals with myelodysplasia has increased dramatically over the past 25 years, and thus the issue of transition has become a primary focus for the continued care of persons with myelodysplasia. Adult multidisciplinary clinics are very rare, and adults must learn to navigate the already complex medical system and piece together their care. This can be daunting and can lead to poor medical care and complications associated with lack of preventive care (Johnson & Dorval, 2001). As in the pediatric multidisciplinary care model, coordinated care is of utmost importance in adults. Primary health care should be directed by providers interested in and committed to working with this high-risk population. This necessary transition of care has been met with reluctance by many adult health care providers for a number of reasons, including lack of familiarity with the complex needs of individuals with myelodysplasia. Providers may perceive this population as having a negative economic effect on their practice.

Coordinated multidisciplinary care, education of health care providers and clients, costs, and promotion of client-directed care are issues that need to be addressed. A few adult programs have been developed in various parts of the United States. Further information can be obtained from the Spina Bifida Association of America.

Family Concerns and Resources

Families of children with myelodysplasia suffer long-term grief for the "loss of the normal child" at birth. This grief is expressed repeatedly as the child fails to achieve developmental milestones.

The risk for sudden death as a result of a shunt malfunction or complications related to the Chiari II malformation is a chronic and intense stress on the family system. This stress, in addition to the other complex needs of these children, often results in families protecting the child and treating the child as a perpetual child (Johnson & Dorval, 2001). Families may be hesitant or fearful of allowing others to care for their child because of the child's special needs. Parents should be encouraged to treat their child as a member of the family, not the center of the family.

The multisystem involvement of this condition requires frequent hospitalizations, surgeries, outpatient services, and multidisciplinary care. These factors, in addition to items such as special equipment or medications that may be needed by these children, place a tremendous financial burden on parents. Many children with myelodysplasia are eligible for social security benefits. Social service involvement with these families is crucial in providing guidance and support (Elias & Hobbs, 1998). The health care system recognizes the many needs of children with myelodysplasia and their families and offers physical, emotional, spiritual, and social care. Nevertheless, no individual understands or feels the problems these children and families face in their day-to-day lives as well as another child or family with the same disorder. Therefore support groups and opportunities available to provide this network of support within the community not only are necessary but also have proven to be a major factor in coping and adaptation for these families. The following are a few support systems available to families. Each region has its own community-based network or local chapter. It is important that the primary care provider be aware of available local resources.

Arnold-Chiari Family Network
c/o Kevin and Maureen Walsh
67 Spring St
Weymouth, MA 02188

Northeast Myelodysplasia Association
c/o New England Regional Genetics Group
Joseph Robinson, coordinator
PO Box 670
Mt Desert, ME 04660
(207) 288-2705

Spina Bifida Association of America
4590 MacArthur Blvd NW, Suite 250
Washington DC 20007-4226
(202) 944-3285 or (800) 621-3141
www.sbaa.org

Summary of Primary Care Needs for the Child with Myelodysplasia

HEALTH CARE MAINTENANCE

Growth and Development

Head size may be enlarged if child is diagnosed with hydrocephalus; measure head each visit.

Motor delays are common.

Obesity is common in these children.

Both precocious puberty and short stature are reported. Growth hormone deficiency may occur.

Diet

Regurgitation, vomiting, and difficulties with gag reflex need to be evaluated for increased intracranial pressure and Chiari II malformation.

Caloric intake should be monitored to minimize potential for obesity.

Diet should include increased fluids to lessen chance of constipation and urinary tract infections.

Children with latex allergies may have allergic reactions to some foods.

Safety

Increased risk of injuries as a result of decreased sensation and mobility is possible.

Proper body positioning, frequent position changes, and proper fit of adaptive equipment are recommended.

Education on emergency care of seizures is recommended.

Increased risk for latex allergy is possible.

Immunizations

Routine immunizations are recommended.

Pertussis vaccine may be deferred in infants with seizures.

Measles vaccine may cause seizures in children with seizure disorder but is recommended because of prevalence of disease.

Screening

Vision. Routine screening is recommended. These children have a high incidence of visual deficits such as ocular palsies, astigmatism, and visual perceptual deficits.

Hearing. Routine screening is recommended. Children may have hypersensitivity to loud noises if they have shunts. If children are exposed to aminoglycosides or have a history of central nervous system (CNS) infection, hearing should be evaluated by an audiologist.

Dental. Routine care is recommended. Latex precautions are required. Antibiotic prophylaxis is not needed in children with ventriculoperitoneal shunts for hydrocephalus but is recommended for children with ventriculoatrial shunts.

Hematocrit. Routine screening is recommended.

Tuberculosis. Routine screening is recommended.

Blood Pressure. Routine monitoring is recommended. Children with renal problems may develop hypertension and should have more frequent monitoring. In rare cases, persistent hypertension may be a sign of shunt malfunction.

Urinalysis. Baseline urinalysis and cultures should be obtained in the newborn period.

Bladder catheterization is recommended for obtaining urine for cultures.

Condition-Specific Screening

Blood Tests. Complete blood counts (CBCs) should be obtained frequently on children treated with sulfonamides. Serum creatinine should be done on newborns and then as indicated when changes appear on renal ultrasound.

Scoliosis. Screening for scoliosis should be done yearly from birth through adolescence.

Latex Allergies. Latex precautions include monitoring for signs and symptoms and educating the patient, family, and other care providers.

COMMON ILLNESS MANAGEMENT

Differential Diagnosis

If the child presents with:

Respiratory difficulties, stridor, croupy cough: rule out Chiari II malformation.

Scoliosis, altered gait pattern, changes in muscle strength and tone, disturbance in urinary and bowel patterns, and back pain: rule out tethered cord.

Headaches: rule out shunt malfunction.

Fevers: rule out shunt or CNS infection, urinary tract infection, and fracture or injury of insensate area.

Gastrointestinal symptoms: rule out increased intracranial pressure with nausea and vomiting, urinary tract infection, and fecal impaction.

Drug Interactions

No routine drug therapy exists, but children are frequently taking daily medications; therefore any interactions are specific to the individual and medications being taken.

DEVELOPMENTAL ISSUES

Sleep Patterns

Apnea, increased stridor, and snoring may occur in children with symptomatic Chiari II malformation. Sleep studies may be indicated.

Children may need to be repositioned during the night to prevent skin irritation resulting in fatigue.

Lethargy may indicate increased intracranial pressure.

Toileting

Aggressive bowel and bladder management should be begun early to avoid delay in continence.

Independence should be encouraged when developmentally and physically appropriate.

Bowel regimens will vary. Antegrade continence enemas (ACE) are being used.

Intermittent catheterization is common, and compliance may be an issue during adolescence.

Continued

Summary of Primary Care Needs for the Child with Myelodysplasia—cont'd

Discipline

These children are at an increased risk of psychosocial adjustment problems.

They have a need for discipline and encouragement toward independence.

Child Care

Special medical needs may be necessary with severe physical involvement.

Early intervention programs are ideal for infants and toddlers.

Latex precautions are necessary.

Schooling

Federal laws protect children with disabilities.

Families need assistance in individualized education plan (IEP) hearings.

Children may have adjustment problems.

Neuropsychologic testing is recommended.

Special provisions may be necessary for adaptive equipment, transportation, and accessibility.

Special physical needs must be tended to during school hours.

Sexuality

Precocious puberty may occur.

Sexual functioning may be altered.

Genetic counseling may be necessary.

In choosing birth control, individuals must consider latex precautions and allergy and blood clots associated with oral contraceptives.

Transition into Adulthood

The following issues depend on the severity of associated problems: primary health care, independent living, vocational training, and socialization.

FAMILY CONCERNS

Parents suffer chronic grief for loss of "normal" child.

Stress is related to frequent hospitalizations, surgeries, and need for multidisciplinary care.

Caring for these children can be a financial burden on families.

REFERENCES

Adams, C.D., Streisand, R.M., Zawacki, T., & Joseph, K.E. (2002). Living with a chronic illness: A measure of social functioning for children and adolescents. *J Pediatr Psychol, 27*(7), 593-605.

American Association of Nurse Anesthetists. (2002). *Latex allergy fact sheet for patients with spina bifida and those who undergo multiple invasive procedures* (press release, April 11, 2002).

Babcook, C.J. (1995). Ultrasound evaluation of prenatal and neonatal spina bifida. *Neurosurg Clin N Am, 6*(2), 203-218.

Bannister & Carys, M. (2000). The case for and against intrauterine surgery for myelomeningoceles. *Eur J Obstet Gynecol Reprod Bio, 92*(1), 109-113.

Brinchmann, B.S. (1999). When the home becomes a prison: Living with a severely disabled child. *Nurs Ethics, 6*, 137-143.

Brown, J.P. (2001) Orthopedic care of children with spina bifida: You've come a long way, baby! *Orthop Nurs, 20*(4), 51-58.

Buran, C.F., McDaniel, A.M., & Brei, T.J. (2002). Needs assessment in a spina bifida program: A comparison of the perceptions by adolescents with spina bifida and their parents. *Clinical Nurse Specialist, 16*(5), 256-262.

Cheng, L. & Lee, D. (1999). Review of latex allergy. *J Am Board Fam Pract, 12*(4), 285-292.

The Children's Hospital of Philadelphia. The Center for Fetal Diagnosis and Treatment. *Fetal diagnosis of spina bifida;* Web site: www.fetasurgery.chop.edu.

Coakley, R.M., Holmbeck, G.N., Friedman, D., Greenley, R.N., & Thill, A.W. (2002). A longitudinal study of pubertal timing, parent-child conflict, and cohesion in families of young adolescents with spina bifida. *J Pediatr Psychol, 27*(5), 461-473.

Cragen, J.D. et al. (1995). Surveillance for anencephaly and spina bifida and the impact of prenatal diagnosis: United States, 1985-94. *MMWR Morb Mortal Wkly Rep CDC Surveill Summ, 44*, 1-13.

Daly, L.E., Kirke, P.N., Molloy, A., Weir, D.G., & Scott, J.M. (1995). Folate levels and neural tube defects: Implications for prevention. *JAMA, 274*, 1698-1702.

Dise, J.E. & Lohr, M.E. (1998). Examination of deficits in conceptual reasoning abilities associated with spina bifida. *Am J Phys Med Rehabil, (7)*3, 247-251.

Edwards-Beckett, J. & King, H. (1996). The impact of spinal pathology on bowel control in children. *Rehabil Nurs, 21*(6), 292-296.

Elias, E.R. & Hobbs, N. (1998) Spina bifida: Sorting out the complexities of care. *Contemp Pediatr, 15*(4), 156-171.

Fletcher, J.M., Barnes, M., & Dennis M. (2002). Language development in children with spina bifida. *Semin Pediatr Neurol, 9*(3), 201-208.

Green, N. (2002). Folic acid supplementation and prevention of birth defects. *Am Soc Nutritional Sci J Nutr, 132*, 2356S-2360S.

Greenberg, M.S. (2001). *Handbook of neurosurgery* (5th ed). Lakeland, Fla.: Greenberg Graphics, Inc.

Hamilton, R.G. (2002). Diagnosis of natural rubber latex allergy. *Methods, 27*(22), 22-31.

Hasenau, S. & Covington, C. (2002). Neural tube defects prevention and folic acid. *MCN Am J Matern Child Nurs, 27*, 87-91.

Hirose, S., Farmer, D., & Albanese, C. (2001). Fetal surgery for myelomeningocele. *Curr Opin Obstet Gynecol, 13*, 215-222.

Hochleitner, B., Menardi, G., Haussler, B., Ulmer, H., Kofler, H., et al. (2001). Spina bifida as an independent risk factor for sensitization to latex. *J Urol, 166*, 2370-2374.

Holmbeck, G.N., Coakely, R.N., Hommeyer, M.A., Shapera, W.E., & Westhoven, V.C. (2002). Observed and perceived dyadic and systemic functioning in families of preadolescents with spina bifida. *J Pediatr Psychol, 27*(2), 177-189.

Holmes, N., Nguyen, H., Harrison, M., Farmer, D., & Baskin, L. (2001). Fetal intervention for myelomeningocele: Effect on postnatal bladder function. *J Urol, 166*, 2383-2386.

Honein, M.A., Paulozzi, L.J., Mathews, T.J., Erickson, J.D., & Wong, L.Y. (2001). Impact of folic acid fortification of the U.S. food supply on the occurrence of neural tube defects. *JAMA, 285*, 2981-2986.

Hudson, M. (2001). Dental surgery in pediatric patients with spina bifida and latex allergy. *AORN J, 74*(1), 57-72.

James, H.E. & Brant, A. (2002). Treatment of the Chiari malformation with bone decompression without durotomy in children and young adults. *Childs Nerv Syst, 180*(5), 202-206.

Johnson, C.P. & Dorval, J. (2001). *Transitions into adolescence. Spina Bifida Association of America fact sheet.* Washington, D.C.: Spina Bifida Association of America.

Joseph, D.B. (2001). *Urologic care and management 2001. Spina Bifida Association of America fact sheet.* Washington, D.C.: Spina Bifida Association of America.

Karpman, E., Das, S., & Kurzrock, E. (2002). Laparoscopic antegrade continence enema (Malone) procedure: Description and illustration of technique. *J Endourol, 16*(6), 325-328.

Kripalani, H.M. (2000). Quality of life in spina bifida: Importance of parental hope. *Arch Dis Child, 83,* 749-758.

Larson, E. (1998). Reframing the meaning of disability to families: The embrace of paradox. *Soc Sci Med, 47,* 865-875.

Little, J. & Elwood, J.M. (1991). Reproductive epidemiology and perinatal epidemiology. In M. Klely (ed). *Epidemiology of neural tube defects.* Boca Raton, Fla.: CRC Press.

Lollar, D. (2001a). *Educational issues among children with spina bifida. Spina Bifida Association of America fact sheet.* Washington, D.C.: Spina Bifida Association of America.

Lollar, D. (2001b). *Learning among children with spina bifida. Spina Bifida Association of America fact sheet.* Washington, D.C.: Spina Bifida Association of America.

Mangels, K.J., Tulipan, N., Tsao, L.Y., Alarcon, J., & Bruner, J.P. (2000). Fetal MRI in the evaluation of intrauterine myelomeningocele. *Pediatr Neurosurg, 32*(3), 124-131.

Manning, S.M., Jennings, R., & Madsen, J.R. (2000). Pathophysiology, prevention, and potential treatment of neural tube defects. *Ment Retard Dev Disabil Res Rev, 6,* 6-14.

Marge, M. & Lollar, D.J. (1994) *Preventing secondary conditions associated with spina bifida or cerebral palsy; proceedings and recommendations of a symposium. Toward a state of well-being; promoting healthy behaviors to prevent secondary conditions.* Washington, D.C.: Spina Bifida Association of America.

Mataro, M., Junque, C., Poca, M.A., & Sahuquillo, J. (2001). Neuropsychological findings in congential and acquired childhood hydrocephalus. *Neuropsychol Rev, 11*(4), 169-178.

Matthews, T.J., Honein, M.A., & Erickson, J.D. (2002). Spina bifida and anencephaly prevalence—United States, 1991-2001. *MMWR Recomm Rep, 13*(51), 9-11.

McAndrew, H.F. & Malone, P.S. (2002). Continent catheterizable conduits: Which stoma, which conduit and which reservoir? *BJU International, 89,* 86-89.

McComb, J.G. (1999). Principles and practice of pediatric neurosurgery. In *Spinal meningoceles.* New York: Thieme Medical Publishers, Inc., pp. 271-289.

McLone, D.G. & Knepper, P.A. (1989). The cause of Chiari II malformation: A unified theory. *Pediatr Neurosci, 15,* 1-12.

Meade, B.J., Weissman, D.N., & Beezhold, D.H. (2002). Latex allergy: Past and present. *Int Immunopharmacol, 2,* 225-238.

Melvin, E. (2001). *Genetics and spina bifida. Spina Bifida Association of America fact sheet.* Washington, D.C.: Spina Bifida Association of America.

Merropol, E. (2001). *Latex (natural rubber) allergy in spina bifida. Spina Bifida Association of America fact sheet.* Washington, D.C.: Spina Bifida Association of America.

Mersereau, P. (2000). Preventing neural tube birth defects: A national campaign. *Division of Birth Defects, Child Development and Disability, Small Talk Article, 2*(12), 1-2, 4-5.

Nainar, H. (2001). Dental management of children with latex allergy. *Int J Paediatr Dentistry, 11,* 322-326.

Natarajan, V., Kapur, D., Sharma, S., & Singh, G. (2002). Pregnancy in patients with spina bifida and urinary diversion. *Int Urogynecol J Pelvic Floor Dysfunct, 13,* 383-385.

Oakes, J. (2001). *Symptomatic Chiari malformation. Spina Bifida Association of America fact sheet.* Washington, D.C.: Spina Bifida Association of America.

Physicians' Desk Reference (ed. 55). (2001). Montvale, N.J.: Medical Economics Co., Inc.

Pit-ten Cate, I.M., Kennedy, C., & Stevenson, J. (2002). Disability and quality of life in spina bifida and hydrocephalus. *Dev Med Child Neurol, 44,* 317-322.

Rintoul, N.E., Sutton, L.N., Hubbard, A.M., Cohen, B., Melchionni, J., et al. (2002). A new look at myelomeningoceles: Functional level, vertebral level, shunting, and the implications for fetal intervention. *Pediatrics, 3*(109), 409-413.

Rotenstein, D. & Reigal, D.H. (1996). Growth hormone treatment in children with neural tube defects: Results from 6 months to 6 years. *J Pediatr, 128*(2), 184-189.

Spina Bifida Association of America. (2002). *Facts about spina bifida.* Washington, D.C.: Author.

Sprangers, M.A., de Regt, E.B., Andries, F., van Agt, H.M., Bijl, R.V., et al. (2000). Which chronic conditions are associated with better or poorer quality of life? *J Clin Epidemiol, 53,* 895-907.

Talwar, D., Baldwin, M.A., & Horbatt, C.I. (1995). Epilepsy in children with meningomyelocele. *Pediatr Neurol, 13*(1), 29-32.

Teo, C., Parker, E.C., Aureli, S., & Boop, F.A. (1997). The Chiari II malformation: A surgical series. *Pediatr Neurosurg, 27,* 223-229.

Trivin, C.F. et al. (2001). Disorders of growth and puberty in children with non-tumoral hydrocephalus. *J Pediatric Endocrinol Metab, 14*(3), 319-327.

Trollman, R. et al. (2000). Does growth hormone (GH) enhance growth in GH-deficient children with myelomeningocele? *J Clin Endocrinol Metab, 85*(8), 2740-2743.

Trute, B. & Heibert-Murphy, D. (2002). Family adjustment to childhood developmental disability: A measure of parent appraisal of family impacts. *J Pediatr Psychol, 27*(3), 271-280.

Walker, M.L. & Dias, M.S. (2001). *Tethering spinal cord. Spina Bifida Association of America fact sheet.* Washington, D.C.: Spina Bifida Association of America.

Walsh, D.S., Adzick, N.S., Sutton, L.N., & Johnson, M.P. (2001). The rationale for in utero repair of myelomeningocele. *Fetal Diagn Ther, 16*(5), 312-322.

Williams, L.J., Mai, C.T., Edmonds, L.D., Shaw, G.M., Kirby, R.S., et al. (2002). Prevalence of spina bifida and anencephaly during the transition to mandatory folic acid fortification in the United States. *Teratology, 66,* 33-39.

Wong, Y.C. & Paulozzi, L. (2001). Survival of infants with spina bifida: A population study, 1979-1994. *Paediatr Perinat Epidemiol, 15,* 374-378.

Youdimk & Kogan, B.A. (2002). Preliminary study of the safety and efficacy of extended-release oxybutynin in children. *Urology, 59,* 428-432.

34 Organ Transplantation

Beverly Kosmach-Park, Melanie Klein, and Kathy S. Lawrence

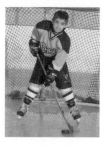

Etiology

Solid organ transplantation has evolved into an effective treatment for a variety of end-stage organ diseases. This complex surgical procedure is followed by a phase of intensive surgical and medical management leading to stable graft function with routine monitoring. The liver, kidney, and heart are the most commonly transplanted solid organs in the pediatric population. Intestine transplantation has recently become an accepted procedure for those children with end-stage short gut syndrome, with nearly 100 intestine transplants being performed annually throughout the world (Grant, 2001). Lung and heart-lung transplants are performed only when other treatments are not viable.

With increased success and survival following solid organ transplantation, the indications for transplantation of the kidney, liver, and heart continue to increase (Table 34-1). The most common causes of renal failure resulting in end-stage renal disease requiring transplantation in children are obstructive uropathy, renal aplasia/hypoplasia/dysplasia, reflux nephropathy, focal segmental glomerulosclerosis, and chronic glomerulonephritis (North American Pediatric Renal Transplant Cooperative Study [NAPRTCS], 2001).

Liver transplantation is a treatment therapy for a variety of end-stage liver diseases (ESLDs) that can generally be categorized as cholestatic disease, metabolic disease, fulminant hepatic failure, hepatitis, and malignancy (Jaskowski, 2002). Biliary atresia, which is an obstructive biliary tract disease, is the most common indication for pediatric liver transplantation in most centers (McDiarmid, 2001). A Kasai portoenterostomy may result in improved bile drainage if performed within an infant's first 60 days of life. About 75% of children, however, will eventually require liver transplantation because of jaundice, recurrent cholangitis, portal hypertension, ascites, growth failure, and decreased synthetic function (Mazeriegos et al, 2000). The most common metabolic disease requiring transplantation is alpha$_1$-antitrypsin deficiency.

Cardiomyopathy and congenital heart disease (CHD) are the leading indications for heart or heart-lung transplantation in children, with more than 50% of those referred for transplant having CHD (Boyle & Fricker, 2000). The most common indication for heart-lung transplantation is either surgically corrected or uncorrected CHD, which is associated with end-stage pulmonary vascular disease, primary pulmonary hypertension, and cystic fibrosis. Fewer children now require heart-lung transplantation as a result of advancements in single- or double-lung transplants and surgery for congenital heart disease.

Known Genetic Etiology

There are many renal diseases with genetic etiologies that can lead to chronic and end-stage renal disease. Genetic etiologies include Alport syndrome, focal segmental glomerulosclerosis (FSGS), Wilms tumor, familial juvenile nephronophthisis, and polycystic kidney disease, either autosomal dominant (ADPKD) or autosomal recessive (ARPKD). Genetic susceptibility to hypertension, diabetes, and immune-mediated diseases such as lupus are genetic factors that may predispose an individual to developing renal disease, but those are less common in the pediatric population.

Although gene therapy is not available at this time, there is promise. Researchers are working not only to develop ways to identify and modify the genes that cause inherited renal diseases but also to modify the susceptibility of an individual to develop hypertension (the predisposition to progress to ESRD) or to modify the immune response in acute transplant rejection (George & Neilson, 2000). The hope is that this research will provide new technology to diagnose, treat, and even prevent renal failure in children. See Chapter 38 for further discussion on genetic etiology for renal disease.

Several etiologies of liver disease requiring transplantation have a genetic predisposition. These include familial cholestasis, Alagille syndrome, Byler syndrome, Wilson disease, and alpha$_1$-antitrypsin deficiency. In addition, some children with cystic fibrosis, an autosomal recessive disorder, may present with secondary liver disease requiring transplantation.

The incidence of cardiomyopathy in children is not well documented and varies according to primary causes (i.e., congenital, acquired) or secondary causes (e.g., infection, systemic disease, toxic exposure, malnutrition). The most common cardiomyopathy in children is of the dilated type. For every 20 cases of cardiomyopathy there is one case with a positive family history indicating a genetic predisposition to develop the cardiovascular changes (Stockwell et al, 1995). See Chapter 21 for additional discussion on the genetic etiology of cardiac conditions leading to transplantation.

Incidence and Prevalence

Transplantation provides an accepted treatment for a variety of end-stage organ diseases with nearly 81,000 adults and children currently listed for solid organ transplantation (www.UNOS.org). According to the United Network of Organ Sharing's (UNOS's) Organ Procurement and Transplantation Network, 22,494 children from birth to 18 years of age have received a solid organ transplant since data were compiled by that agency in 1988. Of that group, renal transplants were

TABLE 34-1
Comparative Indications for Transplantation in Children by Organ*

Renal	Liver	Heart	Dual Transplants
CONGENITAL DISEASE	**CHOLESTATIC DISEASE**	**CARDIOMYOPATHY**	**HEART AND LIVER**
Renal hypoplasia/aplasia	Biliary atresia	Dilated	Familial hypercholesterolemia with ischemic
Renal dysplasia	Familial cholestasis	Hypertrophic	cardiomyopathy
Eagle-Barrett syndrome	Alagille syndrome	Restrictive	Intrahepatic biliary atresia and dilated
Congenital nephrotic syndrome	Byler syndrome	**CONGENITAL HEART DEFECTS**	cardiomyopathy
Wilms tumor	**PARENCHYMAL DISEASE**	**(SELECT LESIONS)**	**LIVER AND KIDNEY**
Obstructive uropathy	Budd-Chiari syndrome		Cystinosis
Reflux nephropathy	Congenital hepatic fibrosis		Oxalosis
ACQUIRED DISEASE	Cystic fibrosis		**HEART AND LUNG**
Glomerulonephritis	Neonatal hepatitis		Primary pulmonary hypertension
Lupus nephritis	Acute fulminant hepatic failure		Congenital heart defects with elevated pulmonary
Membranoproliferative glomerulonephritis,	Hepatitis B		vascular resistance
types I and II	Hepatitis C		Cystic fibrosis
Focal segmental glomerulosclerosis	**METABOLIC DISORDERS**		
IgA nephropathy	Alpha$_1$-antitrypsin deficiency		
Henoch-Schönlein purpura	Wilson disease		
Hemolytic-uremic syndrome	Glycogen storage disease, type IV		
Chronic pyelonephritis	Tyrosinemia		
Renal infarct	**HEPATOMAS**		
Sickle cell nephropathy			
HEREDITARY DISEASE			
Alport syndrome			
Juvenile nephronophthisis			
Polycystic kidney disease			
METABOLIC DISORDERS			
Cystinosis			
Oxalosis			

*This list includes the most common etiologies of end-stage organ failure; it is not all-inclusive.

performed in 9933 children younger than 18 years of age, liver transplants were performed in 7761 children younger than 18 years of age, and 2481 children received heart transplants (http://www.optn.org/latestData/rptData.asp).

See Chapters 21 and 38 for further discussion of the incidence of cardiac and renal conditions leading to transplantation.

Clinical Manifestations at Time of Diagnosis

The presenting symptoms and severity of illness of children with end-stage organ disease vary according to the specific disease and affected organ, as well as the length of illness, age of the child, and effectiveness of treatment. Table 34-2 presents the clinical manifestations of end-stage organ disease in children.

Children with ESRD typically exhibit symptoms related to fluid and electrolyte imbalances and hypertension. Early signs and symptoms may include pallor and fatigue on exertion. Children with renal disease may also present with anorexia, recurrent emesis, edema, anemia, and rickets (Ellis et al, 1997). These children also often exhibit growth failure as a long-term effect of chronic renal disease (Fine, 2002). A complete discussion of the manifestations of chronic renal failure is presented in Chapter 38.

Children with liver disease may have an acute or chronic course of illness depending on the etiology and severity of the liver disease. Some children may remain stable for several years before transplantation with appropriate medical management,

TABLE 34-2
Comparative Clinical Manifestations of End-Stage Renal, Liver, and Heart Disease in Children

Renal	Liver	Heart
Hyperphosphatemia	Jaundice	Tachypnea
Hyperkalemia	Ascites	Congestive heart failure
Elevated BUN and creatinine	Hepatomegaly	Growth retardation
Hyperlipidemia	Splenomegaly	Cardiac murmurs
Metabolic acidosis	Coagulopathies	Arrhythmias
Hypertension	Hyperammonemia	ST- and T-wave
Edema/hypervolemia	Hypercholesterolemia	abnormalities
Congestive heart failure	Hypoalbuminemia	Respiratory distress
Pericarditis	Hypoglycemia	
Peripheral neuropathy	Portal hypertension	
Growth retardation	Malnutrition	
Secondary hyperparathyroidism	Hormone imbalance	
Anemia	Encephalopathy	
Renal osteodystrophy		

BUN, Blood urea nitrogen.

but others may have a moderate to rapid decline in hepatic function requiring emergent transplantation. Symptoms of liver dysfunction, such as those seen with biliary atresia, may include jaundice, hepatomegaly, splenomegaly, ascites, pruritus, xanthomas, and variceal bleeding. Hepatic enzymes, bilirubin, gamma guanosine triphosphate (GTP), and ammonia levels are elevated. Children who have had a Kasai portoenterostomy are also at risk for cholangitis. Other symptoms associated with liver failure may include delayed growth, malnutrition, rickets, osteomalacia with fractures, increased synthetic function, and encephalopathy.

Acute end-stage liver disease secondary to fulminant hepatic failure may have an insidious onset with rapid clinical deterioration over a few days, characterized by encephalopathy and coagulopathy. With progression of hepatic dysfunction, cerebral edema increases, causing neurologic deterioration often with intracranial hemorrhage, a critical situation requiring liver transplantation before the child deteriorates to the point of being ineligible for transplantation.

Complex CHD and cardiomyopathies requiring transplantation may have similar presenting symptoms (see Chapter 21 for a review of CHD). Symptoms of cardiomyopathy vary depending on the child's age at presentation of illness and the type of cardiomyopathy. The clinical manifestations of dilated cardiomyopathy include symptoms of congestive heart failure as a result of decreasing myocardial contractility. Other common clinical signs include an enlarged heart by chest radiography, nonspecific ST-T wave changes and sinus tachycardia on electrocardiography, and a gallop rhythm on auscultation. Nonspecific symptoms may include fever, vomiting, weight loss, or failure to thrive.

Most children discovered to have hypertrophic cardiomyopathy do not have prominent cardiac symptoms because thickening of the left ventricular wall may remain stable or progress slowly. There is usually a positive family history in 30% to 60% of affected individuals (Park, 1996). Children and young adults are at risk for episodes of syncope and sudden death during exercise when the left ventricular demand increases and obstruction to the outflow tract occurs. This diagnosis is sometimes first made on autopsy. The annual incidence of sudden death is 4% to 6% per year in children and adolescents with hypertrophic cardiomyopathy (Park, 1996).

Treatment

Pretransplant Management

Conservative therapy of renal disease consists of managing fluid, electrolyte, and metabolic imbalances, as well as hypertension and anemia (see Chapter 38). When conservative treatment for chronic renal failure is no longer effective, ESRD care consists of hemodialysis, peritoneal dialysis, or renal transplantation (Chan et al, 2002). Because of the deleterious effects of dialysis on children, preemptive renal transplantation, or transplantation before the initiation of dialysis, has become more common. As of 2000, nearly 25% of all renal transplants were preemptive (NAPRTCS, 2001). Because this goal is not always immediately attainable, such as in the cases of acute renal failure or chronic renal failure with no available living donor, dialysis is often initiated. Transplantation is the treatment choice for children with ESRD in order to maximize survival; minimize the sequelae of uremia on growth and development; improve the overall quality of life for the child and family; and reduce the physiologic, psychologic, and financial effects of end-stage disease.

Children with chronic liver disease may be observed on an outpatient basis with medical management designed to optimize and stabilize hepatic function. To meet nutritional requirements, these children may require enteral supplementation, administration of fat-soluble vitamins, and/or total parenteral nutrition (TPN). Synthetic function of the liver, coagulation times, and ammonia levels, as well as electrolytes, fluid balance, and renal function, must be frequently monitored.

Medications may provide symptomatic relief to mitigate the effects of hepatic dysfunction. Ursodiol and phenobarbital may help decrease cholestasis. Pruritus may be lessened with single or combination therapy including ursodiol (Actigall), diphenhydramine (Benadryl), hydroxyzine (Atarax), or rifampin (Rifadin). High ammonia levels may be controlled by lactulose (Cephulac).

Recurrent cholangitis as a result of biliary stasis and bacterial contamination in children who have had a Kasai procedure is common. Symptoms may include a fever of more than 38° C (100.4° F), an elevated white blood cell count, and an increase in serum bilirubin concentration. Diagnosis is confirmed by positive blood cultures. Treatment includes an appropriately sensitive intravenous antibiotic followed by long-term prophylaxis with trimethoprim-sulfamethoxazole (Bactrim, Septra), metronidazole (Flagyl), or ciprofloxacin hydrochloride (Cipro).

Bleeding episodes from esophageal and gastric varices caused by portal hypertension can be temporized by sclerotherapy and band variceal ligation. Peritoneal-venous shunt surgery may also be performed to decrease ascites, and the splenic artery may be embolized to mediate thrombocytopenia. In the event of massive bleeding refractory to sclerotherapy, transcutaneous intrahepatic portosystemic shunting (TIPS) may be required (Reyes et al, 1999). Although this procedure may help stabilize a child during the waiting period, complications may occur and include bleeding from perforation or extrahepatic portal vein puncture, peritonitis, hepatic injury, or biliary injury.

Children with CHD who develop ventricular dysfunction, lethal arrhythmias, and/or irreversible pulmonary hypertension are also managed medically until transplantation. Management is similar to dilated cardiomyopathy but may vary slightly depending on the type of CHD and previous operative or palliative procedures. Some children and adolescents with cyanotic heart defects may have additional management issues related to polycythemia, hypoxemia, and central nervous system (CNS) sequelae (see Chapter 21). In addition, children who have increased pulmonary vascular resistance (PVR) unresponsive to pulmonary vasodilators will require heart-lung transplantation instead of an isolated heart transplant. If the PVR index can be lowered preoperatively to less than 6 units by medication, an isolated heart transplant is possible (Boyle & Fricker, 2000).

In contrast, medical management for hypertrophic cardiomyopathy consists of maintaining a normal preload and afterload while reducing ventricular contractility, usually accomplished with calcium channel blockers as well as betablockers, to decrease the septal muscle from obstructing the left ventricular outflow tract. Antiarrhythmics may be needed for ventricular arrhythmias but have not been shown to prevent sudden death. Automatic implanted defibrillator devices may also be used (Boyle & Fricker, 2000). Surgical intervention can be attempted to remove muscle bundles in the left ventricular outflow tract to relieve obstruction. Surgical intervention is not recommended until medical management has failed because of the possibility of recurrent obstruction.

Medical management of children with dilated cardiomyopathy consists of maximizing cardiac output and controlling symptoms of heart failure with digoxin, diuretics, and afterload reduction. Angiotensin-converting enzyme inhibitors (i.e, captopril [Capoten], enalapril [Vasotec]) for afterload reduction have been beneficial in optimizing cardiac function and decreasing the workload of the heart. Antiarrhythmics may be needed in some children. Anticoagulation therapy may help to prevent thrombus formation in a dilated and poorly contracting heart.

Heart transplantation is the alternative to failed medical and surgical management. Because of the shortage of pediatric donors, however, children at the maximum limits of medical management may not survive until transplantation. The mortality rate for pediatric heart candidates is reported to be nearly 30% (Morrow et al, 2000).

Evaluation for Transplantation

Evaluation for organ transplantation requires a detailed, multidisciplinary approach that includes medical, surgical, nutritional, and psychosocial assessments with multiple diagnostic tests, laboratory data, radiologic testing, and consultant evaluations (Jaskowski, 2002; Kosmach-Park, 2002). The evaluation process is organ specific and institution specific, but usually includes consultations by the transplant surgery staff; specialty medical services (e.g., nephrology, gastroenterology, anesthesiology, cardiology), and infectious disease specialists; nursing services with transplant coordinators, clinical nurse specialists, or nurse practitioners; psychosocial services through social work and psychiatry; nutritional therapists; behavioral medicine involving developmental and child life specialists; and physical and occupational therapists. Although not involved in direct care, financial counselors are also utilized to assist families with insurance and billing questions. Evaluations are usually scheduled on an outpatient basis in specialty clinics, with routine outpatient follow-up facilitated by the transplant coordinator during the waiting period. Children with more advanced disease, however, may be hospitalized during the evaluation and also require long-term hospitalization while waiting for transplantation. Children with rapidly progressive renal disease or end-stage disease diagnosed on initial presentation may be hospitalized until stabilized on dialysis and then sent home with follow-up by the local nephrologist.

Pretransplant surgical procedures may be necessary in some cases to provide corrective or palliative repairs to prepare or stabilize a child for transplantation. For example, a child with uncontrollable hypertension, refractory to medical treatment, may require a preemptive bilateral nephrectomy, preferably at least 6 months before transplantation.

Laboratory data commonly obtained for all children awaiting organ transplant include a complete blood count; a full chemistry profile to assess electrolytes, renal function, and nutritional status; and prothrombin and partial thromboplastin times. Serologic testing is also completed to diagnose previous infections with hepatitis A, B, and C, cytomegalovirus (CMV),

Epstein-Barr virus (EBV), human immunodeficiency virus (HIV), herpes, and varicella zoster. A child's immunization record is reviewed, and every attempt is made to administer delinquent vaccines if the child is well enough to tolerate a vaccination. Live vaccines, such as the MMR (measles, mumps, rubella), and varicella virus vaccine (Varivax) are not administered after transplantation since the child has an increased risk of acquiring the virus from a live vaccine when the immune system is suppressed.

Blood typing to achieve ABO-matched organs is required for heart, kidney, and liver transplantation. In addition, human leukocyte antigen (HLA) matching is necessary in renal transplantation. Cytotoxic antibody cross-match compatibility, percent panel reactive antibody (PRA), and HLA tissue typing are also completed. Children awaiting cardiac transplant with high PRAs are treated before transplant with intravenous immune globulin (IVIG), plasmapheresis, cyclophosphamide (Cytoxan), azathioprine (Imuran), and mycophenolate mofetil (CellCept) in hopes of reducing rejection of the donor heart (Boyle, 2000a).

Although most children with end-stage organ disease are suitable candidates for transplantation, there are some exclusion criteria. These criteria have decreased significantly over the past 2 decades because of innovations in care and advances in surgical techniques. Exclusion criteria vary by institution, but most centers agree that children with systemic sepsis, multisystem organ failure, and metastatic disease are not appropriate candidates. Individuals who are HIV positive, once considered an absolute contraindication to transplantation, are receiving transplants at some centers. Children infected with hepatitis C (HCV) carry the added risk of liver cirrhosis and carcinoma and are not ideal candidates for cardiac transplantation (Boyle & Fricker, 2000). A history of medical noncompliance and poor social support may place the transplant recipient at increased risk for graft failure (Pearlman, 2002a). Referral to Child and Family Services may be necessary if a family is unable or unwilling to provide appropriate care to the child both before and after transplant.

Following acceptance as a transplant candidate, a child is listed with UNOS according to organ-specific criteria. While waiting at home or in a community hospital for transplantation, the child is medically managed by the primary care provider, who must provide regular updates to the transplant center and inform the center of any deterioration or complications in the child's medical status. Because the primary care provider may also have developed a supportive relationship with the child and family during the diagnosis of the illness and pretransplant care, this caregiver may be best able to assess the child and family's coping abilities, responses to stress, level of understanding, and adaptability. This assessment should be communicated to the transplant team to help build on the family's strengths as the family learns to cope with and adapt to the various stressors of the transplant process. The waiting period is variable, depending on the organ or organs needed, as well as the child's blood type, weight, and medical status. Waiting for a cadaveric organ may range from a few days to months and possibly years. It is a highly stressful time for family members as they hope for an organ before their child's condition deteriorates.

Therapeutic Levels of Cyclosporine (CSA) and Tacrolimus (Prograf) (ng/ml) Following Transplantation

Time	Liver CSA*	Liver Tacrolimus	Kidney CSA	Kidney Tacrolimus	Heart CSA	Heart Tacrolimus
<1 mo	500-800	10-15	125-400	10-15	300-700	15-20
1-3 mo	300-500	10	125-250	5-10	300-500	10-15
Long term	200	5-10	60-200	5-10	150-300	5-10

Data from the Children's Hospital of Pittsburgh and Rainbow Babies and Children's Hospital, Cleveland. From Kosmach, B., Webber, S., & Reyes, J. (1998). Care of the pediatric solid organ transplant recipient. *Pediatr Clin North Am, 45*(6), 1399.
*CSA, Cyclosporine, measured by monoclonal TDx in whole blood.

After Transplant

Immunosuppressive Management. Immunosuppressive regimens vary according to the organ transplanted and institution protocol, but the goals are similar: to maintain the lowest acceptable level of drug that results in stable and adequate functioning of the transplanted organ without drug toxicity. The most common immunosuppressive medications used alone or in combination therapy to prevent rejection are cyclosporine (CSA, Neoral), tacrolimus (Prograf), prednisone, sirolimus (Rapamune), mycophenolate mofetil (MMF, CellCept), and azathioprine (Imuran). Therapeutic levels and doses vary according to the organ transplanted, the length of time after transplant, and the presence of infection or rejection (Table 34-3).

Cyclosporine (CSA) has been the mainstay of solid organ transplantation since its introduction in the 1980s. Originally used in conjunction with steroids and azathioprine, this immunosuppressant revolutionized transplantation and resulted in dramatically improved survival rates. CSA inhibits the activity of calcineurin, which triggers transcription factors involved in interleukin-2 (IL-2) and other cytokine gene activation (Vanrenterghem, 2001). Absorption of CSA is bile dependent because it is excreted and reabsorbed from bile through enterohepatic circulation. Consequently, therapeutic drug levels may be difficult to maintain in people receiving liver transplants, in other organ recipients with cholestasis caused by hepatic dysfunction, and in people with external bile drainage. A microemulsion formulation of CSA absorbed independently of bile is available (Neoral) and is commonly used.

Although nephrotoxicity is the most significant side effect of CSA, it is dosage dependent and usually reversible (Table 34-4). Acute nephrotoxicity may present with a sudden increase in the blood urea nitrogen (BUN) level and creatinine. Hyperkalemia, hyponatremia, metabolic acidosis, and hypomagnesemia may also occur. Chronic toxicity can result in permanent vascular changes and renal atrophy (Cronin et al, 2000). Hypertension is common, especially when CSA is given in combination with high-dose corticosteroids, but is usually responsive to antihypertensive therapy with calcium channel blockers (e.g., nifedipine [Procardia], amlodipine [Norvasc], verapamil [Calan]) or beta-adrenergic blockers (e.g., atenolol [Tenormin], propranolol [Inderal], labetalol [Normodyne]). Calcium channel blockers, especially diltiazem (Cardizem), not only treat hypertension but also may offer some protection against posttransplant coronary artery disease in heart recipients. Beta-blockers may exacerbate chronotropic incompetence in people

Toxicity of Cyclosporine and Tacrolimus

Adverse Effect	Cyclosporine (CSA)	Tacrolimus (Prograf)
Neurotoxicity	+	++
Nephrotoxicity	++	++
Hyperkalemia	++	+++
Hypertension	+++	+
Diabetogenicity	+	+
Hypercholesterolemia	++	+
Increased low-density lipoprotein levels	++	+
Hyperuricemia	+	+
Gingival hyperplasia	++	–
Hirsutism	++	–
Alopecia	+	++
Anemia	+	++
Hand tremors	+	+

Data from Jain, A. & Fung, J. (1996). Cyclosporine and tacrolimus in clinical transplantation: A comparative review. *Clin Immunotherapy, 5*, 365.
+ to +++, Increasing frequency and/or severity of each adverse effect; –, adverse effect not observed.

with heart transplants and are generally not used as first-line therapy. Angiotensin-converting enzyme (ACE) inhibitors should be avoided in people with marginal renal function or hyperkalemia. Although nephrotoxicity is a concern in all transplant recipients, it may be more critical in those with renal transplants because renal dysfunction may reflect not only CSA toxicity but also rejection and acute tubular necrosis.

Neurotoxicities, most commonly tremor and headache, are associated with CSA but are usually level dependent and reversible (Cronin et al, 2000). Other neurotoxic side effects include dizziness, photophobia, insomnia, paresthesia, and seizures (Cronin et al, 2000). CSA may also cause gingival hyperplasia, hirsutism, gastrointestinal (GI) disorders, and an increased risk for infection and malignancy. Maintaining a low therapeutic CSA trough level may often decrease the risk and severity of these side effects.

Tacrolimus (Prograf), formerly known as FK-506, is a calcineurin inhibitor that differs chemically from CSA but has a similar mechanism of action. It was first used in 1989 and has been even more effective at preventing and limiting the severity of acute rejection (Chand et al, 2001) as well as treating antibody- and steroid-resistant rejection (Chand et al, 2001; Flynn et al, 2001). Approved for use in 1994, tacrolimus has been used as a primary immunosuppressant and as a treatment for steroid- or antibody-resistant rejection (Flynn et al, 2001; Jain et al, 2002a).

Tacrolimus is up to 100 times more potent in inhibiting the production of cytotoxic T-lymphocytes and IL-2 and gamma interferon production than CSA in vitro (Cronin et al, 2000) and does not depend on bile for absorption, so more stable levels may be seen in recipients with cholestasis or external bile drainage.

Individuals receiving tacrolimus-based immunosuppression have demonstrated lower rates of acute rejection than those on cyclosporine, and the rejection episodes that did occur were less severe (Chand et al, 2001; Jain et al, 2002a). Side effects of tacrolimus are similar to those of CSA, including nephrotoxicity, neurotoxicity, hypertension, infection, hyperglycemia, malignancy, and gastrointestinal disturbances. As with CSA, the severity of these side effects may be decreased or eliminated after transplantation as levels are decreased over time. Posttransplant diabetes mellitus has been reported in up to 20% of people taking tacrolimus (Chand et al, 2001), but it is often transient and related to corticosteroid use. Posttransplant lymphoproliferative disease (PTLD), particularly when associated with a primary Epstein-Barr viral (EBV) infection, has been associated with tacrolimus use (Chand et al, 2001; Jain et al, 2002b; Shapiro, 2000). Hirsutism and gingival hyperplasia are not reported with tacrolimus therapy.

In renal transplantation, triple combination therapy protocols are frequently employed, using cyclosporine (CSA) or tacrolimus (Prograf), prednisone, and a purine synthesis inhibitor, such as azathioprine (Imuran) or mycophenolate mofetil (MMF) (Vanrenterghem, 2001). Mycophenolate has recently replaced azathioprine as a purine synthesis inhibitor in many renal transplant programs (NAPRTCS, 2001). Another calcineurin inhibitor, sirolimus (Rapamune), is being used as an adjunctive or primary immunosuppressant in place of the purine synthesis inhibitors in pediatric clinical trials (Sindhi et al, 2001). An advantage of sirolimus is that it may effectively prevent rejection without the nephrotoxicity seen with calcineurin inhibitors (Sindhi et al, 2001). Studies are underway to determine the safety of these medications in children and evaluate the outcomes when used in conjunction with CSA or tacrolimus as part of steroid-free, calcineurin inhibitor drug regimens (Sindhi et al, 2001; Webber, 2000b).

Corticosteroids (prednisone, methylprednisolone [Solu-Medrol]) are also used for immunosuppressant effects and are part of the immunosuppressive regimen at most transplant centers. The mechanism of action is not completely understood, but corticosteroids affect T-lymphocytes and reduce the production of lymphokines (McGhee et al, 2002). The antiinflammatory effects of steroids may also play a large role in protecting the transplanted organ. Depending on the dose and length of treatment, steroids produce a variety of mild to severe side effects. Stomach irritation, cushingoid facies, mood swings, acne, swelling and weight gain, hypertension, and insomnia are most commonly seen. Side effects of higher, long-term doses may include cataracts, glaucoma, hyperglycemia, delayed growth, osteoporosis, and muscular weakness.

The ability to wean and withdraw steroids from transplant recipients receiving tacrolimus is beneficial for posttransplant health as well as growth and development. Successful steroid withdrawal is more commonly seen in children with liver and heart transplants than in renal transplant recipients (Jain et al, 2000; Shapiro, 2000). With steroid withdrawal, side effects from long-term high-dose steroids (e.g., cushingoid facies, growth failure, osteoporosis, cataract formation, hypertension, diabetes, increased risk of infection) can be minimized or eliminated. An adjunctive agent, such as mycophenolate mofetil or sirolimus, may be added as steroids are weaned (Sindhi et al, 2000; Webber, 2000b).

Mycophenolate mofetil (MMF, CellCept) was approved by the US Food and Drug Administration (FDA) in 1995 for prevention of acute rejection in renal transplantation. It was reported to significantly reduce the rate of treatment failure (i.e., acute rejection, death, graft loss, or early termination from the study for any reason) during the first 6 months after transplantation, when compared with regimens that employed azathioprine (Imuran) (Roche Pharmaceuticals, 2000).

Graft Evaluation. Most transplant centers prefer that pediatric transplant recipients return to the transplant center for an annual evaluation of the graft. Blood work and organ-specific testing are completed as indicated and may include an abdominal ultrasound, echocardiogram, chest x-ray, or renal flow scan. Biopsies of the transplanted organ are not routinely obtained unless there are clinically significant concerns. The evaluation is usually completed on an outpatient basis over 1 to 2 days, although a short-stay admission may be required following an invasive procedure, such as a cardiac catheterization or biopsy.

Although follow-up varies by center, the majority of transplant centers prefer to manage the recipient's immunosuppressive therapy. The child's primary care provider will continue to see the child for routine childhood illnesses and examinations, with any fevers or illnesses reported to the transplant center as well. Although the child may present with what appears to be a community virus, it is also important to assess the child for posttransplant viral infections, such as CMV or EBV. Laboratory results, obtained through a community health center or private practice, are sent to the transplant center for evaluation as well.

Complementary and Alternative Therapies

Mechanical circulatory support as a temporary bridge to transplantation is an option for the failing heart. A variety of mechanical devices are available for adults, but few are designed for long-term pediatric support. If only ventricular support is required, the most common mechanical circulatory support used while an older child is waiting for transplantation is the ventricular assist device (VAD). A right and/or left VAD can be inserted, depending on the child's need. Some success with VADs has been shown in children weighing more than 6 kg during short-term use (Throckmorton, 2002). Extracorporeal membrane oxygenation (ECMO) can also be employed for infants and children requiring both cardiac and pulmonary support (Boyle, 2000b).

VADs have been well documented as a bridge to transplantation in adults, with 60% of the individuals supported going on to transplantation and 89% discharged from the hospital (Hunt & Frazier, 1998). The better outcomes from the VADs can be attributed to improving kidney, liver, and pulmonary function as a result of improved organ perfusion if no sequelae occur while an individual is being supported by the device. Some VADs allow a child to ambulate, which provides physical rehabilitation and places the child in optimal condition before transplantation.

There are risks associated with any mechanical circulatory device. The most frequent complications are bleeding, infection, thromboembolism, hemolysis, technical problems, and neurologic dysfunction (Hunt & Frazier, 1998). The ideal long-term mechanical circulatory support device for children has not yet evolved although current devices on the market are being adapted for pediatric use.

Because the function of the liver is primarily metabolic, the challenge is to develop a device that could duplicate these complex chemical reactions. One type of hepatic-assist device under development consists of growing hepatocytes in the extracapillary spaces of a hollow fiber cartridge. An individual's blood is pumped through this cartridge as a continuous rather than an intermittent process, and the hepatocytes function as if they were in an intact liver (Sechser et al, 2001). Clinical trials are underway for a limited number of cases of fulminant hepatic failure, and preliminary findings are encouraging. This type of "liver dialysis" could be helpful in sustaining liver function until the liver recovers by beginning a regenerative process after injury caused by trauma or disease or by helping to maintain a child with end-stage liver disease awaiting transplantation.

Because not much is known about herbal therapies and the effect of these therapies on the metabolism of medications, herbal remedies are not recommended in children awaiting transplant or with transplants. In addition, herbal remedies are not regulated by the FDA. Limited information is available that reports interference with the absorption or metabolism of immunosuppressants and other medications. Any herbal or natural supplement that affects the activity of cytochrome P-450, the drug-metabolizing enzyme, can affect the metabolism of calcineurin inhibitors cyclosporine and tacrolimus. It is thought that St. John's wort works in this way by either inhibiting the absorption or increasing the metabolism of those medications. Regardless of the mechanism, St. John's wort reduces the serum concentration of cyclosporine or tacrolimus, resulting in decreased immunosuppression and placing the child at risk for rejection and allograft loss. Other medication-herb interactions include ephedra, which interacts with antihypertensives and increases blood pressure; licorice, which reduces the effectiveness of and increases the risk of hypokalemia with diuretics by causing sodium retention and potassium depletion; and echinacea, which stimulates the immune system, interfering with the effects of cyclosporine and tacrolimus (Barone et al, 2001; Mayo Foundation for Medical Education & Research, 2002). In addition, the herbal anxiolytic kava has been associated with hepatic toxicity requiring transplantation (Campo et al, 2002).

Anticipated Advances in Diagnosis and Management

Recipient and graft survival has improved significantly over the past 3 decades because of advances in immunosuppression, surgical techniques, organ preservation, and monitoring for infections, as well as a better understanding of postoperative management and intensive care medicine. New approaches to standard immunosuppressive protocols that result in optimum graft function with minimal side effects are being explored. Ongoing research is focused on immunosuppressive medications that more specifically inhibit the immune system and decrease the incidence of rejection, subsequently placing a child at less risk for long-term infection and nephrotoxicity. Steroid-free regimens, induction therapies, and weaning trials are innovative immunosuppressive protocols that are being investigated with the goal of inducing tolerance of the transplanted organ.

Approved for use in the late 1990s, daclizumab (Zenapax) and basiliximab (Simulect) are monoclonal antibodies used for the prophylaxis of acute organ rejection. They are chimeric antibodies, made of recombinant murine and human DNA, and work by directly inhibiting IL-2–expressing T-lymphocytes (Nissen, 2002). Daclizumab is administered before transplant and then every other week after transplant for a total of five doses, whereas basiliximab is given in two doses over a 5-day period, the first dose immediately before transplant and the second dose on postoperative day 4. Studies have reported a decreased incidence of acute rejection in people receiving daclizumab or basiliximab prophylaxis, with no significant difference between the two preparations (Chan et al, 2001; Luke, 2001).

Induction therapy with antilymphocyte globulin (ATG, thymoglobulin) is being administered preoperatively or intraoperatively with the goals of decreasing rejection, delaying the first episode of rejection, or preventing or delaying the additional use of calcineurin inhibitors and their associated toxicities (Flynn, 2002). Induction therapy is becoming a more accepted treatment with promising early outcomes; however, the advantages of this type of immunosuppression must be balanced with the risk of infection and recurrent disease (Flynn, 2002).

Chimerism and Tolerance

Following transplantation, donor cells migrate throughout the recipient's body with an exchange of leukocytes from the donor organ into recipient tissue and a replacement of the same type of leukocytes from the recipient into the donor tissue. Chimerism, which is the co-existence of donor and recipient cells, depends on effective immunosuppression and is thought to be necessary for the body to accept the transplanted organ (Starzl & Zinkernagel, 2001; Starzl et al, 1993a). It is theorized that if chimerism can be maintained, chronic rejection may be avoided and less immunosuppression will be required over the long term.

Achieving a chimeric state is thought to lead to the development of tolerance. Although it has been presumed that transplant recipients will require lifelong immunosuppression, some individuals may achieve tolerance of the transplanted organ after they have been successfully weaned off maintenance immunosuppression (Ohler & Braym, 2002). Weaning trials have not been attempted in children with heart transplants.

As a result of observations indicating that bone marrow cells were the most effective antigen-presenting cells to produce the donor-specific effect (Padbury et al, 1998), donor bone marrow infusion at the time of solid organ transplantation is being used to augment the process of chimerism and possibly increase the incidence of immunosuppressive withdrawal in recipients of liver transplants.

Xenotransplantation

Cadaveric organ donation is unable to meet the demands of the increasing numbers of individuals requiring organ transplantation for end-stage disease. Split liver techniques and living-related liver and kidney transplantation have been of some use in increasing the donor pool, but the growing demand for organs far exceeds the supply. Xenotransplantation, the cross-species transplantation of organs, has been done experimentally since 1964 (Appel et al, 2002; Starzl et al, 1993b) using non-human primates and pigs. Although xenotransplantation would provide an increased source of organs, significant immunologic barriers have deterred the progress of this strategy (Appel et al, 2002). Pig-to-primate xenotransplantation is currently being studied, although this procedure has not yet proved to be safe or beneficial enough to initiate clinical trials in humans. Preliminary trials involving the transplantation of animal cells and tissues are underway (Appel et al, 2002).

Animal-to-human xenotransplantation includes a few experimental procedures. A heterotopic auxiliary transplant of a pig liver into an individual with fulminant hepatic failure was performed in 1993 as a bridge in waiting for a human liver. The pig liver functioned for about 24 hours as evidenced by lactate clearance, bile production, and improved renal function. A rise in antipig antibodies was observed, however, and thought to be the cause for graft failure. The individual died from cerebral edema before a human liver was available (Makowka et al, 1993, 1994).

Two xenotransplants of the liver from baboon donors to human recipients were performed at the University of Pittsburgh with one person surviving 70 days after transplant. Death was due to a subarachnoid hemorrhage secondary to invasive aspergillosis. The immunosuppressive regimen included tacrolimus, cyclophosphamide, prostaglandin E, and steroids. Although liver function was normal for nearly 2 months, an autopsy revealed biliary stasis with damage of the intrahepatic ducts and infection (Starzl et al, 1993b).

Associated Problems (Box 34-1)

Rejection

Rejection is an inflammatory response of the immune system in which the transplanted tissue is recognized as foreign. Acute cellular rejection most commonly occurs during the first 6 months after transplantation. This type of rejection is a T-cell–mediated event and is usually reversible by increasing the level of immunosuppression. Chronic rejection develops over a longer period of time and is a combination of cellular and humoral immune responses. Increased immunosuppressive therapies may not resolve chronic rejection, and the graft may be lost. Tacrolimus (Prograf) may be helpful as rescue therapy in some cases if the primary immunosuppressive therapeutic agent is CSA (Chand et al, 2001).

Acute rejection is usually reversed if detected early and treated promptly. Treatment varies by center and severity but

BOX 34-1
Associated Problems

IMMUNOSUPPRESSION
Side effects of medications (see treatment section)
Potential for infection
Nephrotoxicity
Lymphoproliferative disease

REJECTION
Acute—first 6 months after transplant
Reversible
Chronic—slower process lasting months to years; leading cause of late graft loss

INFECTION
Bacterial
Viral
Fungal
Protozoan
Symptoms of infection masked by immunosuppressive therapy

usually involves an increased level of baseline immunosuppression, increased corticosteroids, and the addition of an adjunctive immunosuppressant such as azathioprine (Imuran), mycophenolate mofetil, or sirolimus (Rapamune). Children receiving CSA may receive tacrolimus as rescue therapy. Muromonab-CD3 (OKT3), a monoclonal antibody, or antilymphocyte globulin may be used to treat rejection that is refractory to steroids and/or increased baseline immunosuppression. Total lymphoid irradiation is effective in treating more serious refractory rejection, but because of cost, inconvenience, and uncertain long-term side effects, including tumor development, it is reserved for use when all other treatments have been unsuccessful (Chin et al, 2002; Webber, 2000b). Repeat biopsies may be performed to evaluate the effectiveness of treatment and determine changes in immunosuppression.

Presenting symptoms of liver rejection include fever, elevated liver function tests, abdominal tenderness, irritability, and fatigue (Table 34-5). If left untreated, rejection may progress from mild to moderate symptoms to those of hepatic dysfunction: ascites, jaundice, acholic stools, bile-stained urine, pruritus, encephalopathy, decreased synthetic function, and renal dysfunction. A percutaneous liver biopsy may be performed to definitively diagnose rejection since elevated enzymes and fever may also be seen with infectious processes, biliary tract complications, or hepatic artery thrombosis. Chronic rejection is defined by the progressive disappearance of bile ducts with subsequent cholestasis and liver failure (i.e., vanishing bile duct syndrome) and may result in late graft loss (Jain et al, 2002a; Wallot et al, 2002).

Acute rejection occurs in more than 50% of children receiving renal transplants (NAPRTCS, 2001) although most episodes can be reversed with early diagnosis and treatment. Careful assessment is key because a low-grade fever and hypertension may be the only signs of early acute rejection. Other presenting symptoms of rejection may include irritability, malaise, oliguria, increased BUN and creatinine levels, weight gain caused by fluid retention, swelling and tenderness at the graft site, edema of the lower extremities, and anorexia.

TABLE 34-5

Clinical Signs of Organ Rejection

Liver	Kidney	Heart
Fever	Fever	Heart failure with tachycardia and gallop rhythm
Elevated liver enzymes (ALT, AST, GGTP), bilirubin, alkaline phosphatase	Elevated BUN and creatinine	Cardiomegaly
Lethargy, fatigue, malaise, irritability	Lethargy, fatigue, malaise, irritability	Hepatomegaly
Acholic stools and bile-stained urine	Weight gain	Fever (nonspecific)
Jaundice	Edema (particularly of lower extremities)	Poor feeding and irritability (infants)
Abdominal tenderness	Tenderness at the graft site	Abdominal pain, vomiting
Ascites	Anorexia, oliguria, hypertension	Sudden increase in blood pressure (diastolic >100)

ALT, Alanine aminotransferase; *AST,* aspartate aminotransferase; *GGTP,* gamma-glutamyl transpeptidase phosphate; *BUN,* blood urea nitrogen.

Rejection is confirmed definitively through percutaneous renal biopsy and renal flow scan. Treatment varies based on center-specific immunosuppressive protocols and severity of rejection but usually involves an increased level of baseline immunosuppression, increased corticosteroids, and the possible addition of an adjunctive immunosuppressant. In children receiving cyclosporine, tacrolimus has been shown to be an effective rescue therapy for steroid- and antibody-resistant rejection (Chand et al, 2001). Antibody therapy with antilymphocyte globulin (Thymoglobulin), daclizumab (Zenapax), or basiliximab may also be used to reduce the immune response by temporarily blocking IL-2 receptors (Vester et al, 2001). Repeat biopsies may be performed to evaluate the effectiveness of treatment.

Acute and chronic rejection causes more than one half of all graft losses in renal transplantation (NAPRTCS, 2001; Vester et al, 2001). Chronic rejection is a slow process in which the transplant recipient progressively loses renal function, resulting in graft loss in 17% of all renal allograft failures (NAPRTCS, 2001). Of this group, 92% had at least one prior episode of acute rejection (Tejani & Sullivan, 2000).

Unlike rejection of the liver or kidney, children receiving heart transplants usually do not present with symptoms until rejection is severe. Severe rejection results in graft dysfunction that presents as heart failure with tachycardia, tachypnea, arrhythmia, gallop rhythm, hepatomegaly, and cardiomegaly. Other symptoms may include shortness of breath, increased respiratory rate, edema and/or sudden weight gain, and changes in blood pressure. Nonspecific findings may include fever, irritability, and poor feeding, particularly in infants. Abdominal pain and vomiting secondary to decreased cardiac output and perfusion to the gastrointestinal tract may also be seen. Rejection is diagnosed through clinical assessment and echocardiography and confirmed by cardiac biopsy. Surveillance biopsies are performed more frequently in the early postoperative period and then less often as the risk of rejection decreases.

Chronic rejection of the heart allograft is a progressive condition that occurs over many years resulting in graft loss. It is characterized by coronary artery narrowing and detected by arteriography and dobutamine stress echocardiography, which are performed in alternating years. Retransplantation is the primary treatment for chronic rejection although palliative treatment through successful stenting of discrete coronary artery lesions may be attempted in older children with progressive disease. Unfortunately, syncope or sudden death may be the first clinical sign of chronic rejection.

Infection

The dilemma of transplantation is that an adequately suppressed immune system to prevent rejection must be balanced with one that is also competent in resisting infection. This delicate equilibrium can be easily disturbed when immunosuppression is increased to treat or avoid rejection. The common result is infection, which is a significant cause of morbidity and mortality following transplantation.

The most significant infections usually occur within the first 6 months after transplant. During the early postoperative period, the first 30 days, bacterial and fungal infections are most common. These infections are usually the result of a preexisting chronic illness or infection, wound or line infections, pneumonia, surgical complications, urinary tract infections, iatrogenic factors, or nosocomial infections (Cohen & Galbraith, 2001; Green & Michaels, 1997).

During the second through sixth months after transplant, the most common infections are those usually transmitted from the donor, reactivated viruses, or opportunistic infection such as *Pneumocystis carinii* and toxoplasmosis (Cohen & Galbraith, 2001; Green & Michaels, 1997). Lymphoproliferative disorders associated with cytomegalovirus (CMV) and Epstein-Barr virus (EBV) are also seen during this time (Allen et al, 2001; Green, 2001).

Long-term infections are difficult to document because most transplant recipients are receiving care through primary settings where data on infections may not be gathered. At 6 months after transplant, 75% of transplant recipients have satisfactory graft function and are receiving maintenance immunosuppression (Cohen & Galbraith, 2001). Infections in this group are most commonly community acquired (i.e., influenza, respiratory syncytial virus, pneumococcal pneumonia).

Cytomegalovirus. CMV is a common viral infection following transplantation, usually occurring 1 to 3 months after transplant, with a reported incidence of 15% in pediatric liver transplantation (Mazariegos & Reyes, 1999) and from less than

5% to 75% in pediatric renal transplantation, depending on seropositive or seronegative CMV status of the donor and recipient at the time of transplant (Kasiske et al, 2000). CMV accounts for 50% of all viral infections in pediatric heart transplantation but is less common in infants under 6 months of age (Schowengerdt et al, 1997). Children who are CMV seronegative before transplant and receive a seropositive organ are at greater risk of developing primary disease. Additional risk factors include the intensity and duration of immunosuppression, particularly the use of antilymphocyte and antithymocyte therapies, the administration of CMV-seropositive blood products, the presence of other viral infections, acute rejection, and retransplantation (Schowengerdt et al, 1997; Tenney & Sakarcan, 2001). CMV disease may range from an asymptomatic viremia to a life-threatening invasive tissue disease (Pearlman, 2002b). Mild disease may present with fever, chills, diarrhea, malaise, anorexia, myalgias, arthralgias, and hematologic abnormalities including leukopenia and thrombocytopenia. Primary CMV disease can involve the allograft and native organs causing pneumonitis, hepatitis, gastrointestinal tract ulcers, chorioretinitis, and encephalitis (Kasiske et al, 2000). Diagnosis is based on clinical presentation, viral cultures, serology, and histopathology. Newer methods to detect CMV-specific antigens in peripheral blood polymorphonuclear cells include the PP65 tegument protein, a CMV antigenemia assay, and the polymerase chain reaction (PCR). Detecting antigenemia may result in earlier treatment and intervention before the development of clinical symptoms.

There are similarities in the prevention and treatment of CMV after transplant, but protocols are center specific. Ganciclovir (Cytovene) is widely used for the treatment of CMV disease because of its potent ability to inhibit viral DNA replication of the human herpesviruses (Daly et al, 2002). In pediatrics, intravenous ganciclovir is preferred because of the erratic absorption of the oral solution. CMV immune globulin, which contains antibodies against CMV and Epstein-Barr virus (EBV), is also used in combination with ganciclovir to treat severe CMV disease and provides passive immunity to the child. The duration of antiviral therapy is based on the extent of CMV disease, level of immunosuppression, presence of concurrent rejection or other infections, and institution protocols.

EBV-Associated Lymphoproliferative Disorders. EBV and associated posttransplant lymphoproliferative disorders (PTLDs) may range from a self-limiting mononucleosis to PTLD with polyclonal or monoclonal disease and ultimately lymphoma. PTLD is usually triggered by a primary EBV infection and is a serious complication following transplantation. The term is applied to a wide range of abnormal hyperplasias and neoplastic lymphocytic processes (Pearlman, 2002b).

The incidence of EBV/PTLD is 2.6% to 9% in renal transplantation, 6.8% to 13 % in liver transplantation, and 4% to 23% in cardiac transplantation (Collins et al, 2001; Webber & Green, 2000). Risk factors for EBV include young age, EBV-seronegative status before transplant, tacrolimus use, co-existing CMV infection, and intensified immunosuppression including the use of OKT3 (Collins et al, 2001; Dharnidharka et al, 2001). Presenting symptoms may include lymphade-

nopathy, fever, lethargy, tonsillitis, hepatosplenomegaly, or gastrointestinal disturbances (Green, 2001). Tumorlike infiltrates, as well as ulcerations of the gastrointestinal tract with abdominal pain and bleeding, are seen in invasive disease.

Early diagnosis is vital to recovery and is based on clinical presentation, histopathology, laboratory studies, and radiographic findings. A biopsy is often performed on an accessible node, and a computed tomography (CT) scan is obtained to assess the chest and abdomen for enlarged nodes or disseminated disease. The EBV polymerase chain reaction (EBV-PCR) is a sensitive tool that detects the EBV genome in peripheral blood lymphocytes. It is used in some centers to determine the viral load of EBV and to track disease progression in transplant recipients (Collins et al, 2001; Green, 2001).

Treatment and management of EBV and PTLD is controversial, although the reduction or discontinuation of immunosuppression with frequent monitoring of the EBV-PCR is generally accepted. Evaluation of graft function with biopsy is essential to monitor for rejection in the setting of reduced immunosuppression. Other treatments include the use of antiviral agents, chemotherapy, monoclonal anti-B cell antibody, radiation, interferon-alpha, and tumor resection (Allen et al, 2001; Cohen, 2000; Green, 2001).

***Pneumocystis carinii* Pneumonia.** Children who are immunosuppressed are at risk for *Pneumocystis carinii* pneumonia (PCP), a rare but serious infectious complication. Trimethoprim-sulfamethoxazole (TMP-SMX, Bactrim, Septra) is widely accepted as effective prophylaxis. TMP/SMX is generally without serious side effects, with benefits of prophylaxis outweighing the risks, but it can cause a rise in serum creatinine by blocking the tubular secretion of creatinine and transient neutropenia (Kasiske et al, 2000). The recommended lifetime prophylactic dose of TMP-SMX is 5 mg/kg three times per week, with a maximum daily dose of 160 mg (McGhee et al, 2002). If a transplant recipient presents with fever and a lower respiratory tract infection and is not receiving prophylaxis, PCP should always be considered in the differential diagnosis.

Varicella-Zoster Virus. Varicella zoster is a highly contagious childhood disease that can be potentially severe in the child who is immunocompromised. Complications include pneumonia, encephalitis, pancreatitis, hepatitis, disseminated intravascular coagulation (DIC), acute renal failure, rejection, graft loss, and death (Olson et al, 2001; Pandya et al, 2001). Recommended therapy is administration of varicella-zoster immune globulin (VZIG) within 72 hours of exposure as well as a reduction of immunosuppression to help prevent or decrease the severity of the illness. Approximately 50% of children treated with VZIG following direct exposure develop a mild form of the virus and are usually hospitalized to receive intravenous acyclovir until the lesions crust, followed by a course of oral acyclovir (Pearlman, 2002b). Graft function should be monitored closely for rejection for several weeks in the setting of reduced baseline immunosuppression. Following an exposure or outbreak of the disease, transplant recipients should be tested for immunity to varicella zoster to determine whether precautions need to be taken with future exposures. The varicella-zoster vaccine Varivax is routinely administered to immunocompetent children at 1 year of age. However, since this vaccine is a live virus, it is not recommended for use in the immunocompromised child. If the child awaiting transplant is otherwise medically stable and the transplant is not imminent, the vaccine should be administered before transplant if the child is 1 year of age or older (Olson et al, 2001).

Fungal Infections. Fungal infections usually occur during the early postoperative period. *Candida* is the primary causative organism in the majority of fungal infections in children with liver transplants and up to 60% in kidney, lung, or heart-lung recipients (Simon & Levin, 2001). Fungal infections usually present as noninvasive infections of the oropharynx, esophagus, or genitalia caused by high immunosuppressive levels. Invasive disease can develop, however, with the most common risk factors being the presence of a bile leak or hepatic artery thrombosis in the liver transplant recipient, steroid administration, transfusions, prolonged operative time, repeat laparotomies, retransplantation, and renal or respiratory compromise. Noninvasive *Candida* appears as plaques on the oral mucosal or as a papular rash of the genitalia. Treatment with an oral "swish and swallow" solution of nystatin or topical nystatin ointment usually resolves a noninvasive infection. Invasive disease presents with fever, irritability, malaise, decreased appetite, or an erythematous central catheter site and is confirmed by blood, urine, throat, or wound cultures. Fungemia is treated with an intravenous antifungal agent with close monitoring of renal function (Jaskowski, 2002).

Polyomavirus. Human polyomavirus, composed of subgroups BKV, JCV, and SV40, is a DNA virus. Serologic studies have shown the presence of BKV in 50% of children under 3 years of age and nearly 100% by age 9 to 10 years (Lin et al, 2001). Although not much is known about this virus, transmission is thought to be by respiratory secretions. Risk factors include high levels of immunosuppression, BKV-seropositive donors, and a history of rejection (Lin et al, 2001). Infection, typically asymptomatic in persons with an intact immune system, can cause hemorrhagic cystitis, tubulointerstitial nephritis, and ureteral stenosis in renal transplant recipients (Lin et al, 2001). Interstitial nephritis can mimic the symptoms of rejection, making the identification of BKV important when making treatment decisions. A renal biopsy is the current gold standard of diagnosis, although serum and urine assays using PCR are being investigated (Lin et al, 2001). While intensified immunosuppression is used for rejection, a reduction of immunosuppression is appropriate for the treatment of BKV. There is limited anecdotal experience with the antiviral medications vidarabine (Vira-A) and cidofovir (Vistide).

Recurrent Disease

Unique to some causes of renal failure is the recurrence of the original disease that led to end-stage renal disease. Diseases such as hyperoxaluria and focal segmental glomerulosclerosis (FSGS) can both recur rapidly in the transplanted allograft. Recurrence rates of FSGS vary from 20% to 60%. Risk of graft failure secondary to recurrent FSGS is 60% (Mazareigos et al, 2000), and the likelihood of recurrence in a subsequent transplant is 75% to 90% (Tan, 2001). Membranoproliferative glomerulonephritis (MPGN) can also recur, but the risk of recurrence depends on the specific type of MPGN. MPGN type II recurs in 50% to 100% of allografts, whereas type I only

recurs in 20% to 30% (Tan, 2001). Membranous nephropathy, immunoglobulin A (IgA) nephropathy, and hemolytic-uremic syndrome are other renal diseases that may recur following transplantation.

Prognosis

Pediatric transplantation has offered a second chance at life for thousands of children with end-stage organ disease. Although recipient and graft survival is high, long-term graft loss may be associated with late acute rejection, chronic rejection, infection, and noncompliance (Boyle & Fricker, 2000; Jain et al, 2002a; NAPRTCS, 2001).

The first successful clinical trials in renal transplantation were conducted in 1962 at the University of Colorado (Starzl & Demetris, 1997). Before that series, a few isolated cases of renal transplantation between fraternal and identical twins were reported. Renal transplantation has evolved as the treatment choice for end-stage renal disease. Combined graft survival rates for living and cadaver kidney recipients have increased over the past 5 years. The 1-year survival in 1987 and 1995 for cadaveric and living grafts were 81% and 91%, respectively, increasing to 93% in 1996 and 95% in 2000 (NAPRTCS, 2001).

Dr. Thomas Starzl pioneered pediatric liver transplantation, with the first surgery being performed in 1963 (Starzl et al, 1982). Survival in this early period was less than 50% but has greatly improved over the last 30 years. The United Network for Organ Sharing (UNOS) reports a 90% graft survival at 1 year and an 82% graft survival at 3 years (UNOS, 2002), although a higher survival is reported at some individual centers (Deshpande et al, 2002; Jain et al, 2002a; Wallot et al, 2002).

With the demand for donor livers far exceeding the supply, split liver transplantation and living-related liver transplantation (LRLT) have been developed as strategies to increase the donor pool. The split liver procedure involves dividing the liver into two sections using various segments of the right or left lobe depending on the size of the recipients (Depshpande et al, 2002). LRLT usually involves liver donation between a child with ESLD and an ABO-compatible donor, most commonly a biologic parent. Although the timing of LRLT is advantageous, postoperative complications such as postoperative hemorrhage, hepatic artery thrombosis, and rejection are similar to those receiving cadaveric livers (Anselmo et al, 2001; Broering et al, 2001). LRLT also poses the ethical dilemma of placing a healthy donor at risk in order to save the life of a child. The evaluation for LRLT demands a full assessment of the risk/benefit ratio for the child, donor, and family.

Heart transplantation in humans began in the 1960s. The development of successful orthotopic surgical techniques involving the removal of the recipient's ventricles, leaving the posterior atrial walls and the ridge of the interatrial septum intact, was a significant breakthrough (Lower & Shumway, 1960). The first pediatric heart transplant was performed on an 18-day-old infant with Ebstein anomaly; however, this child died 6 hours later from complications (Kantrowitz et al, 1968).

For every 1000 live births in the United States, there are 7.67 children diagnosed with congenital heart disease (Hoffman,

2002). Many of these children can be helped through surgical interventions, yet an estimated 10% who have complex, uncorrectable CHD require heart or heart-lung transplantation. In 1985, neonatal transplantation was introduced as a treatment option for infants with hypoplastic left heart syndrome. Without surgical intervention, this condition is usually fatal within the first few months of life (Morrow et al, 2000). The number of cardiac transplants in infants has decreased because of the limited supply of donors and the advancement in surgical palliation for congenital heart defects (Boyle & Fricker, 2000).

Graft survival at 1 year following pediatric cardiac transplantation is 78% to 87%, depending on the age of the recipient, with the older children having a higher survival. Graft survival at 3 years is 73% to 75%, and at 5 years it is 60% to 62% (UNOS, 2002). Long-term survival exceeds 65% at 5 years and 50% at 10 years at some centers (Boyle & Fricker, 2000).

Although the use of total parenteral nutrition (TPN) has extended the lives of children with end-stage short gut syndrome, associated morbidities are common. These morbidities include TPN-related liver failure; venous access complications related to thrombosis, multiple line insertions, and sepsis; and ultimately a lack of venous access. The financial burdens of daily TPN and associated care, as well as the psychosocial impact of a permanent indwelling line and connection to an infusion pump, are also stressors for these children and their families. Over the last 40 years, intestine transplantation has progressed from an experimental strategy to an accepted treatment for permanent intestinal failure. The International Intestinal Transplant Registry reported that 55 intestinal transplant programs have been established worldwide, with 696 transplants being performed in 656 people since 1985. The majority of people (60%) are 16 years of age or younger. Actuarial graft survival 5 years after transplantation is 45% for isolated intestine, 43% for a composite liver-intestine graft, and nearly 30% for multivisceral transplantation involving the intestine (Grant, 2001).

PRIMARY CARE MANAGEMENT

Health Care Maintenance

Growth and Development

The goal of pediatric organ transplantation is for the child to achieve normal growth and development with an improved quality of life. Growth affects the emotional well-being of children and participation in the routine activities of childhood. Although more severe in children with kidney and liver transplants, growth retardation is seen in all children with solid organ transplants (Fine, 2002). The primary care provider has an essential role in monitoring the child's long-term growth and development. Height and weight should be routinely documented on standardized growth charts and evaluated.

Transplant candidates exhibit symptoms and effects of chronic disease, such as anorexia, vomiting, malnutrition, anemia, and bone problems, that affect growth and development. Although transplantation may preclude some of these complications, immunosuppressive therapy with long-term and/or high-dose steroids also impacts growth. Aggressive

nutritional support and minimization or discontinuation of steroids will contribute to growth. Increased or intensified nutritional support or growth hormone therapy may be required in some cases of growth retardation.

The average child awaiting renal transplant is nearly 2 standard deviations below the mean for height (NAPRTCS, 2001) at the time of transplantation. Growth after renal transplantation is affected by age at transplant (NAPRTCS, 2001), persistent hyperparathyroidism and renal osteodystrophy, graft function, and immunosuppressive medications (Sanchez et al, 2002). Of children transplanted before 15 years of age, 70% remain below the third percentile for height as adults (Sanchez et al, 2002). Catch-up growth has been seen primarily in children who were under 6 years of age at the time of transplant, with children under 2 years of age showing the most improvement (Seikaly et al, 2001). Improvements in growth velocity have been seen with the use of growth hormone for children with chronic renal insufficiency, for children requiring dialysis, and for children with renal transplants (Sanchez et al, 2002). The ability to wean or withdraw steroids may also impact growth and development.

The majority of children with heart transplants demonstrate normal linear growth, although growth falls in the low normal range. Neurologic outcomes and development are also reported as normal (Baum et al, 2000).

Early studies of children with liver transplants reported that nearly two thirds of the children did not achieve normal growth. With maximized nutritional support after transplant and steroid reduction and/or withdrawal within the first 12 months following transplantation, normal growth patterns are being achieved in the majority of children, although the etiology of liver disease may also affect growth after transplant (Kelly, 2000). The Studies of Pediatric Liver Transplantation (SPLIT), a cooperative research network of pediatric liver transplantation centers in the United States and Canada, report that the pediatric liver transplant candidate is on average 1.4 standard deviations below the age- and gender-adjusted height level. Younger children (less than 5 years of age) have even greater height deficits but also have the best catch-up growth within 24 months after transplant (SPLIT Research Group, 2001). Early liver transplantation in children with growth retardation has been found to restore growth potential, although age at time of transplant, gender, onset of puberty, and disease etiology also affected growth (Renz et al, 2001).

Cognitive and emotional functioning of children after transplantation has been evaluated in several studies with variable findings. This population has been difficult to assess because of the unavailability of baseline data before transplant, the subject variables, the measurement issues, and the impact of medical interventions (Kosmach et al, 1998). In addition, studies with sufficient numbers of subjects that analyze the long-term effects of transplantation on cognitive and emotional functioning are severely lacking.

Brain atrophy can be seen in children with chronic renal failure, and has been reported in up to 60% of that population (Qvist et al, 2002). When compared with healthy siblings, children with ESRD were found to have lower IQs (intelligence quotients) and lower school achievement. Some studies have reported that successful renal transplantation in these children can help correct these deficits, particularly in infants (Brouhard et al, 2000; Qvist et al, 2002).

Liver transplantation in children less than 12 months of age is associated with maintenance of normal development although social skills and eye-hand coordination were reported to decline temporarily, possibly from the effects of the hospital environment or neurotoxicity related to cyclosporine (van Mourik et al, 2000). In addition, health-related quality of life for children from the parents' perspective is lower than that of healthy children but is similar to that of children with other chronic illnesses (Bucuvalas et al, 2003); however, perceptions of quality of life improve over time. The child's psychosocial functioning was predicted by the child's age at the time of transplant and maternal education (Bucuvalas et al, 2003).

After heart or heart-lung transplantation, most children return to school, participate in sports and age-appropriate activities, and are classified as a New York Heart Association Functional Class I with no activity restrictions other than competitive sports. Psychosocial functioning was measured below normal in children with heart and heart-lung transplants when measured on a global assessment of psychosocial functioning (Serrano-Ikkos et al, 1999).

Diet

Optimal nutritional management for children both before and after transplantation is crucial in achieving normal growth and development. Postoperatively, a child's diet is usually liberalized. Renal recipients may have mild to moderate sodium intake restrictions, and cardiac recipients are encouraged to maintain healthy eating habits, avoiding foods high in sodium and cholesterol. In addition, medication side effects may cause hyperkalemia, hypertension, hypomagnesemia, hypophosphatemia, hyperglycemia, or hyperlipidemia necessitating a respective dietary restriction or supplement. Hyperlipidemia not controlled by diet and exercise, particularly in cardiac recipients, is treated with lipid-lowering agents (Boyle, 2000a).

Some children may require enteral supplementation because of an inability to ingest adequate calories or meet fluid requirements as a result of anatomic space limitations, taste changes, side effects of oral medications, long-standing feeding aversions, and difficulty in accepting new textures after formula feeds (Kelly, 1997; Wren & Tarbell, 1998). Nasogastric (NG) tube feedings, particularly in young children, are not uncommon in the early postoperative period. Initiation of NG feedings is based on postoperative complications and length of time with nothing by mouth, high caloric requirements for wound healing and catch-up growth, transient oral aversion or anorexia, and gastrointestinal disturbances.

Safety

As with all routine pediatric visits, counseling about safety issues (e.g., the proper use of car seats, seat belts, bicycle helmets; child proofing the home) at a child's age and developmental level is necessary for all families with a child who has had an organ transplant. Because most children have good graft function and are prescribed maintenance doses of immunosuppression, good hand-washing techniques and avoidance of others with obvious infections are sound guidelines to decrease the risk of infection.

Activity. In children with a heart or heart-lung transplant, it is important to understand that the incisions in the heart sever the sympathetic and parasympathetic nerves, which ordinarily regulate the heart rate. This lack of neural connections is known as denervation. Without direct control of the CNS, the transplanted heart will beat faster in a resting state (e.g., 90 to 110 beats/min). This faster than normal rate is associated with normal cardiac function and the capability of sustaining vigorous physical activity. The transplanted heart depends on circulating adrenalin and related hormones produced by the adrenal gland, instead of a direct impulse from the brain, to change its rate. The transplanted heart may take up to 10 minutes before an increase in heart rate is seen in response to exercise, and up to 1 hour may pass after stopping exercise before a decrease in rate is seen (Webber, 2000a). Another effect of denervation is that chest pain or angina pectoris cannot be perceived if coronary artery disease develops; however, some recipients may regrow these nerves and will experience the typical symptoms of coronary artery blockage if it develops. Consequently, coronary arteriograms and dobutamine stress echocardiograms are obtained at the individual's yearly follow-up examination.

Pediatric heart and heart-lung recipients are activity restricted for the first 6 to 8 weeks after surgery to allow the sternum to heal. Recipients should avoid bike riding, climbing, sit-ups, push-ups, roller skating, and contact sports and should also refrain from lifting, pushing, or pulling heavy objects during this period. After 8 weeks, all activities, as well as physical education class at school, may be resumed. Teens who are licensed drivers may also resume driving at 2 months after transplant. A physical therapist should instruct children on an exercise program before discharge from the hospital. This program consists of a 5-minute warm-up and cool-down period before and after peak physical activity. If a child shows signs of increased shortness of breath or fatigue, then the cool-down period should begin. Exercise should also be decreased during periods of graft rejection. Physical education teachers should be informed of the heart recipient's additional exercise considerations.

Children who have received liver or kidney transplants are encouraged to resume previous activities, although there are some limitations in the early postoperative period. Push-ups or sit-ups, as well as activities that stretch or put pressure on the abdomen and incision, are to be avoided for 3 to 6 months. Recipients should avoid heavy lifting for at least 6 months. Although some centers discourage contact sports, most children can participate in age-appropriate activities as they develop greater endurance and fitness, such as soccer, softball, basketball, bicycling, skating, swimming, dancing, and gymnastics.

Some centers prefer that families notify the transplant center when they plan to travel for an extended period of time or to a foreign country. This notification is particularly important for children awaiting an organ transplant so that a means of communication is available in case an organ becomes available. Medication doses and schedules should always be maintained while a child is on vacation, and an adequate supply of medication should be taken with the child. Medications should be carried on to airplanes rather than being checked with luggage. Parents are encouraged to obtain Medic-Alert bracelets for their child to identify the child as a transplant recipient and provide the name and telephone number of the transplant center in case of an emergency. In addition, infectious disease precautions need to be taken with foreign travel to certain areas where immunizations may not be available for all children and adults.

Immunizations

Because of the inconsistent rates of serologic conversion of many vaccines after transplant, care should be taken to complete the schedule for routine immunizations before transplantation whenever possible. Children older than 1 year and who have been previously immunized should have serologic testing for antibodies to measles, mumps, rubella, and varicella. Those children who are susceptible should be reimmunized, (Committee on Infectious Disease, 2000).

After transplant, primary care practitioners should follow the guidelines established for immunosuppressed children (Committee on Infectious Disease, 2000; Molrine & Hibbard, 2001). Live-bacterial and live-virus vaccines are contraindicated in this population, and only inactivated vaccines (e.g., the inactivated polio vaccine) should be administered. Siblings of the child should also receive the inactivated polio virus to avoid transmitting the disease to the recipient. Unfortunately, no inactivated form of vaccination exists for measles, mumps, and rubella (MMR). For those children who received the MMR before transplant, yearly serum titers should be drawn to verify immunity (Committee on Infectious Disease, 2000). Siblings of the child should receive the MMR.

Because children are more highly immunosuppressed in the early postoperative period, no immunizations should be given during this time. The immunization schedule for children who are immunosuppressed is followed when the recipient is receiving maintenance immunosuppression, usually by 3 to 6 months. If a child is receiving augmented immunosuppression to treat rejection, any scheduled immunizations should be postponed for at least 1 to 3 months.

The influenza vaccine should be administered annually to children with organ transplants who are 3 or more months after transplant. All family members living within the household should also receive the vaccine.

The live-attenuated varicella virus vaccine (Varivax) may be administered to children 1 year of age or older before transplantation if they are medically stable. This vaccine has been shown to decrease the severity and frequency of varicella in healthy children as well as transplant recipients who received the vaccine before transplant (Donati et al, 2000; Pandya et al, 2001; Vessey et al, 2001). All siblings should also receive this vaccine at 1 year of age. Parents are encouraged to contact the school nurse to be aware of any outbreaks of varicella in the child's or siblings' schools so that prompt treatment may be given in the event of exposure to the virus.

Hepatitis B is an infrequent but significant cause of decreased graft survival, morbidity, and mortality. Children awaiting transplant, particularly children with end-stage renal disease receiving dialysis, should be vaccinated against hepatitis B since it can be acquired through contact with blood products. Children may receive the hepatitis B vaccine 3 months after transplantation following posttransplant guidelines. This vaccine is also recommended for siblings, caretakers, and household contacts.

Immunization policies vary by transplant center, so the primary care provider should contact the transplant center for specific immunization guidelines for the child and family.

Screening

Vision. Routine screening is recommended. Because cataracts, glaucoma, and pseudotumor cerebri may be side effects of long-term steroid use, an annual ophthalmologic examination should be performed on children at risk for these conditions. CMV retinitis may occur as a result of a CMV infection and requires ophthalmologic follow-up until resolution. Children with no prior exposure to toxoplasmosis who receive organs from toxoplasmosis-positive donors require periodic ophthalmologic examinations. These children receive prophylaxis with pyrimethamine (Daraprim) and leucovorin (Wellcovorin) for 6 months after transplant (Michaels, 2000).

Hearing. Routine screening is recommended. In addition, transplant recipients who received intravenous ototoxic medications (i.e., gentamicin, vancomycin) frequently before and after transplant are at risk for hearing deficits and should be referred to an audiologist for screening. Audiograms are recommended to determine the extent of hearing loss and to recommend interventions.

Dental. Biannual dental visits and good oral hygiene practices are recommended for children following organ transplantation. Gingival hyperplasia is commonly seen in children receiving cyclosporine or calcium channel blockers. In severe cases, gingivectomy may be necessary to reduce gum overgrowth and related swelling, pain, or infection. Antibiotic prophylaxis per standard endocarditis protocols is recommended for invasive dental procedures. Heart transplant recipients require antibiotic coverage for all dental procedures as well as all other surgical procedures as outlined by the American Heart Association guidelines for prevention of bacterial endocarditis (Ferrieri et al, 2002) (see Chapter 21). This treatment is continued for the first 6 months after transplantation. A prolonged course of antibiotics may be required if there is regurgitation of blood flow at the heart valves.

Blood Pressure. Since hypertension is a common side effect of some immunosuppressants, blood pressure measurement should be a part of all discharge teaching plans. If antihypertensive medications are prescribed, parents are instructed to measure the child's blood pressure before administering these medications. Administration guidelines, based on blood pressure parameters, should be clearly delineated for the child and family. Parents are also advised to maintain a record of blood pressure readings and administered antihypertensive medications so that the primary care provider and transplant team can monitor treatment and adjust medications. Antihypertensive medications are usually not required for the long term after transplant if the child is steroid free or if immunosuppressive levels are maintained at a low level.

Hematocrit. The hematocrit is obtained with routine laboratory tests as recommended by the transplant center during the early postoperative period and through the primary care provider if the child is discharged from the transplant area. Laboratory tests are obtained frequently, up to weekly or twice weekly, during the first 3 months after the transplant and then with decreasing frequency over time. Children with renal transplants may develop anemia secondary to progressive renal dysfunction from recurrent disease or chronic rejection.

Urinalysis. Nephrotoxicity is a well-recognized complication of both tacrolimus and cyclosporine immunosuppressive therapy in all solid organ transplantation. BUN and creatinine are monitored frequently, and the glomerular filtration rate is measured periodically (Boyle, 2000a). In addition, urine samples are obtained for urinalysis and culture in renal transplant recipients as a part of posttransplant management. Routine monitoring of the serum creatinine and albumin, as well as a urinalysis, is essential to screen for recurrent renal diseases, such as focal segmental glomerulosclerosis or membranoproliferative glomerulonephritis.

In children with liver and heart transplantation, urinalysis is obtained to monitor for nephrotoxicity caused by immunosuppressive therapies. Otherwise, a urinalysis is obtained only if the child is symptomatic or as part of an evaluation of fever. Fever in the posttransplant period is usually diagnostic of rejection or infection. If rejection is ruled out, infection is likely, and cultures of urine, blood, stool, and sputum are obtained.

Tuberculosis. Some transplant centers may recommend a Mantoux purified protein derivative (PPD) with an anergy panel in addition to chest radiography to evaluate a child for exposure to tuberculosis (TB) before transplantation. Risk factors for developing TB after the transplant include prior exposure to the disease, living in an area endemic for TB, and having a high level of immunosuppression and/or a concurrent HIV infection (Green & Michaels, 1997). Treatment is with isoniazid, which is administered for 6 to 12 months after transplant, although it is recommended as maintenance therapy by some experts (Green & Michaels, 1997).

Condition-Specific Screening

Posttransplant Blood Tests. Laboratory blood testing is usually obtained at weekly to biweekly clinic visits after discharge from the hospital. Laboratory tests vary depending on the organ transplanted, the length of time after transplant, current complications, and center-specific protocols. The most commonly obtained laboratory tests include a complete blood cell count with differential, a full chemistry profile including glucose, BUN, creatinine, magnesium, phosphorus, bicarbonate, uric acid, aspartate aminotransferase (AST), alanine aminotransferase (ALT), gamma-glutamyl transpeptidase phosphate (GGTP), lactic dehydrogenase (LDH), creatine phosphokinase (CPK), cholesterol, and triglycerides.

Medication Levels. Trough levels of CSA, tacrolimus, or sirolimus are usually obtained with these routine tests. In addition, fasting lipids and glycated hemoglobin (HbA_{1C}) are done periodically to screen for hyperlipidemia and diabetes.

Maintenance Laboratory Testing. Laboratory testing decreases over time. By 6 months after transplant, the majority of children have stable graft function and require laboratory testing monthly. Long-term survivors commonly have laboratory testing completed every 2 to 3 months; however, laboratory tests may be required more frequently during episodes of infection and/or rejection as immunosuppressive mediations are

adjusted. Children are followed closely until the episode of rejection or the infectious process resolves.

Common Illness Management
Differential Diagnosis (Box 34-2)

Fever. Children are more highly immunosuppressed for the first 3 to 6 months after transplantation and consequently are at greater risk for infection. As discussed previously, bacterial infections are most commonly seen in the early period related to the preexisting chronic condition, surgical complications, or nosocomial infections. Viruses and opportunistic infections are more common in the intermediate and late periods following transplantation. Fever, especially in the first 3 months after transplant, demands a thorough assessment. The differential diagnoses of rejection or infection must be investigated with each febrile episode, particularly in the early postoperative period. The primary care provider and the transplant specialist work cooperatively to evaluate and manage febrile episodes.

Abdominal Symptoms. Abdominal pain in children with liver transplants during the early postoperative period most commonly indicates a surgical complication, including a postoperative ileus, hepatic artery thrombosis, or portal vein thrombosis. Biliary complications may also present with abdominal pain and may occur in the early postoperative period as well as weeks to months after transplant. Acute rejection of the liver may also cause abdominal pain.

Abdominal pain in renal transplant recipients, as well as tenderness in the kidney area, may be a symptom of a urinary tract infection (UTI), acute pyelonephritis, posttransplant lymphoproliferative disease, CMV infection, or rejection.

Although abdominal pain and vomiting in the child with a heart transplant may be a viral illness, this clinical presentation warrants an echocardiogram to evaluate for the possibility of rejection secondary to decreased cardiac output and decreased perfusion to the gastrointestinal tract.

As with the general pediatric population, the differential diagnoses of abdominal pain may also include intestinal obstruction, peptic ulcer disease, appendicitis, or viral or bacterial gastroenteritis. A definitive diagnosis is determined through clinical presentation, laboratory testing, and radiologic testing.

Vomiting and Diarrhea. Prolonged vomiting or diarrhea caused by a community-acquired virus may result in poor absorption of tacrolimus (Prograf) or cyclosporine (CSA), leading to subtherapeutic blood levels that may place the child at risk for rejection. Parents should contact the transplant center if the child is unable to retain the immunosuppressive medication.

BOX 34-2
Differential Diagnosis

Fever: Common childhood conditions vs. rejection
Abdominal symptoms: Common childhood conditions vs. obstruction in common bile duct, ulcers, small bowel obstruction, peritonitis, or rejection
Vomiting and diarrhea: May result in poor absorption of medications.
Metabolic abnormalities: Hyperkalemia, hyperglycemia, and low CO_2 levels may be related to immunosuppressant medications

The primary care provider will facilitate the transplant center's recommendations for immunosuppression and will supervise medical management of fluids and electrolytes. A protracted course of vomiting or diarrhea may result in hospitalization for intravenous administration of CSA or tacrolimus, fluid management, and any indicated work-up for infection. Children receiving tacrolimus, mycophenolate mofetil, and/or oral magnesium supplements may experience loose stools or diarrhea. However, diarrhea lasting more than 3 days may decrease immunosuppressive levels substantially, requiring routine monitoring of trough levels to maintain an appropriate immunosuppressive level (Mittal et al, 2001).

Metabolic Abnormalities. Children with stable graft function receiving maintenance immunosuppression usually do not experience metabolic abnormalities. Elevated levels of CSA and tacrolimus during the early postoperative period may result in hyperkalemia, hypophosphatemia, hypomagnesemia, or metabolic acidosis.

Drug Interactions

Cyclosporine (CSA) and tacrolimus (Prograf) are metabolized in the liver by the cytochrome P450 III system (McGhee et al, 2002). Metabolism of CSA or tacrolimus depends on liver function and other agents that induce or inhibit this enzyme system, subsequently affecting blood levels. Because primary care providers often prescribe medications for a variety of acute and chronic childhood illnesses, it is important that the family or health care provider contact the transplant center to discuss possible drug interactions. Drugs that interact with CSA or tacrolimus disrupt an otherwise stable level, which may result in drug-related neurotoxicities and nephrotoxicities (Table 34-6). Fluctuating levels may also increase the risk of infection or rejection.

Developmental Issues

Sleep Patterns

Sleep disturbances in children with end-stage organ disease are common and may be caused by the existing chronic condition, symptoms of organ deterioration (e.g., severe pruritus from liver disease), emotional distress, and the psychologic effects of extended hospitalization. In addition, tacrolimus, CSA, and steroids are reported to cause insomnia. During periods of rejection when the child is treated with increased tacrolimus or CSA levels in addition to high-dose oral steroids or intravenous methylprednisolone, sleep patterns may be significantly altered and insomnia and irritability are common.

Parents may find it helpful to maintain familiar home routines and rituals to the fullest extent possible while the child is hospitalized. An improved sleep pattern is usually seen following discharge from the hospital, since the child feels more secure in the home environment and home routines are reestablished. In some cases, professional counseling may help the child and family.

Toileting

Regression in toileting habits is expected in toddlers and preschool-aged children during and after hospitalization. Care providers should be aware of this temporary regression and

TABLE 34-6

Drug Interactions with Cyclosporine and Tacrolimus

Drug	Cyclosporine (CSA) Increase	Decrease	Tacrolimus (Prograf) Increase	Decrease
CALCIUM CHANNEL BLOCKERS				
Diltiazem	X		X	
Nicardipine	X		X	
Nifedipine			X	
Verapamil	X			
ANTIFUNGALS				
Clotrimazole			X	
Fluconazole	X		X	
Itraconazole	X		X	
Ketoconazole	X		X	
ANTIBIOTICS				
Clarithromycin	X		X	
Erythromycin	X		X	
Troleandomycin			X	
Rifabutin		X		X
Rifampin		X		X
Nafcillin		X		
GASTROINTESTINAL AGENT				
Metoclopramide	X		X	
ANTICONVULSANTS				
Carbamazepine		X		X
Phenobarbital		X		X
Phenytoin		X		X
OTHERS				
Octreotide		X		
Ticlopidine		X		
Allopurinol	X			
Bromocriptine	X		X	
Cimetidine	X		X	
Cyclosporine			X	
Tacrolimus	X			
Danazol	X		X	
Protease inhibitors			X	
Grapefruit juice	X		X	
St. John's wort		X		

Data from Novartis Pharmaceuticals Corp. (2001). *2001 Cyclosporine drug interaction manual*; Fujisawa, USA, Inc. (1999). *Fujisawa drug monograph*; Fujisawa Healthcare, Inc. (1999). *Known significant and potential drug interactions for Prograf.*

support children in regaining their toileting skills. Pediatric renal transplant recipients may have specific concerns and issues related to toileting and the establishment or reestablishment of urinary flow and continence. The initiation of urine flow for a child following renal transplantation is often a time of great excitement for the child and family. However, the child may have periods of incontinence while learning to recognize the body cues that signal the need to urinate and to control the urine flow.

Some heart and renal transplant recipients may require diuretic therapy, which may contribute to increased incontinence, consequently affecting toileting routines and new behaviors. When possible, diuretics should be administered early in the day to decrease nighttime incontinence, frequency of nightly urination, and sleep disruption. Incontinence and enuresis are common occurrences in the early posttransplant period and parents should be counseled about the implications of the child's medical management on daily routines, as well as the need for emotional support for their child and consistency of home routines.

Discipline

A child's chronic illness affects the entire family, its system of functioning, and the roles within it. As a child with end-stage organ disease improves significantly after transplantation, former coping mechanisms used by the family, as well as parental roles and family dynamics, may no longer be successful. It is often difficult for families to make the transition from parenting a sick child to parenting a healthier one. Many parents continue to overprotect their child and now have the additional concerns of infection and rejection. Parents may have difficulty encouraging children to develop independence and peer relationships and are often reticent to integrate the child into school and community activities. In contrast, other parents may have trouble setting limits on inappropriate behavior and may overindulge the child.

The primary care provider plays an essential role in evaluating family dynamics and the parents' ability to appropriately discipline and nurture a child after transplantation. The caregiver can help parents achieve a balance between establishing age-appropriate and consistent limits and allowing the child some control in decision making. Encouraging independence helps promote confidence and positive self-esteem. Family counseling can be a highly effective method to help families cope with the ongoing stressors of the transplant process.

Child Care

Attendance at daycare centers is generally not recommended by most transplant centers for 1 to 3 months following transplantation because these children are usually more highly immunosuppressed during that time with a greater risk for infection. As immunosuppressive levels are decreased, routine social contact and participation in group activities and daycare programs may be resumed. Community-acquired viruses are usually tolerated well by children who are receiving lower-dose maintenance immunosuppression. However, parents should be informed by the primary care provider or daycare staff of any outbreaks of varicella or measles in the community or daycare center because these viruses could be potentially serious for the child with a transplant, particularly if the child was unable to be immunized before transplantation.

Schooling

Children are encouraged to return to school as soon as possible after transplantation to resume a normal routine, continue class work, and interact with peers. Although most children can return to the classroom within 3 months after transplantation, some children benefit from gradually increasing school attendance from a few hours daily to a full schedule as tolerated. Tutoring in the home, as provided by the school district, may be an ideal option when children have had an extended absence from school and are significantly behind in class content.

Children who are recuperating at home from extensive complications related to transplantation may also benefit from short-term tutoring until they can attend school. In addition, a high level of tacrolimus or CSA in the early postoperative period may cause mild to moderate hand tremors that may interfere with fine motor activities, such as writing or working on craft activities.

Parents are often hesitant to return their child to school because of concerns about exposure to infections, their perception of the child's fragility and increased demands on the child, and peer influences. Primary care providers should encourage the resumption of routine childhood activities and school while emphasizing the benefits of developmentally appropriate play, social interactions, and instruction. Teachers also have an important role in normalizing the child's school experience by accommodating medical absences and encouraging optimal academic performance (Hangard-Patton & Lawrence, 2000).

The child's medication schedule should be organized to accommodate the school day with minimal interruptions. Medications prescribed on a daily or twice-daily schedule are easily adaptable to the child's schedule. Frequent visits to the health office for medications or having a parent visit daily to administer medications is disruptive to the child's school routine and may emphasize the different needs of the child. Children may be particularly sensitive to these intrusions during adolescence.

School nurses are helpful resources in reintegrating a child into the classroom. In a cooperative effort with the transplant team, the school nurse can facilitate age-appropriate discussions of transplantation to increase classmates' understanding and support.

Children with chronic conditions leading to transplantation and children after transplantation may benefit from special education services, and an individualized education program should be initiated (see Chapter 5).

Sexuality

The majority of children experience significant improvements in physical appearance following successful solid organ transplantation. Older school-aged children and adolescents are very aware of these dramatically positive physical changes: increased energy and strength, a natural skin color following resolution of jaundice or cyanosis, a normal body shape in the absence of ascites or peripheral edema, increased growth and maturation, and/or the absences of appliances such as central venous lines, gastrostomy tubes, oxygen cannulas, or dialysis catheters. In addition, daily care routines, laboratory testing, clinic visits, and medical routines may be considerably minimized with stable graft function.

Recipients may also experience some negative effects to appearance and body image. The physical stigmata of immunosuppressive therapy with CSA and steroids include hirsutism, cushingoid facies, gingival hyperplasia, obesity, and short stature. Steroids may also intensify outbreaks of acne in adolescents and cause mood swings. Physical stigmata as a result of immunosuppressive therapy with tacrolimus are very rare, although a small percentage of children experience transient alopecia. Scarring from multiple surgeries, invasive lines and catheters, and other procedures is unavoidable. Parents and children are advised about skin care issues as they recuperate from surgery. Some adolescents are interested in minimizing scarring and any keloid formations and may benefit from a plastic surgery consultation. Professional counseling and support groups are also encouraged for this population because these children may be at risk for depression, noncompliance, or increased risk-taking behaviors.

Transplant education for adolescents should include information about puberty, sexual development, sexual activity/abstinence, birth control, and sexually transmitted diseases. Adolescents with chronic organ disease often experience delayed pubertal development. Following transplantation and stable graft function, there may be a rapid onset and progression through puberty. Pretransplant and posttransplant counseling and education will help the adolescent prepare for and adapt to these sudden changes. Adolescent women should be referred to a gynecology practitioner for routine gynecologic examinations and birth control counseling as indicated. Sexual activity may resume at 6 to 8 weeks after transplantation. Recommendations for planning a pregnancy may include discontinuation of teratogenic medications at least 3 months before suspending birth control, achievement of stable graft function with low levels of immunosuppression, and genetic counseling for recipients with an inherited etiology of organ disease.

With increased long-term survival and a significantly improved physical status, pregnancy is now a more frequent occurrence for women with transplants. Successful pregnancies in recipients of solid organ transplants are possible but are not without certain risks and complications. The pregnancy should be carefully monitored with close assessment of graft function and fetal development. In addition to routine prenatal care, the pregnant woman requires frequent monitoring to assess immunosuppressive levels and specific laboratory tests to evaluate for rejection caused by the physiologic changes of pregnancy. Routine surveillance to assess for gestational diabetes and hypertension is also essential since diabetes and hypertension may occur with administration of cyclosporine, tacrolimus, or prednisone. Hypertension and preeclampsia are the most common complications of the mother, and the incidence of rejection is similar to that in the nonpregnant population of women with transplants. When compared with the general population, there is a high incidence of prematurity and low birth weight in infants of women with transplants but generally favorable outcomes (Armenti et al, 2000a, 2000b). Men with transplants who have fathered infants are not as well studied as females; however, these outcomes have been satisfactory and similar to the general population (Armenti et al, 2000b).

Transition into Adulthood

Adolescents with transplants struggle with the same issues of separation and developing independence and identity as their peers but within the context of adapting to the chronicity of transplantation (Aley, 2002). Because of a suppressed immune system, the transplant recipient has an increased risk of developing sexually transmitted diseases if safe sex practices are not followed. Drugs, alcohol, and cigarette smoking affect the transplanted organs and may possibly interfere with the metabolism of immunosuppressive medications. Tattoos and body piercings, which are popular with this age-group, also place

transplant recipients at risk for infection. Noncompliance with medications and care routines can jeopardize the graft, resulting in rejection and ultimately graft loss and death.

Supporting adolescents during this transition may be difficult for parents as they help their child achieve the developmental tasks of adolescence and as the adolescent assumes a greater responsibility for routine care. Individual and family counseling is recommended and encouraged. Consistent and routine communication with the transplant center may also help provide parents with strategies and advice in working through these complex issues within the context of transplantation. In addition, as the adolescent progresses chronologically and developmentally into adulthood, a gradual transition to an adult transplant center should be planned to better meet the needs of an adult transplant recipient.

Family Concerns and Resources

Transplantation is an exchange of end-stage organ disease for the long-term condition of transplantation. Although most families and recipients believe this is an acceptable trade-off, anxiety and apprehensions about the future may be ongoing. Long-term survival, the child's transition into adulthood, noncompliance with care, fear of rejection, late infections, possible retransplantation, and the child's future employment and quality of life are major concerns.

Securing employment and obtaining insurance are significant concerns for the late adolescent entering college or the job force. An employer may be fearful of possible physical limitations and potential absences from work. Young adults eventually lose their parents' insurance coverage and must find health insurance through a private carrier or apply for medical assistance. Private insurance may be difficult to obtain because of a preexisting condition and/or employment issues. Although the expenses of transplantation decrease in the long term, an ongoing financial obligation remains for the recipient's lifetime. Medications, laboratory tests, and physical examinations are routinely required. Additional invasive testing and hospitalization may be necessary if the individual acquires an infection or has an episode of acute rejection. Transplant financial counselors and social workers from the transplant center offer counseling about insurance options, medication programs, and grants. In addition, support groups and Web sites established by a variety of foundations, pharmaceutical companies, private individuals, and community groups also provide information about the transplant process and resources.

Noncompliance is a major cause of late rejection and other complications in solid organ transplantation, with a pattern of decreasing compliance during the first few months after transplant being highly predictive of later rejection (Nevins, 2002). Because noncompliance is such a significant problem following transplantation, adherence to medication and care routines should be discussed with the child and family throughout the transplant process, from the pretransplant evaluation through ongoing care follow-up. More than 60% of pediatric renal transplant recipients are reported to be noncompliant, resulting in increased financial and emotional costs (Fennell et al, 2001; Tucker et al, 2002). These children require repeated hospitalizations for rejection and ultimately may face graft loss and death (Fennell et al, 2001). More than 50% of pediatric heart and heart-lung recipients have demonstrated unsatisfactory adherence to their treatment regimen (Serrano-Ikkos et al, 1998). Similarly, repeated episodes of noncompliance with a 14% graft loss have been seen in adolescents with liver transplants (Molmenti et al, 1999).

Noncompliance should always be considered in the differential diagnosis of rejection, particularly if the child is an adolescent and a long-term survivor. Factors or symptoms suggestive of noncompliance may include the following: unexpectedly low or erratic tacrolimus or CSA levels indicating missed doses or drug loading, inconsistencies between the dose and trough level, stabilization of tacrolimus or CSA levels when given in the hospital setting, poor follow-up with the transplant center or community physician, behavior changes, lack of support, dysfunctional family or parental functioning, poor school performance, or decreased socialization (Kosmach et al, 1998). The transplant team must work closely with the adolescent to ensure that the outcome and consequences of poor adherence to medical routines are understood. Repeated education about medications, rejection, infection, and chronic care requirements is essential and must be reinforced. Counseling with a psychologist or medical social worker may help the adolescent recognize the underlying causes of noncompliance and lead to changes to increase adherence. The transplant team should also make every effort to help by minimizing medication requirements and the number of daily dosages while working with the child to create a schedule that is supported by the child's daily routine, is easy to adhere to, and does not interfere with other activities. A system for routinely obtaining laboratory tests and communicating with the transplant coordinator is also imperative.

In repeated cases of noncompliance, a contract may be helpful to delineate the responsibilities of the child and the transplant center, the adherence plan, and the consequences of breaking the contract. Ultimately, a referral to Family Services may be needed in some extreme cases.

The financial impact of transplantation may be another significant concern for families. The transplant surgery and initial hospitalization, possible repeat admissions, an array of medications, living expenses while at the transplant center, and ongoing expenses at home amass an enormous financial burden for many families. Financial support can come from third-party health insurance payers, community fund raising, state funding, or the family's own resources.

Ongoing communication, updated information, and emotional support from the transplant team and primary care providers will help families cope with the fears and uncertainty they may have about their child's future as they progress and adapt to life after transplantation.

RESOURCES AND ORGANIZATIONS

Alpha₁ Antitrypsin Disease
http://www.alpha1.org

American Association of Kidney Patients (AAKP)
http://www.aakp.org

American Heart Association (AHA)
http://www.Americanheart.org

American Liver Foundation
http://www.liverfoundation.org

Children's Liver Association for Support Services
www.classkids.org

Children's Organ Transplant Association (COTA)
http://www.cota.org

Coalition on Donation
http://www.shareyourlife.org

Fujisawa, Inc.
http://www.fujisawa.com

Healthfinder Kids
http://www.healthfinder.gov/kids

International Transplant Nurses Society
http://www.itns.org

The James Redford Institute for Transplant Awareness
http://www.jrifilms.org

The Kids Organ Donor Education Program
http://www.kodeprogram.org

Minority Organ Tissue Transplant Education Program
http://www.mottep.org

National Foundation for Transplant
http://www.transplants.org

National Kidney Foundation, Inc.
http://www.kidney.org

National Transplant Assistance Fund (NTAF)
http://www.transplantfund.org

North American Transplant Coordinators' Organization
http://www.Natco1.org

Novartis
http://www.pharma.us.novartis.com

Roche Pharmaceuticals
http://www.rocheusa.com

The Thomas Starzl Transplant Institute
http://www.sti.upmc.edu

Transplant Health
http://www.Transplanthealth.com

The Transplant Pharmacy
http://www.TransplantRx.com

Transplant Recipients' International Organization (TRIO)
http://www.trioweb.org

Transplant Speakers International
http://www.transplant-speakers.org

Transweb
http://www.transweb.org

United Network for Organ Sharing (UNOS)
http://www.unos.org

Wilson's Disease Association
http://www.wilsonsdisease.org

Wyeth-Ayerst
http://www.wyeth.com

Summary of Primary Care Needs for the Child with a Solid Organ Transplant

HEALTH CARE MAINTENANCE

Growth and Development

Measure height and weight at each visit.

Measure head circumference for children <3 years old at each visit.

Linear growth may be affected by long-term use of corticosteroids.

Catch-up growth may be attained after transplantation.

Growth hormone may be advised for children <1 year before renal transplantation and for children >1 year following renal transplantation.

Improved physical development after transplantation has a positive effect on psychosocial development.

Cognitive functioning should be monitored at regular intervals.

Screening for depressive symptoms related to body image changes, side effects of medications, and adaptation to chronic illness may be advisable.

Diet

A regular oral diet without restrictions is common following stable graft function, although cardiac and renal recipients may have sodium restrictions.

Enteral supplements may be needed to meet caloric requirements for catch-up growth and wound healing, particularly in younger children.

Dietary restrictions are instituted when indicated for electrolyte imbalances or hyperglycemia.

Children with heart transplant are on a heart-healthy diet.

Safety

Good hand washing and avoidance of people with infection are recommended to decrease the risk of toxoplasmosis or other potential infections.

Medic-Alert bracelets are recommended.

The transplant center should be contacted before travel outside the United States or to report extended travel arrangements to give contact information.

Activity and exercise are usually restricted for 6 to 8 weeks after transplant. Activity may also be limited during periods of rejection or infection.

Age-appropriate safety issues should be addressed as in the healthy pediatric population: seat belts, helmets, Mr. Yuk stickers, electrical outlet covers, and so on.

Immunizations

All recommended immunizations should be administered at least 1 month before the transplant whenever possible.

Interrupted immunization schedules can usually be resumed 3 months after transplantation.

Live-virus vaccines are contraindicated in transplant recipients. Transplant recipients should receive inactivated vaccines when available.

The inactivated polio virus (IPV), measles mumps rubella (MMR), and varicella vaccines should be given to siblings and other close contacts.

Transplant recipients and family members within the household should get the annual influenza vaccine.

Screening

Vision. Routine vision screening and ophthalmologic exams are completed as in the general population. Pediatric transplant recipients receiving high-dose long-term steroid therapy are at risk for developing glaucoma and cataracts and may require more frequent examinations.

Hearing. Routine audiograms may be obtained to evaluate hearing loss in children who have received ototoxic drugs.

Dental. Biannual dental visits, as in the general pediatric population, are recommended.

CSA may cause gingival hyperplasia. Antibiotic prophylaxis is indicated for invasive dental procedures for renal and liver transplant and for all dental procedures for cardiac transplants.

Blood Pressure. Blood pressure measurement should be obtained at each check-up.

If antihypertensive medications are prescribed, blood pressure should be checked and recorded before administration of each dose. A record of blood pressure results should be kept and assessed at each check-up. Further evaluation may be required for long-term hypertension.

Hematocrit. Screening should be done per transplant center routine.

Anemia may occur as a result of renal dysfunction or recurrent disease.

Urinalysis. Nephrotoxicity is a complication of cyclosporine and tacrolimus.

Additional screening is necessary in children with kidney transplants.

Immunosuppression may mask symptoms of urinary tract infection (UTI). Urinalysis should be obtained in children with fever and possible UTI.

Tuberculosis. Routine screening with a PPD and anergy panel is recommended. Chest radiography is obtained if indicated. A lifetime course of isoniazid (IHN) is recommended in patients with a positive PPD and chest films.

Condition-Specific Screening

Blood Work. Routine laboratory testing is obtained at regular intervals, usually weekly to monthly, depending on the time after transplant and any current episodes of infection or rejection. Tacrolimus, CSA, and/or sirolimus levels are also monitored regularly and adjusted as indicated per transplant center protocols.

Continued

Summary of Primary Care Needs for the Child with a Solid Organ Transplant—cont'd

COMMON ILLNESS MANAGEMENT

Differential Diagnosis

Fever. The risk of bacterial, fungal, and viral infections is highest during the first 3 months after a transplant and whenever immunosuppression is maximized

Immunosuppression will mask symptoms, so careful assessment of any fever is very important.

Normal childhood illnesses should be ruled out.

Fever may indicate organ rejection or infection.

Abdominal Symptoms. Abdominal pain should be investigated to rule out appendicitis or intestinal obstruction, ulcers, peritonitis, rejection, or posttransplant lymphoproliferative disorder (PTLD).

Abdominal pain in liver transplant recipients may be a sign of rejection or surgical complications.

Abdominal pain and/or vomiting may be a sign of rejection in heart transplant recipients.

Vomiting and diarrhea may lower therapeutic blood levels of immunosuppressant drugs.

Metabolic Abnormalities. Hyperkalemia can result from drug therapy.

Hyperglycemia may result from immunosuppressant medications.

Drug Interactions

CSA and tacrolimus absorption is altered by phenytoin, phenobarbital, ketoconazole, fluconazole, erythromycin, diltiazem, and other drugs.

When administered with anticonvulsants, higher doses of CSA may be needed to achieve a therapeutic range.

Acetaminophen should be used instead of aspirin or ibuprofen.

If the child is hypertensive, decongestants should be avoided.

It is important for the primary care provider to contact the transplant center before prescribing any medication.

DEVELOPMENTAL ISSUES

Sleep Patterns

End-stage organ disease, hospitalization, or drugs may alter sleep patterns.

Familiar routines and rituals should be maintained when possible.

Toileting

Regression in toddlers and preschoolers is to be expected.

Children with renal transplantation may need to relearn body cues to achieve toilet training.

Children taking diuretics may have difficulty with urinary continence and training.

Emotional support is required as children learn skills.

Discipline

Parental overprotectiveness is likely; parents may need help to promote independence in their children.

Family counseling may be helpful.

Child Care

Children may attend daycare by 3 months after surgery if immunosuppression requirements have been reduced.

Precautions should be taken to limit exposure to communicable diseases.

Schooling

Normal schooling should be resumed 1 to 3 months after transplantation.

Additional academic help may be needed to attain grade level skills because of time lost.

An individual education plan (IEP) should be initiated if school problems develop.

Sexuality

The transplant experience may affect body image and self-esteem.

Barrier methods of birth control are recommended.

Childbearing is possible after transplantation.

Physiologic strain on the maternal system must be monitored.

Affects of immunosuppression on the fetus must be monitored.

Transition into Adulthood

Many individuals have difficulty attaining independence.

Body image and intimacy may be negatively affected.

Concerns about employment and health insurance develop.

FAMILY CONCERNS

Family concerns include the fear of rejection, search for a new organ, organ donor issues, and finances.

Securing employment and continued health insurance may be difficult.

Noncompliance with immunosuppressive therapy is a major problem that can result in graft loss. Counseling may be helpful.

REFERENCES

Aley, K. (2002). Developmental approach to pediatric transplantation. *Prog Transplant, 12*(2), 86-91.

Allen, U., Hebert, D., Moore, D., Dror, Y., & Wasfy, S. (2001). Epstein-Barr virus-related post-transplant lymphoproliferative disease in solid organ transplant recipients, 1988-97: A Canadian multi-centre experience. *Pediatr Transplant, 5*, 198-203.

Anselmo, D.M., Baquerizo, A., Geevarghese, S., Ghobrial, R.M., Farmer, D.G., et al. (2001). Liver transplantation at Dumont-UCLA Transplant Center: An experience with over 3000 cases. *Clin Transpl, 2001*, 179-186.

Appel, J., Alwayn, I., & Cooper, D. (2002). Xenotransplantation: The challenge to current psychosocial attitudes. *Prog Transplant, 10*(4), 217-225.

Armenti, V.T., Herrine, S.K., Radomski, J.S., & Moritz, M.J. (2000a). Pregnancy after liver transplantation. *Liver Transpl, 6*(6), 671-685.

Armenti, V.T., Radomski, J.S., Moritz, M.J., Philips, L.Z., McGrory, C.H., et al. (2000b). Report from the National Transplantation Pregnancy Registry (NTPR): Outcomes of pregnancy after transplantation. *Clin Transpl, 2000*, 123-134.

Barone, G.W., Gurley, B.J., Ketel, B.L., & Abul-Ezz, S.R. (2001). Herbal supplements: A potential for drug interactions in transplant recipients. *Transplantation, 71*(2), 239-241.

Baum, M., Freier, K., & Chinnock, E. (2000). Growth and cognitive development. In A. Tejani, W. Harmon, & R. Fine (Eds.). *Pediatric solid organ transplantation.* Copenhagen: Munksgaard, pp. 433-439.

Boyle, G. (2000a). Other complications. In A. Tejani, W. Harmon, & R. Fine (Eds.). *Pediatric solid organ transplantation.* Copenhagen: Munksgaard, pp. 411-416.

Boyle, G. (2000b). Pretransplant management. In A. Tejani, W. Harmon, & R. Fine (Eds.). *Pediatric solid organ transplantation.* Copenhagen: Munksgaard, pp. 334-341.

Boyle, G. & Fricker, F. (2000). Indications for heart transplantation. In A. Tejani, W. Harmon, & R. Fine (Eds.). *Pediatric solid organ transplantation.* Copenhagen: Munksgaard, pp. 321-327.

Broering, D.C., Mueller, L., Ganschow, R., Kim, J.S., Achilles, E.G., et al. (2001). Is there still a need for living-related liver transplantation in children? *Ann Surg, 234*(6), 713-721.

Brouhard, B.H., Donaldson, L.A., Lawry, K.W., McGowan, K.R., Drotar, D., et al. (2000). Cognitive functioning in children on dialysis and post-transplantation. *Pediatr Transplant, 4*(4), 261-267.

Bucuvalas, J.C., Britto, M., Krug, S., Ryckman, F.C., Atherton, H., et al. (2003). Health-related quality of life in pediatric liver transplant recipients: A single-center study. *Liver Transpl, 9*(1), 62-71.

Campo, J.V., McNab, J., Perel, J.M., Mazariegos, G.V., Hasegawa, S.L., et al. (2002). Kava-induced fulminant hepatic failure. *J Am Acad Child Adolesc Psychiatry, 41*(6), 631-632.

Chan, J.C, Williams, D.M., & Roth, K.S. (2002). Kidney failure in infants and children. *Pediatr Rev, 23*(2), 47-60.

Chan, L., Gaston, R., & Hariharan, S. (2001). Evolution of immunosuppression and continued importance of acute rejection in renal transplantation. *Am J Kidney Dis, 38*(S6), 52-59.

Chand, D.H., Southerland, S.M., & Cunningham III, R.J. (2001). Tacrolimus: The good, the bad, and the ugly. *Pediatr Transplant, 5*(1), 32-36.

Chin, C., Hunt, S., Robbins, R., Hoppe, R., Reitz, B., et al. (2002). Long term follow-up after total lymphoid irradiation in pediatric heart transplant recipients. *J Heart Lung Transplant, 21*(6), 557-673.

Cohen, D. & Galbraith, C. (2001). General health management and long-term care of the renal transplant recipient. *Am J Kidney Dis, 38*(S6), S10-S24.

Cohen, J.I. (2000). Epstein-Barr virus infection. *N Engl J Med, 343*(7), 481-492.

Collins, M.H., Montone, K.T., Leahey, A.M., Hodinka, R.L., Salhany, K.E., et al. (2001). Post-transplant lymphoproliferative disease in children. *Pediatr Transplant, 5*(4), 250-257.

Committee on Infectious Diseases. (2001). *Report of the Committee On Infectious Diseases* (24th ed.). Elk Grove, Ill.: The American Academy of Pediatrics.

Cowan, S.W., Coscia, L.C., Philips, L.Z., Wagoner, L.E., Mannion, J.D., et al. (2002). Pregnancy outcomes in female heart and heart-lung transplant recipients. *Transplant Proc, 34*(5), 1855-1856.

Cronin II, D.C., Faust, T.W., Brady, L., Conjeevaram, H., Jain, S., et al. (2000). Modern immunosuppression. *Clin Liver Dis, 4*(3), 619-655.

Daly, J.S., Kopasz, A., Anandakrishnan, R., Robins, T., Mehta, S., et al. (2002). Preemptive strategy for ganciclovir administration against cytomegalovirus in liver transplantation recipients. *Am J Transplant, 2*(10), 955-958.

Deshpande, R.R., Bowles, M.J., Vilca-Melendez, H., Srinivasan, P., Girlanda, R., et al. (2002). Results of split liver transplantation in children. *Ann Surg, 236*(2), 248-253.

Dharnidharka, V.R., Sullivan, E.K., Stablein, D.M., Tejani, A.H., & Harmon, W.E. (2001). Risk factors for posttransplant lymphoproliferative disorder (PTLD) in pediatric kidney transplantation: A report of the North American Pediatric Renal Transplant Cooperative Study (NAPRTCS). *Transplantation, 71*(8), 1065-1068.

Donati, M., Zuckerman, M., Dhawan, A., Hadzic, N., Heaton, N., et al. (2000). Response to varicella immunization in pediatric liver transplant recipients. *Transplantation, 70*(9), 1401-1404.

Ellis, D. et al. (1997). Renal transplantation in infants and children. In R. Shapiro & T. Starzl (Eds.). *Renal transplantation.* Stamford, Conn.: Appleton & Lange.

Ettenger, R.B. & Grimm, E.M. (2001). Safety and efficacy of TOR inhibitors in renal transplant recipients. *Am J Kidney Dis, 38*(4, suppl. 2), S2, S22-S28.

Fennell, R.S., Tucker, C., & Pedersen, T. (2001). Demographic and medical predictors of medication and compliance among ethnically different pediatric renal transplant patients. *Pediatr Transplant, 5*(5), 343-348.

Ferrieri, P., Gewitz, M.H., Gerber, M., Newburger, J.W., Dajani, A.S., et al. Committee on Rheumatic Fever, Endocarditis, & Kawasaki Disease of the American Heart Association Council on Cardiovascular Disease in the Young. (2002). Unique characteristics of infective endocarditis in childhood. *Circulation, 105*(17), 2115-2126.

Fine, R.N. (2002). Growth following solid-organ transplantation. *Pediatr Transplant, 6*(1), 47-52.

Flynn, B. (2002). Liver transplantation. In S. Cupples & L. Ohler (Eds.). *Transplantation nursing secrets.* Philadelphia: Hanley & Belfus, pp. 151-172.

Flynn, J.T., Bunchman, T.E., & Sherbotie, J.R. (2001). Indications, results, and complications of tacrolimus conversion in pediatric renal transplantation. *Pediatr Transplant, 5*(6), 439-446.

George Jr., A.L. & Neilson, E.G. (2000). Genetics of kidney disease. *Am J Kidney Dis, 35*(4, suppl. 1), S160-S169.

Grant, D. (2001). Report of the International Intestine Transplant Registry; Web site: www.lhsc.on.ca/itr.

Green, M. (2001). Management of Epstein-Barr virus induced post-transplant lymphoproliferative disease in recipients of solid organ transplantation. *Am J Transplant, 1*(2), 103-108.

Green, M. & Michaels, M. (1997). Infections in solid organ transplant recipients. In S. Long, L. Pickery, & C. Prober (Eds.). *Principles and practice of pediatric infectious diseases.* New York: Churchill-Livingstone.

Hangard-Patton, L. & Lawrence, K. (2000). Psychosocial implications of heart transplantation. In A. Tejani, W. Harmon, & R. Fine (Eds.). *Pediatric solid organ transplantation.* Copenhagen: Munksgaard, pp. 440-443.

Hoffman, J. (2002). Incidence, mortality and natural history. In R.H. Anderson, E.J. Baker, F.J. Macartney, M.L. Rigby, E.A. Shinebourne, et al. (Eds.). *Pediatric cardiology.* Edinburgh: Churchill Livingstone.

Hunt, S.A. & Frazier, O.H. (1998). Mechanical circulatory support and cardiac transplantation. *Circulation, 97*(20), 2079-2090.

Jain, A., Mazariegos, G., Kashyap, R., Green, M., Gronsky, C., et al. (2000). Comparative long-term evaluation of tacrolimus and cyclosporine in pediatric liver transplantation. *Transplantation, 70*(4), 617-625.

Jain, A., Mazariegos, G., Kashyap, R., Kosmach-Park, B., Starzl, T.E., et al. (2002a). Pediatric liver transplantation: A single center experience spanning 20 years. *Transplantation, 73*(6), 941-947.

Jain, A., Nalesnik, M., Reyes, J., Pokharna, R., Mazariegos, G., et al. (2002b). Posttransplant lymphoproliferative disorders in liver transplantation: A 20 year experience. *Ann Surg, 236*(4), 429-436.

Jaskowski, S. (2002). Pediatric liver transplantation. *Prog Transplant, 12*(2), 136-154.

Kantrowitz, A., Haller, J.D., Joos, H., Cerruti, M.M., & Carstensen, H.E. (1968). Transplantation of the heart in an infant and adult. *Am J Cardiol, 22*(16), 782-790.

Kasiske, B.L., Vazquez, M.A., Harmon, W.E., Brown, R.S., Danovitch, G.M., et al. (2000). Recommendations for the outpatient surveillance of renal transplant recipients. *J Am Soc Nephrol, 11*(suppl. 15), S1-S86.

Kelly, D. (2000). Post transplant rehabilitation. In A. Tejani, W. Harmon, & R. Fine (Eds.). *Pediatric solid organ transplantation.* Copenhagen: Munksgaard, pp. 306-311.

Kelly, D.A. (1997). Nutritional factors affecting growth before and after liver transplantation. *Pediatr Transplant, 1*(1), 80-83.

Kosmach, B., Webber, S.A., & Reyes, J. (1998). Care of the pediatric solid organ transplant recipient. The primary care perspective. *Pediatr Clin North Am, 45*(1), 1395-1418.

Kosmach-Park, B. (2002). Intestinal transplantation in pediatric patients. *Prog Transplant, 12*(2), 97-113.

Lin, P.L., Vats, A.N., & Green, M. (2001). BK virus infection in renal transplant recipients. *Pediatr Transplant, 5*(6), 398-405.

Lower, R.R.& Shumway, N.E. (1960). Studies on orthotopic transplantation of the canine heart. *Surg Forum, 11*, 18-19.

Luke, P.P. & Jordan, M.L. (2001). Contemporary immunosuppression in renal transplantation. *Urol Clin North Am, 28*(4), 733-750.

Makowka, L., Cramer, D., & Hoffman, A. (1993). Pig liver xenografts as a temporary bridge for human allografting. *Xenotransplantation, 1*, 27-29.

Makowka, L., Wu, G.D., Hoffman, A., Podesta, L., Sher, L., et al. (1994). Immunohistopathologic lesions associated with the rejection of pig to human liver xenograft. *Transplant Proc, 26*, 1074-1075.

Mayo Foundation for Medical Education and Research. (2002). Herb and drug interactions; Web site: www.mayoclinic.com.

Mazariegos, G.V., Boucek, M.M., & Bartosh, S.M. (2000). Pediatric issues in solid organ transplantation. Medscape: Medical Educational Collaborative; Web site: www.medscape.com.

Mazariegos, G.V. & Reyes, J.R. (1999). What's new in pediatric organ transplantation? *Pediatr Rev, 20*(1), 363-375.

McAlister, V.C, Gao, Z., Peltekian, K., Domigues, J., Mahalati, J., et al. (2000). Sirolimus-tacrolimus combination immunosuppression. *Lancet, 355*, 376-377.

McDiarmid, S.V. (2001). Update from studies of pediatric liver transplantation. *Transplant Proc, 33*(8), 3604-3605.

McGhee, W., Howrie, D., Schmitt, C., & Dice, J. (Eds.). (2002). *Pediatric drug therapy handbook and formulary.* Dept. of Pharmacy, Children's Hospital of Pittsburgh. Hudson, Ohio: Lexicon, Inc.

Michaels, M. (2000). Infectious complications. In A. Tejani, W. Harmon, & R. Fine (Eds.). *Pediatric solid organ transplantation.* Copenhagen: Munksgaard, pp. 404-410.

Mittal, S., Thompson, J.F., Kato, T., & Tzakis, A.G. (2001). Tacrolimus and diarrhea: Pathogenesis of altered metabolism. *Pediatr Transplant, 5*(2), 75-79.

Molmenti, E., Mazariegos, G., Bueno, J., Cacciarelli, T., Alasio, T., et al. (1999). Noncompliance after pediatric liver transplantation. *Transplant Proc, 31* (1-2), 408.

Molrine, D.C. & Hibberd, P.L. (2001). Vaccines for transplant recipients. *Infect Dis Clin North Am, 15*(1), 273-305.

Morrow, W.R., Frazier, E., & Naftel, D.C. (2000). Survival after listing for cardiac transplantation in children. *Prog Pediatr Cardiol, 11*(2), 99-105.

Nevins, T.E. (2002). Non-compliance and its management in teenagers. *Pediatr Transplant, 6*(6), 475-479.

Nissen, D. (Ed.). (2002). *Mosby's drug consult.* St. Louis: Mosby.

North American Pediatric Renal Transplant Cooperative Study. (2001). *Annual report.* Rockville, Md.: Emmes Corporation.

Ohler, L. & Bray, R. (2002). Immunology. In S. Cupples & L. Ohler (Eds.). *Transplantation nursing secrets.* Philadelphia: Hanley & Belfus, pp. 9-15.

Olson, A.D., Shope, T.C., & Flynn, J.T. (2001). Pretransplant varicella vaccination is cost-effective in pediatric renal transplantation. *Pediatr Transplant, 5*(11), 44-50.

Padbury, R.T., Toogood, G.J., & McMaster, P. (1998). Withdrawal of immuno-suppression in liver allograft recipients. *Liver Transpl Surg, 4*(3), 242-248.

Pandya, A., Wasfy, S., Hevert, D., & Allen, U. (2001). Varicella-zoster infection in pediatric renal-solid organ transplant recipients: A hospital-based study in the prevaricella vaccine era. *Pediatr Transplant, 5,* 153-159.

Park, M. (1996). Primary myocardial disease. In *Pediatric cardiology for practitioners* (3rd ed). St. Louis: Mosby.

Pearlman, L. (2002a). Pediatric solid organ transplantation. In S. Cupples & L. Ohler (Eds.). *Transplantation nursing secrets.* Philadelphia: Hanley & Belfus, pp. 235-245.

Pearlman, L. (2002b). Postransplant viral syndromes. *Prog Transplant, 12*(2), 116-124.

Qvist, E., Pihko, H., Fagerudd, P., Valanne, L., Lamminranta, S., et al. (2002). Neurodevelopmental outcome in high risk patients after renal transplantation in early childhood. *Pediatr Transplant, 6*(1), 53-62.

Renz, J.F., de Roos, M., Rosenthal, P., Mudge, C., Bacchetti, P., et al. (2001). Posttransplantation growth in pediatric liver recipients. *Liver Transpl, 7*(12), 1040-1055.

Reyes, J., Mazariegos, G.V., Bueno, J., Cerda, J., Towbin, R.B., et al. (1999). The role of portosystemic shunting in children in the transplant era. *J Pediatr Drug, 34*(1), 117-122.

Roche Pharmaceuticals. (2000). *Cellcept. Roche product monograph.* Nutley, N.J.: Author.

Sanchez, C.P., Kuizon, B.D., Goodman, W.G., Gales, B., Ettenger, R.B., et al. (2002). Growth hormone and the skeleton in pediatric renal allograft recipients. *Pediatr Nephrol, 17*(5), 322-328.

Schowengerdt, K.O., Naftel, D.C., Seib, P.M., Pearce, F.B., Addonizio, L.J., et al. (1997). Infection after pediatric heart transplant: Results of a multi-institutional study. *J Heart Lung Transplant, 16*(12), 1207-1216.

Sechser, A., Osorio, J., Freise, C., & Osorio, R.W. (2001). Artificial liver support devices for fulminant liver failure. *Clin Liver Dis, 5*(2), 415-430.

Seikaly, M., Ho, P.L., Emmett, L., & Tejanie, A. (2001). The 12th annual report of the North American Pediatric Renal Transplant Cooperative Study: Renal transplantation from 1987 through 1998. *Pediatr Transplant, 5*(3), 215-231.

Serrano-Ikkos, E., Lask, B., Whitehead, B., & Eisler, I. (1998). Incomplete adherence after pediatric heart and heart-lung transplantation. *J Heart Lung Transplant, 17*(12), 1177-1183.

Serrano-Ikkos, E., Lask, B., Whitehead, B., Rees, P., & Graham, P. (1999). Heart or heart-lung transplantation: Psychosocial outcomes. *Pediatr Transplant, 3*(4), 301-308.

Shapiro, R. (2000). Tacrolimus in renal transplantation—a review. *Graft, 3*(2), 64-80.

Simon, D.M. & Levin, S. (2001). Infectious complications of solid organ transplantations. *Infect Dis Clin North Am, 15*(2), 521-549.

Sindhi, R., Webber, S., Venkataramanan, R., McGhee, W., Phillips, S., et al. (2001). Sirolimus for rescue and primary immunosuppression in transplanted children receiving tacrolimus. *Transplantation, 72*(5), 851-855.

SPLIT Research Group. (2001). Studies of Pediatric Liver Transplantation (SPLIT): Year 2000 outcomes. *Transplantation, 72*(3), 463-476.

Starzl, T. & Demetris, A. (1997). History of renal transplantation. In R. Shapiro, R. Simmons, & T. Starzl (Eds.). *Renal transplantation.* Stamford, Conn.: Appleton & Lange.

Starzl, T. et al. (1993a). The role of cell migration and chimerism in organ transplant acceptance and tolerance induction. *Transplant Sci, 3*(1), 47-50.

Starzl, T.E., Fung, J., Tzakis, A., Todo, S., Demetris, A.J., et al. (1993b). Baboon-to-human liver transplantation. *Lancet, 341*(8837), 65-71.

Starzl, T.E., Iwatsuki, S., Van Thiel, D.H., Gartner, J.C., Zitelli, B.J., et al. (1982). Evolution of liver transplantation. *Hepatology, 2*(5), 614-636.

Starzl, T.E. & Zinkernagel, R.M. (2001). Transplantation tolerance from a historical perspective. *Natl Rev Immunol, 1*(3), 233-239.

Stockwell, J., Tobias, J., & Greeley, W. (1995). Noninflammatory, noninfiltrative cardiomyopathy. In D.H. Nichols, D.E. Cameron, W.L. Greeley, D. Lappe, R.M. Ungerleider, & R.C. Wetzel (Eds.). *Critical heart disease in infants and children.* St. Louis: Mosby.

Straatman, L.P. & Coles, J.G. (2000). Pediatric utilization of rapamycin for severe cardiac allograft rejection. *Transplantation, 70*(3), 541-543.

Tan, J.C. (2001). *Recurrent disease after kidney transplantation.* Palo Alto, Calif.: Grand Rounds presentation, Division of Nephrology at Stanford University.

Tejani, A. & Sullivan, E.K. (2000). The impact of acute rejection on chronic rejection: A report of the North American Renal Transplant Cooperative Study. *Pediatr Transplant, 4*(2), 107-111.

Tenney, F. & Sakarcan, A. (2001). Fatal cytomegalovirus disease in a high-risk renal transplant recipient. *Pediatr Nephrol, 16*(1), 8-10.

Throckmorton, A.L., Allaire, P.E., Gutgesell, J.H., Matherne, J.G., Olsen, D.B., et al. (2002). Pediatric circulatory support systems. *ASAIO J, 48*(3), 216-221.

Tucker, C.M., Fennell, R.S., Pederson, T., Higley, B., Wallack, C., et al. (2002). Associations with medication adherence among ethnically different pediatric patients with renal transplants. *Pediatr Nephrol, 17*(4), 251-256.

United Network of Organ Sharing (UNOS). (2002). *Scientific registry data; transplant patient.* Available: www.UNOS.org.

van Mourik, I.D., Beath, S.V., Brook, G.A., Cash, A.J., Mayer, A.D., et al. (2000). Long-term nutritional and neurodevelopmental outcome of liver transplantation in infants aged less than 12 months. *J Pediatr Gastroenterol Nutr, 30*(3), 269-275.

Vanrenterghem, Y.F. (2001). Tailoring immunosupressive therapy for renal transplant recipients. *Pediatr Transplant, 5*(6), 467-472.

Vessey, S.J., Chan, C.Y., Kuter, B.J., Kaplan, K.M., Waters, M., et al. (2001). Childhood vaccination against varicella: Persistence of antibody, duration of protection, and vaccine efficacy. *J Pediatr, 139*(2), 297-304.

Vester, U., Kranz, B., Testa, G., Malago, M., Beelen, D., et al. (2001). Efficacy and tolerability of interleukin-2 receptor blockade with basiliximab in pediatric renal transplant recipients. *Pediatr Transplant, 5*(4), 297-301.

Wallot, M.A., Mathot, M., Janssen, M., Holter, T., Paul, K., et al. (2002). Long-term survival and late graft loss in pediatric liver transplant recipients: A 15 year single center experience. *Liver Transplant, 8*(7), 615-622.

Webber, S. (2000a). Allograft physiology, exercise performance, and rehabilitation. In A. Tejani, W. Harmon, & R. Fine (Eds.). *Pediatric solid organ transplantation.* Copenhagen: Munksgaard, pp. 427-432.

Webber, S. (2000b). Diagnosis, prevention, and treatment of acute rejection. In A. Tejani, W. Harmon, & R. Fine (Eds.). *Pediatric solid organ transplantation.* Copenhagen: Munksgaard, pp. 396-403.

Webber, S. & Green, M. (2000). Post transplant lymphoproliferative disorders: Advances in diagnosis, prevention, and management in children. *Prog Pediatr Cardiol, 11,* 145-157.

Wren, F. & Tarbell, S. (1998). Feeding and growth disorders. In R. Ammerman & J. Campo (Eds.). *Handbook of pediatric psychology and psychiatry: Disease, injury, and illness* (vol. 2). Boston: Allyn & Bacon.

Wyeth-Ayerst Laboratories. (1999). *Rapamune: Practical guide to clinical use.* Philadelphia: Wyeth-Ayerst Pharmaceutical Inc.

35 Phenylketonuria

Catherine Yetter Read and Renee M. Charbonneau

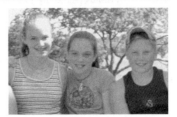

Etiology

Phenylketonuria (PKU) is an autosomal recessive biochemical genetic disorder that results in elevated plasma phenylalanine (Phe) levels. High levels of phenylalanine are toxic to the developing nervous system, and untreated individuals experience mental retardation and other complications. PKU is caused by a mutation of the phenylalanine hydroxylase (PAH) gene on chromosome 12 and exposure to dietary phenylalanine, an essential amino acid found in most protein foods. Absence or deficiency of PAH halts the conversion of Phe to tyrosine (Tyr) and results in hyperphenylalaninemia (HPA). Individuals with HPA caused by deficient PAH are historically classified as having classic PKU if their Phe levels are consistently greater than 1200 μmol/L (20 mg/dl),* mild PKU (sometimes referred to as variant PKU) for Phe levels between 600 μmol/L (10 mg/dl) and 1200 μmol/L (20 mg/dl), or mild HPA for Phe levels below 600 μmol/L (10 mg/dl) (Weglage et al, 2001). Offspring of women with PKU, who generally do not have PKU themselves, may be exposed to toxic levels of Phe in utero and experience the effects of maternal PKU syndrome (Nussbaum et al, 2001).

The metabolic pathway for Phe is mainly in the liver. Phe not used for new protein synthesis is converted to Tyr for use in the biosynthesis of protein, melanin, thyroxine, and the catecholamines. Loss of PAH activity in PKU results in an increase in the concentration of Phe relative to that of Tyr in the blood and causes an accumulation of Phe metabolites such as phenylpyruvic acid, phenylacetic acid, and others. A high level of Phe inhibits the transport of large neutral amino acids into the brain, which disrupts the synthesis of essential substances such as myelin, neurotransmitters, and other proteins. These deficiencies all contribute to the neuropathology of PKU, although the exact mechanisms of neurologic damage remain poorly understood (Rezvani, 2000; Scriver & Kaufman, 2001).

The Phe hydroxylation system is a complex biochemical reaction that requires the presence of oxygen and the co-factor tetrahydrobiopterin (BH₄). A deficiency in any enzyme involved in the synthesis or regeneration of BH₄ will result in HPA. BH₄ disorders, found in approximately 1% to 2% of individuals with HPA, are phenotypically and genotypically distinct from PKU, require different modes of therapy, and have a different prognosis. Testing for BH₄ disorders should be done in all newborns with HPA and in any child with microcephaly, mental retardation, seizure disorders, developmental delays, disturbances of tone and posture, movement disorders, hyperpyrexia, or other unexplained neurologic findings (Smith & Lee, 2000).

Known Genetic Etiology

More than 400 mutations (allelic variations) in the human PAH gene have been described and compiled in the PAH mutation database at http://www.pahdb.mcgill.ca. Mutations result from a variety of mechanisms, including insertions, deletions, missense and nonsense mutations, and DNA (deoxyribonucleic acid) splicing defects. Mutations change the DNA code for PAH, resulting in an unstable enzyme with loss of normal activity (Scriver & Kaufman, 2001). All individuals inherit two PAH alleles—one from each parent—at the PAH locus. Since PKU is an autosomal recessive disorder, an individual with one normal allele and one mutant allele will produce adequate PAH and will be an asymptomatic carrier of the disease.

Most cases of PKU result from allelic heterogeneity, whereby a different mutation is inherited from each parent. Figure 35-1 depicts a family pedigree in which the affected child has inherited one allele for mild HPA and one allele for PKU. The R408W PKU allele is one of the six mutations responsible for about two thirds of PKU in populations of European descent; most mutations that account for PKU in Asian populations are entirely different (Nussbaum et al, 2001).

The degree of hyperphenylalaninemia in the affected child depicted in Figure 35-1 cannot be accurately predicted from genotype information at the current time. Correlation of genotype with biochemical and metabolic phenotype has been established for many of the common genotypes (Guttler & Guldberg, 2000), but allelic heterogeneity complicates the analysis. Genotype-phenotype correlation is an important area of research, but there are many challenges owing to the number of known mutations and the probable influence of modifier genes and environmental factors. For example, variations in transport of Phe into the brain may explain the existence of siblings with the same genotype at the PAH locus who exhibit different clinical phenotypes and the existence of the rare individuals with PKU who experience no neurologic damage (National Institutes of Health [NIH], 2000).

Direct DNA analysis of the PAH gene is performed to determine the specific mutation present in a child with HPA or to rule out mutations in potential sperm or egg donors. For fetal diagnosis, a combination of mutation analysis and identification of polymorphisms in the PAH gene is usually necessary. All individuals in the world have identifiable normal variations in the DNA surrounding the PAH locus on chromosome 12 called restriction fragment length polymorphisms (RFLPs).

---

*To convert Phe from μmol/L to mg/dl, multiply μmol/L by .0165. To convert Phe from mg/dl to μmol/L, multiply mg/dl by 60.53.

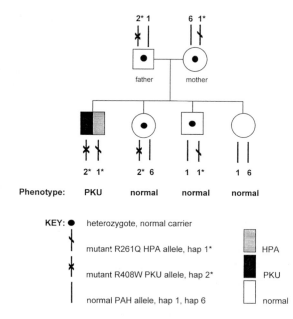

FIGURE 35-1 Hypothetical family pedigree showing segregation of mutant PKU and mutant HPA alleles with haplotype.

TABLE 35-1

Incidence of Phenylketonuria by Racial or Ethnic Group

Population	Approximate Incidence
Whites	
In the United States	1 in 17,000
In Ireland and Scotland	1 in 6,000
In (former) West Germany	1 in 9,000
In Italy	1 in 16,000
Yemenite Jews	1 in 6,000
Ashkenazi Jews	1 in 60,000
Chinese and Japanese	1 in 60,000
African Americans	1 in 127,000
Hispanics in the United States	1 in 60,000
Native Americans	1 in 15,000

Data from the American Academy of Pediatrics (1996) and The National Institutes of Health (2000).

Because specific RFLPs segregate with the PKU mutation on the PAH gene, they act as markers for PKU and are called PKU haplotypes (haps). Analysis of the parental haplotypes in association with the PAH mutation enables prenatal genetic counseling (Scriver & Kaufman, 2001).

Incidence and Prevalence

In the United Sates, the incidence of PKU is 1 in 10,000 to 1 in 25,000; the incidence of non-PKU HPA is estimated to be 1 in 48,000. There are no gender differences, although there is significant racial and ethnic variability, with an increased incidence in certain European white populations, as shown in Table 35-1 (American Academy of Pediatrics, 1996; NIH, 2000). For autosomal recessive disorders, carrier (heterozygote) frequency is calculated from disease incidence (Nussbaum et al, 2001), so

carrier frequency for PKU also varies among populations. For a population with a PKU incidence of 1 in 10,000, the carrier frequency is calculated to be 2%; that is, 1 in 50 persons in that population possesses one copy of the mutated PKU gene. The nonuniform distribution of cases of PKU and its major alleles may be explained by migration, genetic drift, recurrent mutation, and intragenic recombination over the past 100,000 years (Scriver & Kaufman, 2001).

The incidence of PKU is calculated from data collected through mandated newborn screening programs. An NIH consensus development panel on PKU (NIH, 2000) reviewed the Council of Regional Networks for Genetic Services National Newborn Screening Report (Newborn Screening Committee, 1999) and found several factors that confound incidence estimates of PKU. States do not uniformly report the number of infants born, the number of infants screened, the gender or race of the infant, or data about non-PKU HPA. In addition, there are wide variations in the blood phenylalanine levels considered diagnostic of PKU and HPA. For example, most states or provinces (22 of 53) define classic PKU as blood Phe above 20 mg/dl, but four states use 10 mg/dl as the cutoff value. In addition to altering estimates of incidence, such discrepancies lead to state-to-state differences in referrals for follow-up testing and treatment.

Maternal PKU syndrome (MPKU) is becoming a cause for concern, since large numbers of healthy young women with PKU are now reaching childbearing age. There are approximately 4000 women of reproductive age in the United States with PKU who are at high risk for giving birth to infants with maternal PKU syndrome if they fail to restrict dietary phenylalanine before and throughout pregnancy (Centers for Disease Control and Prevention, 2002). Despite the recommendation that all individuals with PKU follow a Phe-restricted diet for life, discontinuance during adolescence is common. The success of dietary therapy in arresting the neurologic deficits caused by PKU has inadvertently produced an increasing number of mentally retarded offspring with maternal PKU syndrome; the possibility exists that in one generation the incidence of PKU-related mental retardation could return to the level it was before newborn screening and treatment were available.

Clinical Manifestations at Time of Diagnosis
Identification of Phenylketonuria

Mass screening of newborn infants for PKU is conducted in all US states, Puerto Rico, the Virgin Islands, all provinces in Canada, and many other countries. Guthrie's method of detecting elevated Phe in a blood spot on a piece of filter paper became widely used in the 1960s. Applications of the method have changed over the years and have included the Guthrie Bacterial Inhibition Assay, automated fluorometric analysis, and high-performance liquid chromatography. In recent years, many states have begun to use tandem mass spectrometry (TMS or MS/MS) to screen newborn blood spots. TMS allows detection of elevated Phe and a large number of other metabolic disorders simultaneously, and it has been shown to reduce the incidence of false-positive results. Nevertheless, the cost, technical complexity, and need for sophisticated interpretation of the results obtained by TMS demand cautious adoption of the technology (NIH, 2000).

Screening refers to efforts to distinguish persons who probably do have a disease from those who do not. Newborns with positive newborn screening tests for PKU may or may not actually have PKU; further testing is always required. Parents of a newborn with a positive screening test are notified in various ways, depending on the policy of the regional screening laboratory. Every effort should be made to avoid delays in the diagnostic process, since dietary treatment of the child with PKU should ideally begin no later than 7 to 10 days after birth (NIH, 2000).

Despite screening efforts, some cases of PKU and HPA are diagnosed late or undiagnosed. False-negative screening results may occur if the blood is collected before the infant is 24 hours old. Early discharge of newborns from the hospital necessitates a second test, although there is a lack of uniformity in state policies related to repeat testing. Others at risk for a missed diagnosis of PKU include premature infants who are transferred to neonatal intensive care units shortly after birth, those whose parents refuse the screening test, or those born outside of a health care institution or who immigrate to the United States at a young age. Primary care providers should be alert to the possibility of PKU in any of these situations or when the child has unexplained signs and symptoms associated with untreated PKU. In addition, maternal PKU syndrome should be suspected in a child with unexplained microcephaly, cardiac defects, or other dysmorphology or developmental delay, since some women have asymptomatic forms of PKU or HPA.

Clinical Manifestations of Untreated Phenylketonuria

For more than 40 years, newborn screening has been successful in the prevention of clinical manifestations in children with PKU (Box 35-1). Nevertheless, there remain a number of persons who experience the consequences of misdiagnosis, late

---

BOX 35-1

Clinical Manifestations of Untreated Phenylketonuria

Normal appearance at birth
Fair pigmentation
Irritability
Neonatal vomiting
Infantile spasms
Generalized epilepsy
Microcephaly
Atopic dermatitis
Mousy odor of urine and sweat
Plantar responses variable
Tailor's sitting position
Fine, rapid, irregular tremor
Parkinson's-like movements
Bony changes with altered growth patterns
Delayed motor skills
Delayed intellectual skills
Delayed speech and language skills
Hyperphenylalaninemia

---

diagnosis, or lack of metabolic control. Infants with PKU generally appear normal at birth, but they may present with feeding difficulties, vomiting, and irritability soon after birth. Approximately one third of infants with untreated PKU demonstrate lack of increase in head circumference and infantile spasms with hypsarrhythmia on electroencephalogram (EEG) after the first few months of life (Smith & Lee, 2000). Infantile spasms (West syndrome) often occur as the first clinical sign of untreated PKU (Zhongshu et al, 2001).

As the infant gets older, there are noticeable developmental delays and an unpleasant "mousy" or "musty" odor from the excretion of phenylacetic acid, a metabolite of the accumulated Phe. Mental retardation is generally severe, with a drop in developmental quotient to 50 points by 1 year of age and to 30 points by 3 years of age (Koch & Wenz, 1987). Neurologic features may include seizures (25%), EEG abnormalities (50%), tremors, tics, abnormalities of gait and posturing, and hypertonicity with hyperactive deep tendon reflexes (Rezvani, 2000). Excitability, autism, schizophrenia-like behaviors, and self-destructiveness have also been described in untreated individuals with PKU (Smith & Lee, 2000).

Children with untreated PKU have lighter skin, eyes, and hair than their unaffected siblings because of impaired melanin synthesis in the absence of sufficient levels of tyrosine. In ethnic backgrounds where black hair is expected, this feature will be expressed as hair that is brown or even reddish. Other physical manifestations of untreated PKU include eczema (20% to 40%), prominent maxilla with widely spaced teeth, enamel hypoplasia, and growth retardation that is more evident in boys (Rezvani, 2000; Smith & Lee, 2000).

Clinical Manifestations of Maternal Phenylketonuria Syndrome

Children of women with PKU are obligatory heterozygotes who can only have PKU if their father is a carrier; thus the vast majority do not have PKU. The greatest risk to these infants is prenatal exposure to high levels of Phe in the mother's blood. Until the 1980s it was common to discontinue the diet in middle childhood, and lack of adherence to the recommended diet remains problematic. Return to diet once it has been discontinued is very difficult, even for women planning a pregnancy, and many pregnant women with PKU do not achieve dietary control before conception (Centers for Disease Control and Prevention, 2002).

Infants born to women with PKU who do not adhere to a low Phe diet before and during pregnancy have a high incidence of mental retardation (93%), microcephaly (72%), and heart defects (14%) (Levy et al, 2001; Rouse et al, 2000). Other features of maternal PKU syndrome include intrauterine and postnatal growth delay and dysmorphic facial features that resemble fetal alcohol syndrome (Figure 35-2). There is also a higher incidence of other birth defects in infants with maternal PKU syndrome, including dysgenesis of the corpus callosum (Nissenkorn et al, 2001), tracheoesophageal fistula, bowel malrotation, bladder exstrophy, orofacial clefting, and eye abnormalities such as coloboma and cataracts (Smith & Lee, 2000).

In a pregnant woman with PKU, a transplacental gradient that favors the fetus results in a fetal/maternal ratio of Phe of

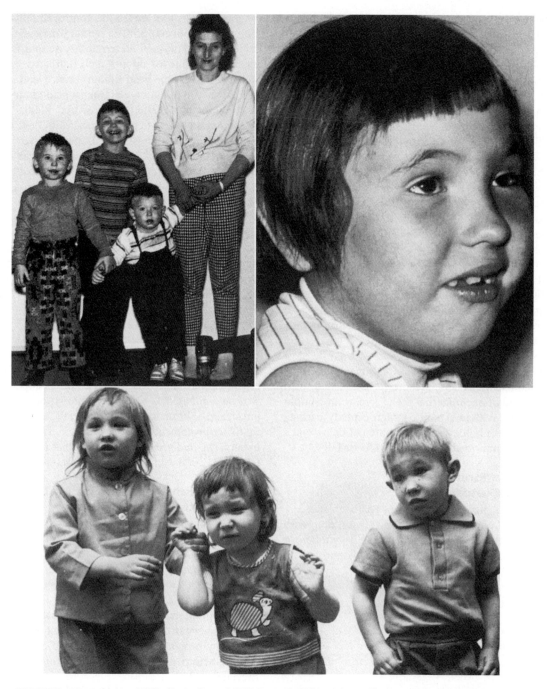

FIGURE 35-2 Maternal PKU effects. *Upper left*, Mother with PKU and three offspring with maternal PKU. The children do not have PKU. *Upper right*, Girl with maternal PKU. *Lower*, Three children of PKU mother. In addition to the relative microcephaly, note the subtle similarity in the facies, including the poorly defined philtrum. (From Jones, K.L. (1997). *Smith's recognizable patterns of human malformation* [5th ed.]. Philadelphia: W.B. Saunders. Courtesy of Dr. Witheld Zaleski, University of Saskatoon, Department of Pediatrics, Saskatoon, Saskatchewan. Reprinted with permission.)

about 1.5, although that ratio may be as high as 2.9 (Scriver & Kaufman, 2001). Thus studies of MPKU rely on maternal Phe levels, and these may not be valid indicators of the fetal level. Nevertheless, many studies document a dose-dependent teratogenic effect of maternal Phe on a developing fetus, which is more pronounced in the early weeks of pregnancy. Rouse et al (1997) determined that at maternal Phe levels of 900 μmol/L (15 mg/dl), 85% of infants had microcephaly, 51% had

postnatal growth retardation, and 26% had intrauterine growth retardation, compared with 6%, 4%, and 0%, respectively, if the maternal Phe level was less than 360 μmol/L (6 mg/dl). Levy et al (2001) found that a basal maternal Phe level above 900 μmol/L (15 mg/dl) may be the threshold for congenital heart disease in the fetus and that a level above 1800 μmol/L (30 mg/dl) poses a significant risk of congenital heart disease. Consequently, clinicians must counsel women of childbearing

BOX 35-2
Treatment

Phe-restricted diet to maintain levels
　For children <12 years and for women before and throughout
　　pregnancy: 120 μmol/L (2 mg/dl) to 360 μmol/L (6 mg/dl)
　>12 years: 120 μmol/L (2 mg/dl) to 900 μmol/L (15 mg/dl), although an
　　upper limit of 600 μmol/L (10 mg/dl) strongly encouraged
Supplement tyrosine and other nutrients as needed

age with PKU or HPA to have their blood levels checked and to achieve metabolic control of Phe before becoming pregnant.

Treatment

Dietary modification is the primary treatment (Box 35-2) for PKU and for prevention of maternal PKU syndrome. It is well established that a Phe-restricted diet can prevent the severe neurologic consequences associated with untreated PKU. However, metabolic control in PKU may be difficult to achieve in practice; it requires frequent monitoring of blood Phe levels, maintaining a highly restrictive diet, careful monitoring of food intake, frequent visits to a PKU clinic, and supplementation with formula that many persons find unpalatable.

The NIH Consensus Statement (NIH, 2000) on the management of PKU recommends that treatment of the neonate with PKU be initiated as soon as possible but no later than 7 to 10 days after birth. Blood Phe levels should be maintained between 120 μmol/L (2 mg/dl) and 360 μmol/L (6 mg/dl) up until the age of 12 years. After age 12 years, Phe levels should be between 120 μmol/L (2 mg/dl) and 900 μmol/L (15 mg/dl), although 600 μmol/L (10 mg/dl) as an upper limit is strongly encouraged. For women of childbearing age, a Phe level between 120 μmol/L (2 mg/dl) and 360 μmol/L (6 mg/dl) should be achieved at least 3 months before conception and maintained throughout the pregnancy. Individuals with mild HPA whose Phe levels remain below 400 μmol/L (6.6 mg/dl) may remain on a natural protein diet.

The diet for PKU is far more involved than simple restriction of Phe. Since all naturally occurring food proteins contain (on average) 5% Phe and must be avoided, supplements are required to ensure adequate nutrient intake for optimum growth and development. The diet is prescribed by the PKU treatment center team, who continually monitor the child's Phe tolerance. An individual's Phe and other nutrient requirements depend on many factors, including PAH activity, age, growth rate, adequacy of energy and protein intake, and state of health. The precise tolerance for Phe varies, but for most individuals with PKU it is between 200 and 500 mg/day. Phe tolerance may change over time, so careful and continuous monitoring of individuals whose Phe intake is restricted is necessary to avoid both elevations and deficiencies of Phe. Long-term deficiencies of Phe from excessive restriction are also associated with adverse outcomes (Scriver & Kaufman, 2001).

In the neonate, breast milk supplemented with Phe-free formula is recommended. If the infant is bottle fed, one of the commercially available elemental medical foods (EMFs) should be used and continued throughout life. These products are modified protein hydrolysates in which Phe is removed, or they are mixtures of free amino acids that do not contain Phe. EMFs provide the essential amino acids in suitable proportions for the given age of the individual. As the infant begins to eat solid foods, the Phe content must be calculated and the amount of EMF adjusted to ensure that all nutrients are ingested in proper amounts and the desired blood Phe level is maintained. Parents invariably require the assistance of a nutritionist to accomplish these goals.

There is much controversy over the need for supplementation of certain nutrients for individuals on Phe-restricted diets. Tyrosine deficiency is a consequence of inadequate Phe metabolism in PKU, and it has been postulated that low Tyr levels may be responsible for learning difficulties in well-treated individuals with PKU. EMFs are enriched with Tyr, and clinicians often prescribe additional Tyr supplements. However, tyrosine supplementation in PKU has not been found to improve neuropsychologic function in recent studies, and this is thought to be related to nonsustained plasma Tyr elevations after ingestion of the supplement with inadequate levels reaching the brain (Kalsner et al, 2001). The potential dangers of fluctuating Tyr levels have prompted some researchers to recommend against additional supplementation and advocate reduction of the Tyr content in EMFs and the development of slow-release Tyr dietary compounds (Van Spronsen et al, 2001).

Long-chain polyunsaturated fatty acids, including docosahexanoic (DHA) and arachidonic acid (AA), may be reduced in the blood of individuals treated for PKU, and blood lipid monitoring with supplementation of DHA and AA in deficient individuals is recommended (Moseley et al, 2002). There is also evidence that supplementation with omega-3 long-chain polyunsaturated fatty acids from fish oil improves visual evoked potentials in children with treated PKU (Beblo et al, 2001). Other dietary components commonly monitored and supplemented in individuals with PKU include vitamin B$_{12}$, folic acid, calcium, zinc, iron, calcium, phosphate, and selenium (NIH, 2000; Van Bakel et al, 2000).

Children with late-diagnosed PKU should also be placed on the Phe-restricted diet no matter how late they are identified. Improvements in behavior and neurologic status have been seen in individuals with severe retardation who had untreated PKU (Baumeister & Baumeister, 1998). In a study of 57 late-diagnosed persons with a mean IQ (intelligence quotient) of 44 at the time of diagnosis, institution of the Phe-restricted diet improved their mean IQ to 73 (Koch et al, 1999). In addition, return to diet for adults with PKU who have discontinued it has been shown to improve a variety of conditions, including brain magnetic resonance imaging (MRI) changes, agoraphobia, panic attacks, and recurrent headaches (Koch et al, 1999).

Complementary and Alternative Therapies

Complementary therapies for PKU must be administered in conjunction with conventional dietary treatment. A person with PKU should not take dietary supplements or herbal remedies without the approval of the metabolic practitioner, since many of these contain high protein or aspartame. However, affected children and their families may derive significant benefit from relaxation training, spirituality, imagery, and therapies involving art, music, and touch. PKU, like any chronic condition requiring constant care and vigilance, places enormous stress on all involved. Support groups and E-mail mailing lists for families with PKU may provide practical information and act as a resource for relevant complementary therapy programs.

Anticipated Advances in Diagnosis and Management

Although diet therapy is an effective treatment for PKU, some individuals have difficulty adhering to the strict regimen and experience poor outcomes as a result. Potential alternative treatments that are being investigated include somatic enzyme substitution and gene therapy. One promising therapy involves oral administration of recombinant phenylalanine ammonia lyase (PAL), an enzyme that degrades phenylalanine in the intestinal tract. Animal studies and limited human studies suggest that PAL has the potential to make the PKU diet less restrictive for humans (Sarkissian et al, 1999; Scriver & Kaufman, 2001). Oral supplementation with tetrahydrobiopterin (BH_4), a coenzyme to PAH, has been shown in some cases to cause a 50% reduction in blood Phe levels (Schuett, 2002).

Phenylalanine tolerance was restored to a 10-year-old boy with PKU who received a liver transplant for concurrent active cirrhosis, although liver transplants are unlikely to become standard therapy for a condition treatable by diet therapy (Scriver & Kaufman, 2001). Hepatocyte transplantation is under consideration for PKU; in this scenario, the person's own liver cells are removed, the normal PAH gene is inserted into the cells, and the cells are then reinserted into the person. Techniques for insertion of the PAH gene into skin, lymphocytes, or other human cells may eventually be able to restore normal Phe metabolism in people with PKU, but at the present time there are many obstacles to overcome in the field of gene therapy (Scriver & Kaufman, 2001; Spirito et al, 2001).

Research on foods and supplements also shows promise for improving the lives of persons with PKU. Gamma zein, a protein in corn, may be genetically modified to remove Phe. This substance could be incorporated into foods and provide high-quality, low-Phe protein (Hainline & Ems-McClung, 1999). Glycomacropeptide (GMP) is the only known protein free of Phe; efforts are under way to develop an economic process to purify GMP from whey so it can be used in food products (Etzel, 2002). Phe-free milk protein may one day be available through production by genetically modified cows (Ayares & D'Arcy, 1999).

There is some evidence that large neutral amino acids (LNAAs) lower the brain Phe level by competing with phenylalanine for transport across the blood-brain barrier. Brain Phe levels may now be measured using MRI (Giewska et al, 2001; Pietz et al, 1999). One European company is currently marketing a pill form of LNAAs called PreKUnil, but further study will be required to determine the appropriateness of this product for long-term use.

Regular blood Phe monitoring is an important aspect of care in PKU. Home monitoring devices are being developed (Andrade, 2002), and the possibility of a noninvasive monitoring device is being investigated (Miller, 2002). Such technologies would give the individual greater autonomy and potentially improve Phe control.

BOX 35-3

Potential Clinical Manifestations of Treated Phenylketonuria (Associated with Poor Dietary Control)

Neurologic changes
    Cerebral white matter changes on magnetic resonance imaging (MRI)
    Abnormal visual and auditory evoked potentials
    Hyperactive tendon reflexes
    Intention tremor
    Electroencephalogram (EEG) abnormalities
Cognitive and behavioral deficits
    Poorer performance on IQ (intelligence quotient) tests
    Poorer performance on school achievement measures
    Cognitive difficulties related to planning, problem solving, and self-regulation
    Tendency toward depression, anxiety, phobias
    Attention deficit hyperactivity disorder
Physical problems
    Decreased bone mineral density
    Atopic dermatitis

Associated Problems

Potential Clinical Manifestations of Treated Phenylketonuria (Box 35-3)

Although dietary treatment has largely eliminated the severe problems associated with untreated PKU, questions remain about subtle manifestations people with PKU may have within neurologic functions, cognitive development, behavioral adjustment, school achievement, and physical health (NIH, 2000). Unfortunately, it is difficult to determine precisely which factors account for impairments. High Phe levels are presumed to cause the pathophysiologic changes in body systems, but low tyrosine, low fatty acid levels or imbalances in other substances may also play a role. However, it is generally agreed, based on all the available evidence, that early and consistent Phe control is associated with better outcomes in all domains.

Neurologic Changes

Parents and children must be apprised of the lifelong vulnerability of the nervous system to high levels of Phe. Abnormal findings in cerebral white matter on MRI have been observed in some individuals with PKU, likely related to a myelin defect. The clinical significance of white matter abnormalities remains unclear, and the severity of signs and symptoms may not reflect the degree of visualized abnormality. Reversal of cerebral white matter change has been observed when Phe restriction is resumed. Some researchers believe that there are individual differences in the brain's vulnerability to Phe and that this vulnerability varies throughout the life span. Recent evidence suggests that maintaining Phe levels below 600 µmol/L minimizes cerebral white matter changes (Weglage et al, 2001). Abnormal visual and auditory evoked potentials have been identified in some individuals with treated PKU. Other signs of impaired nerve conduction found in some individuals who relax their dietary Phe restriction include hyperactive tendon reflexes, intention tremor, and abnormal EEG findings (NIH, 2000; Smith & Lee, 2000; Welsh & Pennington, 2000).

Cognitive and Behavioral Deficits

The NIH (2000) Consensus Development Panel summarized recent literature on the intellectual outcomes of individuals with PKU. This review of 48 studies supported the following conclusion of Welsh & Pennington (2000, p. 285):

Studies of intelligence provide evidence of the effectiveness of dietary treatment when initiated very early in development. Early-treated PKU children exhibit intellectual levels well within the normal range (low to high 90s). However, it is also clear that their intellectual functioning does not achieve the levels predicted by their parents' and siblings' intelligence, and that IQ declines with age during the school years in some children. Declining mental abilities appear to be related to elevations in Phe caused by poor or absent dietary control.

Dietary discontinuation before age 8 is associated with poorer performance on IQ tests; adults on relaxed diets have stable IQ scores but may have poorer performance on measures of attention and speed of processing.

The NIH Consensus Panel also reviewed 37 studies reporting outcomes that involved school achievement, behavioral adjustment, or cognitive functions other than IQ tests. Poorer performance among persons with PKU was found in 29 of these studies, with the most prominent findings being diminished school achievement and greater difficulty on achievement tests. Cognitive difficulties reported included executive functions (planning, problem solving, self-regulation) and attention. The panel noted that many of these studies were limited by small sample sizes and inconsistent use of comparison groups but concluded that levels of Phe show moderate relationships to performance on measures of cognitive function and the presence of behavioral difficulties.

Both anecdotal evidence and scientific evidence support the conclusion that certain neuropsychiatric and psychologic deficits are more frequent in persons with PKU and that these may sometimes be relieved by a return to a strict diet. Anxiety, depression, anorexia, and agoraphobia may be associated with high blood Phe levels that decrease dopamine and serotonin in the brain. A link between PKU and autism (see Chapter 13) has also been noted, especially in late-treated individuals (NIH, 2000). Smith & Knowles (2000) reviewed 34 studies related to behavioral problems in people with treated PKU and found good evidence they are more prone to depression, anxiety, phobic tendencies, and isolation from peers; the authors suggested that these findings are related to a combination of the stress of maintaining the diet and the degree of neurobiologic impairment.

Attention deficit hyperactivity disorder (ADHD; see Chapter 12) may be more common in children with early-treated PKU than in the general population (Antshel, 2001). Welsh & Pennington's review of related studies (2000, p. 287) led to the following conclusion:

On average, an early treated child will present with the symptoms of mild ADHD; that is, there will be evidence of hyperactivity, impulsivity, and less task persistence . . . completing self-directed academic tasks especially those that require more planning and organization may be problematic. These children would be more likely to have problems with mathematics than they would have with reading.

A recent explanation for some of the attention deficits noted in children with early-treated PKU was posited by Banich et al (2000), who found that interhemispheric interaction is compromised in the brains of these children as compared with normal controls.

Evaluation of the relationship between various Phe levels and cognitive functioning remains an active area of research. Weglage et al (2001) reported normal intellectual and educational outcomes in 31 adolescent subjects with mild HPA (persistent Phe levels between 360 and 600 μmol/L) when compared with healthy controls. Griffiths et al (2000) found that verbal intelligence in the primary school years tends to normalize if blood Phe is maintained below 360 μmol/L in infancy, but spatial intelligence may remain poor. Huijbregts et al (2002) found that people with PKU with Phe levels above 360 μmol/L exhibited lower speed of information processing, less ability to inhibit task-induced cognitive interference, less consistent performance, and a stronger decrease in performance level over time compared with control subjects.

Physical Problems

Reports of increased incidences of congenital heart disease, cataracts, and peptic ulcer in people with treated PKU have appeared in the literature, although the data are inconclusive. Decreased total bone mineral density and spine bone mineral density may occur in prepubertal children and adults with treated PKU; these changes are associated with an increased incidence of fractures. PKU has been reported to co-exist in the same individual with other genetic conditions, including cystic fibrosis, galactosemia, Duchenne muscular dystrophy, and cystinuria, but these are chance events (Scriver & Kaufman, 2001).

Scaling eczematous dermatitis is more prevalent in children with PKU, presumably because of the toxic effects of phenylalanine and its metabolites. Skin and muscle indurations resembling scleroderma have been reported, especially on the arms and buttocks of young children with PKU. These skin manifestations have been noted to improve with better dietary control (NIH, 2000).

Prognosis

Early-treated individuals with PKU may be expected to grow and develop normally. The lifelong outcome for children with well-treated PKU is yet to be observed, since the oldest treated individuals are currently in their 40s. Several factors affect the prognosis for PKU, including age at time of diagnosis and Phe restriction, degree of metabolic control, and the specific mutation responsible. Adherence to the treatment regimen, a primary predictor of overall health in PKU, is undoubtedly affected by psychosocial factors.

PRIMARY CARE MANAGEMENT

Health Care Maintenance

Growth and Development

Growth and development are generally normal for children with PKU on a controlled, Phe-restricted diet. Careful monitoring of heights, weights, and head circumference on growth charts as well as body mass index is an especially important aspect of primary care of a child with PKU, since efforts to limit Phe may result in inadequate protein or calorie intake. Head circumference, weight, and length should be measured at scheduled monthly intervals for the first year, then every 3 months until after the prepubertal growth spurt, and then every 6 months throughout adolescence to monitor adequacy of diet.

Since diet for life is the primary treatment for PKU, it is important to initiate self-management at an early age. The child must be taught to make low-Phe food choices and to understand the importance of doing so. At the same time, great care must be taken not to make the child feel stigmatized by "different" eating habits. Overemphasizing the restrictions may instill undue fear or guilt in a young child. Establishing a balance between a healthy Phe-restricted diet and making the child feel normal takes a tremendous amount of effort and sensitivity on the part of parents and caregivers.

Diet

"Diet for life" is the primary treatment for PKU. The goals of diet therapy are to maintain blood Phe levels in the safe range and provide adequate amounts of all other nutrients to support growth and prevent protein catabolism. The requirements for the PKU diet vary among individuals and throughout their lifetimes, and Phe levels must be monitored on a regular basis. Blood Phe levels should be maintained between 120 μmol/L (2 mg/dl) and 360 μmol/L (6 mg/dl) up until the age of 12 years (and for women with PKU who may become pregnant) and between 120 μmol/L (2 mg/dl) and 600 μmol/L (10 mg/dl) for all others. The level must not go below 120 μmol/L (2 mg/dl), since some Phe is essential for growth, development, and body processes. Since children with PKU lack PAH, the enzyme that catalyzes the conversion of Phe to tyrosine, Tyr deficiency must be avoided; some practitioners recommend that the ratio of Phe

to Tyr be maintained at less than 4 (Acosta & Yannicelli, 2001; NIH, 2000).

Consultation with a professional nutritionist experienced with PKU is an essential part of care. Dietary management of PKU is simple in theory but very difficult in reality. Parents are often overwhelmed to learn that their child has PKU, yet they must begin to make modifications immediately. Most parents have never heard of PKU at the time their newborn is diagnosed, so they have numerous concerns about the implications of having a genetic condition in the family, the child's prognosis, and the details of the treatment. It takes time for parents to adjust to the diagnosis and to the knowledge that this is a condition that will require lifelong attention and management.

Although the decision to breastfeed is a personal one, clinicians should inform women of the particular advantages of human breast milk for a newborn with PKU. Mature human breast milk has a mean Phe content of 48 mg/dl, which is lower than the mean Phe content of cow's milk (164 mg/dl) and common infant formulas such as Isomil (88 mg/dl) and Similac (59 mg/dl) (Acosta & Yanicelli, 2001). Bottle-fed infants generally accept one of the commercially available Phe-free infant formulas. Since some Phe is essential in the diet, infants are also given a prescribed amount of a Phe-containing formula. Table 35-2 gives the recommended daily nutrient intakes for persons with PKU; these values provide general guidelines but cannot be a substitute for monitoring of Phe levels and nutritional indices. Frequent diet adjustments are necessary throughout life but especially in periods of rapid growth.

Solid foods should be introduced to infants with PKU as they would be for any infant, but parents must monitor and adjust the child's Phe intake. In general, protein foods are high in Phe, so foods to avoid include cheese, eggs, meat, milk,

TABLE 35-2

Recommended Daily Nutrient Intakes (Ranges) for Infants, Children, and Adults with Phenylketonuria

Age	Nutrient				
	Phe	Tyr	Protein	Energy	Fluid
INFANTS	mg/kg	mg/kg	g/kg	kcal/kg	ml/kg
0-3 mo	25-70	300-350	3.50-3.00	120 (95-145)	160-135
3-6 mo	20-45	300-350	3.50-3.00	120 (95-145)	160-130
6-9 mo	15-35	250-300	3.00-2.50	110 (80-135)	145-125
9-12 mo	10-35	250-300	3.00-2.50	105 (80-135)	135-120
GIRLS AND BOYS	mg/day	g/day	g/day	kcal/day	ml/day
1-4 yr	200-400	1.72-3.00	>30	1300 (900-1800)	900-1800
4-7 yr	210-450	2.25-3.50	>35	1700 (1300-2300)	1300-2300
7-11 yr	220-500	2.55-4.00	>40	2400 (1650-3300)	1650-3300
WOMEN					
11-15 yr	250-750	3.45-5.00	>50	2200 (1500-3000)	1500-3000
15-19 yr	230-700	3.45-5.00	>55	2100 (1200-3000)	1200-3000
>19 yr	220-700	3.75-5.00	>60	2100 (1400-2500)	2100-2500
MEN					
11-15 yr	225-900	3.38-5.50	>55	2700 (2000-3700)	2000-3700
15-19 yr	295-1100	4.42-6.50	>65	2800 (2100-3900)	2100-3900
>19 yr	290-1200	4.35-6.50	>70	2900 (2000-3300)	2000-3300

From Acosta, P.B. & Yannicelli, S. (2001). *The Ross metabolic formula system nutrition support protocols* (4th ed.). Columbus, Ohio: Ross Products Division/Abbott Laboratories. Reprinted with permission.

poultry, nuts, dried beans and peas, most breads, seeds, and peanut butter. Foods that are low in protein include fruits, fats, vegetables, sweets, and some cereals. Special low-protein breads, pasta, and cereal should be encouraged, since they will become an important part of the lifelong diet. Such products are commercially available, although many families prefer to prepare their own.

One common method for calculating Phe intake involves the use of exchanges, where one exchange is equal to 15 mg of Phe. Other practitioners prefer to instruct parents to calculate milligrams of Phe and to maintain a daily intake that will keep their blood level in the desired range. Some clinics recommend the use of a gram scale or use standard scoops and household measures. The protein content is listed on food products; as a general rule, 1 g of protein contains approximately 50 mg of Phe (Smith & Lee, 2000). Detailed lists of the Phe content in foods are available from the US Department of Agriculture (USDA) Nutrient Database at www.nal.usda.gov/fnic/cgi-bin/nut_search.pl, medical food companies, the nutritionist at the metabolic clinic, or the National PKU News Web site at www.pkunews.org. Parents may be asked to weigh or measure all the food the child eats for 3 days before the clinic visit and blood test. This diet record allows the nutritionist to calculate necessary adjustments.

All persons with PKU require some elemental medical food (EMF) to maintain proper nutrition. A typical individual requires three servings of EMF per day, and these generally accompany regular meals. In any case, optimal growth and Phe homeostasis are best maintained by distributing the protein intake throughout the day. The EMF products look and taste very different from milk, and many individuals find them unpalatable. Since EMF ingestion is critical for the health of the child with PKU, parents and significant others need to be very careful not to communicate any distaste for the product. Most children readily accept the EMF if it is started early and if the family has a positive attitude about it. The use of straws and "sippy cups" often facilitates EMF ingestion. Some children prefer to have flavorings added to the formula, such as Tang, Kool-aid mixes, chocolate syrup, concentrated fruit juice, or flavor packets available from the EMF company. The nutritionist must approve such flavorings, and great care must be taken to avoid any product containing aspartame, which is converted to Phe in the gastrointestinal tract. Older children may choose to take their EMF in the form of a capsule or bar. Scientific Hospital Supplies (www.shsna.com) makes Phe-free protein capsules that replace formula; however, more than 100 capsules per day may be required. Many states require that insurance companies or state agencies provide formula and/or low-protein foods for individuals with PKU (www.pkunews.org).

Parents should follow the instructions supplied by the manufacturer when preparing EMF products. The amount of powder to be ingested should be carefully measured, although the volume of liquid to be used may be adjusted according to individual preferences. Some children prefer a more concentrated mixture so they have to drink less. It is important that all the powder is ingested, and this may necessitate further dilution of any remaining "sludge" in the bottom of the container. Most people prefer to mix a 24-hour supply of the EMF and

store it in the refrigerator for use the following day. These products should not be heated beyond 54.5° C (130.1° F) to avoid a chemical reaction that alters their protein structure. The shelf life of EMF products is limited, and parents should note the expiration date on the can.

Many children exhibit feeding problems at some point in their development, and children with PKU are no different. However, parents may be more concerned about such problems when they know that their child's health depends on adherence to a strict diet. Parents may be reassured that 1 or 2 days of poor intake will not harm the child, nor will occasional nonsustained elevations in Phe. As with any child, parents should not force feed. It is often useful to offer smaller portions; the child can always ask for more but may feel overwhelmed by large helpings. The EMF should be served first. Giving the child some choice in selection of foods and having large amounts of "free" foods available also are useful strategies (Castiglioni & Rouse, 1995). In an older child, extra protein-free foods may be necessary to meet calorie and energy requirements. These should be monitored carefully, however, since they often contain large amounts of sugar and fat and may lead to obesity if used in excess. There are anecdotal reports of increased incidence of eating disorders in children with PKU. The idea of a young child being on a "diet" may cause confusion or abnormal perceptions about the meaning of food. As one young adult with PKU so aptly put it, "My main advice for parents of children with PKU is to try not to make PKU a big deal or a central issue in the child's life. What you eat is not even remotely close to being the most important aspect of life" (Beck, 1999).

Safety

The only safety concerns particular to PKU are related to nutritional imbalances. Overrestriction resulting in long-term Phe deficiency may lead to aminoaciduria, hypoproteinemia, bone changes, decreased growth, anemia, mental retardation, and hair loss (Acosta & Yannicelli, 2001). Ingestion of Phe that exceeds the individual's tolerance leads to the complications associated with hyperphenylalaninemia. Occasional ingestion of a high-Phe substance such as aspartame is less deleterious than chronic lapses of the restricted diet. Teaching the child and significant others about the importance of a Phe-restricted diet is the best prevention against this hazard. Siblings or others without PKU should not ingest Phe-free formulas, since this may lead to nutritional deficiencies, although occasional or accidental ingestion would have no adverse effects.

Immunizations

Immunizations are administered to children with PKU on the recommended schedule.

Screening

Vision. Routine screening is recommended.
Hearing. Routine screening is recommended.
Dental. The diet for PKU includes a high proportion of carbohydrates to meet the daily requirement for calories. Dietary sugars are known to increase the risk for dental caries, although one recent study found no greater incidence in tooth decay in children with PKU (Lucas et al, 2001). To promote dental

health, parents should be cautioned not to put the baby to bed with a bottle. Infants should be weaned to a cup as early as 6 months of age. Free foods such as fruits should be offered in place of more retentive forms of refined sugars, as well as liquid forms of carbohydrate that promote oral clearance. Fluoride supplementation is recommended if it is not added to the local water supply. Oral hygiene and dentist visits should be implemented soon after the teeth erupt. Children with PKU who were diagnosed late may require specialized dental care if they have enamel hypoplasia or abnormal tooth spacing.

Blood Pressure. Routine screening is recommended.

Hematocrit. Children on protein-restricted semisynthetic diets are at risk for inadequate intake of iron and other trace elements. Hematocrit monitoring and related tests are part of the biochemical nutritional assessment done at the metabolic clinic. Primary care practitioners should communicate with the metabolic practitioner to determine the need for additional tests.

Urinalysis. Routine screening is recommended.

Tuberculosis. Routine screening is recommended.

Condition-Specific Screening (Box 35-4)

Newborn Screening and Testing. A positive newborn screening test for elevated Phe is not a positive diagnosis for PKU. Fewer than 30% to 50% of infants identified through newborn screening will ultimately be diagnosed with PKU or HPA (Wilcox & Cederbaum, 2002). An infant with a positive screening test should be referred to a metabolic specialty center for a diagnostic work-up as soon as possible. This evaluation will reveal false-positive results or identify the specific enzyme defect responsible for the hyperphenylalaninemia. Although 98% to 99% of cases of PKU result from phenylalanine hydroxylase (PAH) deficiency, it is essential to rule out defects in the biopterin synthase group of enzymes, dihydropterin reductase (DHPR) deficiency, or PAH with decreased affinity for BH_4, since these require different therapies. For newborns with a positive screening test, blood Phe and tyrosine should be quantified. If the blood Phe elevation persists and Tyr is within normal limits, pterin metabolites in the urine and DHPR in the blood will be evaluated (Acosta & Yannicelli, 2001; Smith & Lee, 2000; Wilcox & Cederbaum, 2002).

Blood Phe Monitoring. Plasma Phe and Tyr levels are evaluated twice weekly in newborns with PKU until concentrations are stabilized and approximate dietary Phe and Tyr requirements are known. Thereafter, blood Phe is evaluated weekly until age 1 year, twice monthly until age 12 years, monthly after age 12 years, and twice weekly for pregnant women (NIH, 2000). Parents may be taught to collect the capillary blood samples at home and return them to the metabolic clinic or other laboratory. These results are evaluated by the PKU treatment center team, and dietary adjustments are made as needed.

Nutritional Indices Monitoring. Nutrient intake is recorded on provided forms for 3 days before each blood Phe test and evaluated for Phe, Tyr, protein, and energy intake by the nutritionist on the PKU treatment team. Protein status is evaluated by plasma transthyretin, albumin, or prealbumin levels every 3 months in infants and every 6 months in children and adolescents. The metabolic treatment team also monitors for insufficient intake of iron, folate, vitamin B_{12}, and other nutrients (Acosta & Yannicelli, 2001).

Mutation Analysis. DNA analysis to determine the specific PKU mutation may be suggested by the PKU specialty center. At the present time this information is not required for routine diagnostic or therapeutic decisions, but it may be useful for genetic counseling.

Common Illness Management

Differential Diagnosis

Well-nourished children with PKU respond to infection and trauma in the same way as any child. Children with chronically elevated Phe levels may exhibit the associated signs and symptoms of PKU, including eczematous skin lesions, musty body odor, and cognitive and neurologic sequelae.

Management During Illness and Surgery. Minor uncomplicated surgery with general anesthesia does not cause a major alteration in the blood Phe level. Febrile illness and trauma are normally accompanied by protein catabolism, which may result in elevation of plasma Phe concentrations. These elevations are generally transient and do not require additional Phe monitoring. Supportive measures should be undertaken to limit protein catabolism. Liberal volumes of fruit juices, liquid gelatin, caffeine-free soft drinks, or electrolyte formulas (e.g., Pedialyte) without aspartame should be allowed. Polycose powder or liquid or a Phe-free additive recommended by the medical food company may be mixed with the fluids. Acetaminophen, ibuprofen, antibiotics or other medications may be recommended or prescribed as for any child, but the Phe content of these substances must be taken into consideration. EMFs are reinstituted as soon as possible, initially at half strength. If parenteral amino acid solutions are indicated for any reason, involvement of a specialist familiar with PKU is necessary (Acosta & Yannicelli, 2001).

Drug Interactions

Aspartame. Aspartame (L-aspartyl-L-phenylalanine methyl ester [APM]) is contraindicated in individuals with PKU because it is converted to phenylalanine in the gastrointestinal tract. Currently marketed under the brand names NutraSweet,

TABLE 35-3
Phe Content of Selected Medications*

Product	Phe content
Children's Tylenol chewable tablets	
80-mg Fruit Burst flavor	5 mg/tablet
80-mg Great Grape flavor	3 mg/tablet
160-mg Fruit and Grape flavors	6 mg/tablet
Dimetapp Cold & Allergy chewable tablet	8 mg/tablet
TheraFlu Flu & Cold Medicine	25 mg/packet
Flintstones Complete chewable tablets	2 mg/tablet
Amoxicillin, 250-mg chewable tablets (Warner-Chilcott)	2 mg/tablet
Pedialyte freezer pops	16 mg/pop

*NOTE: This information was taken from pkunews.org, updated January 2002. It is provided only as an example and must be confirmed with the manufacturer, since formulations change frequently.

Equal, Sweetmate, or Canderal, aspartame must be identified on the label of all products with the statement "Phenylketonurics: Contains phenylalanine." This popular artificial sweetener is used in numerous foods, chewing gums, drinks, and liquid medicines. A quart of aspartame-sweetened fruit drink contains 280 mg of Phe, more than one half the daily allowance for a child with PKU (Scriver & Kaufman, 2001).

Parents should be cautioned about aspartame in over-the-counter medications or vitamins or any product labeled "sugar free." The exact amount of Phe in medications must be calculated as part of a child's daily Phe intake. A variety of resources are available for information about the Phe content of medications, including the manufacturer, the product information, a pharmacist, or the *Physicians' Desk Reference* (*PDR*) (Medical Economics Staff, 2003). The National PKU News Web site (www.pkunews.org) has a frequently updated list of the Phe content of over-the-counter and prescription medications; a few of the common ones are listed in Table 35-3.

Developmental Issues

Sleep Patterns

There are no particular sleep disturbances associated with PKU. Routine counseling about establishing and maintaining healthy sleep habits is recommended.

Toileting

Children with PKU achieve bowel and bladder control at the same age as children without PKU. If Phe levels are chronically elevated, the child may be more prone to eczematous skin lesions that are associated with an increased risk for diaper rash. There is a characteristic musty smell to urine containing Phe metabolites, but this does not occur in well-treated PKU.

Discipline

Parenting strategies for the child with PKU are the same as for any child. Positive reinforcement of good behavior is always more effective than negative reinforcement of undesirable behavior. Limit setting and consistent expectations are essential, even if the parent has ambivalent feelings because the child has a chronic condition.

Food is an important social factor in any child's life, and how it is managed from the very beginning by parents can determine the success of the therapy. A major pitfall in disciplining children with PKU is to use food as a reward system and the need for blood tests as punishment. It is critical to establish strict habits when the child is very young, since the child must begin to make the right food choices independently once school age is reached.

Child Care

All individuals in the child's home environment should be knowledgeable about the Phe-restricted diet and the preparation of the EMF products. Grandparents and other caregivers play an essential role in supporting the diet and should be included in educational sessions at the metabolic clinic or in primary care. Significant others must support the parents' efforts to provide the diet and resist the temptation to "treat" the child to ice cream or other restricted foods. Most daycare providers will feed the child whatever the parents send but will need to be educated about the importance of dietary restrictions and the potential hazards of sharing protein foods with other children in the daycare. Parents devise creative ways to make their child feel "normal," such as preparing low-Phe "look-alike" treats to take to birthday parties or other activities that involve food. As the child's primary advocates, parents find themselves teaching others in the community about PKU on a constant basis.

Schooling

Children with PKU are likely to progress in school just like other children. Although there is some evidence of an increased risk for attention deficit hyperactivity disorder or mild cognitive dysfunction, most experts agree that these may be minimized with good control of Phe. If a child needs to be evaluated for an individualized educational plan (IEP), the primary care or metabolic care provider may be involved in reviewing the plan or communicating information about the child. Children with PKU generally undergo psychologic testing at the PKU treatment center, including developmental assessments, language development tests, intelligence tests, and tests of executive functioning or attention. Testing is begun around 6 months of age, continued every 6 months until 2 years of age, and done at annual or 3-year intervals thereafter. For optimal performance, it is important that the child's blood Phe level be in maintenance range on the day of testing.

School personnel may have little or no knowledge of or experience with PKU. It is often necessary for the professionals at the metabolic clinic or the primary care practice or the parents to educate teachers, cafeteria personnel, and school administrators about the child's special needs. The school nurse may be enlisted to assist with these efforts. A useful publication, "A Teacher's Guide to PKU," is available through the Texas Department of Health at www.tdh.state.tx.us/newborn/teach-pku.htm. This booklet explains PKU and gives teachers specific guidelines related to dietary restrictions. Since diet is the primary aspect of life affected by PKU, cafeteria personnel can be of great help in preventing the child from feeling different. Many parents report that their children have positive experiences with school meals thanks to the willingness of the personnel to provide detailed information about weekly cafeteria menus, to heat meals sent from home, to weigh portions, or to give the child specially prepared items. Open and frequent communication between the family and the school is essential.

Sexuality

Sexual development and curiosity are no different for children with PKU than for any other child. Females with PKU must be educated from an early age about strict Phe control before and throughout pregnancy. The best approach to prevention of maternal PKU is to foster adherence to diet at all times. Numerous educational materials are available for parents and adolescents related to sexuality and PKU. These may be obtained from the metabolic center or through links at the National PKU News Web site (www.pkunews.org). Discussions of contraception and the implications of being a woman with PKU should be individualized and approached with sensitivity. PKU peer support groups, online chat rooms, and written materials and videos designed specifically for adolescents with PKU are available.

Transition into Adulthood

All adolescents face the challenges of peer pressure, desire for independence from authority figures, and social and emotional change. Adolescents with conditions such as PKU or diabetes need much support to adhere to a restricted diet and to take their medical foods. Despite clinic recommendations to adhere to the diet for life, studies have shown that adolescents often discontinue the diet (NIH, 2000). Pediatric metabolic clinics may not routinely follow individuals with PKU after the age of 18 years since many individuals transfer their care to practitioners who care for adults. It is not unusual for persons in this age-group to abandon routine medical care for a variety of reasons. Every effort must be made to ensure that individuals with PKU receive continuing primary care given the recent compelling evidence of the benefits of lifelong therapy and the need to prevent the growing problem of maternal PKU syndrome.

Before the 1980s, most adults with PKU relaxed or discontinued Phe restriction. Consequently, many adults with PKU are currently attempting to reinstitute the diet. This has proved to be very difficult, and individuals may benefit from the guidance of professionals who can promote adherence, primary care providers, family counseling, and peer support mechanisms. Previously untreated adults with PKU may show improvement in behavior, neurologic status, and IQ (Koch et al, 1999) after institution of a low-Phe diet, and specific protocols are available (Acosta & Yannicelli, 1997).

Special Concerns of Women of Childbearing Age. Since contact with a metabolic clinic is often lost in adulthood, primary care practitioners have an essential role in the prevention of maternal PKU syndrome. Women of childbearing age must prevent pregnancy or maintain Phe levels between 120 µmol/L (2 mg/dl) and 360 µmol/L (6 mg/dl) before conception to prevent birth defects in the fetus. This should be reinforced at every opportunity by practitioners who care for adolescents and women with PKU or HPA.

Pregnancy in women with PKU is a medical challenge. Phe must be restricted, but adequate tyrosine, vitamins, and other nutrients must be supplied. Ideally, a practitioner familiar with PKU or one who is in close association with such an expert will provide prenatal care. Special EMF products and detailed guidelines for nutrition management are available (Acosta & Yannicelli, 2001).

Several factors affect a woman's adherence to a Phe-restricted diet in pregnancy, including age, socioeconomic status, and social support. Women with higher intellectual levels are more likely to follow dietary guidelines; thus women with late-diagnosed or inadequately treated PKU are at greater risk for having affected offspring. Strategies that have improved dietary adherence in pregnant women include the use of specially trained resource mothers and maternal PKU camps. Internet-based and other methods for tracking and communicating with women at risk are currently being developed.

Phenylketonuria in Men. Although much emphasis had been placed on adherence to diet in women with PKU owing to the grave effects of Phe on the fetus, young men should also be counseled about the importance of diet for life and supported in this endeavor by their primary care practitioner. The benefits of Phe level maintenance include decreased depression, agitation, and aggressiveness and improved attention span, concentration, and skin condition.

Family Concerns and Resources

Despite strong evidence of the effectiveness of dietary treatment of PKU, many affected individuals fail to adhere to the recommendations. Barriers to adherence include the complexity of the treatment regimen, poor palatability and cost of the medical food, and psychosocial factors. Cultural practices have an impact on the family's acceptance and management of PKU. Beliefs about disease causality, customs related to parenting, and dietary preferences are just some of the factors a practitioner must consider in order to provide comprehensive care. Families often have a difficult time adjusting to the frequent clinic visits, blood draws, and rigid diet control required to care for a child with PKU.

Successful treatment of a child with PKU requires the support and commitment of everyone involved with the child. More than one individual in the home should be knowledgeable about the Phe-restricted diet, preparation of EMF products, and obtaining blood samples. It is not necessary or advisable for the entire family to adopt the eating habits of the child with PKU, although children in vegetarian families may have less difficulty adhering to the protein-restricted PKU diet. The focus of mealtime discussions should be on topics other than the food.

Raising a child with PKU can be very expensive. The financial burden of PKU is variable, owing to inconsistent policies on the part of third-party payers, Medicare/Medicaid, and other entities regarding funding for medical and supportive care, formula, and low-protein foods. A list of state laws and policies related to reimbursement for formula and foods is posted on the National PKU News Web site (www.pkunews.org). Although most states require coverage for infant formula, many do not cover the cost of foods. The primary care provider may need to intercede on behalf of the parents in negotiating coverage of the expenses of EMF, low-protein medical foods, and blood Phe monitoring.

The diagnosis of PKU has implications for blood relatives of the affected child. Parents with a child with PKU are obligate carriers of the disorder and face a 25% recurrence risk in subsequent pregnancies. Other children in the family, grandparents, and the child's aunts and uncles may also carry the gene. Genetic counseling can be provided by a metabolic physician, a genetic counselor, or a specially trained nurse, social worker, psychologist, or other provider. Carrier testing is available for families whose mutations are known, although some individuals prefer not to know, since there is some psychologic burden associated with genetic information. Parents with a child with PKU may choose to prevent another affected pregnancy through contraception, prenatal diagnosis with pregnancy termination, or preimplantation genetic diagnosis. Factors shown to have the greatest impact on reproductive decisions of parents with a child with a metabolic disorder include stress, worry about the child's future, difficulty meeting the child's needs, and lower functional level of the child (Read, 2002).

RESOURCES

Numerous supports are available for families with PKU. The metabolic clinic will provide information and referrals, but parents increasingly use the World Wide Web as a resource. This has led to a change in health care, whereby consumers come to clinicians with questions about information they have gathered. Many levels of information are available to consumers on the Internet, from full-text articles in leading medical journals to informal discussions in chat rooms. Providers have a responsibility to assist clients to evaluate such resources. PKU is a rare disease, and parents quickly become informed consumers who educate others about their child's condition. Two organizations provide comprehensive guides to current information and resources.

National PKU News

This nonprofit organization is dedicated to providing accurate and up-to-date information to families and professionals. The Web site (www.pkunews.org) provides direct information and links to a wide variety of resources related to PKU. The organization also publishes a newsletter three times per year. Membership in the organization, subscriptions to the newsletter, and additional information may be obtained by contacting the following:

Virginia Schuett, MS, RD, Director and Editor
National PKU News
6869 Woodlawn Ave NE, #116
Seattle, WA 98115-5469
206-525-8140
schuett@pkunews.org

The following are some items of interest on the PKU News Web site:
- Articles about all aspects of PKU, including personal stories written by parents and teens
- Diet information, including low-protein food companies, lists of Phe content in foods and medicines, order forms for PKU cookbooks, screening and treatment guidelines, practical information about dietary adherence for all age-groups

- Information about legislation to cover PKU costs
- Summaries of current research related to PKU
- Information about support groups, PKU treatment centers, meetings, camps, and other events
- A comprehensive list of audiovisual and written materials about PKU; includes materials appropriate for professionals, parents, siblings
- Instructions for joining the PKU E-mail mailing list

There are more than 1000 subscribers to this mailing list from more than 20 countries. Its purpose is to provide a vehicle for communication among families of children with PKU, young adults with PKU, and professionals treating PKU. This busy mailing list often has as many as 25 entries per day, with a wide range of comments and inquiries about cooking tips, low-protein recipes, issues related to diet management, low-protein food sources, and information about other support groups. It is not intended to be a source of medical information or advice, although professionals occasionally respond to questions.

Children's PKU Network

This national nonprofit organization aims to address the special needs and concerns of children and families with PKU. The Web site (www.pkunetwork.org) provides information and links to multiple resources. Materials may also be obtained by contacting the following:

Children's PKU Network
3970 Via De La Valle, Ste 120
Del Mar, CA 92014
(800) 377-6677(toll-free); (858) 509-0767; fax: 858-509-0768
pkunetwork@aol.com

Some items of interest on the Children's PKU Network Web site include the following:
- General information about the disorder
- Information about how to obtain free "Express Packs" that contain booklets, videos, and other materials about PKU; available both for families of a newborn with PKU and women with PKU of childbearing age who are at risk for having a fetus with maternal PKU syndrome
- Crisis intervention programs
- Scholarship information
- Research clearinghouse
- Information about food scales
- A comprehensive list of low-protein food companies and links to other PKU-related publications and resources

Other Web Sites

www.tdh.state.tx.us/newborn/teachpku.htm
Texas Department of Health
"A Teacher's Guide to PKU," a booklet that explains PKU and gives teachers specific guidelines related to dietary restrictions

www.nal.usda.gov/fnic/cgi-bin/nut_search.pl
USDA Nutrient Database
Detailed lists of Phe content in foods

www.pahdb.mcgill.ca
An on-line database of the mutations in the human PAH gene

Acknowledgement The authors gratefully acknowledge the contribution of Kathleen Schmidt Yule, the author of this chapter in previous editions.

Summary of Primary Care Needs for the Child with Phenylketonuria

HEALTH CARE MAINTENANCE

Growth and Development

Growth and development are normal on a Phe-restricted diet.

Careful monitoring of growth charts is necessary to ensure adequate nutrient intake and to avoid obesity from high-carbohydrate, high-fat foods.

Diet

Breast-feeding is recommended for infants.

Involvement of a professional nutritionist is essential.

Phe-restricted diet is for life.

Dietary modifications are dictated by blood Phe and Tyr levels.

Self-management of Phe-restricted diet should be initiated early in childhood.

Elemental medical food (EMF) products should be prepared as prescribed and taken with meals.

Avoid overemphasis on the diet as the central issue in one's life.

Safety

Only individuals with a diagnosis of PKU should ingest EMF products as prescribed.

Occasional high Phe levels are unlikely to be detrimental.

Immunizations

Routine immunizations are recommended.

Screening

Vision. Routine screening is recommended.
Hearing. Routine screening is recommended.
Dental. Early evaluation is recommended because of the high-carbohydrate diet.
Blood Pressure. Routine screening is recommended.
Hematocrit. Hematocrit is part of the nutritional assessment at metabolic clinic; routine screening is as for any child.
Urinalysis. Routine screening is recommended.
Tuberculosis. Routine screening is recommended.

Condition-Specific Screening (see Box 35-4)

COMMON ILLNESS MANAGEMENT

Catabolic state related to common childhood illness should be prevented with adequate hydration and caloric intake. Transient Phe increases during periods of illness are expected. Analgesics, antipyretics, and antibiotics should be used as for any child, but formulations with the lowest Phe content should be sought.

Drug Interactions

Aspartame ingestion is contraindicated.

Check Phe content of all medications.

DEVELOPMENTAL ISSUES

Sleep Patterns

Routine counseling is recommended.

Toileting

Routine counseling is recommended.

Discipline

Expectations are normal based on age and developmental level.

Avoid use of food as a reward system and blood tests as punishment.

Child Care

All care providers must be aware of dietary modifications.

Schooling

Children with good Phe control generally progress normally.

Developmental testing should be done at the metabolic clinic.

School personnel must be made aware of child's dietary restrictions.

Sexuality

Young women with PKU should be educated about the risks of maternal PKU syndrome.

Transition into Adulthood

All individuals should remain on a Phe-restricted diet for life.

Participation in PKU support groups and professional counseling as needed are recommended for adults with PKU and their families.

FAMILY CONCERNS

Many barriers exist that prevent persons with PKU from adhering to the diet, including complexity and inconvenience, poor palatability and cost of the foods, and psychosocial factors.

Multiple supports are available and should be promoted by the practitioner.

Genetic counseling for all family members is advisable.

REFERENCES

Acosta, P.B. & Yannicelli, S. (1997). Ross metabolic formula system: Nutrition support protocol for previously untreated adults with phenylketonuria. Columbus, Ohio: Ross Products Division/Abbott Laboratories.

Acosta, P.B. & Yannicelli, S. (Eds.). (2001). Ross metabolic formula system: Nutrition support protocols (4th ed.). Columbus, Ohio: Ross Products Division/Abbott Laboratories.

American Academy of Pediatrics. (1996). Committee on Genetics: Newborn screening facts sheets. *Pediatrics, 98,* 473-501;
Web site: http://www.aap.org/policy/01565.html.

Andrade, J.D. (2002). ChemChip project at the University of Utah. *National PKU News, 14*(1), 1.

Antshel, K. (2001). ADHD and PKU. *National PKU News, 13*(2), 3.

Ayares, D. & D'Arcy, A. (1999). Alpha-Lac: Another diet supplement on the horizon. *National PKU News, 10*(3), 2.

Banich, M.T., Passarotti, A.M., White, D.A., Nortz, M.J., & Steiner, R.D. (2000). Interhemispheric interaction during childhood. II. Children with early-treated phenylketonuria. *Dev Neuropsychol, 18*(1), 53-71.

Baumeister, A. & Baumeister, A. (1998). Dietary treatment of destructive behavior associated with hyperphenylalaninemia. *Clin Neuropharmacol, 21*(1), 18-27.

Beblo, S., Reinhardt, H., Muntau, A.C., Mueller-Felber, W., Roscher, A.A., et al. (2001). Fish oil supplementation improves visual evoked potentials in children with phenylketonuria. *Neurology, 57*(8), 1488-1491.

Beck, T. (1999). My life with PKU. *National PKU News, 10*(3), 11-12; Web site: http://www.astro.sunysb.edu/tracy/mystory.html.

Castiglioni, L. & Rouse, B. (1995). *The child with PKU*. Galveston, Tex.: Department of Pediatrics, University of Texas Medical Branch; Web site: www.tdh.state.tx.us/newborn/childpku.htm.

Centers for Disease Control and Prevention. (2002). Barriers to dietary control among pregnant women with phenylketonuria—United States, 1998-2000. *MMWR Morb Mortal Wkly Rep, 51*, 117-120.

Etzel, M.R. (2002). Glycomacropeptide (GMP) update. *National PKU News, 14*(1), 2.

Giewska, M., Cyryowski, L., Jowiak, I., Bich, W., Romanowska, H., et al. (2001). A diet with large neutral amino acids supplementation as a combined treatment for difficult to control or late diagnosed patients with PKU—preliminary data. *J Inherit Metab Dis, 24*(suppl. 1), 22 (abstract).

Griffiths, P.Y., Demellweek, C., Fay, N., Robinson, P.H., & Davidson, D.C. (2000). Wechsler subscale IQ and subtest profile in early treated phenylketonuria. *Arch Dis Child, 82*(3), 209-215.

Guttler, F. & Guldberg, P. (2000). Mutation analysis anticipates dietary requirements in phenylketonuria. *Eur J Pediatr, 159*(suppl. 2), S150-S153.

Hainline, B.E. & Ems-McClung, S.C. (1999). Gamma zein: A new high protein Phe-free diet supplement under development. *National PKU News, 10*(3), 1-2.

Huijbregts, S.C., de Sonneville, L.M., Licht, R., van Spronsen, F.J., Verkerk, P.H., et al. (2002). Sustained attention and inhibition of cognitive interference in treated phenylketonuria: Associations with concurrent and lifetime phenylalanine concentrations. *Neuropsychologica, 40*(1), 7-15.

Kalsner, L.R., Rohr, F.J., Strauss, K.A., Korson, M.S., & Levy, H.L. (2001). Tyrosine supplementation in phenylketonuria: Diurnal blood tyrosine levels and presumptive brain influx of tyrosine and other large neutral amino acids. *J Pediatr, 139*(3), 421-427.

Koch, R., Moseley, K., Ning, J., Romstad, A., Guldberg, P. et al. (1999). Long-term beneficial effects of the phenylalanine restricted diet in late diagnosed individuals with phenylketonuria. *Mol Genet Metab, 67*(2), 148-155.

Koch, R. & Wenz, E. (1987). Phenylketonuria. *Ann Rev Nutr, 7*, 117-135.

Levy, H.L., Guldberg, P. Guttler, F., Hanley, W.B., Matalon, R., et al. (2001). Congenital heart disease in maternal phenylketonuria: Report from the Maternal PKU Collaborative Study. *Pediatr Res, 49*(5), 636-642.

Lucas, V.S., Contreras, A., Loukissa, M., & Roberts, G.J. (2001). Dental disease and caries related oral microflora in children with phenylketonuria. *ASDC J Dent Child, 68*(4), 263, 267, 229.

Medical Economics Staff (Eds.). (2003). *Physicians' desk reference* (57th ed.). Oradell, N.J.: Medical Economics Co.

Miller, D. (2002). Acoint works on non-invasive phenylalanine monitoring device. National *PKU News, 14*(1), 1-2.

Moseley, K., Koch, R., & Moser, A.B. (2002). Lipid status and long-chain polyunsaturated fatty acid concentrations in adults and adolescents with phenylketonuria on phenylalanine-restricted diets. *J Inherit Metab Dis, 25*(1), 56-64.

National Institutes of Health. (2000). Phenylketonuria (PKU): Screening and management. *NIH Consensus Statement, 17*(3); Web site: www.nichd.nih.gov/publications/pubs/pku/index.htm.

Newborn Screening Committee. (1999). The Council of Regional Networks for Genetics Services (CORN). National newborn screening report—1994. Atlanta: CORN.

Nissenkorn, A., Michelson, M., Ben-Zeev, B., & Lerman-Sagie, T. (2001). Inborn errors of metabolism: A cause of abnormal brain development. *Neurology, 56*(10), 1265-1272.

Nussbaum, R., McInnes, R., & Willard, H. (2001). *Thompson & Thompson genetics in medicine* (6th ed.). Philadelphia: W.B. Saunders.

Pietz, J., Kreis, R., Rupp, A., Mayatepek, E., Rating, D., et al. (1999). Large neutral amino acids block phenylalanine transport into brain tissue in patients with phenylketonuria. *J Clin Invest, 103*(8), 1169-1178.

Read, C.Y. (2002). Reproductive decisions of parents of children with metabolic disorders. *Clin Genet, 61*, 268-276.

Rezvani, I. (2000). Defects in metabolism of amino acids: Phenylalanine. In R.E. Behrman, R.M. Kliegman, & H.B. Jenson (Eds.). *Nelson textbook of pediatrics* (16th ed.). Philadelphia: W.B. Saunders.

Rouse, B., Azen, C., Koch, R., Matalon, R., Hanley, W., et al. (1997). Maternal phenylketonuria collaborative study (MPKUCS) offspring: Facial anomalies, malformations, and early neurological sequelae. *Am J Med Genet, 69*, 89-95.

Rouse, B., Matalon, R., Koch, R. Azen, C., Levy, H., et al. (2000). Maternal phenylketonuria syndrome: Congenital heart defects, microcephaly, and developmental outcomes. *J Pediatr, 136*(1), 57-61.

Sarkissian, C.N., Shao, Z., Blain, F., Peevers, R., Su, H., et al. (1999). A different approach to treatment of phenylketonuria: Phenylalanine degradation with recombinant phenylalanine ammonia lyase. *Proc Natl Acad Sci USA, 96*, 2339-2344.

Schuett, V. (2002). BH4 may help "hyperphe." *National PKU News, 14*(1), 3.

Scriver, C.R. & Kaufman, S. (2001). Hyperphenylalaninemia: Phenylalanine hydroxylase deficiency. In C.R. Scriver et al (Eds.). *The metabolic and molecular bases of inherited disease*, vol. II (8th ed.). New York: McGraw-Hill, pp. 1667-1724.

Smith, I. & Knowles, J. (2000). Behaviour in early treated phenylketonuria: A systematic review. *Eur J Pediatr, 159*(suppl. 2), S89-S93.

Smith, I. & Lee, P. (2000). The hyperphenylalaninemias. In J. Fernandes, J.M. Saudubray, & G. Van den Berghe (Eds.). *Inborn metabolic disease: Diagnosis and treatment* (3rd ed.). New York: Springer.

Spirito, F., Meneguzzi, G., Danos, O., & Mezzina, M. (2001). Cutaneous gene transfer and therapy: The present and future. *J Gene Med, 3*(1), 21-31.

Van Bakel, M.M., Printzen, G., Wermuth, B., & Weismann, U.N. (2000). Antioxidant and thyroid hormone status in selenium-deficient phenylketonuric and hyperphenylalaninemic patients. *Am J Clin Nutr, 72*(4), 976-981.

Van Spronsen, F.J., van Rijn, M., Bekhof, J., Koch, R., & Smit, P.G. (2001). Phenylketonuria: Tyrosine supplementation in phenylalanine-restricted diets. *Am J Clin Nutr, 73*(2), 153-157.

Weglage, J., Pietsch, M., Feldmann, R., Koch, H.G., Zschocke, J., et al. (2001). Normal clinical outcome in untreated subjects with mild hyperphenylalaninemia. *Pediatr Res, 49*(4), 532-536.

Welsh, M.C. & Pennington, B.F. (2000). Phenylketonuria. In K.O. Yeats, D. Ris, & H.G. Taylor (Eds.). *Pediatric neuropsychology: Research, theory, and practice*. New York: Guilford Press, pp. 275-299.

Wilcox, W.R. & Cederbaum, S.D. (2002). Amino acid metabolism. In J.M. Connor, R. Pyeritz, B. Korf, & D.L. Rimoin (Eds.). *Emery & Rimoin's principles and practice of medical genetics* (4th ed) Philadelphia: W.B. Saunders, pp. 2405-2440.

Zhongshu, Z., Weiming, Y., Yukio, F., Cheng-Lning, Z., & Zhixing, W. (2001). Clinical analysis of West syndrome associated with phenylketonuria. *Brain Dev, 23*(7), 552-557.

36 Prematurity

Patricia Jackson Allen and Mary E. Lynch

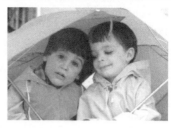

Etiology

Premature, low birth weight (LBW) infants are a heterogeneous group. At one end of the spectrum are extremely low birth weight (ELBW) infants who are critically ill and require prolonged neonatal intensive care and if they survive often experience chronic pulmonary, gastrointestinal, and/or neurologic sequelae. At the other end of the spectrum are premature infants who have little or no neonatal health complications and require no special long-term care. Historically the term *low birth rate* has been used almost synonymously with the term *premature,* but this can be misleading. For example, some term infants have birth weights less than 2,500 g (these infants are termed *small for gestational age* [SGA]), and some premature infants have birth weights greater than 2500 g (these infants are termed *large for gestational age* [LGA]). *Appropriate for gestational age* (AGA) infants have a birth weight within the normal range for their gestational age whether they are full-term or preterm (Kenner & Lott, 2003).

Premature, or preterm infants, are born before 37 completed weeks of gestation (Gardner et al, 2002). LBW refers to infants whose birth weight is less than 2,500 g and comprise 7% to 8% of all births (MacDorman et al, 2002b); very low birth weight (VLBW) refers to infants weighing less than 1,500 g at birth, approximately 1% of all births; and ELBW refers to infants weighing less than 1,000 g at birth (Kliegman, 2002). Although the infant mortality rate has improved in the United States, there has been no improvement in the LBW rate and this is one of the major reasons the infant mortality rate has remained high compared with other industrialized countries (Kliegman, 2002).

The causes of preterm birth are varied, and many are interrelated. There are two primary phenomena associated with preterm birth: (1) the infant may need to be delivered preterm because of maternal and/or fetal problems, i.e., maternal hypertension, maternal infection, fetal distress, or multiple gestation, or (2) the infant is born because of spontaneous preterm labor or preterm rupture of fetal membranes (Abrahams & Katz, 2002; Kliegman, 2002). Some of the known causes or risk factors are listed in Box 36-1. Assisted reproductive technology (ART) (i.e., in vitro fertilization) is associated with an increased incidence of multifetal preterm births when compared with either singleton or multiple spontaneous pregnancies (Centers for Disease Control and Prevention [CDC], 2000; Kogan et al, 2000) and with the increased use of ART, there has been the consequential higher incidence of multiple preterm births. Delayed childbearing beyond 35 years of age has also contributed to increasing the preterm birth rate and LBW

(Tough et al, 2002; MacDorman et al, 2002a). In many cases a specific cause or risk factor cannot be identified, or the etiology potentially begins preconceptually (Abrahams & Katz, 2002). Until there is a better understanding of the causes of preterm birth, particularly in relation to maternal infection, it is unlikely that a substantial reduction in the preterm birth rate will occur (MacDorman et al, 2002b; Martin et al, 2002).

Known Genetic Etiology

To date there have been no specific genetic disorders that have been directly linked to preterm birth. In addition, although preterm infants do not experience an increased risk for congenital malformations, genetic syndromes or inborn errors of metabolism, congenital anomalies are often associated with preterm delivery (Matthews & Robin, 2002). Preterm infants who experience intrauterine growth restriction from unknown etiology and/or who demonstrate dysmorphic features should be referred for genetic evaluation.

Incidence and Prevalence

Birth certificate gestational data reveal that the preterm birth rate dropped from 11.8% of all births in 1999 to 11.6% in 2000 (MacDorman et al, 2002a). This was the first decline in the preterm birth rate since 1992, which had previously risen steadily from 9.4% in 1981 and 10.6% in 1990. A greater time interval is needed to determine if this first nominal decrease in the preterm birth rate will continue through this decade. The very preterm birth rate (<32 weeks' gestation) remained at 1.9% of all live births in 1999-2000. Multifetal pregnancies contributed to the preterm birth rate and measures of infant health with approximately 50% of all twins and the majority of triplet and higher-order births resulting in preterm or LBW infants (Martin et al, 2002; MacDorman et al, 2002b).

There has been no improvement in specific birth weight rates in relation to preterm birth in 2000. The LBW rate has remained at 7.6% since 1997 and has risen steadily from 6.7% in 1984 (CDC, 2002). The VLBW rate remains steady at 1.43% having risen from 1.15% of births in 1980 (CDC). In addition to the initial health care risks at birth, the risk of infant death in 2000 was 6 times higher for LBW infants and 98 times higher for VLBW infants in comparison to infants weighing ≥2,500 g (MacDorman et al, 2002b; Mathews et al, 2002). A racial disparity in birth weight continues. The incidence of LBW among black infants is approximately two times that among white infants and is primarily attributed to a preterm birth rate of 17.3% in black infants as compared with 10.6% in white infants and 11.2% in Hispanic infants (Alexander et al, 2003;

BOX 36-1
Causes of Preterm Birth

INDICATIONS FOR PRETERM DELIVERY
Maternal indications
   Severe preeclampsia
   Infection placing mother or infant at risk
   Bleeding (previa, abruption)
   Cardiovascular instability
   Uncontrolled diabetes

Fetal indications
   Poor growth (IUGR)
   Death of an identical twin
   Unstable biophysical profile
   Hydrops
   Severe alloimmunization and hemolysis

SPONTANEOUS PRETERM DELIVERY
Maternal risk factors
   Prior premature birth
   Prior abortion
   Pariety = 0 or >4
   Incompetent or abnormal cervix
   Abnormal placenta
   Infection (bacterial vaginosis)
   Drug use (alcohol, cocaine, tobacco, etc.)
   Preterm rupture of membranes
   Short interval since last live born
   Previous cesarean section
   Uterine anomaly
   Poor nutrition
   Anemia (Hbg <10 g/dl)
   Inadequate prenatal care
   Poor social environment
   Age <18 years

Fetal risk factors
   Multiple gestation
   Fetal anomalies

BOX 36-2
Treatment

PREVENTION OF PREMATURITY
   Ensure prenatal care
   Avoid drugs, tobacco, and alcohol
   Prolong gestation (tocolytics)
   Identify early signs of labor

TREATMENT IN UTERO
   Corticosteroids given to mother to increase fetal lung maturation
   Prevent infection (antenatal antibiotics)
   Birth at a center for high-risk pregnancies

TREATMENT OF COMPLICATIONS OF PREMATURITY
   Metabolic
   Infections
   Respiratory
   Neurologic
   Hematologic
   Cardiovascular
   Gastrointestinal
   Nutritional

Instruments that have been developed for the clinical assessment of gestational age take advantage of the multiple physical and neurologic changes that occur in the fetus during the last trimester. For example, a preterm infant of 24 weeks' gestation is extremely hypotonic, with fragile, thin, gelatinous skin (Houska-Lund & Durand, 2002). Because the chest wall is so flexible at this gestational age, respiratory effort results in substernal retractions (Hagedorn et al, 2002). As the fetus matures there is a global increase in resting tone, a flexed posture develops, the skin thickens, and the bone and cartilage become firmer (Houska-Lund & Durand, 2002) (see Figure 36-1 for maturational assessment of gestational age and Table 36-1, New Ballard Scoring System).

Treatment (Box 36-2)
Prevention

Prevention of preterm birth is the most desirable therapy. Tertiary strategies for prevention of preterm birth and the associated problems include use of tocolytic drugs to slow or prevent the progression of labor while enhancing lung maturity with steroids to decrease the effect of respiratory distress syndrome (RDS) and chronic lung disease (CLD). Secondary strategies attempt to identify women at high risk for preterm birth and institute preventive measures such at decreased strenuous physical activity, bed rest, cervical cerclage, or treatment of asymptomatic urinary tract infections and bacterial vaginosis. Controversy exists as to the consistency in benefits associated with various therapies (e.g., use of tocolytic drugs, treatment of urinary tract infections and bacterial vaginosis, or cervical cerclage) to prevent preterm birth (Amon et al, 2000; Goldenberg & Rouse, 1998). Primary prevention will be enhanced when there is a better understanding of the mechanisms of preterm labor and delineation of the interrelationship of risk factors contributing to preterm birth (Hall, 2000). Preterm birth prevention programs, educational materials, and technology

MacDorman et al, 2002b). The reasons for this continued racial disparity are not well understood but are probably multifactorial, composed of maternal medical and past pregnancy history, socioeconomic and demongraphic factors, access to health care, and lifestyle habits (Gilbert & Harmon, 2003).

Clinical Manifestations at the Time of Diagnosis (Figure 36-1, Table 36-1)

The degree of gestational immaturity is most accurately assessed using reliable maternal history. When the date of the last menstrual period is uncertain, the gestational age can be estimated using measurements obtained at early ultrasound examinations. In the absence of reliable dates or conflicting data, the physical and neurologic findings within the first few hours of life in the preterm neonate can be used to estimate gestational age to within 2 weeks (American Academy of Pediatrics [AAP] and American College of Obstetrics and Gynecology [ACOG], 2002; Ballard et al, 1991; Dubowitz et al, 1970).

Neuromuscular Maturity

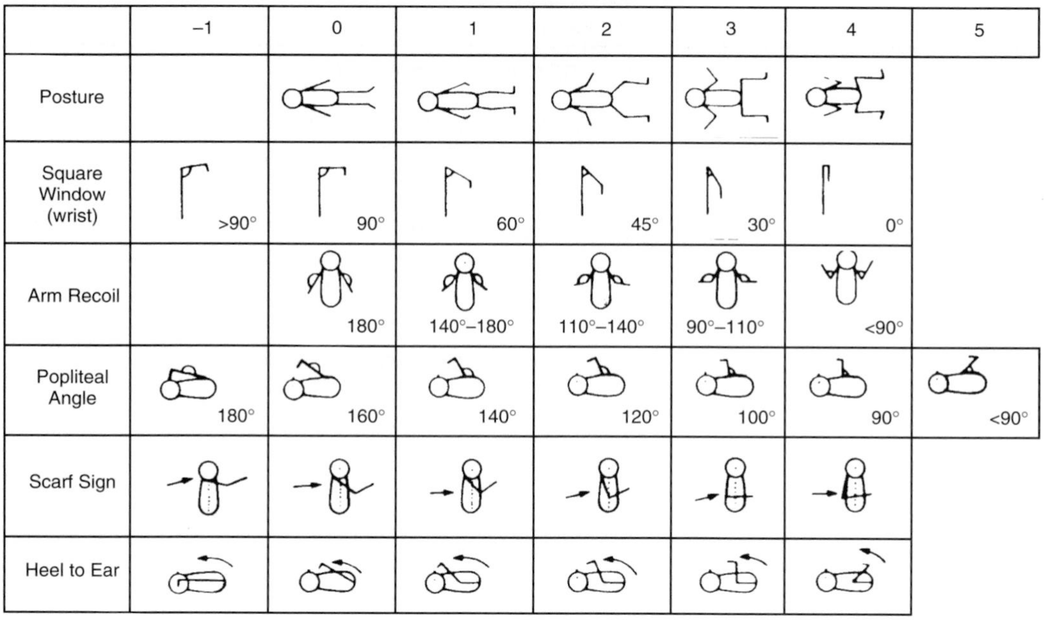

	−1	0	1	2	3	4	5
Posture							
Square Window (wrist)	>90°	90°	60°	45°	30°	0°	
Arm Recoil		180°	140°–180°	110°–140°	90°–110°	<90°	
Popliteal Angle	180°	160°	140°	120°	100°	90°	<90°
Scarf Sign							
Heel to Ear							

Physical Maturity

Skin	sticky friable transparent	gelatinous red, translucent	smooth pink, visible veins	superficial peeling &/or rash few veins	cracking pale areas rare veins	parchment deep cracking no vessels	leathery cracked wrinkled
Lanugo	none	sparse	abundant	thinning	bald areas	mostly bald	
Plantar Surface	heel–toe 40–50mm: −1 <40mm: −2	>50mm no crease	faint red marks	anterior transverse crease only	creases ant. 2/3	creases over entire sole	
Breast	imperceptible	barely perceptible	flat areola no bud	stippled areola 1–2mm bud	raised areola 3–4mm bud	full areola 5–10mm bud	
Eye/Ear	lids fused loosely: −1 tightly: −2	lids open pinna flat stays folded	sl. curved pinna;soft; slow recoil	well–curved pinna; soft but ready recoil	formed &firm instant recoil	thick cartilage ear stiff	
Genitals male	scrotum flat, smooth	scrotum empty faint rugae	testes in upper canal rare rugae	testes descending few rugae	testes down good rugae	testes pendulous deep rugae	
Genitals female	clitoris prominent labia flat	prominent clitoris small labia minora	prominent clitoris enlarging minora	majora & minora equally prominent	majora large minora small	majora cover clitoris & minora	

Maturity Rating

score	weeks
−10	20
−5	22
0	24
5	26
10	28
15	30
20	32
25	34
30	36
35	38
40	40
45	42
50	44

FIGURE 36-1 Maturational assessment of gestational age: New Ballard scoring system. (From Ballard, J.L., et al. [1997]. New Ballard Score, expanded to include extremely premature infants. *J Pediatr, 119*, 417-423. Reprinted with permission.)

(e.g., home uterine activity monitors and telemetry) can be used by clinicians and pregnant women so that the signs of preterm labor in high-risk women can be identified and potentially managed to prevent preterm delivery (Creasy & Iams, 1999).

Fetal fibronectin and transvaginal ultrasonography measurements of cervical length are two interventions that give the obstetric provider more information regarding the impending risk of preterm delivery. When present in the cervicovaginal mucus, fetal fibronectin, which is an extracellular matrix protein normally found in fetal membranes and decidua, has been shown to be a good predictor of spontaneous preterm delivery within 7 days of presentation (Lopez et al, 2000). Cervical shortening observed through transvaginal ultrasonography, is also predictive of preterm birth particularly in women

TABLE 36-1
New Ballard Scoring System

Component	Assessment Technique	Effect of Maturity	Comments
NEUROMUSCULAR MATURITY			
Posture	Observe infant while baby is unrestrained and supine; note amount of flexion and extension of extremities.	Extensor tone is replaced by flexor tone in a cephalocaudal progression.	Knees may be hyperextended in a frank breech delivery.
Square window	Flex wrist; measure minimum angle formed by ventral surface of forearm and palm.	Angle decreases; at term no space exists between palm and forearm.	Response depends on muscle tone and intrauterine position.
Arm recoil	Place infant in supine position with head in midline. Flex elbow and hold forearm against arm for 5 seconds; fully extend elbow, then release; note time required for infant to resume flexed position.	Angle decreases and recoil becomes more rapid.	
Popliteal angle	Flex hips, placing thighs on abdomen; keeping hips on surface of bed, extend knee as far as possible until resistance is met; estimate popliteal angle.	Popliteal angle decreases.	Amount of extension can be overestimated if knee is extended beyond point where resistance is first met; this assessment also is affected by intrauterine position and hip dislocation.
Scarf sign	With head in midline, pull hand across chest to encircle neck; note position of elbow relative to midline.	Increased resistance to crossing the midline.	Reflects muscle tone; response is altered by obesity, hydrops, or fractured clavicle.
Heel to ear	Keep infant supine with pelvis on mattress; press feet as far as possible toward head, allowing knees to be positioned beside abdomen; estimate angle created by arc from back of heel to mattress.	Angle decreases; hip flexion decreases toward term.	Reflects muscle tone.
PHYSICAL MATURITY			
Skin	Observe translucency of skin over abdominal wall.	Skin becomes thicker and ultimately dry and peeling; pigmentation increases.	Skin becomes drier hours after birth; phototherapy or sunlight enhances pigmentation.
Lanugo	Assess for presence and length of hair over back.	Lanugo emerges at 19 to 20 weeks and is most prominent at 27 to 28 weeks; it then gradually disappears, first from the lower back and then from at least half of the back.	The degree of pigmentation and quantity of hair are related to race, gender, and nutritional status.
Plantar surface	Measure length of foot; determine presence or absence of true deep creases (not merely wrinkles).	Early in gestation, foot length correlates with fetal growth; creases develop from toes to heel, and absence of creases correlates with immaturity.	Plantar creases also reflect intrauterine fetal activity; accelerated creasing is seen with oligohydramnios; diminished creasing suggests lack of activity in a mature fetus.
Breast	Estimate diameter of breast bud; assess color and stippling of areola.	Definition and stippling of areola and pigmentation are evident near term; bud size increases because of maternal hormones and fat accumulation.	With intrauterine growth restriction, breast tissue may be diminished, but development of areola proceeds regardless of malnutrition.
Ear cartilage	Fold top of auricle; observe speed of recoil.	Cartilage becomes stiff, and auricle thickens.	Compression in utero and absence or dysfunction of auricular muscles diminishes firmness.
Eyelid opening	Without attempting to separate eyelids, evaluate degree of fusion.	Opening begins at 22 weeks; lids are completely unfused by 28 weeks.	Fused eyelids should not be considered a sign of nonviability; lids may be fused at term with anophthalmia.
EXTERNAL GENITALIA			
Male	Palpate scrotum to assess degree of descent of testes; observe rugae and suspension of scrotum.	At 27 to 28 weeks; testes begin to descend into scrotum; rugae formation begins at about 28 weeks; by term rugae are well defined, and scrotum is pendulous.	Rugae are decreased with scrotal edema; testes may be absent (cryptorchidism).
Female	Assess size of labia minora and labia majora.	Labia minora increase in size before labia majora; at term labia majora cover labia minora completely.	Size of labia majora depends on amount of body fat; with malnutrition, size may be diminished; edema may increase size of labia majora.

From Kenner, C. & Lott, J.W. (2003). *Comprehensive neonatal nursing* (3rd ed.). Philadelphia: W.B. Saunders. Reprinted with permission. Data from Fletcher, M.A. (1998). *Physical diagnosis in neonatology*. Philadelphia: Lippincott-Raven; and Southgate, W.M. & Pittard, W.B. (2001). *Classification and physical examination of the newborn infant.*

with a prior history of preterm labor and/or preterm birth (Owen, 2001). When preterm delivery cannot be entirely prevented, prolonging the pregnancy and achieving advancement of gestational age may decrease the risk of neonatal mortality or the attendant morbidities associated with extreme preterm birth (Amon et al, 2000; Challis, 2000; McGrath et al, 2000).

Treatment in Utero

If a preterm birth appears inevitable, treatment should begin in utero. Antenatal corticosteroids will accelerate fetal lung maturation and decrease the incidence and severity of RDS and associated morbidities including chronic lung disease (CLD), intraventricular hemorrhage (IVH), and necrotizing enterocolitis (NEC) for infants born prior to 32 weeks' gestation (ACOG, 1998; National Institute of Health [NIH], 1995; NIH Consensus Statement, 2000). The optimal benefit for antenatal corticosteroid administration is within 7 days preceding delivery (ACOG, 1998). Controversy exists regarding the use of multiple courses of antenatal corticosteroids particularly if delivery has been delayed beyond 7 days of administration of the steroids (Guinn and BMZ Study Group, 2000; NIH Consensus, 2000). Multiple courses of antenatal corticosteroids have inconsistently demonstrated a decreased severity in RDS, and impaired growth and psychomotor delay may occur due to excess fetal exposure to the corticosteroids (Bolt et al, 2001; Caughey & Parer, 2002; Fausett et al, 2000; Sinervo & Lange, 2000). If prolonged rupture of the membranes occurs or choreoamnionitis is suspected, prenatal administration of antibiotics improves neonatal survival and outcome (Goldenberg et al, 2000).

When it is safe for the pregnant woman and fetus, they should be transferred to a center with expertise in the management of preterm labor, high-risk deliveries, and care of high-risk infants. In a recent comparison of neonatal mortality and the level of neonatal care at the hospital of birth for LBW infants, it was determined that the lowest risk-adjusted mortality for preterm infants less than 2,000 g at birth was associated with hospitals having regional neonatal intensive care units (NICUs) in comparison with institutions having small or community NICUs (Cifuentes et al, 2002). Neonatal transport to a regional center after delivery had minimal benefit over the disadvantage of being born in a smaller or community center.

Treatment of Complications of Prematurity

After the preterm infant is born, treatment is tailored to existing or anticipated complications. Prophylactic treatment modalities are often used in infants at highest risk. Synthetic or natural exogenous surfactant can be given to the preterm neonate through an endotracheal tube immediately after delivery to prevent or lessen the severity of RDS (Curley, 2001; Malloy & Freeman, 2000). In addition, prevention and treatment of cold stress and hypovolemia reduce the risk of RDS and its severity (Kliegman, 2002). Sepsis with pneumonia can be difficult to distinguish from RDS; therefore, broad-spectrum parental antibiotics are administered for 72 hours pending the results of blood cultures (Kliegman). Indomethacin may be given before or soon after manifestations of patent ductus arteriosus (PDA) are clinically apparent (Narayanan

et al, 2000; Quinn et al, 2002), and respiratory stimulants such as caffeine may be given to prevent or treat apnea of prematurity (Gannon, 2000).

Complementary and Alternative Therapies

There have been no documented investigations that have identified complementary therapies that prevent/reduce the likelihood of preterm birth or physiologic complications experienced in preterm infants. Because stress has been associated with early onset of labor in some women, stress-reduction therapies such as meditation, imagery, massage, and mild exercise may be of some benefit. Use of alcohol and other recreation drugs is strongly discouraged because of the potential teratogenic effects on the fetus, and abuse of these drugs may interfere with maternal nutrition, resulting in an SGA fetus or premature labor, such as with cocaine use. Herbal preparations and folk medicines that are often composed of variable amounts of substances, are also discouraged. Herbal remedies sold in the United States do not need to prove efficacy, safety, potency, or standardization from preparation to preparation. Some herbal preparations, i.e., angelica, juniper, mugwort, nutmeg, pennyroyal, raspberry tea, saffron, and sage in high doses, can act as an abortifacient (Bright, 2002; Fetrow & Avila, 1999). In addition, there are herbal agents that are contraindicated in breast milk and therefore must be avoided in lactating mothers (Box 36-3).

The preterm infant is vulnerable to environmental stimuli. Sensory stimulation may result in increased difficulty with oxygenation (Kenner & Lott, 2003). Controlling the environment, i.e., temperature, noise, lights, touch, both in the hospital and at home, and allowing the infant periods of uninterrupted rest will support stable oxygenation and growth. Massage therapy of preterm infants has been shown to increase weight gain and decrease the time spent in the hospital (Field, 1995). There is controversy regarding the effect of massage on promoting better developmental outcomes in premature infants, and further study is needed (Vickers et al, 2002). Massage can be taught to parents to use after the infant is discharged to reduce stress in the infant and promote bonding/attachment between

---

BOX 36-3

Herbal Preparartions Contraindicated in Breast-feeding Mothers

Aloe
Buckthorn bark
Buckthorn berry
Caraway oil
Cascara sagrada bark
Coltsfoot leaf
Indian snakeroot
Kava kava
Peppermint oil
Petasites root
Rhubarb root
Senna leaf
Uva ursi

From Mattison, D. Herbal supplements: Their safety, a concern for health care providers. Available at www.marchofdimes.com/professionals/681_1815.asp. Reprinted with permission.

infant and parent. Kangaroo care, the practice of carrying the infant with skin-to-skin contact with the parent's chest, has shown the infant's breathing, oxygenation, and heart rate become more regular, tone and flexion improve, and the infant's sleep pattern becomes less disorganized (Gale, 1993). Additional study of kangaroo care in preterm infants is needed (Eichel, 2001).

Parents must be asked about the use of home remedies and cultural practices with their preterm infant. Primary care providers must be open to exploring the therapeutic potential of complementary and alternative therapies with the safety of the infant as their primary concern. Aloe vera has been used to protect the fragile skin of the preterm infant, chamomile, fennel, aniseed, and cardamom are gastrointestinal antispasmodics and may be beneficial in small amounts to treat colic, and caffeine, the most commonly used herb therapy in the United States, is used in preterm infants with apnea or bradycardia (Kenner & Lott, 2003). Parents of infants with complications or disabilities, such as bronchopulmonary dysplasia (see Chapter 16), cerebral palsy (see Chapter 18), or epilepsy (see Chapter 25) may use complementary or alternative therapies directed toward these conditions. Many therapies may not demonstrate efficacy but may not be harmful. Others may interfere with prescribed treatment plans, be a financial burden to families without obvious gain, or be potentially harmful. Primary care providers must question families as to their use of complementary and alternative medicines, weigh their risks and benefits, and provide balanced advice to families about therapeutic options for their child (Committee on Children with Disabilities, 2001).

Anticipated Advances in Diagnosis and Management

Preterm birth does not cause long-range problems for affected infants; however, the complications associated with preterm birth cause, in some cases, irreparable damage. In general, VLBW and ELBW infants have a higher incidence of long-range problems (Horbar et al, 2002; McGrath et al, 2000). In addition, the complex ethical decisions presented with health care for previable infants (e.g., <24 weeks' gestation and <500 g at birth) who have neonatal death rates in excess of 50% will continue to challenge providers to determine what is in the best interests for the child.

Decreasing the incidence of preterm births has been a consistent objective of the national health agenda, *Healthy People 2000* and *2010*. However, only a minimal reduction in preterm births rate occurred from 1999 to 2000 (11.8% to 11.6%), the first decline since 1992 (MacDorman et al, 2002). Despite the increased number of women seeking prenatal care, there has not been a consequential reduction in the incidence of preterm births. The phenomenon of preterm labor and delivery is a complex interaction of multiple intrinsic and extrinsic factors that will require greater exploration to develop strategies to meet this national health challenge (Abrahams & Katz, 2002). The National Institute of Child Health and Development (NICHD) Preterm Prediction Study is collecting data in a prospective population-based study to identify markers that might predict preterm delivery (Creasy & Iams, 1999). Two

markers in this prediction study, elevated alkaline phosphatase and alphafetoprotein, have recently been linked to spontaneous preterm birth in asymptomatic pregnant women at 24 and 28 weeks' gestation, and elevated levels of corticotropin-releasing hormone at 28 weeks was associated with preterm birth prior to 35 weeks' gestation (Moawad et al, 2002). Further empirical investigation of these potentially predictive markers for spontaneous preterm labor is needed before implementation in clinical practice.

Medical advances in managing the complications associated with preterm birth are likely to lessen the incidence of poor outcomes for these vulnerable infants. Improved techniques to support ventilation in the preterm neonate, such as continuous positive airway pressure (CPAP) or high-frequency ventilation, decrease the lung damage seen with conventional ventilation (Ho et al, 2002). Limiting supplemental oxygen decreases the risk of hyperoxia and associated risks of retinopathy of prematurity (ROP) and bronchopulmonary dysplasia (BPD) (see Chapter 16) (Chow et al, 2003; Cole & Fiascone, 2000; Piuze et al, 2000). Laser therapy for prevention of advanced ROP has proved successful in reducing the risk of blindness (DeRoo-Merritt, 2000; STOP-ROP Multicenter Study Group, 2000).

Low-dose prophylactic indomethacin may be useful in prevention of severe periventricular and intraventricular hemorrhage (Ment et al, 2000; Paige & Carney, 2002) and closure of a PDA (Allen et al, 2001). However, in a recent report from the Trial of Indomethacin Prophylaxis in Preterms, it was determined that the routine use of prophylactic indomethacin did not improve long-term neurologic outcomes nor did it increase the likelihood of survival for ELBW infants (Schmidt et al, 2001). Ethamsylate, an agent that promotes platelet aggregation, is under investigation to reduce the incidence of hemorrhage (Papile, 2002). The use of erythropoietin has been determined to stimulate erythropoiesis in preterm infants with birth weights ≤1250 g; however there are conflicting outcomes on the likelihood of reducing the need for erythrocyte transfusions during the initial hospitalization in the NICU (Ohls et al, 2001). The addition of the long-chain polyunsaturated fatty acids, docosahexaenoic acid (DHA) and arachidonic acid (AA) to infant formulas is being investigated for safety in preterm infants during the first year of life, and improved cognitive and visual outcomes in preterm infants have been observed with the addition of these nutrients to infant formulas (O'Connor et al, 2001; Klein, 2002).

Future therapies and management strategies for preterm infants are likely to be influenced by the development in the past decade of two innovative collaborative database efforts (Vermont Oxford Network and National Institute of Child Health and Human Development Neonatal Network) with the primary goals of research, education, and collaborative quality improvement for neonatal intensive care. These databases reflect all infants with birth weights ≤1,500 g hospitalized in tertiary care NICUs, and multiple investigators have used these data sources to examine similarities and differences in clinical management and outcomes for preterm infants (Horbar et al, 2002; Lemons et al, 2001). In addition to examining infant outcomes from collaborative database efforts, it is likely that future randomized clinical trials will go beyond short-term or proxy outcomes for preterm infants and include long-term efficacy and safety of specific treatment strategies to improve the scope of evidence-based neonatal practice (Harrold & Schmidt, 2002).

Associated Problems (Box 36-4)

There are multiple clinical complications that may develop in the preterm infant. The associated cost of caring for premature infants in the United States is estimated to be $5 to $6 billion annually (Challis, 2000). There can be a progression of complications, and one complication increases the risk for additional complications. For example, a preterm infant with severe RDS is more apt to develop an IVH than an infant without RDS; a preterm infant who experiences a prolonged interference in the establishment of enteral feedings because of feeding intolerance or necrotizing enterocolitis (NEC) is more likely to develop osteopenic fractures or rickets (Dabezies & Warren, 1997; Klein, 2002; Krug-Wispe, 1998). It is important for clinicians to recognize the risk of these complications and institute therapy to potentially prevent their occurrence and long-term sequelae.

Intraventricular Hemorrhage

IVH occurs in an estimated 20% to 40% of preterm infants. The associated risk of complications from IVH can be negligible to catastrophic depending upon the degree of neurologic injury (Volpe, 2001). IVH often begins with bleeding into the subependymal germinal matrix, which can subsequently extend into the ventricular system or the nearby brain parenchyma. The germinal matrix is a metabolically active, highly vascularized area that persists until term and is predisposed to hemorrhage. Because there is poor autoregulation of blood flow to this area in preterm infants, the delicate capillaries of the germinal matrix are vulnerable to damage from acute changes in sys-

temic arterial or venous pressure (Gleissner et al, 2000). Perinatal asphyxia and metabolic or respiratory problems can also damage the capillary bed and further predispose the preterm infant to an IVH (Paige & Carney, 2002). The classification of IVH, originally described by Papile et al (1978), includes the following four grades of hemorrhage: grade I or subependymal or germinal matrix hemorrhage; grade II, intraventricular hemorrhage; grade III, intraventricular hemorrhage with ventricular dilation; and grade IV, intraventricular hemorrhage with extension of bleeding into the brain parenchyma. The American Academy of Neurology and the Practice Committee of the Child Neurology Society recommend that routine cranial ultrasound be performed on all infants less than 30 weeks' gestation once between 7 and 14 days of age and repeated between 36 and 40 weeks' postmenstrual age (Ment et al, 2002)

Treatment for IVH is supportive. Minimizing fluctuations in blood pressure and cerebral blood flow are important because these vascular alterations may contribute to further hemorrhage (Paige & Carney, 2002). Follow-up ultrasound examinations are performed to examine the resolution of a hemorrhage or the development of complications including hydrocephalus or periventricular leukomalacia (PVL). If hydrocephalus develops, treatment must be instituted to minimize brain damage (see Chapter 29). Mortality from IVH is related to severity. Although there is typically no mortality associated with minimal hemorrhage, some infants with the most extensive hemorrhage do not survive. Those who do survive with higher grades of IVH, posthemorrhagic hydrocephalus, and PVL have significant neurologic sequelae (McGrath et al, 2000; Volpe, 2001).

PVL is generally a result of symmetric, nonhemorrhagic ischemic injury to the cerebral white matter of preterm infants and is usually—but not always—a neuropathologic accompaniment of grades 3 and 4 IVH (Volpe, 2001). This white matter injury may not be limited to the periventricular area and has a high incidence of neurologic sequelae, including cerebral palsy. PVL can be diagnosed with neural ultrasound.

Respiratory Problems

Lung Damage. An inverse relationship exists between birth weight and gestational age and risk of respiratory complications in the neonate. The smallest and lowest gestational age infants have the highest incidence of RDS due to immature pulmonary function and surfactant deficiency (Bolt et al, 2001; Fitzgerald et al, 2000). However, the combined use of antenatal steroids and exogenous surfactant administration in the immediate newborn period have substantially reduced the severity of RDS in preterm infants and have also reduced the risk of chronic lung disease (CLD) (Suresh & Soll, 2001; Stevens et al, 2002).

Most preterm infants require only supplemental oxygen given through a hood or nasal cannula; however, some ELBW infants with RDS may require nasal continuous positive airway pressure (NCPAP), variable-flow CPAP, or mechanical ventilation through an endotracheal tube (Ho et al, 2002). High-frequency mechanical ventilation has been used successfully to support respiratory function in the extremely preterm infant. It has been associated with a lower risk of acute and chronic complications such as pneumothorax or CLD in comparison with use of traditional modes of mechanical ventilation but may

---

BOX 36-4
Associated Problems

INTRAVENTRICULAR HEMORRHAGE
RESPIRATORY PROBLEMS
　Lung damage
　Apnea
CARDIAC PROBLEMS
PATENT DUCTUS ARTERIOSUS
CONGENITAL HEART DISEASE
SEPSIS
NUTRITION
　Parenteral nutrition
　Enteral feeding
　Necrotizing enterocolitis
　Gastroesophageal reflux
RETINOPATHY OF PREMATURITY
ANEMIA
GENITOURINARY PROBLEMS
　Reduce renal function
　Undescended testicles
　Inguinal hernias

be associated with an increased incidence of severe IVH (Moriette et al, 2001). Postnatal glucocorticoids, such as dexamethasone, have been used on a limited basis with caution and with parental permission for preterm infants with severe RDS to reduce pulmonary inflammation, decrease the risk of CLD, and support extubation. Concerns regarding impaired growth and neurodevelopmental delay in preterm infants receiving steroids have resulted in a recent recommendation that systemic dexamethasone for prevention or treatment of CLD in infants with very low birth weight not be used (American Academy of Pediatrics, Committee on Fetus & Newborn. Canadian Paediatric Society: Fetus & Newborn Committee, 2002; Romagnoli et al, 2002).

Supplemental oxygen and positive pressure, although lifesaving, may damage the lungs and airways from hyperoxia and barotrauma (Jobe & Ikegami, 1998; Speer & Groneck, 1998). This damage must be viewed as a continuum ranging from minor changes in lung function to chronic lung changes associated with bronchopulmonary dysplasia (BPD) (see Chapter 16). Lung damage in preterm infants is demonstrated primarily through abnormalities in pulmonary function testing and reflected clinically in increased airway reactivity and/or increased pulmonary infections in the first years of life (Hansen & Corbet, 1998). Children with a history of prematurity and BPD were also found to be at higher risk to have lower receptive language skills during the preschool years (Singer et al, 2001).

Apnea. Approximately 25% to 30% of LBW infants have apnea that is primarily attributable to immaturity of the respiratory center (i.e., apnea of prematurity). The incidence increases with decreasing gestational age. In most cases, apnea resolves by the time an infant reaches 36 to 40 weeks' maturational age (Di Fiore, 2001; Ramanathan et al, 2001). Apnea of prematurity may persist beyond term gestation in infants born <28 weeks' gestational age and is usually associated with CLD (Eichenwald & Stark, 1997). An association between apnea and gastroesophageal reflux in preterm infants has been challenged and requires further investigation (Kikkert, et al, 2000; Peter et al, 2002).

There is no evidence that apnea of prematurity increases the risk for sudden infant death syndrome (SIDS) (Di Fiore, 2001). Preterm infants, particularly LBW infants, however, are at much higher risk for SIDS (Task Force on Infant Sleep and Suddent Infant Death Syndrome, 2000), whereas SIDS rates are declining for all other infants (Mathews et al, 2000). This risk appears to be magnified by other factors such as BPD, maternal substance use (especially nicotine and cocaine), and prone or side-sleeping position (Pollack, 2001). Unfortunately there is no way to predict which preterm infant will develop SIDS. Although many centers perform pneumograms on LBW infants as a diagnostic tool to determine which infants should be sent home with a cardiorespiratory monitor, their usefulness is controversial (Zupancic et al, 2003).

Most neonatologists require a 3- to 10-day apnea-free period after discontinuing caffeine or theophylline before discharge for preterm infants who have significant apnea near the time of discharge. The cost-effectiveness of a predischarge monitoring period has been examined in infants with apnea of prematurity and differences were observed across gestation (Zupancic et al, 2003). These investigators recommend that better outcomes and decreased costs could be obtained through monitoring lower gestational age infants <30 weeks for longer intervals and higher gestational age infants ≥30 weeks for shorter intervals. If an infant requires home apnea monitoring, families are taught the use of the equipment and cardiopulmonary resuscitation prior to discharge from the NICU. Monitoring must be maintained during infant sleep, when the infant is in the car seat, and when the infant is away from the caregiver (Ritchie, 2002). Recording of heart rate and chest wall movement in addition to documentation of bradycardia and/or apnea episodes are downloaded and examined by the primary care provider working in conjunction with pulmonary specialists. Decisions regarding discontinuation of apnea monitoring are based on the respiratory health of the infant and apnea monitoring equipment reports and/or pneumocardiogram evaluations (Bernbaum, 2000).

Preterm infants less than 50 to 60 weeks' postconceptional age are at high risk for postanesthesia apnea and require monitoring for prolonged periods after surgery. This risk must be taken into consideration before performing outpatient surgery after discharge from the NICU (Hansen & Corbet, 1998).

Cardiac Problems

Patent Ductus Arteriosus (PDA). The ductus arteriosus is a fetal shunt that connects the pulmonary artery with the descending aorta and facilitates blood return to the placenta (Allen et al, 2001). For the majority of term infants, the ductus arteriosus functionally closes within the first 24 hours of life as arterial oxygenation improves. However, this functional closure can be delayed in preterm infants due to an altered response to oxygen, increased pulmonary vascular resistance, and the size of the lumen of the ductus. Persistent ductal patency occurs in approximately 50% of LBW infants and 80% of preterm infants weighing <1,000 g and results in increased pulmonary blood flow and volume overload in the left ventricle (Park, 2003). Most preterm infants with PDA will have clinical symptomatology including systolic murmur, bounding peripheral pulses, and pulmonary venous congestion by the third postnatal day.

The preterm infant with symptomatic PDA is initially managed with indomethacin, a prostaglandin synthetase inhibitor, which facilitates ductal closure. The likelihood for successful ductal closure in preterm infants may vary in response to the standard three-dose course of indomethacin (Narayanan et al, 2000), and recommendations for prolonged treatment with six doses have been associated with greater likelihood of ductal closure (Lee et al, 2001; Quinn et al, 2002). Indomethacin works best during the early postnatal period; it is not effective 4 to 6 weeks after birth (Kenner & Lott, 2003). For many preterm infants, indomethacin will result only in ductal constriction and not permanent closure, and a surgical ligation of the ductus will be necessary to prevent further cardiopulmonary compromise (Allen et al, 2001). Conservative management prior to surgery includes fluid restrictions and diuretics to control pulmonary congestion.

Congenital Heart Disease. Preterm infants may have congenital heart disease (CHD) (see Chapter 21) that complicates their neonatal course and increases their risk of developing complications associated with prematurity. Maintenance of adequate oxygenation, normal vascular pressure gradients, and fluid volume are all more complicated when the preterm infant has a CHD. The risks of increased pulmonary vascular resistance and pulmonary hypertension are increased in infants with left-to-right shunts and will compromise the infant's respiratory status. For these reasons, corrective cardiac surgery is often performed in the early postnatal period.

Sepsis

The preterm infant is extremely susceptible to a wide array of bacterial, viral, and fungal infections and the incidence of sepsis in approximately 1 case per 250 preterm infants (Kliegman, 2002). Intrauterine, perinatal, and postnatal infectious exposures can precipitate acute and potentially fatal infections or be associated with chronic organ damage. Prevention of infection is the primary goal in the care of the preterm infant; however, immunologic limitations, physiologic stress, inadequate nutrition, and nosocomial infectious exposures in the NICU constantly challenge this goal (Merenstein et al, 2002).

Preterm infants are at an increased risk for both early- and late-onset sepsis (Escobar et al, 2000). The preterm infant born prior to 32 weeks' gestation receives a limited quantity of maternal antibody IgG, which normally crosses the placenta in greater quantities late in the third trimester (Merenstein et al, 2002). In addition, the preterm infant has limited ability to generate IgG, which coupled with deficiencies in complement, neutrophil, and phagocytic function place the preterm infant at greater risk for sepsis. Early-onset sepsis may begin in utero or occur with exposure to infectious agents at the time of delivery. Organisms including group B streptococcus *Escherichia coli, Klebsiella,* and *Listeria monocytogenes* are frequent causative agents for early-onset sepsis (White et al, 2000; Remington & Klein, 2001; Wendel, 2002). In addition to preterm birth, obstetric complications including premature and prolonged rupture of membranes, choreoamnionitis, maternal genitourinary tract infection, and maternal fever increase the likelihood of early-onset sepsis (Committee on Fetus & Newborn, 1998; Remington & Klein, 2001).

The preterm infant can initially present within the first week of life with nonspecific symptoms including respiratory distress, temperature instability, poor feeding, jaundice, and seizures and rapidly progress to potentially fatal multiorgan system disease including respiratory failure, disseminated intravascular coagulopathy (DIC), and shock (Thilo & Rosenberg, 2001). Identification of the specific causative organism through cultures may be difficult to determine due to a poor yield of organism growth. Management with broad-spectrum antibiotics to cover the common organisms found in the preterm infant is instituted in addition to multiorgan system support for the preterm infant with early-onset sepsis (Kliegman, 2002).

Late-onset sepsis, or nosocomial infections, typically occur in preterm infants from 7 days of life to the time of discharge from the NICU and reflect infections from multiple organisms including *Staphylococcus aureus, E. coli, Klebsiella,* and *Enterobacter* and *Candida* species (Merenstein et al, 2002; Zafir, 2001). Preterm infants who have required surgical interventions, received broad-spectrum antibiotic therapy, or post-

natal steroid therapy (Pera et al, 2002) are at increased risk of infection. Infants who have had prolonged management with vascular catheters, endotracheal tubes, and indwelling monitoring devices are at risk for bloodstream infections and late-onset sepsis (Rubin et al, 2002). Approximately 25% of LBW infants hospitalized in NICUs experience late-onset sepsis (Beck-Sague et al, 1994). The presentation and progression of symptoms in late-onset sepsis is similar to that observed with early-onset sepsis. Hematogenous seeding may result in urinary tract infections, meningitis, or osteomyelitis (Kliegman, 2002). Management with appropriate antibiotics or antifungals and multiorgan system support are the mainstay for management of the preterm infant with late-onset sepsis (Merenstein et al, 2002).

Nutrition

Nutrition can be a significant challenge in the care of the smallest preterm infants. Generally preterm infants with birth weights of more than 1,250 g and without significant medical problems easily tolerate enteral feedings. The caloric intake of 120 kcal/kg/day from enteral feedings should result in a net weight gain of approximately 10 to 30 g/day (Thilo & Rosenberg, 2001).

Parenteral Nutrition. For those infants with acute health conditions and for VLBW infants, however, enteral feedings are often delayed for days or weeks. Preterm infants relying on parenteral nutrition may receive only 85 to 100 kcal/kg/day, and those infants requiring surgery or experiencing cardiac and/or pulmonary dysfunction may need in excess of 30% greater caloric intake above maintenance calories for growth (Embleton etal, 2001; Kilbride et al, 2002). In a report from the Workshop on Nutrition of the Extremely Low Birthweight Infant, it was highlighted that there is a significant need for large long-term investigations to examine the short- and long-term metabolic, growth, and neurodevelopmental responses to early and aggressive nutritional management for these vulnerable preterm infants (Hay et al, 1999).

Parenteral nutrition consisting of carbohydrate, lipids, amino acids, electrolytes, and other micronutrients is the primary caloric source for ELBW infants; however, there is an associated risk of complications with this therapy. Physiologic complications of parenteral nutrition include hyperglycemia, protein intolerance reflected by hyperammonemia or acidosis, elevated triglycerides, and platelet dysfunction. Difficulties related to prolonged intravenous access, including tissue infiltrates, catheter misplacement, and catheter infections, may also occur (Committee on Nutrition, 1998; Kilbride et al, 2002). Late complications of parenteral nutrition include cholestatic jaundice, hyperlipidemia, and fungal infections and are more likely to occur with prolonged use of parenteral nutrition in ELBW infants (Berseth & Abrams, 1998).

The process of weaning parenteral nutrition and slowly introducing breast milk or formula can be frustrating. Feedings are often "not tolerated," a catchall phrase that includes vomiting, abdominal distention, and large gastric residuals. Because these nonspecific symptoms may also represent early signs of NEC, feeding is often temporarily discontinued. This on-again, off-again phase of enteral feeding results in a period of poor nutrition unless adequate calories are maintained by continuing supplementation with parenteral nutrition (Embleton et al, 2001). Feeding patterns of continuous versus intermittent feedings and/or rapid versus slow advancement of volume and caloric intake may also influence the preterm infant's feeding tolerance and subsequent weight gain (Rayyis, 1999).

Enteral Feeding. Enteral feeding practices have changed substantially over the past decade, particularly with the introduction of small-volume trophic or minimal enteral feedings, which increase production of gastric hormones, including gastrin and motilin, and support gut maturation (Anderson & Loughead, 2002; McClure, 2001; Klein, 2002). Because preterm infants have unique nutritional needs (i.e., increased need for protein, calcium, phosphorus, sodium, and potassium) (Klein, 2002; Anderson et al, 2002), formulas and breast milk supplements have undergone many changes to meet as many of these needs as possible while maintaining an acceptable caloric density and low osmolality and solute load. Preterm mother's milk supplemented with human milk fortifiers has been shown to be highly suited to a preterm infant's nutritional needs and extremely beneficial for immunologic protection, growth potential, and personal connectivity for the mother (Hay et al, 1999; Reis et al, 2000). In the absence of breast milk, infant formulas are effective nutritional substitutes (Berseth, 2001). Preterm formulas with a base of protein from cow's milk are available in varying caloric densities. Soy protein–based formulas are not recommended for preterm infants because of concerns of aluminum toxicity and their failure to achieve equivalent growth and bone mineralization when compared with fortified human milk or cow protein formulas (Committee on Nutrition, 1998). Despite the availability of parenteral nutrition, fortified breast milk, and complex formulas, some preterm infants do not receive adequate calcium and phosphorus intake and are risk for bone demineralization, fractures, and rickets (Embleton et al, 2001). Serial serum analyses are done to assess for the risk of these complications and long-bone radiographs are done to examine for bony demineralization.

Necrotizing Enterocolitis

Necrotizing enterocolitis (NEC) is a gastrointestinal complication characterized by ischemic damage to the submucosal layer of the bowel, primarily in the terminal ileum or proximal colon. This complication has a typical onset at 3 to 12 days after birth and occurs in about 10% of VLBW infants (Caplan & Jilling, 2001). The highest mortality rates are seen in preterm infants with birth weights less than 1000 g (Lemons et al, 2001), and mortality is higher when other organ systems are involved. The exact etiology of NEC is unknown and is likely multifactorial. Risk factors that may precipitate NEC in the preterm infant include umbilical vessel catheterization, exchange transfusion, polycythemia, recurrent apnea and bradycardia, and enteral feedings. Necrotizing enterocolitis is more common in infants who have been fed than in those who have not been fed and more common in infants fed formula than in those fed breast milk (Singh & Sinha, 2002). In a recent comparison of preterm infants given small amounts of enteral feedings versus preterm infants who received increasing volumes of enteral feedings, Berseth and colleagues (2003) closed the study early due to the

increased numbers of infants who developed NEC in the advanced volumes group. More research is needed to determine the safe progression of enteral feeding volumes to support caloric intake needs while minimizing the risk of NEC.

The diagnosis of NEC is often suspected on clinical findings (i.e., abdominal distention, gastric residuals or emesis, and heme-positive or bloody stools) and confirmed radiographically with the presence of dilated bowel loops, thickened walls of the lumen, and intraluminal gas pockets called pneumatosis intestinalis. In severe cases, evidence of bowel perforation can be seen (Bensard et al, 2002; Kenner & Lott, 2003). Approximately 50% of infants with NEC respond to medical management consisting of bowel rest, gastric decompression, fluid and electrolyte management, and broad-spectrum antibiotics. Serial abdominal radiographs are performed to document the progression or resolution of the disease and to determine if intestinal perforation has occurred. Most infants with perforation are treated with surgery after stabilization; however, management by peritoneal drainage for VLBW and ELBW infants may result in lower mortality and fewer long-term gastrointestinal complications including short bowel syndrome (Dimmit & Moss, 2001).

Whether or not perforation occurs, strictures and obstruction, along with symptoms of abdominal distention and vomiting can occur weeks later in approximately 20% of infants with NEC. Infants who require surgical intervention show higher rates of prolonged poor growth and an increased risk of neurodevelopmental delay within the first 2 years of life (Sonntag et al, 2000). Permanent nutritional challenges and deficiencies may occur in infants who require substantial bowel resection resulting in short bowel syndrome (Bensard et al, 2002).

Gastroesophageal Reflux

Gastroesophageal reflux (GER) refers to the retrograde passage of gastric contents from the stomach into the esophagus and is caused by decreased lower esophageal sphincter (LES) tone. Approximately 3% to 10% of preterm infants are diagnosed with GER, and infants with chronic lung disease account for up to 70% of neonatal cases (Jadcheria, 2002). Methylxanthines (aminophylline, theophylline) and caffeine therapy, used to prevent or reduce the likelihood of apnea and bradycardia episodes in preterm infants, may worsen GER due to a further reduction in lower esophageal tone and stimulation of gastric acid secretion. The clinical presentation of GER may be subtle and reflect nonbilious vomiting or progress to coughing, choking, wheezing, apnea, or pneumonitis (Bensard, 2002). Preterm infants may need prolonged treatment for GER, and this gastrointestinal complication is associated with increased length of hospital stay and delayed achievement of full feedings (Jadcheria, 2002). Treatment depends on the clinical findings and degree of severity and may include elevated head and chest positioning, monitoring, thickened feedings, and prokinetic agents such as metoclopramide or erythromycin and gastric acid modifiers including ranitidine (Zantac) or aluminum hydroxide (Gaviscon) (Thompson, 2000). Most infants respond to medical management; however, a surgical fundoplication procedure to wrap the gastric fundus around the distal esophagus may be necessary for infants with recurrent aspiration pneumonia, persistent apnea, and/or failure to thrive due to GER (Thompson, 2000).

Retinopathy of Prematurity

Retinopathy of prematurity (ROP) is a vascular disorder of the retina that develops in approximately 85% of preterm infants born prior to 28 weeks' gestation (STOP-ROP Multicenter Study Group, 2000). Vascularization of the retina may not be complete until after approximately 42 to 44 weeks' postconceptional age. For reasons that are not clear, abnormal vascularization of the retina develops in some preterm infants. In most cases the retinopathy resolves with little or no sequelae, but in a few infants a proliferative neovascularization accompanied by fibrosis and retinal detachment and subsequent vision loss can develop (O'Connor et al, 2002). The stages of ROP are stage 1, demarcation line between vascularized and avascular retina; stage 2, ridge or raised demarcation line; stage 3, ridge with extraretinal fibrovascular proliferation; stage 4, partial retinal detachment; and stage 5, total retinal detachment (International Committee on Classification of ROP, 1984).

The majority of the cases resolve without visual loss; however, the incidence of severe ROP ranges from 4% to 18% in NICUs in the United States. The risk factors for development of ROP have been identified (Hussain et al, 1999), but clear cause-and-effect relationships remain to be confirmed. The most important risk factors appear to be preterm birth and the length of time supplemental oxygen is used (Chow et al, 2003; Tin et al, 2001). Other factors that may increase risk are sepsis, apnea, and transfusion with adult blood. In a comparison of oxygen saturation levels and threshold retinopathy, Tin and associates (2001) noted that the lowest rates (6.2%) for retinopathy occurred in preterm infants having an oxygen saturation range of 70% to 90%; the highest rates (27.7%) occurred in infants with oxygen saturation ranges of 88% to 98%. Investigation into the optimal oxygenation of preterm infants resulting in minimal sequelae continues to be needed (Harrold & Schmidt, 2002). Over the past 15 years there has been a significant decrease in the rate and severity of ROP (McGregor et al, 2002).

Treatment of neovascularization with laser photocoagulation has been effective in preventing progression of the retinopathy in most cases (STOP-ROP Multicenter Study Group, 2000). This treatment appears to have fewer side effects than cryotherapy, with less pain and swelling, and is less likely to cause damage to the eye. Recent data have suggested that laser photocoagulation also results in better visual acuity and less myopia when compared with cryotherapy (O'Connor et al, 2002).

Anemia

Preterm infants are born with reduced iron stores and are particularly vulnerable to developing anemia. Because no single, specific definition for anemia exists in this population, the hemoglobin level or hematocrit value must be assessed in light of an infant's age. For example, a hematocrit value of below 40% at term birth is considered anemic; it is normal, however, for the hematocrit value to be below 40% at very early gestation and to rise with advancing gestational age. All hematocrit values then decrease over the weeks after birth, leading to physiologic anemia (Manco-Johnson et al, 2002). Anemia of prematurity is thus an exaggeration of this process, and the responsible mechanisms remain undefined. Shortened erythrocyte survival, hemodilution from rapidly increasing body mass, hemolysis due to birth trauma or blood incompatibility, and low serum erythropoietin concentrations, despite diminished available oxygen to tissues, may contribute to anemia of prematurity (Ohls, 1998).

Infants found to have anemia at birth should be evaluated for hemolysis, chronic blood loss in utero, or acute perinatal blood loss. Common causes of anemia that develop in preterm infants after the immediate perinatal period are iatrogenic blood loss and anemia of prematurity (Ohls et al, 2001). The blood volume of a preterm infant is only 80 to 100 ml/kg. Even with microtechniques, repeated laboratory tests in sick preterm infants can easily deplete this blood volume, resulting in the need for blood transfusion to restore the circulating blood volume.

Tachycardia, tachypnea, poor growth, increased oxygen requirement, and acidosis are nonspecific symptoms of anemia. The presence of any of these symptoms in conjunction with a low hematocrit value may indicate the need for a transfusion of red blood cells (Manco-Johnson et al, 2002). Treatment is not without risk; however, transfusion reactions are rare. With improved screening and DNA- and/or RNA-directed assays of donor blood for virus detection for agents such as human immunodeficiency virus (HIV) (Mofenson & Committee on Pediatric AIDS, 2000), cytomegalovirus (CMV), and hepatitis B and C, infectious complications from transfusions have decreased significantly.

Recombinant human erythropoietin may be used to treat anemia in preterm infants because physiologic erythropoietin levels are anticipated to be low for a prolonged period. Given with oral elemental iron and vitamin E, or in combination with parenteral iron, exogenous erythropoietin stimulates erythropoiesis in LBW infants (Manco-Johnson et al, 2002; Ohls et al, 2001). However, routine use of recombinant human erythropoietin is not recommended because this therapy is not associated with decreased need for blood transfusions in preterm infants (Goodnough, 2000; Ohls et al, 2001).

Genitourinary Problem

Preterm infants have reduced renal function when compared with term infants or older children, and extreme care must be given in the administration of fluids and medication to avoid toxic levels of drugs and other chemicals. Preterm male infants have a higher rate of undescended testes than full-term newborns, but in most of these infants the testes descend during the first year of life. Medical and surgical intervention is indicated soon after 1 year of age for males with undescended testes because there is evidence of decreased spermatogonia if the testes remain in the abdomen (Hawtrey, 1990). The incidence of inguinal hernias has been found to be upward of 11% in VLBW and 17% in ELBW infants in the nursery and is inversely related to infant gestational age (Kumar et al, 2002). Males, SGA infants, and infants with CLD or BPD have a higher incidence of inguinal hernias, and this risk extends into their early school years (Kumar et al, 2002). Approximately 50% of the male infants will have bilateral inguinal hernias.

Preterm infants with inguinal hernia may have an increased risk of bowel incarceration with possible testicular injury from obstruction of blood flow. Surgical repair of inguinal hernias should be accomplished as soon as possible by a qualified pediatric surgeon before these infants are discharged from the NICU or when identified postdischarge (Kapur et al, 1998). Postoperative complications include recurrent apnea; therefore, outpatient surgical procedures are not recommended in the first few months of life.

PROGNOSIS

In 2001 the infant mortality rate was 6.9 per 1,000 live births with infants of black mothers having 2.5 times the mortality rate of infants of non-Hispanic white or Hispanic mothers (MacDorman et al, 2002b). More than 11.5% of all births were preterm births with 17.3% of black infants being born preterm as compared with 10.6% of white infants and 11.2% of Hispanic infants. The majority of infant deaths (66%) occurred in the 7.6% of infants who were born with low birth weights, and 52% of all infant deaths occurred in the 1.4% of infants born VLBW (MacDorman et al, 2002b). The higher infant mortality rate for black infants can be largely explained by the higher incidence of preterm and LBW and VLBW births in black mothers. A similar, but not as dramatic, pattern was seen for Hispanic LBW infants.

Survival rates for even the smallest preterm infants continue to improve. The number of multiple births has also increased since the 1980s (adding to the increase in LBW infants), in large part because of increased use of reproductive technology and an increase in the number of older mothers. Approximately half of all twins and the majority of triplets are born preterm or LBW (MacDorman et al, 2002b). Infants weighing 501 to 750 g at birth have a survival rate of 49%, infants weighing 751 to 1000 g 85%, infants 1,001 to 1,250 g 93%, and 96% of infants weighing 1,251 to 1,500 g at birth survive. Even if the preterm infant survives the first month of life, preterm and LBW infants have a three to seven times greater chance of dying after discharge from the hospital (Hulsey et al, 1994), and the risk is highest for those of lowest gestational age (23 to 27 weeks) (Doyle, 2001).

A national analysis of morbidity and mortality data for VLBW infants born between 1991 and 1999 determined that major improvements in obstetric and neonatal care (e.g., antenatal steroid use and surfactant postnatally) during the first half of the decade decreased morbidity and mortality for these vulnerable preterm infants. However, since 1995 there has been no additional improvement in morbidity and mortality (Horbar et al, 2002). The exact etiology for this leveling of morbidity and mortality in VLBW infants is unknown; subsequent examination of practice variations in NICUs and infant outcomes may explain this change in health outcomes for VLBW infants. Some preterm infants will have persistent health problems beyond discharge from the NICU (D'Angio et al, 2002; Doyle, 2001; McGrath et al, 2000). Infants with birth weights between 1,500 and 2,499 g are twice as likely as infants >2,500 g to require subsequent hospitalizations and preterm infants <1,500 g are four times more likely to be hospitalized (Svenson & Schopflocher, 1997).

A body of outcome data now available for preterm infants consistently indicates that the smaller the baby, the lower the survival rate and the higher the morbidity in relation to medical status, cognitive ability, behavior regulation, and social competence. On average, most VLBW infants do well, but a small yet significant proportion of them develop disabilities of varying degrees of severity (Hack et al, 1995; Kliegman, 2002). Socioeconomic status, parental education, childrearing environment, or postdischarge medical morbidity contributes to—and may be more predictive of—later outcome than interventions and complications in the NICU (Resnick et al, 1999; Singer et al, 2001).

PRIMARY CARE MANAGEMENT

Health Care Maintenance

Growth and Development

When plotted by corrected age (postnatal age less the number of weeks the infant was born preterm), the growth pattern of preterm AGA infants follows a different pattern from that of full-term infants. Preterm infants who experience minimal health problems exhibit catch-up growth earlier than those with serious medical problems. Heights and weights should be plotted at each office visit. Preterm infants should grow 25 cm in length over the first year of life and weight gains of 25 to 30 g per day are expected in preterm infants from birth to 3 months, 12 to 21 g per day in preterm infants from 3 to 6 months, and 10 to 13 g per day from 6 to 12 months postnatally (Klaus & Fanaroff, 2001). Failure to gain height and weight within these parameters, or a decrease in growth percentiles, may indicate a need to alter the nutritional management of the infant or a need to evaluate the infant for physiologic stress interfering with expected height and weight attainment (Olsen et al, 2002). VLBW and ELBW infants demonstrate growth patterns in the lowest percentiles during the first 12 months and remain smaller as a group than term children at 3 years of age (Hirata & Bosque, 1998). These children may catch up to the general population, however, by school age and can reach their genetic potential in stature by adolescence (Hirata & Bosque, 1998).

Preterm SGA infants tend to have poor neonatal growth, with the period of rapid catch-up growth occurring between 40 weeks' corrected age and 8 months of age. These children generally have lower rates of catch-up growth when compared with AGA preterm infants of the same birth weight (Strauss & Dietz, 1997).

The head circumference in preterm infants must be followed closely. Catch-up growth, which usually occurs in the first 6 weeks after birth and continues until 6 to 8 months, may result in disproportionately high head circumference percentiles, especially in the first 3 months after term. The head circumference often grows 2 cm per month from birth to 3 months, then slows to 1 cm per month from 4 to 6 months and 0.5 cm per month from 7 to 12 months (Klaus & Fanaroff, 2001). Increases in head circumference beyond these parameters, especially when the infant has a history of IVH, may indicate delayed development of hydrocephalus (see Chapter 29) (Sifuentes, 2000). Early postnatal head growth is an indicator of positive neurodevelopmental outcome. Lack of catch-up growth or initial catch-up growth followed by slow head growth are ominous signs of neurologic dysfunction (Sifuentes, 2000).

Development. Preterm infants with birth weights less than 1,500 g are at greatest risk for developmental morbidity. Outcomes have improved over time for VLBW infants, particularly for ELBW infants. There has been a dramatic increase in survival without an increase in the incidence of disabilities (D'Angio et al, 2002; Doyle, 2001). If adjustments are made for severity of associated complications of prematurity, there is also significant improvement in the disability rate. Neonatal medical status and associated morbidities are important variables predicting neurocognitive and school performance outcomes (McGrath et al, 2000; Ment et al, 2003).

Major developmental disabilities associated with VLBW infants include cerebral palsy, mental retardation, sensorineural hearing loss, and visual impairment related to ROP. These conditions are two to five times more frequent in LBW infants than in term infants. In addition, low to average intelligence, static motor disorders other than overt cerebral palsy (CP) (i.e., including motor clumsiness and incoordination), seizure disorders, and behavior disorders are prevalent. Educational disabilities, school failure, and speech delay are found in a high percentage of VLBW children (Bennett & Scott, 1997; Leonard & Piecuch, 1997). Many children have multiple problems, with the most pervasive and global disabilities becoming evident early.

Preterm infants are more vulnerable to environmental deprivation, resulting in more abnormal developmental outcomes in infants of lower socioeconomic status (SES) (Engleke et al, 1995; Resnick et al, 1999). Premature infants show significantly lower scores in social competence and significantly higher rates of behavior problems. Ross and colleagues (1990) showed that intelligence quotient (IQ) test scores best explained social competence scores, and family stability and socioeconomic status have explained behavior problem outcomes. Educational and cognitive disabilities of these infants are influenced differently by perinatal and sociodemographic variables. Both of these sets of variables must be considered to ascertain their contributions to the long-term risk of educational disabilities (Leonard & Piecuch, 1997; Resnick et al, 1999).

Intervention, as early as in the NICU, may maximize the developmental potential of high-risk preterm infants. Education and parental intervention in the first few years of life enhance early development, particularly in preterm children from disadvantaged environments (Committee on Children with Disabilities, 2001; McCormick et al, 1993; Ramey et al, 1992); this effect attenuates over time, however, if not reinforced (McCarton et al, 1997). The majority of preterm infants born prior to 32 weeks' gestation and less than 1,500 g and who required complex care in the NICU (i.e., resuscitation or prolonged mechanical ventilation) and/or who experienced complications (i.e., grade 3 or 4 IVH) are referred for regional developmental services and enrolled in infant follow-up programs prior to discharge from the NICU. It is crucial for primary care providers to work with these developmental specialists to understand the infant and family needs for early intervention services and to follow the infant's progress.

An essential component of primary care for preterm infants is developmental assessment and anticipatory guidance concerning developmental expectations. It is often difficult to perform formal testing in an office setting, but the Denver Developmental Screening Test II can help clinicians effectively screen and formulate a clinical impression of an infant's developmental capabilities. For VLBW infants, corrected age should be used for the first year of life and until 3 years of age. Using chronologic age to assess gross motor abilities will lead to overdiagnosis of neurologic abnormality in VLBW preterm infants. Corrected age should be used when specific and comprehensive developmental tests are used. Assessment of motor milestones during sequential visits can be a multistep screening process for neurologic complications including cerebral palsy (Allen & Alexander, 1997; Sifuentes, 2000). Further evaluation is necessary when a delay is evident or parents are extremely worried about their child's development. Referrals can be made to high-risk infant follow-up clinics, child development centers, regional developmental services, Easter Seal centers, or developmental pediatricians with training in assessing preterm infants.

Preterm infants often show signs of neuromuscular abnormalities that resolve during the second year of life and therefore do not carry the same prognostic importance as in the full-term infant. The most common neurologic abnormalities include increased extensor tone of the lower extremities, shoulder retractions caused by hypertonicity of the shoulder girdle and trapezius muscles, mild or transient asymmetry in tone, mild to moderate hypotonicity, and hypertonicity of the upper or lower extremities or trunk (Dubowitz, 1988). Primary care providers must perform thorough neurologic assessments during the first 2 years of life to determine the presence and progress of abnormalities. To ensure early identification of CP, careful examination for abnormal motor patterns and motor delay should be noted, but at the same time one must be cautious about labeling a child as having CP before 18 months' corrected age (Allen & Alexander, 1997; Morgan, 1996) (see Chapter 18).

Diet

Feeding the preterm infant in the immediate newborn period is a complex process. The immature gastrointestinal (GI) tract with decreased levels of bile salts, pancreatic lipase, lactase levels and reduced motility often prevent the preterm infant from being able to obtain adequate nutrition for growth through oral feedings (Anderson, 2002). In addition, the processes of sucking, swallowing, and breathing are not well coordinated in infants less than 32 weeks' gestation. Oral aversion can also occur in infants who have had endotracheal tubes or prolonged gavage feedings. For all of these reasons, many of the smallest preterm infants will require parental feeding for a time after birth.

When enteral feedings are initiated small amounts of fortified formula or breast milk with added oils containing long-chain polyunsaturated fatty acids, arachidonic acid (AA), and docosahexaenoic acid (DHA) are used (Fewtrell et al, 2002; O'Connor et al, 2001). When nutrient-enriched formulas or breast milk is continued postdischarge, growth parameters improve as compared with preterm infants fed standard term formula or breast milk (Carver et al 2001; Cooke et al, 2001; Lucas et al, 2001).

BOX 36-5
Advantages of Mother's Milk

ANTIINFECTIVE PROPERTIES
Antimicrobial factors
 IgA
 Lactoferrin
 Lysozyme
 B_{12} and folate-binding proteins
 Complement
 Antiviral factors
Live cells
 Macrophages
 Polymorphonuclear leukocytes
 T and B lymphocytes

GROWTH-ENHANCING PROPERTIES
Hormones and hormone releasors
Growth factors
Enzymes
Nucleotides
Docosahexaenoic acid (DHA) (essential fatty acid)
Arachidonic acid
Preterm mother's milk, which has a higher content of protein, Na, Cl, Mg,
 Fe, Cu, Zn, and IgA, is adapted to preterm infants.

Primary care providers should encourage breast feeding by providing the family information about the advantages of this form of nutrition (Box 36-5). The use of an electric pump on each breast every 3 hours helps mothers of preterm infants maintain an adequate milk supply while their infants are hospitalized and enables transition to breast feeding. Giving preterm infants the opportunity to suckle, as early as 32 weeks' gestational age, engenders positive effects for both mother and infant and encourages breast feeding after discharge (Morton, 2002). In addition to well-known antiinfective properties and enhanced iron absorption, breast feeding has also been associated with psychologic, socioeconomic, and environmental benefits. The presence of DHA and AA in breast milk, which are required for optimal brain and eye development, enhances visual acuity (O'Conner, 2001). These findings should encourage health care providers to ensure that parents are given information and support.

Certain maternal viral infections may result in transmission of virus to the infant via breast milk feedings, and therefore breast milk is not recommended. Such viruses include human immunodeficiency virus 1 (HIV-1) and human T-cell lymphotrophic virus type 1 (HTLV-1). CMV may be shed intermittently in breast milk, but disease does not usually develop in a term infant, presumably because of passively transferred maternal antibodies. Preterm infants, however, are at a greater potential risk because of low levels of transplacental antibodies, particularly if mothers become CMV-positive during lactation. Preterm infants are at risk for systemic disease and sensorineural hearing loss from CMV infection (Arnold & Radkowski, 1997). Pasteurization of human milk appears to inactivate the CMV virus and allow CMV-positive mothers to provide breast milk for their infants (Committee on Infectious

Disease, 2000). There are many preterm infant formulas available for mothers who cannot or choose not to provide breast milk.

Feeding preterm infants can be difficult because their mouths are small, oral musculature is weak, and the sucking mechanism is disorganized. Preterm infants may benefit from any or all of the following interventions: frequent, small-volume feedings; soft bottle nipples; support of head, neck, and hips in slight flexion; avoidance of excessive sensory stimuli; and observing and responding to infant cues (Kenner & Lott, 2003). Nonnutritive sucking may have beneficial effects on gastrointestinal function and growth and may facilitate nutritive sucking. Restricted-flow devices (i.e., through which milk only flows when the infant sucks) have been shown to facilitate oral feeding in infants of 26 to 29 weeks' gestational age (Lau et al, 1997). Prolonged skin-to-skin contact between mother and baby with opportunity for suckling at any time has been used as a means to promote successful breast feeding of hospitalized preterm infants. Caretakers must also be counseled on the need for an identified number of feedings or schedule of feedings because preterm infants may not demand feedings frequently. Regular feedings around the clock are required to maintain adequate caloric intake for growth. Frequent weight checks during the first year of life will help to identify problems early and institute change in the feeding program.

Abnormal feeding behaviors such as tonic bite reflex, tongue thrust, hyperactive gag reflex, or oral hypersensitivity can be seen. Hypersensitivity secondary to intubation, repeated suctioning, or use of nasogastric or orogastric tubes can make infants resistant to any type of oral stimulation, including nipples, spoons, and cups, and this oral aversion may last months to years after discharge. It is important for primary care providers to continually assess an infant's feeding capabilities and parental concerns about feeding. Referral to an oral-motor therapist (i.e., speech, physical, or occupational) familiar with feeding disorders is warranted when a significant or prolonged problem is recognized.

A multivitamin supplement should be given until preterm infants are ingesting more than 32 ounces of formula per day or until their body weight exceeds 2.5 kg. If breast fed, an infant should receive a multivitamin supplement until 1 year of age. Infants with poor growth because of recurrent or chronic illness or poor caloric intake should continue to receive a multi-vitamin supplement until they are consuming a well-balanced diet (Committee on Nutrition, 1998). Iron supplementation (2 to 4 mg/kg/day to maximum of 15 mg/day), as either an iron-fortified formula or a ferrous sulfate liquid if breast feeding, should be given by 2 months' chronologic age and continue for 12 to 15 months until a child is regularly eating iron-rich solid foods (Committee on Nutrition, Nutrition Handbook, 1998. If iron deficiency is anticipated because of the infant's history or VLBW status, iron supplementation can begin by 2 to 3 weeks of age when full oral feedings are established (Krug-Wispe, 1998). Vitamin E and folic acid supplementation should also continue until an infant is at least 40 weeks' postconceptional age. Multivitamin preparations containing vitamin E should satisfy this requirement. When iron deficiency is proven by laboratory testing, an

---

BOX 36-6

Safe Transportation of Premature Infants

Place the infant in the rear car seat with observation by an adult.
Infants <1 year of age or weighing <20 lb must ride facing the rear.
Infants ≥1 year of age and >20 lb should ride in rear seats approved for higher weights.
Blanket rolls should be used inside the car seat for head and lateral trunk control.
Rolls should be placed between the crotch strap and infant to reduce slouching.
If the infant's head drops forward, the seat should be tilted back and/or a cloth roll wedged under the safety seat base.
The seat should be reclined at a 45-degree angle to avoid the head dropping forward.
Use of convertible car seats with shields, abdominal pads, or arm rests that would contact the infant's face or neck during impact should be avoided.
The car seat's retainer clip should be positioned on the infant's chest.
A car seat for young children should never be placed in the front passenger seat of any vehicle with a passenger-side airbag.
An infant should never be left unattended in a car seat.

From Committee on Injury and Poison Prevention and Committee on Fetus and Newborn. (1996). Safe transportation of premature and low birth weight infants. *Pediatrics, 97,* 758-760. Adapted with permission.

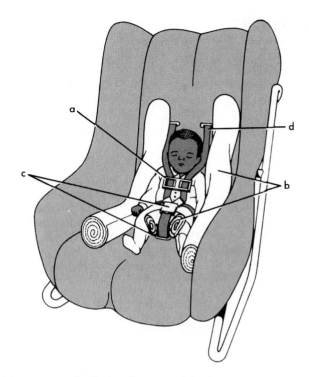

FIGURE 36-2 Positioning of premature infant in car seat. **A,** Retainer clip positioned on child's chest. **B,** Blanket rolls on both sides of trunk and between crotch strap and infant. **C,** Distance of 5½ inches or less from crotch strap to seat back. **D,** Distance of 10 inches or less from lower harness strap to seat bottom.

infant may require increased iron supplementation (i.e., up to 6 mg/kg/day).

Solid foods can be introduced to preterm infants when any one of the following criteria is met: (1) the infant consistently consumes more than 32 ounces of formula per day for 1 week, (2) the infant weighs 6 to 7 kg, or (3) the infant's corrected age is 6 months. The American Academy of Pediatrics (AAP) does not recommend feeding solids before 4 months of age. Cow's milk should not be introduced before 12 months past an infant's due date (Committee on Nutrition, 1998).

Safety

Anticipatory guidance about safety must be adjusted to a child's developmental level, not chronologic age. Because many parents continue to consider their child weak or vulnerable, they must be encouraged not to restrict activities but to allow exploration and social interaction in a safe setting.

Recommendations for the safe transportation of premature infants are shown in Box 36-6 and Figure 36-2 (Committee on Injury and Poison Prevention and Committee on Fetus and Newborn, 1996).

Safety must be ensured during air travel because of the decreased environmental oxygen concentration in commercial aircraft. Specific recommendations regarding travel for infants at risk for respiratory problems are shown in Box 36-7.

Parents of preterm infants at higher risk for apnea or SIDS should be taught infant cardiopulmonary resuscitation (CPR) before the infant is discharged from the hospital. Home cardiorespiratory monitoring needs to be decided on an individual basis. If parent education and reliable methods of recording events are instituted, home monitoring can reduce hospitalizations for apparent life-threatening events (ALTE). Home monitoring for apnea in preterm infants can initially increase caretaker stress, depression, and hostility but over time these

---

BOX 36-7

Recommendations for Traveling with High-Risk Infants

Families should be counseled to minimize travel for infants at risk for respiratory compromise.
An appropriate hospital staff person should observe the infant in a car seat before discharge to monitor for possible apnea, bradycardia, or oxygen desaturation for infants of <37 weeks' gestation.
Infants with documented apnea, bradycardia, or oxygen desaturation should travel in a supine or prone position in an alternative safety device (e.g., an approved car bed).
Infants with home cardiac and apnea monitors should use this equipment during travel with portable self-contained power for twice the expected transport duration.
All portable medical equipment should be restrained with adjacent seat belts or wedged on the floor or under the seats.
Air travel should be postponed until maturation of the respiratory control center occurs (at least 6 to 8 weeks past the infant's due date).
Pulmonary function or hypoxia or carbon dioxide challenge tests should be considered to determine safety of air travel.

Data from Trachtenbarg, D.E. & Golemon, T.B. (1998). Care of the premature infant: Part I. Monitoring growth and development. *Am Fam Physician, 57,* 2383-2390.

decrease (Abendroth et al, 1999). But with anticipatory education, guidance regarding false alarms and technical aspects of monitoring, and reassurance that with development the infant will outgrow apnea spells, most caretakers find the monitor reassuring.

Immunizations

The recommendations of the AAP Committee on Infectious Disease (2000) should be used for immunizing preterm infants. Precautions and contraindications for vaccine use designated for term infants also apply to preterm infants. All inactivated vaccines used during infancy, including the recently introduced pneumococcal vaccine (Prevnar), should be administered according to the preterm infant's chronologic age. Hepatitis B vaccine should be given to infants of hepatitis B surface antigen (HbsAg)-negative mothers when the infant weighs 2 kg or is 2 months of age, whichever comes first. If the mother is surface antigen positive, or her antigen status is unknown, both hepatitis B vaccine and hepatitis immunoglobulin (HBIG) should be given immediately after birth regardless of the infant's weight. Inactivated vaccines can be administered while the infant is hospitalized and in a recovery state from any acute health condition. Measles, mumps, and rubella and varicella live-virus vaccines should be administered on or after the preterm infant's first birthday as with infants born at term. These vaccines are live-virus vaccines and therefore should not be given if the infant is still in the hospital due to the theoretical risk of exposing other infants to shed live virus. Because of the poor transfer of antibodies across the placenta early in pregnancy, all preterm infants born before 28 weeks' gestation (or weighing ≤1,000 g) who are still hospitalized and exposed to varicella should receive varicella-zoster immune globulin (125 units). The recommendation also applies to preterm infants born after 28 weeks' gestation whose mothers have a negative history of infection (Committee on Infectious Disease, 2000).

Parents and caretakers of preterm infants younger than 6 months of age and all preterm infants with pulmonary or cardiac problems should be immunized yearly with influenza vaccine to decrease the viral exposure to the infant (Committee on Infectious Disease, 2002). Preterm infants less than 1,500 g at birth and/or less than 32 weeks' gestation at birth are recommended to receive the monoclonal antibody vaccine palivizumab (Synagis), to prevent infections associated with the respiratory syncytial virus (RSV). This vaccine is typically given monthly during the fall and winter months of the first 2 years of the preterm life (Committee on Infectious Disease and Committee on Fetus and Newborn, 1998).

Screening

Vision. Ophthalmologic problems, as a consequence of ROP—particularly stage 3 or higher—include myopia, amblyopia, and rarely retinal detachment and blindness. Strabismus also occurs with increased frequency among preterm infants (O'Conner et al, 2002). All oxygen-exposed infants with birth weights less than 1,500 g (or ≤38 weeks of gestation) or those weighing more than 1,500 g at birth with an unstable clinical course and at high risk for ROP should have an ophthalmologic examination 4 to 6 weeks after birth, from 31 to 33 weeks' postconceptional age, or before discharge to assess for ROP. Those who are still at risk for ROP by virtue of their immature retinas should receive close ophthalmologic follow-up after discharge. The follow-up examinations should occur at 1- to 4-week intervals, depending upon the immaturity of the retinal vessels, until the retina is mature (Ophthalmology and Strabismus, American Academy of Ophthalmology, 1997). Infants with ELBW may benefit from earlier examinations due to their increased risk of ROP (Subhani et al, 2001).

Eye examinations of preterm infants by the primary care provider should include assessments of vision, the fundus, and alignment of the eyes. Visual assessment includes the infant's ability to fixate and follow objects. This response should be present by 6 weeks' corrected age. Continued yearly assessment of visual acuity in preterm infants is important to identify strabismus, early myopia, and more subtle refractive errors that may affect scholastic achievement.

Hearing. The incidence of sensorineural hearing loss in preterm infants is reported to be 1% to 3%. Risk factors associated with preterm birth including hypoxia, mechanical ventilation for 5 days or longer, hyponatremia, metabolic acidosis, hyperbilirubinemia, environmental noise levels, concomitant antibiotic and diuretic therapy, and congenital infections place LBW infants at particular risk for hearing problems (Joint Committee on Infant Hearing, 2000). Significantly better language development is associated with early identification of hearing loss and early intervention (i.e., at less than 6 months of age).

The AAP Task Force on Newborn and Infant Hearing (1999) recommends implementation of universal newborn hearing screening. VLBW infants or preterm infants with any other risk factors should be screened under the supervision of an audiologist. Screening should optimally be performed before discharge from the newborn nursery—never later than 3 months of age. The gold standard for assessment of hearing sensitivity in newborns is the auditory brainstem response (ABR) (Sokol & Hyde, 2002). If the results of an initial screening are equivocal, the infant should be referred for general medical, otologic, and audiologic follow-up, which should include a repeat ABR and a behavioral auditory testing when the child is 4 to 6 months of corrected age. Ongoing testing is necessary when there are conditions that increase the probability of progressive hearing loss, such as family history of delayed onset of hearing loss, degenerative disease, craniofacial anomalies, stigmata associated with hearing loss, meningitis, or intrauterine infections (Task Force on Newborn and Infant Hearing, 1999). Health care providers should be alerted to children who have delays in speech development, poor attentiveness, and absent or abnormal responses to sound. These findings may indicate hearing loss and necessitate more thorough investigation.

Dental. Prolonged orotracheal intubation affects the palate and possibly the dentition; very high arched palates and deep palatal grooves have also been observed. In mild cases these deformities usually resolve within the first year of life. Abnormally shaped teeth with notching have been observed in some infants. Dental eruption is usually mildly delayed in premature infants (even allowing for corrected age), with greater delays seen in chronically ill infants. Staining of deciduous teeth as a result of neonatal illness (e.g., hyperbilirubinemia and cholestasis) may be evident. Consultation with a pediatric dentist may be required. Specific guidelines for fluoride use in preterm infants do not exist, but routine fluoride supplementation is not recommended for the first 6 months of life (Committee on Nutrition, 1995).

Blood Pressure. Preterm infants may be particularly at risk for developing hypertension, possibly because of complications of umbilical arterial catheters. Occult renal disease and BPD are also associated with hypertension. Hypertension screening should be done several times in the first year of life and then routinely in childhood. Normal blood pressures, adjusted for height, are within the 90th percentile on the blood pressure tables and graphs produced by the National High Blood Pressure Education Program (NHBPEP, 1996) and should be used for accuracy of diagnosis. Infants with blood pressures above the 95th percentile for age on three separate visits should be considered hypertensive, and the cause should be identified (NHBPEP, 1996). Children with blood pressures between the 90th and 95th percentiles warrant careful follow-up.

Hematocrit. At each visit, hematocrit screening should be tailored to individual preterm infants and the health care provider index of suspicion about the infant's hemoglobin status. History of general nutrition, iron and vitamin intake, use of exogenous erythropoietin, and birth weight will help determine the need to check a blood count before the signs and symptoms of anemia (tachycardia, tachypnea, pallor, lethargy, poor feeding, poor weight gain, and apnea with bradycardia) develop. Routine hematocrit determinations should be performed on preterm infants with hemolytic diseases (e.g., ABO or Rh incompatibility) or those whose vitamin and iron intake is poor. Although hematocrit levels below 25% are not well tolerated, the need for transfusion should be determined by signs and symptoms of anemia rather than a defined hematocrit level (Kliegman, 2002).

Urinalysis. Routine screening is recommended.

Tuberculosis. Routine screening is recommended.

Condition-Specific Screening

Hernia and Testicular Screening. At each primary care visit the preterm infant's caretaker must be asked about the presence of inguinal swelling that increases in size with coughing or crying. The inguinal area and canal must be palpated for any swelling or masses. Because of the increased incidence of undescended testicles in preterm male infants, a thorough testicular examination is warranted.

Common Illness Management

Differential Diagnosis (Box 36-8)

Respiratory Infections. Respiratory infections are frequent causes of rehospitalization in preterm infants, and viral respiratory disease is particularly dangerous for infants with residual lung disease. These infants must be monitored closely by the primary care provider for signs of respiratory distress (see Chapter 16, Bronchopulmonary Dysplasia [BPD]). The risk of acquiring lower respiratory tract infection is related to an infant's age at acquisition of the primary infection, with highest morbidity in the first year and lower morbidity in the second and third years of life. Because older siblings and adults usually bring viral pathogens into the home, direct contact with the infant by symptomatic individuals should be minimized, especially during the infant's first year of life. Respiratory viruses (e.g., RSV, parainfluenza viruses, and influenza viruses) are a major cause of morbidity and late mortality (Committees on

---

BOX 36-8

Differential Diagnosis

RESPIRATORY INFECTIONS
Increased susceptibility to viral respiratory illnesses, especially RSV
Increased incidence of wheezing and bronchiolitis
RSV immune globulin prophylaxis

OTHER VIRAL INFECTIONS
Herpes simplex virus types 1 and 2

BACTERIAL INFECTIONS
Group B *Streptococcus, Chlamydia, Staphylococcus aureus,* and *Escherichia coli* require appropriate antibiotics
Increased risk for *Streptococcus pneumoniae* and *Haemophilus influenzae* type b
Need early identification of possible sepsis

Infectious Disease and Fetus and Newborn, 1998). Synagis is recommended during the fall and winter months for preterm infants in the first 2 years of life to prevent RSV infections. Parents should also be counseled to avoid exposing infants to environmental tobacco smoke, which is known to cause or exacerbate respiratory illness and middle ear effusions in the infant.

Other Viral Infections. The incubation period for infants with perinatal exposure to herpes simplex virus (HSV) is variable, ranging from 2 days to 6 weeks. Because the attack rate for HSV increases with preterm birth and is associated with significant morbidity and mortality, the diagnosis of HSV should be considered in high-risk premature infants who have any symptoms compatible with HSV, including lethargy, poor feeding, herpetic (vesicular) lesions, respiratory distress, or seizures. A maternal history of herpes infection or vesicular lesions increases the suspicion. Because the effects of HSV type 1 can be as devastating as HSV type 2, parents must be advised to avoid exposing their infant to individuals with fever blisters, cold sores, or any vesicular lesions suspected to be caused by HSV (Committee on Infectious Disease, 2000). Appropriate cultures should be taken and treatment should be begun with acyclovir when an infant is suspected of being infected with HSV.

Bacterial Infections. Organisms such as *Chlamydia,* group B *Streptococcus, Staphylococcus aureus,* or *Escherichia coli* can colonize in an infant during birth or hospitalization and become invasive, causing serious infection characterized by sepsis and/or meningitis after discharge, particularly in the first month of life. In addition, preterm infants may be at special risk for organisms such as *Streptococcus pneumoniae (pneumococcus)* and *Haemophilus influenzae* type b (Hib). The major sites of infection are the respiratory system, CNS, bones, and joints.

Healthy preterm infants who have unexplained fever should be assessed according to their corrected ages. This investigation is similar to that for term infants but with a higher degree of suspicion. In early stages, close follow-up is critical to the evaluation because signs and symptoms may be nonspecific and subtle. Empiric antibiotic therapy must be given immediately after cultures are taken because infection can spread rapidly because of the relative immunodeficiency of preterm infants if the provider awaits culture results. Antibiotic selection must take into account possible neonatal sources of infection (e.g., *S. aureus*), resistant bacteria from the NICU (e.g., *Enterococcus* or *Enterobacter*), or organisms recovered from or known to inhabit the maternal genital tract (e.g., group B *Streptococcus*). An infant with obtundation, hypothermia, poor color, respiratory distress, seizures, or apnea is a medical emergency, and immediate hospitalization and treatment must be achieved. Parents should be instructed about the possible early signs and symptoms of infection, which may include lethargy, poor feeding, irritability, fever, respiratory distress, skin lesions, and bowel changes. Because some of these symptoms in milder form may be characteristics of a well premature infant's baseline behavior, awareness of changes in this baseline may help to identify illness.

Developmental Issues

Sleep Patterns

The sleep patterns of preterm infants may differ from those of full-term infants in the first weeks after hospital discharge. Nutritional needs of preterm infants may entail night feedings and establish a pattern of night waking. Some preterm infants may be hypersensitive to sights and sounds and, conversely, some have become habituated to the noise and lights of the NICU and have difficulty adjusting to the quiet and dark of the home environment. Preterm infants do, however, develop circadian sleep-wake rhythms after exposure to an environment with daily routines and time cues (Shimada et al, 1999) and do not appear to have more sleep problems than term infants beyond the first few months (Wolke et al, 1995). Although an individual infant's ability to sleep through the night is determined by factors such as age, temperament, previous sleep patterning, and type of feeding, more night waking is seen with breast feeding than with bottle feeding (Wolke et al, 1998), and more support and education by the provider is necessary to prevent early termination of breast feeding.

Parents should be encouraged to follow current recommendations regarding sleep positioning and environmental factors believed to decrease the risk of sudden infant death syndrome (SIDS) (Task Force on Infant Sleep Position and Sudden Infant Death Syndrome, 2000). Preterm infants are at increased risk of SIDS, with the risk increasing with decreasing gestational age. Infants should be placed on their back to sleep or securely on their sides; sleeping surfaces should be firm without soft pillows, quilts, or comforters; the environment should not be overheated or the infant overclothed; and the environment should be free of secondhand smoke (Task Force on Infant Sleep Position and Sudden Infant Death Syndrome, 2000).

Toileting

Signs of toileting readiness are more likely to appear at the appropriate corrected—chronologic—age. Abnormal neurologic findings (e.g., increased muscle tone) may have a negative effect on the toilet training process, and training may be effective when muscle tone has decreased.

Discipline

The stress of having a preterm infant in the NICU leaves many parents and their infants prone to a vulnerable child syndrome. These attitudes about the child may result in the compensatory parenting of overindulgence and overpermissiveness (Miles & Holditch-Davis, 1997). Families often have difficulties setting limits, which can interfere with normal development; these children may exhibit dependent, demanding, or uncontrolled behavior. Guidelines on effective discipline from the AAP Committee on Psychological Aspects of Child and Family Health (1998) are helpful for primary care providers to impart to parents.

Some preterm infants are more difficult to care for than full-term infants and reciprocity or parent-infant interactions may be limited particularly during the first few months of life. Preterm infants may become agitated or nonresponsive to what is considered average stimulation. These infants are often difficult to soothe, have trouble eating and delayed milestones, and require more care and patience from their parents. It is important that parents learn to read the preterm infant regarding satisfaction versus distress and that the parent-infant relationship be supported as an evolving relationship. Children born preterm may be more prone to child abuse than term children due to altered parent-infant relationships and the stress of having a preterm infant.

Primary care providers should assess the parent-infant relationship with each visit and offer anticipatory counseling to parents regarding the unique needs of the preterm infants. Maternal mental health, infant security of attachment, family cohesion, family adaptability, and family adequacy of income have all been found to affect mental health problems in children (Weiss & Seed, 2002). Externalizing behaviors of mental health problems can lead to behavior problems at home and in the community.

Child Care

Many studies have shown the increased incidence of infectious diseases, particularly diarrheal and respiratory illnesses in infants and children attending daycare centers as compared with children cared for in the home. Because preterm infants have more prolonged immune deficiencies, the transmission of infectious diseases within daycare centers may affect the morbidity of preterm infants attending these facilities. Based on these considerations, child care at home is preferable to other daycare situations, at least for the infant's first year of life (Committee on Infectious Disease, 2000). Parents must also consider their role in educating daycare providers about the special needs of LBW infants (e.g., nutrition, stimulation, and sleep habits).

Schooling

Many studies have documented an increased frequency of educational problems in premature children. Children who were born preterm are more likely to have lower school achievement and greater need for special class placements. These problems are often manifested as subtle visual-motor, perceptual, language, and reading difficulties or hyperactive behavior (D'Angio et al, 2002; Doyle, 2001; Leonard & Piecuch, 1997; Resnick et al, 1998; Resnick et al, 1999). School readiness is often delayed in VLBW infants (particularly in boys), and early school problems may be prevented by starting these children in school a year behind their full-term peers.

The prevalence of learning problems in preterm infants of normal intelligence emphasizes the need for early identification and implementation of individual intervention programs (see Chapter 5) (Committee on Children with Disabilities, 1998). Ideally these children should be longitudinally followed into their school years in high-risk clinics. If these services are not available, primary care providers should assess the neurodevelopmental progress of a child, including the presence of soft signs, which may indicate poor academic performance. School performance and progress should be discussed with parents and school personnel; referral for educational testing should be initiated if a problem is suspected.

Sexuality

Children who were born preterm do not appear to have problems in becoming parents. Both male and female survivors have had normal progeny (Hirata, 1999). Undescended testicles in preterm infants must be followed and corrected it they persist to ensure normal spermatogenesis. Women who were born SGA have been found to be at increased risk for giving birth to both growth-restricted and preterm infants (Klebanoff et al, 1989). Appropriate counseling and early prenatal referral for parents and adolescents are necessary with regard to these findings.

Transition to Adulthood

Transition to adolescence and adulthood may be more difficult for children born preterm, depending on earlier developmental and behavioral problems. Fortunately although growth continues to be compromised, most VLBW and ELBW children experience more rapid catch-up growth during adolescence and reach stature closer to their genetic potential (Saigal et al, 2001). ELBW survivors continued to have substantial morbidity but with a reduction in the prevalence of acute health problems and decreased utilization of medical resources (Saigal et al, 2001). Saigal (1996) found that a majority of ELBW infants 12 to 16 years of age viewed their own health status and quality of life as quite satisfactory, although as a whole this cohort suffered a greater burden of morbidity than the control group. Many VLBW children, however, appear to have lower social competence and more behavior problems in their school years when compared with their peers (Ross et al, 1990).

In preterm children any preexisting developmental or behavioral problems may be exaggerated during the turbulence of adolescence. Feelings of not measuring up to their peers may surface if growth has been poor and health problems have interfered with their quest for independence. Parental overprotection may add to low self-esteem. During adolescence children are more sensitive about personal appearance, and any cosmetic deformities and scars from their hospital experience (e.g., IV, chest tube, and surgery scars) may cause anguish. Efforts toward cosmetic repair of more pronounced problems should be made.

If a child's concerns during adolescence are addressed with good parental communication, support, and encouragement, the transition to adulthood should be less problematic and more comparable with that of their full-term peers. In some cases professional psychologic intervention may need to be provided.

Family Concerns and Resources

Families with preterm infants have multiple issues to address. Parents must deal with the grief of delivering a preterm infant while going through the attachment process. The transition from hospital to home is a period of extreme anxiety; parents are faced with caring for their infant without the support of hospital staff. Parents have financial issues as well as concerns involving the health and developmental outcome of the infant. It is often difficult to appreciate the progress of their preterm infant while friends, relatives, and strangers continually make comparisons with full-term infants. Education and support from primary care providers may enable parents to create an environment that will encourage infants to attain their full potential. Understanding the preexisting and concurrent personal and family factors that influence the family's experience of having a premature infant may provide opportunities for support and intervention, both during hospitalization and after discharge to home (Miles & Holditch-Davis, 1997).

Today new approaches and programs aid families with high-risk infants after discharge. There is growing evidence that early intervention programs have a positive effect on both the infant's development and the family's adjustment (Committee on Children with Disabilities, 2001). Early and appropriate referral of infants to community-based, coordinated, multidisciplinary, and family-centered programs for at-risk infants and families is an important responsibility of the primary care provider. Anticipatory guidance can help parents deal with premature infants who behave differently from full-term infants. Parents should be educated about behavioral cues and a developmentally supportive environment, including consistency in caregiving, a structured routine, pacing of caregiving in accordance with the infant's cues for interaction versus rest, and an individualized feeding plan (Berger et al, 1998).

Resources are available for families with premature infants. Many hospitals have parent support groups that work with families during hospitalization and after discharge. Many NICUs have a follow-up clinic that employs an interdisciplinary team for ongoing evaluation of infants considered to be at high risk for physical, developmental, and psychologic problems. Government agencies and regional developmental centers provide funding for evaluation and treatment of the developmental needs of these infants. Ancillary support services are listed below.

Support Organizations

Family Voices
(888) 835-5669
www.familyvoices.org
National family support group and lobbying organization for families with children with special health care needs.

The Federation for Children with Special Needs
(800) 331-0688
www.fcsn.org
Center for parent organizations to work together to improve care for children with disabilities.

March of Dimes
(888) MODIMES (888-663-4637)
Spanish speaking number: (800) 925-1855
www.marchofdimes.com
Supports education and research to decrease birth defects.

National Organization of Mothers of Twins Club, Inc.
(800) 243-2276
www.nomotc.org
National organization to support parents of twins or higher multiple births.

The Preemie Store . . . and More!
(800) 676-8469
www.preemie.com
Shopping for preterm infants. Also has parent support activities and chat rooms.

Zero to Three
(202) 638-1144
www.zerotothree.org
Parent and professional resource center for early childhood development.

Summary of Primary Care Needs for the Premature Infant

HEALTH CARE MAINTENANCE

Growth and development

Use corrected age to plot height, weight, and head circumference.

Preterm infants who are AGA follow growth patterns similar to those of full-term infants.

Infants who are SGA tend to be smaller children.

"Catch-up" growth occurs within the first year to after 3 years of age and may be prolonged to adolescence in ELBW infants.

Head circumference should be monitored for abnormal growth.

VLBW and ELBW infants are at high risk for neurologic, cognitive, or learning abnormalities.

The incidence of abnormal development increases with decreasing birth weight.

Corrected age should be used to assess development.

Transient neuromuscular abnormalities can be present in the first year.

Diet

Breast feeding is recommended

There are special concerns regarding viral transmission of HIV, CMV, and hepatitis B in breast milk.

Feeding problems such as oral hypersensitivity and gastroesophageal reflux are common.

Fortification of breast milk or higher-caloric formula may be needed for ELBW and SGA infants for several weeks after hospital discharge.

Multivitamins should be given for infants who weigh <2.5 kg or those who have chronic illness or poor growth.

All preterm infants should receive 2 to 4 mg of iron/kg/day for the first year of life.

Safety

Anticipatory guidance is based on developmental age.

Recommendations for car seat use include using blanket rolls for support, observing while driving, and avoiding models with lap pads or shields.

Air travel should be delayed until an infant tolerates lower environmental oxygen concentrations.

Parents should be trained in CPR for infants at high risk for apnea.

Immunizations

All immunizations should be administered at the chronologic ages recommended by the AAP.

Infants should be given IPV while still in hospital.

The effectiveness of the hepatitis B vaccine is unknown in infants <2 kg.

Preterm infants with long-term pulmonary or cardiac problems and their caretakers should receive the influenza vaccine each fall.

Varicella-zoster immune globulin should be given to infants born at <28 weeks who are exposed to varicella while hospitalized.

Breast-feeding infants of mothers who are hepatitis B surface-antigen positive should receive hepatitis B immune globulin.

Screening

Vision. Assessment of fixation following alignment and funduscopic examination is recommended. Ophthalmologic follow-up is necessary for infants with ROP or positive visual finding.

Hearing. Screening is recommended for all infants—particularly for those with identified risk factors before hospital discharge—and repeated within 3 months of age if abnormal or equivocal.

Dental. Prolonged intubation affects palate and dentition.

Tooth eruptions may be delayed, and teeth may be abnormally shaped or discolored.

Routine fluoride supplementation is recommended after 6 months' corrected age.

Blood pressure. Hypertension screenings should be done at 1, 2, 6, 12, and 24 months of age, and then routinely in childhood.

Children with BP >95% for 3 screenings should be considered hypertensive and the reason identified.

Hematocrit. Hematocrit values should be checked based on history, nutritional status, and symptoms.

Urinalysis. Routine screening is recommended.

Tuberculosis. Routine screening is recommended.

Condition-Specific Screening

Hernia and testicular screening: Infants should be screened for inguinal hernia and undescended testicles.

COMMON ILLNESS MANAGEMENT

Differential Diagnosis

Risk of infection—particularly respiratory infection—is increased.

RSV, HSV, *Chlamydia*, group B *Streptococcus, S. aureus,* and *E. coli* must all be considered possible pathogens.

Risk for *Streptococcus pneumoniae* and *H. influenzae* type b infections must be evaluated.

Possible sepsis must be identified early.

Continued

Summary of Primary Care Needs for the Premature Infant—cont'd

DEVELOPMENTAL ISSUES

Sleep Patterns

Children may have disorganized sleep patterns.

Toileting

Toileting readiness is based on developmental age.
Increased muscle tone may impede toilet training.

Discipline

Children should be assessed for vulnerable child syndrome.
Limits should be set as with any other child.
The incidence of child abuse is higher than with other children.

Child care

Home care or small daycare programs are recommended.

Schooling

These children have an increased incidence of educational problems. School readiness should be ascertained before a child enters kindergarten.
Psychometric testing is indicated for poor school performance.

Sexuality

Preterm children have normal offspring.
Standard developmental counseling is advised. There is an increased incidence of SGA and prematurity in the offspring of women who were SGA at birth.

Transition to Adulthood

Preexisting developmental or behavior problems may become more exaggerated. Concerns of parental overprotection, adolescent low self-esteem, correction of cosmetic deformities, and parental communications should be addressed.
These child's self-perception of quality of life is good.

FAMILY CONCERNS

Family concerns include grief, attachment issues as a result of prolonged hospitalization, financial considerations, and concerns about developmental outcomes.

REFERENCES

Abendroth, D., Moser, D.K., Dracup, K., & Doering, L.V. (1999). Do apnea monitors decrease emotional distress in parents of infants at high risk for cardiopulmonary arrest? *J Pediatr Health Care, 13*(2), 50-57.

Abrahams, C. & Katz, M. (2002). A perspective on the diagnosis of preterm labor. *J Perinat Neonat Nurs, 16*(1), 1-11.

Affonso, D., Bosque, E., Wahlberg, V., & Brady, J.P. (1993). Reconciliation and healing for mothers through skin to skin contact provided in an American tertiary level intensive care nursery. *Neonatal Network, 12*(3), 25-32.

Alexander, G.R., Kogan, M., Bader, D., Carlo, W., Allen, M., et al. (2003). US birth weight/gestational age-specific neonatal mortality: 1995-97 rates for Whites, Hispanics and Blacks. *Pediatrics, 111*(1), e61-66. Available at: http://www.pediatrics.org/cgi/content/full/111/1/e61.

Allen, H.D., Gutgesell, H.P., Clark, E.B., & Dirscoll, D.J. (2001). *Moss and Adams: Heart disease in infants, children, and adolescents* (6ᵗʰ ed.). Philadelphia: Williams and Wilkins.

Allen, M.C. & Alexander, G.R. (1990). Gross motor milestones in preterm infants: correction for degree of prematurity. *Pediatrics, 116*, 955-959.

Allen, M.C. & Alexander, G.R. (1997). Using motor milestones as a multistep process to screen preterm infants for cerebral palsy. *Dev Med Child, 39*, 12-16.

Als, H., Lawhon, G., Duffy, F.H., McAnulty, G.B., Gibes-Grossman, R., et al. (1994). Individualized developmental care for the very low birth weight preterm infant. *JAMA, 272*, 853-858.

American Society of Parenteral and Enteral Nutrition (ASPEN). (1993). Section VII: nutrition support for low-birth-weight infants. *J PEN, 17*(4), 33S-38SA.

American Academy of Pediatrics. American Association for Pediatric Ophthalmology and Strabismus and the American Academy of Ophthalmology. (1997). Screening examination of premature infants for retinopathy of prematurity. *Pediatrics, 100*, 273.

American Academy of Pediatrics (AAP) & American College of Obstetricians and Gynecologists (ACOG). (2002). *Guidelines for perinatal care*. Washington, DC: Author.

American Academy of Pediatrics. Committee on Nutrition. (1998). Soy protein-based formulas: recommendations for use in infant feedings. *Pediatrics, 101*, 148-152.

American College of Obstetricians and Gynecologists (ACOG). (1998). Antenatal Corticosteroid Therapy for Fetal Maturation. ACOG Committee Opinion. Washington, DC: Author.

Amon, E., Midkiff, C., Winn, H., Holcomb, W., Shumway, J., et al. (2000). Tocolysis with advanced cervical dilation. *Obstet Gynecol, 95*(3), 358-362.

Anderson, D.M. & Loughead, J.L. (2002). Feeding the Ill or preterm infant. *Neonatal Netw, 21*(7), 7-14.

Anderson, M.S., Johnson, C.B., Townsend, S.F., & Hay Jr., W.W. (2002). Enteral nutrition. In G.B. Merenstein & S.L. Gardner (Eds.). *Handbook of neonatal intensive care* (5ᵗʰ ed.). St Louis: Mosby.

Anderson, J.E. & Radkowski, D. (1997). Hearing loss in the newborn infant. In A.A. Fanaroff & R.J. Martin (Eds.), *Neonatal-perinatal medicine: diseases of the fetus and infant* (6ᵗʰ ed.). St Louis: Mosby.

Arnold, J.E. & Radkowski, D. (1997). Hearing loss in the newborn infant. In A.A. Fanaroff & R.J. Martin (Eds.).

Aziz, K., Vickar, D.B., Sauve, R.S., Etches, P.C., Pain, K.S., et al. (1995). Province-based study of neurologic disability of children weighing 500 through 1249 grams at birth in relation to neonatal cerebral ultrasound findings. *Pediatrics, 95*, 837-844.

Ballard, J.L., Khoury, J.C., Wedig, K., Wang, L., Eilers-Walsman, B.L., et al. (1991). New Ballard score, expanded to include extremely premature infants. *J Pediatr, 119*, 417-423.

Beck-Sague, C.M., et al. (1994). Bloodstream infections in neonatal intensive care unit patients: results from a multicenter study. *Pediatric Infectious Disease Journal, 13*, 1110-1116.

Bennett, F.C. & Scott, O.T. (1997). Long term perspective on preterm infant outcome and contemporary intervention issues. *Semin Perinatol, 21*, 190-201.

Bensard, D.D., Calkins, C.M., Patrick, D., & Price, F.N. (2002). Neonatal surgery. In G.B. Merenstein & S.L. Gardner (Eds.), *Handbook of neonatal intensive care* (5ᵗʰ ed.). St Louis: Mosby.

Bernbaum, J.C. (2000). *Preterm infants in primary care: A guide to office management*. Columbus, Ohio: Ross Products Division, Abbott Laboratories.

Berger, S.P., Holt-Turner, I., Cupoli, J.M., Mass, M., & Hageman, J.R. (1998). Caring for the graduate from the neonatal intensive care unit. *Ped Clin North Am, 45*(3), 701-712.

Berseth, C.L. (2001). Feeding methods for the preterm infant. *Semin Neonatol, 6*, 417-424.

Berseth, C.L. & Abrams, S.A. (1998). Special gastrointestinal concerns. In H.W. Taeusch & R.A. Ballard (Eds.), *Avery's diseases of the newborn* (7th ed.). Philadelphia: W.B. Saunders.

Berseth, C.L., Bisquera, J.A., & Paje, V.U. (2003). Prolonged small feeding volumes early in life decreases the incidence of necrotizing enterocolitis in very low birth weight infants. *Pediatrics, 111*(3), 529-534.

Blondis, T., Snow, J., & Accardo, P. (1990). Integration of soft signs in academically normal and academically at-risk children. *Pediatrics, 85*(suppl)421-425.

Bolt, R.J., van Weissenbruch, M.M., Lafeber, H.N., & Delemarre-van de Waal, H.A. (2001). Glucocorticoids and lung development in the fetus and preterm infant. *Pediatr Pulmon, 32*, 76-91.

Bosque, E.M., Brady, J.P., Affonso, D.D., & Wahlberg, V. (1995). Physiological measures of kangaroo versus incubator care in a tertiary level nursery. *JOGNN, 24*(3), 219-226.

Bright, M.A. (2002). *Holistic Health and Healing*. Philadelphia: F.A. Davis Co.

Canadian Paediatric Society: Fetus & Newborn Committee. (2002). Postnatal corticosteroids to treat or prevent chronic lung disease in preterm infants. *Pediatrics, 109*(2), 330-338.

Caplan, M.S. & Jilling, T. (2001). New concepts in necrotizing enterocolitis. *Curr Opin Pediatr, 13*(2), 111-115.

Capone, A. Jr., Diaz-Rohena, R., Sternberg, P. Jr., Mandell, B., Lambert, H.M., et al. (1993). Diode-laser photocoagulation for zone 1 threshold retinopathy of prematurity. *Arch Ophthalmol, 110*(12), 1714-1716.

Carver, J.D., Wu, P.Y., Hall, R.T., Ziegler, E.E., Sosa, R., et al. (2001). Growth of preterm infants fed nutrient-enriched or term formula after hospital discharge. *Pediatrics, 107*(4), 683-689.

Casey, P.H., Kraemer, H.C., Bernbaum, J., Yogman, M.W., & Sells, J.C. (1991). Growth status and growth rates of a varied sample of low birth weight, preterm infants: a longitudinal cohort from birth to three years of age. *J Pediatr, 119*, 599-605.

Caughey, A.B. & Parer, J.T. (2002). Recommendations for repeat courses of antenatal corticosteroids: A decision analysis. *Am J Obstet Gynecol, 186*(6), 1226-1229.

Centers for Disease Control and Prevention. (1997). Births and deaths: United States—1996. *MMWR, 46*(1), 1-44.

Centers for Disease Control and Prevention (2000). Contribution of assistive reproductive technology and ovulation-inducing drugs to triplet and higher order multiple births-United States, 1980-1997. *MMWR, 41*, 3-11.

Centers for Disease Control and Prevention (2002). Infant mortality and low birth weight among black and white infants: United States, 1980-2000. *MMWR, 51*, 589-592.

Challis, J. (2000). Mechanism of parturition and preterm labor. *Obstet & Gynecol Surv, 55*(10), 650-660.

Chathas, M.K. & Paton, J.B. (1997). Meeting the special nutritional needs of sick infants with a percutaneous central venous catheter quality assurance program. *J Perinat Neonat Nurs, 10*(4), 72-87.

Chow, L.C., Wright, K.W., & Sola, A. (2003). Can changes in clinical practice decrease the incidence of severe ROP in very low birth weight infants. *Pediatrics, 111*(2), 339-335.

Cifuentes, J., Bronstein, J., Phibbs, C.S., Phibbs, R.H., Schmitt, S.K., et al. (2002). Mortality in low birth wieght infants according to level of neonatal care at hosptial of birth. *Pediatrics, 109*(5), 745-751.

Clark, R.H., Gerstmann, D.R., Null, D.M. Jr., & deLemos, R.A. (1992). Prospective randomized comparison of high frequency oscillatory and conventional ventilation in respiratory distress syndrome. *Pediatrics, 89*, 5-12.

Clyman, R. (1996). Recommendations for the postnatal use of indomethacin: an analysis of four separate treatment strategies. *J Pediatr, 128*, 601-607.

Cole, C. & Fiascone, J. (2000). Strategies for prevention of neonatal chronic lung disease. *Semin Perinatol, 24*, 445.

Cole, F.S. (1998a). Bacterial infections in the newborn. In H.W. Taeusch & R.A. Ballard (Eds.), *Avery's diseases of the newborn* (7th ed.). Philadelphia: W.B. Saunders.

Cole, F.S. (1998a). Viral infections of the fetus and newborn. In H.W. Taeusch & R.A. Ballard (Eds.), *Avery's diseases of the newborn* (7th ed.). Philadelphia: W.B. Saunders.

Committee on Children with Disabilities. American Association for Pediatric Ophthalmology and Strabismus, American Academy of Ophthalmology. (1998). Learning disabilities, dyslexia, and vision: subject review. *Pediatrics, 100*, 1217-1219.

Committee on Children with Disabilities. (2001). Counseling families who choose complementary and alternative medicine for their child with chronic illness or disability. *Pediatrics, 107*, 598-601.

Committee on Children with Disabilities. (2001). Role of the pediatrician in family-centered early intervention services. *Pediatrics, 107*(5), 1155-1157.

Committee on Classification of Retinopathy of Prematurity. (1984). An international classification of Retinopathy of Prematurity. *Arch Ophthalmol, 102*, 1130-1134.

Committee on Infectious Disease. (2000). *Report of the Committee on Infectious Disease* (24th ed.). Elk Grove Village, IL: Author.

Committee on Infectious Disease and Committee on Fetus & Newborn. (1998). Prevention of respiratory syncytial virus infections: indications for the use of palivizumab and update on the use of RSV-IVIG. *Pediatrics, 102*, 1211-1216.

Committee on Infectious Disease. (1998). Prevention of rotavirus disease: guidelines for use of rotavirus vaccine. *Pediatrics, 102*, 1483-1491.

Committee on Infectious Disease. (1999). Recommended childhood immunization schedule—United States, January-December 1999. *Pediatrics, 103*, 182-185.

Committee on Injury, Violence, & Poison Prevention and Committee on Fetus & Newborn. (1996). Safe transportation of premature and low birth weight infants. *Pediatrics, 97*, 758-760.

Committee on Nutrition. (1998). Nutritional needs of preterm infants. In R.E. Kleinman (Ed.), *Pediatric Nutrition Handbook* (4th ed.). Elk Grove Village, IL: The American Academy of Pediatrics.

Committee on Nutrition. (1995). Fluoride supplementation for children: interim policy recommendations. *Pediatrics, 95*, 777.

Committee on Psychological Aspects of Child and Family Health. (1998). Guidance for effective discipline. *Pediatrics, 101*, 723-728.

Connolly, B.P., McNamara, J.A., Sharma, S., Regillo, C.D., & Tasman, W. (1998). A comparison of laser photocoagulation with trans-scleral cryotherapy in the treatment of threshold retinopathy of prematurity. *Ophthalmology, 105*, 1628-1631.

Cooke, R.J., Embleton, N.D., Griffin, I.J., Wells, J.C., & McCormick, K.P. (2001). Feeding preterm infants and hospital discharge: Growth and development at 18 months of age. *Pediatr Res, 49*(5), 719-722.

Corbet, A., Gerdes, J., Long, W., Avila, E., Puri, A., et al. (1995). Double-blind, randomized trial of one versus three prophylactic doses of synthetic surfactant in 826 neonates weighing 700 to 1100 grams: effects on mortality rate. *J Pediatr, 126*, 969-978.

Creasy, R.K. & Iams, J.D. (1999). Preterm labor and delivery. In R.K. Creasy & R. Resnick (Eds.), *Maternal-fetal medicine*. Philadelphia: W.B. Saunders.

Curley, A. & Halliday, H. (2001). The present status of exogenous surfactant for the newborn. *Early Hum Dev, 61*, 67.

Dabezies, E.J. & Warren, P.D. (1997). Fractures in very low birth weight infants with rickets, *Clin Orthop, 335*:233–239.

D'Angio, C.T., et al. (2002). Longitudinal, 15-year follow-up of children born at less than 29 weeks gestation after introduction of surfactant therapy into a region: neurologic, cognitive and education outcomes. *Pediatrics, 110*(6), 1094-1102.

Darnall, R.A., Kattwinkel, J., Nattie, C., & Robinson, M. (1997). Margin of safety for discharge after apnea in preterm infants. *Pediatrics, 100*, 795-801.

Day, S. (1988). The eyes of the ICN graduate. In R. Ballard (Ed.), *Pediatric care of the ICN graduate*. Philadelphia: W.B. Saunders.

DeRoo-Merritt, L. (2000). Lasers in medicine: Treatment of retinopathy of prematurity. *Neonat Netw, 19*, 21-26.

Desmond, M.M., Wilson, G.S., Alt, E.J., & Fisher, E.S. (1980). The very low birth infant after discharge from intensive care: anticipatory health care and developmental course. *Curr Probl Pediatr, 10*, 1-59.

Di Fiore, J.M., Arko, M.K., Miller, M.J., Krauss, A., Betkerur, A., et al. (2001). Cardiorespiratory events in preterm infants referred for apnea monitoring studies. *Pediatrics, 108*(6), 1304-1308.

Dimmitt, R.A. & Moss, R.L. (2001). Clinical management of necrotizing enterocolitis. *NeoRev, 2*(5), 110-116.

Doyle, L.W. (2001). Outcome at 5 years of age of children 23 to 27 weeks' gestation: Refining the prognosis. *Pediatrics, 108*(1), 134-140.

Dubowitz, L.M. (1988). Neurologic assessment. In R. Ballard (Ed.). *Pediatric care of the ICN graduate*. Philadelphia: W.B. Saunders.

Dubowitz, L.M., Dubowitz, V., & Goldberg, C. (1970). Clinical assessment of gestational age in the newborn. *J Pediatr, 77*, 1-10.

Eichel, P. (2001). Kangaroo care. *Newborn and infant nursing reviews, 1*(4), 224-228.

Eichenwald, E.C., Aina, A., & Stark, A. (1997). Apnea frequently persists beyond term gestation in infants delivered at 24 to 28 weeks. *Pediatrics, 100*, 354-359.

Ein, S.H., Shandling, B., Wesson, D., & Filler, R.M. (1990). A 13-year experience with peritoneal drainage under local anesthesia for necrotizing enterocolitis perforation. *J Pediatr Surg, 25*, 1034.

Embleton, N.E., Pang, N., & Cooke, R.J. (2001). Postnatal malnutrition and growth retardation: An inevitable consequence of current recommendations in preterm infants. *Pediatrics, 107*(2), 270-273.

Engleke, et al. (1995). Cognitive failure to thrive in high-risk infants: the importance of the psychosocial environment. *J Perinatol, 15,* 325-329.

Escobar, G.J., Li, D.K., Armstrong, M.A., Gardner, M.N., Folck, B.F., et al. (2000). Neonatal sepsis workups in infants >/= 2000 grams at birth: A population-based study. *Pediatrics, 106*(2), 256-263.

Fanaroff, A.A., Wright, L.L., Stevenson, D.K., Shankaran, S., Donovan, E.F., et al. (1995). Very-low-birth-weight outcomes of the National Institute of Child Health and Human Development Neonatal Research Network, May 1991 through December 1992. *Am J Obstet Gynecol, 173,* 1423-1431.

Fausett, S.M., et al. (2000). Multiple courses of antenatal steroids are associated with a delay in long-term psychomotor development in children with birthweights less than 1500 grams. *Am J Obstet Gynecol, 182*(1), S24.

Fetrow, C.W. & Avila, J.R. (1999). *Professional Handbook of Complimentary and Alternative Medicines.* Springhouse, PA: Springhouse.

Fewtrell, M.S., Morley, R., Abbott, R.A., Singhal, A., Isaacs, E.B., et al. (2002). Double-blind, randomized trial of long-chain polyunsaturated fatty acid supplementation in formula fed to preterm infants. *Pediatrics, 110*(1), 73-82.

Field, T.M. (Ed.) (1995). *Touch in early development.* Mahwah, NJ: Lawrence Erlbaum Associates.

Fielder, A.R., Robinson, J., Shaw, D.E., Ng, Y.K., & Moseley, M.J. (1992). Light and retinopathy of prematurity: does retinal location offer a clue? *Pediatrics, 89,* 648-653.

Fitzgerald, D., Mesianom, G., Brosseau, L., & Davis, G.M. (2000). Pulmonary outcome in extremely low birthweight infants. *Pediatrics, 105,* 1209-1214.

Fonkalsrud, E.W. (1998). Surgical treatment of gastroesophageal reflux in children: A combined hospital study of 74677 patients. *Pediatrics, 101*(3), 419-422.

Gale, G., Franck, L., & Lund, C. (1993). Skin-to-skin (kangaroo) holding of the intubated premature infant. *Neonatal network, 12*(6), 49-57.

Gannon, B. (2000). Theophylline or caffeine: Which is best for apnea of prematurity? *Neonat Netw, 19,* 33-38.

Gardner, S.L., Johnson, J.L., & Lubchenco, L.O. (2002). Initial nursery care. In G.B. Merenstein & S.L. Gardner (Eds.), *Handbook of neonatal intensive care* (5th ed.). St Louis: Mosby.

Garland, J.S., Buck, R., & Leviton, A. (1995). Effect of maternal glucocorticoid exposure on risk of severe intraventricular hemorrhage in surfactant-treated preterm infants. *J Pediatr, 126,* 272-279.

Gerstmann, D.R., Minton, S.D., Stoddard, R.A., Meredith, K.S., Monaco, F., et al. (1996). The Provo multicenter early high-frequency oscillatory ventilation trial: improved pulmonary and clinical outcome in respiratory distress syndrome. *Pediatrics, 98,* 1044-1057.

Gilbert, E. & Harmon, J. (2003). *Manual of high-risk pregnancy and delivery,* 3rd ed. St Louis: Mosby.

Gleissner, M., Jorch, G., & Avenarius, S. (2000). Risk factors for intraventricular hemorrhage in a birth cohort of 3271 premature infants. *J Perinat Med, 28,* 104-110.

Goddard-Finegold, J., Mizrahi, E.M., & Lee, R.T. (1998). The newborn nervous system. In H.W. Taeusch & R.A. Ballard (Eds.), *Avery's diseases of the newborn* (7th ed.). Philadelphia: W.B. Saunders.

Goldenberg, R.L., Hauth, J.C., & Andrews, W.W. (2000). Intrauterine infection and preterm delivery. *N Engl J Med, 342*(20), 1500-1507.

Goldenberg, R.L. & Rouse, D.J. (1998). Prevention or preterm birth. *N Engl J Med, 339*(5), 313-320.

Goldman, A.S., Chheda, S., Keeney, S.E., Schmalstieg, F.C., & Schanler, R.J. (1994). Immunologic protection of the premature newborn by human milk. *Sem Perinatol, 18,* 495-501.

Gorski, P.A. (1988). Fostering family development after preterm hospitalization. In R. Ballard (Ed.), *Pediatric care of the ICN graduate.* Philadelphia: W.B. Saunders.

Goodnough, L.T., Skikne, B., & Brugnova, C. (2000). Erythropoietin, iron and erythropoiesis. *Blood, 96,* 823-833.

Green, M. & Solnit, A. (1964). Reactions to the threatened loss of a child: a vulnerable child syndrome. *Pediatrics, 34,* 58-66.

Guignard, J.P. (1998). Renal morphogenesis and development of renal function. In H.W. Taeusch & R.A. Ballard (Eds.), *Avery's diseases of the newborn* (7th ed.). Philadelphia: W.B. Saunders.

Guinn, D.A. & BMZ Study Group. (2000). Multicenter randomized trial of single versus weekly courses of antenatal corticosteroids (ACS): Interim Analysis. *Am J Obstet Gynecol, 182*(1), S12.

Guyer, B. (1998). Annual summary of vital statistics—1997. *Pediatrics, 102,* 1333-1349.

Hack, M. & Fanaroff, A. (1999). Outcomes of children of extremely low birth weight and gestational age in the 1990s. *Early Hum Dev, 53,* 193-218.

Hack, M. & Fanaroff, A. (1988). Growth patterns in the ICN graduate. In R. Ballard (Ed.), *Pediatric care of the ICN graduate.* Philadelphia: W.B. Saunders.

Hack, M., Friedman, H., & Fanaroff, A.A. (1996). Outcomes of extremely low birth weight infants. *Pediatrics, 98,* 931-937.

Hack, M., Weissman, B., & Borawski-Clark, E. (1996). Catch-up growth during childhood among very-low-birth-weight children. *Arch Pediatr Adolesc Med, 150,* 1122-1129.

Hack, M., Wright, L.L., Shankaran, S., Tyson, J.E., Horbar, J.D., et al. (1995). Very low birth weight outcomes of the NICHD neonatal network, November 1989-October 1990. *Am J Ob Gyn, 172,* 457-464.

Hagedorn, M.I., Gardner, S.L., & Abman, S.H. (2002). Respiratory diseases. In G.B. Merenstein & S.L. Gardner (Eds.), *Handbook of neonatal intensive care* (5th ed.). St Louis: Mosby.

Hall, R.T. (2000) Prevention of premature birth: Do pediatricians have a role?. *Pediatrics, 105*(5), 1137-1140.

Hansen, T. & Corbet, A. (1998). Chronic lung disease. In H.W. Taeusch & R.A. Ballard (Eds.), *Avery's diseases of the newborn* (7th ed.). Philadelphia: W.B. Saunders.

Harris, T.R. & Wood, B.R. (1996). Physiologic principles. In J.P. Goldsmith & E.H. Karotkin (Eds.), *Assisted ventilation of the neonate.* Philadelphia: W.B. Saunders.

Harrold, J. & Schmidt, B. (2002). Evidence-based neonatology: Making a difference beyond discharge from the neonatal nursery. *Current Opin Pediatr, 14,* 165-169.

Hawtrey, C. (1990). Undescended testis and orchiopexy: recent observations. *Pediatric Rev, 11,* 305-308.

Hay Jr., W., Lucas, A., Heird, W.C., Ziegler, E., Levin, E., et al. (1999). Workshop summary: Nutrition of the extremely low birth weight infant. *Pediatrics, 104*(16), 1360-1368.

Heird, C. & Gomez, M.R. (1993). Parenteral nutrition. In R.C. Tsang (Ed.), *Nutritional needs of the preterm infant. Scientific basis and practical guidelines.* Baltimore: Williams & Wilkins.

Hewlett, I.K. & Epstein, J.S. (1997). Food and Drug Administration conference on the feasibility of genetic technology to close the HIV window in donor screening. *Transfusion, 37,* 346-351.

Hirata, jT. & Bosque, E. (1998). When they grow up: the long-term growth of extremely low birth weight infants from birth to adolescents. *J Pediatr, 132,* 1033-1035.

Hirata, T. (1999). Unpublished data.

Ho, J.J., Henderson-Smart, D.J., & Davis, P.G. (2002). *Early versus delayed initiation of continuous distending pressure for respiratory distress syndrome in preterm infants (Cochrane Review).* In the Cochrane Library, Issue 2. Oxford: Update Software.

Horbar, J.D., Badger, G.J., Carpenter, J.H., Fanaroff, A.A., Kilpatrick, S., et al. (2002). Trends in morbidity and mortality in very low birth weight infants, 1991-1999. *Pediatrics, 110*(1), 143-151.

Horwood, J.L. & Fergusson, D.M. (1998). Breastfeeding and later cognitive and academic outcomes. *J Pediatr, 101*(1), 9S (abstract).

Houska-Lund, C. & Durand, D.J. (2002). Skin and skin care. In G.B. Merenstein & S.L. Gardner (Eds.), *Handbook of neonatal intensive care* (5th ed.). St Louis: Mosby.

Hulsey, T.C., Hudson, M.B., & Pittard, III W.B. (1994). Predictors of hospital postdischarge infant mortality: implications for high risk infant follow-up efforts. *J Perinatol, 14,* 219-225.

Hunt, J.V., Cooper, B.A., & Tooley, W.H. (1988). Very low birth weight infants at 8 and 11 years of age: role of neonatal illness and family status. *Pediatrics, 82,* 596-603.

Hurwitz, E.S., Gunn, W.J., Pinsky, P.F., & Schonberger, L.B. (1991). Risk of respiratory illness associated with day-care attendance: a nationwide study. *Pediatrics, 87,* 62-69.

Hussain, N., Clive, J., & Bhandari, V. (1999). *Current incidence of retinopathy of prematurity 1986-1997.* Available at: www.pediatrics.org/chi/content/full/104/3/e26.

Iams, J.D., Casal, D., McGregor, J.A., Goodwin, T.M., Kreaden, U.S., et al. (1995). Fetal fibronectin improves the accuracy of diagnosis of preterm labor. *Am J Obstet Gynecol, 173,* 141-145.

Iams, J.D., Goldenberg, R.L., Mercer, B.M., Moawad, A., Thom, E., et al. (1998). The preterm prediction study: recurrence risk of spontaneous preterm birth. *Am J Obstet Gynecol, 178,* 1035-1040.

International Committee for the Classification of the Late Stages of Retinopathy of Prematurity. (1987). An international classification of retinopathy of prematurity II, the classification of retinal detachment. *Arch Ophthalmol, 105,* 906-912.

Jadcheria, S.R. (2002). Gastroesophageal reflux in the neonate. *Clin Perinatol, 29*(1), 135-158.

Jobe, A. & Ikegami, M. (1998). Mechanisms initiating lung injury in the preterm. *Early Human Dev, 53*, 81-90.

Jobe, A.H., Mitchell, B.R., & Gunkel, J.H. (1993). Beneficial effects of the combined use of prenatal corticosteroids and postnatal surfactant on preterm infants. *Am J Obstet Gynecol, 168*, 508-513.

Joint Committee on Infant Hearing. (1995). 1994 position statement. *Pediatrics, 95*, 152-156.

Joint Committee on Infant Hearing. (2000). 2000 position statement. *Audiology Today 2000, special issue*, 6-27.

Kaplan, M.D. & Mayes, L.C. (guest editors) (1997). Outcomes of low birth-weight premature infants. *Sem Perinatol, 21*(3).

Kapur, P., Caty, M.G., & Glick, P.C. (1998). Pediatric hernias and hydroceles. *Ped Clinic North Am, 45*(4), 773-784.

Kari, M.A., Hallman, M., Eronen, M., Teramo, K., Virtanen, M., et al. (1994). Prenatal dexamethasone treatment in conjunction with rescue therapy of human surfactant: a randomized placebo-controlled multicenter study. *Pediatrics, 93*, 730-773.

Keith, C.G. & Doyle, L.W. (1995). Retinopathy of prematurity in extremely low birth weight infants. *Pediatrics, 95*, 42-45.

Kenner, C., Lott, J.W., & Wright, J.W. (2003). *Comprehensive neonatal nursing: A physiologic perspective* (3rd ed.). Philadelphia: W.B. Saunders.

Khalak, R., Pichichero, M.R., & D'Angio, C.T. (1998). Three-year follow-up of vaccine response in extremely preterm infants. *Pediatrics, 101*, 597-603.

Kikkert, M., et al. (2000). Apnea and gastroesophageal reflux in preterm and term infants: A retrospective study. *Pediatrics Res, 47*, 407A.

Kilbride, H.W., Leick-Rude, M.K., & Allen, N. (2002). Total parenteral nutrition. In G.B. Merenstein & S.L. Gardner (Eds.), *Handbook of neonatal intensive care* (5th ed.). St Louis: Mosby.

Kilpatrick, S.J., Schlueter, M.A., Piecuch, R., Leonard, C.H., Rogido, M., et al. (1997). Outcome of infants born at 24-26 weeks' gestation: I, survival and cost. *Obstet Gynecol, 90*, 803-808.

Klaus, M.K. & Fanaroff, A.A. (2001). *Care of the high-risk neonate* (5th ed.). Philadelphia: W.B. Saunders.

Klebanoff, M., Meirik, O., & Berendes, H. (1989). Second generation consequences of small-for-dates birth. *Pediatrics, 84*, 343-347.

Klein, C.J. (2002). Nutrient requirements for preterm infant formulas. *J Nutr, 132*, 1395S-1577S.

Kliegman, R.M. (2002). Fetal and neonatal medicine. In R.E. Behrman & R.M. Kliegman (Eds.), *Nelson: Essentials of pediatrics* (4th ed., pp. 179-249). Philadelphia: Saunders.

Kogan, M.D., Alexander, G.R., Kotelchuck, M., MacDorman, M.F., Buekens, P., et al. (2000). Trends in twin birth outcomes and prenatal care utilization in the United States, 1981-1997. *JAMA, 284*(3), 335-341.

Koo, W.W. & Tsang, R.C. (1993). Calcium, magnesium, phosphorus and vitamin D. In R.C. Tsang (Ed.), *Nutritional needs of the preterm infant: scientific basis and practical guidelines*. Baltimore: Williams & Wilkins.

Kopelman, A.E. & Mathew, O.P. (1995). Common respiratory disorders of the newborn. *Pediatr Rev, 16*, 209-217.

Kossel, H. & Versmold, H. (1997). 25 years of respiratory support of newborn infants. *J Perinat Med, 25*, 421-432.

Krug-Wispe, S.K. (1998). Vitamins, minerals and trace elements. In S. Groh-Warg, M. Thompson, & J.H. Cox (Eds.), *Nutritional care for high risk newborns* (3rd ed.). Chicago: Precept Press.

Kumar, H.S., Clive, J., Rosenkrantz, T.S., Bourque, M.D., & Hussain, N. (2002). Inguinal hernia in preterm infants. *Pediatr Surg, 18*, 147-152.

Kumar, P., Shankaran, S., & Krishnan, R.G. (1998). Recombinant human erythropoietin therapy for treatment of anemia of prematurity in very low birth weight infants: a randomized, double-blind, placebo-controlled trial. *J Perinatol, 18*, 173-177.

Landers, M.B. 3rd, Semple, H.C., Ruben, J.B., & Serdahl, C. (1990). Argon laser photocoagulation for advanced retinopathy of prematurity. *Am J Ophthalmol, 110*(4), 429-431.

Lau, C., Sheena, H.R., Shulman, R.J., & Schanler, R.J. (1997). Oral feeding in low birth weight infants. *J Pediatr, 130*, 561-569.

Leach, C.L., Greenspan, J.S., Rubenstein, S.D., Shaffer, T.H., Wolfson, M.R., et al. (1996). Partial liquid ventilation with perfluoron in premature infants with severe respiratory distress syndrome. *N Engl J Med, 335*, 761-767.

Lee, J., et al. (2001). Comparing two Indomethacin dosing regimes for treating Patent Ductus Arteriosus: A randomized clinical trial. *J Pediatr, 49*, 387-390.

Lemons, J.A. (2001). *Very low birth weight infant outcomes of the National Institute of Child Health and Human Development Neonatal Research Network, January, 1995 through December, 1996*. Available at: www.pediatrics.org/cgi/content/full/107/1/e1.

Leonard, C.H., Clyman, R.I., Piecuch, R.E., Juster, R.P., Ballard, R.A., et al. (1990). Effect of medical and social risk factors on outcome of prematurity and very low birth weight. *J Pediatr, 116*, 620-626.

Leonard, C.H. & Piecuch, R.E. (1997). School age outcomes of low birth weight preterm infants. *Sem Perinatol, 21*(3), 240-253.

Long, W.A., Zucker, J.A., & Kraybill, E.N. (guest editors) (1995). Symposium on synthetic surfactant II: health and developmental outcomes at one year. *J Pediatr, 126*(suppl 5), part 2.

Lopez, R.L., Francis, J.A., Garite, T.J., & Dubyak, J.M. (2000). Fetal fibronectin detection as a predictor of preterm birth in actual clinical practice. *Am J Obstet Gynecol, 182*(5), 1103-1106.

Lou, H.C., Lassen, N.A., & Friss-Hansen, B. (1979). Impaired autoregulation of cerebral blood flow in the distressed newborn infant. *J Pediatr, 94*, 118-121.

Lucas, A. (1993). Enteral nutrition. In R.C. Tsang, et al. (Eds.), *Nutritional needs of the preterm infant: scientific basis and practical guidelines*. Baltimore: Williams & Wilkins.

Lucas, A., Fewtrell, M.S., Morley, R., Singhal, A., Abbott, R.A., et al. (2001). Randomized trial of nutrient-enriched formula versus standard formula for postdischarge preterm infants. *Pediatrics, 108*(3), 703-711.

Lucas, A., Morley, R., Cole, T.J., Lister, G., & Leeson-Payne, C. (1992). Breast milk and subsequent intelligence quotient in children born preterm. *Lancet, 339*, 261-264.

Lucas, A., Lockton, S., & Davies, P.S. (1992). Randomized trial of nutrition for preterm infants after discharge. *Arch Dis Child, 67*, 324-327.

MacDorman, M.F., Mathews, T.J., Martin, J.A., & Malloy, M.H. (2002a). Trends and characteristics of induced labor in the United States, 1989-1998. *Paediatr Perinat Epidemiol, 16*, 263-273.

MacDorman, M.F., Minino, A.M., Strobino, D.M., & Guyer, B. (2002b) Annual Summary of vital statistics-2001. *Pediatrics, 110*(6), 1037-1052.

Makrides, M., Neumann, M., Simmer, K., Pater, J., & Gibson, R. (1995). Are long-chain polyunsaturated fatty acids essential nutrients in infancy? *Lancet, 345*, 1463-1468.

Malloy, M. & Freeman, D. (2000). Respiratory distress syndrome mortality in the United States, 1987-1995. *J Perinatol, 20*, 414.

Manco-Johnson, M., Rodden, D.J., & Collins, S. (2002). Newborn hematology. In G.B. Merenstein & S.L. Gardner (Eds.), *Handbook of neonatal intensive care* (5th ed.). St Louis: Mosby.

Martin, J.L., Hamilton, B.E., Ventura, S.J., Menacker, F., & Park, M.M. (2002). Births: Final data for 2000. *Natl Vital Stat Rep, 50*(8), 1-101.

Martin, R.J., Fanaroff, A., & Klaus, M. (1993). Respiratory problems. In M. Klaus & A. Fanaroff (Eds.), *Care of the high-risk neonate*. Philadelphia: W.B. Saunders.

Martinez, J.C., Garcia, H.O., Otheguy, L.E., Drummond, G.S., & Kappas, A. (1999). Control of severe hyperbilirubinemia in full-term newborns with the inhibitor of bilirubin production snmesoporphyrin. *Pediatrics, 103*, 1-5.

Matthews, A.L. & Robin, N.H. (2002). Genetic disorders, malformations, and inborn errors of metabolism. In G.B. Merenstein & S.L. Gardner (Eds.), *Handbook of neonatal intensive care* (5th ed). St Louis: Mosby.

Matthews, T.J., Menacker, F., & MacDorman, M.F. (2002). Infant mortality statistics from the 2000 Period Linked Birth/Infant Death Data Set. *National Vital Statistics Reports, 50*(12). Hyattsville, MD: National Center for Health Statistics.

Matthews, T.J., Curtin, S.C., & MacDorman, M.F. (2000). Infant mortality statistics from the 1998 period linked birth/infant death data set. *National Vital Statistics Report, 48*, 1-25.

McCain, G.C. (1990). Family functioning 2 to 4 years after preterm birth. *J Pediatr Nurs, 5*, 97-104.

McClure, R.J. (2001). Trophic feeding of the preterm infant. *Acta Paediatr Suppl, 90*(436), 19-21.

McCarton, C.M., Wallace, I.F., Divon, M., & Vaughan, H.G. Jr. (1996). Cognitive and neurologic development of the premature SGA infant through age 6. *Pediatrics, 98*, 1167-1178.

McCarton, C.M., Brooks-Gunn, J., Wallace, I.F., Bauer, C.R., Bennett, F.C., et al. (1997). Results at age 8 years of early intervention for low-birth-weight premature infants. *JAMA, 277*, 126-132.

McCormick, M.C., Gortmaker, S.L., & Sobol, A.M. (1990). Very low birth weight children: behavior problems and school difficulty in a national sample. *J Pediatr, 117*, 687-693.

McCormick, M.C., McCarton, C., Tonascia, J., & Brooks-Gunn, J. (1993). Early educational intervention for very low birth weight infants: results from the Infant Health and Development Program. *J Pediatr, 123*, 527-533.

McCormick, M.C., Workman-Daniels, K., Brooks-Gunn, J., & Peckham, G.J. (1993). Hospitalization of very low birth weight children at school age. *J Pediatr, 122*, 360-365.

McCourt, M.F. & Griffin, C.M. (2000). Comprehensive primary care follow-up for premature infants. *J Pediatr Health Care, 14*(6), 270-279.

McGrath, M.M., Sullivan, M.C., Lester, B.M., & Oh, W. (2000). Longitudinal neurologic follow-up in neonatal intensive care unit survivors with various neonatal morbidities. *Pediatrics, 106*(6), 1397-1405.

McGregor, M.L., Bremer, D.L., Cole, C., McClead, R.E., Phelps, D.L., et al. (2002). Retinopathy of Prematurity and oxygen saturation >94% in room air: The High Oxygen Percentage in Retinopathy of Prematurity Study. *Pediatrics, 110*(3), 540-544.

McMillen, I.C., Kok, J.S., Adamson, T.M., Deayton, J.M., & Nowak, R. (1991). Development of circadian sleep-wake rhythms in preterm and full term infants. *Pediatr Res, 29,* 381-384.

Meis, P.J., Goldenberg, R.L., Mercer, B.M., Iams, J.D., Moawad, A.H., et al. (1998). The preterm prediction study: risk factors for indicated preterm births. *Am J Obstet Gynecol, 178,* 562-567.

Ment, L.A., Vohr, B., Allan, W., Katz, K.H., Schneider, K.C., et al. (2003). Change in cognitive function over time in very-low-birth-weight infants. *JAMA, 289*(6), 705-711.

Ment, L.R., Bada, H.S., Barnes, P., Grant, P.E., Hirtz, D., et al. (2002). Practice parameters: Neuroimaging of the neonate: Report of the Quality standards subcommittee of the American academy of neurology and the practice committee of the child neurology society. *American Academy of Neurology, 58,* 1726-1738.

Ment, L.R., Oh, W., Ehrenkranz, R.A., Philip, A.G., Vohr, B., et al. (1994). Low-dose indomethacin and prevention of intraventricular hemorrhage: a multicenter randomized trial. *Pediatrics, 93,* 543-550.

Ment, L.R., Vohr, B., Allan, W., Westerveld, M., Sparrow, S.S., et al. (2000). Outcome of children in the Indomethacin intraventricular hemorrhage prevention trial. *Pediatrics, 105*(3 pt 1), 485-491.

Mentzer, W.C. & Glader, B.E. (1998). Erythrocyte disorders in infancy. In H.W. Taeusch & R.E. Ballard (Eds.), *Avery's diseases of the newborn.* Philadelphia: W.B. Saunders.

Mentzer, W.C. & Shannon, K.M. (1995). The use of recombinant human erythropoietin in preterm infants. *Int J Pediatr Hematol Oncol, 2,* 97.

Merkatz, I.R. & Merkatz, R.B. (guest editors) (1995). Social interventions in perinatology. *Sem Perinatol, 19,* 241-242.

Merenstein, G.B., Adams, K., & Weisman, L.E. (2002). Infection in the neonate. In G.B. Merenstein & S.L. Gardner (Eds.), *Handbook of neonatal intensive care* (5th ed). St Louis: Mosby.

Miles, M.S. & Haditch-Davis, D. (1997). Parenting the prematurely born child: pathways of influence. *Sem Perinatol, 21,* 254-265.

Moawad, A.H., Goldenberg, R.L., Mercer, B., Meis, P.J., Iams, J.D., et al. (2002). The Preterm Prediction Study: The value of serum alkaline phosphatase, alpha-fetoprotein, plasma corticotrophin-releasing hormone, and other serum markers for the prediction of spontaneous preterm birth. *Am J Obstet Gynecol, 186*(5), 990-996.

Mofenson, L.M. & Committee on Pediatric AIDS. (2000). *American Academy of Pediatrics: Technical Report: Perinatal HIV testing and prevention of transmission.* Available at: www.pediatrics.org/cgi/content/full/106/6/e88.

Morgan, A.M. (1996). Early identification of cerebral palsy using a profile of abnormal motor patterns. *Pediatrics, 98,* 692-697.

Morgan, J.L., Shochat, S.J., & Hartman, G.E. (1994). Peritoneal drainage as primary management of perforated NEC in the very low birth weight infant. *J Pediatr Surg, 29,* 310-315.

Moriette, G., Paris-Llado, J., Walti, H., Escande, B., Magny, J.F., et al. (2001). Prospective randomized multicenter comparison of high-frequency oscillatory ventilation and conventional ventilation in preterm infants of less than 30 weeks with respiratory distress syndrome. *Pediatrics, 107*(2), 363-372.

Morton, J.A. (2002). Strategies to support extended breastfeeding of the preterm infant. *Advances in Neonatal Care, 2*(5), 267-282.

National High Blood Pressure Education Program. (1996). Update on the task force report on high blood pressure in children and adolescents: a working group report from the National High Blood Pressure Education Program. National Institutes of Health Publication No. 96-3790, September 1996, National Heart, Lung and Blood Institute.

Narayanan, N.M. (2000). Prophylactic Indomethacin: Factors determining permanent ductus arteriosus closure. *J Pediatr, 136,* 414.

National Institutes of Health. (2000). Antenatal corticosteroids revisited: Repeat courses. *NIH Consensus Statement, 17*(1).

O'Connor, A.R., Stephenson, T., Johnson, A., Tobin, M.J., Moseley, M.J., et al. (2002). Long-term ophthalmic outcomes of low birth weight children with and without retinopathy of prematurity. *Pediatrics, 109*(1), 12-18.

O'Connor, D.L., Hall, R., Adamkin, D., Auestad N., Castillo M., et al. (2001). Growth and development in preterm infants fed long-chain polyunsaturated fatty acids: a prospective, randomized controlled trial. *Pediatrics, 108*(2), 359-371.

Ohls, R.K. (1998). Developmental erythropoiesis. In R.A. Polin & W.W. Fox (Eds.), *Fetal and neonatal physiology.* Philadelphia: W.B. Saunders.

Ohls, R.K., Ehrenkranz, R.A., Wright, L.L., Lemons, J.A., Korones, S.B., et al. (2001). Effects of early erythropoietin therapy on the transfusion requirements of preterm infants below 1250 grams birth weight: A multicenter, randomized, controlled trial. *Pediatrics, 108*(4), 934-942.

Olsen, I.E., Richardson, D.K., Schmid, C.H., Ausman, L.M., & Dwyer, J.T. (2002). Intersite differences in weight growth velocity of extremely premature infants. *Pediatrics, 110*(6), 1125-1131.

Owen, J., Yost, N., Berghella, V., Thom, E., Swain, M., et al. (2001). Mid-trimester endovaginal sonography in women at risk for spontaneous preterm birth. *JAMA, 282*(11), 1340-1348.

Oyen, N., Markestad, T., Skaerven, R., Irgens, L.M., Helweg-Larsen, K., et al. (1997). Combined effects of sleeping position and perinatal risk factors in sudden infant death syndrome: the Nordic epidemiologic SIDS study. *Pediatrics, 100,* 613-621.

Paige, P.L. & Carney, P.R. (2002). Neurologic disorders. In G.B. Merenstein & S.L. Gardner (Eds.), *Handbook of neonatal intensive care* (5th ed.). St Louis: Mosby.Pandit, P.B., Courtney, S.E., Pyon, K.H., Salslow, J.G. & Habib, R.H. (2001) Work of breathing during constant and variable-flow nasal continuous positive airway pressure in preterm neonates. *Pediatrics, 108*(3), 682-686.

Paneth, N., et al. (Eds.). (1994). *Brain damage in the preterm infant.* Lavenham Suffolk: MacKeith Press (Cambridge University Press).

Papile, L. (2002). Intracranial hemorrhage. In A.A. Fanaroff & R.J. Martin (Eds.), *Neonatal-perinatal medicine* (7th ed.). Mosby: St. Louis.

Papile, L.A., Munsick-Bruno, G., & Schaefer, A. (1983). Relationship of cerebral intraventricular hemorrhage and early childhood neurologic handicaps. *J Pediatr, 103,* 273-277.

Papile, L., Burstein, J., Burstein, R., & Koffler, H. (1978). Incidence and evolution of subependymal and intraventricular hemorrhages: A study of infants with birthweights less than 1500 grams. *J Pediatr, 92*(4), 529-534.

Park, M.K. (2003). *Pediatric cardiology handbook* (3rd ed.). Philadelphia: Mosby.

Pera, A., Byun, A., Gribar, S., Schwartz, R., Kumar, D., et al. (2002). Dexamethasone therapy and Candida sepsis in neonates less than 1250 grams. *J Perinatol, 22*(3), 204-208.

Peter, C.S., Byun, A., Gribar, S., Schwartz, R., Kumar, D., et al. (2002). Gastroesophageal reflux and apnea of prematurity: No temporal relationship. *Pediatrics, 109*(1), 8-11.

Piuze, G., et al. (2000). Etiologic factors for the development of chronic lung disease in infants less than 30 weeks gestation. *Pediatr Res, 47,* 462A.

Poets, C.F., Stebbens, V.A., Alexander, J.R., Arrowsmith, W.A., Salfield, S.A., et al. (1991). Oxygen saturation and breathing patterns in infancy, 2: preterm infants at discharge from special care. *Arch Dis Child, 66,* 574-578.

Pollack, H.A. (2001). Sudden Infant Death Syndrome: Maternal smoking during pregnancy and the associated cost-effectiveness of smoking cessation interventions. *Am J Pub Hlth, 91,* 432-436.

Quinn, D., Cooper, B., & Clyman, R.I. (2002). Factors associated with permanent closure of the ductus arteriosus: A role for prolonged Indomethacin therapy. Available at: www.pediatrics.org/cgi/content/full/111/1/e10.

Ramanathan, R., Corwin, M.J., Hunt, C.E., Lister, G., Tinsley, L.R., et al. (2001). Cardiorespiratory events recorded on home monitors: Comparison of healthy infants and those at increased risk for Sudden Infant Death Syndrome. *JAMA, 285,* 12199-2207.

Ramey, C.T., Bryant, D.M., Wasik, B.H., Sparling, J.J., Fendt, K.H., et al. (1992). Infant health and development program for low birth weight, premature infants: program elements, family participation, and child intelligence. *Pediatrics, 89,* 454-465.

Rayyis, S.F., et al. (1999). Randomized trial of "slow" versus "fast" feed advancements on the incidence of necrotizing enterocolitis in very low birth weight infants. *J Pediatr, 134,* 293-297.

Reis, B.B., Hall, R.T., Schanler, R.J., Berseth, C.L., Chan, G., et al. (2000). Enhanced growth of preterm infants fed a new powdered human milk fortifier: A randomized controlled trial. *Pediatrics, 106,* 581-585.

Remington, J.S. & Klein, J.O. (2001). *Infectious diseases of the newborn* (5th ed.). Philadelphia: Saunders.

Resnick, M.B., et al. (1999). The impact of low birth weight, perinatal conditions, and sociodemographic factors on educational outcome in kindergarten. www.pediatrics.org/cgi/content/full/104/6/74.

Resnick, M.B., et al. (1998). Educational disabilities of neonatal intensive care graduates. *Pediatrics, 102,* 308-314.

Ritchie, S.K. (2002). Primary care of the premature infant discharged from the NICU. *MCN, 27*(2), 75-86.

Romagnoli, C., Zecca, E., Luciano, R., Torrioli, G., & Tortorolo, G. (2002). Controlled trial of early dexamethasone treatment for the prevention of chronic lung disease in preterm infants: A 3-year follow-up. www.pediatrics.org/cgi/content/full/109/6/e85.

Ross, G., Lipper, E.G., & Auld, P.A. (1990). Growth achievement of very low birth weight premature children at school age. *J Pediatr, 117*, 307-309.

Ross, G., Lipper, E.G., & Auld, P.A. (1990). Social competence and behavior problems in premature children at school age. *Pediatrics, 86*, 391-397.

Ross Products Division, Abbott Laboratories. (1994). *IHDP Growth charts for LBW and VLBW boys and girls.* Columbus, OH: Abbott Laboratories.

Rubin, L.G., Sanchez, P.J., Siegel, J., Levine, G., Saiman, L., et al. (2002). Evaluation and treatment of neonates with suspected late-onset sepsis: A survey of neonates with suspected late-onset sepsis: A survey of neonatologists' practices. Available at: www.pediatrics.org/cgi/content/full/110/4/e42.

Ruff, A.J. (1994). Breast milk, breastfeeding and transmission of virus to the neonate. *Sem Perinatol, 18*(6), 510-516.

Sacher, R.A., Luban, N.L., & Strauss, R.G. (1989). Current practice and guidelines for the transfusion of cellular blood components in the newborn. *Transfusion Med Rev, 3*(1), 39-54.

Saigal, S., Stoskopf, B.L., Streiner, D.L., & Burrows, E. (2001). Physical growth and current health statgus of infants who were of extremely low birth weight and controls at adolescence. *Pediatrics, 108*(2), 407-415.

Saigal, S., Feeny, D., Rosenbaum, P., Furlong, W., Burrows, E., et al. (1996). Self perceived health status and health related quality of life of extremely low-birth-weight infants at adolescence. *JAMA, 276*, 453-459.

Schmidt, B., Davis, P., Moddemann, D., Ohlsson, A., Roberts, R.S., et al. (2001). Long-term effects of Indomethacin prophylaxis in extremely low birth weight infants. *N Engl J Med, 344*, 1966-1972.

Shimada, M., Takahashi, K., Segawa, M., Higurashi, M., Samejim, M., et al. (1999). Emerging and entraining patterns of sleep-wake rhythm in preterm and term infants. *Brain Dev, 21*, 468-473.

Sifuentes, M. (2000). Well-child care for preterm infants. In C.D. Berkowitz (Ed.), Pediatrics: a primary care approach (2 ed.). Philadelphia: W.B. Saunders.

Sinervo, K. & Lange, I. (2000). Maternal and neonatal outcomes following single vs. multiple courses of antenatal corticosteroids. *Am J Obstet Gynecol, 182*(1), S52.

Singer, L.T., Siegel, A.C., Lewis, B., Hawkins, S., Yamashita, T., et al. (2001). Preschool language outcomes of children with history of bronchopulmonary dysplagia and very low birth weight. *J Dev Behav Pediatr, 22*(1), 19-26.

Singh, J. & Sinha, S. (2002). Necrotizing enterocolitis: An unconquered disease. *Indian Pediatr, 39*(3), 229-237.

Sokol, J. & Hyde, M. (2002). Hearing screening. *Pediatr Rev, 23*(5), 155-161.

Sonntag, J., Grimmer, I., Scholz, T., Metze, B., Wit, J., et al. (2000). Growth and neurodevelopmental outcome of very low birth weight infants with necrotizing enterocolitis. *Acta Paediatr, 89*(5), 528-532.

Speer, C. & Groneck, B. (1998). Oxygen radicals, cytokines, adhesion molecules and lung injury in neonates. *Semin in Neonatol, 3*, 712-720.

Stevens, T.P., Blennow, M., & Soll, R.F. (2002). *Early surfactant administration with brief ventilation vs. selective surfactant and continued mechanical ventilation for preterm infants at risk for respiratory distress syndrome (Cochrane Review).* In the Cochrane Library, Issue 2. Oxford: Update Software.

Stockman, J.A. 3rd., Graeber, J.E., Clark, D.A., McClellan, K., Garcia, J.F., et al. (1984). Anemia of prematurity: determinants of the erythropoietin response. *J Pediatr, 105*, 786-792.

STOP-ROP Multicenter Study Group: Supplemental therapeutic oxygen for pre-threshold retinopathy of prematurity (2000) (STOP-ROP): A randomized controlled trial of primary outcomes. *Pediatrics, 105*, 295.

Strauss, R.G. (1997). Recombinant erythropoietin for the anemia of prematurity: still a promise, not a panacea. *J Pediatr, 131*, 653-655.

Strauss, R.S. & Dietz, W.H. (1997). Effects of intrauterine growth retardation in premature infants on early childhood growth. *J Pediatr, 130*, 95-102.

Subhani, M., Combs, A., Weber, P., Gerontis, C., & DeCristofaro, J.D. (2001). *Pediatrics, 107*(4), 656-659.

Suresh, G.K. & Soll, R.F. (2001). Current surfactant use for premature infants. *Clin Perinat, 28*, 671-694.

Svenson, L. & Schopflocher, D. (1997). Hospitalizations by birth weight: Results from the Alberts Children's Health Study. *Graph of the Week*, 44. Edmonton, Alberta, Canada: Alberta Health.

Task Force on Infant Sleep Position and Sudden Infant Death Syndrome. (2000). Changing concepts of sudden infant death syndrome: implications for infant sleeping environment and sleep position. *Pediatrics, 105*(3), 650-656.

Task Force on Newborn and Infant Hearing. (1999). Newborn and infant hearing loss: detection and intervention. *Pediatrics, 103*, 527-530.

Thilo, E.H. & Rosenberg, A.A. (2001). The newborn infant. In W.W. Hay, A.R. Hayward, M.J. Levin, & J.M. Sondheimer (Eds.), *Current pediatric diagnosis and treatment* (15th ed.). New York: Lange Medical Books.

Thompson, M. (2000). Gastroesophageal reflux. In S. Groh-Wargo, M. Thompson, & J. Cox (Eds.). *Nutritional care for high-risk newborns* (3rd ed.). Chicago: Precept Press.

Tin, W., Milligan, D.W., Pennefather, P., & Hey, E. (2001). Pulse oximetry, severe retinopathy and outcome at one year in babies less than 28 weeks gestation. *Arch Dis Child Fetal Neonatal Ed, 84*, F106-F110.

Tintoc, E., et al. (1994). Early indomethacin permanently closes the ductus in 88% of infants, 1000 grams, *Ped Res (abstract) 35,* 43A, 1994.

Tough, S.C., Newburn-Cook, C., Johnston, D.W., Svenson, L.W., Rose, S., et al. (2002). Delayed childbearing and its impact on population rate changes in LBW, multiple birth and preterm delivery. *Pediatrics, 109*(3), 399-403.

Valaes, T., Petmezaki, S., Henschke, C., Drummond, G.S., & Kappas, A. (1994). Control of jaundice in preterm newborns by an inhibitor of bilirubin production: studies with tin-mesoporphyrin. *Pediatrics, 93*, 1-11.

Vanderhoof, J.A. (1996). Short bowel syndrome. *Clin Perinatol, 23*(2), 377-386.

Vickers, A., Ohlsson, A., Lacy, J.B., & Horsley, A. (2002). *Massage for promoting growth and development of preterm and/or low birth-weight infants.* The Cochrane Library (Oxford) 2002 (CCD000390).

Vohr, B.R. & Msall, M.E. (1997). Neuropsychological and functional outcomes of very low birth weight infants. *Semin Perinatol, 21*(3), 202-220.

Volpe, J.J. (1995). Intracranial hemorrhage: germinal matrix-intraventricular hemorrhage of the premature infant. In J.J. Volpe (Ed.), *Neurology of the Newborn* (3rd ed.). Philadelphia: W.B. Saunders.

Volpe, J.J. (1997). Brain injury in the premature infant-from pathogenesis to prevention. *Brain Dev, 19*, 519-534.

Volpe, J.J. (1998). Neurologic outcome of prematurity. *Arch Neurol, 55*, 297-300.

Volpe, J.J. (2001). *Neurology of the newborn* (4th ed.). Philadelphia: Saunders.

Weiss, S.J. & Seed, M. (2002). Precursors of mental health problems for low birth weight children: the salience of family environment during the first year of life. *Child Psychiatry and Human Development 33*(1), 3-27.

Wellborn, et al. (1990). Postoperative apnea in former preterm infants: prospective comparison of spinal and general anesthesia. *Anesthesiology, 72*, 838-842.

Wendel, G.D., Leveno, K.J., Sanchez, P.J., Jackson, G.L., McIntire, D.D., et al. (2002). Prevention of neonatal Group B streptococcal disease: A combined intrapartum and neonatal protocol. *Am J Obstet Gynecol, 186*(4), 618-626.

Whitaker, A.H., Feldman, J.F., Van Rossem, R., Schonfeld, I.S., Pinto-Martin, J.A., et al. (1996). Neonatal cranial ultrasound abnormalities in low birth weight infants: relation to cognitive outcomes at six years of age. *Pediatrics, 98*, 719-729.

White, K., et al. (2000). Early onset Group B streptococcal disease-United States, 1998-1999. *MMWR, 49*(35), 793-796.

Wolke, D., Sohne, B., Riegel, K., Ohrt, B., & Osterlund, K. (1998). An epidemiologic longitudinal study of sleeping problems and feeding experience of preterm and term children in southern Finland: comparison with a southern German population sample. *J Pediatr, 133*, 224-231.

Wolke, D., Meyer, R., Ohrt, B., & Riegel, K. (1995). The incidence of sleeping problems in preterm and term infants discharged from special neonatal care units: an epidemiological longitudinal study. *J Child Psychol Psychiatry, 36*, 203-223.

Work Group on Breastfeeding. (1997). Breastfeeding and the use of human milk. *Pediatrics, 100*, 1035-1039.

World Health Organization (WHO). (1969). *Prevention of perinatal morbidity and mortality, public health papers No. 42.* Geneva: The Organization.

Zafir, N., et al. (2001). Improving survival of vulnerable infants increases neonatal intensive care nosocomial infection rate. *Archiv Ped Adoles Med, 155*, 1098-1104.

Zupancic, J.A., Richardson, D.K., O'Brien, B.J., Eichenwald, E.C., & Weinstein, M.C. (2003). Cost-effectiveness analysis of predischarge monitoring for apnea of prematurity. *Pediatrics, 111*(1), 146-152.

37 Prenatal Cocaine Exposure

Elizabeth A. Kuehne and Marianne W. Reilly

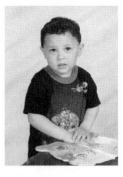

Etiology

Substance abuse during pregnancy is a long-standing problem within our society. It was not until 1973, however, that the term fetal alcohol syndrome was first used to describe a distinctive pattern of malformations in infants born to alcoholic mothers (Jones et al, 1973), that these problems began to receive attention from health care professionals and the general public. Since then the effects of alcohol, opiates, marijuana, and other noncocaine substances on the developing fetus have been extensively studied and described. Since the mid-1980s, cocaine has emerged as a widely used recreational drug and is often used in combination with other substances.

According to the 2001 National Household Survey on Drug Abuse, 15.9 million Americans are users of illicit drugs. Currently 1.7 million Americans use cocaine, and 406,000 use "crack" (Substance Abuse and Mental Health Services Administration [SAMHSA], 2002). With cocaine's rise in popularity among the general public has come a rise in use by women of childbearing age. Cocaine and marijuana are now the illicit substances most often used by pregnant women and are commonly used in combination with tobacco and alcohol (National Pregnancy and Health Survey [NPHS], 1996, SAMHSA 2002) (Box 37-1).

Cocaine can be administered in a variety of ways: intranasal snorting, intravenous (IV) injection, and smoking (National Institute on Drug Abuse [NIDA], 1998). Crack is a popular form of cocaine that consists of alkaloid crystals of cocaine that are smoked in a water pipe. Crack became available in the mid-1980s, and its popularity shows no signs of diminishing (SAMHSA, 2002). Crack differs from cocaine hydrochloride (i.e., the preparation used intranasally) in the following three ways: (1) because crack is smoked and not sniffed, the "high" is reached within 10 seconds and lasts approximately 5 to 15 minutes; (2) it is absorbed more effectively from the highly vascular surface of the lung, creating a more intense and powerful high; and (3) it is relatively inexpensive, costing a few dollars per "rock" (Eyler et al, 1998; NIDA, 1998). These factors and elimination of the need for IV injection are believed to contribute to crack's popularity among both young people and women of childbearing age.

Because of crack's dramatic effects on users, a few maternal patterns of abuse have emerged. Many women use crack to abort an unwanted pregnancy or because they think that it will ease their deliveries. Some women use crack to induce labor, thinking that early delivery will prevent further fetal exposure to cocaine. In addition, many women addicted to crack begin prostituting themselves or their children to support their habit. This situation has many grave social and public health implications, including sexually transmitted diseases (STDs), congenital infections, unwanted pregnancies, and the abandonment and/or physical and sexual abuse of children.

Known Genetic Etiology

Children of substance abusers are the highest risk group of children for becoming alcohol and drug abusers for both genetic and family environment reasons (Kumpfer, 1999). A relationship between parental substance abuse and subsequent alcohol problems in their children has been documented extensively (Johnson & Leff, 1999). Adoption and twin studies have led researchers to support a genetic theory of alcoholism transmission. Less information is available regarding the genetic etiology of illicit drug use. Recent review articles (Johnson & Leff, 1999; Kodjo & Klein 2002) suggest that genetics might play a role in drug use, and that dependence, regardless of substance type, may be hereditary. Males have higher rates of substance abuse than do females (Kodjo & Klein, 2002). Reinherz and colleagues (2000) found parental substance use disorder to be a specific risk factor for drug disorders in boys only. The combination of a possible genetic predisposition with other risk factors such as living with a drug-using parent, poor school performance, stress, and hyperactivity make children of drug-using parents at high risk for substance abuse themselves.

Another genetic consideration when dealing with drug-exposed children is that sensitive individuals could be more susceptible to the damaging effects of cocaine (Plessinger & Woods, 1998). This may account for some of the differences in outcome seen in infants and children prenatally exposed to cocaine.

Incidence and Prevalence

Each year in the United States it is estimated that between 212,000 and 956,000 infants are exposed to one or more illicit substances (National Center on Addiction and Substance Abuse at Columbia University, 1996). The National Pregnancy and Health Survey (NPHS, 1996), based on maternal self-report, estimates that 5.5% of all pregnant women use illicit drugs during pregnancy and that 45,000 cocaine-exposed children are born each year. The 2001 National Household Survey on Drug Abuse (NHSDA) (SAMHSA 2002) estimated that 3.7% of pregnant females used illicit drugs, with rates of illicit drug use being similar for white, black, and Hispanic pregnant women. Recent reports have found prevalence rates ranging from 4.6% (Chasnoff et al, 2001) to 10.7% (Lester et al, 2001). In general, use of alcohol and tobacco was strongly linked to use of illicit drugs.

BOX 37-1
Effects of Drug Use on Fetal Development

COCAINE
Cocaine causes placental and uterine vasoconstriction, resulting in fetal hypoxia. Associated problems include prematurity, low birth weight, hypertonicity, irritability, tremors, CNS abnormalities, neurodevelopmental problems, and congenital anomalies.

HEROIN
Newborns undergo a true withdrawal syndrome that includes irritability, tremors, hypertonicity, and fever. Infants have increased risk for SIDS and are vulnerable to many neonatal infections, including HIV.

ALCOHOL
Infants undergoing withdrawal from alcohol may have tremors, irritability, hypertonicity, muscle twitching, and restlessness. The term fetal alcohol syndrome (FAS) is used to describe a similar pattern of malformations noted in the offspring of alcohol-abusing women. Features of this syndrome include intrauterine growth retardation, slow postnatal growth, microcephaly, mental retardation, and craniofacial abnormalities.

MARIJUANA
Infants may have tremors, altered visual responses, low birth weight, growth retardation, and neurobehavior abnormalities. Severity of symptoms is probably related to the amount of the drug used by the mother.

BARBITURATES
Severe and prolonged withdrawal syndrome may occur. Symptoms include hyperactivity, restlessness, excessive crying, and hyperreflexia. Sudden withdrawal by the mother or infant can result in seizures.

TOBACCO
Smoking in pregnancy is associated with spontaneous abortion, low birth weight, prematurity, increased perinatal mortality, and SIDS.

Illicit drug use should be addressed with all pregnant women. Users often deny drug use, so clinicians can accordingly expect an underestimation of drug use when relying entirely on maternal self-report. Other maternal factors that may help clinicians identify children who have been exposed to cocaine in utero are history of drug use, previous birth of a drug-exposed infant, STD, signs of intoxication, lack of prenatal care, physical indications of drug use, and suspicious or erratic behavior. Because of the unreliability of maternal self-report, many hospitals in communities with known drug abuse problems routinely screen all high-risk mothers and their newborns for prenatal drug exposure.

Screening for cocaine and its metabolites using a biologic marker enhances identification of newborns exposed to cocaine in utero. Maternal and infant urine screening has been the marker most widely used. Urine assay can detect benzoylecgonine (a cocaine metabolite) for 24 to 72 hours after use but cannot detect earlier use or quantify the dose. Because urine toxicologic screening of newborns is feasible only during the immediate postpartum period, primary care providers will find its usefulness limited. Because of the rapid metabolism and excretion of cocaine, it is important to remember that a negative urine assay is not conclusive evidence of lack of prenatal exposure.

Meconium has been shown to be a sensitive biologic marker for determining prenatal drug exposure (Ostrea et al, 2001). Drug metabolites are excreted into meconium during the latter part of the pregnancy, so a meconium drug screen will reflect drug use during that time. Studies show that meconium testing can detect significantly more cocaine-exposed infants than urine testing (Ryan et al, 1994). Additionally, meconium may be useful in quantifying drug use during pregnancy and in clarifying issues of dose-response relationship (Delaney-Black et al, 1996). More widespread use of meconium screening will help primary care providers identify children prenatally exposed to drugs.

Other biologic markers under evaluation are hair, amniotic fluid, sweat, and cord blood, but the clinical usefulness of these tests has not been determined. For clinicians working in the newborn nursery, toxicologic screening must be performed within institutional policy and protocol.

Clinical Manifestations at Time of Diagnosis
Pharmacology and Physiologic Effects of Cocaine

Cocaine is benzoylmethylecgonine, which is a local anesthetic and central nervous system (CNS) stimulant prepared from the extract of the leaves of the coca plant *(Erythroxylon coca)*. Cocaine readily crosses from maternal to fetal circulation and, because of metabolic differences, may remain in the fetal system long after it has been excreted by the mother. Cocaine is metabolized by liver and plasma cholinesterases into several major metabolites that are excreted in the urine: benzoylecgonine, ecgonine, and ecgonine methyl ester (Plessinger & Woods, 1998; Drug Facts and Comparisons, 2002).

Three additional biologically active cocaine metabolites have been identified: norcocaine, cocaethylene, and methylecgonine (MEG). Norcocaine is water soluble with a high level of CNS penetration. Because of these characteristics, norcocaine does not reenter the maternal circulation, so the fetus may continue to be exposed to this metabolite by ingestion of the amniotic fluid (Wootton & Miller, 1994). Cocaethylene is formed in the liver when cocaine and alcohol are simultaneously ingested. It is a potent stimulant and dopamine uptake blocker that is more cardiotoxic and longer acting than cocaine alone (Frank et al, 1998; Plessinger & Woods, 1998). MEG is a substance formed when cocaine is heated, as with crack. It has been shown to reach the fetus and is thought to contribute to adverse neonatal outcomes in infants of crack-using mothers (Plessinger & Woods, 1998) (Box 37-2).

Cocaine is a CNS stimulant that can cause feelings of well-being, euphoria, restlessness, and excitement. Overdosage can lead to convulsions, CNS depression, and respiratory failure. Cocaine inhibits the reuptake of neurotransmitters at the adrenergic nerve terminals, producing increased levels of norepinephrine, dopamine, and serotonin. These elevated levels of catecholamines result in increased blood pressure, tachycardia, and vasoconstriction. Cocaine also causes elevations in body temperature. Large doses are directly toxic to the myocardium and may result in cardiac failure (Drug Facts and Comparisons, 2002).

BOX 37-2

Clinical Manifestations at Time of Diagnosis

PHARMACOLOGIC AND PHYSIOLOGIC EFFECTS OF COCAINE
Local anesthetic
CNS stimulant
   Euphoria
   Restlessness
   Excitement
   Convulsions
   CNS depression
   Respiratory failure

PRENATAL EFFECTS OF COCAINE
Decreased uterine blood flow
Decreased fetal oxygenation
Increased blood pressure and heart rate

MANIFESTATIONS AT BIRTH
Prematurity

INTRAUTERINE GROWTH RETARDATION
MICROCEPHALY
LOW BIRTH WEIGHT
CNS ABNORMALITIES
POOR FEEDING
INCREASED NECROTIZING ENTEROCOLITIS

BOX 37-3

Treatment

Narcotic withdrawal therapy if indicated
Pacification techniques
Assessment of safety and competence of caretaker
Close home follow-up

Bandstra et al, 2001; Singer et al, 2002); (2) CNS abnormalities, such as jitteriness, tremors, seizures, electroencephalographic (EEG) abnormalities, hypertonicity, abnormal reflexes, cerebral infarct, and intraventricular hemorrhage (Kramer et al, 1990; Coles et al, 1992; Cohen et al, 1994; Singer et al, 1994; Datta-Bhutada et al, 1998; Richardson, 1998; Scher et al, 2000; Morrow et al, 2001); (3) poor feeding (Barton, 1998); and (4) a higher incidence of necrotizing enterocolitis (NEC) (Czyrko et al, 1991; Porat & Brodsky, 1991). The adverse effects manifested in infants exposed to cocaine are probably not indicative of a true withdrawal syndrome as seen with infants exposed to narcotics. Some believe that these signs of cocaine exposure represent either CNS hyperexcitability as a result of the direct effects of cocaine or indications of CNS damage.

Treatment (Box 37-3)

Infants who have been exposed to cocaine in utero can be identified based on maternal history, urine or meconium toxicologic screening, and clinical presentation. Although pharmacologic therapy (including the use of phenobarbital, paregoric, and tincture of opium) has been advocated for narcotic withdrawal (Committee on Drugs, 1998; Wagner et al, 1998), infants who have been prenatally exposed only to cocaine do not usually require such therapy. Pacification techniques such as swaddling and decreasing environmental stimuli are used to treat the symptoms of irritability and tremors seen in these infants. Infants exposed to multiple drugs may require treatment if the mother used opiates or methadone in addition to cocaine.

Details of discharge planning for infants with prenatal exposure to cocaine depend on who their caretakers will be after discharge. Planning for discharge is generally done in conjunction with family members and hospital social service staff, as well as child protective workers, in some cases. Once the caretaker has been identified, he or she must be provided with routine discharge information and information on behavioral patterns to expect and pacification techniques to use. A referral to or consultation with a primary care provider familiar with drug misuse and addiction and its associated problems is ideal. The same provider should see these infants often—perhaps monthly—for at least the first year.

Prenatal Effects of Cocaine

Because cocaine readily crosses the placenta, its physiologic effects (e.g., CNS stimulation, vasoconstriction, tachycardia, and blood pressure elevations) are thought to occur in both the mother and the fetus. Maternal administration of cocaine consistently results in decreased uterine blood flow and impaired fetal oxygenation and elevated fetal blood pressure and heart rate (Wagner et al, 1998). In addition, the hormonal milieu of pregnancy may increase the hypertensive and cardiovascular effects of cocaine (Plessinger & Woods, 1998). Prenatal manifestations of maternal cocaine use are spontaneous abortion, preterm labor, precipitous labor, fetal distress, meconium staining, in utero intracranial hemorrhage, and abruptio placentae (Cohen et al, 1991; Robins & Mills, 1993; Nair et al, 1994; Wootton & Miller, 1994; Plessinger & Woods, 1998; Sherer et al, 1998).

Studies in cocaine-exposed rabbits and mice suggest that high levels of neurotransmitters are pooled into the cell spaces of the nervous system, causing the developing brain to undergo permanent changes. When exposed to cocaine, the anterior cingulate cortex, which is involved in attention and learning, develops dendrites that are 30% to 50% longer than normal and formed in a woven configuration. In unexposed brains, dopamine bound to protein receptors inhibits the growth of these neuronal extensions (Vogel, 1997).

Manifestations at Birth

A growing body of research describes the manifestations of intrauterine cocaine exposure exhibited at birth, including the following: (1) prematurity, intrauterine growth retardation, microcephaly, and low birth weight (Datta-Bhutada et al, 1998; Eyler et al, 1998; Richardson, 1998; Chiriboga et al, 1999;

Complementary and Alternative Therapies

Infant massage may be a beneficial adjunct to traditional therapy for the cocaine-exposed infant. Problems such as muscle tone abnormalities, irritability, poor oral motor skills, and sensitivity to sensory stimulation may be addressed through this type of therapy (Drehobl & Fuhr, 1991).

Anticipated Advances in Diagnosis and Management

Over the past decade the issues surrounding prenatal exposure to cocaine have received attention in both the medical literature and the mass media. Initial media reports described a "lost" generation of children who were "permanently damaged" and would never function well in society. The term "crack baby" was coined, and urban schools braced themselves for classrooms full of disturbed children.

Since the mid-1980s, much has been learned about prenatal cocaine exposure, including the following: (1) fetal growth is affected by the continued use of cocaine during pregnancy; (2) most women who use cocaine do so in combination with other drugs, such as alcohol, tobacco, opiates, and marijuana; and (3) small differences in IQ scores, behavior and self-regulation problems, and attention difficulties may influence long-term outcomes for these children. This subtle brain damage may eventually lead to a substantial educational burden to society (Lester et al, 1998).

What we now know is that cocaine alone is not responsible for all of the problems reported in exposed children. Frank and associates (2001), in reviewing 36 articles published between 1984 and 2000, conclude that prenatal cocaine exposure is not associated with any severe developmental effects. It is helpful to view maternal cocaine use as a "marker" for other health and developmental risk factors, including inadequate prenatal care, poor nutrition, polydrug use, poverty, violence, foster-care placement, inadequate parenting, and a chaotic home environment.

Associated Problems (Box 37-4)

Prematurity

Infants exposed to cocaine in utero have an increased risk of preterm birth and consequently require appropriate neonatal intervention and long-term follow-up (see Chapter 36).

Congenital Infections

The general use of illicit drugs is associated with infectious diseases, STDs, and acquired immunodeficiency syndrome (AIDS) (Wagner et al, 1998). Therefore the offspring of women using drugs can be expected to have increased rates of congenitally acquired infections. Congenital syphilis reached epidemic proportions during the early 1990s. However, recent data (CDC, 2001) show that rates of congenital syphilis declined 51% between 1997 and 2000. Despite this encouraging trend, several major cities faced dramatic increases in infection rates between 1999 and 2000 (CDC, 2002). Practitioners need to remain vigilant regarding the threat of congenital syphilis.

Many crack users will exchange sex for drugs, resulting in frequent sexual activity with multiple partners, which places the mother and infant at increased risk for STDs and human immunodeficiency virus (HIV) infection. Many crack users also inject cocaine or use heroin to bring themselves down from periods of prolonged cocaine use, thus increasing their risk of HIV infection from contaminated needles.

In addition to syphilis and HIV infection, primary care providers must consider infectious diseases such as hepatitis B, hepatitis C, tuberculosis, TORCH (toxoplasmosis, other viruses, rubella, cytomegalovirus, herpes) infections, and other STDs (e.g., gonorrhea and chlamydia) when assessing the health status of an infant or child of a cocaine-abusing mother.

Growth Retardation and Microcephaly

Fetal growth, birth weight, and head circumference are affected by continued use of cocaine throughout the pregnancy (Eyler et al, 1998; Bandstra et al, 2001; Behnke et al 2001). These effects are thought to be related to chronic uterine and placental hypoxia secondary to cocaine-induced vasoconstriction. Poor maternal nutrition is probably also a factor, especially in light of the anorectic effects of cocaine. A potentially worrisome finding of prenatal cocaine exposure is that of microcephaly. Early data suggest that the head circumference of cocaine-exposed children remains smaller than that of unexposed children for at least 6 years (Chasnoff et al, 1998). More recent studies have not demonstrated this finding (Bandstra et al, 2001).

Congenital Anomalies

Cocaine has been associated with congenital malformations, the most common being those involving the genitourinary (GU) tract. Other malformations include congenital heart disease, skull defects, limb reduction defects, intestinal atresia, and ocular defects—specifically strabismus (Bingol et al, 1987; Chavez et al, 1989; Hoyme et al, 1990; Lipschultz et al, 1991; Ho et al, 1994; Block et al, 1997). It is thought that vascular compromise or fetal hypoxia resulting from cocaine-induced vasoconstriction may be responsible for the apparently increased rate of congenital malformations in these infants (Bingol et al, 1987; Hoyme et al, 1990). In contrast to these studies, a recent blinded, prospective longitudinal study of cocaine-exposed infants showed no increase in number or consistent pattern of abnormalities (Behnke et al, 2001).

Sudden Infant Death Syndrome (SIDS)

It is not clear whether infants exposed to cocaine prenatally are at an increased risk for sudden infant death syndrome (SIDS). Kandall and associates (1993) reviewed SIDS cases among 1.2 million infants born in New York City between 1979 and 1989. After controlling for high-risk variables such as ethnicity, maternal age, parity, maternal smoking, and low birth weight, the authors found that opiate use was associated with a 2.3- to 3.7-fold increase in SIDS. They also demonstrated a significant yet more modest increase in the rate of SIDS after intrauterine exposure to cocaine.

A metaanalysis (Fares et al, 1997) of 10 published articles found that an increased risk of SIDS was specific to intrauterine drug exposure, in general. Furthermore, cocaine exposure had a significant effect on risk when exposed infants were compared with drug-free infants, but not when cocaine-exposed infants were compared with polydrug-exposed infants. In contrast, Ostrea and associates (1997) studied mortality rates among 3000 infants in Michigan and found no increased risk for SIDS among infants who were drug-positive. Klonoff-Cohen and Lam-Kruglick (2001) found no association between maternal recreational drug use and SIDS. However, they found that paternal marijuana use during conception, pregnancy, and postnatally was significantly associated with SIDS. Although no causative relationship between drugs and SIDS has been established, clinicians should be aware that infants of substance-abusing mothers seem to be at an increased risk for SIDS and may have other risk factors (e.g., prematurity and exposure to cigarette smoke). The practitioner must stress the importance of the supine sleep position as it relates to the prevention of SIDS. This message should be reinforced at health supervision visits.

Neurologic and Developmental Effects

The effects of intrauterine cocaine and/or polydrug exposure on the developing CNS that have been reported include seizures and perinatal cerebral insults. Neurodevelopmental abnormalities described include irritability, tremulousness, and hypertonicity. These unusual patterns of behavior, combined with inconsolability and irritability, may interfere with appropriate caregiver-infant interactions, potentially hindering the process of bonding and attachment. Early studies by Delaney-Black and associates (1996) reported significant differences in autonomic stability using the Brazelton Neonatal Behavioral Assessment Scale (BNBAS) and suggested that a dose-response relationship was evident as measured by cocaine concentration in meconium.

Motor behavior in these infants is characterized by an increase in extensor tone, which interferes with their ability to explore the environment and their own bodies. When supine, these children often lie in an extended posture and, when held upright, stiffen and extend their ankles, knees, and hips, placing their toes in a weight-bearing position. These children have difficulty bringing their arms to midline and are poorly coordinated. Children with truncal hypertonicity often have difficulty with balance and may not be able to sit. These motor findings are mild or transient in some children and persistent in others. Morrow and associates (2001) using the BNBAS on 334 cocaine-exposed infants during the first week postpartum found evidence of subtle cocaine-associated deficits in neurobehavioral functioning. Infants exposed to cocaine during all three trimesters exhibited more pronounced deficits. Singer and associates (2000) studied 158 cocaine-exposed infants (58 heavily exposed and 76 lightly exposed) using the Neurobehavioral Assessment (NB Assessment) at 43 weeks postconception. Heavily exposed infants were four times more likely to be jittery and twice as likely to have other abnormalities. Cocaethylene and benzolyecgonine (metabolites of cocaine) were related to higher incidence of tone abnormalities, jitteriness, and attentional abnormalities.

Chiriboga and associates (1999) studied 104 infants who were exposed to cocaine as documented by maternal hair analysis. Newborns were assessed at ages 1 and 7 days using the Neurological Examination for Children (NEC). When compared with unexposed controls, the newborns exposed to cocaine exhibited higher rates of global hypertonia, coarse tremor, and extensor leg posture. Fetters and associates (1996) studied cocaine-exposed and unexposed infants and evaluated neuromotor development at 1, 4, 7, and 15 months using the Alberta Infant Motor Scale (AIMS), Movement Assessment of Infants (MAI), and the Peabody Developmental Motor Scales (PDMS). They concluded that cocaine exposure was associated with poor motor performance at 4 and 7 months but was no longer evident at 15 months. Arendt and associates (1999) used the PDMS to examine 98 toddlers exposed to cocaine. Their findings indicate that abnormalities in fine and gross motor movements may persist at 2 years of age. Children exposed to cocaine had the most difficulty with hand use and eye-hand coordination. Hurt and associates (2001), however, found no difference in neurologic examination findings at age 6 years comparing 52 cocaine exposed and 63 control subjects.

Early reports in the press predicted devastating neurodevelopmental outcomes for children exposed to cocaine. After more than a decade of research and study the effects of cocaine exposure remain controversial. Researchers must control for confounding variables such as small sample size, multidrug exposure, environmental factors, and poor parenting skills. Following is a literature review of the most pertinent studies on behavior, language, and cognitive effects.

Using the Stanford-Binet Intelligence Scales, Richardson (1998) reported decreased attention span, more difficulty focusing, and restlessness during testing in 3-year-old children who were prenatally exposed to cocaine. Chasnoff and associates (1998) studied cocaine and/or polydrug-exposed subjects at 4, 5, and 6 years using the Child Behavior Checklist (CBCL) and concluded that these children had problems with self-regulation and an inability to manage their behaviors and impulses. Previous studies have suggested early problems with state regulation. In a blinded controlled study, teachers using the Connors Teacher Rating Scale (CTRS) and the Problem Behaviors Scale (PROBS 14) identified significantly more problem behaviors in cocaine-exposed first graders than in the unexposed group (Delaney-Black, 1998). Delaney-Black and associates (2000) reported gender-specific behavioral effects related to prenatal cocaine exposure. Using the Achenbach Teacher's Report Form (TRF) cocaine-exposed boys were found to have clinically significant scores for "total externalizing aggressive and delinquent behaviors." Mayes (1998) followed a group of prenatally cocaine-exposed children from infancy to preschool. She found that these children were more likely to exhibit problems with disrupted arousal regulation across all ages. These findings have important implications for learning and memory.

In terms of cognitive and language development, results are conflicting. Lewkowicz and associates (1998) studied the auditory visual response in 4- and 10-month-old infants who were exposed to cocaine. These infants showed an arousal response difference to "infant directed talk" at 10 months, suggesting a decline in developmental performance beginning at that age.

Hurt (1997) found no differences in cocaine-exposed and matched controls of inner-city children at age 4 years using the Wechsler *Preschool and Primary Scale of Intelligence-Revised (WPPSI-R)*. Chasnoff's 4- to 6-year outcome study (1998) found IQ scores using the WPPSI-R at 4 and 5 years and the *Wechsler Intelligence Scales for Children-III (WISC-III)* at 6 years to be at the low end of the normal range in cocaine- and/or polydrug-exposed children, but these results were not statistically significant. In Toronto 23 children who were prenatally exposed to cocaine and then adopted by middle-class families were tested using the Bayley Infant Scales of Development, the McCarthy Scales (Koren et al, 1998), and the Reynell Language Test. Findings were statistically significant for language delay. The McCarthy Scales showed a trend toward lower IQ scores, but the results were not statistically significant. This study—unlike others—controlled for maternal IQ and socioeconomic status. Singer and associates (2001) administered the Preschool Language Scale-3 at 1 year of age to 131 nonexposed subjects, 66 heavily cocaine exposed and 68 lightly exposed. They found that the infants who were heavily exposed to cocaine had lower auditory comprehension scores and lower total language scores. Auditory comprehension scores are precursors for receptive language. Kilbride and associates (2000) reported a higher 6-month score on the Bayley Mental Developmental Index score in cocaine-exposed infants who received special case management. By 36 months there were no statistically significant differences in cognitive, psychomotor, or language quotients between cocaine-exposed and nondrug-exposed infants. Verbal scores, however, were significantly higher in the case-managed group at 36 months. Bandstra and associates (2002) followed a large sample of full-term children (236 cocaine exposed and 207 noncocaine exposed) through age 7 years as part of the Miami Prenatal Cocaine Study. Language function was measured at 3 and 5 years using the Clinical Evaluation of Language Fundamentals—Preschool (CELP-P) and at 7 years Core Language Domain of NEPSY: A developmental neuropsychologic assessment. This study reveals a cocaine-associated deficit in language functioning across the span of 3 to 7 years. Singer and associates (2002) also looked at cognitive and motor outcomes using the Bayley Scales of Infant Development—1993 at 6.5, 12, and 24 months. This cohort consisted of 218 cocaine-exposed and 197 nonexposed infants. Significant cognitive deficits were found throughout the first 2 years of life. This is the first study to use the revised Bayley Scales of Infant Development, which are predictive of later cognitive development. In this study cocaine had no significant effect on motor outcomes.

Lester and associates (1998) performed a metaanalysis of 101 published studies analyzing the effects of intrauterine cocaine exposure on IQ and reported a statistically significant variation of 3.26 IQ points between the cocaine-exposed and contrast groups. The authors concluded that the prenatal cocaine exposure did not cause devastating brain damage but instead subtle damage that may lead to substantial costs in special education. Frank and associates (2001) reviewed 36 articles published from 1984 to October 2000 related to prenatal cocaine exposure. They did not find a consistent negative effect on physical growth, developmental test scores, or receptive/expressive language. They concluded that there is no convincing evidence to date that cocaine exposure alone is associated with adverse developmental outcomes.

Research is ongoing and it is hoped that it will provide definitive data concerning the intellectual functioning of cocaine-exposed children and school performance when more complex cognitive skills are necessary for learning. Other problems, such as learning disabilities or attention deficit hyperactivity disorder (ADHD), may be uncovered (see Chapter 12).

Feeding Difficulties

Feeding difficulties and gastrointestinal (GI) symptoms, such as poor suck-swallow coordination, vomiting, diarrhea, and constipation, have been reported in infants exposed to cocaine in utero (Barton, 1998; Committee on Drugs, 1998). Wagner and associates (1998) report that infants born to drug-using women may take in excess of 300ml/kg/day in an attempt to achieve catch-up growth that is necessary for normal development.

Continued Exposure to Drugs

Children of parents who use cocaine can be exposed to cocaine after, as well as before, birth. Cocaine, cocaethylene, and other metabolites are detectable in breast milk, and infants can be exposed to large doses of cocaine by breast feeding. Irritability, tremulousness, and other signs of CNS stimulation are seen in infants who ingest cocaine via breast milk (Bailey, 1998; Committee on Drugs, 2001). Children who have been passively exposed to crack smoke have manifested neurologic symptoms such as seizures, obtundation, delirium, dizziness, drooling, and ataxia (Mott et al, 1994). Furthermore, ingestion of crack cocaine by a child can be fatal (Havlick & Nolte, 2000). Lustbader and associates (1998) documented cocaine metabolites in 36.3% of urine samples from infants younger than 1 year of age brought to Yale-New Haven hospital's emergency department. Among these infants, upper and lower respiratory symptoms significantly correlated with a positive urine toxicology. Practitioners should consider the possibilities for later cocaine exposure via breast feeding, passive inhalation, and accidental ingestion when caring for the children of drug-using parents. Because of the known frequency of polydrug and tobacco use, primary care providers should be mindful of signs and symptoms of exposure to other drugs, including secondhand smoke.

Parenting Issues

Parents dealing with their own addiction may have multiple health and social problems that interfere with their ability to care for their children. They may also have been children of substance-abusing parents. These parents, who are often single, may have had few positive parenting experiences in their own lives. If interventions such as preventive social service supports are inadequate, the courts may move to terminate parental rights so that a permanency plan can be made for the young child.

Prognosis

Long-term studies about the prognosis for children with prenatal exposure to cocaine are inconclusive at this time. Two correlates of prenatal drug exposure—HIV infection and preterm birth—however, significantly affect morbidity and mortality and must be considered when determining the prognosis for these children. Ostrea and associates (1997) did not find drug exposure to be associated with an increased risk of mortality within the first 2 years of life. A significantly higher mortality rate, however, was observed among low birth weight infants who were positive for both cocaine and opiates.

PRIMARY CARE MANAGEMENT

Health Care Maintenance

Growth and Development

Primary care providers must closely monitor the physical growth of these infants and young children. Monthly evaluations are prudent during infancy. Accurate measurements for weight, length, and head circumference necessitate use of the same scale and measuring tools at each visit. It is especially important that head size be measured accurately because of the reported incidence of microcephaly. Data should be plotted on the revised CDC/National Center for Health Statistics growth chart. Data for infants with a history of prematurity should be plotted using the corrected age. Recent data indicate that by the age of 2 years, infants exposed to cocaine catch up in height and weight when compared with nondrug-exposed children from a similar background. Children prenatally exposed to cocaine, however, have smaller head circumferences than unexposed children for at least 6 years (Chasnoff, 1998).

Developmental assessment of infants exposed to cocaine poses a challenge to primary care providers. Routine office screening tools, such as the Denver Developmental Screening Test II, may be helpful. The validity of such tests depends on the stability of the infant's state control during testing. In addition, these infants may exhibit problems with motor development that can affect results.

It is useful to monitor the infant's development at monthly intervals during the first 6 months of life and every 2 months during the second 6 months of life. Frequent assessments by the same provider offer valuable information about the child's developmental progress. Early referral to infant stimulation programs for high-risk infants is recommended. Early referrals for a more detailed evaluation by a developmental psychologist and speech therapist may be useful before school entry or if problems are suspected.

For some infants, simultaneous visual and voice stimuli may be too stressful and interfere with parent-infant interaction. Without appropriate guidance, bonding and attachment may be jeopardized. Parents should be advised to make full use of the infant's quiet and alert states and should also be informed that the attainment of developmental milestones can be unpredictable and is generally slower in these fragile infants.

When infants who were exposed to cocaine are evaluated, a complete physical assessment is essential. Abnormal neurologic findings are common in these young children. Examiners should observe for irritability, tremors, extended postures, limb stiffness, hyperreflexia, clonus, persistence of primitive reflexes, subtle signs of infantile spasms, jerky eye movements, and the inability to track visually and respond to sound. A neurologic consultation is necessary if seizures or other withdrawal symptoms (e.g., persistent hypertonicity, irritability, or disturbance in the sleep-wake state) are noted in newborns. Moreover, early assessment and intervention by a neurodevelopmentally trained physical therapist can provide parents with helpful advice about handling and positioning "stiff" infants.

Diet

Breast feeding is not recommended for women using cocaine because cocaine and cocaethylene are secreted in breast milk (Committee on Drugs, 2001). Because cocaine-exposed infants often have low birth weights, careful monitoring of caloric intake and feeding behavior is required. Infants suffering from withdrawal should receive 150 to 250 calories/kg/day and use of a hypercaloric formula (24 calories/oz) may be necessary (Committee on Drugs, 1998). In addition, caretakers may tend to overfeed or inappropriately feed irritable infants. These infants tend to have poor coordination of sucking and swallowing reflexes, tongue thrusting, and tongue tremors, as well as general oral hypersensitivity.

Parents need continued support in introducing solid foods to infants because their tongue thrust and oral hypersensitivity may persist beyond 6 months. Forced feeding is not appropriate and should be avoided. Primary care providers should encourage parents to give food and fluids that are well tolerated.

Proper positioning and handling are essential for satisfactory feeding. Parents should have a gentle, calm approach and use a soothing voice while maintaining the infant in a relaxed, flexed posture to assist with feeding. If vomiting or spitting up occurs after feeding, frequent feedings of small amounts may be better tolerated. A side-lying swaddled position is recommended after feeding.

Safety

Because the chronic use of mind-altering drugs by a parent can interfere with memory, attention, and perception, the safety of children is a major concern for providers. Home visits by health or social service professionals facilitate assessment of the home situation and limit parental supervision for these vulnerable children.

The primary interest of parents who are addicted to drugs—especially those using crack—is often the drug, not their children. When these parents are high, they may be completely unaware of their child's presence. In addition, these children may be living in unstable, dangerous environments with parents who are unable to function as protectors. Therefore it is important to keep children visible in the community. Social service case workers can recommend infant-stimulation programs, daycare programs, and after-school and weekend recreational programs that are appropriate for these children and will allow community workers to regularly assess a child's health and emotional status. All reported and suspected injuries should be assessed to determine if they were unintentional or suspicious of abuse or neglect. When necessary, findings should be reported to Child Protective Services for further evaluation. Substance-abusing parents should also be warned about the danger of their children's passive inhalation or accidental ingestion of the drugs.

Immunizations

The recommendations published yearly by the American Academy of Pediatrics (AAP) should be followed when caring for a cocaine-exposed child.

Hepatitis B. Hepatitis B infection is a common problem among cocaine-using parents. Mothers are generally tested during the prenatal or immediate postpartum period. Dosages and timing of these vaccines should be based on the mother's hepatitis B surface antigen (HBsAg) status and AAP recommendations.

Unfortunately a child's health care maintenance may not be a high priority for drug-using parents. Every effort should be made to encourage these parents to keep their child's immunizations up-to-date, as well as to keep the immunization record intact and in a safe place. Clinicians may choose to administer several immunizations when a child is seen for health care because there may be no guarantee of compliance with follow-up visits. The AAP guidelines should be followed in doing this.

Screening

Vision. The corneal light reflex should be evaluated from birth; the cover test should be performed when a child is able to cooperate. Routine screening for visual acuity is recommended.

Hearing. Routine screening is recommended unless there is a speech delay, in which case a complete audiologic evaluation is warranted.

Dental. Routine screening is recommended.

Blood Pressure. Four extremity blood pressures at birth and yearly screenings are recommended as a result of the possibility of renal vascular abnormalities.

Hematocrit. Routine screening is recommended.

Urinalysis. Routine screening is recommended.

Tuberculosis. There is a higher incidence of tuberculosis among people using drugs, especially if infected with HIV. Yearly screening with purified protein derivative (PPD), 0.1 ml intradermally, is recommended starting at age 12 months.

Condition-Specific Screening (Box 37-5)

Developmental and/or Speech and Language. Developmental and/or language delays are often seen. Refer the child for a complete evaluation if a problem is suspected.

Toxicology Screens. If a mother is suspected of substance abuse or has not received prenatal care, the newborn's urine and/or meconium can be screened for drugs.

Congenital Infections. Because women who abuse drugs are also at high risk for contracting infectious diseases, it may be wise to obtain TORCH titers to rule out congenital infections. A maternal syphilis serologic test, HIV test, and hepatitis B and C screens may also be helpful.

Genitourinary Abnormalities. The urologist may recommend a renal ultrasonogram or a voiding cystourethrogram (VCUG) to evaluate the urologic system.

Cardiac Abnormalities. The cardiologist may recommend an electrocardiogram (ECG) and echocardiogram (ECHO) to evaluate for heart disease if signs and symptoms indicate possible abnormality.

BOX 37-5

Condition-Specific Screening

Developmental and/or speech and language
Toxicology screens
Congenital infections
Genitourinary abnormalities
Cardiac abnormalities
Neurologic abnormalities

BOX 37-6

Differential Diagnosis

Infections
Gastrointestinal problems
Neurologic symptoms
Potential for child abuse and/or neglect
Continued exposure to drugs

Neurologic abnormalities. The neurologist may recommend any of the following studies: brainstem auditory–evoked response (BAER), magnetic resonance imaging (MRI), EEG, and skull radiographic studies to evaluate the nervous system and developmental/neurologic testing to monitor neurologic and cognitive effects of cocaine exposure.

Common Illness Management

Differential Diagnosis (Box 37-6)

Infections. During the first 3 months of life it is often difficult to diagnose illness because of the subtle signs and symptoms newborns exhibit when ill. A change in behavior is often a key factor in the assessment of a child, which complicates diagnosing illness in infants prenatally exposed to cocaine because of the great variability in their sleep-wake state control. Primary care providers should carefully assess irritable or deeply sleeping infants for signs of concomitant illness. Practitioners must be aware of the increased risk of TORCH, HIV, hepatitis B or hepatitis C infections, or sexually transmitted diseases in this population. Accordingly, frequent infections may warrant an immunologic consultation.

Parents should be taught how to take temperatures and encouraged to call the pediatric office or clinic with any concerns. Frequent telephone contact will help parents manage the child at home. If a parent is a poor historian or seems overly concerned on the telephone, the child should be seen in the office or clinic.

Gastrointestinal Symptoms. Gastrointestinal symptoms (e.g., poor feeding, vomiting, diarrhea, or constipation) are common in the first 6 to 9 months of life (Barton, 1998, Committee on Drugs, 1998). Parents should be advised to report any GI symptoms to their primary care provider. Once serious illness is ruled out, routine advice for handling these problems is helpful.

Neurologic Symptoms. Passive exposure to cocaine can cause neurologic symptoms such as seizures, obtundation, delirium, dizziness, and unsteady gait (Mott et al, 1994). Practitioners should include cocaine exposure in the differential diagnosis of children with these symptoms. Seizures may occur in neonates. Parents must be advised of injury prevention when a child is having a seizure, as well as the importance of having the child immediately evaluated by the provider (see Chapter 25). As children enter preschool or school, an evaluation for learning disabilities should be undertaken if there is any indication of difficulty processing information or attending to tasks. These children are considered "at risk" and therefore are eligible for evaluative services under Public Laws 99-457 and 101-476 (see Chapter 5).

Child Abuse. These potentially difficult children are at increased risk for child abuse. Providers should be alert to this possibility and take a complete history and thoroughly examine the skin for marks or bruises. Parents who did not have appropriate parenting role models may have difficulty knowing how to care for themselves and may have no understanding of how to care for an irritable infant. Using the Child Abuse Potential Inventory (CAPI) administered to a group (with and without histories of substance abuse disorders [SUD]) of mothers and fathers of 10- to 12-year-old boys, it was found that those with a history of SUD had higher abuse scale scores. The authors concluded that a history of SUD increases child abuse potential. (Ammerman et al, 1999).

Parental Drug Use. Providers should also keep in mind that parents who are high on drugs may not follow directions appropriately. Therefore any potentially serious condition warrants an office visit, and children who are ill may need to be hospitalized or placed in temporary foster care to ensure appropriate medical management.

Drug Interactions

If a child is taking anticonvulsants for seizure activity or medications for ADHD, the same precautions outlined in Chapters 12 and 25 should be followed.

Developmental Issues

Sleep Patterns

Establishing regular sleeping patterns can be difficult in the cocaine-exposed infant. Techniques that assist parents with sleep problems include swaddling, slow rhythmic rocking, offering a pacifier, and holding the infant in a relaxed, flexed position. Keeping the lights low and reducing environmental noise are also helpful. Fortunately, few sleep problems are reported after the first year. Because drug-exposed infants may have an increased risk of SIDS, they, like all infants, should be placed on their backs for sleep.

Toileting

Persistent motor delays, hyperactivity, and behavioral problems may cause difficulty with toilet training. Parents need a great deal of patience and support for their efforts with the child. Early counseling may help parents avoid potential difficulties. Children with persistent enuresis may require urologic evaluation because of the increased incidence of urinary tract anomalies in cocaine-exposed children.

Discipline

Irritability, excessive crying, and hyperactivity may characterize behavior in these infants and young children. Primary care providers need to assess the parents' ability to parent and their potential for using inappropriate discipline techniques. Suggesting techniques for pacifying these children (e.g., swaddling, offering pacifiers, and decreasing environmental distractions) may be helpful. Older children—especially slow learners—require patient limit setting, and discipline must be developmentally appropriate. Few resources exist that provide expertise in managing children with difficult behaviors. Primary care providers will need to assess the mental health and developmental services in their communities for appropriate referrals.

Child Care

Parents often place children in daycare and preschool nursery programs. There is no clear evidence that children with a history of drug exposure need to be placed in special or therapeutic settings.

Schooling

Children who are prenatally exposed to drugs may be at risk for behavior and/or learning problems. It is wise to make early referrals to Head Start or licensed preschool programs. Head Start programs also have parenting programs to support parents wishing to improve their skills. Enrollment in these programs gives children the added benefit of daily supervision by child care professionals. Problems such as abuse, neglect, or poor academic performance can be addressed in a timely fashion.

Substance-abusing parents may be unable to assist their children with homework assignments and are sometimes lax about making sure their children attend school regularly. Referrals to after-school and tutorial programs will encourage these children to recognize their strengths, increase their self-esteem, and develop appropriate peer relationships, as well as provide ongoing supervision during the school years.

Any children with behavioral problems or who are performing below grade level should be evaluated for learning disabilities, ADHD, and other psychological co-morbidities. A specialized educational program should be developed to meet these children's needs. Primary care providers can use instruments such as the Achenbach Child Behavior Checklist, teacher report form, and youth self-report form to assess anxiety, depression, and ADHD. A team approach in evaluation is most helpful (Simkin, 2002). Sensitive listening to children's concerns is encouraged (Reinherz et al, 2000). Substance-exposed children have difficulty calming themselves, suffer sensory and emotional overload, and are highly sensitive to frustration. Teaching strategies that help children with self-regulation provide a stable structured school environment, predictable day-to-day outcomes, and consistent response to behavior problems (Chasnoff et al, 1998). As early as age 6, childhood behavior problems have been shown to predict later drug disorders for both sexes (Reinherz et al, 2000). For children with early conduct problems, The Incredible Years offers a videotape training series designed to help parents (Hawkins, 2002).

Sexuality

Besides giving routine advice to adolescents, primary care providers must be aware of the potential for desperate drug users to prostitute their children for drugs. In addition, there is the added risk of sexual abuse in these highly dysfunctional families. Providers should be alert to any physical or psychologic indications of sexual abuse and, if suspected, report the situation to the appropriate authorities. Although no published studies describe the sexual behavior of adolescents exposed to cocaine, these teens may be vulnerable to problems such as high-risk sexual activity and teen pregnancy. Illicit drug use during adolescence can lead to early sexual activity, and this behavior can lead to STDs and HIV infection (Guo et al, 2002). Over the past decade, however, there has been a decrease in adolescent sexual activity and an increase in condom use (McManus, 2002).

Transition to Adulthood

Children of substance abusers are more likely than other children to develop addictions and other problem behaviors. Adolescents often engage in risky behavior. Experimenting with drugs is especially dangerous. Many adolescents use drugs as a form of self-medication or mood elevation. Teens who live in poor neighborhoods may witness drug sales and be solicited to buy drugs (Kodjo & Klein, 2002). Risk factors for adolescent substance abuse include parental or sibling alcohol and/or drug use, learning problems, low self-esteem, depression, anxiety, early persistent behavior problems, undetected psychiatric disorders, ADHD with conduct disorder, bulimia, family conflicts, lack of family closeness and stability, and having young parents (Simkin, 2002). Accordingly, teens exposed to cocaine may be at risk for failure in school and delinquency (Kodjo & Klein, 2002). These problems may lead to higher dropout rates, future unemployment, and incarceration.

In the past decade, adolescent use of cigarettes, marijuana, and cocaine have been increasing (McManus, 2002). Males are at a higher risk of drug use than females, and African-American adolescents report lower rates of illicit drug use than white adolescents. The typical pattern begins with use of alcohol or tobacco followed by marijuana and other illicit drugs (Guo et al, 2002).

In a large California study the authors looked at childhood stressors such as growing up with a substance-abusing parent. They found that these stressors adversely affect adult health behaviors like substance abuse and chronic diseases such as diabetes and heart disease (McManus, 2002). Strong family ties, low family conflict, close parental supervision, and clear family rules may significantly reduce the risk of adolescent drug use (Guo et al, 2002). Prevention is a key component of adolescent primary care. Motivational enhancement therapy, which has six components—feedback on personal impairment, emphasis on personal responsibility, clear advice to change, menu of alternative options, empathy as a counseling style, and self-efficacy—may be helpful when confronting adolescents who are suspected of substance abuse (Simkin, 2002).

Adolescents in foster care should be encouraged to use "independent living" programs that focus on smoothing the transition between foster care and life on their own. When providing anticipatory guidance for these teens, primary care providers should discuss reducing their health risk, taking responsibility for their own health, and accessing health care. These young adults should also be encouraged to apply for Medicaid or private health insurance before being discharged from foster care, as well as to locate an appropriate primary care provider. Discharge with a medical summary and a current immunization record will promote continuity of care.

Children treated for congenital syphilis will continue to have a positive serum treponemal test (i.e., fluorescent treponemal antibody absorption [FTA-ABS] or microhemagglutination assay for *Treponema pallidum* [MHA-TP]), which is thought to persist into adulthood. Adolescents should be made aware of this fact and have documentation of treatment on their permanent medical record or immunization card.

Family Concerns and Resources

The family court system may deem parents of a drug-exposed infant to be unfit. In some states the result of a neonatal drug screen test that is positive for illicit drugs triggers a report to the Child Welfare Administration as evidence of neglect. Delaney-Black and associates (2000) reported that 59% of cocaine-exposed children studied always lived with a biological parent, 8% never lived with a biological parent, and 32% had experienced custody changes by age 6. This situation forces relatives, often elderly grandparents, to assume full responsibility for infants who are drug addicted and their siblings while parents seek treatment in the limited number of available programs. Few drug treatment programs will accept pregnant women who are addicted to drugs. Low-income women and women of African-American and Latino descent may be more likely to be tested for illicit substances during their pregnancies, but drug use crosses ethnic and socioeconomic boundaries. All women should be treated respectfully, and judgments about their drug use and fitness as a parent should not be based solely on their ethnicity or economic status.

Before being placed in either a kinship or temporary foster home, these infants may stay in the hospital for 2 to 4 weeks in the boarder nursery. The court will mandate requirements such as drug treatment, parenting classes, and supervised family visits. In cases in which parents cannot meet these requirements, children should be quickly moved to adoptive homes.

Parents and foster parents should be role models for these vulnerable children by providing a loving, supportive family life. Parenting programs such as Preparing For Drug Free Years developed by the American Medical Association Guidelines for Adolescent Preventive Services (GAPS) can provide parents and foster parents with useful information and appropriate parenting skills (Hawkins, 2002).

Despite careful counseling by health care professionals, adoptive parents often have expectations about the infant or child that they accept into their home. Because long-term outcomes are unknown in the cocaine-exposed population, adoptive parents must be advised accordingly. Many of these infants who have had a difficult first few months look "normal" to adoptive parents who so eagerly want a child. It is important for primary care providers to follow a child's progress with adoptive parents while remaining objective and realistic about the outcome.

Across the nation, communities are responding to the devastating problems associated with drug addiction. Many government and private agencies have substance abuse hotlines and Internet Web sites.

ORGANIZATIONS

National Council on Alcoholism and Drug Dependency, Inc.
20 Exchange Place, Suite 2902
New York, NY 10005
(212) 269-7797; hopeline: (800) NCA-CALL

National Institute on Drug Abuse (NIDA)
(800) 662-HELP; Infofax: (888) 644-6432 (access science-based facts on drug abuse)
800-DRUGHELP, 24-hour confidential information and referral service

INTERNET RESOURCES:

The National Center on Addiction and Substance Abuse at Columbia University
www.casacolumbia.org

National Council on Alcoholism and Drug Dependence, Inc
www.ncadd.org

National Center for Infants, Toddlers and Families
www.zerotothree.org

American Council for Drug Education
800-488-DRUG
www.acde.org

American Society of Addiction Medicine
www.asam.org

Substance Abuse and Mental Health Services Administration
www.samhsa.gov

National Clearinghouse on Drug and Alcohol Information (NCDAI)
www.health.org

National Institute on Drug Abuse
www.drugabuse.gov
www.nida.nih.gov

Web of Addictions
www.well.com/user/woa

National Substance Abuse Web Index
http://nsawi.health.org

Substance abuse treatment facility locator
www.findtreatment.samhsa.gov

Summary of Primary Care Needs for the Child with Prenatal Cocaine Exposure

HEALTH CARE MAINTENANCE
Growth and Development

Growth parameters, particularly weight and head circumference, should be monitored closely.

Developmental assessment should be performed every 1 to 2 months during the first year of life.

Early referral to infant-stimulation programs is recommended.

Speech and language delays are common.

Motor problems are common in the first year of life.

Neurologic assessment is important to monitor effects of exposure.

Guidance on handling infants with increased tone, irritability, and poor feeding is necessary.

Diet

Breast feeding is not recommended for cocaine-using women because cocaine metabolites are present in breast milk.

Caloric intake and feeding behavior should be monitored.

To enhance feeding, parents should be taught proper positioning and handling techniques.

Safety

Home visits are recommended if parents are suspected substance abusers.

Social service involvement and referrals to after-school and recreational programs are recommended to keep the child visible in the community.

Parents should be warned about the dangers of passive inhalation of crack fumes and the potential for accidental ingestion of drugs by the children.

Injuries should be evaluated for abuse and/or neglect.

Immunizations

Routine immunizations are recommended.

Hepatitis B immune globulin is given if the mother is infected with hepatitis.

If parents who use drugs are not compliant with well-child care visits or if the child has inconsistent health care, the clinician should assess immunization status of each visit and may choose to give several immunizations at one visit.

Screening

Vision. The corneal light reflex should be tested from birth, and the cover test should be administered when the child is able to cooperate. Routine screening for visual acuity is recommended.

Hearing. Routine office screening is recommended unless there is a speech delay, in which case a complete audiologic evaluation is warranted.

Dental. Routine screening is recommended.

Blood pressure. A four-extremity screening is recommended for neonates.

Hematocrit. Routine screening is recommended.

Urinalysis. Routine screening is recommended. The high incidence of urologic abnormalities in these children may require referral to a urologist for testing.

Continued

Summary of Primary Care Needs for the Child with Prenatal Cocaine Exposure—cont'd

Tuberculosis. Yearly screening with PPD beginning at 12 months is recommended.

Condition-Specific Screening

Developmental and/or Speech and Language. Problems are common. Progress should be monitored closely, and the child referred for evaluation if a problem is suspected.

Toxicology. Urine toxicologic screening should be done if the mother is a suspected substance abuser or did not receive prenatal care.

Infections. Syphilis serologic testing and TORCH titers should be considered.

Genitourinary Screening. Renal ultrasound and/or VCUG may be done in infancy because of questionable increased anomalies.

Cardiac Screening. Both ECG and ECHO may be obtained if a heart murmur is detected.

Neurologic Screening. If neurologic problems are suspected, BAER, MRI, EEG, and skull films may be obtained.

Developmental and neurologic testing may be indicated.

COMMON ILLNESS MANAGEMENT

Differential Diagnosis

Infections. Irritable or deeply sleeping infants should be carefully assessed.

Parents should be taught to take temperatures.

An office visit should be scheduled if there are any questions about the child's condition.

These children are at high risk for contracting congenital infections, including HIV, TORCH, and STDs.

GI Problems. GI symptoms such as vomiting, diarrhea, and constipation may persist for the first 6 to 9 months. Other illnesses need to be ruled out.

Neurologic Problems. The child should be evaluated immediately if a seizure occurs.

These children may experience academic difficulties and school failure.

Child Abuse. Behavior should be observed and skin checked closely for signs of abuse.

Parental Drug Use. If the parents are abusing drugs, the child may need to be hospitalized or placed in temporary foster care during periods of illness to ensure medical management.

Drug Interactions

No routine medications are prescribed. If the child is taking seizure medication or medications for ADHD, see Chapters 12 and 28.

DEVELOPMENTAL ISSUES

Sleep Patterns

Infant massage, pacification techniques, low lighting, and a relatively quiet environment are helpful.

Infants should be placed on their backs to sleep.

Toileting

Persistent motor delays, hyperactivity, and behavior problems may interfere with toilet training.

Children with persistent enuresis may need genitourinary workup.

Discipline

Parents should be encouraged to be consistent, firm, and patient in their disciplinary efforts.

Child Care

Routine placement is advised and may help improve later school performance.

Schooling

Early identification of behavior problems and referrals to Head Start or therapeutic programs may be helpful.

These children may be at high risk for learning and/or behavior problems.

School attendance and performance should be evaluated.

Referrals for specialized education programs may be necessary.

Sexuality

These children are at high risk for sexual abuse and high-risk sexual activity.

Transition to Adulthood

Teens exposed to cocaine may be at risk for failure in school and delinquency.

Drugs may be used to self-medicate for depression.

Children of substance abusers are at high risk for substance abuse themselves.

Teens in foster care should be enrolled in independent living programs.

Access to health care, risk reduction, and health insurance should be discussed.

Treatment for congenital syphilis should be documented on immunization card.

Family Concerns

Parents with illicit drug use may be ruled as unfit to care for their children often shifting care responsibilities to other family members or the foster care system.

Adoptive parents require ongoing counseling because long-term outcomes are generally unknown.

Health care providers must try to remain empathic and nonjudgmental.

REFERENCES

Ammerman, R.T., Kolko, D.J., Kirisci, L., Blackson, T.C., & Dawes, M.A. (1999). Child abuse potential in parents with histories of substance use disorders. *Child Abuse Negl, 23*, 1225-1238.

Arendt, R., Angelopoulos, J., Salvator, A., & Singer, L. (1999). Motor development of cocaine-exposed children at age two years. *Pediatrics 103*, 86-92.

Bailey, D.N. (1998). Cocaine and cocaethylene binding to human milk. *Am J Clin Pathol 110*, 491-494.

Bandstra, E.S., et al. (2001). Intrauterine growth of full term infants: impact of prenatal cocaine exposure. *Pediatrics, 108*, 1309-1319.

Bandstra, E.S., et al. (2002). Longitudinal influence of prenatal cocaine exposure on child language functioning. *Neurotoxicol Teratol, 24*, 297-308.

Barton, S.J. (1998). Foster parents of cocaine exposed infants. *J Pediatr Nurs, 13*, 104-112.

Behnke, M., Eyler, F.D., Garvan, C.W., & Wobie, K. (2001). The search for congenital malformations in newborns with fetal cocaine exposure. *Pediatrics, 107*, e74.

Bingol, N., Fuchs, M., Diaz, V., Stone, R.K., & Gromisch, D.S. (1987). Teratogenicity of cocaine in humans. *J Pediatr 110*, 93-96.

Block, S.S., Moore, B.D., & Scharre, J.E. (1997). Visual anomalies in young children exposed to cocaine. *Optom Vis Sci, 74*, 28-36.

Centers for Disease Control and Prevention. (2002, March). Media release, Gonorrhea rates increased in two-thirds of hardest hit U.S. cities [online]. Available: www.cdc.gov/std/media/2002ConfTrends.htm.

Centers for Disease Control and Prevention. (2001, July). Press release, Syphilis among infants down more than half in three years [online]. Available: www.cdc.gov/std/press/presscsyph7-2001.htm.

Chasnoff, I.J., et al. (1998a). Prenatal exposure to cocaine and other drugs: outcome at four to six years. *Ann N Y Acad Sci, 846*, 314-328.

Chasnoff, I.J., Neuman, K., Thornton, C., & Callaghan, M.A. (2001). Screening for substance abuse in pregnancy: a practical approach for the primary care physician. *Am J Obstet Gynecol, 184*, 752-758.

Chavez, G.F., Mulinare, J., & Cordero, J.F. (1989). Maternal cocaine use during early pregnancy as a risk factor for congenital urogenital anomalies. *JAMA 262*, 795-798.

Chiriboga, C.A., Brust, J.C., Bateman, D., & Hauser, W.A. (1999). Dose-response effect of fetal cocaine exposure on newborn neurologic function. *Pediatrics, 103*, 79-85.

Cohen H.L., et al. (1994). Neurosonographic findings in full term infants born to maternal cocaine abusers: visualization of subependymal and periventricular cysts. *J Clin Ultrasound 22*, 327-333.

Cohen, H.R., Green, J.R., & Crombleholme, W.R. (1991). Peripartum cocaine use: estimating risk of adverse pregnancy outcome. *Int J Gynaecol Obstet 35*, 51-54.

Coles, C.D., Platzman, K.A., Smith, I., James, M.E., & Falek, A. (1992). Effects of cocaine and alcohol use in pregnancy on neonatal growth and neurobehavioral status. *Neurotoxicol Teratol 14*, 23-33.

Committee on Drugs. (1998). Neonatal drug withdrawal. *Pediatrics, 101*, 1079-1088.

Committee on Drugs. (2001). The transfer of drugs and other chemicals into human milk. *Pediatrics, 108*, 776-789.

Czyrko, C., et al. (1991). Maternal cocaine abuse and necrotizing enterocolitis: outcome and survival. *J Pediatr Surg, 26*, 414-421.

Datta-Bhutada, S., Johnson, H.L., & Rosen, T.S. (1998). Intrauterine cocaine and crack exposure: neonatal outcome. *J Perinatol, 18*, 183-188.

Delaney-Black, V., et al. (1998). Prenatal cocaine exposure and child behavior. *Pediatrics, 102*, 945-950.

Delaney-Black, V., et al. (1996). Prenatal cocaine and neonatal outcome: evaluation of dose-response relationship. *Pediatrics, 98*, 735-740.

Delaney-Black, V., et al. (2000). Teacher-assessed behavior of children prenatally exposed to cocaine. *Pediatrics, 106*, 782-791.

Drehobl, K.F. & Fuhr, M.G. (1991). *Pediatric massage* (pp. 7-20). Tucson: Therapy Skill Builders a division of Communication Skill Builders, Inc.

Drug facts and comparisons. (2002). *Topical local anesthetics* (pp. 1811-1812). St. Louis: Facts and comparisons.

Eyler, F.D., Behnke, M., Conlon, M., Woods, N.S., & Wobie, K. (1998). Birth outcome from a prospective matched study of prenatal crack/cocaine use: I. Interactive and dose effects on health and growth. *Pediatrics, 101*, 229-236.

Fares, I., McCulloch, K.M., & Raju, T.N. (1997). Intrauterine cocaine exposure and the risk for sudden infant death syndrome: a meta analysis. *J Perinatol, 17*, 179-182.

Fetters, L., et al. (1996). Neuromotor development of cocaine-exposed and control infants from birth through 15 months: Poor and poorer performance. *Pediatrics, 98*, 930-943.

Frank, D.A., Augustyn, M., & Zuckerman, B.S. (1998). Neonatal neurobehavioral and neuroanatomic correlates of prenatal cocaine exposure: problems of dose and confounding. *Ann N Y Acad Sci 846*, 40-50.

Frank, D.A., Augustyn, M., Knight, W.G., Pell, T., & Zuckerman, B. (2001). Growth, development, and behavior in early childhood following prenatal cocaine exposure a systematic review. *JAMA, 285*, 1613-1625.

Guo, J., Hill, K.G., Hawkins, J.D., Catalano, R.F., & Abbott, R.D. (2002). A developmental analysis of sociodemographic, family, and peer effects on adolescent illicit drug initiation. *J Am Acad Child Adolesc Psychiatry, 4*, 838-45.

Hawkins, J.D., Smith, B.H., & Catalano, R.F. (2002). Delinquent behavior. *Pediatr Rev, 23*, 387-392.

Havlick, D.M. & Nolte, K.P. (2000). Fatal "crack" cocaine ingestion in an infant. *Am J Forensic Med Pathol, 21*, 245-248.

Ho, J., Afshani, E., & Stapleton, F.B. (1994). Renal vascular abnormalities associated with prenatal cocaine exposure. *Clin Pediatr, 32*, 155-156.

Hoyme, H.E., et al. (1990). Prenatal cocaine exposure and fetal vascular disruption. *Pediatrics, 85*, 743-747.

Hurt, H., et al. (1997). Children with in utero exposure do not differ from control subjects on intelligence testing. *Arch Pediatr Adolesc Med, 151*, 1237-1241.

Hurt, H., Giannetta, J., Brodsky, N.L., Malmud, E., & Pelham, T. (2001). Are there neurological correlates of in utero cocaine exposure at age 6 years? *J Pediatr, 138*, 911-913.

Johnson, J.L. & Leff, M. (1999). Children of substance abusers: overview of research findings. *Pediatrics, 103*, 1085-1099.

Jones, K.L., Smith, D.W., Ulleland, C.N., & Streissguth, P. (1973). Pattern of malformation in offspring of chronic alcoholic mothers. *Lancet 1*, 1267-1271.

Kandall, S.R., Gaines, J., Habel, L., Davidson, G., & Jessop, D. (1993). Relationship of maternal substance abuse to subsequent sudden infant death syndrome in offspring. *J Pediatr, 123*, 120-126.

Kilbride, H., Castor, C., Hoffman, E., & Fuger, K.L. (2000). Thirty-six month outcome of prenatal cocaine exposure for term or near-term infants: impact of early case management. *J Dev Behav Pediatr, 21*, 19-26.

Klonoff-Cohen, H. & Lam-Kruglick, P. (2001). Maternal and paternal recreational drug use and sudden infant death syndrome. *Arch Pediatr Adolesc Med, 155*, 765-770.

Kodjo, C.M. & Klein, J.D. (2002). Prevention and risk of adolescent substance abuse: the role of adolescents, families and communities. *Pediatr Clin North Am, 49*, 257-268.

Koren, G., et al. (1998). Long-term neurodevelopmental risks in children exposed in utero to cocaine: the Toronto adoption study. *Ann N Y Acad Sci, 846*, 306-312.

Kramer, L.D., Locke, G.E., Ogunyemi, A., & Nelson, L. (1990). Neonatal cocaine-related seizures. *J Child Neurol, 5*, 60-64.

Kumpfer, K.L. (1999). Outcome measures of interventions in the study of children of substance abusing parents. *Pediatrics, 103*, 1128-1144.

Lester, B.M., LaGasse, L.L., & Seifer, R. (1998). Cocaine exposure and children: the meaning of subtle effects. *Science, 282*, 633-634.

Lester, B.M., et al. (2001). The maternal lifestyle study: drug use by meconium toxicology and maternal self report. *Pediatrics, 107*, 309-317.

Lewkowicz, D.J., Karmel, B.Z., & Gardner, J.M. (1998). Effects of prenatal cocaine exposure on responsiveness to multimodal information in infants between 4 and 10 months of age. *Ann NY Acad Sci, 846*, 408-411.

Lipschultz, S.E., Frassica, J.J., & Orav, E.J. (1991). Cardiovascular abnormalities in infants prenatally exposed to cocaine. *J Pediatr, 118*, 44-51.

Lustbader, A.S., Mayes, L.C., McGee, B.A., Jatlow, P., & Roberts, W.L. (1998). Incidence of passive exposure to crack/cocaine and clinical findings in infants seen in an outpatient service. *Pediatrics, 102*, e5.

Mayes, L.C., Grillon, C., Granger, R., & Schottenfeld, R. (1998). Regulation of arousal and attention in preschool children exposed to cocaine prenatally. *Ann N Y Acad Sci, 846*, 126-143.

McManus, R.P. (2002). Adolescent care: reducing risk and promoting resilience. *Prim Care, 29*, 557-569.

Morrow, C.E., et al. (2001). Influence of prenatal cocaine exposure on full-term infant neurobehavioral functioning. *Neurotoxicol Teratol, 23*, 523-544.

Mott, S.H., Packer, R.J., & Soldin, S.J. (1994). Neurologic manifestations of cocaine exposure in childhood. *Pediatrics, 93*, 557-560.

Nair, P., Rothblum, S., & Hebel, R. (1994). Neonatal outcome in infants with evidence of fetal exposure to opiates, cocaine, and cannabinoids. *Clin Pediatr 33*, 280-285.

National Center on Addiction and Substance Abuse at Columbia University. (1996). Illicit drug use during pregnancy, substance abuse and the American woman [online]. Available: www.casacolumbia.org/usr_doc/5894.pdf.

National Institute on Drug Abuse. (1998). Crack and cocaine: NIDA Infofax [online]. Available: www.nida.nih.gov/Infofax/cocaine.html.

National Institute on Drug Abuse. (1996). National Pregnancy and Health Survey—drug use among women delivering live births: 1992, HHS, National Institute on Drug Abuse, NIH Publication #96-3819.

Ostrea, E.M., Ostrea, A.R., & Simpson, P.M. (1997). Mortality within the first two years in infants exposed to cocaine, opiates, or cannaboid during gestation. *Pediatrics, 100*, 79-83.

Ostrea, E.M. Jr., et al. (2001). Estimates of illicit drug use during pregnancy by maternal interview, hair analysis and meconium analysis. *J Pediatr, 138*, 344-348.

Plessinger, M. & Woods, J. (1998). Cocaine in pregnancy recent data on maternal and fetal risks. *Obstet Gynecol Clin North Am, 25*, 99-118.

Porat, R. & Brodsky, N. (1991). Cocaine: a risk factor for necrotizing enterocolitis. *J Perinatol 11*, 30-32.

Richardson, G.A. (1998). Prenatal cocaine exposure: a longitudinal study of development. *Ann N Y Acad Sci, 846*, 144-152.

Reinherz, H.Z., Giaconia, R.M., Hauf, A.M., Wasserman, M.S., & Paradis, A.D. (2000). General and specific childhood risk factors for depression and drug disorders by early adulthood. *J Am Acad Child Adolesc Psychiatry, 39*, 223-31.

Robins, L.N. & Mills, J.L. (1993). Effects of in utero exposure to street drugs. *Am J Public Health Suppl, 83*, 17.

Ryan, R.M., et al. (1994). Meconium analysis for improved identification of infants exposed to cocaine in utero. *J Pediatr, 125*, 435-440.

Scher, M.S., Richardson, G.A., & Day, N.L. (2000). Effects of prenatal cocaine/crack and other drug exposure on electroencephalographic sleep studies at birth and one year. *Pediatrics, 105*, 39-48.

Sherer, D.M., Anyaegbunam, A., & Onyeije, C. (1998). Antepartum fetal intracranial hemorrhage, predisposing factors and prenatal sonography: a review. *Am J Perinatol, 15*, 431-441.

Simkin, D.R. (2002). Adolescent substance use disorders and comorbidity. *Pediatr Clin North Am, 49*, 463-477.

Singer, L.T., et al. (1994). Increased incidence of intraventricular hemorrhage and developmental delay in cocaine-exposed very low birthweight infants. *J Pediatr, 124*, 765-771.

Singer, L.T., Arendt, R., Minnes, S., Farkas, K., & Salvator, A. (2000). Neurobehavioral outcomes of cocaine-exposed infants. *Neurotoxicol Teratol, 22*, 653-666.

Singer, L.T., et al. (2001). Developing language skills of cocaine-exposed infants. *Pediatrics, 107*, 1057-1064.

Singer, L.T., et al. (2002). Cognitve and motor outcomes of cocaine exposed infants. *JAMA , 287*, 1952-1960.

Substance Abuse and Mental Health Service Administration, Office of Applied Statistics. (2002). Preliminary results from the 2001 National Household Survey on Drug Abuse, Washington, DC, U.S. Dept. of Health and Human Services [online]. Available: www.samhsa.gov/oas/nhsda/2k1nhsda/vol1/higlights.htm.

Vogel, G. (1997). Cocaine wreaks subtle damage on developing brains. *Science, 278*, 38-39.

Wagner, C.L., Katikaneni, L.D., Cox, T.H., & Ryan, R.M. (1998). The impact of prenatal drug exposure on the neonate. *Obstet Gynecol Clin, 25*, 169-194.

Wootton, J. & Miller, S.I. (1994). Cocaine: a review. *Pediatr Rev 15*, 89-92.

38 Renal Failure, Chronic

Melanie Klein and Alicia Namrow

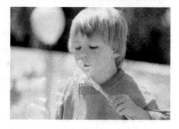

Etiology

Causes of chronic renal failure (CRF) are varied and can be broadly categorized as congenital, hereditary, or cystic diseases; obstructive uropathy; glomerulonephritis; secondary glomerulonephritis and vasculitis; interstitial nephritis and pyelonephritis; diabetes; hypertension; and malignancies (Figure 38-1). Hypertensive nephrosclerosis and diabetic nephropathy, the most common causes of renal failure in adults, are rarely seen in children. Glomerulonephritis accounts for the largest single group of children with end-stage renal disease (ESRD), followed by congenital and other hereditary and/or cystic diseases. Race-related patterns are present, with incidence rates of ESRD being more common among black children (as in adults). Glomerulonephritis is the most common diagnosis for ESRD in black, Native American, and Asian children, regardless of age, and congenital or hereditary diseases are more common in young white children (USRDS, 2001).

Staging of Chronic Renal Failure (CRF)

Assessment of the glomerular filtration rate (GFR) is the most important test for determining kidney function. A low or declining GFR is a good indicator for chronic renal failure (Holloway, 2001). In children the Schwartz formula is used to determine GFR. This formula takes into account the child's age and weight in addition to the serum creatinine level.

CRF is a broadly used term and may be described in four stages. Stage 1 is asymptomatic and corresponds to a GFR of 50% to 75% of normal. Stage 2 is referred to as chronic renal insufficiency; children in this stage experience increases in serum urea nitrogen, creatinine, and parathyroid hormone (PTH). Significant but asymptomatic proteinuria is often seen. A GFR of 25% to 50% correlates to this stage. Stage 3 is CRF. The GFR in this stage is 10% to 25% of normal. Laboratory features of this stage include metabolic acidosis, hyperphosphatemia, hypocalcemia, and anemia. Renal osteodystrophy and rickets can also be noted. Stage 4 is the final stage and is commonly called ESRD. It correlates with a GFR of <10%. Severe clinical, laboratory, and radiologic abnormalities can be seen, and renal replacement therapy (RRT) by dialysis or transplantation is initiated (Chan et al, 2002).

Children with congenital disorders or whose renal disease begins in infancy are at greatest risk for significant growth failure and progression to ESRD. Children with congenital renal anomalies often have abnormalities of other organ systems, as well, according to the period of embryonic development and gestational stage at which the problem occurred. Genetic counseling is recommended for family planning.

Early detection of renal failure and the establishment of the exact cause of CRF is important for the following reasons: (1) timely surgical intervention, as early in utero as possible in some congenital obstructive disorders, may minimize the amount of renal damage acquired prenatally; (2) disorders may require different treatments and have varying prognoses; (3) genetic counseling and early diagnosis and treatment of similarly affected siblings should be initiated if a hereditary or metabolic disease is involved; and (4) the timing and donor selection for renal transplantation may be altered in diseases with a high incidence of recurrence in renal allografts. Unfortunately it is not always possible to determine the cause, especially when a child is already experiencing CRF. A renal biopsy may be indicated for diagnosis and/or prognosis and treatment recommendations.

Known Genetic Etiology

In recent years academic research has focused on the study of the genetic origin and expression of a variety of diseases. The goal of genetic research is to provide new opportunities for diagnosis, treatment, and ultimately prevention of certain medical conditions. Research is being focused on determining the genetic basis for certain renal diseases in both children and adult populations. Examples of pediatric kidney diseases on which genetic research has been focused include but are not limited to the following: Wilms' tumor, focal segmental glomerulosclerosis (FSGS), Alport syndrome, and polycystic kidney disease (PKD).

Wilms' tumor, a rapidly developing tumor of the kidney, usually affects children 3 to 4 years of age and is now thought to be associated with the expression of the WT1 gene (Watkins et al, 1999). WT1 gene has also been named the Wilms' tumor suppressor gene; mutations of the WT1 gene may be responsible for the development of this invasive malignancy (Neville & Ritchey, 2000). Renal researchers hope to ultimately prevent the development of this pediatric disease by altering WT1 gene expression (Ito et al, 2001).

FSGS is a major cause of glomerular disease in children and results in irreversible glomerular scarring (Devarajan & Spitzer, 2002). Individuals affected by FSGS display variable disease progression and responses to treatment. Identification of genetic differences between children affected with FSGS has led researchers to believe that genetic factors may play a role in the various clinical courses of this disease (Frishberg et al, 2000).

Alport syndrome is a form of congenital glomerulonephritis that arises from mutations in the gene responsible for developing basement membranes in type IV collagen. Research has

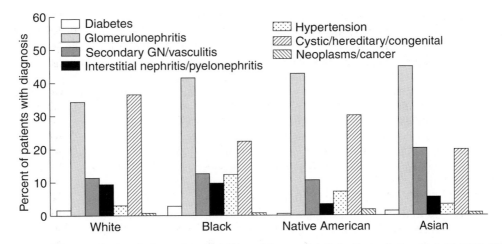

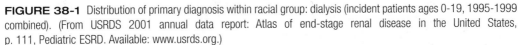

FIGURE 38-1 Distribution of primary diagnosis within racial group: dialysis (incident patients ages 0-19, 1995-1999 combined). (From USRDS 2001 annual data report: Atlas of end-stage renal disease in the United States, p. 111, Pediatric ESRD. Available: www.usrds.org.)

been focused on new genetic diagnostic techniques for Alport syndrome that may someday decrease the need for invasive kidney biopsies (Kashtan, 1999).

Polycystic kidney disease is a heritable disorder that takes two major forms: autosomal dominant polycystic kidney disease (ADPKD) and autosomal recessive polycystic kidney disease (ARPKD). Both forms can result in pediatric renal failure secondary to cyst formation (McDonald et al, 1999). Unlike ADPKD, the genetic mutation responsible for ARPKD has not yet been identified (Davis et al, 2001). The identification of a gene mutation seen in an individual with polycystic kidneys may identify which form of the disease is present. In addition, differentiating between ADPKD and ARPKD has important implications for genetic counseling of the affected families. Also, scientists are using genetic research to identify specific therapies that might slow the actual disease progression (Davis, et al, 2001).

Active research involving the genetic link between these and other renal diseases is under way. This research will hopefully provide new diagnostic, therapeutic, and preventive approaches to managing children with renal failure.

Incidence and Prevalence

In the most comprehensive collection of data available, the United States Renal Data System (USRDS) (2001) identified 89,252 newly diagnosed individuals with ESRD in 1999. Children up to 19 years of age beginning treatment for ESRD were 1.4% (i.e., 1,292) of this total. Over the past decade the incidence rates of ESRD in children have increased 2% to 3%. Incidence also increases with age. In the 1990s, there was little variation in the incidence and prevalence rates of ESRD per million population in children younger than than 10 years of age. During that same period, the prevalence rates in children older than 10 years of age had increased, most likely evidence of improved survival rates posttransplant. Males have a higher incidence and prevalence of CRF than females in all age

groups, but especially in the age group of children younger than 5 years because congenital renal disorders are more common in males. As of December 1999, point prevalence counts listed 344,094 people of all ages with ESRD, with children up to 19 years of age representing 1.8% of the total (USRDS, 2001).

Clinical Manifestations at Time of Diagnosis

Symptoms at the time of diagnosis vary depending on the primary renal disease and the amount of residual renal function (RRF). Children with CRF may exhibit a few or many common signs and symptoms of renal failure (Box 38-1).

Fluid, Electrolyte, and Acid-Base Abnormalities

As renal function decreases, solute, fluid, and toxins accumulate in the blood (i.e., uremia). Alterations in calcium,

---

BOX 38-1
Clinical Manifestations

FLUID AND ELECTROLYTE AND ACID-BASE ABNORMALITIES
Alterations in calcium and phosphorus
Hyperkalemia
Fluid volume overload
Slow adjustment to sodium loads

HORMONE ALTERATION
Increased secretion of parathyroid hormone
Decreased production of erythropoietin
Blood pressure may be elevated

UREMIA
Decreased energy, increased fatigue
In severe uremia: CHF, pericarditis, somnolence, and seizures may occur

GROWTH RETARDATION

phosphorus, and acid-base metabolism begin to develop. Impairment of bicarbonate resorption and decreased acid and ammonia excretion lead to metabolic acidosis. Hyperkalemia occurs as a result of tissue breakdown, acidosis, and reduced renal excretion and—if untreated—is fatal, causing peaked T waves, long P-R interval, and widened QRS complex, which typically signal the onset of ventricular fibrillation and, potentially, cardiac arrest (Bergstein, 2000). Hypokalemia, although less common, can result from the use of diuretics, including osmotic diuretics and carbonic anhydrase inhibitors or by tubular defects, such as renal tubular acidosis or Fanconi syndrome (Wassner & Baum, 1999).

Children with CRF maintain the ability to adjust sodium excretion in response to changes in intake, but lose the ability to make these changes quickly. A rapid increase in sodium intake is excreted at a slower rate, causing an acute increase in extracellular fluid (ECF) (Wassner & Baum, 1999). This rapid increase in ECF volume can lead to edema, hypertension, or heart failure. Conversely an acute reduction in intake leads to ECF contraction. Congenital renal abnormalities (e.g., hypoplasia, dysplasia, and obstructive uropathy) can produce a "salt-wasting state" so severe that it impairs growth. In children with salt-losing nephropathy, serum sodium levels may remain within normal limits because of volume contraction.

Decreased GFR and tubular defects result in retention of phosphate wastes that result in elevated serum phosphorus levels and cause a correlative decrease in serum calcium.

Hormone Alteration

Hyperphosphatemia causes calcium resorption from bone and increased stimulation by the parathyroid gland to secrete more parathormone (PTH) to enhance phosphate excretion. Renal conversion of 25-hydroxycholecalciferol to the active vitamin D, 1,25-dihydroxycholecalciferol becomes impaired. Active vitamin D deficiency decreases intestinal calcium absorption and impairs the skeletal response to PTH, further promoting hypocalcemia. This circular mechanism ultimately results in secondary hyperparathyroidism. Vitamin D deficiency also promotes PTH secretion, causing additional bone resorption. Disturbance in the calcium-phosphorus-bone metabolism relationship causes renal osteodystrophy (ROD). In children ROD resembles rickets. ROD is manifested as delayed bone growth, bone deformities, bone pain, muscle weakness, slipped capital femoral epiphyses, and uremic calcifications. Of particular concern is the deposition of calcium into coronary arteries, leading to early (<30 years of age) development of atherosclerosis and cardiovascular disease breakdown. Hyperlipidemia can accompany chronic renal failure, as well, further increasing the risk of early cardiovascular disease (Warady et al, 1999; Goodman, 2000).

At least 90% of all erythropoietin (EPO) is produced in the kidney; consequently, renal failure causes a deficiency in EPO. This deficiency coupled with a shorter life span of red blood cells, as seen in renal failure, results in anemia and its manifestations (Van Damme-Lombaerts & Herman, 1999). Excessive renin production, coupled with sodium and fluid imbalance, may lead to hypertension in children with chronic renal failure (Bergstein, 2000).

Uremia

The inability of the kidneys to rid the body of nitrogenous wastes leads to a syndrome called uremia. Though serum urea nitrogen levels may be significantly elevated and other electrolyte and hormonal levels impressively disturbed, clinical signs usually to not appear until GFR is 15% to 20% of normal (Wolfson & Maenza, 2002). A child with CRF may initially exhibit a loss of normal energy and increased fatigue on exertion. Such fatigue often develops gradually and goes unnoticed. These children may prefer sedentary activities to active play. Physical examination may reveal a slightly listless, pale child whose hemoglobin is low. Blood pressure may be elevated or normal. Secondary amenorrhea is common in adolescent girls. Urine output may remain normal or decrease in volume but with decreased solute clearance.

As renal failure worsens, its manifestations become more pronounced. Children become more fatigued and uninterested in play, have a poor appetite, and are less capable of accomplishing schoolwork as their attention span diminishes and memory becomes erratic from toxin accumulation. Anemia worsens, calcium-phosphorus levels become increasingly unbalanced, accelerating the development of renal osteodystrophy. Symptoms of severe uremia can include congestive heart failure, pericarditis, uremic pleuritis, malaise, somnolence, and seizures (Wolfson & Maenza, 2002).

Growth Retardation

Growth retardation is a significant consequence of CRF in children and is the symptom that occasionally leads to the diagnosis of renal disease. Impairment of growth begins when the GFR is <50% and becomes more pronounced as GFR falls to <25% (Vimalachandra, 2001). At the time of dialysis initiation, children with ESRD are, on average, approximately 1.6 standard deviations (SDs) below the mean height for their age and worsen to almost 2 SDs below the mean at 24 months after starting dialysis. Growth retardation is more pronounced in younger children and males with ESRD (North American Renal Transplant Cooperative Study [NAPRTCS], 2001). Other factors associated with poor growth in CRF include inadequate nutrition and manifestations of uremia such as anorexia, electrolyte imbalance, and renal osteodystrophy (Warady et al, 1999).

Treatment

Treatment goals include restoring and maintaining the child's health and improving growth and developmental level of function to the highest degree possible. As significant psychosocial, emotional, and financial stressors accompany chronic medical conditions, the child and family should be provided with psychologic and emotional support from a specialized and multidisciplinary renal team. Treatment is based on the severity of the clinical manifestations of CRF. Approaches include conservative medical management and—eventually—RRT (Box 38-2).

Conservative Management Therapy

Fluid, Electrolyte, and Blood Pressure Control. Early recognition and management of biochemical imbalances may prevent

Treatment

CONSERVATIVE MANAGEMENT
Fluid, electrolyte, and blood pressure control
Anemia management
Metabolic control and calcium and phosphate homeostasis
Managing growth retardation

RENAL REPLACEMENT THERAPY (RRT)
Peritoneal dialysis (APD or CAPD)
Hemodialysis
Transplantation

adverse consequences. Fluid overload and hypertension may be controlled by limiting total fluid intake to total output volume plus insensible losses, restricting salt intake, and using diuretic and antihypertensive medications. The control of hypertension limits damage to the renal arterioles and slows the progression of CRF. Diuretics help control the volume-dependent hypertension seen in CRF, although this is effective only in children with a GFR >30% of normal (Chan et al, 2002). Although beta-adrenergic blockers, alpha-adrenergic antagonists, peripheral vasodilators, calcium channel blockers, and angiotensin-converting enzyme (ACE) inhibitors are groups of drugs available for CRF-associated hypertension, some of these drugs are not acceptable for use in young children. Hypertension must be controlled primarily by, or in consultation with, a pediatric nephrologist.

Hyperkalemia can be controlled through dietary restriction of high-potassium foods, use of bicarbonate for intracellular mobilization and acidosis prevention, and use of polystyrene sulfonate (Kayexalate) 1 g/kg/dose to remove potassium from the body (Bergstein, 2000). Metabolic acidosis may be controlled by use of alkalizing medications (e.g., sodium citrate [Bicitra] or sodium bicarbonate tablets).

Anemia Management. Treatment for anemia is aimed at increasing red blood cell (RBC) production and decreasing RBC loss. Iron supplementation is prescribed if the serum ferritin is <20 ng/L or the serum iron level is <100 g/dl, or both (National Kidney Foundation, 2000). Blood transfusions are not indicated in asymptomatic children with a hemoglobin >6 g/dl because this would further suppress EPO production. Transfusions also increase the risk of acquiring bloodborne pathogens and sensitization to histocompatibility antigens, making transplantation with an immunologically compatible kidney more difficult (Warady et al, 1999). If transfusions are required, filtered and washed leukocyte-poor RBC mass is usually preferred over whole blood.

Administration of synthetic human recombinant erythropoietin (r-HuEPO, epoetin alfa, EPO, Epogen, Procrit) produced by recombinant DNA technology is the gold standard for treatment of anemia associated with CRF. Multicenter studies report variations in frequency (one to three times weekly) and starting dose (25 to 150 U/kg/week) according to the current stage of renal failure and desired hematocrit. The dosage must be carefully titrated to prevent a rapid rise in hematocrit and possible hypertensive crisis. As the desired erythropoiesis is achieved, iron stores become depleted. Certain foods (e.g., tea,

coffee), medications (e.g., phosphate binders), and inadequate dietary intake related to uremia-induced anorexia, contribute to iron depletion. Iron supplementation (oral or intravenous) is usually required. Oral therapy is often the initial route of iron supplementation, but a lack of therapeutic response secondary to decreased gut absorption caused by the uremia of renal failure may warrant a change to intravenous iron therapy (Tenbrock et al, 1999). Transferrin saturation and ferritin levels should be monitored, along with RBC indices. Expected results include an increase in an individual's appetite and energy, as well as improvement in concentration ability and school performance (Van Damme-Lombaerts & Herman, 1999; Chan et al, 2002). Improvement in cognitive function has been reported in adults, but pediatric studies have not been consistently able to prove this (Warady et al, 1999). The present recommendation is toward earlier use of r-HuEPO in children with renal insufficiency before ESRD and significant anemia develop (Warady et al, 1999). Refer to the anemia section of the National Kidney Foundation's (NKF) Kidney Disease Outcome Quality Initiative (K/DOQI) Guidelines for further discussion (NKF, 2000).

Metabolic Control and Calcium Homeostasis. Control of calcium and phosphate balance prevents renal osteodystrophy and secondary hyperparathyroidism. Dietary phosphate restrictions significantly limit a child's intake of dairy products. Medications used include phosphate binders to remove excess phosphate from the blood, calcium supplements, and vitamin D replacement therapy with calcitriol (Rocaltrol) or dihydrotachysterol (DHT) to allow available calcium to be better used (Warady et al, 1999).

Managing Growth Retardation. Supplementation with sodium chloride improves growth (Wassner & Baum, 1999). Dietary manipulations to avoid exacerbation of uremic symptoms (e.g., protein restrictions) can further compromise growth. Unfortunately even with optimal renal care, children with renal disease continue to have issues with growth retardation and short stature (Wassner, 2001). Recombinant human growth hormone (rhGH) has significant potential for safely and effectively improving the stature of CRF children with growth retardation. On average, the use of rhGH can potentially provide the child with an additional 3 to 4 inches of height over 2 years (Chan et al, 2002).

Blood levels of growth hormone (GH) are normal to elevated in CRF secondary to uremia, but free levels of insulin-like growth factor-1 (IGF-1) are decreased (Wassner, 2001). IGF-1 acts at the growth plate of the long bones to stimulate growth. Impaired expression of IGF-1, growth hormone receptor mRNA inhibition, and an increased concentration of IGF-binding proteins, all thought to be secondary to uremia, contribute to growth retardation (Wassner, 2001; Chan et al, 2002). Before starting rhGH, optimal nutritional management and dialysis efficacy should be achieved, the PTH should be normal or reduced if very high, and the baseline parameters should be established for biochemical assays and hip radiographs.

Renal Replacement Therapy (RRT)

As GFR drops to 5% to 10% of normal, conservative management is no longer adequate and treatment with either dialysis or transplantation is required. As ESRD approaches, it is

---

BOX 38-3

Timing for Initiating Renal Replacement Therapy

RELATIVE INDICATORS
Age of child
GFR <10%
Primary renal disease and co-morbidity
Failure to thrive
Developmental delay
Inability to function at school
Inadequate electrolyte and metabolic control
Poor nutritional status

ABSOLUTE INDICATORS
Congestive heart failure
Uncontrollable hypertension, hyperkalemia, or acidosis
Pericarditis
Uremic encephalopathy
Uremic peripheral neuropathy

---

important to have ongoing discussions about the future and options for dialysis and transplantation with the child (if of suitable age) and parents. Educating the family about the different modalities of therapy, touring the pediatric dialysis center, and introducing the child and parent to one or more well-adjusted families on dialysis or experiencing a transplant are helpful ways to prepare children and families.

Indications for the timing of renal replacement therapy (RRT) are individualized, with consideration given to the following clinical and psychosocial factors: (1) GFR <10%, or creatinine clearance <10 ml/min/1.73 m^2; (2) inadequate control of blood pressure, fluid, electrolyte, and metabolic parameters despite aggressive medical management; (3) primary renal disease and effect of comorbid conditions; (4) child's age; (5) nutritional status; (6) failure to attain developmental milestones; and (7) fatigue and general weakness, causing a decline in school performance or an increase in school absenteeism (Warady et al, 1999; Mendley et al, 2001). Absolute indicators include uncontrollable hypertension, hyperkalemia, or acidosis; congestive heart failure; uremic encephalopathy and pericarditis; and peripheral neuropathy (Ahya & Coyne, 2001) (Box 38-3).

The many special needs of children help determine the modality of RRT selected. Because of the problems associated with small blood vessels for vascular access, hemodialysis (HD) in young children may not be practical. If a family is supportive and lives a long distance from the pediatric dialysis center, peritoneal dialysis may be preferred. Middle to older adolescents are more apt to be on HD. Transplantation is by far the preferred modality, however, because it offers a more normal lifestyle and greater potential for linear growth than either type of dialysis (Wassner, 2001). In 1998 the mean time (in days) to first transplant, cadaveric or living donor, was 510 and 302, respectively (USRDS, 2001). Children may have more live related kidney donors—especially parents—available to them, which may allow for preemptive transplant, forgoing the need for prolonged dialysis. Improved technology and more effective medications promote better survival (i.e., of both child and graft) with transplantation and offer both the child and family greater potential to live a less restricted life. There are positive and negative aspects for all treatment modalities. The child and family must understand that a kidney transplant is not a cure for CRF but is another treatment and can only be successful through carefully guided immunosuppression management with frequent clinical assessment (see Chapter 34).

The preference among pediatric nephrology practitioners is to initiate RRT early, before the development of severe malnutrition and symptoms of uremia occurs (Warady et al, 1999). Initiation of dialysis or transplantation is traumatic for the child and family, even with pre-ESRD counseling, but is worse if the child is very ill. Denial is a strong coping mechanism, however, and is supported when a child feels "well" despite a significantly elevated creatinine level.

Peritoneal Dialysis
Approximately 60% of children with ESRD are treated by peritoneal dialysis (PD), with 74% using automated PD (APD) (NAPRTCS, 2001) (Figure 38-2).

PD is the dialysis modality of choice in the pediatric population. PD uses the peritoneum as a filtering membrane to remove waste products and excess fluid from the vascular system. The surface area of the peritoneal membrane in children is relatively large in relation to their body surface area (BSA) compared with adults. Transport of solutes across the membrane is also more efficient in children than adults (Mendley et al, 2001). Access to the peritoneal membrane is through a catheter placed in the child's abdomen. There are two categories of peritoneal dialysis catheters, acute and chronic. Acute peritoneal catheters are fairly rigid and are either straight or slightly curved. They are made to be placed at the bedside. Acute catheters are used infrequently in pediatrics because any delays secondary to surgical concerns such as procedural or placement issues may place the child at risk by impeding the initiation of treatment in acute renal failure. Because the acute catheters are stiffer, there is an increased risk of bowel injury. To avoid this, the child must be immobilized while the catheter is in place, difficult with children. Another concern is the risk of peritonitis, which increases after only 3 days of use. For these reasons, chronic catheters are most frequently used.

Chronic peritoneal catheters are created with either silicone or polyurethane and have one or two Dacron cuffs, which elicit an inflammatory response in the tissue to form granulation tissue. This tissue secures the catheter into position and prevents bacterial migration into the peritoneum. Through the catheter, a sterile solution (dialysate) of electrolytes and glucose is instilled into the peritoneal space. Dialysate volume is calculated at 1,100 to 1,500 ml/m^2/cycle. Because the size of the peritoneal membrane correlates with the body surface area of the child, volume calculations should be based on BSA rather than weight and should take into consideration any residual renal function the child may have (Warady et al, 1999; Holloway, 2001). Waste particles are removed from the blood across the peritoneal membrane by diffusion, and excess water is removed by osmosis. Ultrafiltration is regulated by the amount of glucose in the dialysis solution in concentrations of 1.5%, 2.5%, and 4.25%. The amount of ultrafiltrate that can be removed is dependent on the glucose concentration of dialysis solution used and the transport characteristics of the peritoneal

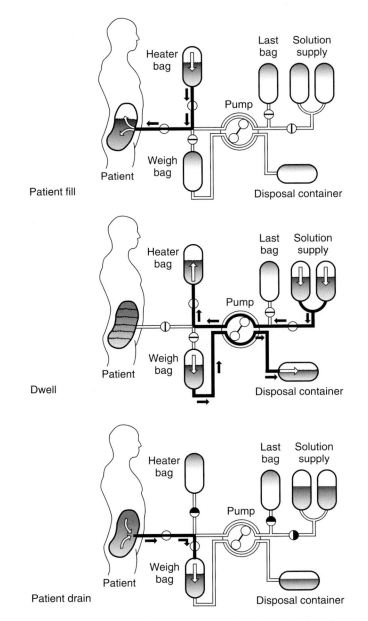

FIGURE 38-2 An example of a system used for cycler-assisted peritoneal dialysis. Solution is heated before use and weighed after use. The last bag of solution may have a different concentration to last throughout the day. (From National Institutes of Health, National Institute of Diabetes and Digestive and Kidney Diseases, and National Publication on No. 01-4688, April, 2001. Reprinted with permission.)

membrane, classified as high, high average, low average, or low. The amount and duration of cycles prescribed are individualized for each child according to their transport classification. In other words, a child who is a "high-transporter" would benefit from short, frequent cycles and a "low-transporter" from slower, fewer cycles with a last fill (fluid left in the abdomen for an entire day) or a midday exchange (an exchange done manually in the middle of the day) (Chadha & Warady, 2001). Higher transporters have faster diffusion of glucose and consequently are at increased risk for obesity, hyperlipidemia, and cardiovascular disease (Ahmad, 1999; Holloway, 2001).

Continuous ambulatory peritoneal dialysis (CAPD) delivers 4 or 5 dialysate bag exchanges daily into the peritoneum, with dwell times of 3 to 4 hours during the day and a long dwell overnight. CAPD affords greater freedom because no machine is required. Performing 4 or 5 exchanges during the day is time consuming, however, and inconvenient at work and school. Automated peritoneal dialysis (APD) uses a similar concept, but by using an automated cycler, all exchanges can be performed at night while the child and parents sleep, so the daytime is free of exchanges.

With both CAPD and APD, meticulous care is crucial to prevent contamination and infection at the catheter exit site and within the peritoneum. Clinical diagnosis of peritonitis, the most common complication of PD, is made by the presence of two or more of the following: signs and symptoms of peritoneal inflammation, such as abdominal or referred chest or back pain, nausea, vomiting, fever, and/or rebound tenderness; cloudy effluent with white blood cells (WBCs) >100/mm^3 and 50% neutrophils; and positive gram stain or positive culture of microorganism (Ahmad, 1999). Peritonitis episodes are highest in individuals up to 1 year of age and decrease in frequency with age. Most peritonitis is experienced by a few children who have repeated episodes (NAPRTCS, 2001). Data from NAPTRCS (2001) indicate that placement of double-cuffed catheters with a curved tunnel and downward exit site direction helps prevent peritonitis. The most common type of pediatric catheter in use is a single-cuffed Tenckhoff that is curled with a straight tunnel and a lateral exit site orientation. After placement, the catheter should be flushed periodically to maintain patency but not used for full-volume maintenance PD for 2 to 4 weeks, to allow healing and decrease the risk of complications such as leaking at the catheter site (Brandt & Brewer, 2001).

More than 50% of peritonitis is caused by *Staphylococcus aureus* or coagulase-negative staphylococci (Haffner, 2001). Though no formal studies have been done in children, eradication of nasal *S. aureus* carriage decreases peritonitis and exit site infections in adults (Mendely et al, 2001). In response to these data in adults, topical antibiotic treatment, applied intranasally and at the catheter exit site, of children and caregivers with nasal cultures positive for *S. aureus* is being performed in some pediatric centers.

Early use of intraperitoneal antibiotics for suspected peritonitis usually resolves the infection without catheter replacement. Most commonly used antibiotics are the cephalosporins and vancomycin. Though treatment courses vary from center to center, daily dosing of intraperitoneal antibiotics for 10 to 14 days, or until effluent is clear and cultures are negative, is common. Repeated or persistent peritonitis can result in catheter colonization and require the replacement of the catheter. Multiple episodes of infection can also lead to the loss of membrane permeability by scarring, often requiring a change to HD. Other clinical problems associated with PD include hernia development, bleeding or leaking, catheter exit-site or tunnel infection, catheter displacement, cuff extrusion, and catheter obstruction by fibrin or omentum (Ahmad, 1999; Brandt & Brewer, 2001).

PD has many advantages over hemodialysis (HD). Because PD is performed either continuously, as in CAPD, or over 8 to

10 hours every night with APD, better control of blood pressure and volume status can be maintained and there are fewer dietary restrictions, leading to better growth and development. Though caregivers must be taught how to technically perform dialysis, it is a relatively simple procedure. Vascular access required for HD can be difficult to achieve and maintain in young children. This is not of concern with PD (Mendely et al, 2001; Neu, 2001). Treating a child with home PD also offers educational and psychological advantages. Seventy-seven percent of children on PD attend school full time and 10% attend part time, compared with 51% and 28% of those children on hemodialysis (NAPRTCS, 2001). PD is a simple and safe procedure that can be carried out at home without the psychologic trauma associated with repeated fistula venipunctures. Perhaps the most attractive features of CAPD and APD are that they interfere less with normal daily activities and offer more control to the child and family. A child on peritoneal dialysis can attend school every day with little or no interruption, and family vacations are easier to arrange. There is, however, a downside.

A common reason for PD failure is family burnout from the repetitive daily regimen of PD. Providing respite care may provide a solution in some cases. Noncompliance, particularly in the adolescent population, is common. The presence of an external catheter can have an effect on body image. In children with excessive glucose absorption, obesity further complicates self-esteem issues. By preventing peritonitis and exit-site infections, promoting good nutrition, and assisting with the psychosocial aspects of chronic peritoneal dialysis, PD can be considered a potential long-term therapy (Holloway, 2001; Mendely et al, 2001).

Hemodialysis

Usually performed three or four times per week, HD has the advantage of more rapid correction of fluid, electrolyte, and metabolic abnormalities over PD. HD requires vascular access, dialyzer and blood lines, an HD delivery system with a blood pump and many monitoring devices, heparin to prevent clotting, pediatric nephrologists, and the specialized skills of nurses, social workers, and nutritionists. As the blood passes through the filtering membrane, waste particles diffuse across the membrane out of the blood while excess water is ultrafiltrated by negative pressure into the waste dialysate. The 3- to 5-hour process is constantly monitored for pressure changes, air detection or leaks, chemical imbalance, and temperature, in addition to the child's vital signs. Blood flow rates, medications, and fluid volumes are calculated based on the weight of the child (refer to the hemodialysis adequacy sections of the NKF's 2002 DOQI guidelines) (NKF, 2000). Complications associated with HD include hypotension, nausea and vomiting, headache, muscle cramps, flushing of face, increased pruritus, fever, chills, blood loss from frequent blood sampling or accidental clotting of the dialyzer system, chest pain, air embolism, pyrogenic or hemolytic reactions related to dialysate problems, dialysis disequilibrium syndrome, arrhythmia, hypoxemia, dialyzer membrane reaction, sepsis, and septic shock secondary to an access infection (Ahmad, 1999).

Maintaining a patent and infection-free vascular access is the greatest challenge of HD. Internal or external vascular access is necessary to deliver blood to the extracorporeal dialysis circuit for solute and fluid removal (Figures 34-3 and 34-4). Access is categorized in two types: permanent and temporary. Permanent access is created surgically and includes the arteriovenous (AV) fistula, AV graft, and dual-lumen catheters with Dacron cuffs. A maturation time of at least 2 weeks for a graft or 2 months for a fistula is required before the access can be used. Then the fistula or graft is accessed through a special fistula-needle cannulation (Ahmad, 1999). The catheter can be accessed immediately after placement. An internal fistula or graft is preferred for all children because it affords them less risk for complications and lower rates of access failure (Sharma et al, 1999). NAPRTCS data (2001) show 79% of children on HD receive their treatments through an external catheter, whereas only 12% are accessed through AV fistulas and 9% through AV grafts. Children 12 to 18 years of age were shown to have better dialysis adequacy using an AV fistula or graft when compared with a catheter (Health Care Financing Administration, 2001). Unfortunately many small children do not have the extremity blood flow to maintain a fistula or graft, and must have a central venous catheter placed (Haffner, 2001). Temporary access is accomplished through an indwelling central venous catheter that can be placed at the bedside and is used for emergent dialysis or in children who require dialysis for a short time, as in acute reversible renal failure (Ahmad, 1999). Failure of access, external or internal, is common secondary to infection, obstruction of the access device, fibrin sheath formation around an external catheter, thrombosis, vascular stenosis, or failure of the AV fistula to mature (Ahmad, 1999; Sharma et al, 1999; Brandt & Goldstein, 2001). Access sites are at a premium and must be preserved because these children will eventually require multiple vascular accesses. Potential problems warrant early assessment and intervention.

PD is technically easier to perform than HD in infants and small children. In many cases, however, PD may be medically contraindicated. Though morbidity and mortality are high, even very small infants can be successfully hemodialyzed, using central venous, umbilical, or femoral catheters for vascular access and specialized equipment and supplies adaptable to neonatal volume requirements. Infants and small children are hemodynamically more fragile. They respond more quickly to fluid depletion or excess and more commonly develop seizures as a consequence of the disequilibrium syndrome associated with dialysis procedures (Al-Hermi et al, 1999; Ellis, 2001; Mendely et al, 2001). All medications and fluid volumes in pediatric HD are calculated based on a child's weight and medical condition. Pediatric HD should be performed in a pediatric dialysis center. If distance to a pediatric dialysis center is a problem, adolescents may be dialyzed in adult centers but risk the lack of comprehensive assessment and therapies provided by a pediatric center. In such cases the pediatric primary care provider's role becomes more important in ensuring continuity of care for a child with ESRD. Very stable older children might be considered, on an individual basis, for home HD. HD takes time away from normal activities, such as school and play, and procedures and access care can be threatening to both the child and family. The child-life specialists, art, and music therapists employed to emotionally support and teach the child coping skills by instituting play, art, or musical therapy and social

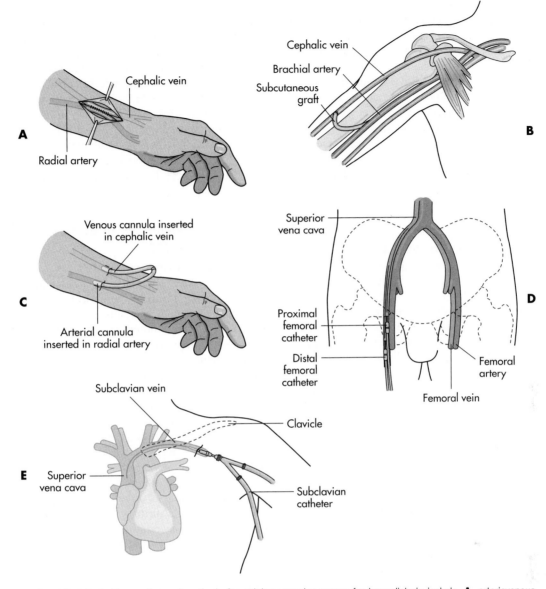

FIGURE 38-3 Frequently used methods for gaining vascular access for hemodialysis include, **A,** arteriovenous fistula; **B,** arteriovenous graft; **C,** external arteriovenous shunt; **D,** femoral vein catheterization; and **E,** subclavian vein catheterization. (From Phipps, W.J., Sands, J.K., & Mack, J.F. [1999]. *Medical-surgical nursing: concepts and clinical practice* [6th ed.]. St. Louis: Mosby. Reprinted with permission.)

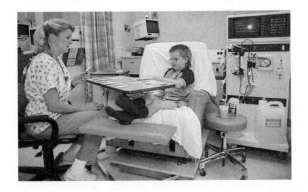

FIGURE 38-4 Child undergoing hemodialysis. (From Wong, D.L. et al. [1999]. *Whaley & Wong's nursing care of infants and children* [6th ed.]. St. Louis: Mosby. Reprinted with permission.)

workers for family counseling, both emotional and financial, are all important members of the treatment team.

Renal Transplantation

Renal transplantation is usually preferred for children with ESRD and, with careful planning, may be a primary therapy, bypassing the need for dialysis. Preemptive transplants account for 24% of primary transplants. Children as young as 3 months of age have been transplanted. Live related donor sources accounted for 52% of all pediatric transplants reported in the NAPRTCS group since 1995 (NAPRTCS, 2001). Because transplantation is the preferred option and donor kidneys are scarce, eligible donors include live immediate family members; live related donors outside the immediate family; as well as live unrelated donors. Ten confirmed transplants across ABO-compatible barriers have been done to date. This area of inquiry is worthy of further study as the early data suggest that graft outcomes are excellent in those recipients whose anti-A titer history is positive (NAPRTCS, 2001). Adult kidneys may be transplanted into small children with intraabdominal placement and parents make up the majority of live donors (83%) for pediatric recipients (NAPRTCS, 2001). The increasing use of laparoscopic nephrectomy can allow live donors to return to work and regular activities sooner and may increase overall use of live donors. Apart from surgical techniques, careful medical management is the key to maintaining a successful kidney transplant (see Chapter 34). With a successful renal transplant, children have a better chance of achieving desired growth and development, attending school regularly, and leading a more normal life.

Complementary and Alternative Therapies

The most common complementary therapy used in renal diseases is the use of fish oil (omega-3 fatty acids) for treatment of immunoglobin A (IgA) nephropathy. IgA nephropathy is one of the most common types of glomerulonephritis and can result in proteinuria, an elevated serum creatinine, and/or hypertension (Dillon, 2001). A 1994 study found that the use of fish oil reduced the risk of elevated creatinine by 82% and the risk of death or ESRD by 67% (Dillon, 2001). It is thought that the omega-3 fatty acids have an antiinflammatory effect. A study by Kutner (2002) showed that individuals on dialysis who reported fish intake were associated with higher survival rates. It has also been discovered that fish oil can prolong bleeding times, without the gastrointestinal side effects of aspirin, inhibit intimal hyperplasia in autogenous vein grafts, decrease turbulence in the bloodstream, and decrease shear stress within the endothelial cells. These effects introduced the thought that the use of fish oil may reduce the rate of graft thrombosis in individuals on hemodialysis (Schmitz, 2002).

Though no comprehensive studies have been completed, preliminary evidence suggests that a diet rich in phytoestrogens, such as soy protein and flaxseed, can slow the progression of renal disease (Velasquez, 2001). The mechanism of action is unknown, but the theory is that phytoestrogens may act as antioxidants, reduce proteinuria and hyperlipidemia, and stabilize the GFR (Velasquez, 2001).

Many herbs have been anecdotally documented to be beneficial to individuals with chronic renal failure. A case study by Bradley and colleagues (1999) discussed the hematopoietic effect of the Chinese herb Dang qui on an individual on hemodialysis that suffered from anemia refractory to treatment with recombinant human erythropoietin. An article from the *Journal of Traditional Chinese Medicine* (Wei et al, 1999) describes the use of the following: modified Renshen Yangrong Tang for anorexia and hypoproteinemia, Siwu Tang for cutaneous pruritus, and Guishao Sijunzi Tang for anemia.

Not all complementary therapies are considered beneficial, and are potentially harmful to individuals with chronic renal failure. Drug-herb interactions are abundant and usually unknown to the individual seeking alternative therapy. Garlic, ginger, ginseng, and gingko potentiate the anticoagulant effects of aspirin and warfarin. St. John's wort affects the metabolism of antidepressants, digoxin, and cyclosporin. Ephreda alone can lead to hypertension and seizures, but becomes even more dangerous when taken with caffeine, antidepressants, and decongestants (Mayo Clinic, 2002), particularly in individuals with preexisting hypertension. Cayenne can increase the absorption of ACE inhibitors, increasing the likelihood of developing a cough as a side effect and potentially causing hypotension (Mayo Clinic, 2002). Noni juice, made from the fruit of the noni tree has a concentration of potassium similar to that of orange and tomato juice and has been associated with hyperkalemia in individuals with chronic renal failure (Mueller et al, 2000). Much study is needed in this area to provide safe, alternative choices for the treatment of the effects of chronic renal failure.

Anticipated Advances in Diagnosis and Management

Early Detection and Referral

The primary care provider's early detection of potential renal problems and referral of the child to a pediatric nephrologist can often prevent irreversible renal damage. Early and close monitoring of vesicoureteral reflux, including periodic urine cultures, voiding cystourethrograms to monitor degree and any improvement of reflux, and renal scans to detect scarring, can sometimes prevent permanent damage. Renal deterioration and failure may be prevented with the use of antibiotic prophylaxis to prevent recurrent urinary tract infections. Surgical intervention is indicated in some children with severe reflux and recurrent urinary tract infections, despite antibiotic prophylaxis. The condition of posterior urethral valves, which occurs in 1 of 8,000 boys, may be detected by a prenatal sonogram. Percutaneous placement of a stent, while in utero, or open fetal surgery, can be performed in order to decrease fetal hydronephrosis and early postnatal urinary diversion until surgical correction of valves can be accomplished, although the outcomes of these procedures are understudied and are still considered experimental (Elder, 2000).

Significant technical advances in the treatment of infants and children with CRF have occurred over the past decade. More children are receiving dialysis or transplant for ESRD and surviving longer and living with a higher quality of life. This longevity and improved quality can be credited to some of the following developments: use of recombinant human erythropoietin and GH in children with CRF via subcutaneous, intravenous, and intraperitoneal routes; greater adherence to kinetic modeling calculations, biochemical parameters, and clinical responses to individually tailor the adequacy of dialysis and improve efficiency; early and aggressive correction of electrolyte and metabolic imbalances; and prevention of associated consequences of ESRD.

Because children are such a small percentage of the overall ESRD population, it is not cost effective for manufacturers to produce dialysis supplies geared to small children. Therefore pediatric supplies are very standardized and costly, and their continued availability is in jeopardy. Pediatric dialysis nurses must be creative and innovative to "rig" adult devices for use with children. Peritoneal dialysis innovations include various disconnect methods and design of smaller and simpler, computer-driven, suitcase-size portable PD cyclers that propose to

BOX 38-4
Associated Problems

Electrolyte abnormalities
Anemia
Hypertension
Cardiovascular disorders
Neurologic problems
   Aluminum toxicity
   Uremic neuropathy
   Encephalopathy
Calcium and/or phosphate disorders
   Renal osteodystrophy
Dermatologic manifestations
Gastrointestinal manifestations
Intercurrent illness

decrease risk for infection, promote easier PD exchanges, and improve quality of life. HD equipment now has computerization capabilities, allowing for individualization of treatment to be more refined. A greater dependence on computerization will guide the future of education, communication, data collection and analysis, and research.

The Internet has opened many doors for both professionals and lay individuals to access education, peer consulting, continuing education sites for licensure and certification updates, and discussion groups (see sources at end of chapter). Nutritional information and recipes can be downloaded, and dialysis and transplant medications can be researched. Electronic journals related to nephrology are available for professionals and interested individuals.

Many new medications to treat problems associated with CRF—especially immunosuppressive therapy for transplantation—are being tested, approved, and released for use. Improved immunosuppression may reduce selected side effects of current medications and prolong graft survival.

Associated Problems (Box 38-4)

Electrolyte Abnormalities

Electrolyte disturbances are probably the most common abnormalities found in renal failure. Hyperkalemia (i.e., potassium >5.5) is a frequent problem in CRF management, even after initiation of dialysis. Aggressive infant nutrition to improve brain growth and developmental potential may provide higher dietary potassium than desired. Infant formulas specifically designed for infants with renal failure can be treated with sodium polystyrene sulfonate (Kayexalate) prior to use. Kayexalate leaches the potassium from the formula and replaces it with sodium. Children often find it difficult to adhere to a low-potassium diet. In children on dialysis, overall electrolyte control can be better established by CAPD or APD because of the continuous steady state of dialysis clearance as opposed to the intermittent clearance of HD.

Anemia

The primary cause of anemia (hematocrit <30) in CRF is decreased red blood cell (RBC) production as a result of decreased production and release of erythropoietin. Other contributing factors include shorter RBC life span because of retained uremic toxins, microcytic anemia caused by aluminum toxicity, iron and folate deficiency, severe hyperparathyroidism, hemolysis, and blood loss associated with HD treatments and lab testing (Van Damme-Lobaerts & Herman, 1999). Treatment includes iron supplementation and administration of recombinant human erythropoietin. Goal of treatment is to maintain a hemoglobin of 11 to 12 g/dl (National Kidney Foundation, 2000).

Hypertension

Hypertension secondary to CRF accounts for approximately 5% of all hypertension, regardless of age group. In children, that number increases to two thirds. Hypertension becomes more common as renal failure progresses until nearly all children become hypertensive by the time they reach end stage (Galla & Luke, 2000).

Aside from treating the primary renal disease, proper control of hypertension is the most helpful task in slowing the progression of renal disease and reducing the risk of cardiovascular complications. Managing hypertension in children on dialysis includes nonpharmacologic interventions such as exercise, reducing obesity, smoking cessation, restricting fluid and dietary salt, and ultrafiltrating excess fluid from the child through dialysis. Antihypertensive medications are used when nonpharmacologic methods are unsuccessful (Norwood, 2002). ACE inhibitors help to slow the rate of renal tissue injury by minimizing glomerular hyperfiltration, though renal function must be monitored closely as ACE inhibitors can quickly reduce function in some children. Though a rare cause of renal failure in children, the development of diabetic nephropathy can be delayed by use of calcium channel blockers. Other classes of medications used include alpha- and beta-blockers, diuretics, and vasodilators (Fang, 2000).

Cardiovascular Disorders

Abnormal cardiac function associated with CRF can be attributed to hypertension, anemia, and uremia, and vascular calcifications. Congestive heart failure can occur as a result of fluid overload, severe hypertension, or uremic myocardiopathy. The presence of anemia and arteriovenous shunting (from the vascular access) can increase the cardiac workload and contribute to congestive heart failure. As with the general population, cardiovascular disease advances with age, but the risk for cardiovascular disease is significantly higher for individuals with ESRD than in the general population. Approximately 50% of deaths in individuals on dialysis can be attributed to cardiovascular disease (Block & Port, 2000). Heart murmurs are common in children with CRF as a result of anemia, hypertension, and volume overload. Electrocardiogram (ECG) abnormalities are associated with left ventricular hypertrophy and hyperkalemia. Uremic pericarditis is a less common manifestation, seen with long-standing severe renal failure. It is caused by pericardial irritation secondary to the metabolic imbalances seen in uremia. It can result in recurrent hypotension during hemodialysis (Bernstein, 2000). Treatment of uremic pericarditis includes daily dialysis with ultrafiltration and surgical drainage of the pericardium.

Neurologic Disorders

Neurologic manifestations are attributed to retention of uremic toxins. Multiple studies have noted neuropsychologic abnormalities in children with chronic renal failure. Such abnormalities include poor school performance, mental retardation, myoclonus, and seizures. Aluminum toxicity and malnutrition may be contributing factors in developmental delay (Warady et al, 1999). Initiation of chronic dialysis improves many neurologic symptoms of CRF.

Aluminum Toxicity. A syndrome of progressive neurologic deterioration in children with CRF has been linked to aluminum toxicity, which induces bone disease and anemia. Aluminum toxicity is indistinguishable from the dialysis dementia of adults and is characterized by regression of verbal and motor skills, speech disorders, seizures, myoclonic jerks, and dementia. Using calcium-based rather than aluminum-based phosphate binders to control hyperphosphatemia is safer and more effective and may reduce the incidence of aluminum poisoning. Children absorb larger amounts of aluminum from the gut than do adults; therefore, aluminum-based phosphate binders or antacids should not be used (D'Hease & DeBroe, 2001). Other agents possibly contributing to aluminum toxicity include total parenteral nutrition (TPN) and repeated administration of albumin. In addition to removing any aluminum-based medications from the child's regimen, deferoxamine (DFO) can be administered intravenously. DFO causes the release of tissue-bound aluminum in its dialyzable form into the bloodstream. DFO also increases the excretion of aluminum through the feces (D'Hease & DeBoe, 2001).

Uremic Neuropathy. Uremic neuropathy symmetrically affects the distal portions of the extremities and involves both motor and sensory function (Chan et al, 2002). Signs of neuropathy caused by uremia include muscle weakness and cramps; restless legs syndrome, a syndrome of persistent neurologic discomfort of the legs that is only relieved by movement; and alterations in distal sensorimotor function (Wolfson & Maenza, 2002). Uremic neuropathy may be improved with adequate dialysis and relieved by successful transplantation.

Encephalopathy. Encephalopathy may be seen in advanced renal failure. Children may exhibit early symptoms including headache, depression, fatigue, and listlessness. Hiccups, myoclonic twitching, memory loss, decreased attention span, drowsiness, impaired speech, and psychosis appear as deterioration in renal function progresses (Chan et al, 2002; Wolfson & Maenza, 2002). Rapid reduction of urea from blood through highly efficient HD may cause cerebral edema, which results in the syndrome of dialysis disequilibrium. When a very high BUN level is present, the rate of urea clearance must be reduced until control of BUN is obtained. Mannitol can be given through the dialysis circuit to minimize the osmotic changes and this syndrome from occurring (Ellis, 2001).

Calcium and/or Phosphorus Disorders and Renal Osteodystrophy

Growth retardation and renal osteodystrophy are significant problems for children with ESRD. Loss of renal function has a profound effect on calcium and phosphorus homeostasis and thus on bone integrity (Sanchex et al, 1999). Bones contain 99% of the body's total calcium. Dietary phosphorus restriction in children with renal problems is difficult because it curtails intake of dairy products and meat. It is especially difficult to provide adequate nutrition to infants with CRF because of this restriction. Phosphorus restriction and use of calcium-based phosphorus binders, however, help to keep the serum concentration of phosphorus within the normal range in an attempt to prevent or curtail the development of renal osteodystrophy and secondary hyperparathyroidism (Stapleton, 2001).

Renal osteodystrophy occurs in approximately 20% of children and adolescents in ESRD (Salusky & Goodman, 2001) and is a significant complication in growing children because of their open epiphyses and rapid bone mineralization. Renal osteodystrophy varies along a continuum from low turnover bone lesions, or osteomalacia, to high turnover bone lesions, or osteitis fibrosa, secondary to hyperparathyroidism (Sanchez et al, 1999). High turnover is the most common bone lesion in renal failure that can lead to actual reduction in bone mass or osteoporosis (Sanchez et al, 1999). These children do not usually complain of bone pain but often restrict their physical activity to protect a painful extremity and may develop subtle gait abnormalities. Clinical manifestations include valgus deformities, fractures, rickets, myopathy, growth retardation, bone pain, extra skeletal calcifications in soft tissues and organs, and—in severe bone disease—epiphyseal slipping of the femoral head and metaphyseal fractures (Chan et al, 2002). Development of renal osteodystrophy can be lessened by early and aggressive calcium and vitamin D therapy with dihydrotachysterol (DHT), 25-hydroxy vitamin D, calcitriol or vitamin D_3, 1,25-dihydroxy vitamin D (Rocaltrol), as well as adequate metabolic control by diet, medication, and adequate dialysis (Warady et al, 1999). A relatively new drug, paricalcitol injection (Zemplar), has been approved for use in adults and older children to reduce the PTH level and renal osteodystrophy (Llach & Yudd, 2001). Paricalcitol has been shown to control PTH levels but results in less hypercalcemia and hyperphosphatemia than calcitriol (Sprague et al, 2001). However, its injection form has limited paricalcitol's use to those children on hemodialysis where intravenous access is readily available.

Dermatologic Manifestations

Retention of uremic toxins, which are deposited in skin and soft tissue, may contribute to dry, scaly, itchy skin that is characterized by broken skin and scratch marks. Pallor and sallow complexion can be improved by anemia control. As a child progresses toward ESRD, calcium and phosphorus imbalances can lead to metastatic calcifications of the skin (Robinson-Bostom & DiGiovanna, 2000). In fact some researchers have identified a phenomenon called *renal itch*, a localized or generalized itch that is not associated with severe uremia levels (Murphy, 2000). This etiology of this itch remains unclear.

Gastrointestinal Manifestations

Uremic symptoms of anorexia, nausea, vomiting, stomatitis, and halitosis improve with adequacy of dialysis and control of anemia. Many children gain weight after starting dialysis, and most who are well dialyzed and have normal hemoglobin and hematocrit levels have a good appetite and high energy level.

Intercurrent Illness

The development of intercurrent illnesses in children with CRF must be thoroughly assessed and appropriately managed to prevent further complications and promote optimal health. Infection, especially of the vascular access and peritoneum, is a frequent and common complication. Heart failure, pericarditis, pulmonary edema, and gastrointestinal disease may occur with uremia. Children on immunosuppressive therapy, whether it is because they have received a renal transplant or have conditions such as lupus or nephrotic syndrome, are much more susceptible to infections (Simon & Levin, 2001).

Prognosis

Although medical reasons often dictate the preferred treatment modality, infants and children can be treated by either PD or HD. With recent technical advances, small children can be more safely and effectively treated with HD conducted at pediatric dialysis centers. The use of newer medications may delay the onset of CRF in some diseases and more effectively treat problems children may encounter during HD and PD.

Children in all age groups are more likely to receive a transplant than to be treated with dialysis (USRDS, 2001). Of children younger than 17 years of age, 85% to 90% have a functioning transplant graft after 2 years of receiving their transplanted kidney (USRDS, 2001). Advances in medical technology have resulted in the development of better antirejection management for renal transplant recipients with fewer adverse reactions or side effects. If a transplant is rejected, children must return to either PD or HD while waiting for another transplant. Unfortunately many children develop high percentages of reactive antibodies to a large potential donor pool. Therefore the wait for a second or third transplant may be long.

Recent advances in equipment, expendable supplies technology, and medications have improved the potential quality of life for children on HD, PD, or those who have received a transplant, allowing them to pursue a more normal lifestyle. The self-esteem of children affects their quality of life and prognosis of morbidity and mortality. Many factors may contribute to poor self-esteem in children with ESRD. Every effort should be made to provide interventions that enhance the self-esteem of children of all ages.

From 1994 to 1996 the mortality rate among children (up to 9 years of age) with ESRD was considerably lower than that among the 20- to 44-year age group. Children on dialysis had a death rate nine times higher than those with transplants, which is partly explained by the fact that the dialysis group included children waiting for transplants and those too ill to receive one. Cardiac problems and infections remain some of the leading causes of death among children with ESRD (USRDS, 2001). Early recognition and aggressive treatment should help reduce morbidity and mortality in children with CRF.

PRIMARY CARE MANAGEMENT

Health Care Maintenance
Growth and Development
Incorporating developmental and behavioral assessments into primary health care evaluations can result in significant advances in early identification and intervention. Children with renal disease may not have any clinical signs besides retarded growth. Many children exhibit growth retardation at the time of referral to a pediatric nephrologist, but inadequate growth remains a problem for many individuals, including those undergoing dialysis. With aggressive nutritional supplementation, infants have achieved better but suboptimal growth (Tom et al, 1999). Besides infancy, the next greatest physical growth stage is during puberty. Children with CRF often have delayed linear growth and development of secondary sexual characteristics. Decreased estrogen and testosterone levels may occur.

Accurate growth measurements should be taken at the initial visit and at least every 3 to 6 months thereafter and plotted on appropriate growth charts. Following head circumference growth every 3 to 6 months on all children younger than 3 years of age assesses neurologic potential. The weight-height index provides a measure of a child's weight relative to height, with a low index suggesting malnutrition, and should be performed at each visit. At the onset of puberty, staging using the Tanner scale (Kasiske et al, 2000) should be determined every 6 to 12 months for school-aged children until adult staging is reached.

Developmental assessment should be done with the onset of CRF and repeated at 2- to 9-month intervals, depending on a child's age and disease severity. Although the timing may be delayed, children with CRF have the same developmental needs as healthy children and must progress through the same developmental stages. To best help a child attain developmental milestones, the level of development attained must be assessed. Assessment tools (see Chapter 2) are useful in obtaining objective data. The effect of the disease process on the child's psychologic status, school attendance, intellectual performance, and social development should be assessed every 6 to 9 months.

Adolescence can be a time of turbulence that is associated with transition, maturational crises, and adjustment (Holmbeck, 2002). Table 38-1 highlights some of the differences, problems, and interventions related to cognitive, physical, and psychosocial development in adolescents with ESRD.

Diet
Although protein restriction may delay progression of CRF, it is not acceptable in children. In addition to growth and developmental delay in children, poor nutrition—especially with low serum albumin levels—is associated with increased morbidity and mortality (Meireles, 1999). Nutritional problems are manifested long before ESRD is reached and continue after RRT is initiated. It has been known for many years that many children with renal failure suffer malnutrition ranging from the very mild to the severe (Warady et al, 1999).

Children on PD experience a feeling of fullness soon after eating small amounts because of abdominal distention from the volume of peritoneal fluid, which may be more apparent with CAPD and daytime dwells than with nightly APD. In addition, with PD there are obligatory protein losses through the peritoneum because the pore size is easily permeable to albumin transfer (National Kidney Foundation, 2000). Children on PD have increased protein requirements (i.e., 2.3 to 3 g/kg in infants, 1.7 to 2 g/kg in toddlers and children, and approximately 1.5 g/kg in adolescents) (National Kidney Foundation, 2000).

Energy requirements are based on the recommended dietary allowance for children with increased physical activity and

TABLE 38-1

Characteristics of Adolescents with ESRD by Developmental Domain

Expected Difference from Normal Development	Manifestations or Potential Problems	Prevention and Interventions
COGNITIVE ASPECTS: Should move from concrete to abstract thinking at 12 to 15 years of age. May have excessive school absences for medical reasons and slower or accelerated learning, which must be individualized. Academic achievement is less affected with later CRF onset. RF affects acquisition of new skills, attention, and speed of processing data.	Advanced education requires greater ability to abstract, which is reflected in competency or scholastic testing and academic scores. Concrete thinkers lack ability to apply general principles from one event to another. Academic delay may result in school disinterest and dropout. Hearing and/or vision problems may be CRF related More difficulty in learning new skills. Attention and responses aided by good biochemical control and worsened by nonadherence.	Concrete thinkers need care plan that realizes immediate goals; abstract thinkers can work with long-range goals. Incorporate results from academic and/or neuropsychomotor skills testing to guide improvement. Encourage school attendance and participation in extracurricular activities. Encourage adherence to care plan. Encourage opportunities for responsible decision making, problem solving, and development of own beliefs and values. Help prepare for transition into adulthood.
PHYSICAL ASPECTS: Linear growth retardation is affected by treatment modality and steroids. Decreased effect and/or production of growth and sex hormones. Delayed puberty onset (refer to Tanner staging, 1962): Girls—10.5 to 14 years of age, with menarche onset at about 13 years. Boys—12 to 16.5 years. Delay in development of secondary sexual characteristics and sexually active behavior. Nutritional needs vary with age: Protein—0.8–1 g/kg needed; Calories—38 to 60 cal/kg needed. Phosphorus restricted. Anemia present.	Short stature (i.e., 1–3 SD below norm). Does not follow height-weight curve pattern of puberty. Compares size to peers. Girls—delay in breast enlargement, pubic hair, menarche onset (hallmark of womanhood) Boys—delay in testes and/or scrotal growth, pubic hair, penile size and ability to erect and ejaculate, muscle mass increase, voice change to deeper pitch May be under or overweight. May rebel at ESRD treatment regimen through dietary indiscretions, especially in peer groups. May be nonadherent with medications, especially those causing visible side effects. May develop ROD with rickets or fractures; hypocalcification by bone radiographs. Fatigue or SOB from anemia.	Early diagnosis and RRT. Child and family education about normal growth and/or development and expected alterations. Encourage diet and medication adherence, physical activities and exercise, and physical independence. Consider use of growth hormone; teach self-administration. Encourage self-participation in care plan. Provide sexuality education at individual level of understanding. Encourage optimal nutrition to promote best growth potential. Encourage dietary adherence; work with dietitian to include as many favorite foods as possible. Consider meal pattern of school lunches, fast-food stops with peers. Focus on positive—not negative—nutrition. Encourage taking phosphate binders. Consider early use (preRRT) of epoetin alfa; teach self-administration; monitor.
PSYCHOSOCIAL ASPECTS: Interruption or inability in mastery of adolescent developmental tasks; dependency vs. independency conflict; identity quest; body image dissatisfaction; peer group identity desired; future planning Self-esteem influenced by actual and perceived image and peer response. Risk for lower self-esteem greater with negative body image, poor peer and family relationships, strong family dependence Delayed psychosexual development	Coping behaviors used include denial, regression, projection, displacement, anger, acting out, increased risk taking, being disruptive, resentment, being argumentative, challenging authority. Vacillates between child-compliant and rebel-noncompliant. May sublimate poor academic performance with physical prowess. Fears peer rejection, loneliness, depression, and withdrawal despite strong need for friends and social support. May avoid sexual relationships and activity or experiment to prove sexual worth	Promote achievement of developmental tasks; foster independence and autonomy. Allow controlled choices. Encourage activities that enhance positive self-esteem and self-worth. Encourage healthy group activities in community, school, church, camps, support groups. Evaluate self-concept through assessment tools. Encourage ventilation of feelings of sexuality and provide education for understanding. Assist in preparation for transition into adulthood.

From Taylor, J.H. (1994). Enhancing development in the adolescent with ESRD. Presentation at ANNA symposium, Dallas, Adapted with permission.

range from 98 to 108 kcal/kg in infants to 40 to 50 kcal/kg in adolescents (National Kidney Foundation, 2000). Glucose absorption from the dialysate in both HD and PD provides calories, occasionally resulting in obesity. Anemia control via r-HuEPO injections results in increased appetite and energy level and eventual weight gain. This helps reduce the incidence of malnutrition in children with CRF. Intradialytic parenteral nutrition (IDPN) is provided in some dialysis centers, but reimbursement problems present obstacles to this approach. Lipids increase caloric content significantly but must be monitored closely by lab tests because children on dialysis tend to have higher lipid levels (Harmon, et al, 1999).

Parents of infants and small children soon become frustrated with unsuccessful efforts to get children to eat the recommended calories and protein. Children with renal failure are often poor eaters. Supplemental tube feedings by orogastric, nasogastric, or gastrostomy tube or button may be instituted early in renal insufficiency as an important and useful therapy to ensure better nutritional intake with less stress to the family (National Kidney Foundation, 2000). Unpalatable additives of corn or safflower oil and Polycose can easily be instilled by tube along with medications as needed to supplement a child's oral feedings. The formula calculation for supplemental feedings should be determined with the help of a nutritionist familiar with the special needs of children with renal failure. The current recommendation is to aggressively treat infants with caloric and protein intake above the recommended daily allowance (RDA) to help improve physical and cognitive growth.

Dietary restrictions change with ESRD modality. In HD, potassium and phosphorus generally govern the dietary prescription. There is greater dietary freedom with PD, and protein may be increased. The posttransplant diet also has restrictions of no added salt, low fat, and low cholesterol to prevent hypertension and obesity. Because eating is a social custom in our society and not just for sustenance, pizza may be the favorite food of a child with CRF, making dietary restrictions difficult. Phosphorus restriction limits dairy products, and most children are expected to drink milk. Fluid restriction depends on a child's urinary output volume and is calculated by intake volume allowed being equal to output plus 500 to 600 ml (insensible loss). The primary care provider should obtain the dietary management plan from the nephrology team to reinforce family education.

Safety

Although children with CRF should be encouraged to pursue normal childhood activities, some considerations and limitations must be kept in mind. Delay in cognitive and gross motor development may result in these children being academically and physically slower than classmates, as well as smaller in size. Attempting to keep up with larger and faster children in active play may result in injury to a child with CRF. Children with CRF may become the brunt of jokes and unkind comments. In response to a challenge, these children may retaliate and attempt to accomplish something of which they are not capable, possibly injuring themselves in the process.

Some children require special occupational and physical therapy programs to enhance their physical ability and improve skills and stamina. Bike helmets and kneepads can be used to help prevent easy bruising. Children should be encouraged to wear a Medic-Alert bracelet or necklace to notify other health care providers of their CRF status, medication needs, and other possible complications.

Children on immunosuppressive therapy are more at risk for infections and heal more slowly. Children with an HD internal vascular access (i.e., AV fistula or graft) must be cautioned against allowing blood pressure measurement or venipuncture in their affected arm, wearing restrictive clothing or accessories that can lead to venostasis and clotting, and engaging in activities that may cause bleeding soon after dialysis while they are still heparinized. Children with indwelling central venous catheters should not be allowed to swim to prevent serious infection through the catheter (Berkoben & Schwab, 1995). Swimming with PD catheters is controversial and may require special catheter and exit site care procedures.

Renal osteodystrophy may predispose children to fractures or cause bone pain on exertion. Physical activity, however, should be encouraged to promote physical and mental health. Group aerobic exercise programs, camping, group games at picnics, and other fun outings are excellent ways to promote controlled exercise, encourage independence, and help raise self-esteem.

Immunizations

Routine immunizations should be given to children with CRF except for a few specific disease conditions and therapies. Immunosuppressive therapy is used not only with transplantation but also to treat some renal conditions, including glomerulonephritis, nephrotic syndrome, and lupus nephritis. Immunosuppression is generally an indication for withholding live virus immunizations, including the measles-mumps-rubella (MMR) and varicella vaccine (Committee on Infectious Diseases, 2001). Immunizations should be withheld until a child is in remission and off therapy for 6 months; exceptions are determined by weighing the risks versus the benefits on an individual basis for children who are steroid resistant or have frequent relapses. Inactivated polio vaccine (IPV) is preferred for immunosuppressed children (Committee on Infectious Diseases, 2000). Disease-specific immunoglobulins may be given after known exposure. Because varicella-zoster reactions can be severe in children with a transplant (5% to 25% mortality rate with a high potential for graft loss), children without positive antibody titer should be immunized before transplant or immunosuppressive therapy if possible. Seroconversion, although not as effective as in healthy children, in children with renal failure is still relatively high and therefore vaccination is recommended (Webb, 2000). Children should continue to receive varicella-zoster immune globulin (VZIG) after exposure to minimize adverse occurrences (Committee on Infectious Diseases, 2001).

Pneumococcal and influenza vaccines are recommended for children with CRF and active nephrotic syndrome because of their increased susceptibility to infections (Committee on Infectious Diseases, 2001; Pesanti, 2001).

Even though r-HuEPO has decreased the need for blood transfusions in children with ESRD, hepatitis B is still a risk. If a child is negative for hepatitis B antigen, the hepatitis vaccine series should be started as soon as possible so it can be completed before possible transplant. Because the antibody response to the hepatitis B vaccine may be diminished with CRF, these children may require repeated doses until seroconversion is achieved (Pesanti, 2001). Hepatitis B and C viral screening are also recommended in individuals on dialysis or awaiting transplantation (Tokars et al, 2001). As part of the transplant evaluation process, extensive immunologic screening is performed to determine exposure to a variety of infectious diseases including HIV.

Screening

Vision. A yearly eye examination by a pediatric ophthalmologist is recommended. Eyes should be examined for scleral calcification caused by hypercalcemia or uncontrolled hyperphosphatemia. The fundus should be examined for arterial narrowing, hemorrhages, exudates, and papilledema secondary to hypertension. Cataract assessment should be included for any child having been treated with steroid therapy.

Hearing. An annual assessment by an audiologist is recommended. High-frequency sensorineural deafness is characteristic of Alport syndrome (Kashtan, 1999). Hearing loss can also result from use of ototoxic drugs (e.g., furosemide and gentamicin).

Dental. Routine dental care (every 6 months) is recommended for children with CRF. Dental procedures may cause breaks in the skin and mucous membranes with bleeding and release of microorganisms into the bloodstream, causing infective endocarditis or colonization of the vascular access

(Durack & Phil, 1995). A pediatric nephrologist should be consulted to prescribe prophylactic antibiotic coverage prior to dental procedures for children who are immunosuppressed or have a vascular access. (See Chapter 17 for prophylaxis protocols.)

Children with congenital renal disease often have enamel defects. Poor nutritional intake may lead to poor mineralization of teeth. In an effort to improve nutrition, small children with CRF may be allowed to use a bottle for a longer time, resulting in deformities of the primary teeth. Use of oral iron for anemia may stain teeth; liquid preparations should be placed in the mouth past the teeth.

Drug-induced gingival hyperplasia may occur in children with CRF receiving drugs such as phenytoin (Dilantin) for seizures, calcium channel blockers (e.g., nifedipine [Procardia] or verapamil [Calan]) for hypertension, and cyclosporine (Neoral) for immunosuppression in transplant, lupus, and nephrotic syndrome treatment. Good dental and oral hygiene with mechanical stimulation by daily brushing and flossing, gingival massaging, and plaque control is recommended. Gingivectomy treatment by surgical excision or laser may be needed periodically (Cohen & Galbraith, 2001).

Blood Pressure. Blood pressure measurements should be taken at each visit and at periodic intervals, depending on a child's clinical condition. Initiation and follow-up of anti-hypertensive therapy should be done in consultation with the pediatric nephrologist. The "white coat phenomenon" (i.e., blood pressure being higher in clinics) is reduced by use of automated monitoring devices (Sorof & Portman, 2000a). Small, computerized blood pressure monitors are available to be worn for 24 to 48 hours and can give better insight to the true daily overall blood pressure at rest and during activity and facilitate more ideal medical management (Sorof & Portman, 2000b).

Hematocrit. Routine screening may be deferred if a recent complete blood cell count (CBC) is included with the other renal function tests. Anemia is a chronic problem that is usually followed by the nephrology team.

Urinalysis. Routine screening is not necessary because of the frequent urinalysis done by the renal team. Some children with CRF have little to no urine output, so urinalysis is not indicated.

Tuberculosis. Yearly screening with PPD testing is recommended.

Condition-Specific Screening

Blood Work. The nephrology team regularly monitors the CBC, serum ferritin, iron, transferrin, folate, and reticulocyte counts to assess the anemia management. Serum electrolyte, blood urea nitrogen (BUN), creatinine, calcium, phosphorus, alkaline phosphatase, protein, albumin, cholesterol, and liver function tests help monitor renal function and treatment efficacy. Metabolic acidosis must be promptly identified and treated to prevent bone demineralization and growth retardation. Parathyroid hormone (PTH) levels should be monitored every 3 to 6 months and correlated with radiologic findings for prevention and/or management of renal osteodystrophy. Fasting blood levels are best for monitoring cholesterol and triglycerides, which is difficult in small children or infants. Viral titers for Varicella zoster virus (VZV), cytomegalovirus (CMV), herpes simplex virus (HSV), Epstein Barr virus (EBV), hepati-

tis profile (i.e., hepatitis A, hepatitis C, and hepatitis B viruses, antibody to HBV), rubella, rubeola, and human immunodeficieny virus (HIV) should initially be monitored as a baseline, then before transplant and periodically as determined by the pediatric nephrologist.

Cardiac Screening. A chest radiograph and baseline electrocardiogram and echocardiogram should initially be performed and then again at 6- to 12-month intervals to assess the cardiovascular status of children with CRF.

Radiologic Screening. Radiologic bone studies can show evidence of secondary hyperparathyroidism, rickets or osteomalacia, osteosclerosis, and delayed bone age as distinct patterns in children with renal osteodystrophy (Sanchex et al, 1999). Examination of the hands and knees should initially be obtained and then again at 6-month intervals to assess for improvement or worsening of renal osteodystrophy and compare bone age with chronologic age to determine growth potential. Bone density studies and bone biopsies are helpful but less commonly used methods of assessing bone mineralization in children.

Common Illness Management

Differential Diagnosis

Infections. Because of a compromised immune system, children with CRF may be at greater risk for routine infections and their sequelae. Primary care providers should evaluate and manage routine pediatric problems (e.g., influenza, urinary tract or gastrointestinal infections, and fever), consulting the pediatric nephrologist about a child's hydration status and residual renal function, as well as antibiotic selection and dosage related to a child's renal disease and residual function. Temporary alterations in a child's dialysis program may be necessary during illness. If other common benign causes of fever have been ruled out, fever related to a dialysis access infection or peritonitis should be managed directly by the pediatric nephrologist.

Gastrointestinal Symptoms. Nausea and vomiting are common symptoms in childhood. Decreasing renal function must be ruled out in children with mild renal failure, especially in the absence of associated fever.

Headaches. Uncontrolled hypertension should be ruled out in children with CRF complaining of frequent headaches.

Drug Interactions

The most important factors to consider in pharmacokinetics are the extent to which the drug is excreted by the kidney, the degree of renal impairment, and the drug's interactions with various other medications needed in the ESRD treatment regimen.

In general if the GFR is greater than 50 ml/minute, drug dosage regimens do not need to be altered (Wassner, 2001). The initial loading dosage of drugs (especially antibiotics) excreted by the kidney, however, is usually the same as it is for children without renal failure. Maintenance dosages must be adjusted by either lengthening the interval between doses or reducing individual doses (Suzuki, 2000). CRF may predispose children to bleeding and easy bruising; therefore, acetaminophen is preferred over aspirin for pain and fever control.

Anticonvulsants may require dosage adjustments and often interfere with trough drug levels in transplant immunosuppression. Children with anemia and CRF receiving a calcium (not aluminum)-based phosphate binder given with food or within 30 minutes after eating should wait at least 1 hour before taking oral iron because the two medications are antagonistic to each other, compromising the desired effect (Lacy et al, 1999). All pediatric medication calculations should be based on the weight—not the age—of a child with CRF. Medications that are removed by dialysis (i.e., vitamins, some antihypertensive medications, and aminoglycoside antibiotics) should be given after dialysis (i.e., at night with CAPD or in the morning with APD). The pediatric nephrologist should be consulted for appropriate medication selection and dosage adjustment.

Children with CRF may have up to 40 pills to take daily, which requires much determination and perseverance for them as well as their parents. Transplant medications can total up to six or seven different medications (and comprise 30 to 40 pills) and are critical to the life of the transplant; even one missed dose can cause a rejection episode. Avenues to promote therapeutic adherence must be explored with the child and family (Ringewald et al, 2001). (Refer to Developmentally Based Teaching Strategies, in Vol. 23, No.6 of *Pediatric Nursing* [November-December 1997] for an excellent reference table for teaching medications.)

Developmental Issues

Sleep Patterns

Infants and young children should be encouraged to assume a normal sleep pattern at night. Most children can sleep undisturbed with nocturnal APD treatment. An increased need for sleep and lethargy or depression may indicate increasing renal failure and should be reported to the pediatric nephrology team. Restlessness, insomnia, or cramps may indicate the need for more dialysis time or physical activity to promote rest.

Toileting

Children with CRF may be oliguric, anuric, or have normal urine output, determined largely by the cause of the renal disorder. Some congenital abnormalities require bladder augmentation or creation of a type of urinary diversion with an appliance worn over the stoma (Garvin, 1994). The adolescent with a urinary stoma and appliance may have difficulty emotionally accepting the diversional system and participating in peer activities. Families and children need instruction in care of the stoma and supportive care as indicated.

Even after corrective urologic surgery, some children may be unable to achieve urinary continence. Toilet training for urinary continence is often deferred until after transplant if a child is capable of urinary continence (DeKernion & Trapasso, 1996). Female children and their parents should be taught to wipe properly to prevent urinary tract infections. Bowel training should be initiated when a toddler is developmentally ready.

Discipline

Parental anxiety, guilt, and despondency over their child's chronic condition may lead to ambivalent feelings toward child rearing or the treatment program, resulting in child behavior problems or nonadherence to the treatment regimen. Parental overprotection of a child with CRF may further reinforce a lack of discipline. Parents need honest answers to questions about their child, as well as encouragement and support in setting and holding limits and behavioral expectations for their child. Children with CRF need the same behavior control and discipline set for their siblings and other healthy children (Gilman & Frauman, 1998).

Children on HD can have difficulty accepting the painful procedure of venipuncture required for each treatment. For pain associated with procedures, management techniques (e.g., play therapy, guided imagery, hypnosis, and progressive muscle relaxation) can be taught to children and their parents. Topical anesthetics (e.g., EMLA cream [Astra Pharmaceutical Company]) are commonly used in many pediatric dialysis centers. Play therapy helps children work through these difficult situations and lets parents or other caregivers know their unexpressed thoughts. A firm but loving disciplinary approach helps to make a positive difference in a child's life (Richardson, 1997).

Children should be encouraged to participate in their care by performing achievable tasks and making decisions. Cooperation can be gained by allowing even 3-year-olds to help select the venipuncture site, remove the tourniquet, rotate the blood tubes, and help place the tape. Singing and other diverting activities also elicit cooperation. Many children on HD self-cannulate their needles or set up their own dialysis machines for treatment. These children can compete with one another in the dialysis center to complete tasks independently and exercise self-control. Children on APD can learn to do their own exchanges and care for their exit site. Children may also be taught to subcutaneously self-administer their r-HuEPO or GH (Gilman & Frauman, 1998).

Child Care

Children with CRF are not restricted from daycare. Because children receiving corticosteroid therapy are more susceptible to infections, home care or small group child care is recommended. Daycare and preschool settings provide stimulation for learning and sharing with other children and may be a positive situation, especially if classes are small. When child care is used, the caregiver must be taught about the child's dietary restrictions, medications, and any special treatment regimen. Specific instructions should be given in writing, with a phone contact in case of questions. The nephrology team should encourage children on CAPD and their parents to arrange the dialysis schedule around the child care hours whenever possible. If a child has a vascular or peritoneal dialysis access, those entrusted as caregivers must be given instructions on potential emergencies and actions to be taken.

Schooling

School-age children must be encouraged to attend school full time. CAPD exchanges should be scheduled around school activities with the least interference possible, or else nocturnal APD might be preferable for school-age children. Changes in schedules to accommodate after-school activities can be discussed with the pediatric nephrology team. Pediatric HD centers should include a schoolteacher or tutor to help children with missed schoolwork. A dual school-home educational program may be established with both teachers communicating with each other for continuity of the child's learning. Children with renal disease may need a note to be allowed extra trips to the bathroom because of a small bladder capacity or infection, to perform intermittent catheterization, to drink more or fewer fluids, or receive assistance with ureterostomy or central venous catheter care. Some children need to be assigned to a school with a nurse in attendance daily, which does not mean that the child needs to be in special education classes. The pediatric nephrology team may need to provide educational materials on specific CRF management and inservice presentations on a child's physical or emotional needs to school personnel, in addition to participating in a child's Individualized Educational Program (IEP) conference. Parents need to be informed about laws protecting their child's education rights (Vessey, 1997) (see Chapter 5).

Poor school performance must be evaluated for contributing factors, including family disharmony. Cognitive deficits have been correlated with more advanced CRF and congenital etiologies (Warady et al, 1999).

Sexuality

Delayed sexual development is common among children with CRF as a result of insufficient production of gonadal steroid and elevated gonadotropin levels (Shaefer & Mehls, 1999). More than half of female adolescents with ESRD have delayed development of secondary sex characteristics and menarche. Although menstrual abnormalities (e.g., amenorrhea, oligomenorrhea, and menorrhagia) and infertility have been described, successful pregnancies in women who were on dialysis have been reported (Owens & Honebrink, 1999). Adolescent males with ESRD may show delayed development of genitalia, pubic hair, and testicular size and decreased sperm counts. Erectile dysfunction (ED) is common among males on dialysis, but it is unknown with what frequency it actually occurs in this population (Rosas et al, 2001). Impotence usually improves after transplant. Males have been able to achieve erection through testosterone supplementation, use of penile injections (Caveject), suppositories (Muse), sildenafil (Viagra), or penile prosthesis (Rosas, et al, 2001). A successful transplant usually returns hormonal function and fertility capability to normal. These are important issues in adolescent sexuality and preparation for adulthood, as well as for families of small children concerned about the ability of their child to have a normal life.

Adolescents with CRF must be counseled about birth control, sexually transmitted diseases, and acquired immunodeficiency syndrome (AIDS). The aspects of physical and emotional intimacy that are tied to sexual relationships are also important issues to be discussed with these adolescents.

Transition to Adulthood

Children with CRF eventually become adults with CRF. The road to independence and career development begins before a child reaches adulthood. Consequences of childhood noncompliance with phosphate binders is evidenced by renal osteodystrophy in adult life. Individuals with short stature from growth retardation or bone disease may require assistive devices to drive. Hypertension, diabetes, and impaired vision may result in other long-term health problems. Individuals must be encouraged to eat a healthy diet and avoid drug, alcohol, and tobacco abuse. One model that has been suggested for helping adolescents with chronic illnesses transition into the adult health care system is in which the primary pediatric care provider acts as the care coordinator who actually facilitates this slow change over time (Biggs, 2000). In addition, care plans that emphasize self-care can help teens through this stage. Most of all, a successful transition is achieved through a positive mental attitude of overcoming adverse situations into successful lives. The American Association of Kidney Patients (AAKP) can supply dozens of adult role models (see list of resources at end of chapter).

Family Concerns and Resources

The effect of CRF on a child is felt by the child's entire family. Parents may have to deal with the following: (1) feelings of shock and disbelief, (2) anger, (3) loss, (4) guilt at causing renal failure, (5) depression, (6) fatigue and burnout associated with constant care and appointments, (7) inadequacy at not being able to heal or fix the problem, (8) frustration with the medical establishment for no cure, (9) overprotection versus being too lenient, (10) marital stress, and (11) financial worries. Frequent trips to the dialysis center or clinic, daily or nightly PD treatments, and additional physical care interfere with family schedules, school, extracurricular activities, and outings.

Family coping and adaptation are improved through maintaining open communication, active participation in care planning and decision making, and the presence of supportive extended family, friends, church members, or renal-focused support or advocacy groups (Travis et al, 1984). Providing networking sessions is often helpful; new children and families should be grouped with a client who has adjusted well to the dialysis or transplant routine and is willing to share information (Gilman & Frauman, 1998). Families should be encouraged to continue normal activities (e.g., family outings, camps for children, and vacations) with previously arranged transient dialysis scheduling at a pediatric dialysis center if necessary.

A family's belief system must be taken into account. Religious practices may prohibit blood transfusions, even in life-threatening situations, or challenge that healing by faith alone is all that is needed. With children who are Jehovah's Witnesses, it may be advisable to start r-HuEPO administration early (before renal failure reaches end stage), use micro blood tubes for lab tests whenever possible, and use cell-saver reinfusion during surgery. An understanding of the family's background, religious and cultural beliefs and practices, dietary beliefs associated with health care, and identification of the "primary leader" of the family (e.g., a great-grandmother) is valuable to health care professionals when effective interventions require altering a child or family's health care practices (Richie et al, 1995).

Some renal diseases are linked to race and ethnicity. Overall statistics show increased morbidity and mortality in blacks with

ESRD and renal transplants, especially in the early posttransplant period (USRDS, 2001). Some black and Hispanic children wait longer on dialysis for an acceptable transplant match because of ABO compatibility and major histocompatibility complex matching difficulties. The possibility of a better match is secured with a member of the same race for both live related and cadaveric transplantation.

Families need support as they make decisions about their child's care that will have long-range implications. Even the smallest, very ill infant might be treated with life-sustaining dialysis—but at a high cost. Extracorporeal membrane oxygenation (ECMO) with integrated hemofiltration is more widely performed today with positive results. Equipment, supplies, and professional expertise are more costly for infants with ESRD. Many of these infants have other congenital anomalies; morbidity and mortality are high in this early period. Children with mental retardation are being dialyzed and transplanted. Quality of life issues and the rights of parents versus rights of minor children are being discussed with no black-and-white answers (Levine, 2001). Some infants will not become productive members of society, but others have demonstrated adequate growth and development with early and aggressive RRT and are attending regular school full time and living fairly normal lives. Children with severe developmental or mental delays require considerable comprehensive and long-term care. Repeated noncompliance of some adolescents to prescribed therapy may result in loss of the transplanted kidney. All of these issues have a significant effect on the families. In addition, families must deal with members of medical and legislative committees who would argue that many children should not receive all ESRD services because of cost containment. Technologic advances in dialysis and transplant have improved the quality of life and increased life expectancy for thousands with ESRD while pacing the resources. For every kidney donor that becomes available, there are four or five individuals waiting. Tighter selection criteria may appear for transplantation. Research continues with porcine xenotransplantation as the logical resource. Both of these options carry strong ethical consideration (Cummings, 1997).

The cost of ESRD treatment is very expensive, ranging from $20,000 to $35,000 or higher per individual per year. On July 1, 1973, the Social Security Act was amended to provide Medicare benefits for people younger than 65 years of age who were certified to have chronic kidney failure and require dialysis or transplantation (HR-1, Public Law 92-603, section 2001). The total of all ESRD costs paid by Medicare in 1996 was $10.96 billion for 225,000 individuals with ESRD, compared with $6.03 billion in 1992 (Evans & Kitzman, 1998). Total ESRD costs are much higher because Medicare is considered as secondary payor for the first 30 months of RRT for individuals with private insurance. Because the payment process becomes quite complicated, families should be referred to the nephrology social worker for assistance in accessing available services. Additional financial assistance information is available through the National Kidney Foundation affiliates, the American Kidney Fund, and the American Association of Kidney Patients.

RESOURCES

American Nephrology Nurses Association (ANNA)
East Holly Drive, Box 56
Pitman, NJ 08071-0056
(856) 256-2320
(888) 600-2662
anna@mail.ajj.com; http://anna.inurse.com

American Association of Kidney Patients (AAKP)
3505 E. Frontage Road, Suite 315
Tampa, FL 33607
(800) 749-AAKP
info@aakp.org; www.aakp.org

National Kidney Foundation (NKF)
30 East 33rd Street
New York, NY 10016
(800) 622-9010
info@kidney.org; www.kidney.org
Contact the local chapter for educational assistance, summer camps, support groups, and financial information.

American Kidney Fund (AKF)
6110 Executive Boulevard, Suite 1010
Rockville, MD 20852
(800) 638-8299
helpline@akfinc.org; www.akfinc.org

Free educational materials are available.

HCFA ESRD Networks

Divided into geographic regions, these networks are assigned to coordinate and review dialysis and transplant facilities to ensure the best possible care for individuals. Call the AAKP or NKF for the location of the network for your state.

Renal Physicians Association (RPA)
4701 Randolph Road, Suite 102
Rockville, MD 20852
(301) 468-3515
www.renalmd.org

Other Online Resources

Medical Matrix—Pay for service directory of patient education documents on the Internet:
www.medmatrix.org

United Network of Organ Sharing (UNOS)
www.unos.org

RENALNET—Comprehensive renal-related site, the Kidney Information Clearinghouse:
www.renalnet.org

TransWeb—A site for transplant and organ donation information:
www.transweb.org

United States Renal Data System (USRDS)
www.usrds.org

Summary of Primary Care Needs for the Child with Chronic Renal Failure

HEALTH CARE MAINTENANCE

Growth and Development

Despite advances in medical management, dialysis, and transplant, growth retardation is a major problem in children with CRF (most are at least two SDs below the mean height for their age).

Accurate growth measurements should be taken at initial visit and every 3 to 6 months.

Achievement of developmental milestones (all ages) is delayed; sexual maturation is delayed.

Developmental assessment and Tanner staging should be monitored.

Adolescent characteristics differ between early, middle, and late adolescence; areas of growth, cognition, identity, sexuality, emotionality, family, and peer relationships across the age span should be assessed.

Ventilation of emotions; physical activity for emotional health, independence, and support groups should be encouraged.

Aggressive nutrition, adequate dialysis efficiency, and growth hormone injections may improve growth.

Diet

Protein and caloric needs in children with CRF are greater than the normal RDA to enhance growth and development and offset losses (protein in PD). Glucose is absorbed in PD.

Supplemental oral, nasogastric (NG), or gastrostomy-tube feedings should be considered to improve nutrition.

Dietary restrictions differ with change in ESRD modality.

Safety

Children with CRF should be encouraged to live as normal and active lives as possible, with modifications as necessary. Occupational and physical therapy may improve skills and stamina.

Medic-Alert bracelets are recommended

Immunosuppression and renal osteodystrophy increase risk of infection and fracture.

Immunizations

Routine immunizations are recommended. Live virus vaccines are prohibited in the immunosuppressed child.

Influenza, pneumococcal, varicella, and hepatitis vaccines are recommended. Immunoglobulin is given after known exposure to virus (i.e., hepatitis, varicella-zoster)

Screening

Vision. Routine annual exams by a pediatric ophthalmologist are recommended to assess for calcification, arterial hemorrhages, and cataracts (if child is on steroid therapy), as well as vision testing.

Hearing. Routine annual exams are recommended; hearing should be monitored when a child is using ototoxic drugs.

Dental. Routine dental care at 6-month intervals; child with vascular access or immunosuppression is at risk for endocarditis and needs prophylactic antibiotic coverage for dental procedures.

Gingival hyperplasia, enamel defects, and poor mineralization should be monitored.

Blood Pressure. Blood pressure should be taken at all medical visits; frequency of measurement depends on BP value. Correctly sized cuff should be used.

Antihypertensive therapy should be managed by the pediatric nephrologist. Goal is normal BP.

Hematocrit. Anemia is a chronic problem. CBC is monitored by the pediatric nephrology team.

Urinalysis. Routine screening is done by pediatric nephrology team if indicated.

Tuberculosis. Yearly screening by mantoux purified protein derivative testing is done.

Condition-Specific Screening

Bloodwork. CBC and RBC indices and folate studies, electrolytes, BUN, creatinine, calcium, phosphorus, alkaline phosphatase, albumin, ferritin, PTH, and iron are monitored regularly. Cholesterol, triglycerides, and viral titers periodically.

Cardiac Screening. Monitor chest x-ray, ECG, and echocardiogram every 6 to 12 months.

Radiologic Screening. Monitor bone radiographs for skeletal growth and renal osteodystrophy.

COMMON ILLNESS MANAGEMENT

Differential Diagnosis

Routine pediatric care should be provided by a pediatric provider in collaboration with the pediatric nephrologist.

Fever should always be assessed for etiology; fever related to a vascular access or PD catheter infection or peritonitis should be managed by the pediatric nephrologist. Gastrointestinal (GI) symptoms should be assessed for decreasing renal function.

Headaches should be assessed for hypertension; blood pressure (BP) should be controlled to normal.

Drug Interactions

For all medications in CRF management, the route of excretion, degree of renal impairment, and interaction with other medications in CRF management should be known.

Dosage of all medications should be calculated by weight—not age—of the child.

Renal-excreted drugs may require dosage adjustment.

Calcium-based—not aluminum-based—phosphate binders should be used.

Acetaminophen rather than aspirin should be used for pain or fever.

Absolute medication compliance is key to a successful kidney transplant; many graft losses are because of noncompliance, especially in adolescents.

Medication teaching should be related to child's developmental level.

DEVELOPMENTAL ISSUES

Sleep Patterns

Increased fatigue and need for sleep may indicate decreasing renal failure.

Summary of Primary Care Needs for the Child with Chronic Renal Failure—cont'd

Restlessness, insomnia, or cramps may indicate need for increased dialysis time or more physical activity.

Toileting

Children with CRF may have normal urine output, oliguria, or anuria. Urinary diversion may present greater difficulty for adolescent.

Not all children can achieve urinary continence.

Bowel training should begin when a child is developmentally ready.

Proper wiping direction should be taught to female children and their parents.

Discipline

Parents' own emotions may interfere with discipline of the child, (e.g., overprotective or too lenient without discipline).

Parents need honest answers and encouragement.

Nonadherence with plan of care is source of conflict.

Children with CRF should learn self-discipline and begin taking responsibility for self-care as possible.

Child Care

The child care provider must be taught about diet, medications, special treatment regimen, and emergency measures.

The dialysis schedule should be arranged around child care hours.

Children may be exposed to more infections in daycare.

School

School attendance, when possible, should be encouraged or an alternative (home bound, tutor, teacher in dialysis) provided.

Teachers should be instructed about child's care plan and needs.

Children may need additional school-based services to perform catheterizations, take medication, or deal with fatigue.

An IEP should be established

Poor school performance should be evaluated for physical versus psychologic factors contributing to cause.

Sexuality

Delayed sexual development is common.

Erectile dysfunction is common in males but may resolve with transplantation

Counseling on birth control, STDs, human immunodeficiency virus (HIV) exposure should be provided.

Responsibility toward transition to adulthood should be promoted.

Transition to Adulthood

CRF makes independence difficult.

Hypertension, diabetes, and impaired vision result in long-term health problems.

Positive mental attitude is important.

FAMILY CONCERNS

CRF affects entire family; the goal is to strengthen the total family unit.

Networking with the other families of children with CRF should be provided.

Religious, ethnic, cultural, and racial factors affect adjustment to CRF and care.

Ethical issues are closely related to economics and highly controversial.

Health care team should practice patient advocacy.

Cost containment has an effect on care.

REFERENCES

Ahmad, S. (1999). Manual of clinical dialysis. London: Science Press.

Ahya, S.N. & Coyne, D.W. (2001). Renal diseases. In S.N. Ahya, K. Flood., & S. Prarnjothi. (Eds.), The Washington manual of medical therapeutics (30th ed., pp. 262-263), Philadelphia: Lippincott Williams & Wilkins.

Al-Hermi, B.E., Al-Saran, K, Secker, D., & Geary, D.F. (1999). Hemodialysis for end-stage renal disease in children weighing less than 10 kg. Pediatr Nephrol, 13, 401-403.

Bergstein, J.M. (2000). Potassium. In R. Behrman, R. Kliegman, & H. Jenson (Eds.) Nelson textbook of pediatrics (16th ed., p.197). Philadelphia: W.B. Saunders.

Berkoben, M. & Schwab, S.N. (1995). Maintenance of permanent hemodialysis vascular access patency. ANNA J, 22(1),17-24.

Bernstein, D. (2000). Diseases of the pericardium. In R. Behrman, R. Kliegman, & H. Jenson (Eds.), Nelson textbook of pediatrics. (16th ed., p. 1438). Philadelphia: W.B. Saunders.

Biggs, W.S. (2000). The family physician's challenge: Guiding the adolescent with chronic disease to adulthood. Clinics in Family Practice, 2(4), 823-836.

Block, G.A. & Port, F.K. (2000). Re-evaluation of risks associated with hyperphosphatemia and hyperparathyroidism in dialysis patients: Recommendations for a change in management. Am J Kidney Dis, 35(6), 1226-1237.

Bradley, R.R., Cunniff, P.J., Pereira, B.J., & Jaber, B.L. (1999). Hematopoietic effect of Radix angelicae sinesis in a hemodialysis patient. Am J Kidney Dis, 34(2), 349-354.

Brandt, M.L. & Goldstein, S. (2001). Vascular access in children. In A.R. Nissenson, & R.N. Fine (Eds.), Dialysis therapy (3rd ed.). Philadelphia: Hanley & Belfus.

Brandt, M.L. & Brewer, E.D. (2001). Peritoneal catheter placement in children. In A.R. Nissenson, & R.N. Fine (Eds.), Dialysis therapy (3rd ed.). Philadelphia: Hanley & Belfus.

Chadha, V. & Warady, B.A. (2001). Adequacy of peritoneal dialysis in pediatric patients. In A.R. Nissenson, & R.N. Fine (Eds.), Dialysis therapy (3rd ed.). Philadelphia: Hanley & Belfus.

Chan, J.C.M., Williams, D.M., & Roth, K.S. (2002). Kidney failure in children. Pediatr Rev, 23(2), 47-60.

Cohen, D. & Galbraith, C. (2001). General health management and long-term care of the renal transplant recipient. Am J Kidney Dis, 38(6), S10-24.

Committee on Infectious Diseases. (2001). Report of the Committee on Infectious Diseases (24th ed.), Elk Grove Village, IL: The American Academy of Pediatrics.

Cummings, N.B. (1997). Ethical and legal considerations in end-stage renal disease. In R.W. Schrier, & C.W. Gottschalk (Eds.), Diseases of the kidney, vol. III (6th ed.). Boston: Little Brown.

Devarajan, P. & Spitzer, A. (2002). Towards a biological characterization of focal segmental glomerulosclerosis. Am J Kidney Dis, 39(3), 626-636.

Davis, I.D., MacRae Dell, K., Sweeney, W.E., & Avner, E.D. (2001). Can progression of autosomal dominant or autosomal recessive polycystic kidney disease be prevented? *Semin Nephrol, 21*(5), 430-440.

DeKernion, J.B. & Trapasso, J.G. (1996). Urinary diversion and continent reservoir. In J.Y. Gillenwater, S.S. Howards, J.T. Grayhack, & J.W. Duckett (Eds.), *Adult and pediatric urology* (3rd ed.). St Louis: Mosby.

D'Hease, P.C., & DeBroe. M.E. (2001). Aluminum toxicity. In J.T. Daugirdas, P.G. Blake, & T.S. Ing (Eds.), *Handbook of dialysis*. Philadelphia: Lippincott Williams & Wilkins.

Dillon, J.J. (2001). Treating IgA nephropathy. *J Am Soc Nephrol, 12*(4), 846-847.

Durack, D.T. & Phil, D. (1995). Prevention of infective endocarditis. *N Engl J Med, 332*, 37-44.

Elder, J.S. (2000). Obstructions of the urinary tract. In R. Behrman, R. Kliegman, H. Jenson (Eds.), *Nelson textbook of pediatrics* (16th ed., p. 1636). Philadelphia: W.B. Saunders.

Ellis, E.N. (2001). Infant hemodialysis. In A.R. Nissenson, & R.N. Fine (Eds.), *Dialysis therapy* (3rd ed.). Philadelphia: Hanley & Belfus.

Evans, R.W. & Kitzman, D.J. (1998). An economic analysis of kidney transplantation, *Surgical Clinics of North America, 78*(1), 149-172.

Fang, L.S. (2000). Management of the patient with chronic renal failure. In A.H. Goroll, & A.G. Mulley (Eds.), *Primary care medicine: Office evaluation and management of the adult patient* (4th ed., p. 809). Philadelphia: Lippincott Williams & Wilkins.

Frishberg, Y., Toledano, H., Becker-Cohen, R., Feigin, E., & Halle, D. (2000). Genetic polymorphism in paraoxonase is a risk factor for childhood focal segmental glomerulosclerosis. *Am J Kidney Dis, 36*(6), 1253-1261.

Galla, J.H. & Luke, R.G. (2000). Hypertension in renal parenchymal disease. In B.M. Brenner & S.A. Levine (Eds.), *Brenner & Rector's: the kidney* (6th ed., pp. 2037, 2041). Philadelphia: W.B. Saunders.

Garvin, G. (1994). Caring for children with ostomies. *Nurs Clin North Am, 29*(4), 645-654.

Gilman, C. & Frauman, A.C. (1998). The pediatric patient. In J. Parker (Ed.), *Contemporary nephrology nursing ANNA*. Pitman, NJ: AJ Jannetti, Inc.

Goodman, W.G., et al. (2000). Coronary artery calcification in young adults with end-stage renal disease who are undergoing dialysis. *N Engl J Med, 342*, 1478-1483.

Haffner, J.C. (2001). The technology-dependent child. *Pediatr Clin North Am, 48*, 751-764.

Harmon, W.E., Jabs, K.L. & Alexander, S.R. (1999). Pediatric dialysis. In W.F. Owen, B.J.G. Pereira, & M.H. Sayegh (Eds.), *Dialysis and transplantation: A companion to Brenner's & Rector's the kidney* (pp. 319-336). Philadelphia: W.B. Saunders.

Health Care Financing Administration. (2001). A study of pediatric (≥ 12 < 18 years old) in-center hemodialysis patients: Results from the 2000 end stage renal disease clinical performance measures project. Supplemental report #1, 2000 ESRD clinical performance measure project. Washington, DC: HCFA.

Holloway, M.S. (2001). Peritoneal dialysis orders in children. In A.R. Nissenson & R.N. Fine (Eds.), *Dialysis therapy* (3rd ed.). Philadelphia: Hanley & Belfus.

Holmbeck, G.N. (2002). A developmental perspective on adolescent health and illness: An introduction to the special issues. *J Pediatr Psychol, 27*(5), 409-416.

Ito, S., et al. (2001). Clinical and laboratory observations: Isolated diffuse mesangial sclerosis and Wilms tumor suppressor gene. *J Pediatr, 138*(3), 425-427.

Kashtan, C.E. (1999). Alport syndrome. An inherited disorder of renal, ocular, and cochlear basement membranes. *Medicine, 78*(5), 338-350.

Kasiske, B.L., et al. (2000). Recommendations for the outpatient surveillance of renal transplant recipients. *J Am Soc Nephrol, 11* (S 15), 1-86.

Kutner, N.G. (2002). Association of fish intake and survival in a cohort of incident dialysis patients. *Am J Kidney Dis, 39*,1018-1024.

Lacy, C.F., Armstrong, L.L., Ingrim, N.B., & Lance, L.L. (1999). *Drug information handbook*. Hudson, OH: Lexi-Comp Inc.

Levine, D.Z. (2001). Discontinuing immunosuppression in a child with a renal transplant: Are there limits to withdrawing life support? *Am J Kidney Dis, 38*(4), 901-915.

Llach, F. & Yudd, M. (2001). Paricalcitol in dialysis patients with calcitriol-resistant secondary hyperparathyroidism. *Am J Kidney Dis, 38*(5), 545-550.

Mayo Foundation for Medical Eduaction and Research. (2002). Herb and drug interactions [online]. Available: www.mayoclinic.com.

McDonald, R.A., Watkins, S.L., & Avner, E.D. (1999). Polycystic kidney disease. In Barratt, T.M., Avner, E.D., & Harmon, W.E. (Eds.), *Pediatric Nephrology* (pp. 459-474). Baltimore: Lippincott Williams & Wilkins.

Meireles, C.L. (1999). Nutrition and chronic renal failure in rats: What is an optimal dietary protein? *J Am Soc Nephrol, 10*(11), 2367-2373.

Mendley, S.R., Fine, R.N., & Tejani, A. (2001). Dialysis in infants and children. In J.T. Daugirdas, P.G. Blake, & T.S. Ing, *Handbook of dialysis* (3rd ed.). Philadelphia: Lippincott Williams & Wilkins.

Mueller, B.A., Scott, M.K., Sowinski, K.M., & Prag, K.A. (2000). Noni juice *(Morinda citrifolina):* Hidden potential for hyperkalemia? *Am J Kidney Dis, 35*, 310-312.

Murphy, M. (2000). Renal itch. *Clinical experimental dermatology, 25*(2), 103-106.

National Kidney Foundation. (2000). Dialysis outcome quality initiative (DOQI) guidelines [online]. Available: www.kidney.org/professional/doqi/index.cfm.

Neu, A.M. (2001). Infant and neonatal peritoneal dialysis. In A.R. Nissenson, & R.N. Fine (Eds.), *Dialysis therapy* (3rd ed.). Philadelphia: Hanley & Belfus.

Neville, H.L. & Ritchey, M.L. (2000). Wilms' tumor: Overview of national Wilms' tumor study group results. *Urology Clinics of North America, 27*(3), 435-442.

North American Pediatric Renal Transplant Cooperative Study (NAPRTCS). (2001). *2001 annual report*. Rockville, MD: The Emmes Corp.

Norwood, V.F. (2002). Hypertension. *Pediatr Rev, 23*(6), 197-209.

Owens, K. & Honebrink, A. (1999). Gynecologic care of medically complicated adolescents. *Pediatr Clin North Am, 46*(3), 631-642.

Pesanti, E.L. (2001). Immunologic defects and vaccination in patients with chronic renal failure. *Infect Dis Clin North Am, 15*(3), 813-832.

Richardson, D.C. (1997). Discipline and children and chronic illness: strategies to promote positive patient outcomes. *ANNA J, 24*(1), 35-40.

Richie M.F., Mapes D., & Dailey F.D. (1995). Psychosocial aspects of renal failure and its treatment. In L.E. Lancaster (Ed.), *Core curriculum for nephrology nursing* (3rd ed.). Pitman, NJ: AJ Jannetti.

Ringewald, J.M., Gidding, S.S., Crawford, S.E., Backer, C.L., Mavroudis, C. & Pahl, E. (2001). Nonadherence is associated with late rejection in pediatric heart transplant recipients. *J Pediatr, 139*(1), 75-78.

Robinson-Bostom, L. & DiGiovanna, J. J. (2000). Cutaneous manifestations of end-stage renal disease. *J Am Acad Dermatol, 43*(6), 975-986.

Rosas, S.E., Wasserstein, A.L., Kobrin, S., & Feldman, H.I. (2001). Preliminary observations of sildenafil treatment for erectile dysfunction in dialysis patients. *Am J Kidney Dis, 37*(1), 134-137.

Salusky, I.B. & Goodman, W.B. (2001). Adynamic renal osteodystrophy: Is there a problem? *J Am Soc Nephrol, 12*, 1978-1985.

Sanchex, C.P., Goodman, W.G., & Salusky, I. B. (1999). Osteodystophy. In T.M. Barrett, E.D. Avner, & W.E. Harmon (Eds.), *Pediatr Nephrol* (pp. 1231-1239). Baltimore: Lippincott Williams & Wilkins.

Schaefer, F. & Mehls, O. (1999). Endocrine and growth disturbances. In T. Barratt, E. Avner, W. Harmon (Eds.), *Pediatric Nephrology* (pp. 1197-1230). Baltimore: Lippincott Williams & Wilkins.

Schmitz, P.G. (2002). Prophylaxis of hemodialysis graft thrombosis with fish oil: Double-blind, randomized, prospective trial. *J Am Soc Nephrol, 13*, 184-190.

Sharma, A., Zillereulo, G. Abitbol, C., Montane, B., & Strauss, J. (1999). Survival and complications of cuffed catheters in children on chronic hemodialysis. *Pediatr Nephrol, 13*, 245-248.

Simon, D.M. & Levin, S. (2001). Infectious complications of solid organ transplantion. *Infect Dis Clin North Am, 15*(2), 521-549.

Sorof, J.M. & Portman, R.J. (2000). Ambulatory blood pressure monitoring in the pediatric patient. *J Pediatr, 136*(5), 578-586.

Sorof, J.M. & Portman, R.J. (2000). White coat hypertension in children with elevated casual blood pressure. *J Pediatr, 137*(4), 493-497.

Sprague, S.M., Lerma, E., McCormmick, D., Abraham, M., & Battle, D. (2001). Suppression of parathyroid hormone secretion in hemodialysis patients: Comparison of paricalcitol with calcitriol. *Am J Kidney Dis, 38*(5), 551-556.

Stapleton, F.B. (2001). Advances in pediatric nephrology: The serenity to accept the things we cannot change versus the courage to try. *J Pediatr, 138*(4), 606-607.

*The data here have been supplied by the United States Renal Data System (USRDS). The interpretation and reporting of these data are the responsibility of the author(s) and in no way should be seen as an official policy or interpretation of the US government.

Suzuki, M.M. (2000). Drugs in renal failure. In G.K. Siberry & R. Iannone (Eds.), *The Harriet Lane handbook: A manual for the pediatric house officers* (15th ed.). St. Louis: Mosby

Tenbrock, K., Müller-Berghaus, J., Michalk, D., & Querfeld, U. (1999). Intravenous iron treatment of renal anemia in children on hemodialysis. *Pediatr Nephrol, 13,* 580-582.

Tokars, J.I., Arduino, M.J., & Alter, M.J. (2001). Infection control in hemodialysis units. *Infect Dis Clin North Am, 15*(3), 797-812.

Tom, A., et al. (1999). Growth during maintenance hemodialysis: impact of enhanced nutrition and clearance. *J Pediatr, 134*(4), 464-471.

United States Renal Data System. (2001). *USRDS 2001 annual data report: Atlas of end-stage renal disease in the United States,* The National Institutes of Health, National Institute of Diabetes and Digestive and Kidney Diseases, Bethesda, MD [online]. Available: www.med.umich.edu.usrds/chapters/html.

Van Damme-Lombaerts, R. & Herman, J. (1999). Erythropoietin treatment in children with renal failure. *Pediatr Nephrol, 13,* 148-152.

Velasquez, M.T. (2001). Dietary phytoestrogens: A possible role in renal disease protection. *Am J Kidney Dis, 37,* 1056-1068.

Vessey J.A. (1997). School services for children with chronic conditions. *Pediatr Nurs, 23*(5), 507-510.

Vimalachandra, D, et al. (2001). Growth hormone treatment in children with chronic renal failure: A meta-analysis of randomized controlled trials. *J Pediatr, 139,* 560-567.

Warady, B.A., Alexander, S.R., Watkins, S., Kohaut, E., & Harmon, W.E. (1999). Optimal care of the pediatric end-stage renal disease patient on dialysis. *Am J Kidney Dis, 33,* 567-583.

Wassner, S. J. (2001). Growth in children with ESRD. In A.R. Nissenson & R.N. Fine (Eds.), *Dialysis therapy* (3rd ed.). Philadelphia: Hanley & Belfus.

Wassner, S.J. & Baum, M. (1999). Physiology and management. In T. Barratt, E. Avner, & W. Harmon (Eds.), *Pediatric Nephrology* (4th ed.). Baltimore: Lippincott Williams & Wilkins.

Watkins, S.L., McDonald, R.A., & Avner, E.D. (1999). Renal dysplasia, hypoplasia, and miscellaneous cystic disorders. In T.M. Barratt, E.D. Avner, & W.E. Harmon (Eds.), *Pediatric Nephrology* (pp. 415-425). Baltimore: Lippincott Williams & Wilkins.

Webb, N. J. (2000). Immunization against varicella in end stage and pre-end stage renal failure. *Arch Dis Child, 82*(2), 141-143.

Wei, L., Chen, B., Ye, R., & Li, H. (1999). Treatment of complications due to peritoneal dialysis for chronic renal failure with traditional Chinese medicine. *J Tradit Chin Med, 19* (1), 3-9.

Wolfson, A.B. & Maenza, R.L. (2002). Renal failure. In J.S. Marx, R. Hockberger, & R.M. Walls (Eds.), *Rosen's emergency medicine: Concepts and clinical practice* (5th ed., pp.1374-1387). St. Louis: Mosby.

39 Sickle Cell Disease

Barbara A. Carroll and Elizabeth O. Record

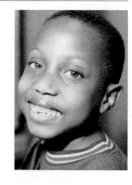

Etiology

Sickle cell disease (SCD) is a term used to describe several inherited, sickling hemoglobinopathy syndromes, including sickle-β-thalassemia (Hb Sβ° thal or Hb Sβ+ thal), sickle-C disease (Hb SC), and—most commonly—sickle cell anemia (Hb SS). Adult hemoglobin contains two pairs of polypeptide chains, alpha (α) and beta (β). Each of these hemoglobinopathy syndromes involves the mutated sickle hemoglobin (Hb S), which differs from normal hemoglobin (Hb A) by the substitution of a single amino acid, valine, for glutamic acid at the sixth position of the β-globin chain.

Red blood cells (RBCs) that contain normal hemoglobin are pliable, biconcave disks with a life span of approximately 120 days. When deoxygenated, RBCs containing predominantly Hb S polymerize and form microtubules (i.e., rods) that distort the shape of the cell, characteristically to a crescent or sickle shape. In this form the cell is rigid and friable. Hypoxia and acidosis, which may be caused by fever, infection, dehydration, or other factors, are known to induce this change in shape (Figure 39-1). Many times, however, the RBC changes shape without apparent provocation. To a limited degree this change in shape is reversible, though not indefinitely. These cells eventually become irreversibly sickled cells (ISCs) with a life span of approximately 10 to 20 days. The fragility and shortened life span of these RBCs lead to chronic anemia, which serves as a stimulus for the bone marrow to create new RBCs, resulting in an elevated reticulocyte count.

The sickle "prep" is a solubility test often used to screen infants and children for SCD. This test is inexpensive and rapidly performed but is not very specific. A sickle prep result will be positive for sickle cell trait, sickle cell anemia, and other sickle hemoglobinopathies but will not distinguish one from another. The definitive diagnosis of SCD is made by performing a complete blood count (CBC), peripheral blood smear, and—most important—a quantitative hemoglobin electrophoresis. Measurement of hematologic indices is often important in the differential diagnoses of thalassemia syndromes and hemoglobinopathies. It is occasionally helpful to perform hematologic studies on a child's parents to confirm the diagnosis. Fetal hemoglobin (Hb F) predominates from 10 weeks after conception through the remainder of gestation and normally begins to decline at 34 weeks. Hb F comprises 60% to 80% of the total hemoglobin at birth and declines to normal adult levels (1% to 2%) by 6 to 9 months of age. In premature infants, however, the falloff in Hb F is somewhat slower. The remaining 20% to 40% of hemoglobin found at birth has the adult electrophoresis forms, Hb A and Hb A₂ or Hb S if found

to be affected. Hb F does not sickle, so it is unusual to find clinical manifestations of the disease with significant amounts of Hb F. Because of this phenomenon, manifestations of SCD may not be clinically apparent until 4 to 6 months of age or later.

Known Genetic Etiology

SCD has an autosomal recessive inheritance pattern. Both parents must carry some type of abnormal hemoglobin (i.e., one or both of them must carry sickle hemoglobin) for the disease to be manifested in their child. Carriers of SCD are described as having sickle cell trait (Hb AS). When two individuals, each of whom has sickle cell trait, elect to have a child, there is a 25% chance that they will have a child with sickle cell anemia (Hb SS). These individuals also have a 50% chance of having a child with sickle cell trait (Hb AS) and a 25% chance of having a child with entirely normal hemoglobin (Hb AA) with each pregnancy (Figure 39-2). Forty-four states, the District of Columbia, the Virgin Islands, and Puerto Rico are performing routine newborn screening for hemoglobinopathies, and screening is available upon request by the other six states. Newborn screening identifies approximately 2,000 infants/year with sickle cell hemoglobinopathies (Lane & Buchanan, 2002). Most screening programs use isoelectric focusing (IEF) of an elute from paper impregnated with blood that is used to screen for phenylketonuria, hypothyroidism, and other disorders, whereas other states rely on high-performance liquid chromatography (HPLC), or cellulose acetate electrophoresis. Most programs require a second test to ensure accuracy of the diagnosis.

Incidence and Prevalence

SCD is one of the most common genetic diseases seen in individuals of African descent but is also found in other ethnic groups, including those from the Caribbean, Mediterranean, Arabian Peninsula, and India. In the United States, 1 in 12 African-Americans is a carrier of the sickle cell gene, and 1 in 600 actually manifests the disease.

Prenatal diagnosis is available to couples known to be carriers of hemoglobinopathies. Diagnosis may be accomplished via chorionic villus sampling during the first trimester or amniocentesis during the second trimester. The method depends on the risks and benefits of the techniques involved; both are adequate to determine the diagnosis. To be beneficial, screening, follow-up, and diagnosis of sickle cell disease must be followed with prompt referral to knowledgeable providers of comprehensive care (National Institutes of Health [NIH], 2002).

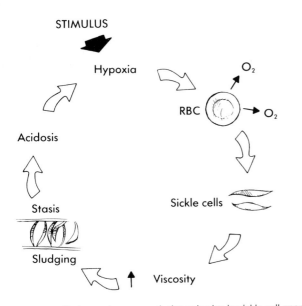

STIMULUS

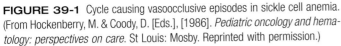

FIGURE 39-1 Cycle causing vasoocclusive episodes in sickle cell anemia. (From Hockenberry, M. & Coody, D. [Eds.], [1986]. *Pediatric oncology and hematology: perspectives on care.* St Louis: Mosby. Reprinted with permission.)

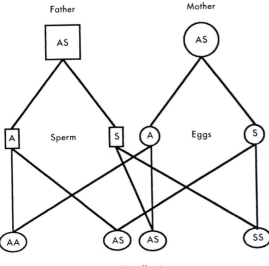

FIGURE 39-2 Genetics of sickle cell anemia. Both parents possess one gene for normal hemoglobin (A) and one for sickle hemoglobin (S). With each pregnancy, there is a 25% statistical chance that the child will have normal hemoglobin (AA) and a 25% chance that the child will have sickle cell anemia (SS); 50% of the children will have the sickle cell trait. (From Miller, D. & Baeher, R. [1990]. *Blood diseases of infancy and childhood: in the tradition of CH Smith* [6th ed.]. St Louis: Mosby. Reprinted with permission.)

Clinical Manifestations at Time of Diagnosis

As a result of current newborn screening programs for hemoglobinopathies, infants are now identified before the onset of acute symptoms (Table 39-1 and Box 39-1). The anemia from which sickle cell anemia derives its name is broadly characterized as an uncompensated hemolytic anemia, in which a markedly shortened overall RBC survival (i.e., an increased rate

---

Clinical Manifestations of Sickle Cell Anemia

NEONATES
Normal birth weight
No evidence of hemolytic anemia
Hemoglobin electrophoresis shows no evidence of Hgb A production
Neonatal jaundice (when present) related to ABO hemolytic disease of the newborn, not to SCD

INFANTS AND TODDLERS
Development of anemia
Coliclike symptoms, often associated with feeding difficulties
Generalized episodes of bone or abdomen pain preceded by acute-like, febrile infectious disease
Hand-foot syndrome associated with heat, pain, swelling, erythema
Splenic hypofunction marked by presence of Howell-Jolly bodies in the blood smear
Autosplenectomy preceded by splenomegaly in 73% of infants, followed by decrease in size
Splenomegaly noted frequently during febrile episodes

EARLY CHILDHOOD
Generalized vasoocclusive crisis (VOC) of bone or abdomen that may or may not be preceded by acute, febrile infection; seemingly triggered by emotional stress or abrupt weather changes
Usually nonpalpable spleen but sometimes retained in Hbg SC disease
Males may develop priapism
Biliary colic caused by stasis and gallstones
Development of cerebral vasculopathy with cerebral infarction

LATE CHILDHOOD
Gallstones with or without symptoms
Delayed pubescence
Females may have increased incidence of VOC with menses, presumably due to hormonal changes
Males may develop priapism
Early signs of sickle retinopathy
Early signs of sickle nephropathy

---

of RBC destruction) is insufficiently balanced by the increase in production (i.e., erythropoiesis) to maintain normal levels of total RBC and hemoglobin.

The Natural History Study on Sickle Cell Disease (Powars, 1975), indicated that in the first two decades of life, sickle cell anemia is marked by periods of clinical quiescence and relative well-being, interspersed with episodes of acute illness. This classic study supports that these acute episodes are treatable by state-of-the-art medical care and are often preventable. The expression of untreated sickle cell anemia is often characterized by septicemia and/or meningitis during infancy, followed by cerebral vasculopathy with cerebral infarction during early childhood. Splenic hypofunction is present in nearly 30% of infants with sickle cell anemia by their first birthday and in 90% by age 6 years. Splenic hypofunction accounts for the high risk of sepsis by polysaccharide-encapsulated organisms.

Treatment
Supportive Symptomatic Care
There is no cure for SCD short of bone marrow transplantation (BMT) (see Chapter 15). Despite the thorough understanding

TABLE 39-1

Differential Diagnosis of Common Hemoglobinopathies

Diagnosis	Clinical Severity	Hemoglobin (g/dl)	Hematocrit (%)	Mean Corpuscular Volume (MCV) (μ^3)	% of Reticulocytes	RBC Morphology*	Solubility Test	Electrophoresis (%)	Distribution of Hbg F
SS	Moderate -severe	7.5 (6-11)	22 (18-30)	>80	11 (5-20)	Many ISCs, target cells, nucleated RBCs, normochromic H-J bodies	Positive	>90 S <10 F <3.6 A_2	Uneven
SC	Mild-moderate	10 (10-15)	30 (26-40)	75-95	3 (5-10)	Many target cells, aniso-/ poikilocytosis	Positive	50 S 50 C <5 F	Uneven
S/B° thal	Moderate -severe	8.1 (6-10)	25 (20-36)	<80	8 (5-20)	Marked hypochromia, microcytosis and target cells, variable ISCs	Positive	>80 S <20 F >3.5 A_2	Uneven
S/B + thal	Mild-moderate	11 (9-12)	32 (25-40)	<75	3 (5-10)	Mild microcytosis, hypochromia, rare ISCs	Positive	55-75 S 15-30 A <20 F >3.5 A_2	Uneven
S/HPFH†	Asymptomatic	14 (12-14)	40 (32-48)	<80	1.5 (1-2)	No ISCs, occasional target cells, and mild hypochromia	Positive	<70 S >30 F <2.5 A_2	Even
AS	Asymptomatic	Normal	Normal	Normal	Normal	Normal	Positive	38-45 S 60-55 A 1-3 A_2	Uneven

*ICSs, Irreversibly sickled cells.
†S/HPFH, Sickle hereditary persistence of fetal hemoglobin.
From Charche, S., Lubin, B., & Reid, C.D. (1995). *Management and therapy of sickle cell disease, NIH publication no. 95-2117.* Washington, DC: U.S. Government Printing Office.

that exists among researchers and clinicians about the inheritance, diagnosis, and pathophysiology of SCD, treatment is essentially supportive and symptomatic. This therapy is aimed at aggressive treatment of infection and maintenance of optimal hydration and body temperature to prevent hypoxia and acidosis. Standard care implies bed rest, hydration, transfusions, analgesics, oxygen, and folic acid administration to prevent megaloblastic anemia.

Drug Therapy with Hydroxyurea

Treatment has moved from care during specific crises to the prevention of sickling episodes by inducing production of Hb F with hydroxyurea (HU) (NIH, 2002) (Box 39-2). HU, which is a derivative of urea, has been used for neoplastic diseases. For individuals with SCD it increases production of Hb F through mechanisms that remain unclear. Expression of Hb F, in combination with the native Hb S, forms a diluted pool of RBCs with Hb F and Hb S. This combination reduces both the polymerization of the cells and the rate of hemolysis. Other observers note HU decreases production of WBCs and reticulocytes, while increasing RBC survival time (Ballas, 1999). Additionally HU has been demonstrated to be a nitric oxide generator, which in turn decreases adhesion of platelets and leukocytes to the endothelium, and increases microvascular perfusion (Space et al, 2000). Researchers recognize the complex interplay of sickle erythrocytes, leukocytes, vascular endothelium, platelets, plasma clotting factors, and certain mediators of inflammation in producing tissue ischemia and

BOX 39-2

Treatment

SUPPORTIVE CARE (SEE ASSOCIATED PROBLEMS)
Aggressive treatment of infection
Maintenance of optimal hydration
Maintenance of body temperature
Penicillin prophylaxis
Pneumococcal immunization

DRUG THERAPY WITH HYDROXYUREA

SELECTIVE USE OF TRANSFUSIONS
CORD BLOOD TRANSFUSIONS/BONE MARROW TRANSPLANT

end-organ damage. Clinical trials aimed at modulating the effect of these various players are being studied (Ware et al, 2002).

Pediatric trials of HU therapy report significant improvement in Hb F production, mean corpuscular volume (MCV), and a mild to moderate increase in hemoglobin, which in turn reduces the number of sickle cell crises. Growth failure in children with SCD has long been identified, probably secondary to their hypermetabolic state. Treatment with HU decreases the resting energy expenditure, thus improving the hypermetabolic state with better growth parameters than expected (Fung et al, 2001). Children with more than three hospitalizations a year for vasoocclusive crisis (VOC), priapism, or acute chest syndrome are potential candidates for this therapy (Lane & Buchanan, 2002). They are generally started on 15 mg/kg of HU per day, with doses escalating by 5 mg/kg every 8 weeks if no signs or symptoms of toxicity are noted. The maximum dose is usually 35 mg/kg/day (NIH, 2002).

Administration of HU should be managed in a research-oriented practice because questions of long-term toxicity, carcinogenesis, growth retardation, and chromosomal damage are unanswered. At the present time, the only FDA-approved use of HU has been for selected adults willing to comply with hematologic monitoring and strict contraceptive use. A recent 2-year pilot study of HU use in very young children indicates that this drug is very well tolerated, effective, and may delay functional asplenia (Wang, 2001). Most centers using HU with children require an informed consent prior to trial because of non-FDA approval. Although HU has the potential of reducing the incidence of both hemolytic and vasoocclusive manifestations of the disease, it is not an option for treatment of these acute complications.

Selective Use of Transfusions

The Cooperative Study of Sickle Cell Disease (CSSCD) group completed an important study evaluating perioperative transfusion needs of children with SCD. It is well known that general anesthesia places an individual with SCD at risk for stroke. Standard protocol was to transfuse these individuals to a hemoglobin of 11 g/dl with an Hb S level of 30%. In the Preoperative Transfusion Study, individuals were transfused to a preoperative level of 10 g/dl with an Hb S level of 60%. Results suggest that stable individuals with Hb SS who are undergoing major elective surgery should be transfused to the lower level of 10 g/dl. Transfusion with limited phenotypic units of packed red blood cells (PRBCs) would most likely eliminate the alloimmunization observed from E, K, C, and Fy^a RBC phenotypes. Definitive data to not recommend preoperative transfusion in SCD are not available.

Because frequent transfusion carries the risk of chronic iron overload, an approach is transfusion by erythrocytapheresis. In this method, sickled cells are selectively removed and replaced with normal red cells via a rapid, continuous flow system that is similar to the production of pheresed units of platelets. Because normal erythrocytes are exchanged for sickled erythrocytes, the net gain of iron is greatly reduced or eliminated. Although this approach has merit, its application is limited to a few sickle cell centers in the United States because it is costly.

A study group of the CSSCD, Stroke Prevention in Sickle Cell Anemia (STOP I), looked at genetic markers, laboratory and radiographic indicators, and clinical findings that were predictive of stroke in this population (Adams et al, 1998). More than 2,000 children, between the ages of 2 and 16, with Hb SS and S $\beta°$ thal were screened by transcranial doppler (TCD) ultrasound. This noninvasive technique reliably demonstrates flow abnormalities. In particular, TCD demonstrates that high velocities (i.e., 200 cm/sec) in either the distal intracerebral or middle cerebral arteries are associated with an increased risk of subsequent stroke. Those identified with abnormal velocities were randomized to receive either monthly transfusions or no treatment at all. The risk of stroke, about 10% in SCD, was reduced by 90% in those children treated with transfusions

(Adams, 2000). This dramatic finding caused early termination of this study and a recommendation by the National Heart, Lung and Blood Institute (NHBI) that all children with Hb SS and Hb S $\beta°$ thal be screened with TCD. Children identified with high velocities are offered scheduled transfusions as a means of preventing stroke and its subsequent consequences. Further studies have indicated that those children with abnormal TCD should also be screened with magnetic resonance imaging (MRI). Silent infarcts are seen on MRI in a substantial minority of children with SCD, even those with normal neurologic function. The combination of abnormal TCD and silent infarct on MRI further increases the risk of stroke or silent infarcts (Pegelow et al, 2001). These children should be aggressively treated with scheduled transfusion therapy.

Positron-emission tomography (PET) has confirmed areas of irregular brain metabolism in children with SCD. A study by Powars and associates (1999) confirms areas of irregular brain metabolism by assessing functional glucose metabolism and microvascular blood flow and has confirmed the effectiveness of PET by comparing it with MRI or magnetic resonance angiography (MRA). Powars and associates concluded the following: (1) the addition of PET to MRI identified a much greater proportion of children with SS neuroimaging abnormalities, particularly in children with no history of overt neurologic events; (2) lesions identified via PET are more extensive (i.e., often bihemispheric) when compared with abnormalities identified via MRI; (3) PET may be useful as a management tool to evaluate metabolic improvement after therapeutic interventions (i.e., chronic transfusions); and (4) the correlation of PET abnormalities to subsequent stroke or progressive neurologic dysfunction necessitates further study.

Cord Blood Transfusion.   From a preventive point of view, providing genetic counseling for those individuals with sickle cell trait, prenatal diagnosis for pregnant women who are at risk for delivering a child with SCD, and education for parents of children newly diagnosed, is the standard of care. As awareness has grown as to the benefits of umbilical cord blood salvage, large-scale banking has begun in Europe and the United States (Walters, 1999). The Sickle Cell Center in Oakland, California, offers free storage of cord blood for families considering the option of cord blood transplant. Transplant could offer a cure for their child's disease, and pregnant families may wish to consider this option.

Complementary and Alternative Therapies

Researchers and those affected by SCD have long pondered as to why the severity of VOC seems to be more virulent in modern countries as compared to the disease evidenced by native Africans. Reports of a native African yam as holding modulating powers to reduce the pain suffered by those afflicted with VOC have been anecdotally reported. Some community organizations thus suggest ingestion of yams as a preventive effort despite lack of scientific studies. Part of the confusion regarding its effectiveness is confounded by the steep infant mortality experienced by African populations either from SCD, human immunodeficiency virus (HIV), or other infectious agents.

Families coming from Caribbean countries are reported to use noni juice, a derivative of native herbs, as a preventive

Data from NIH, pub. 02-2117, 2002.

```
┌─────────────────────────────────────────────────────┐
│  BOX 39-3                                             │
│  Sickle Cell Disease                                  │
├─────────────────────────────────────────────────────┤
│  ELIGIBILITY FOR TRANSPLANT                           │
│  Inclusions                                           │
│  Children <16 years of age with sickle cell anemia    │
│    (SCD-SS, SCD-S β°                                   │
│    thalassemia)                                       │
│  One or more of the following complications:          │
│    Stroke or central nervous system event lasting     │
│      longer than 24 hours                             │
│    Impaired neuropsychologic function and abnormal    │
│      cerebral MRI                                     │
│    Recurrent acute chest syndrome of Stage I or II    │
│      sickle lung disease                             │
│    Recurrent vasoocclusive painful episodes           │
│    Sickle nephropathy (GFR—30%-50% of predicted       │
│      normal)                                          │
│    Osteonecrosis of multiple joints                   │
│                                                       │
│  Exclusions                                           │
│  Children >16 years of age                            │
│  HLA nonidentical donor                               │
│  One or more of the following conditions:             │
│    Karnofsky performance score <70%                   │
│    Acute hepatitis or biopsy evidence of cirrhosis    │
│    Renal impairment with GFR <30% of predictive       │
│      normal                                          │
│    Stage III or IV of sickle lung disease             │
└─────────────────────────────────────────────────────┘
```

```
┌─────────────────────────────────────────────────────┐
│  BOX 39-4                                             │
│  Associated Problems                                  │
├─────────────────────────────────────────────────────┤
│  Functional asplenia                                  │
│  Splenic sequestration                                │
│  Neurologic problems                                  │
│  Vasoocclusive crisis                                 │
│  Acute chest syndrome                                 │
│  Transient red cell aplasia                           │
│  Hemolysis                                            │
│  Renal problems                                       │
│  Priapism                                             │
│  Skeletal changes                                     │
│  Ophthalmologic changes                               │
│  Audiologic problems                                  │
│  Leg ulcers                                           │
│  Reactions to contrast mediums, anesthesia            │
│  Cardiac problems                                     │
│  Hepatobiliary problems                               │
│  Transfusion complications                            │
│    Formation of antibodies                            │
│    Iron overload                                      │
│    Bloodborne pathogens                               │
└─────────────────────────────────────────────────────┘
```

agent for VOC. As with African yams, no studies have been recorded.

Massage, acupuncture, and relaxation techniques are effective as complementary therapies for pain associated with SCD.

Anticipated Advances in Diagnosis and Management

BMT has effectively cured a small but growing number of individuals with sickle cell anemia (Walters et al, 2000). This approach is limited because only 24% of individuals have an HLA-matched donor sibling. The National Marrow Donor Program is attempting to expand its minority representation with extensive recruitment. New researchers are investigating the use of umbilical cord blood, unrelated donor cord blood, and mismatched related donors as alternative avenues for seeking donors (Reed & Vichinsky, 2001) (see eligibility criteria in Box 39-3). At present, approximately 175 individuals with SCD have been treated with hematopoietic stem cell transplant worldwide. The survival rate is 91% with 82% surviving and remaining disease free. Graft rejection occurred in 9% of these children. Recent results with umbilical cord blood transplants in children with SCD indicated excellent survival (100%), low graft-versus-host disease (GVHD), but only 49% were cured (Walters, 1999). Hematopoietic mixed chimerism, whereby a mix of donor cells and host cells remains after transplant may be effective in ameliorating or eliminating the symptoms of SCD, and is under study. This technique in mice was effective in curing SCD without evidence of GVHD or significant toxicities (Kean et al, 2002). In general, children selected for transplant demonstrate a morbid course of disease but not to the extent of irreversible organ damage, which would reduce chances for success (see eligibility criteria in Box 39-3).

Another consideration that limits this approach is the morbidity associated with BMT, including risks for death, organ impairment, curtailed sexual function, and impaired motor and psychologic function. Other considerations include disturbance of family systems, cost-benefit ratios, the rights of siblings, and client compliance. BMT options must be decisions shared by the health care workers and the family; differences in cultural background between the two, however, may impede the ability to negotiate informed consent. External factors (e.g., educational level, economic conditions of the family, and quality of life) are often more critical in minority communities than in other settings.

Gene therapy continues to be studied as a means to inactivate the sickle gene, to increase expression of the gene for Hb F, or to introduce genes whose products can inhibit the polymerization of Hb S (Wethers, 2000). Curative gene therapy continues to be investigational at the level of the test tube and transgenic mouse models (Ballas, 2002). Chimeric oligonucleotides designed to direct a site-specific nucleotide exchange in the human β-globin gene were microinjected into normal human cells. A sufficient percentage of transduced cells demonstrated gene conversion (Liu et al, 2002). The transgenic mouse model utilized a β-A gene variant capable of preventing Hb S polymerization through use of a lentiviral vector (Pawliuk et al, 2001). The results in the mouse model achieved correction of red blood cell dehydration and sickling. Other strategies directed toward the elevation of Hgb F expression through gene therapy manipulation have been suggested.

Associated Problems

Associated problems are primarily caused by the following: (1) blockage of small blood vessels secondary to the clumping of sickled RBCs that cause tissue ischemia, and (2) hemolytic anemia and its sequelae (Figure 39-3 and Box 39-4).

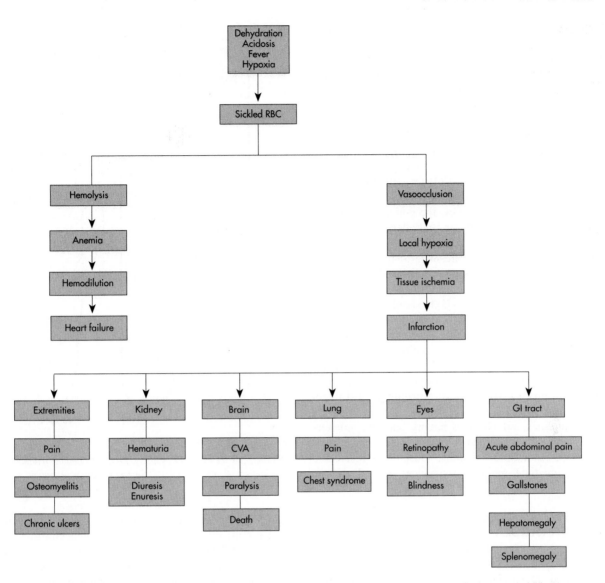

FIGURE 39-3 Tissue effects of sickle cell anemia. (From Wong, D. [1995]. *Nursing care of infants and children* [5th ed.]. St Louis: Mosby. Reprinted with permission.)

Functional Asplenia

Splenic function is normal at birth in infants with SCD, but by 6 months of age a state of splenic dysfunction develops, most likely a result of massive infarction. Palpation of the spleen on physical examination is no indication of splenic function. A palpable spleen in older children is thought to be the result of fibrosis and is almost exclusively found in individuals with Hb SC disease. The presence of Howell-Jolly bodies (e.g., "pocked cells") on blood smear confirms the condition of functional asplenia.

Functional asplenia occurs when the level of "pocked cells" is greater than 3.5% and the Hgb F level falls below 20%. Thus splenic malfunction and failure to make specific IgG antibodies to polysaccharide antigens contribute to unusual susceptibility (NIH, 2002). Without adequate splenic function, children with SCD are at high risk for infection from organisms, such as *Streptococcus pneumoniae, Haemophilus influenzae,* and *Neisseria meningitidis.* Less common causes of bacteremia include other streptococci, *Escherichia coli, Staphlococcus aureus,* and gram-negative bacteria such as *Klebsiella* sp., *Salmonella* sp., and *Pseudomonas aeruginosa.* Other organisms associated with frequent infections in sickle cell anemia include *Mycoplasma* and *Chlamydia pneumoniae* for symptoms of pneumonia and/or acute chest syndrome, and parvovirus B19 for aplastic anemia (Wong, 2001).

Furthermore, those children chronically transfused have iron overload, become more susceptible to organisms such as *Yersinia enterocolitica* as well as other bloodborne pathogens seen in other transfused populations.

Intervention should be threefold: (1) aggressive management of infectious episodes, (2) timely immunization (including pneumococcal vaccines, i.e., Prevnar and Pneumovax), and (3) antibiotic prophylaxis. Because current pneumococcal vaccines do not cover all pathogenic strains, antibiotic prophylaxis is the standard of care for all young children with SCD and should be started at the time of diagnosis—preferably by 2 months of age (Lane & Buchanan, 2002). The usual doses for penicillin V or G are 125 mg twice daily for children less than 3 years of age, and 250 mg twice daily for those more than 3 years of age. For children who are not compliant with oral antibiotic therapy at home, 1.2 million units of a long-acting penicillin may be given intramuscularly every 3 weeks (NIH, 2002). If an individual is allergic to penicillin, erythromycin (20 mg/kg) may be substituted. Some experts have recommended amoxicillin (20 mg/kg/day) or trimethoprim-sulfamethoxazole (4 mg/kg/day trimethoprim [TMP] to 20 mg/kg/day sulfamethoxazole [SMX]) for children less than 5 years of age (Committee on Infectious Diseases, 2000). As with other children taking antibiotics, the potential for fungal infections, gastrointestinal (GI) upset, and allergy exists.

The number of cases of penicillin-resistant invasive pneumococcal infections and the presence of nasopharyngeal carriage on penicillin prophylaxis may indicate that penicillin is no longer as effective at preventing invasive pneumococcal infections. The age at which prophylaxis should be discontinued is often an empirical decision (Committee on Infectious Diseases, 2000). The report of the Prophylactic Penicillin Study II established guidelines for discontinuing prophylaxis at 5 years of age (Falletta et al, 1995). These guidelines include the following: (1) children receiving regular medical attention, (2) those with no history of prior severe pneumococcal infection, and (3) those without surgical splenectomy. Consistent with these guidelines, all children having surgical splenectomies or history of pneumococcal sepsis must continue penicillin prophylaxis indefinitely. Parents must be counseled to always seek immediate medical assistance with all febrile episodes.

Acute Splenic Sequestration Complication (ASSC)

In this condition, blood flow into the spleen is adequate, but the vascular outflow system from the spleen to the systemic circulation is occluded. This occlusion results in a large collection of blood pooling in the spleen, causing significant enlargement. The systemic circulation may then be deprived of its needed blood volume, causing shock and cardiovascular collapse. The acute illness is associated with an Hb 2 g/dl or more below the child's baseline value with an acutely enlarged spleen (Lane & Buchanan, 2002). Children with Hb SS are susceptible to this at an early age (i.e., at less than 5 years). Those with other variants of the disease may continue to be at risk until their teenage years because they maintain splenic circulation longer than children with Hb SS. Parents can be taught to palpate and measure their child's spleen using a simple measuring device such as a calibrated tongue blade (Figure 39-4). Knowledge of the child's steady state spleen size is essential in determining appropriate diagnosis and treatment during an acute event.

Management of ASSC necessitates hospitalization with immediate therapy, including transfusion. If shock is present, systemic circulation must be supported with fluids. Once adequate circulation is reestablished, however, the volume of fluid previously sequestered in the spleen is returned to the circulation, and circulatory overload must be avoided. In children with life-threatening episodes, splenectomy is recommended or else these children are placed on a chronic transfusion program

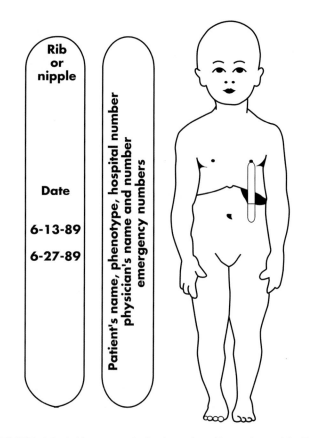

FIGURE 39-4 Measurement of spleen size with a spleen stick. (From Eckman, J.R. & Platt, A.F. [1991]. *Problem oriented management of sickle syndromes.* Atlanta: Georgia NIH Sickle Cell Center. Reprinted with permission.)

(NIH, 2002). Splenectomy, however, places a child at increased risk for infection. It is optimal to splenectomize a child after the age of 2 years and after the pneumococcal vaccines have been received. Many institutions offer the meningococcal vaccine when splenectomy is planned. In contrast to the acute episodes, some children develop chronic massive splenomegaly. Splenectomy is indicated in these children when pressure or pain from the enlarged spleen is evident or accompanied by thrombocytopenia, neutropenia, or severe anemia.

Neurologic Problems

The vasculature of the brain is subject to vasoocclusive episodes in children with SCD; by age 14 years the incidence of stroke in children with SCD is 8%, but stroke may occur during infancy. The estimated age of the first cerebrovascular accident (CVA) differs significantly for children with Hb SS and Hb SC. The chances of a child with Hb SS having a first stroke by age 20 years is estimated at 11%, but the estimated risk for a child with Hb SC is 2% (Ohene-Frempong et al, 1998). Of note, the higher incidence of CVA in the 1- to 9-year age group—as opposed to the 10- to 19-year age group—suggests that a subset of children may have additional risk factors for stroke (Ohene-Frempong et al, 1998). These risk factors include all-aged children with more severe anemia, and older children with high reticulocyte and white blood cell counts (Blumenthal & Glenn, 2002). The Cooperative Study of Sickle Cell Disease found that both the recency and frequency of acute chest syndrome (ACS) [discussed further in later section] due to pulmonary infection were associated with stroke, suggesting that repeated damage to the vascular endothelium may be predictive of damage to the cerebral vasculature (Jenkins, 2002).

When a blood vessel is partially occluded by a small embolus or vessel spasm, the manifestations may be focal and last less than 24 hours without residual deficit. This is classified as a transient ischemic attack (TIA) and is a predictor of stroke. Accordingly, the general recommendation is that all children with TIAs receive the appropriate therapy for stroke prevention, chronic transfusion therapy. When the affected vessel is completely occluded by thrombus or embolus—with or without narrowing of the vessel lining—a CVA occurs. Intracranial hemorrhage is a rare but usually fatal complication that occurs when blood vessel walls are thinned by intravascular sickling and then dilate and rupture. Computed tomography (CT), MRI, and magnetic resonance angiography (MRA) can show infarcts and areas of hemorrhage. In the early hours following symptoms, CT may be negative and or show only subtle signs, but treatment should be initiated nevertheless (NIH, 2002). Symptoms include hemiparesis, aphasia, visual disturbances, seizures, and altered sensation, alertness, and mentation. Unless the diagnosis is in doubt, the MRI should be deferred until treatment is initiated (NIH, 2002). MRI provides better detail of ischemia and can also show the patchy white matter abnormal signals that are present in individuals with SCD—both with and without neurologic deficits—and are thought to be due to disease in penetrating arterioles. MRA may show large vessel occlusive disease or aneurysms.

Initial treatment consists of an exchange transfusion and hydration. Hyperthermia increases cerebral metabolism and therefore should be treated. Hypotension is treated to prevent further ischemia. Admission to an intensive care unit (ICU) facilitates the treatment and observation that these children require. Chronic transfusion (every 3 to 4 weeks) is usually conducted until the child is 5 years past CVA or reaches 18 years of age.

Multiple studies have implicated silent infarcts with decreased neurocognitive development of children with SCD. School-age children with SCD who do not show silent infarcts on MRI nevertheless show declining IQ scores in verbal and math achievement scores with increasing age (Wang & Enos, 2001). Assessment of neurocognitive development is warranted at an early age with ongoing evaluation of cerebral vessels by TCD for primary stroke prevention with children with Hb SS or Sβ°thal. Examining flow velocities in the cerebral arteries with TCD (see discussion of new therapies earlier in this chapter) can be diagnostic of impending stroke. Those identified with abnormal velocities (>200) are offered chronic transfusion therapy as a stroke preventative.

Chronic transfusion secondary to stroke is usually conducted until the child is 5 years past CVA or reaches 18 years of age. Stoppage carries with it the ever-present risk of re-stroke. Recent research (Scothorn et al, 2002) concluded that the absence of an antecedent or concurrent medical event associated with an initial stroke was a major risk factor for subsequent stroke despite receiving regular transfusions and must be considered prior to cessation of transfusion therapy.

STOP II, utilizing the population identified with abnormal TCD findings, is a study of the length of transfusion therapy needed in order to normalize and retain normalization of the TCD and determine if transfusions may be stopped after some period of time when risk of stroke has diminished (NIH, 2002). Chronic transfusion (either for stroke or for abnormal TCD findings) induces iron overload. Chelation therapy to manage this complication must be addressed at the initiation of transfusions and again when the child shows evidence of iron overload.

Vasoocclusive Crisis (VOC)

Painful, vasoocclusive episodes are the most common cause of emergency department visits and hospital admissions for individuals with SCD. Vasoocclusion is a physiologic process, but the resultant pain is a complex biopsychosocial event. Physiologic factors combined with social considerations (e.g., developmental stage, pain history, and family and child coping skills) contribute to the expression of vasoocclusion. Each child exhibits an individualized pattern of duration, frequency, severity, and location of vasoocclusive crises. The hallmark of these crises is their unpredictability. A few children state that they are always in pain, but approximately one third of children and adolescents rarely seek hospital-based treatment. There are two major kinds of assessment: rapid assessment of the acute episode to focus on pain intensity, prompt treatment, and relief, and comprehensive assessment of chronic pain induced by bony changes (NIH, 2002).

Precipitation of painful episodes in SCD has been related to numerous factors, including weather changes (i.e., warm to cold), stress, and menstrual cycles in females. The frequency of painful episodes is indirectly related to the Hb F level and numerous painful crises are a prognostic sign for further complications as a result of sickling.

VOCs typically affect the chest, abdomen, and long bones, although any area in the body or organ is subject to sickling episodes. In long bones, infarcts are most common in the shaft and are usually confined to the medulla. Muscular infarcts occasionally occur with secondary hemorrhage and myonecrosis and are clearly seen on CT and MRI scans.

The optimal treatment for VOCs is multimodal and includes treating any antecedent causes, improving circulation, and providing analgesia. Treatment of antecedent causes includes correcting fever, hypoxia, and acidosis, as well as treating infection and dehydration. History taking includes effective treatments at home, usual drugs, dosages, and side effects during acute pain and medications and timing since the onset of acute pain. Primary care providers must be aware that an extraneous illness possibly precipitated a painful episode and the child has two independent problems.

Hydration is an important part of improving circulation to the affected area. Children may be hydrated orally or intravenously with an electrolyte solution. Options for oral hydration include juice, bouillon, water, milk, sports drinks, Pedialyte, or Infalyte. Fluids given intravenously may include a normal saline bolus with care being taken not to tax the cardiovascular system with too large or rapid a bolus.

Maintenance fluids of 5% dextrose with 0.45% normal saline with 20 mEq KCL/L, adjusted for serum chemistry results should follow (NIH, 2002). The rate of fluids given should be approximately 1.5 times the maintenance dosage, or $2,500 \, \text{ml/m}^2$ daily. Circulation to infarcted areas may also be improved by the local application of heat (e.g., heating pad, warm bath, or whirlpool). Once comfort has been established, passive range of motion and massage may be initiated. These children should be encouraged to be as active as possible.

Severe pain should be considered a medical emergency that prompts timely and aggressive management (NIH, 2002). Initial assessment includes measurement of pain intensity utilizing a simple pain intensity rating tool. Analgesia may take several forms, including nonpharmacologic agents, nonsteroidal antiinflammatory drugs (NSAIDs), and oral or parenteral narcotics. Multimodal therapy, which includes several of these approaches, is more effective than single agents because each agent increases analgesia. NSAIDs act on peripheral inflammatory pain receptors, and narcotics act centrally. This combination therapy may also contravene the "ceiling effect" that occurs with nonsteroidals and acetaminophen, as well as have a significant narcotic-sparing effect. There are multiple narcotic agents from which to choose, and each child, health care provider, and institution is likely to have a preference. Readers are referred to the *Guideline for the Management of Acute and Chronic Pain in Sickle-Cell Disease* published by the American Pain Society (1999) for a full discussion of pain agents. Placebos are never appropriate because they erode the trusting relationship between the health care provider and child. The dosage given should begin at a standard therapeutic dosage or a dosage known to be therapeutic for a given child and then adjusted as needed.

Many narcotics have very brief half-lives, and care must be taken to administer them often enough for analgesic effect. For example, when a medication with a 12-hour half-life is used, dosing should be approximately every 2 hours to maintain consistent pain relief. Early in the course of a vasoocclusive episode, the vascular occlusion is constant—not intermittent. Therefore early in the course of a painful episode, as needed (i.e., prn), dosing is inappropriate. Scheduled doses of narcotics should be given over the first 24 hours after admission for VOC. Later in the course, collateral circulation may develop or the occlusion may have decreased, improving circulation to the infarcted area. It is preferable to control a child's pain early in the course of the illness and maintain control by frequent reassessment.

It is inappropriate to administer intramuscular injections to children for pain relief because an injection alone can be quite painful unless it is for a single dose and a longer half-life is desired (e.g., for outpatient management) or IV access has not been obtained. Intrathecal catheters have been suggested as a route for analgesic administration for children who are hospitalized with severe, intractable pain but should not be considered before an adequate trial of maximal doses of systemic opioids and adjuvant medications are given. Patient-controlled analgesia (PCA) is also recommended if institutions are familiar with its use in children.

Because all pain episodes cannot be prevented, children and their families should be taught to manage mild pain and recognize symptoms that suggest serious problems. For mild pain,

nonnarcotic medicines including acetaminophen, aspirin (provided there is no concurrent viral process or other contraindication), ibuprofen, and ketorolac are appropriate and may be given at the standard recommended doses. Caution should be exercised with the use of NSAIDs in children with renal or liver complications. Optimal management requires adequate education of the child, family, and health care providers. Nonpharmacologic forms of pain relief are useful adjuncts to pharmacologic therapy. Self-hypnosis, biofeedback, and distraction are particularly helpful, but must be taught to the child prior to a pain episode.

When children become significantly uncomfortable they experience anxiety and, consequently, a heightened perception of pain. They may ultimately develop dysfunctional illness behavior as a result of inadequately treated pain. It is important for the child, family, and health care providers to have realistically attainable goals related to pain control. The goal of pain management should be prompt pain relief to a functional level. Relief could be defined as a pain intensity reduction of at least 50% to 60% from the upper end of the pain scale. The alleviation of pain provided by narcotics must be balanced against known side effects such as pruritus, nausea, constipation, and respiratory depression. Hospitalized children are routinely started on stool softeners and laxatives at the onset of opioid therapy and given standing orders for antihistamines for pruritus and antinausea medications. Side effects, such as respiratory depression, should be closely monitored by scheduled visual observations and pulse oximetry.

Several studies document the low prevalence of drug addiction within this population. Despite these studies, health care providers continue to believe that drug addiction is a major problem among people with SCD, which is unfortunate because this misperception can interfere with the provision of adequate health care. Tolerance and physical dependence are expected pharmacologic consequences of long-term opioid use and should not be confused with addiction (NIH, 2002).

Acute Chest Syndrome (ACS)

ACS ranks second as a cause for hospitalization and is responsible for 25% of all deaths from SCD. ACS is a frequent cause of death in both children and adults. Pulmonary problems not directly related to sickle cell VOC, such as pneumonia or asthma, can worsen SCD because local or systemic hypoxia increases the rate of sickle polymerization (NIH, 2002). ACS is a life-threatening complication that results from occlusions in the pulmonary vasculature, resulting in areas of infarcted lung tissue. The occlusion is caused by localized sickling, thromboembolism, or embolism with collections of sickled cells, bone marrow, or marrow fat. The occlusion can also be induced by respiratory depression caused by narcotics. Special instructions for deep-breathing exercises before surgery can prevent certain episodes.

Acute chest pain, a nonproductive cough, leukocytosis, fever, and respiratory distress characterize ACS. Fever, cough, and tachypnea are often the only findings in children. ACS may be difficult to differentiate from, and actually may be concurrent with, pneumonia. Physical examination usually reveals tachypnea, but there may also be evidence of pulmonary consolidation, pleural effusion, a new pulmonary infiltrate, or pleural friction rub. Chest radiographic studies may be normal for the first few days, especially if a child is dehydrated.

ACS may be a fulminant process; admission to the intensive care unit may be necessary for close monitoring. Arterial blood gas (ABG) levels and pulse oximetry should be followed closely; supplemental oxygen and further respiratory support should be provided as needed. All children should be encouraged to use scheduled incentive spirometry in order to fully aerate their lungs. Early transfusion may be necessary to prevent progressive problems because hypoxia will induce further sickling; partial or complete exchange transfusion may be needed (NIH, 2002).

One episode of ACS promotes another with possible progressive lung scarring. In any event, frequent ACS and painful events are associated with shorter life spans (NIH, 2002). Because there are no clear clinical or laboratory parameters that differentiate vasoocclusive disease from pneumonia, primary care providers should empirically use antibiotics directed against *S. pneumoniae, H. influenzae, S. aureus,* and other pathogens commonly seen in community-acquired pneumonia.

Transient Red Cell Aplasia (TRCA) (Formerly Aplastic Crisis)

Periodically the bone marrow does not respond to a fall in hemoglobin and hematocrit values caused by the rapid turnover of RBCs. The hemoglobin and hematocrit values drop, and there is a lack of compensatory rise in the reticulocyte count, which usually happens during or following a viral infection. Symptoms include fever, more severe anemia than usual, headache, fatigue, and dyspnea, and the child may have signs of respiratory involvement and/or gastrointestinal involvement. Human parvovirus B19 has been implicated in 70% to 100% of episodes of TRCA (NIH, 2002). Children being cared for during and shortly after a viral illness should be observed for unusual pallor or prolonged lethargy after the symptoms of the viral illness have subsided. Therapy includes slow transfusion to a hemoglobin level slightly above the baseline hemoglobin level. Recovery is indicated by a return of reticulocytosis.

Hemolysis

Hemolysis in SCD is usually of only moderate severity. The symptoms of anemia (e.g., pallor, fatigue, dyspnea) are not the hallmarks of this disorder. Hemolysis is generally noted by scleral icterus, tea-colored urine, and elevated bilirubin and urobilinogen levels. One long-term consequence of hemolysis is the high prevalence of gallstones. Increased hemolysis may be triggered by bacterial infections, poisons, or glucose 6-phosphate dehydrogenase (G6PD) deficiency. Hemolysis accompanied by a brisk reticulocytosis requires no treatment.

Renal Problems

The environment within the renal medulla is characterized by low oxygen tension, acidosis, and hypertonicity. Therefore intravascular sickling occurs more rapidly in the kidney than in any other organ. Persistent proteinuria, beginning early in life, is the hallmark of sickle nephropathy that occurs in all forms of SCD, and is associated with severity of disease (Wigfall

et al, 2000). This intravascular sickling leaves the kidney with a relative inability to concentrate urine (i.e., hyposthenuria) or adequately acidify urine, which is an early sign of end-stage renal disease. The relative inability to concentrate urine often leads to enuresis or nocturia and also results in a relative inability to excrete potassium and uric acid. Gross hematuria may occur in children with SCD or sickle trait. Blood loss is usually minimal, resolving within 1 to 3 days with bed rest and hydration and does not require transfusion. As with all individuals with gross hematuria, diagnoses of glomerulonephritis, tumor, renal stones, urinary tract infection, and bleeding disorders must be excluded. When other diagnoses have been eliminated, hematuria is often attributed to areas of ischemia or necrosis caused by sickled cells. Renal papillary necrosis, renal infarction, and perinephric hematoma (secondary to infarction) are all described. Progressive medullary and cortical infarction leads to the development of chronic renal failure, resulting in death of affected adults older than age 40 years. Early detection of proteinuria may indicate therapy to prevent progressive renal insufficiency (Wigfall et al, 2000).

Priapism

Males with sickle cell anemia are subject to episodes of priapism. Priapism occurs when an accumulation of sickled cells obstructs the venous drainage of the corpora cavernosa of the penis, causing a prolonged and exquisitely painful erection. Priapism is not associated with sexual desire or excitement. In addition, micturition is often difficult, and urinary retention may occur. MRI is useful in demonstrating corporal destruction with development of intracorporal fibrosis and hemosiderin deposition.

According to one study, the mean age at presentation is 12 years. By the age of 20, approximately 89% of all males with sickle cell disease will have experienced one or more episodes of priapism (Mantadakis et al, 1999). The following four general patterns of priapism are described:

1. Recurrent (i.e., "short stuttering") attacks lasting less than 3 hours several times a week for 4 weeks
2. Acute (i.e., "major") attacks lasting less than 24 hours, followed by partial or complete impotence
3. Chronic, persistent, usually painless enlargement or induration that persists weeks to years, which develops after a major episode and is associated with partial or complete impotence
4. Acute-on-chronic priapism, which is a chronic induration with a superimposed acute attack that may affect only part of the penile shaft

At the onset, the child should be counseled to urinate (a full bladder aggravates priapism), drink extra fluids, and use oral analgesics. Treatment of major episodes begins with conservative measures including hospitalization, hydration, transfusions, and pain management. Application of ice is inappropriate because it promotes vasoconstriction. Surgical intervention is considered if there is no detumescence after 4 to 6 hours of conservative treatment (NIH, 2002). Surgical measures aim to reestablish adequate venous outflow and circulation of the corporal body via aspiration and—if not successful—placement of a shunt. Prophylactic regimens include the addition of vasodilatory drugs including hydralazine and pseudoephedrine, α-agonists and β-agonists and 6-month transfusion programs. Despite intervention, impotence is a frequent complication of priapism.

Skeletal Changes

SCD involves both hematologic and osseous abnormalities because it affects the two major functions of bone tissue: hematopoiesis and osteogenesis. Skeletal changes as a result of expansion of the bone marrow and recurrent infarction are often seen in children with SCD. Symptoms of dactylitis (i.e., hand-foot syndrome) include pain and swelling of the tarsals, metatarsals, carpals, and metacarpals and are often the first symptoms seen in severely affected infants. Because erythropoiesis is critical, the marrow within these small reservoirs is stimulated to produce red cells in these infants. The average age of onset is 9 months, and the risk extends to age 2 years. After this age red cell production is shifted to the marrow within the long bones and axial skeleton.

Dactylitis causes pain and requires frequent hospitalizations for IV administration of fluid. Infants in pain refuse to drink adequate fluids, so hospitalization is necessary to avoid acidosis. These crises do not cause permanent orthopedic problems but are frightening to parents. Back pain is common in older children and is recognized on radiographs by "fish-mouthed" vertebrae, which have decreased vertical height and increased width (Brinker et al, 1998). Sudden infarction causes acute symptoms of pain and must be differentiated from those of bacterial origin. Common sites include the long bones and vertebral bones. Common symptoms consist of pain, warmth, and swelling, as well as limitation of motion to the affected area.

The pathophysiology of bone "erosions" in sickle cell anemia results from necrosis produced by repeated microinfarction. Repeated infarction may lead to avascular necrosis. This pathophysiology most commonly involves the head of the femur but may also occur in the head of the humerus or fibula. Treatment initially includes avoidance of weight bearing on or bracing of the joint for up to 6 months. Judicious use of local heat and analgesics for pain relief may be employed. If pain persists along with radiographic progression, treatment consists of surgical core decompression of the femoral head. A newer technique, the injection of acrylic cement, has been used to restore the spherical shape of the femoral head. Both of these procedures are seen as temporary measures to forestall an eventual total hip replacement. There have been no prospective randomized studies to assess safety or efficacy of these measures (NIH, 2002).

Ophthalmologic Changes

Ophthalmologic complications are a direct result of the vasoocclusive process within the eye. Because early stages of eye disease do not result in visual symptoms, they may go undiagnosed unless an eye examination is performed by an ophthalmologist. Most screenings begin at age 8 or 9, when the child is able to cooperate, although most defects occur during the second decade of life. These complications include nonproliferative retinopathy, proliferative retinopathy, or elevated intraocular pressure in the presence of hyphema. Nonproliferative retinopathy may not affect visual acuity. Proliferative sickle retinopathy can cause vitreous hemorrhage and subsequent retinal detachment and blindness. The occurrence of proliferative sickle retinopathy depends on an individual's age and type of hemoglobinopathy, and is progressive. Proliferative sickle retinopathy is more common in people with Hb SC but also occurs with other forms of SCD. Individuals with sickle hemoglobinopathies who sustain blunt trauma and subsequent hyphema to the eye may quickly develop increased intraocular pressure, which is an ophthalmologic emergency (NIH, 2002).

Audiologic Problems

Vasoocclusive episodes within the circulation of the inner ear and the administration of ototoxic drugs may cause sensorineural hearing loss. This loss may be unilateral or bilateral but is generally manifested as a high-frequency deficit. A 12% failure rate in hearing (as opposed to a 1.6% rate in normal controls) was shown by Gentry and Dancer (1997a). As expected with hearing loss, speech screening should be implemented. Their findings showed that 10% of children with SCD had either an articulation disorder or a fluency disorder at a rate higher than expected.

Leg Ulcers

Leg ulcers are experienced by 10% to 20% of older children and adults with SCD, and are painful, indolent, and disfiguring (NIH, 2002). These ulcers usually begin as a bite or scratch on the lower portion of the leg or the medial or lateral malleolus. These ulcers typically form a shallow depression with a smooth and slightly elevated margin and often have a surrounding area of edema. Bacteria are virtually always recovered from the base of an ulcer; although this may represent colonization of devitalized tissue, clinical observation suggests that infection contributes to enlargement and maintenance of ulcers. Ulcers can produce significant pain and limit movement. These ulcers may take 6 weeks to 6 months to heal, and—despite aggressive treatment—a recurrence rate of 75.4% in 2 years is reported (Cackovic et al, 1998). Early, prompt treatment includes bed rest, elevation, and wound care with antibiotics for cellulitic areas, but skin grafting and transfusion therapy may also be needed. The specific type of wound care is controversial and should be directed by a competent plastic surgeon.

Preparation for Anesthesia or Contrast Medium (Surgery or Radiologic Studies)

General anesthesia and hyperosmolar contrast medium are both known to induce sickling. If an operative or diagnostic procedure using these agents is anticipated, most hematologists suggest that children with SCD receive transfusion to a hemoglobin of 10 g/dl. Children with Hb SC usually carry this high a Hb at baseline and would most likely not require a transfusion. Unusually high-risk children are the exception to this rule. All children receiving tonsillectomies and adenoidectomies should be transfused because this surgery appears to be more serious for the child with SCD due to associated blood loss, fluid loss, and inability to orally hydrate (NIH, 2002). Additional measures such as warming the operating room, warming the IV fluids, or placing the child on a warming blanket during surgery are warranted. Aggressive hydration of 1 to 1½ times maintenance fluids given 8 to 24 hours before surgery is recommended.

Cardiac Problems

Over time the cardiovascular system accommodates to chronic anemia with increased cardiac output. This chronic volume overload causes cardiac enlargement. Although dilation and hypertrophy often occur, systolic and diastolic performance of the left ventricle in the resting state are usually preserved (NIH, 2002). Cardiac enlargement is often apparent on chest radiograph, the precordium is hyperactive, and a low-grade systolic ejection murmur may be heard in the second and third left intercostal spaces on exam. Cardiomegaly is an adaptation to anemia and alone should not be considered pathologic. Children with sickle cell anemia are subject to the same medical conditions as other children; therefore, findings suggestive of congenital, rheumatic, or underlying heart disease should be investigated. In such cases an echocardiogram and cardiac consultation are recommended. Several studies of children and adolescents document a cardiac endurance of 60% to 70% of normal (Covitz, 1994). Electrocardiogram depression in the ST segment occurs during exercise in 15% of children with SCD, suggesting endocardial ischemia.

Hepatobiliary Problems

The ongoing elevated rate of RBC hemolysis generates an increase in serum bilirubin. Likewise, elevations of the serum alkaline phosphatase and lactic dehydrogenase levels as a result of bone metabolism and hemolysis are often seen. Gallstones of bile or calcium bilirubinate are a common finding and easily seen via ultrasound. These gallstones are found in 14% to 30% of children with SCD and are most common in individuals with Hb SS (NIH, 2002). Ultrasonography indicates the onset of cholelithiasis as early as 2 to 4 years with increasing symptoms with age.

Surgeons should be aware of the finding that concomitant common bile duct (CBD) stones have been reported in individuals with SCD and cholelithiasis. Both laparoscopy and open cholecystectomies are approved for individuals with SCD.

A hepatic crisis (sometimes known as right upper quadrant [RUQ] syndrome) may be indistinguishable from acute cholecystitis. RBC sequestration in the liver causes hepatocellular dysfunction, which decreases bilirubin excretion. Children who have RUQ pain, increased jaundice, and fever need careful evaluation and management. Crisis pain involving the liver is often indistinguishable from acute cholecystitis (Box 39-5). Transfused children are at risk for viral hepatitis and hepatic hemosiderosis, which can result in hepatic injury and fibrosis. Hepatic failure resulting from massive sickling has been reported.

Transfusion Complications

Individuals with SCD may need transfusions emergently, episodically, or chronically. Performing RBC phenotyping before transfusion avoids the problems associated with the development of RBC antibodies. Children requiring RBC transfusions should be given phenotypically matched units.

BOX 39-5
Common Sources of Abdominal Pain in Sickle Cell Anemia

Gallstones
Hepatitis
Biliary sludge
Small bowel necrosis
Pancreatic sickling
Cirrhosis of various causes
Intrahepatic cholestasis

Several centers have been successful in recruiting minority donors for extended matching for RBC antigens. This matching has markedly decreased the occurrence of alloimmunization and should be the standard for children needing chronic transfusions. The complications of transfusions include possible exposure to bloodborne infectious agents, formation of alloantibodies, and (with chronic or multiple transfusion) iron overload. Individuals with iron overload experience progressive organ dysfunction, leading to iron-induced cardiac damage and death. Iron chelation with subcutaneous or intravenous deferoxamine is a difficult but essential treatment. An efficient, easily administered oral chelating agent does not currently exist.

Prognosis

In a classic study done more than 20 years ago, a group of adults and children were longitudinally followed to determine the natural history of SCD. The disease effects in the adults tended to be chronic and organ related and the problems in the children were acute and often infectious. Overall there was a 10% expected death rate during the first decade of life and 5% or less during any subsequent decade (Powars, 1975). New findings (Reed & Vichinsky, 2001) indicate that the overall mortality rate (at least in some regions of the United States, has decreased to <2% by age 10. The average longevity in people with Hb SS genotype is 42 years for men and 48 years for women, whereas men and women with Hb SC genotype live to age 60 and 68 years, respectively.

It is now known that 20% of all children with Hb SS will develop the severe form of the disease, which is characterized by frequent pain crises and ultimate end-organ damage; 40% will display moderate symptomatology; and the rest will have a more indolent course (Powars, 1975). Three easily identifiable manifestations of SCD that may appear in the first 2 years of life (dactylitis, severe anemia, and leukocytosis) can help predict the severity of sickle cell disease in later life (Miller et al, 2000). This striking variability between genotypes provides another example of the variable presentation of symptoms and complications that must be considered by the primary care provider. All children with a given genotype (i.e., SS) will not present with either the same symptoms or frequency. Sickle thalassemia is reported to have lower rates of complications and mortality in children who inherit this genetic variant. The β-globin gene cluster haplotypes reported by Powars and associates (1994) further modulate the severity of the disorder.

This information on genotypes assumes urgency in prenatal diagnosis and in making decisions about potentially life-threatening procedures (e.g., BMT). In the former case, the decision to continue a pregnancy can rest on the perceived future clinical course of a child. Factors determining the extremely variable clinical course include the following: (1) genetic factors (e.g., α-thalassemia, β-globin gene haplotypes, heterocellular hereditary persistence of Hb F, and high total hemoglobin) and (2) adherence to suggested clinical guidelines (e.g., penicillin prophylaxis, pneumococcal vaccinations, adequate hydration, and early recognition of life-threatening complications) (Chui, 2001).

Because of penicillin prophylaxis, the mortality rate for children with SCD in the first decade of life has decreased from 10% to 1%. Compliance with prophylactic recommendations is critical in early years. Davis and associates (1997) report that the survival of children with SCD has markedly improved since 1968, but that a substantial number of deaths continue to occur outside the hospital. This finding raises concerns about whether care for acute illness is promptly sought and readily accessible. Improving parental knowledge (Logan et al, 2002) about SCD has proven to correlate with increased use of appropriate and timely medical intervention. As early intervention decreases or eliminates deaths from sepsis, ACS, and splenic sequestration, the primary issue will be chronic organ damage, notably renal, neurologic, and pulmonary changes.

PRIMARY CARE MANAGEMENT

Health Care Maintenance

Growth and Development

When matched with controls of similar socioeconomic status, children with SCD have comparable physical parameters at birth, including weight, length, and head circumference, as well as similar 1- and 5-minute Apgar scores. Classic studies (Modege & Ifenu, 1993) show that—starting at approximately 6 months of age and being clearly defined by the preschool years—those children with Hb SS and Hb Sβ° thal, demonstrate a pattern of physical growth that is divergent from that of their unaffected peers. These children are shorter, weigh less, and have a smaller percentage of body fat and delayed bone age. Their muscle mass and head circumference, however, are comparable with that of their unaffected peers. Weight is affected more than height, and males are affected more than females. Later studies concur that physical delays in growth and development are common (Lawrence, 2000). Pubertal changes are also delayed for both boys and girls.

These changes are coincident with the usual physiologic waning of Hb F levels. It has also been noted that the growth of children who, for unknown reasons, persist in producing Hb F is usually not as growth retarded as that of other children with SCD. Children receiving chronic transfusions, however, show significant increased growth, which suggests that hemolytic anemia plays a major role in the growth retardation in children with sickle cell anemia.

As with standard well-child care, physical growth parameters should be measured and plotted on standardized growth charts every 3 to 4 months (Lane & Buchanan, 2002). The pattern of growth of an individual child, however, is more important than comparison with unaffected children.

Psychosocial researchers have studied the learning abilities, coping skills, anxieties, and self-concepts of unaffected children and those with SCD. Most studies conclude that children with SCD are well adjusted but vulnerable to experiencing psychosocial stresses because of the chronicity of their condition. Rates of mental illness in children and adolescents with SCD noted no difference than other children from similar backgrounds but without SCD.

Beyond the expected significant psychosocial and intellectual deficits experienced by children with a history of stroke, researchers are now focusing on the incidence of subclinical deficits resulting from cerebral microvascular occlusion that are not apparent on routine neurologic examinations. DeBaun and associates (1998) have explored various neurocognitive tests in order to determine instruments sensitive and specific for identifying children with silent cerebral infarcts. Selected test results thus far indicate impairment with fine and visual motor tasks, as well as with short-term memory skills.

Standardized tools such as the Denver Developmental Screening Test II are helpful when screening for developmental delay. Children found to be at developmental risk should be referred for a more thorough developmental assessment. The involvement of a consistent caregiver and the caregiver's rapport with a consistent health care provider are invaluable tools for monitoring developmental progress in children with SCD.

Diet

A child's diet should be well balanced with a generous amount of fluid. Diet during illness or disease exacerbation may include whatever nutritive dense solid foods children desire with oral fluids at 1.5 times their usual fluid intake. Maintenance of daily fluid intake is essential in maintaining homeostasis in children with SCD. A fluid sheet, outlining times to increase fluids and amounts of oral fluids to be given, provides a handy reference to parents (Box 39-6).

Because of increased metabolic demands, children with SCD have a relative deficiency of energy, protein, and several micronutrients, so the recommended daily allowances for the normal population may not be applicable. Limited metabolic studies support the hypothesis that chronic hemolysis leads to a state of high protein turnover and increased metabolic requirements. One controlled study measuring energy expenditure in postpubertal males cited reduced physical activity as the compensatory mechanism for low energy intake that is inadequate to meet their higher metabolic demands, which led to a suboptimal nutritional state. Although reduced physical activity may allow the energy balance to be maintained short term, a persistent energy deficit leads to growth retardation.

Pica, the compulsive ingestion of certain nonfood items or nonnutritive substances, is an unusual behavior that has been classically associated with iron deficiency and lead poisoning. There appears to be an unusually high incidence of pica in children with SCD especially those with low hemoglobin levels and high reticulocyte counts (Ivascu et al, 2001). Further studies to determine the etiology of pica in SCD are under way.

BOX 39-6

Aflac Children's Cancer and Blood Disorders Service: Sickle Cell Fluid Requirements

A CHILD NEEDS MORE FLUIDS WHEN:
1. He or she has a fever.
2. He or she has pain.
3. It's hot outside.
4. He or she is very active.
5. He or she is traveling.

AMOUNT OF CLEAR FLUIDS A CHILD NEEDS EACH DAY DURING SPECIAL TIMES

Child's Weight	Number of 8 oz Cups Per Day
10 lb (4.5 kg)	2 cups
15 lb (6.8 kg)	3 cups
20 lb (9 kg)	4 cups
25 lb (11.3 kg)	5 cups
30 lb (13.6 kg)	5-6 cups
35 lb (15.9 kg)	6-7 cups
40 lb (18.1 kg)	7 cups
50 lb (22.7 kg)	8 cups
60 lb (27.2 kg)	9 cups
More than 60 lb (27.2 kg)	10 or more cups

From Earles, A. (1991). *A parent's handbook for sickle cell disease (birth to 6 years).* Vienna, VA: National Maternal and Child Health Clearinghouse. Adapted with permission.

TABLE 39-2

Recommended Schedule of Pneumococcal Immunizations in Previously Unvaccinated Children with Sickle Cell Disease

Product Type	Age at First Dose	Primary Series	Additional Doses
PCV (Prevnar)	2-6 mo	3 doses 6-8 wk apart	1 dose at 12 to <16 mo
	7-11 mo	2 doses 6-8 wk apart	1 dose at 12 to <16 mo
	≥12 mo	2 doses 6-8 wk apart	—
PPV23 (Pneumovax)	≥24 mo	1 dose at least 6-8 wk after last PCV7 dose	1 dose, 3-5 yr after 1st PPV23 dose

Folic acid therapy, although controversial, is recommended (NIH, 2002). Supplemental iron therapy should not be prescribed unless a child is documented to have reduced iron stores as measured by serum iron, serum ferritin, and iron binding capacity.

Safety

Most children with sickle cell anemia regularly take oral medicines (e.g., folic acid, antibiotics, and narcotics) at home. Ingestion of narcotics beyond the prescribed amount could lead to lethargy and respiratory depression or death. All medicines should be safely stored. Adolescents should be cautioned about driving a car or using machinery while taking narcotics and be counseled that alcohol may potentiate the depressant effects of narcotics. Alcohol should also be avoided because it can cause dehydration and subsequent sickling. Smoking is strongly discouraged because it leads to vasoconstriction and concomitant problems. Parents should be cautioned about allowing exposure to reptiles as pets, due to risk of salmonella exposure (Lane & Buchanan, 2002).

Recreational activities that involve prolonged exposure to cold, prolonged exertion, or exposure to high altitudes (i.e., >10,000 feet) in an unpressurized aircraft should be avoided. Sports injuries should not be treated with ice because this can cause localized sickling.

Adolescents with SCD often demonstrate the same limit-testing and risk-taking behaviors as their unaffected peers. Parents must balance their child's need for safety with their child's need to become self-sufficient. An information card or Medic-Alert bracelet is often helpful in emergency situations.

Immunizations

The conventional schedule may be used for diphtheria-tetanus-acellular pertussis (DTaP) vaccine, inactivated poliomyelitis vaccine (IPV), measles-mumps-rubella (MMR) vaccine, varicella vaccine, and hepatitis B and Hib vaccines.

Pneumovax immunization against pneumococcal sepsis should be given at age 2 and 5 years with a booster 5 years after the last immunization (Lane & Buchanan, 2002). It is important to emphasize that even with vigilant immunization and antibiotic prophylaxis, episodes of pneumococcal septicemia have occurred.

Pneumovax may be given concurrently with the DTaP, IPV, MMR, influenza, and hepatitis B and Hib vaccines. Prevnar, the 7 valent pneumococcal vaccine, is now available to provide additional protection against pneumococcal sepsis for children with SCD younger than the age of 2 years. This vaccine should be given at age 2, 4, 6, and 12 months (Ledwith, 2001). Catch-up schedules for older children up to age 16 are noted in Table 39-2. Recent tests on children with SCD have demonstrated the efficacy of this vaccine by achieving antibody concentration comparable to antibodies in children without SCD (O'Brian et al, 2000).

Children with hemoglobinopathies are identified as being at risk for influenza-related complications. Children with SCD are also known to be at high risk for bacterial infection, which could occur associated with concurrent viral infection. Therefore it is recommended that all children with SCD receive influenza vaccine on an annual basis (Committee on Infectious Disease, 2000). Opinions on the use of meningococcal vaccine are divergent. Some centers suggest administering the vaccine to children older than 2 years of age, but this is not uniform among all comprehensive care centers. The AAP Committee on Infectious Diseases (2000) recommends the meningococcal vaccine for all individuals with asplenia.

Screening

Vision. During their first decade of life, children with SCD require routine screening. Thereafter they need an annual retinal examination by an ophthalmologist to screen for sickle retinopathy and possible intervention. If a child sustains any eye trauma, referral to an ophthalmologist for evaluation of increased intraocular pressure or retinal detachment is necessary.

Hearing. Routine audiologic evaluations are recommended to screen for hearing loss related to vasoocclusion or hyperviscosity in the inner ear. Sensorineural hearing loss has been occasionally described in this population.

Dental. Routine screening is recommended. Children with implanted venous devices, or history of rheumatic fever, mitral valve prolapse, diastolic murmurs or orthopedic prosthesis should receive prophylactic doses of amoxicillin prior to invasive procedures, including aggressive oral hygiene (Committee on Infectious Disease, 2000).

Blood Pressure. Blood pressure should be measured every year after 2 years of age. Although common in African-Americans, hypertension is uncommon in individuals with SCD. The reason for this is unclear. Most individuals have blood pressures lower than those of their unaffected peers, with differences increasing with age. The risk for occlusive stroke increases with rises in systolic—but not diastolic—pressure. Children with high blood pressure values relative to this population (e.g., 140/90) should be evaluated and considered for treatment (Pegelow et al, 1997).

Hemoglobin. Routine hemoglobin testing is deferred because CBC and reticulocyte counts are required as scheduled: every 4 to 6 months (every 3 to 4 months for SS and S β° thalassemia, and every 6 to 12 months for SC and S b+ thalassemia).

Urinalysis. Routine urinalysis screening is deferred because of condition-specific screening.

Tuberculosis. Routine screening is recommended.

Condition-Specific Screening

Pulse Oximetry. Readings should be obtained at every visit, noting changes from baseline. As children with sickle cell disease are susceptible to infections that may progress to ACS, a baseline reading is invaluable in determining divergence from the norm.

Sleep Apnea. Notation of snoring and a history of restless sleep should be obtained at each visit, noting episodes of daytime sleepiness. Enlarged tonsils or adenoids may be the culprit in inducing episodes of sleep apnea, and if found on sleep study, is an indication for surgical removal. Oxygen desaturation occurs during these episodes and is a trigger for sickling events.

Hematologic Screening. A CBC with differential, RBC smear, and reticulocyte count is useful in establishing baseline data and ascertaining bone marrow function. Determining the RBC phenotype of a well child who has not had a transfusion can expedite any future transfusions. Quantitative hemoglobin electrophoresis is obtained at 1 year to determine presence of fetal hemoglobin. Some comprehensive sickle cell centers test children during this time to correlate Hb F levels with clinical severity.

Renal Function Tsting. A urinalysis should be done and blood urea nitrogen (BUN) and creatinine levels checked annually after 3 years of age to monitor renal function. An inability to concentrate or acidify urine may be evident in the urinalysis and is commonly seen in children with SCD. Urobilinogen, a by-product of bilirubin metabolism, is also a frequent finding. Hematuria may be a manifestation of renal dysfunction secondary to SCD or other unrelated pathologic conditions.

These children should be referred to a nephrologist for further evaluation and treatment if the hematuria is severe or casts are present in the urine. Proteinuria is the most common and early clinical manifestation of glomerular injury to the kidney. Follow-up requires a urine culture and sensitivity, and—if negative—a 24-hour collection of urine for protein quantitation. An elevation requires referral to a nephrologist.

Lead Poisoning. Determining erythrocyte protoporphyrin (EP) levels to screen children who may be at high risk for lead intoxication is not valid for children with SCD. Total EP levels may be elevated with iron deficiency, lead intoxication, or reticulocytosis. In a child with SCD, an elevated EP level may reflect the process of accelerated reticulocytosis rather than lead intoxication. Free erythrocyte protoporphyrin (FEP) levels are elevated in children with SCD even in the absence of iron deficiency or lead poisoning. Furthermore, children with Hb SS have significantly higher FEP levels when compared with children with Hb SC, suggesting that higher rates of hemolysis may contribute to higher levels of FEP.

Scoliosis. Scoliosis screenings should be done through late adolescence because of the delayed growth spurts of children with SCD.

Cardiac Function. Electrocardiography (ECG) and echocardiography (ECHO) may be performed every 1 to 2 years after age 5 to evaluate the impact of chronic anemia on ventricular function. Efforts should be made to establish whether symptoms of chest pain, dyspnea, or decreased exercise tolerance have occurred, and significant symptoms should be evaluated with exercise testing. Functional murmurs are frequently heard in these children due to chronic anemia, and parents should be counseled as to their compensatory mechanism.

Liver Function. Yearly liver function studies are helpful to evaluate RBC metabolism and liver function. Bilirubin is often elevated as a consequence of hemolysis, as well as liver disease. Bilirubin levels rise gradually until the third decade of life. Scleral icterus and tea-colored urine are indicative of bilirubin produced by the chronic hemolysis and are frequently seen. Alkaline phosphatase levels fall after periods of most rapid growth in adolescence and reach lower levels in females than in males. Children on chronic transfusion programs are screened yearly for HIV and hepatitis C.

Common Illness Management
Differential Diagnosis (Box 39-7)

Fever. As a result of functional asplenia, bacterial infection is a significant cause of morbidity and mortality in children with SCD. The incidence of bacteremia in children with SCD is highest among those younger than 2 years of age and declines from age 2 to 6 years. The most common pathogen in children younger than 6 years of age is *Streptococcus pneumoniae*. Antibiotic resistance to *S. pneumoniae* has been reported (Committee on Infectious Disease, 2000). Some children with SCD have cultured *S. pneumoniae* from the tonsillar beds despite appropriate doses of prophylactic penicillin. Caregivers must be alert to these exceptions and closely monitor antibiotic effectiveness and compliance with penicillin prophylaxis. The course of *S. pneumoniae* sepsis is often fulminant, with mortality reaching 24% to 50%.

BOX 39-7
Criteria for In-patient Management

Seriously ill appearance
Hypotension
Severe abdominal pain
Poor perfusion
Temperature >40° C (>104° F)
Hemoglobin <5 g/dl
Leukocyte count >30,000/mm³ or <5,000/mm³
Platelet count <100,000/mm
Pain crisis that is unrelieved in 48 hours with home pain remedies
Dehydration by examination or history
Pulmonary infiltrate
Prior history of sepsis
No telephone or immediate access to the hospital
Poor or no track record with previous prescriptions or appointments
No prior training on monitoring for early signs of complications
Pulse oximeter ≤ lowest baseline reading

From Platt, O.S. (1997). The febrile child with sickle cell disease: a pediatricians' quandary. *J Pediatr, 130*, 693-694. Adapted with permission.

Escherichia coli bacteremia is often associated with urinary tract infection and *Salmonella* sp. bacteremia with osteomyelitis. Capillary blockage by sickle cells causes gut infarction, which—combined with defective function of the liver and spleen—allows for invasion by *Salmonella* sp. This invasion combined with expanded bone marrow and poor blood flow provides an ischemic focus for *Salmonella* sp. localization.

Fever is a common finding during vasoocclusive episodes, as well as during infectious episodes. There is no test or diagnostic tool to differentiate fever of an infectious origin from fever that results from inflammation secondary to infarction. Primary care providers must be aware of the fact that children may have two independent problems (e.g., infection and vasoocclusion), both of which require aggressive treatment and management. Some health care workers order CRP (C-reactive proteins), which might indicate an inflammatory reaction.

Any child having a temperature elevation (at or above 38.5° C) should be given appropriate antibiotic coverage and treated as an outpatient, provided that a probable source of temperature elevation can be identified, the child is stable, and looks well clinically. Careful follow-up at clinic visits in 24 and 48 hours with assurance of parental compliance is necessary for outpatient management.

Current treatment consists of prompt assessment of the child, followed by blood and urine cultures and administration of ceftriaxone or cefotaxime to all-ages children. These cephalosporins have a half-life of 8 to 9 hours (Wong, 2001), and effective bactericidal levels persist for 24 hours after a single dose. They are the ideal antibacterials for most of the bacterial pathogens likely to be associated with septic episodes in SCD, including *S. pneumoniae, Haemophilus* spp., and *Salmonella* spp. Children who appear toxic, have an extremely high fever and/or an unreliable caretaker, or to whom close outpatient follow-up is not possible should be hospitalized (see Box 39-7).

Fever is usually high with septicemia, but in as many as 20% of cases, the fever may be less than 39° C. All children with SCD should be considered at risk for fatal sepsis regardless of whether they are on penicillin prophylaxis and have received pneumococcal vaccinations.

An aggressive search for the cause of the fever should include a CBC count, blood culture, urinalysis, urine culture, chest radiograph, and possibly sinus radiographs if symptoms are suggestive of infection. Lumbar puncture should be performed if meningitis is suspected. Clinicians are increasingly aware of the development of penicillin-resistant organisms, which contribute to the difficulty of treating the child with a fever. Bacterial meningitis, suspected or proven to be caused by *S. pneumoniae,* should be treated with combination therapy of vancomycin and cefotaxime or ceftriaxone on all children at least 1 month of age. Based on culture and sensitivity results, penicillin or ceftriaxone should be continued and vancomycin discontinued if not needed. Rifampin is used if found to be sensitive to the offending organism (Committee on Infectious Diseases, 2000).

Even common infections such as otitis media or sinusitis may precipitate a vasoocclusive crisis if fluid intake is reduced and dehydration and acidosis result. During periods of illness, a child must be assessed frequently for early signs of crisis. Maintaining fluid intake and controlling fever are critical.

Urinary Tract Infections. Asymptomatic bacteriuria, symptomatic urinary tract infection, and pyelonephritis occur much more commonly in individuals with SCD than in the general population. A child with a urinary tract infection or pyelonephritis should have a blood culture obtained because bacteremia is present in at least 50% of those with a urinary tract infection. Appropriate antibiotic therapy should be instituted and adequate follow-up—including a repeat culture—arranged. Further diagnostic studies (e.g., renal ultrasound or voiding cystourethrogram) should be done to exclude treatable conditions in children with pyelonephritis or recurrent urinary tract infection.

Orthopedic Symptoms. Areas of bone infarction may be easily confused with osteomyelitis or rheumatologic disorders. Even after the diagnosis of SCD is made, it is important to differentiate areas of infarction from areas of infection because children with SCD have an increased incidence of osteomyelitis. With both pathologic processes, a child may have an elevated white blood cell count, fever, and equivocal radiographic findings. Osteomyelitis, however, is more often associated with an increased number of immature granulocytes, bacteremia, and a purulent joint aspirate. Bone scans may be useful in differentiating osteomyelitis from areas of bone infarction. Bone marrow scans have also been used to further discriminate areas of infection from those of infarction, especially when a bone scan is equivocal. Opinions on the use of bone marrow scans are somewhat divergent, however, and largely depend on the level of expertise available at a given facility.

Acute Gastroenteritis. Vomiting and diarrhea must be carefully evaluated and managed in children with SCD because these children lack the ability to concentrate urine to compensate for decreased fluid intake or excess losses. Significant dehydration may quickly occur and lead to metabolic acidosis and increased sickling. If a child's oral fluid intake is less than that needed to maintain hydration, the child must receive IV hydration.

Abdominal Pain. Episodes of infarction of the abdominal organs (e.g., the liver, spleen, and abdominal lymph nodes) occur and may be quite painful. These abdominal crises should be differentiated from problems that would require surgical intervention (e.g., appendicitis).

Abdominal pain and cramps found commonly in young children are possibly related to mesenteric ischemia. Normal bowel sounds and lack of ileus support nonoperative management with adequate pain control. The duration may last days to weeks, with fluctuations in the severity of the pain. Abdominal pain triggered by constipation is a common presenting complaint and may be treated with a combination of stool softeners and laxatives. Use of narcotics to treat VOC increase the risk of constipation, and bowel prophylaxis should be concurrent with pain management efforts.

Paralytic ileus is common during acute abdominal pain, making the diagnosis problematic. RUQ pain creates further complications because intrahepatic sickling mimics cholecystitis. Neither ultrasound nor laboratory values aid in defining the process. Leukocytosis of 30,000 can be seen with both infarction and infection. Most children find that their sickle cell pain has a unique quality or character and they can often report whether their pain is typical of vasoocclusive pain. Deviation from a characteristic pattern (i.e., lower abdominal pain with persistent local tenderness) with symptoms lasting several hours suggests a surgical problem.

Anemia. Virtually all children with SCD are anemic at baseline. A child with SCD may periodically have acute lethargy and pallor. CBC and reticulocyte counts should be obtained. If these reveal a significant drop in the hemoglobin and hematocrit levels, a child is probably experiencing an aplastic crisis or splenic sequestration. A fall in the hemoglobin and hematocrit values is usually a stimulus to the bone marrow, which then produces new RBCs in the form of reticulocytes. If the reticulocyte count is low in the presence of low hemoglobin and hematocrit levels, a child is experiencing an aplastic crisis. If a child has an enlarged spleen, pallor, lethargy, and an associated drop in hemoglobin, he or she is likely to be experiencing splenic sequestration. Regardless of exact diagnosis, the child will require immediate hospitalization with close observation and transfusion.

Respiratory Distress. Increased respiratory rate and effort, chest pain, fever, rales, and dullness to percussion may indicate pneumonia or ACS. Infiltrates on chest radiograph may reflect either process. With ACS the chest radiograph may be clear in the first few days, but a pleural effusion is often seen. These children should receive antibiotics, hydration, analgesics, and oxygen as needed. Transfusion or partial exchange transfusion may be indicated, depending on the degree of respiratory distress. ACS is a medical emergency and necessitates hospitalization.

Neurologic Changes. A child who has a seizure, hemiparesis, blurry or double vision, or changes in speech, gait, or level of consciousness should have expedient neurologic and radiologic evaluation for the presence of stroke. These neurologic changes are a medical emergency and require exchange transfusion as soon as possible.

Drug Interactions

Antihistamines and barbiturates given concurrently with narcotics may cause respiratory depression, hypoxia, and further sickling. Diuretics and some bronchodilators, which have a diuretic effect, may cause dehydration and sickling and should be used with caution in children with SCD. Children receiving narcotics for pain control should be given stool softeners and cautioned about the use of alcohol or other sedatives.

Developmental Issues

Sleep Patterns

Because of chronic anemia, some children with SCD may fatigue more easily than their unaffected peers and may desire extra sleep. Parents often report that their child with SCD naps after coming home from school—a routine that can be encouraged. Snoring, in combination with daytime sleepiness, is an indication for a sleep study to determine if obstruction from enlarged tonsils or adenoids exists, particularly if pulse oximetry readings are less than 90%.

Toileting

Toilet training should be initiated using the conventional guidelines to assess readiness for training. Bowel training usually progresses without difficulty. Bladder training progresses along normal lines in toddlers. Older children, however, may have difficulty concentrating urine and thus produce a large volume of dilute urine. This symptom is usually not seen until the second decade. Nevertheless, all children may need the opportunity to go to the toilet every 2 to 3 hours during the day. Primary enuresis often occurs in young children and commonly continues into the teenage years. It is especially troublesome when a child requires extra fluids during a vasoocclusive episode. Some children who previously achieved nighttime continence may develop secondary enuresis as subtle insults to the kidney occur. A pattern of enuresis typically emerges as a child begins having more "wet" than "dry" nights. This pattern may reflect the gradual loss of the kidneys' ability to concentrate urine. Daytime continence is unaffected by these renal changes.

Routine counseling regarding enuresis should be offered. Young children may initially use diapers. By the time a child reaches preschool or school age, however, the use of diapers often adversely affects the child's self-esteem and sense of mastery. Many families choose to wake the child once or twice during the night to urinate, but severe restriction of fluids is not wise because hydration needs must be met. Avoidance of caffeine ingestion during the evening hours may help prevent enuresis. Careful questioning by the primary care provider may point to a subclinical infectious process that can be treated.

Discipline

Expectations for the behavior of children with SCD should vary little from those held for their unaffected siblings or peers. These expectations should be as clear and consistent as possible. Likewise, parents should strive to make discipline fair and consistent. Many parents are fearful of disciplining or setting limits for their child with SCD, especially because emotional stress is thought to possibly precipitate a vasoocclusive crisis.

Primary care providers can point out to parents that a lack of or inconsistency in setting limits may be more stressful to a child than consistently set limits. Parents should also be encouraged to note which behaviors their child consistently demonstrates when in pain, (e.g., a certain pitch to his or her cry, a change in activity level, or changes in appetite) to help them discriminate episodes of pain from other behavior.

Child Care

Children with SCD can participate in normal daycare centers, although small group or home-centered daycare may be preferable because it provides less exposure to infections. Caregivers must be informed of a child's need for extra fluids and frequent need to void. They may also need to administer medications during daycare hours and must be instructed in this regard. Caregivers must be able to contact a parent or quickly seek medical care for the child in the event of fever, painful vasoocclusive crisis, respiratory distress, or symptoms of stroke, all of which may be life-threatening. Children attending daycare centers are at higher risk for acquiring community-based resistant infections (Armitage et al, 1999), so health care workers must take this into consideration when prescribing antibiotic coverage.

Schooling

Parents are encouraged to meet with school officials before the beginning of each school year to allow them to communicate about the usual symptoms their child has relative to SCD. A plan should be developed for absences, make-up work, intermittent home-bound study (if necessary), and transfer of assignments from school to the home. These children are frequently eligible for special education services (see Chapter 5).

Many primary care providers play an active role in educating school officials about the needs of children with SCD. Some visit schools and give presentations, and others provide written materials (see the list of resources at the end of this chapter). The needs for adequate hydration, frequent bathroom breaks, rest, physical education, and appropriate dress are all subjects for discussion by the health care team. School officials, in turn, can provide information about learning abilities and behavior. This open exchange of information helps to ensure a successful school year for the student. Knowing whom to call when parents cannot be reached reduces anxiety on the part of school staff.

As previously discussed, some children with SCD have declining IQs with increasing age. The conclusions of recent research support the need for early evaluation of *all* children with SCD because of their high risk for cognitive impairment (Thompson & Gustafson, 2002). Children with SCD who have had strokes should be referred for an individualized education program (IEP) (see Chapter 5). Children with splenomegaly should be cautioned about the risks for injury with contact sports. Modified physical education classes should be offered to keep these children engaged in group activities, which are important to their overall adjustment and well-being. Finally, school personnel should be counseled about the needs of children affected with chronic orthopedic problems (e.g., osteomyelitis or avascular necrosis of the femoral head). These

children may need additional time to get to classes, or may need to obtain an elevator key during times of bone healing.

Sexuality

Children with SCD progress through the Tanner stages in an orderly and consistent manner but usually experience puberty several years later than their unaffected peers, which can have significant adverse effects on their self-concepts. Once sexual maturation has occurred, fertility and contraception are important issues that must be addressed by primary care providers. For men, impotence is often a problem after a major episode of priapism. For female adolescents, menarche is often delayed by 2 to $2\frac{1}{2}$ years, but fertility is normal. Decisions about contraception must take into account the attitudes, lifestyle, and maturity of the adolescent, as well as the hematologic ramifications of the method chosen.

Various contraceptive choices are available to adolescents with SCD, including all barrier forms of contraception (e.g., condoms for men, and foam and diaphragms for women). Women may also use oral contraceptives, preferably those brands containing low levels of estrogen.

Progesterone-only pills are useful because progestins stabilize the red cell membrane. Medroxyprogesterone (Depo-Provera) has also been used in this population and is the method of preference (American College of Obstetrics and Gynecology [ACOG], 2000). Adolescents with SCD should receive careful, repeated genetic counseling before puberty and during adolescence. They need to understand the pattern of transmission of SCD and the availability of testing for partners before conceiving a child.

Transition to Adulthood

Early vocational counseling should be offered to children and adolescents with SCD. Consideration should be directed toward the child or adolescent's interests and intellectual abilities. Work in a climate-controlled environment is preferred over rigorous outdoor work, which might trigger a crisis. SCD excludes a person from military service, so technical and academic training is encouraged. Many community-based sickle cell organizations offer scholarships for skilled and academic work. The Sickle Cell Disease Association of America, Inc. can direct families to local resources.

Families should be counseled about the progressive organ damage that develops as a child ages. Continuity of care by a knowledgeable primary care provider will afford the best quality of life and should be encouraged.

Insurance companies may deem individuals with SCD uninsurable. Local Sickle Cell Foundation chapters can provide counseling to such people about options and resources.

Family Concerns and Resources

The families of children with SCD experience the same psychologic ramifications as other families of children with chronic conditions, often in the context of limited resources. These families bear the additional burden of knowing that this disease is genetically transmitted. This knowledge can prompt feelings of overwhelming guilt and responsibility.

Exacerbations of the condition often occur without provocation, prompting feelings of helplessness. One study found 49% of parents of children with SCD surveyed to be clinically depressed (Kramer & Nash, 1995). Many manifestations of the condition are not objectively visible or measurable; therefore, children with SCD can appear to be well when they are potentially extremely ill. Many parents are fearful that the therapeutic effects of narcotics and blood transfusions will be outweighed by their potentially deleterious effects. Genetic counseling should be offered to the parents of a child with SCD at the time of the child's diagnosis and when subsequent pregnancies are contemplated. Beyond the African-American population, permeations of sickle hemoglobinopathies are found in Hispanics, Central Americans, Greeks, Arabs, Asians, and Caribbean natives. Each of these individuals brings his or her own view of health, coping, and wellness. Primary care providers must be mindful of the differences within and between cultures. Emphasis should focus on the different strengths families bring with them. For example, extended family support is a dominant feature in the African-American community and should play a role during crisis episodes.

Researchers show that African-American families prefer to use their family members as sources of support instead of using formal support groups. Among many minorities, close friends are considered kin and fulfill some functions of extended family members. When working with minority families, primary care providers need to explore and understand the effects of ethnicity on the family's daily life. Such understanding seeks out cultural practices (e.g., male and female roles and African-American language, communication styles, and family rituals). Instructions should be delivered to the head of the household. In contrast to the matriarchal leadership found in many African-American households, Muslim families center their decision making on the father or male head of the household. Strong church affiliations are often in place and offer consolation and hope, leading to greater acceptance and improved quality of life.

Individuals espousing the Jehovah's Witnesses religion will deny blood transfusions to their children, placing stress on the primary care provider. Sensitive open communication and vigilant intensive care management may prevent the need for transfusions and thereby support the religious beliefs of the family. In all instances, members of a particular ethnic or minority group should be consulted when actions or choices conflict with those of the medical care team.

RESOURCES

Note that these listings are not all inclusive. Additional material may be available from your own state or local health department, sickle cell agency, or community agency.

A Parents' Handbook for Sickle Cell Disease, Part I: Birth to 6 Years and Part II: 6 to 18 Years.
Books available from National Maternal and Child Health Clearinghouse
8201 Greensboro Drive
McLean, VA 22102
(703) 821-8955

Sickle Cell Disease Association of America (SCDAA)
200 Corporate Pointe, Suite 495
Culver City, CA 90230-7633
(800) 421-8453
www.sicklecelldisease.org
Sickle Cell Disease—How to Help Your Child to Take It in Stride
A Parent/Teacher Guide
Viewpoints

Also available from this organization are brochures on recent advances; a newsletter on chapter activities; fact sheets; brochures on sickle cell trait, anemia, and other topics; home study kits; games; and a video on parenting.

March of Dimes Birth Defects Foundation
1275 Mamaroneck Avenue
White Plains, NY 10605
(888) 663-4637
www.marchofdimes.com
Thalassemia Information Sheet
Sickle Cell Anemia Public Health Information Sheet
Anemia de células falciformes

National Heart, Lung and Blood Institute Information Center
PO Box 30105
Bethesda, MD 20824-0105
(301) 592-8573
www.nhlbi.nih.gov
Facts about Sickle Cell Anemia
The Management of Sickle Cell Anemia
Hydroxyurea in Pediatric Patients with Sickle Cell Disease

National Organization for Rare Disorders, Inc. (NORD)
PO Box 8923
New Fairfield, CT 06812-8923
(800) 999-6673
www.rarediseases.org

Hemoglobin S Allele and Sickle Cell Disease
Centers for Disease Control and Prevention
www.cdc.gov

The Child with Sickle Cell Disease: A Teaching Manual
Vedro, D. & Morrison, R. Texas Dept. of Health.
New Patient and Parent Guidebook: Hope and Destiny.
Georgia Sickle Cell Center
www.SCInfo.org

Sickle Cell Tutorial
The Sickle Cell Slime-orama Game
www.starbright.org

NIH Science Education Partnership Award Program
www.ncrr.nih.gov/clinical/cr_sepa.asp

Kids Health from the Nemours Foundation
Kids site: www.kidshealth.org

Children's Hospital Oakland Research Institute
5700 Martin Luther King Jr. Way
Oakland, CA 94609-1673
(510) 450-7605

Sibling Cord Blood
www.chori.org/siblingcordblood/index.html

Summary of Primary Care Needs for the Child with Sickle Cell Disease

HEALTH CARE MAINTENANCE

Growth and Development

Children with SCD tend to weigh less and be shorter than their peers. Weight is affected more than height, and males are affected more than females. Weight and height should be checked and plotted every 3 to 4 months.

Puberty is delayed for both sexes with Hb SS.

Developmental impairment varies. Microvascular occlusion may produce subclinical deficits. Fine motor and visual motor tasks often are affected. Developmental delays found on screening must be assessed further.

Diet

Diet should be well balanced with a generous amount of fluid; fluid intake should be increased during febrile illness, times of increased activity, dehydration, traveling, hot weather, or in pain crisis.

Increased metabolic demands require additional protein, micronutrients, and food for energy. Increased metabolic demands often result in reduced physical activity.

Pica more common in children with SCD than other children.

Folic acid supplements are encouraged.

Safety

Ingestion of narcotics could lead to respiratory depression. All medications must be safely stored.

Alcohol may dehydrate and potentiate narcotics.

Narcotics may impair driving or safe use of machinery.

Smoking or exposure to secondhand smoke will increase vasoconstriction and should be avoided.

Reptile pets increase risk of salmonella exposure.

Recreational activities that involve prolonged exposure to cold, prolonged exertion, or exposure to high altitudes should be avoided. Ice should not be used to treat injuries.

Adolescent risk-taking behavior may increase complications.

A Medic-Alert bracelet may be helpful.

Immunizations

Routine schedule for immunizations is recommended.

Prevnar should be given as scheduled. Pneumovax (23 valent) vaccine should be given at 24 months, with a single booster given at 5 years.

An annual influenza vaccine is strongly recommended.

Meningococcal vaccine is recommended for all children with asplenia.

Screening

Vision. Routine screening is recommended until 8 years of age, and then annual retinal examinations are recommended to rule out sickle retinopathy. If a child sustains eye trauma he or she must be referred to an ophthalmologist to rule out increased intraocular pressure or retinal detachment.

Hearing. Routine audiology examination is recommended. Children with SCD have a higher incidence of hearing loss, and failure on the screening examination warrants a referral for further testing.

Dental. Routine screening is recommended.

Blood Pressure. Blood pressure should be measured yearly after 2 years of age. Lower pressure readings for age are expected. An increase in systolic pressure increases risk of stroke.

Hematocrit. Hematocrit is deferred because of condition-specific screening.

Urinalysis. Urinalysis is deferred because of condition-specific screening.

Tuberculosis. Routine screening is recommended.

Condition-Specific Screening

Pulse Oximetry. Readings should be obtained at every visit to establish baseline and to note changes.

Sleep Apnea. Sleep apnea may lead to decreased oxygenation, which can trigger a sickling event. Children with a history of snoring or daytime sleepiness should be evaluated.

Hematologic Screening. A CBC with differential, platelet count, reticulocyte count, and RBC smear should be checked every 6 to 12 months.

Renal Function Screening. BUN and creatinine levels should be checked and a urinalysis done yearly. A child should be referred to a urologist if severe hematuria or casts are found in urine.

Lead Poisoning. Lead screening using the EP level is unreliable; the serum lead level must be determined.

Scoliosis. Screening should be extended to the late teens because of delayed puberty.

Cardiac Function. Both ECG and ECHO should be used every 1 to 2 years after age 5 years.

Liver Function. Serum liver function tests should be done yearly. The gallbladder should be assessed via ultrasound every 2 years after age 10 and then as necessary.

Transfused children should be tested for hepatitis C.

COMMON ILLNESS MANAGEMENT

Differential Diagnosis

Fever. If a child is younger than age 5 years and has a temperature below 38.5° C, outpatient management may be considered if the source of the fever can be identified, appropriate antibiotics are given, follow-up is ensured, and child does not appear toxic.

If a child is younger than 5 years of age and has a temperature above 38.5° C, he or she should be promptly assessed, cultures taken, and ceftriaxone administered IM or IV; the child should be reassessed in 24 and 48 hours.

If a child is older than 5 years of age, the child's condition, compliance with therapy, and ability to obtain follow-up determine whether the child should receive in- or outpatient care.

Even common infections may precipitate a vasoocclusive crisis. All children with SCD should be considered at risk for fatal sepsis.

Urinary Tract Infections. Asymptomatic bacteriuria, urinary tract infections, and pyelonephritis are more common with SCD.

Blood cultures should be done to rule out bacteremia if a urinary tract infection is diagnosed.

Treatment must cover cultured organisms, and follow-up is essential.

Continued

Summary of Primary Care Needs for the Child with Sickle Cell Disease—cont'd

Orthopedic Symptoms. It is difficult to differentiate bone infarction from osteomyelitis or rheumatologic disorders. MRI studies are used to identify bone marrow infarction.

Acute Gastroenteritis. Significant dehydration may occur quickly and lead to acidosis and sickling. If oral intake is inadequate, IV hydration is needed.

Abdominal Pain. Abdominal pain crises may be differentiated from surgical problems by evaluating fever, hematologic changes, peristalsis, and response to symptomatic, supportive therapy.

Anemia. Hemoglobin and hematocrit levels significantly lower than baseline may reflect aplastic crisis, hyperhemolytic crisis, or splenic sequestration. Splenic sequestration and aplasia may be life-threatening.

Respiratory Distress. It is important that individuals are evaluated for ACS, which may be fulminant and require exchange transfusion.

Neurologic Changes. Neurologic changes may indicate stroke. Rapid, thorough evaluation is critical. Exchange transfusion should be performed as quickly as possible if stroke occurs.

Drug interactions

Antihistamines, alcohol, and barbiturates may potentiate sedation with narcotics.

Diuretics and bronchodilators, which may have diuretic effects, may cause dehydration and sickling. Stool softeners are useful while on narcotics.

DEVELOPMENTAL ISSUES

Sleep Patterns

Children may require naps through school age. History of snoring and daytime sleepiness is indication for sleep apnea studies.

Toileting

Enuresis is often a long-term issue because of the kidneys' inability to concentrate urine. Fluids should not be restricted. Nocturia may persist.

Discipline

Expectations should be consistent, fair, and similar to those of unaffected peers and siblings.

Parents often fear emotional stress will stimulate a vasooclusive crisis.

Child Care

Small daycare programs decrease exposure to infections.

Caregivers must be mindful of fluid requirements and the importance of maintaining normal body temperature. Child care personnel must be able to administer medicines and contact parents for emergent symptoms of crisis.

Schooling

These children may have frequent, unpredictable absences. A plan should be established to assist child with schoolwork missed. Children with SCD are eligible for special education services.

They need access to fluids and liberal bathroom privileges.

They may participate in mainstream physical education but should be cautioned about abdominal injury if they have splenomegaly.

Sexuality

Puberty may be delayed. Women usually have normal fertility but have some special contraceptive concerns. Men are often impotent after an episode of priapism.

Genetic counseling is important.

Transition to Adulthood

Early vocational counseling is recommended.

Continuity of care is important due to gradual organ failure. Insurance problems may be encountered.

FAMILY CONCERNS AND RESOURCES

Because SCD is genetically transmitted, there is a need for genetic counseling, as well as support for feelings of guilt and responsibility.

Support for cultural beliefs and family structure are important components of long-term care.

REFERENCES

Adams, R.J., et al. (1998). Prevention of a first stroke by transfusion in children with sickle cell anemia and abnormal results on transcranial doppler. *New Engl J Med, 33*, 5-11.

Adams, R.J. (2000). Lessons from the Stroke Prevention Trial in Sickle Cell Anemia (STOP) study. *J Child Neurol, 15*(5), 344-349.

Adams-Graves, P., et al. (1997). Rheoth Rx (Poloxamer 188) injection for the acute painful episode of sickle cell disease: a pilot study. *Blood, 90*(5), 2041-2046.

American College of Obstetrics and Gynecology. (2000). ACOG practice bulletin: the use of hormonal contraception in women with coexisting medical conditions. No. 18, 93-106. Washington, DC: Author.

Armitage, K., et al. (1999). Respiratory infections: which antibiotics for empiric therapy? *Patient Care for the Nurse Practitioner, 2*(1), 30-46.

Ballas, S. & Saidi, P. (1997). Thrombosis, megaloblastic anaemia and sickle cell disease: a unified hypothesis. *Brit J Haemotol, 96*(4), 879-880.

Ballas, S.K. (1999). Erythropoietic activity in patients with sickle cell anemia before and after treatment with hydroxyurea. *Brit J Haemotol, 105*(2), 491-496.

Ballas, S.K. (2002). Sickle cell anemia: progress in pathogenesis and treatment. *Drugs, 62*(8), 1143-1172.

Benjamin, L.J., et al. (1999). *Guideline for the management of acute and chronic pain in sickle-cell disease.* Jacox, Phd Rd (Ed.), APS Guideline Series, No. 1 Glenview, IL.

Blumenthal, D.T. & Glenn, M.J. (2002). Neurological manifestations of systemic disease. *Neurologic Clin, 20*(1), 265-281.

Brinker, M.R., et al. (1998). Bone mineral density of the lumbar spine and proximal femur is decreased in children with sickle cell anemia. *Am J Orthop*, 43-49.

Buchanan, G.R. (1994). Infection. In S.H. Embury, R.P. Hebbel, & N. Mohandas (Eds.), *Sickle cell disease: basic principles and clinical practice.* Philadelphia: Raven Press.

Cackovic, M., Chung, C., Bolton, L.L., & Kerstein, M.D. (1998). Leg ulceration in the sickle cell patient. *J Am Coll Surg, 187*(3), 307-309.

Charache, S. (1996). Experimental therapy. *Hematol/Oncol Clin North Am, 10*(6), 1373-1382.

Charahe, S., Lubin, B., & Reid, C.D. (1995). *Management and therapy of sickle cell disease, NIH publication no. 95-2117.* Washington, DC: U.S. Government Printing Office

Chui, D. & Dover, G. (2001). Sickle cell disease: no longer a single gene disorder. *Curr Opin Pediatr, 13,* 23-37.

Committee on Genetics. (1996). Health supervision for children with sickle cell disease and their Families. *Pediatrics, 98*(3), 467-472.

Committee on Infectious Diseases. (2000). *Red book: Report on the committee on infectious diseases* (25th ed.). Evanston, IL: Author.

Covitz, W. (1994). Cardiac disease. In S.H. Embury, R.P. Hebbel, & N. Mohandas (Eds.), *Sickle cell disease: basic principles and clinical practice.* New York: Raven Press.

Davis, H., Schoendorf, K.C., Gergen, P.J., & Moore Jr., R.M. (1997). National trends in the mortality of children with sickle cell disease, 1968-1992. *Am J Pub Health, 87*(8), 1317-1322.

DeBaun, M.R., et al. (1998). Cognitive screening examinations for silent cerebral infarcts in sickle cell disease. *Neurology, 50*(6), 1678-1682.

Eckman, J.R. & Platt, A.F. (1991). *Problem oriented management of sickle syndromes.* Atlanta: NIH Sickle Cell Center.

Embury, S.H., Hebbel, R.P., & Mohandas, N. (Eds.). (1994). *Sickle cell disease: basic principles and clinical practice.* New York: Raven Press.

Falletta, J.M., et al. (1995). Discontinuing penicillin prophylaxis in children with sickle cell anemia. *J Pediatr, 127,* 685-690.

Ferrera, P.C., Curran, C.B., & Swanson, H. (1997). Etiology of pediatric ischemic stroke. *Am J Emerg Med, 15*(7), 671-679.

French, J.A. 2nd, et al. (1997). Mechanisms of stroke in sickle cell disease: sickle erythrocytes decrease cerebral blood flow in rats after nitric oxide synthase inhibition. *Blood, 89*(12), 4591-4599.

Fung, E.B., et al. (2001). Effect of hydroxyurea therapy on resting energy expenditure in children with sickle cell disease. *J Ped Hematol Oncol, 23*(9), 604-608.

Gentry, B. & Dancer, J. (1997a). Failure rates of young patients with sickle cell disease on a hearing screening test. *Perception and Motor Skills, 84,* 434.

Gentry, B. & Dancer, J. (1997b). Screening the speech of young patients with sickle cell disease. *Perception and Motor Skills, 84,* 662.

Groce, N.E. & Zola, I.K. (1993). Multiculturalism, chronic illness, and disability. *Pediatrics 91*(5 part 2), 1048-1055.

Hakim, L.S., Hashmat, A.I., & Macchia, R.J. (1994). Priapism. In S.H. Embury, R.P. Hebbel, & N. Mohandas (Eds.), *Sickle cell disease: basic principles and clinical practice.* New York: Raven Press.

Hatcher, R.A. (1994). *Contraceptive technology* (16th ed.). New York: Irvinton Press.

Hockenberry, M. & Coody, D. (Eds.). (1986). *Pediatric oncology and hematology: perspectives on care.* St Louis: Mosby.

Ivascu, N.S., et al. (2001). Characterization of pica prevalence among patients with sickle cell disease. *Arch Ped Adol Med, 155*(11), 1243-1247.

Jenkins, T.L. (2002). Sickle cell anemia in the pediatric intensive care unit: novel approaches for managing life-threatening complications. *AACN Clin Issues, 13*(2), 154-168.

Johnson, R.B. (1997). Folic acid: new dimensions of an old friendship. *Adv Pediatr, 44,* 236-238.

Kean, L.S., et al. (2002). A cure for murine sickle cell disease through stable mixed chimerism and tolerance induction after non-myeloablative conditioning and major histocompatibilty complex-mismatched bone marrow transplant. *Blood, 99*(5): 1840-1849.

Kelly, P., Kurtzberg, J., Vichinsky, E., & Lubin, B. (1997). Umbilical cord blood stem cells: application for the treatment of patients with hemoglobinopathies. *J Pediatr, 130*(5): 695-703.

Kramer K. & Nash K. (1995). *The prevalence of depression among a sample of parents of children with sickle cell disease.* Annual Meeting of Sickle Cell Disease Programs, Boston.

Lane, P.A. & Buchanan, G.A. (2002). Health supervision with children with sickle cell disease. *Pediatrics, 109*(3), 526-34.

Lawrence, P.R. & Ryan, K.M. (2000). Sickle cell disease in children. *Advance for NP,* 48-57.

Ledwith, M. (2001). Pneumococcal conjugate vaccine. *Curr Opin Pediatr, 13,* 70-74.

Lee, S.J., Churchill, W.H., & Bridges, K R. (1995). *Bone marrow infarcts of severe atypical pain in sickle cell crisis: diagnosis by magnetic resonance imaging and treatment with exchange transfusion.* Abstract presented at the 20th Annual Meeting of the National Sickle Cell Disease Program. Boston, March 18-21.

Liu, H., Agarwal, S., Kmiec, E., & Davis, B.R. (2002). Target beta globin gene conversion in human hematopoietic CD 34(+) and lin (-)CD38(-) cells. *Gene Ther, 9*(2), 118-126.

Logan, D.E., Radcliffe, J., & Smith-Whitley, K. (2002). Parent factors and adolescent sickle cell disease: associations with patterns of health service use. *J Pediatr Psychol, 27*(5), 475-484.

Mantadakis, E., Cavender, J.D., Rogers, Z.R., Ewalt, D.H., & Buchanan, G.R. (1999). Prevalence of priapism in children and adolescents with sickle cell anemia. *Am J Pediatr Hematol Oncol, 21,* 518-522.

McCune, S.L., Reilly, M.P., Chomo, M.J., Asakura, T., & Townes, T M. (1994). Recombinant human hemoglobins designed for gene therapy of sickle cell disease. *Proc Nat Acad Sci U S A, 91*(21), 9852-9856.

Miller, D.R. & Baehner, R.L. (Eds.) (1990). *Blood diseases of infancy and childhood.* St Louis: Mosby.

Miller, S.T., et al. (2000). Prediction of adverse outcomes of children with sickle cell disease. *N Engl J Med, 342,* 83-89.

Modege, O. & Ifenu, S.A. (1993). Growth retardation in homozygous sickle cell disease: role of caloric intake and possible gender related differences. *Am J Hematol, 44,* 149-154.

National Institutes of Health, Division of Blood Diseases and Resources. (2002). *The management of sickle cell disease, NIH publication 02-2117* (4th ed.). Washington, DC: U.S. Government Printing Office.

O'Brien, K.L., et al. (2000). Safety and immunogenicity of heptavalent pneumococcal vaccine conjugated to crm 197 among infants with sickle cell disease. *Pediatrics, 106*(5), 965-972.

Ohene-Frempong, K. & Smith-Whitley, K. (1997). Use of hydroxyurea in children with sickle cell disease: what comes next? *Sem Hematol, 34*(Suppl. 3), 30-41.

Ohene-Frempong, K., et al. (1998). The co-operative study of sickle cell disease cerebrovascular accidents in sickle cell disease: rate and risk factors. *Blood, 91*(1), 288-294.

Oswaldo, C., Brambilla, D., & Thorington, B. (1994). The cooperative study of sickle cell disease: the acute chest syndrome in sickle cell disease: incidence and risk factors. *Blood, 84*(2), 643-649.

Pawliuk, R., et al. (2001). Correction of sickle cell disease in transgenic mouse models by gene therapy. *Science, 294*(5550), 2368-2371.

Pegelow, C.H., et al. (1997). Natural history of blood pressure in sickle cell disease: risks for strokes and death associated with relative hypertension in sickle cell anemia. *Am J Med, 102*(2), 171-177.

Pegelow, C.H., et al. (2001). Silent infarcts in children with sickle cell anemia and abnormal cerebral artery velocity. *Arch Neurol, 58*(12), 2017-2021.

Platt, O.S. (1997). The febrile child with sickle cell disease: a pediatrician's quandary. *J Pediatr, 130,* 693-694.

Powars, D.R. (1975). Natural history of sickle cell disease—the first 10 years. *Sem Hematol, 12,* 267-281.

Powars, D.R., Meiselman, H.J., Fisher, T.C., Hiti, A., & Johnson, C. (1994). Beta-S gene cluster haplotype modulate hematologic and hemorrheologic expression in sickle cell anemia: use in predicting clinical severity. *Am J Pediatr Hematol Oncol, 16*(1), 55-61.

Powars, D.R., et al. (1999). Cerebral vasculopathy in sickle cell anemia: diagnostic contribution of positron emission tomography. *Blood, 93*(1), 71-79.

Rao, R. & Kramer, L. (1993). Stress and coping among mothers of infants with a sickle cell condition. *Childrens Healthcare, 22,* 169-188.

Rajkumar, K., et al. (1995). *Elevated levels of erythrocyte protoporphyrin (FEP) in children with sickle cell disease in the absence of lead poisoning or iron deficiency.* Abstract presented at the 20th Annual Meeting of the National Sickle Cell Disease Program. Boston, March 18-21.

Reed, W. & Vichinsky, E.P. (2001). Transfusion therapy: a coming-of-age treatment for patients with sickle cell disease. *J Pediatr Hematol Oncol, 23*(4) 197-202.

Richard, H. & Burlew, K. (1997). Academic performance among children with sickle cell disease: setting minimum standards for comparison groups. *Psychol Rep, 81,* 27-34.

Rodgers, G.P. (1994). Pharmacologic modulation of fetal hemoglobin. In S.H. Embury, R.P. Hebbel, & N. Mohandas (Eds.), *Sickle cell disease: basic principles and clinical practice.* New York: Raven Press.

Scothorn, D.J., et al. (2002). Risk of recurrent stroke in children with sickle cell disease receiving blood transfusion therapy for at least five years after initial stroke. *J Pediatr, 140*(3), 348-354.

Serjeant, G.R. (1995). Natural history and determinants of clinical severity of sickle cell disease. *Curr Opin Hematol, 2,* 103-108.

Shapiro, B. & Ballas, S.K. (1994). The acute painful episode. In S.H. Embury, R.P. Hebbel, & N. Mohandas (Eds.), *Sickle cell disease: basic principles and clinical practice.* New York: Raven Press.

Space, S.L., Lane, P.A., Pickett, C.K., & Weil, J.V. (2000). Nitric oxide attenuates normal and sickle red blood cell adherence to pulmonary endothelium. *Am J Hematol, 63*(4), 200-204.

Steinburg, M.H., et al. (1997). Cellular effects of hydroxyurea in Hbg SC disease. *Brit J Haematol, 98*(4), 838-844.

Steinburg, M.H. & Embury, S.H. (1994). Natural history: overview. In S.H. Embury, R.P. Hebbel, & N. Mohandas (Eds.), *Sickle cell disease: basic principles and clinical practice.* New York: Raven Press.

Steinberg, M.H. & Mohandas, N. (1994). Laboratory values. In S.H. Embury, R.P. Hebbel, & N. Mohandas (Eds.), *Sickle cell disease: basic principles and clinical practice.* New York: Raven Press.

Sterling, Y., Peterson, J., & Weekes, D.P. (1997). American families with chronically ill children: oversights and insights. *J Pediatr Nurs, 12*(5), 292-300.

Styles, L. & Vinchinsky, E. (1997). New therapies and approaches to transfusion in sickle cell disease in children. *Curr Opin Pediatr, 9*, 41-45.

Thompson, R.J. & Gustafson, K.E. (2002). Neurocognitive development of young children with sickle cell disease through 3 years of age. *J Pediatr Psych, 27*(3), 235-244.

Vermylen, C. & Cornu, G. (1997). Hematopoietic stem cell transplantation for sickle cell anemia. *Curr Opin Hematol, 4*, 377-380.

Vernacchio, L., et al. (1998). Combined schedule of 7-valent pneumococcal conjugate vaccine followed by 23-valent pneumococcal vaccine in children and young adults with sickle cell disease. *J Pediatr, 133*(2), 275-278.

Vichinsky, E.P. (1991). Comprehensive care in sickle cell disease: its impact on morbidity and mortality. *Semin Hematol, 28*(3), 220-226.

Vichinsky, E.P. (1997a). Hydroxyurea in children: present and future. *Sem Hematol, 34*(Suppl. 3), 22-29, 1997a.

Vichinsky, E.P., et al. (1995). A comparison of conservative and aggressive transfusion regimes in the perioperative management of sickle cell disease. *New Engl J Med, 333*, 206-213.

Walters, M. (1999). Bone marrow transplantation for sickle cell disease: where do we go from here? *J Pediatr Hematol Oncol, 21*(6), 467-474.

Walters, M.C., et al. (2000). Impact of bone marrow transplant for symptomatic sickle cell disease: an interim report. *Blood, 95*, 1918-1924.

Wang, W.C., Grover, R., Gallagher, D., Espeland, M., & Fandal, A. (1993). Developmental screening in young children with sickle cell disease. Results of a cooperative study. *J Pediatr Hematol Oncol, 15*(1), 87-91.

Wang, W.C., et al. (1991). High risk of recurrent stroke after discontinuance of 5 to 12 years of transfusion therapy in patients with sickle cell disease. *J Pediatr, 118*, 377-382.

Wang, W.C., et al. (2001). A 2 yr. pilot trial of hydroxyurea in very young children with sickle cell anemia. *J Pediatr, 139*, 6, 790-796.

Wang, W.C. & Enos, L. (2001). Neuropsychologic performance in school age children with sickle cell disease: a report from the cooperative study of sickle cell disease. *J Pediatr, 139*, 3.

Ware, R.E., et al. (2002). Predictors of fetal hemoglobin response in children with sickle cell anemia receiving hydroxyurea therapy. *Blood, 99*(1), 10-14.

Wethers, D. (2000). Sickle cell disease in childhood: Part II. Diagnosis and treatment of major complications and recent advances in treatment. *Am Fam Physician, 63*, 6.

Wigfall, D.R., Ware, R.E., Burchinal, M.R., Kinney, T.R., & Foreman, J.W. (2000). Prevalence and clinical correlates of glomerulopathy in children with sickle cell disease. *J Pediatr, 136*(6), 749-753.

Wong, D.L. (1995). *Nursing care of infants and children* (5th ed.). St Louis: Mosby.

Wong, W.Y. (2001). Prevention and management of infection in children with sickle cell anemia. *Paediatr Drugs, 3*(11), 793-801.

40 Tourette's Syndrome and Obsessive-Compulsive Disorder

Naomi A. Schapiro

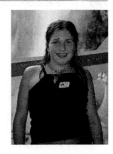

Etiology

Tourette's syndrome (TS) is a neurobiologic condition characterized by vocal and motor tics that change over time and wax and wane in severity. Obsessive-compulsive disorder (OCD) is a neuropsychiatric condition characterized by recurrent and persistent thoughts that are experienced by the individual as intrusive, inappropriate, and distressing and by repetitive behaviors or mental acts that are aimed at preventing or reducing the distress (American Psychiatric Association, 2000). Whereas OCD is usually classified as an anxiety disorder and TS as a movement disorder, there are several reasons for including the two conditions in the same chapter: Recent studies have indicated that the same areas of the brain are involved in both conditions; genetic and family studies have linked the two conditions; and there is a disproportionate number of children who have both diagnoses, suggesting a common or related origin.

TS is part of a spectrum of tic disorders, including transient tic disorder and chronic tic disorder (Table 40-1). Tics can be defined as "sudden, repetitive, stereotyped motor movements or phonic productions that involve discrete muscle groups" (Leckman et al, 1999, p. 24). Tics are exaggerations and repetitions of normal movements, in contrast with other movement disorders, such as chorea or dystonias (Bagheri et al, 1999; Leckman et al, 2001). Primary tics such as TS have no identifiable cause or may be genetic in origin (Jankovic, 2001). Conditions that could cause secondary tics include head trauma, encephalitis, and some medications. There is an increased incidence of tics in children with pervasive developmental disorder (Kiessling, 2001), although tics can sometimes be confused with the stereotypic movements common to children with autism (Rapin, 2001).

If symptoms of either motor or vocal tics, but not both, persist for more than 1 year, the child would be considered to have a chronic tic disorder (Leckman et al, 2001). Children with both vocal and motor tics that persist for more than 1 year generally fulfill the criteria for Tourette syndrome (American Psychiatric Association, 2000). Diagnosis is based on history and observation, with no specific diagnostic tests available (Bagheri et al, 1999; Kiessling, 2001). See Box 40-1 for the DSM-IV-TR criteria for TS.

The DSM-IV-TR (American Psychiatric Association, 2000) defines obsessive-compulsive disorder as obsessions or compulsions that are recognized by the individual as excessive or unreasonable, cause marked distress, interfere with normal functioning and/or take more than 1 hour a day, and are not restricted to symptoms of another disorder (e.g., food in eating disorder). Younger children frequently lack insight into the unreasonableness of their obsessions or compulsions (Geller, 1998), and this insight is not required for the diagnosis of OCD in children (American Psychiatric Association). See Box 40-2 for the DSM-IV-TR criteria for OCD.

As conditions that straddle the boundaries between voluntary and involuntary (Cohen & Leckman, 1999), TS and OCD have been claimed by both neurology and psychiatry. When the

---

TABLE 40-1
Tics and Tic Disorders

	Onset	Description	Prevalence	Diagnostic Criteria	Associations
Transient tics	Usually 3-10 yrs (before age 21)	Motor tics, rarely vocal tics	10%-20% of all children, boys > girls	Duration <12 mo	Possible family history of TS or tic disorders
Chronic tics	Usually 3-10 yrs (before age 21)	Simple & complex motor tics *or* vocal tics (rare); occasionally persist to adulthood	3%-4% of school-age children boys > girls	Duration >12 mo	Possible family history of TS or tic disorders; Possible ADHD, OCD, other behavioral or normal development
Tourette's syndrome	Usually 3-10 yrs (before age 21)	Simple & complex motor & vocal tics	0.05%-0.39% boys > girls	Duration of motor & vocal tics >12 mo; bouts of tics; wax & wane; onset before 18-21 yrs of age	Possible family history of TS or tic disorders; Possible ADHD, OCD, other behavioral **or** normal development

From Schapiro, N.A. (2002). Dude, you don't have Tourette's. *Pediatr Nurs, 22,* 243-253. Reprinted with permission. Data from Bagheri et al, 1999; Zohar et al, 1999; DSM-IV-TR, 2000; Kadesjo & Gillberg, 2000; Leckman et al, 2001.

BOX 40-1

Diagnostic criteria for 307.23 Tourette's Disorder

A. Both multiple motor and one or more vocal tics have been present at some time during the illness, although not necessarily concurrently. (A *tic* is a sudden, rapid, recurrent, nonrhythmic, stereotyped motor movement or vocalization.)

B. The tics occur many times a day (usually in bouts) nearly every day or intermittently throughout a period of more than 1 year, and during this period there was never a tic-free period of more than 3 consecutive months.

C. The onset is before age 18 years.

D. The disturbance is not due to the direct physiological effects of a substance (e.g., stimulants) or a general medical condition (e.g., Huntington's disease or postviral encephalitis).

From DSM-IV-TR, 2000. Reprinted with permission.

---

neurologist Gilles de la Tourette (1857-1904) first described nine individuals exhibiting the unusual movements and sounds of the syndrome that bears his name, he also described their compulsions (Lajonchere et al, 1996). The French psychologist and neurologist Janet (1859-1947) described OCD as a form of "psycholepsy," with neuronal discharges that were like tics of the mind (Rapoport, 1989), and reported success with behavioral treatments (Jenike et al, 1998). Freud, who studied at the same Paris hospital as de la Tourette and Janet, believed in the relationship between neurologic factors and unconscious mental processes (Cohen & Leckman, 1999). Freud described tics in detail in his treatment of Frau Emmy von N (Cohen & Leckman, 1999) and attributed obsessions to overly strict toilet training in his famous Rat Man case, in which the individual was reportedly cured of obsessions by psychoanalysis (Freud, 1909/1973).

Until recently both TS and OCD were felt to have psychiatric origins (Coffey & Park, 1997; Rapoport, 1989). Noting haloperidol's efficacy in reducing tic severity, researchers began to explore the role of dopamine receptors and the limbic system in TS (Coffey & Park, 1997). It is currently felt that there is an underlying defect in TS of either excess dopamine or hypersensitivity of postsynaptic dopamine receptors (Bagheri et al, 1999). Research began to implicate the serotonin system in OCD after clinicians noted that OCD was refractory to traditional psychotherapy, but responded to particular serotonin reuptake inhibitors (SRIs).

Studies suggest that basal ganglia dysfunction may be involved in TS (Sherman et al, 1998) and OCD (Rauch & Savage, 2000). Leckman and Cohen (1999) postulate that specific cortico-striato-thalamo-cortical (CSTC) circuits convey cortical information throughout the basal ganglia and modulate systems that control different aspects of psychomotor behavior (Box 40-3 and Figure 40-1). According to Leckman and Cohen, some of the circuits that convey information from the cortex throughout the basal ganglia are selectively disinhibited in both TS and OCD. In this conceptual model TS is seen as a disorder in which individuals are unable to inhibit premonitory sensory urges, leading to the emergence of motor and phonic behavior. In OCD, individuals are unable to inhibit specific innate worries, leading to the emergence of intense obsessions and compulsions.

BOX 40-2

Diagnostic criteria for 300.3 Obsessive-Compulsive Disorder

A. Either obsessions or compulsions:

Obsessions as defined by (1), (2), (3), and (4):

(1) recurrent and persistent thoughts, impulses, or images that are experienced, at some time during the disturbance, as intrusive and inappropriate and that cause marked anxiety or distress

(2) the thoughts, impulses, or images are not simply excessive worries about real-life problems

(3) the person attempts to ignore or suppress such thoughts, impulses, or images, or to neutralize them with some other thought or action

(4) the person recognizes that the obsessional thoughts, impulses, or images are a product of his or her own mind (not imposed from without as in thought insertion)

Compulsions as defined by (1) and (2):

(1) repetitive behaviors (e.g., hand washing, ordering, checking) or mental acts (e.g., praying, counting, repeating words silently) that the person feels driven to perform in response to an obsession, or according to rules that must be applied rigidly

(2) the behaviors or mental acts are aimed at preventing or reducing distress or preventing some dreaded event or situation; however, these behaviors or mental acts either are not connected in a realistic way with what they are designed to neutralize or prevent or are clearly excessive

B. At some point during the course of the disorder, the person has recognized that the obsessions or compulsions are excessive or unreasonable. **Note**: This does not apply to children.

C. The obsessions or compulsions cause marked distress, are time consuming (take >1 hour a day), or significantly interfere with the person's normal routine, occupational (or academic) functioning, or usual social activities or relationships.

D. If another Axis I disorder is present, the content of the obsessions or compulsions is not restricted to it (e.g., preoccupation with food in the presence of an eating disorder; hair pulling in the presence of trichotillomania; concern with appearance in the presence of body dysmorphic disorder; preoccupation with drugs in the presence of a substance use disorder; preoccupation with having a serious illness in the presence of hypochondriasis; preoccupation with sexual urges or fantasies in the presence of a paraphilia; or guilty ruminations in the presence of major depressive disorder).

E. The disturbance is not due to the direct physiological effects of a substance (e.g., a drug of abuse, a medication) or a general medical condition.

Specify if:

With Poor Insight: if, for most of the time during the current episode, the person does not recognize that the obsessions and compulsions are excessive or unreasonable

From DSM-IV-TR, 2002. Reprinted with permission.

Pediatric autoimmune neuropsychiatric disorders associated with *Streptococcus* (PANDAS)

There has been some research into the association of TS and OCD with streptococcal infections, noting that Sydenham chorea, which involves abnormal movements, OCD-like symptoms, and emotional lability, is thought to be caused by a reaction between antibodies to group A beta-hemolytic *Streptococcus* and neuronal tissue (Müller et al, 2001; Perlmutter et al, 1999). These researchers hypothesize that a subset of children with TS and OCD belong to a category known as PANDAS (Müller et al, 2001). Criteria for PANDAS include abrupt onset of symptoms associated with a streptococcal infection, periods of remission, and exacerbations after additional streptococcal infections (Perlmutter et al, 1999). Müller and colleagues noted that adults with TS have higher levels of specific antibodies to streptococcus than controls without TS. Perlmutter and associates (1999) found that children with TS who fit the PANDAS criteria had their TS and

OCD symptoms significantly reduced after being treated with either intravenous immune globulin or plasma exchange. Studies of the effects of antibiotic treatment have been mixed (Garvey et al, 1999; Murphy & Pichichero, 2002). Researchers have identified a serologic marker, the D18/B17 lymphocyte antigen, which is more commonly found in individuals with rheumatic fever, Sydenham chorea, childhood onset OCD, and TS (Bottas & Richter, 2002). The implications of this area of research for prevention and treatment of TS and OCD are still unclear.

Known Genetic Etiology

Based on extended family studies, most researchers associate TS, chronic tics, OCD, and obsessive-compulsive symptoms as a spectrum of expression of the same underlying genetic disorder (Alsobrook & Pauls, 1997; Peterson et al, 2001). They suggest an autosomal dominant model with sex-specific penetrance, accounting for the higher incidence of TS among boys, but cannot rule out a multifactorial or intermediate mode of inheritance (Alsobrook & Pauls, 1997; Haasstedt et al, 1995). Although some researchers have suggested possible locations for the "TS gene," their findings have not been replicated (Alsobrook & Pauls, 1997).

The onset of OCD has a bimodal distribution, with one mean of onset at age 10 and the other at age 21 (Geller et al, 1998). According to Miguel and associates (2001), younger age at onset is associated with higher incidence of ticlike compul-

---

BOX 40-3

Brain Structures thought to be Involved in TS and OCD

Cerebral cortex—layer of gray matter that covers the surface of each cerebral hemisphere, consists primarily of six-layered neocortex containing functional modules: primary, sensory, and motor areas; unimodal association areas; multimodal association areas; and limbic areas.

Thalamus—acts as the gateway to cerebral cortex; relaying all sensory pathways, as well as circuits used by the cerebellum, basal ganglia, and limbic system.

Basal ganglia—group of subcortical nuclei that modulate output of the frontal cortex. Damage to the basal ganglia can cause disturbance of movement, alterations in muscle tone, and disturbances of cognition and motivation.

Striatum (caudate nucleus, putamen, and ventral striatum)—major point of entry into basal ganglia circuitry, receiving inputs from cortical areas and projecting inhibitory outputs.

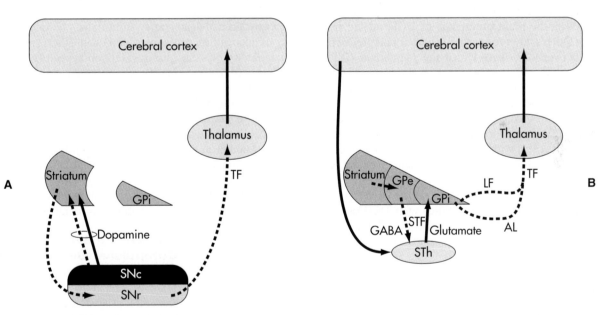

FIGURE 40-1 Two additional ganglia circuits of importance. Excitatory connections are in solid line, inhibitory connections are in dotted line. **A,** The substantia nigra is interconnected with the striatum. The pigmented, compact part of the substantia nigra *(SNc)* projects to the striatum, exciting some striatal neurons and inhibiting others; the striatum projects to the reticular part of the substantia nigra *(SNr)*, which, like GPi, projects to the thalamus via the thalamic fasciculus *(TF)*. **B,** The subthalamic nucleus receives inputs from the cerebral cortex and also is interconnected with the globus pallidus. (As described further in the text, this allows a substantial degree of subthalamic control over pallidal output.) Abbreviations for fiber bundles: *AL,* Ansa lenticularis; *LF,* lenticular fasciculus; *STF,* subthalamic fasciculus; *TF,* thalamic fasciculus. A basal ganglia loop involving the centromedian and parafascicular nuclei of the thalamus is also prominent anatomically, but was omitted from these schematic diagrams because its functional significance is unclear. (From Nolte, J. [2002]. *The human brain: an introduction to its functional anatomy* (5th ed.). St Louis: Mosby. Reprinted with permission.)

sions, tic disorders or TS, sensory phenomena preceding compulsions, poorer short-term response to medication, and higher familial incidence of OCD than the later-onset group. Peterson and associates (2001) found a strong association between tic disorders and OCD, and Zohar and colleagues (1999) suggest that OCD and TS are different expressions of the same underlying genetic abnormality. But Geller and associates (1998) and Hanna (2000) speculate that OCD is a disorder with multiple potential causes. Rosenberg and Hanna (2000) suggest that neuroimaging may be able to clarify the genetic heterogeneity of OCD in the future.

Incidence and Prevalence

A recent study of 11-year-old Swedish schoolchildren revealed an incidence of TS of 1.1% among boys and 0.5% among girls (Kadesjo & Gillberg, 2000). Other population studies of TS have found rates ranging from 0.05% to 0.39% (Peterson et al, 2001; Zohar et al, 1999). In contrast, as many as 10% to 20% of all school-age children have transient motor, and less commonly vocal, tics lasting less than 1 year (Bagheri et al, 1999; Zohar et al, 1999; Peterson et al, 2001; Snider et al, 2002). The relatively high prevalence of transient tic disorder might surprise primary care providers because the tics often resolve before the family seeks medical attention (Leckman et al, 2001). In 3% to 4% of school-age children, symptoms of either motor or vocal tics, but not both, persist for more than 1 year (Leckman et al, 2001).

In the population-based longitudinal study by Peterson and colleagues (2001), the point prevalence of OCD ranged from 1.8% to 5.5%. Other community studies have found prevalence for OCD of between 2% and 4% of the population (Geller et al, 1998), but diagnoses were made on the basis of questionnaires filled out by lay reviewers, which may overidentify cases of OCD (Rapoport et al, 2000). Fireman and associates (2001) found that the 1-year prevalence for pediatric cases of OCD treated in a large health maintenance organization (HMO) was only 0.13%, with the implication that many cases of symptomatically significant OCD are unrecognized and untreated.

Obsessive-compulsive behaviors or OCD has been found in 20% to 60% of children in referral clinics with TS (Coffey & Park, 1997; King et al, 1999; Kadesjo & Gillberg, 2000). Conversely, up to 7% of referred children with OCD have TS and 20% have tics (Coffey & Park, 1997).

Clinical Manifestations at Time of Diagnosis
Tourette's Syndrome (TS)
Motor and Vocal Tics. Tics are commonly classified as simple or complex. Shoulder shrugging, neck twitching, and facial movements are examples of simple motor tics. Touching objects, skipping, and squatting in a rhythmic sequence (such as every four steps) are examples of complex motor tics. Simple vocal tics include sniffing, barking, coughing, yelling, and hiccupping. Complex vocal tics include repeating parts of words or phrases, talking to oneself, assuming different intonations, and uttering obscenities (Bagheri et al, 1999; Leckman et al, 1999).

Most children present first with tics in the head, neck, or upper extremities (Leckman et al, 2001). In children who are eventually diagnosed with TS, almost half report that eye blinking was their initial tic, followed by other head and facial tics. Others report vocal tics such as throat clearing and sniffing to be an early symptom of TS (Jankovic, 1997) and less commonly of transient tic disorder (Leckman et al, 2001.).

Up to 90% of older children and adults with TS report some premonitory sensations related to their tics, whereas children younger than 10 are more likely to view their tics as completely involuntary (Leckman et al, 1999). Although many children are able to suppress their tics for some time, the urge to tic remains, and the tics must eventually be "released." Some children are able to remain relatively tic-free during school hours, only to engage in bouts of tics for several hours at home (Leckman et al, 1997; Packer, 1997). Others report that tics are quiescent while they are engaged in an absorbing mental or physical task (Jankovic, 1997). Stress can exacerbate tics, but they can also increase when a child is in a relaxed state, such as watching television, and can be present during sleep (Jankovic, 1997). Health care providers should keep in mind that most children with TS are able to suppress tics during an office visit (Kiessling, 2001), making it necessary for the provider to ask the child and caretakers about tic and associated symptom severity and their impact on daily life. In specialty practice and research, tic symptoms are measured by self-report, interviews such as the Yale Global Tic Severity Scale, or direct observational methods, such as tic counts from videotapes (Leckman et al, 1989; Scahill et al, 1999).

Coprolalia and Copropraxia. Coprolalia (the involuntary uttering of obscenities, profanities, and racial slurs) and copropraxia (involuntary obscene gestures) tend to appear 4 to 7 years after the onset of tics, peaking during adolescence and greatly diminishing in adulthood (Singer, 1997). Although coprolalia is almost synonymous with TS in the popular media, it is a relatively rare phenomenon. The percentage of children with TS who exhibit these symptoms ranges from 8% in one study of a general pediatric practice, to 60% of children in a referred tertiary care practice. There is a high male to female ratio, ranging from 4.4:1 for coprolalia to 20:1 for copropraxia (Singer, 1997). These particular complex tics can jeopardize a child's safety, ability to stay in school, and ability to socialize (Singer, 1997).

Obsessive-Compulsive Behavior (OCB) and Obsessive-Compulsive Disorder (OCD)
Obsessions typically cluster in contamination themes, harm to self or others, aggressive or sexual themes, scrupulosity or religiosity, forbidden thoughts, or symmetry urges. Some children's obsessions include fears of a catastrophic family event, such as the death of a parent (Geller et al, 1998). Typical compulsions involve washing, checking, repeating, touching, counting, ordering and arranging, hoarding, or praying (March & Mulle, 1998). Compulsions may involve either physical activities or mental rituals (American Psychiatric Association, 2000). Samuels and associates (2002) found that 30% of adults with OCD in a clinical sample included hoarding in their compulsions, and these individuals tended to have an earlier onset of OCD, more associated symmetry rituals, more tics, and more resistance to treatment than those without hoarding.

Onset of OCD is usually gradual, but may be sudden or explosive. A majority of children with OCD will have multiple obsessions and compulsions over time, but there are some younger children who present with compulsions only (Geller et al, 1998). OCD symptoms tend to wax and wane, but persist over time in a majority of children with the condition, although the specific obsessions and rituals may change (Geller et al, 1998). In some instances, parents are intimately involved in the rituals, typically offering the child repeated reassurance (Geller et al, 1998) or helping the child avoid feared objects or situations (Chansky, 2000). Other children and adolescents go to great lengths to hide their symptoms from others, including their parents and health care providers, for fear of being perceived as "crazy" (Geller, 1998; Rapoport, 1989). An older child might be relatively secretive about hoarding, mental rituals, and bedtime rituals, for example. In comparing parent and child reports of OCD in a geographically and ethnically diverse study, Rapoport and associates (2000) found that of 35 identified cases of OCD, only 4 were identified by parent report and 32 by child report, with one overlapping case.

In primary care, the provider can ask the child and caretakers about any unusual habits and their impact on daily functioning. Although they are not used for diagnosis, the current gold standards for measuring the level of functional impairment in specialty care and research are the Yale-Brown Obsessive Compulsive Scale (Y-BOCS) (Goodman et al, 1989) and the Children's Yale-Brown Obsessive Compulsive Scale (CY-BOCS) (Scahill et al, 1997).

Treatment

Behavioral Treatments for Tics

In a review of various behavioral treatments for tics, Piacentini and Chang (2001) found some empirical support for exposure and response prevention (see Cognitive Behavioral Therapy, Table 40-2) for adult subjects who had premonitory sensations before their tics. However, the treatment was longer than for OCD with a more modest response and the sample sizes were small. They note more success with habit reversal training, which consists of increasing awareness of the tic mechanisms, earliest signs of occurrences and situations in which the tic is likely to occur, and then develop a competing and incompati-

ble physical response to the tic. O'Connor and associates (2001) used a habit reversal program with 38 adults with chronic tic disorder and reported that half noted 75% to 100% control over their tics at 2 year follow-up. One small school-based habit reversal study with adolescent boys showed at least moderate success (Clarke et al, 2001). Many clinicians feel that the best approach in children would be to simply allow them to tic (Piacentini & Chang, 2001; Schapiro, 2002).

Cognitive Behavioral Therapy for OCD

Cognitive behavioral therapy (CBT) has become the cornerstone of treatment for OCD (see Table 40-2) (March & Mulle, 1998). Recent open CBT trials of unmedicated children and adolescents have demonstrated a 50% to 60% reduction in symptoms, with many children becoming asymptomatic (Benazon et al, 2002; Waters et al, 2001). Even adolescents who had not responded to medication in the past showed a significant symptom reduction with group cognitive behavioral therapy (Thienemann et al, 2001). March and Mulle generally recommend a treatment plan of between 13 and 20 weekly sessions. Although children may need booster sessions, in general the gains achieved can be maintained after the therapy sessions have ended (Thienemann et al, 2001)

Parental involvement and parent-child teamwork are crucial to the success of treatment, both in initiating the therapy and in helping with the child's "homework" between therapy sessions (Chanksy, 2000; March & Mulle, 1998). Working together with the therapist, the child helps pick the target ritual for extinction. If the target ritual is hand washing, for example, the parent must agree to limit the length of time the child spends washing, to the point of escorting the child out of the bathroom (Chansky, 2000). If the ritual involves checking (for bugs in the bed, for the parent's forgiveness, or for locking the door), the parent must agree to limit the number of times the child is reassured. The parent reminds the child that OCD is playing tricks and trying to control the child. Although such limits may seem cruel in the face of a crying, anxious child, they are necessary in order to reinforce the message that the child can avoid the ritual without catastrophic consequences (Chansky, 2000).

If the child or adolescent with TS and/or OCD is seeing a therapist, the primary care provider should obtain written permission from the parent to communicate with the therapist and assent from the child, particularly if confidential issues such as contraception are involved.

Medication for Tics (Table 40-3)

Pimozide (Orap), a dopamine receptor antagonist, is the only medication approved by the U.S. Food and Drug Administration (FDA) to treat tics in children and adolescents (Riddle & Carlson, 2001). Pimozide has shown efficacy in double-blind, placebo-controlled trials, whereas the studies have been more mixed with haloperidol (Haldol), the original neuroleptic used for TS (Carpenter et al, 1999; Riddle & Carlson, 2001). Potential side effects of these medications, along with other neuroleptics, are extrapyramidal effects, tardive dyskinesia, cognitive dulling, sedation, and weight gain (Carpenter et al, 1999; Riddle & Carlson, 2001). Atypical neuroleptics, such as risperidone (Risperdal), are sometimes used for explosive behavior and tics, and may have fewer side effects than older

TABLE 40-2

Cognitive Behavioral Therapy (CBT)

1. Psychoeducation	Framing OCD in a neurobehavioral model for parents and children, with analogies to medical illnesses
2. Cognitive training	Teaching the child tactics for resisting OCD, such as "bossing back" the OCD symptom
3. Mapping OCD	Detailing the child's specific obsessions and compulsions, particularly identifying the "transition zone" where the child is already able, at times, to win the battle against OCD
4. Graded exposure and response prevention (E/RP)	Either imagined or actual exposures, in which the child is exposed to the feared object, action, or thought without performing the ritual

Data from March, J.S. & Mulle, K. (1998). *OCD in children and adolescents: a cognitive behavioral treatment manual.* New York: The Guilford Press.

TABLE 40-3

Medications Used in the Treatment of Tourette's Syndrome and Obsessive-Compulsive Disorder

Medication Class	Specific Examples	Uses	Notes	Side Effects	Interactions
Alpha-adrenergic receptor agonists	clonidine, guanfacine	Tics, inattention, impulsiveness, hyperactivity	Effects mild, but often tried first; must be tapered off	Sedation, headaches, dry mouth, irritability	Additive sedation with antihistamines, opiates, alcohol
Neuroleptics	haloperidol, pimozide, risperidone	Tics; risperidone used for rages	Beneficial effects on tics noted for >30 yr	Sedation, weight gain, cognitive dulling, tardive dyskinesia, ↑QT interval (pimozide)	Macrolide antibiotics, grapefruit (↑QT interval), additive sedation with other CNS depressants
SSRIs	fluoxetine, fluvoxamine, sertraline	OCD, co-morbid depression	Dosage for OCD higher than antidepressant dosages	GI disturbance, sexual dysfunction, dry mouth, sweating	Additive effects with CNS depressants, may alter metabolism of phenobarbital, desipramine, codeine, rare suicidal ideation
Tricyclic antidepressants	imipramine, desipramine, nortryptyline, clomipramine	ADHD, clomipramine for OCD	Do not worsen tics, may be beneficial with co-morbid depression, anxiety	Dry mouth, sweating, fatigue, dizziness, weight gain, tachycardia, ↑QT interval	Difficult to monitor (same dose produces varying serum levels), hazardous in overdose
Stimulants (controversial)	dexedrine, methylphenidate, pemoline	ADHD	Worsen tics in some children; may be effective alone or combined with neuroleptic or alpha-adrenergic agonist	Headache, anxiety, weight loss, ↑ tics in some children	↑ Cardiac effects with tricyclics, beta blockers

From Schapiro, N.A. (2002). Dude, you don't have Tourette's. *Pediatr Nurs, 22,* 243-253. Adapted with permission. Data from Carpenter, L.L. et al, 1999; Riddle & Carlson, 2001.

neuroleptics; however, there is as yet little evidence, one way or the other, for their efficacy (Findling et al, 1998; Riddle & Carlson, 2001).

The alpha-adrenergic receptor agonists clonidine (Catapres) and guanfacine (Tenex) have been used to treat tics and attention deficit hyperactivity disorder (ADHD), with modest effects on motor tics and less effect on vocal tics (Carpenter et al, 1999). Guanfacine causes less sedation and hypotension than clonidine. Because the medications have fewer adverse effects than neuroleptics, they are often tried first, even though they will help only a portion of children and adolescents with TS. Their primary use is in hypertension, and they can cause hypotension in some children, as well as irritability, insomnia, headache, dry mouth, and depression (Carpenter et al, 1999).

Medications for Obsessions and Compulsions (see Table 40-3)

The first medication to show significant effect for OCD was clomipramine (Anafranil), a tricyclic SRI (Rapoport, 1989). Since then selective serotonin reuptake inhibitors (SSRIs) have largely supplanted clomipramine, due to a greater safety profile, particularly in overdose (Shoaf et al, 2001), and diminished side effects (Bergeron et al, 2002). In a recent double-blind, 6-month study comparing sertraline (Zoloft) and fluoxetine (Prozac), both were 60% efficacious in reducing symptoms at 6 months, with sertraline having a slightly faster onset of efficacy and a slightly higher rate of complete remission (Bergeron et al, 2002) Unfortunately gains do not seem to be maintained after medication has been stopped (Pigott & Seay, 2000; Thienemann et al, 2001). There are no long-term safety studies of SSRIs in children (Shoaf et al, 2001). A concern about growth retardation with long-term SSRI use has recently emerged with the publication of four case studies of children

with TS or OCD and previously identified growth issues. The children showed abnormalities of growth hormone, which resolved when the SSRIs were discontinued in three of the cases (Weintrob et al, 2002).

Medications for Attention Deficit Hyperactivity Disorder (ADHD) with TS and/or OCD

It has been thought that the stimulants used to treat ADHD (see Chapter 12) could exacerbate or even cause tics to appear, but this effect may have been coincidental: ADHD often surfaces before tics in children with both TS and ADHD (Spencer et al, 1998). More recent studies have indicated that many, but not all, children with TS and ADHD can be treated with stimulants without an increase in tic behaviors (Gadow et al, 1999; Tourette's Syndrome Study Group, 2002), and some TS experts are using stimulants, with caution (Walkup, 2002). Alpha-adrenergic receptor agonists such as clonidine seem to decrease impulsivity, but not affect inattention (Tourette's Syndrome Study Group, 2002). Medications used to treat OCD in general do not affect ADHD and vice versa, and some children will benefit from medication for both conditions (Geller et al, 2002).

To Medicate or Not to Medicate?

Because of the relative risk of side effects to modest benefit, most TS experts recommend trying behavioral and environmental measures before using medication, especially for tics, and to consider using medication for OCD or ADHD first (Bagheri et al, 1999; Carpenter et al, 1999; Leckman et al, 1999; Walkup, 2002). Packer (1997) and Kiessling (2001) emphasize the importance of distinguishing between symptoms that bother the child, and symptoms that bother the parent. For example, a parent who is unusually sensitive to environmental noise may be bothered by vocal tics that do not disturb the child (Packer, 1997). Bagheri and associates (1999) note that the use of medication in their practice declined 50% over a 15-year period as they provided increasing written information, referral of parents to support groups, telephone consultation, and inservice training for school staff.

The *Expert Consensus Treatment Guidelines for Obsessive Compulsive Disorder* (March et al, 1997) recommends CBT first for younger children and milder symptoms of OCD. CBT plus SRIs are recommended for moderate symptoms in children and adolescents; for severe OCD, the individual may need to begin medication alone before being able to engage in therapy.

If needed, the goal of medication should be to use the lowest dose possible to bring the target symptom down to acceptable levels and to enhance the child's development (Bagheri et al, 1999). The doses of SSRIs used in OCD are often higher than those used in depression (Pigott & Seay, 2000). Many psychoactive medications have become household words, and children can have relatively sophisticated, if not necessarily accurate, understandings of their uses and reputations. When discussing the possibility of medication with a child and family, it is important to take into account their previous experiences with similar medications in other family members, and the differing concerns and opinions that parents, children, and their siblings may have (Rappaport & Chubinsky, 2000). The recommended medication regimens for target symptoms of TS, OCD, and ADHD are continually evolving, so it is important for the provider to ascertain how, when, and where the family has acquired knowledge about the medications, and for the provider to supply current information (Schapiro, 2002).

Complementary and Alternative Therapies

There are some reports of acupuncture being used for TS (Wu et al, 1996). The National Center for Complementary and Alternative Medicine (2002) reports several studies of the effect of acupuncture on neurobiology in general, but none specifically for TS. Grimaldi (2002) postulates that magnesium deficiency may precipitate a number of conditions, including TS and OCD, but no clinical studies of magnesium supplementation have been conducted to date. German researchers (Müller-Vahl et al, 1999) report a decrease in motor and vocal tics in an adult with delta-9-tetrahydrocannabinol, the major psychoactive ingredient of marijuana, and are planning a double-blind, placebo-controlled crossover study.

Latitudes, a journal that promotes alternatives to medication for a variety of neurologic disorders, reports that controlling allergies and diet can help alleviate symptoms of TS, ADHD, and OCD (Association for Comprehensive NeuroTherapy, 2002). Anecdotal accounts from parents on the *Latitudes* website (*Latitudes,* 2002) report decreasing tic symptoms from homeopathy, magnet therapy, electroencephalograph (EEG) biofeedback, oligomeric proanthocyanidins, B vitamins, flaxseed oil, super blue-green algae *(Aphanizomenon flos-aquae),* amino acid supplements, dimethylaminoethanol (DMAE), and dimethylglycine (DMG). The general difficulties of evaluating the efficacy of any particular treatment for tics are discussed below. In addition, the editors of *Latitudes* note that most parents are trying several modalities at once (e.g., amino acids and vitamins), making it more difficult to disentangle the effect of any one treatment.

There is one study under way on the effect of St. John's wort on social phobias in adults, but none specifically on OCD. Waltz (2000) notes that some adults with OCD feel that their symptoms worsened while taking St. John's wort. In an extensive review of alternative medical approaches and dietary supplements, Waltz found that many could be generally beneficial, but none were yet known to specifically diminish OCD symptoms.

Anticipated Advances in Diagnosis and Management

The significance of the PANDAS criteria for diagnosis and management of OCD and TS is not yet clear. Larger randomized controlled trials of treatment options may clarify diagnosis and management of this possible subtype of TS and OCD in the future (Bottas & Richter, 2002).

Structural neuroimaging studies of untreated children with OCD consistently show abnormalities, including reduced caudate and striatal volumes and increased thalamic volumes (Rosenberg & Hanna, 2000). Additional studies show that abnormalities in glutamate-serotonin interactions may underlie OCD (Rauch et al, 1998). Further studies of the serotonin transporter gene may shed light on OCD and other anxiety disorders responsive to serotonin reuptake inhibitors, as well as provide an increased understanding of the wide variation in treatment response in OCD. Genetic studies of the dopaminergic system may shed more light on TS, as well as tic-related OCD (Rosenberg & Hanna, 2002).

A number of medications are under investigation for control of tics. A recent double-blind trial found that injections of *botulinum* toxin reduced tic severity and urges associated with tics, but that study subjects did not experience subjective benefit from the medication (Marras et al, 2001). In a double-blind, placebo-controlled trial, baclofen did not reduce tic severity, but subjects did experience subjective benefit (Singer et al, 2001). Studies of nicotine (Silver et al, 1999) show that it may potentiate neuroleptics to reduce tics, but side effects of dizziness and nausea may limit its use. Mecamylamine, a nicotinic receptor antagonist, has similar actions with fewer side effects (Silver et al, 2001). Although it is ineffective on its own, future studies may show a benefit as an adjunct to neuroleptics, resulting in reduced dosages of these medications. These studies highlight some of the problems in investigating medications for TS: the symptoms wax and wane, and any improvement may be spontaneous, rather than a medication effect; because tics vary by location, intensity, suppressibility, discomfort, and social impairment, they are difficult to quantify, and there are inherent reliability issues with any established rating scale (Kurlan, 2001).

Research about etiology and treatments for both TS and OCD is quite dynamic, with new findings appearing monthly. Primary care providers who are working with children who have TS and/or OCD are encouraged to check frequently for updated information.

Associated Problems (Box 40-4)

TS and ADHD

In ADHD, children exhibit developmentally inappropriate levels of inattention, impulsivity, and/or overactivity (Sherman et al, 1998) (see Chapter 12). Symptoms of ADHD occur in

BOX 40-4
Associated Problems

ADHD
Rage attacks
Self-injurious behavior
Body dysmorphic disorder and eating disorders
Additional psychiatric diagnoses (anxiety, bipolar)

Data from Nolte, J. (2002). *The human brain: an introduction to its functional anatomy* (5th ed.). St Louis: Mosby.

30% to 90% of children with TS, depending on the sample used (Sherman et al, 1998; Kadesjo & Gillberg, 2000). Recent studies have shown that children with TS plus ADHD exhibit more internalizing and externalizing symptoms, poorer social adaptation, more difficulty sustaining attention, poorer scores on tests of verbal and performance intelligence, and more severe TS symptoms than children with TS alone (Brand et al, 2002; Carter et al, 2000; Sherman et al, 1998).

OCD and ADHD

Hanna (1995) found that up to 30% of children with OCD also meet diagnostic criteria for ADHD, even when children with TS or major depression are excluded. Out of concern that apparent symptoms of ADHD, such as inattention, might be due to unreported intrusive thoughts or compulsions, Geller and associates (2002) compared children from a psychopharmacology clinic who fulfilled DSM-IV criteria for ADHD and for ADHD plus OCD. There were no significant differences in core ADHD symptoms or functional academic impairment between the two groups, suggesting that the ADHD diagnosis represented an additional condition, rather than a variation of OCD presentation. In addition, the onset of ADHD preceded the onset of OCD symptoms in most subjects. The authors note the presence of untreated ADHD might limit the child with OCD's ability to focus on cognitive behavioral treatment.

Rage Attacks

Sudden, explosive outbursts of behavior are reported by approximately 25% of children with TS who are referred to specialty clinics (Budman et al, 2000). These outbursts are described as stereotypic, with abrupt onset or unpredictable and primitive displays of aggression that are grossly out of proportion to provoking stimuli, and that threaten serious self-harm, property destruction, or injury to others (Budman et al, 2000). Outbursts are frequently directed at the child's mother, usually accompanied by autonomic activation, and appear impulsive and poorly modulated, rather than intentional goal-directed expressions of anger or manipulation. Children are typically described as showing empathy between attacks, with immediate remorse after the attack's resolution (Budman et al, 2000; Stephens & Sandor, 1999). Several studies have found rage attacks to occur only in children with TS who have additional conditions, such as ADHD and/or OCD (Budman et al, 2000; Stephens & Sandor, 1999). Currently the etiology of these attacks and their relationship to TS are unknown (Budman et al, 2000). Parents have rated this symptom to be the least common and most distressing of all TS symptoms (Dooley et

al, 1999). Children who present with rage attacks are at risk for deterioration in home and/or school functioning (Budman et al, 2000).

Self-Injurious Behavior

In self-report questionnaires mailed to members of the Tourette Syndrome Association, 34% to 43% of respondents admitted to self-injurious behavior (Robertson, 1992). This behavior ranges from picking at scabs and self-cutting, to touching hot stoves, poking oneself with sharp objects, headbanging, and eye injuries (Robertson, 1992; Jankovic & Sekula, 1998). Self-injurious behavior has been noted before among children and adults with developmental delay and psychotic behavior (Robertson, 1992). According to a review of the literature by Robertson, none of the subjects of the self-injurious behavior studies with TS was found to have coexisting psychosis, and all those in whom intelligence was measured had normal intelligence. Robertson and Bruun and Budman (1997) suggest that the behavior is not intentionally self-injurious, and Jankovic (1997) describes the behavior as straddling the line between a compulsion and a complex tic. Nonetheless, individuals have been known to injure themselves significantly, including fractures (Bruun & Budman, 1997), and detached retinas (Leckman & Cohen, 1999).

Trichotillomania (recurrent pulling-out of one's own hair) has been noted to be more prevalent among individuals with OCD plus TS, than among individuals with OCD or TS alone (Keuthen et al, 1998; Miguel et al, 2001). Trichotillomania may be a symptom of a more heterogeneous group of disorders and more connected to other habit disorders. Individuals report a trancelike state and positive reinforcement from the behavior that is different from the described experience of either a complex tic or a compulsion (Keuthen et al, 1998).

Body Dysmorphic Disorder and Eating Disorders

Phillips (2000) notes similarities in age of onset, gender distribution, symptoms, and response to SRIs between individuals with OCD and with body dysmorphic disorder (BDD), which is a preoccupation with a defect in appearance (American Psychiatric Association, 2000). The joint preoccupation with symmetry and the feeling that something isn't "just right" are striking. In addi-tion there are greater incidences of BDD in individuals and families with OCD (and vice versa) than would be expected to occur by chance (Phillips, 2000). In a study of 237 adults with anorexia or bulimia, Milos and associates (2002) found a 29.5% prevalence of OCD, which was also associated with longer duration of the eating disorder.

Other Psychiatric Symptoms

Coffey and associates (2000) found a greater incidence of non-OCD anxiety disorders, particularly separation anxiety, in children with severe TS. In addition, this study of children with TS in specialty clinics found that 29% of children with severe symptoms qualified for a DSM-III-R diagnosis of bipolar disorder. Almost 95% of the children with mild/moderate TS and 100% of the children with severe TS qualified for some psychiatric co-morbidity (including ADHD and OCD). According to Coffey and associates, the presence of a mood disorder was a better predictor of psychiatric hospitalization than merely the presence of ADHD or OCD.

A number of studies have found equally high rates of associated psychiatric conditions in children with OCD referred to treatment clinics (Geller et al, 1998). These included mood, anxiety, disruptive behavior, developmental disorders, and enuresis (Geller et al, 1998).

There have been some anecdotal accounts of repetitive hallucinations, particularly auditory hallucinations, in non-psychotic children with TS who have other co-morbidities (Bruun & Budman, 1999; Schreier, 1999). Because children may not spontaneously disclose this symptom, some clinicians recommend asking all children with TS about the presence of hallucinations (Bruun & Budman, 1999).

Prognosis

In a cross-sectional study of 36 children with TS who were contacted 7 years after diagnosis, Leckman and associates (1998) found that tics began at a mean of 5.6 years of age, followed by progressive worsening and peaking at age 10. Whereas 22% of the sample had tics that were severe enough to jeopardize or prevent their functioning in school at the peak of symptoms, the tics steadily declined during adolescence, with 50% of the individuals virtually tic-free by age 18. Most of the remaining 18-year-olds experienced minimal to mild symptoms, whereas only 10% reported moderate or marked tics. Spencer and associates (2001) found that tic disorders are overrepresented in adults with ADHD, but the presence of tics does not affect the severity of ADHD; nor does the presence of ADHD affect the course of the tic disorder, which is generally diminished in adulthood.

OCD, in contrast, has a variable course that tends to persist through adulthood (Geller et al, 1998; Miguel et al, 2001). A long-term follow-up study of children seen between 1980 and 1991 in Germany found that 71% of the young adult subjects met the criteria for some form of psychiatric diagnosis, whereas 36% still had OCD (Wewetzer et al, 2001). However, the subjects did not receive either SSRIs or CBT during childhood, and it is possible that future longitudinal studies will have more optimistic outcomes.

Children with TS and OCD can be expected to attain normal developmental milestones and to achieve a normal life span. The lay literature notes that some professional athletes, artists, musicians, actors, professors, and health care professionals have TS and/or OCD (Handler, 1998; Landau, 1998).

PRIMARY CARE MANAGEMENT

Health Care Maintenance

Growth and Development

Children with both TS and OCD are generally thought to achieve normal growth and developmental milestones unless the child has additional conditions, such as pervasive developmental disorder or psychosis. One recent article has raised the concern about growth issues in children on long-term SSRIs (Weintrob et al, 2002), but there were only four children in the study, who had previously identified growth problems. Some medications used for TS or OCD may stimulate appetite, especially neuroleptics (such as haloperidol or pimozide) or alpha-adrenergic agonists (such as clonidine), and some SRIs or SSRIs are associated with weight gain.

Whereas there are some cases of very early onset OCD, most children develop symptoms after age 7 (Leonard et al, 1990; Geller et al, 1998). Parents and some providers may be concerned with distinguishing between developmentally normal rituals and obsessions of early childhood, and the rituals and obsessions associated with OCD, particularly in families with a history of tics or OCD among first-degree relatives. Leonard and associates (1990) suggest that normal childhood rituals bear some similarities to OCD-related rituals: needing things to be "just so," having lucky numbers, and having bedtime rituals. However, in children who are unaffected by OCD, the normal developmental rituals seem to aid in mastering anxiety and enhancing the child's socialization, whereas in OCD the rituals are distressing, isolating, and hinder daily life (Leonard et al, 1990). In addition, whereas ritualized behavior starts to fade in children by age 7 or 8, OCD symptoms often start to increase at this age.

Some parents of young children who were later diagnosed with TS or OCD noted that their children had more separation anxiety than peers or siblings, more aggressive reactions to peers, and more trouble with self-regulation (Papadopoulos et al, 1992).

Diet

Abrupt changes in dietary preferences may be a part of normal development or responses to contamination fears or other obsessions. In addition, children and adolescents with OCD have an increased risk of developing an eating disorder, and individuals with both OCD and eating disorders go to great lengths to hide their preoccupations (Martin & Ammerman, 2002; Milos et al, 2002; Waltz, 2000). Whereas a detailed discussion of food aversion and eating disorders is beyond the scope of this chapter, the growth and body mass index (BMI) charts of children with TS and OCD should be carefully maintained; any failure to make or maintain expected gains in height and weight, failure to progress through puberty, or secondary amenorrhea in the absence of pregnancy should prompt a more careful history, examination, and referral to the appropriate specialists. If the child is already seeing a psychotherapist, close communication between the primary care provider and the therapist is essential.

In looking for alternatives to allopathic medications, parents sometimes try elimination diets or restrict the intake of foods thought to trigger tics or obsessive-compulsive symptoms. In these situations, it is important to work with the family to ensure adequate caloric and nutritional intake.

Safety

Some children with TS feel compelled to touch hot stoves, stand at the edge of precipices, or go through intersections with their eyes closed, risking injury at an age when they would be expected to "know better"(Jankovic, 1997; Landau, 1998; Wilensky, 1999). Self-injurious behavior is associated with both TS and OCD (Jankovic, 1997; Keuthen, O'Sullivan, & Jeffreys, 1998; Miguel et al, 2001). Although parents may not be able to prevent all risky or self-injurious behaviors in older children and adolescents, they should be alert to the possibility of such behaviors, and seek guidance from professionals with expertise in TS and OCD if they occur.

The treatment of self-injurious behaviors can be difficult, depending on whether the behavior is actually a complex tic or a compulsion (Jankovic, 1997; Waltz, 2001). Medications that are intended to control tics can actually make compulsions worse, and medications for OCD don't usually diminish tics (Waltz, 2001). CBT can be quite helpful for compulsions, but the effect on tics is more modest (Piacentini & Chang, 2001).

Adolescents with TS, like other adolescents with chronic conditions, may be more likely than their nonaffected peers to engage in risky behavior (Blum et al, 2001). Unfortunately, aside from first-person accounts by adults with TS and OCD (Colas, 1998; Handler, 1998; Wilensky, 1999), there is a paucity of literature that describes the experience of adolescents with these conditions. There may be additional risks for youth associated specifically with TS. The anecdotal accounts by adults with TS note that tobacco, alcohol, and marijuana use temporarily alleviates a variety of symptoms (Handler, 1998; Wilensky, 1999). The short-term benefits of these substances are confirmed by a few studies (Müller-Vahl et al, 1999; Silver et al, 1999). For adolescents with TS and OCD whose tics, obsessions, and hyperactivity are not declining, symptom relief may be a compelling motivation for experimentation (Schapiro, 2002).

Immunizations

Children with TS and OCD should be vaccinated following the schedule recommended by the American Academy of Pediatrics.

Screenings

Vision. Routine screening is recommended.

Hearing. Routine screening is recommended.

Dental Care. Routine screening is recommended. Some children will note that their tics are set off by the vibrations in dental equipment and may need to have their teeth cleaned by hand.

Blood Pressure. Routine screening is recommended. Children taking medications such as clonidine, guanfacine, or stimulants should have additional screenings when medication is initiated and dosages are changed.

Hematocrit. Routine screening is recommended. Clozapine, an atypical neuroleptic, is associated with blood dyscrasias, and it would be prudent to monitor the complete blood count more frequently of children taking atypical neuroleptics.

Urinalysis. Routine screening is recommended.

Tuberculosis. Routine screening is recommended.

Condition Specific Screening. An electrocardiogram (ECG) is recommended before beginning or increasing doses of tricyclic antidepressants and pimozide, as well as periodic blood tests (depending on the medication) to measure drug levels, blood counts, or liver function tests.

Common Illness Management

Differential Diagnosis (Box 40-5)

Some children with undiagnosed tic disorders present with sniffing and coughing tics (Jankovic, 1997) that may be misdiagnosed as symptoms of a upper respiratory infection (URI) or allergy. Other children with TS notice an increase of symptoms during fevers, viral illnesses, and allergy flare-ups (Bruun & Budman, 1997). OCD and tic symptoms may begin or flare up explosively after a streptococcal infection (see PANDAS section above). At this point, diagnosis and treatment of PANDAS remain experimental, and prophylactic antibiotics are not recommended (Hollenbeck, 2000).

When a child with OCD complains of typical childhood symptoms, such as headaches and stomach aches, it is hard for parents and providers to discern the cause: is the child obsessed with illness? Is there a serotonin imbalance implicated in headaches or stomach aches? Is the child constipated as a side effect of medication? Or is there is a serious health problem? After listening carefully to the child, parents may need to consult with the child's therapist and primary care provider.

Changes in skin condition and musculoskeletal complaints may be due to bruising from tics, holding unusual positions as part of a tic, or self-injurious behavior.

Drug Interactions

Erythromycin and other macrolide antibiotics can interact with medications such as pimozide (a neuroleptic used for tics) to

---

BOX 40-5

Differential Diagnosis

SNIFFING, COUGHING, THROAT CLEARING
Allergy
Upper respiratory infection
Vocal tics

PHARYNGITIS
Streptococcal infection (observe for ↑tics or OCD)
Vocal tics (cough, throat clearing)

HEADACHE
Medication side effect (e.g., clonidine)
Somatic preoccupation or obsession

ABDOMINAL PAIN
Muscle tics (abdominal muscles)
Constipation due to toileting issues (OCD)
Constipation due to medication side effect
Somatic preoccupation or obsession

SKIN-MUCOSA CHANGES
Bruising from tics
Self-injurious behavior
Nail biting
Trichotillomania

MUSCULOSKELETAL COMPLAINTS
Tics (muscle tightness, holding unusual positions)
Injury incurred during tic

prolong the QT interval (Drug Information FullText, 2002a). Dextromethorphan, a cough suppressant commonly found in over-the-counter medications, may interact with fluoxetine to cause increased sedation and hallucinations. SSRIs can interact with codeine to prevent its breakdown to the active metabolite, thereby diminishing its analgesic properties (Oesterheld & Shader, 1998). These examples should alert the provider to keep an accurate list of current medications and updated information about drug-drug interactions, and to ensure that parents and adolescents are aware of them as well.

Given the plethora of vitamins, supplements and complementary and alternative medications available, providers should engage in an open dialog with the child and family about possible drug interactions with any alternative treatments. St. John's wort, dimethylglycine, and trimethylglycine, for example, can interact with SSRIs (Waltz, 2000).

Developmental Issues

Sleep Patterns
Children with TS can have difficulty falling or staying asleep if tics increase as they relax, or the bedclothes don't "feel right." Warm baths or massage can often temporarily diminish the tics, and some children benefit from having a soft mattress pad. Children with OCD, as noted above, tend to have rituals they feel compelled to perform before bedtime, which can often delay sleep for several hours. If the child does not involve the parent in these rituals, the parent may not be aware of them. As with other rituals, bedtime rituals may be diminished with therapy and/or medication.

Toileting
Most children with TS and OCD are not diagnosed until school age, when toilet training is no longer an issue. However, Waltz (2000) notes that children who are later diagnosed with OCD may have had difficulties with toilet training, and often have obsessions and rituals related to toileting. There may be an increased incidence of encopresis and enuresis related to OCD symptoms (for example, wetting or soiling connected to avoiding public bathrooms). As with other OCD symptoms, the combination of CBT and medication may help.

Discipline
The typical cycle of relative suppressibility and release of tics in TS can lead to confusion and misguided attempts on the part of parents and teachers to use discipline or conditioning to stop the tics (Packer, 1997). Part of the family's adjustment to a diagnosis of TS involves learning to understand, reinterpret, and accept their child's unusual behavior—often the very habits they have spent some time and energy encouraging the child to suppress (Leckman et al, 1999). When children with OCD begin treatment, there can be flare-ups of rituals. Parents will have to work with the child and therapist to decide which rituals to limit and which to ignore (Chansky, 2000).

Questions regarding the appropriateness of behavior, fairness to siblings, and consequences for behavior that is only partially under the child's control are complex, and families often benefit from support groups or other contact with parents of children with TS or OCD (Landau, 1998; Schapiro, 2002). Greene (2001) recommends a "basket" system for prioritizing behaviors of explosive children, including children with TS or OCD, with Basket A containing the behaviors needed to maintain safe child and family functioning, Basket B containing behaviors around which there is some room to teach the child negotiation skills, and Basket C containing behaviors the parent is willing to ignore for the time being (such as maintaining a clean room).

In addition to developing an increased flexibility for acceptable behavior standards, parents may have to adjust their systems of consequences and rewards, as well. Most children respond well to positive reinforcement, and children with OCD in particular may need rewards because the acceptable behavior may provoke anxiety rather than being "its own reward" (Waltz, 2000). According to Greene (2001), timeouts are not helpful for children who would like to behave well, but lack the neurologic capability to work through frustrating situations without a meltdown. He recommends instead that parents help children avoid meltdowns by essentially acting as their surrogate frontal lobe: modeling and teaching them flexibility, verbal skills, and the ability to shift gears. For children who are engaging in explosive behavior, a safe place to regroup is important (Waltz, 2000; Waltz, 2001).

Child Care
The combination of structure and flexibility is important for children with TS and OCD. Although children may not be formally diagnosed during the preschool years, they may have increased problems with adaptability and peer relationships, and child care providers can provide important information to parents who have concerns about their child's intellectual and social development.

School
According to Packer (1997), children with TS are more likely to need additional educational support than children without TS, but are not often referred for such support. Even though tics are not directly connected to learning disabilities, they may interfere with school functioning: Arm tics may interfere with handwritten work and eye tics or head movements may interfere with reading (Dornbush & Pruitt, 1995; Packer, 1997). The tics and the effort to suppress them may internally distract the child enough to limit the ability to concentrate in the classroom, and fatigue and irritability increase as the day progresses (Packer, 1997).

Children with TS can have dysgraphia and visual-motor integration problems, affecting all handwritten work and tasks that involve copying from the blackboard or from a test booklet to an answer sheet. Deficits in written expressive language are common, even in children who have no difficulty with reading or oral expression (Dornbush & Pruitt, 1995). Spencer and associates (1998) suggest that some of the learning difficulties attributed to TS may actually be more closely related to ADHD.

Silent rituals associated with OCD, such as counting the number of times a letter occurs in reading, or avoiding the number 3 in math problems, can slow the child down considerably, without being apparent to either teachers or parents (Carter et al, 1999). Conversely, the child's rituals may be disruptive to the class, sometimes leading to the inaccurate labeling of compulsions as symptoms of oppositional defiant disorder (Carter et al, 1999). Children may get stuck on one task, may have rewriting compulsions, or have difficulty making choices. Other children may be able to minimize their OCD symptoms at school, leaving teachers perplexed as to why assignments cannot be completed at home (Adams & Burke, 1999). Individualizing a plan is key, as well as creating alliances with teachers and school personnel whenever possible. Their observations may be invaluable in tracking response to medication and behavioral treatment.

There are two levels of educational support available for children with TS or OCD attending public schools: written plans to provide access to educational programs/protection from discrimination (Section 504), and special education services (Anderson et al, 1997) (see Chapter 5). All children with TS and OCD can qualify for Section 504 protection, which might include preferential seating, parent input into teacher selection, allowing a child to stop an activity if "stuck," permission to leave the classroom to release tics, extra time on tests, and homework modification (Carter et al, 1999; Schapiro, 2002), with only a letter of diagnosis as documentation. Evaluations for services under the Individuals with Disabilities Education Act are more complex (see Chapter 5), but a parent can request an evaluation for an individualized education program (IEP) in writing.

Children with TS often have particular talents in music, sports, the arts, or academic subjects. Some authors suggest that the involvement of children with TS in gifted programs, competitive sports, and drama could aid in school and social success (Edell-Fisher & Motta, 1990; Landau, 1998). For adolescents, time spent practicing or in competition may be protective, providing increased time under adult supervision as well as positive peer interactions (Schapiro, 2002).

Whereas children with TS are reported to have similar self-concepts to children without TS (Edell-Fisher & Motta, 1990), they acknowledge more behavioral difficulties and dysphoric moods, which increase with symptom severity. More recently, Carter and colleagues (2000) found that children with TS without ADHD were similar in social adjustment to unaffected Children, with the exception of school difficulties. ADHD status, obsessional symptoms, and family functioning were all related to social adaptation. In contrast to children with type 1 diabetes mellitus, children with TS tend to have more problems with peer relationships (Bawden et al, 1998).

Children with OCD frequently have difficulty initiating and maintaining friendships. Preoccupation with obsessions often leaves little time or energy for friends. In addition, the desire to hide their obsessions and rituals from peers may lead to social isolation (Adams & Burke, 1999). Children with OCD may benefit from socialization groups, in which social skills are explicitly taught, and from structured activities, such as religious or community youth groups or sports. Other children may find it easier to socialize with just one child, for short periods (Waltz, 2000).

Sexuality

Unless affected by other conditions, physical sexual development and progression through puberty in children with TS and/or OCD are normal. However, the psychosocial aspects of sexuality in children with TS and OCD can be affected in several ways. In some individuals with TS, tics can be set off by touch or may increase during sexual activity (Shimberg, 1995). Adolescents with OCD may avoid any touch, including holding hands and kissing, because of contamination fears (Waltz, 2000). Sexual obsessions are common in OCD (Waltz, 2000; Zohar et al, 1997), including unwanted sexual thoughts, invasive thoughts that disrupt romantic or sexual activity, and obsessions or fears around being homosexual in teens who do not have same-sex attractions (Waltz, 2000). In addition, the medications used for TS and OCD, most notably SSRIs, have some effect on libido and sexual functioning (Drug Information FullText, 2002b), which may be distressing for adolescents and may affect compliance with medications.

Adolescents with TS and OCD may not feel comfortable discussing sexuality with their parents, and may be reluctant to raise the issue to a health care provider. In the urge to prevent teen pregnancy and sexually transmitted diseases, it is important for providers to avoid reducing sexuality to intercourse and reproduction. Sexuality involves how one feels about one's own body, about touch and caring—difficult issues for any teen and even more so for teens with tics and/or compulsions.

Transition to Adulthood

Most adolescents with TS find that their tics have dramatically decreased by adulthood (Leckman et al, 1998). Adults with ongoing motor and vocal tics, but without associated conditions, have few problems with mood, sleep, anger management, or self-injurious behavior (Freeman et al, 2000). However, these individuals may experience discrimination in education or employment (Shimberg, 1995).

A few careers, including the military and some areas of law enforcement, may not be available to youth who have a history of any psychiatric illness or medication, including some of the medications used to treat TS and OCD (Waltz, 2000). Young adults with severe OCD or other associated psychiatric conditions may have limited options for employment, education, housing, and health care. Parents and the adolescent may benefit from hiring a case manager to address transition to adulthood and independent living issues (Waltz, 2000).

Family Concerns and Resources

Mothers of children with TS have expressed lower self-concepts than mothers of controls (Edell-Fisher & Motta, 1990). The child's emotional adjustment to a diagnosis of TS can be predicted by the child's perception of parent-child interaction (Edell & Motta, 1988), and is related to family functioning in general (Carter et al, 2000). These findings and the experience of other clinicians (Packer, 1997) suggest that the child, and the family as a whole, could benefit from parents receiving emotional support after diagnosing a child with TS.

Parents and siblings of children with OCD experience stress in accommodating the child's rituals, and siblings may feel ashamed of the child's bizarre behavior at school (Adams &

Burke, 1999). Chansky (2000) encourages parents to explain OCD as a medical condition to the child's siblings, and to validate the feelings of unfairness or possible embarrassment at their sibling's outbursts. Family meetings with the child's therapist to work out fair house rules may be helpful. The resource section lists books and videos about TS and OCD that may help the child or siblings to understand and cope with their unique circumstances.

Neuropsychiatric conditions have historically been associated with stigma, and are difficult for family members to explain to friends, relatives, and school personnel. Parents may not be used to the role of advocate for their child, and may not even be sure whether to disclose the diagnosis of TS or OCD. Families can benefit from sympathetic guidance by their primary providers, as well as referral to the organizations and resources listed below.

RESOURCES

Organizations

Tourette Syndrome Association, Inc. (TSA)
42-40 Bell Boulevard
Bayside, NY 11361
(718) 224-2999
www.tsa-usa.org

Obsessive-Compulsive Foundation, Inc. (OCF)
377 Notch Hill Road
North Branford, CT 06471
(203) 315-2190
www.ocfoundation.org

Books for Adults and Older Adolescents

Chansky, T.E. (2000). *Freeing your child from obsessive-compulsive disorder: a powerful, practical program for parents of children and adolescents.* New York: Crown Publishers.
Colas, E. (1998). Just checking: scenes from the life of an obsessive-compulsive. New York: Atria Books.
Dornbush, M.P. & Pruitt, S.K. (1995). Teaching the tiger: a handbook for individuals involved in the education of students with attention deficit disorders, Tourette syndrome or obsessive-compulsive disorder. Duarte, CA: Hope Press.
Greene, R.W. (2001). The explosive child: a new approach for understanding and parenting easily frustrated, chronically inflexible children (2nd ed.). New York: HarperCollins.
Haerle, T. (Ed.). (1992). Children with Tourette syndrome: a parents' guide. Rockville, MD: Woodbine House.

Handler, L. (1998). Twitch and shout: a Touretter's tale. New York: Dutton.
Landau, E. (1998). Tourette syndrome. New York: Franklin Watts.
Rapoport, J.L. (1989). The boy who couldn't stop washing: the experience and treatment of obsessive-compulsive disorder. New York: E.P. Dutton.
Seligman, A.W. & Hilkevich, J.S. (Eds.). (1992). Don't think about monkeys: extraordinary stories written by people with Tourette syndrome. Duarte, CA: Hope Press.
Shimberg, E.F. (1995). Living with Tourette syndrome. New York: Simon & Schuster.
Waltz, M. (2000). Obsessive-compulsive disorder: help for children and adolescents. Sebastopol, CA: O'Reilly & Associates.
Waltz, M. (2001). Tourette's syndrome: finding answers and getting help. Sebastopol, CA: O'Reilly & Associates.
Wilensky, A.S. (1999). Passing for normal: a memoir of compulsion. New York: Broadway Books.

Books for Children

Buehrens, A. (1991). Hi, I'm Adam: a child's story of Tourette syndrome. Duarte, CA: Hope Press.
Buehrens, A. & Buehrens, C. (1991). Adam and the magic marble: a magical adventure. Duarte, CA: Hope Press.
Byalick, M. (2002). Quit it. New York: Delacorte Press.
Hesser, T.S. (1998). Kissing doorknobs. New York: Delacorte Press.

Videos

Chiten, L. Twitch and shout. Ho-ho-kus, NJ: New Day Films.
The Obsessive-Compulsive Foundation. (1993). The touching tree. Milford, CT: The Obsessive-Compulsive Foundation.
Tourette Syndrome Associates. Tourette teacher's guide: a regular kid . . . that's me. Bayside, NY: Tourette Syndrome Association.
Tourette Syndrome Associates. (1996). Stop It I Can't. New York: Mediatech.

Internet Resources

www.tourettesyndrome.net
(Tourette Syndrome Plus, Leslie Packer PhD)

www.tsa-usa.org
(Tourette Syndrome Association)

www.vh.org/Patients/IHB/Psych/Tourette/HomePage.html
(Virtual Hospital Iowa)

www.ocfoundation.org/
(Obsessive Compulsive Foundation)

www.latitudes.org
(Association for Comprehensive NeuroTherapy)

http://nccam.nih.gov
(National Center for Complementary and Alternative Medicine)

Summary of Primary Care Needs for the Child with Tourette's Syndrome or Obsessive-Compulsive Disorder

HEALTH CARE MAINTENANCE

Growth and Development

Growth is generally normal, although some recent concerns about growth of children on long-term medication, such as SSRIs. If growth slows or weight falls in older child/adolescent, consider eating disorder.

Development generally normal. Some parents report decreased flexibility and increased difficulties with regulation, even before emergence of specific symptoms. Rituals with OCD associated with isolation and distress, increase when normal childhood rituals are starting to diminish.

Diet

Abrupt changes in dietary preference may be due to obsessions/compulsions, especially around contamination.

Increased risk of eating disorders in children with OCD.

Parents may restrict intake in attempt to eliminate triggers from foods or food additives.

Continued

Summary of Primary Care Needs for the Child with Tourette's Syndrome or Obsessive-Compulsive Disorder

Safety

Excessive risk taking sometimes associated with complex tic behavior.

Self-injurious behavior in both TS and OCD

Adolescents may self-medicate with alcohol and/or recreational drugs for symptom relief

Immunization

Children with TS and OCD should be vaccinated following the schedule recommended by the American Academy of Pediatrics.

Screening

Vision. Routine screening is recommended.

Hearing. Routine screening is recommended.

Dental Care. Routine screening is recommended. Clean teeth by hand if tics set off by vibrations.

Blood Pressure. Routine screening is recommended. Children taking some medications may need increased frequency of screening.

Hematocrit. Routine screening is recommended. Additional frequency if taking atypical neuroleptics.

Urinalysis. Routine screening is recommended.

Tuberculosis. Routine screening is recommended.

Condition-Specific Screening. An ECG is recommended before beginning or increasing doses of tricyclic antidepressants and pimozide, as well as periodic measurement of blood counts and liver function, depending on the medication.

COMMON ILLNESS MANAGEMENT

Differential Diagnosis

Sniffing, coughing, throat clearing: allergy, upper respiratory infection, vocal tics

Pharyngitis. Streptococcal infection (observe for ↑tics or OCD), vocal tics (cough, throat clearing)

Headache. Medication side effect (e.g., clonidine), somatic preoccupation or obsession

Abdominal Pain. Muscle tics (abdominal muscles), constipation due to toileting issues (OCD), or medication side effect, somatic preoccupation or obsession

Skin-Mucosa Changes. Bruising from tics, self-injurious behavior, nail biting, trichotillomania

Musculoskeletal Complaints. Tics (muscle tightness, holding unusual positions), injury incurred during tic

Drug Interactions

Pimozide interacts with macrolide antibiotics to prolong the QT interval.

Dextromethorphan interacts with fluoxetine to increase cholinergic symptoms.

SSRIs reduce the effectiveness of codeine for analgesia.

St. John's wort and other supplements interact with SSRIs.

DEVELOPMENTAL ISSUES

Sleep Patterns

Tics can increase as children relax, making falling asleep more difficult. Bedtime rituals can delay sleep for several hours; parents may not be aware of extent of rituals.

Toileting

Some obsessions and rituals related to toileting. Some medications cause constipation. Avoidance of public toilets may lead to constipation and encopresis.

Discipline

Difficulty distinguishing between tics and more voluntary behaviors. Flexibility needed to accept unusual behavior may be difficult for parents. Children with OCD may need rewards for avoiding rituals. Timeouts may not be effective for children with rage attacks.

Child Care

Need combination of structure and flexibility. Daycare providers can give valuable feedback about socialization skills.

Schooling

Tics and obsessions can interfere with concentration and written work. TS is associated with dysgraphia, visual-motor integration problems, and written expressive language. OCD may not be apparent to teachers, or child may disrupt class. All children are eligible for Section 504 accommodations, some for IEPs. Peer relations may be impaired.

Sexuality

Tics may increase with touch or during sexual activity. Adolescents may avoid touch due to contamination fears. Sexual obsessions may interfere with relationships. SSRIs may decrease sexual desire and function.

Transition to Adulthood

Tics often diminish significantly in adulthood. Individuals with TS and without other conditions have few behavioral problems, but may experience educational, employment, and housing discrimination. Severe OCD may limit educational, work, and independent living options.

FAMILY CONCERNS AND RESOURCES

Decisions about disclosure of TS and OCD can be difficult. Siblings may feel that child's behavior is embarrassing, and families may need professional help to work out fair house rules.

REFERENCES

Adams, G.B. & Burke, R.W. (1999). Children and adolescents with obsessive-compulsive disorder: a primer for teachers. *Childhood Education, 76*, 2-7.

Alsobrook, J.P. & Pauls, D.L. (1997). The genetics of Tourette syndrome. *Neurol Clin North Am, 15*, 381-393.

American Psychiatric Association. (2000). *Diagnostic and statistical manual of mental disorders* (4th text revision ed.). Washington, DC: American Psychiatric Association.

Anderson, W., Chitwood, S., & Hayden, D. (1997). *Negotiating the special education maze: a guide for parents and teachers.* Rockville, MD: Woodbine House.

Association for Comprehensive NeuroTherapy (ACN). (2002). *Latitudes* [online]. Available: www.latitudes.org

Bagheri, M.M., Kerbeshian, J., & Burd, L. (1999). Recognition and management of Tourette's syndrome and tic disorders. *Am Fam Phys, 59* [online]. Available: www.aafp.org/afp/990415ap/2263.html

Bawden, H.N., Stokes, A., Camfield, C.S., Camfield, P.R., & Salisbury, S. (1998). Peer relationship problems in children with Tourette's disorder or diabetes mellitus. *J Child Psychol Psychiatry, 39*, 663-668.

Benazon, N.R., Ager, J., & Rosenberg, D.R. (2002). Cognitive behavior therapy in treatment-naive children and adolescents with obsessive-compulsive disorder: an open trial. *Behav Res Ther, 40*, 529-539.

Bergeron, R., et al. (2002). Sertraline and fluoxetine treatment of obsessive-compulsive disorder: results of a double-blind, 6-month treatment study. *J Clin Psychopharmacol, 22*, 148-154.

Blum, R.W., Kelly, A., & Ireland, M. (2001). Health-risk behaviors and protective factors among adolescents with mobility impairments and learning and emotional disabilities. *J Adolesc Health, 28*, 481-490.

Bottas, A. & Richter, M.A. (2002). Pediatric autoimmune neuropsychiatric disorders associated with streptococcal infections (PANDAS). *Pediatr Infect Dis J, 21*, 67-71.

Brand, N., et al. (2002). Brief report: cognitive functioning in children with Tourette's syndrome with and without comorbid ADHD. *J Pediatr Psychol, 27*, 203-208.

Bruun, R.D. & Budman, C.L. (1997). The course and prognosis of Tourette syndrome. *Neurol Clin North Am, 15*, 291-298.

Bruun, R.D. & Budman, C.L. (1999). Hallucinations in nonpsychotic children. *J Am Acad Child Adolesc Psychiatry, 38*, 1328-1329.

Budman, C.L., Bruun, R.D., Park, K.S., Lesser, M., & Olson, M. (2000). Explosive outbursts in children with Tourette's disorder. *J Am Acad Child Adolesc Psychiatry, 39*, 1270-1276.

Carpenter, L.L., Leckman, J.F., Scahill, L., & McDougle, C.J. (1999). Pharmacologic and other somatic approaches to treatment. In J.F. Leckman & D.J. Cohen (Eds.), *Tourette's syndrome— tics, obsessions, compulsions: developmental psychopathology and clinical care* (pp. 370-398). New York: Wiley & Sons.

Carter, A.S., et al. (1999). Recommendations for teachers. In J.F. Leckman & D.J. Cohen (Eds.), *Tourette's syndrome—tics, obsessions, compulsions: developmental psychopathology and clinical care* (pp. 360-368). New York: Wiley & Sons.

Carter, A.S., et al. (2000). Social and emotional adjustment in children affected with Gilles de la Tourette's syndrome: associations with ADHD and family functioning. *J Child Psychol Psychiatry, 41*, 215-223.

Chansky, T.E. (2000). *Freeing your child from obsessive-compulsive disorder: a powerful, practical program for parents of children and adolescents.* New York: Crown Publishers.

Clarke, M.A., Bray, M.A., Kehle, T.J., & Truscott, S.D. (2001). A school-based intervention designed to reduce the frequency of tics in children with Tourette's syndrome. *School Psych Rev, 30*, 11-22.

Coffey, B.J. & Park, K.S. (1997). Behavioral and emotional aspects of Tourette syndrome. *Neurol Clin North Am, 15*, 277-289.

Coffey, B.J., et al. (2000). Anxiety disorders and tic severity in juveniles with Tourette's disorder. *J Am Acad Child Adolesc Psychiatry, 39*, 562-568.

Cohen, D.J. & Leckman, J.F. (1999). Introduction: the self under siege. In J.F. Leckman & D.J. Cohen (Eds.), *Tourette's syndrome: tics, obsessions, compulsions* (pp. 1-19). New York: John Wiley & Sons.

Colas, E. (1998). *Just checking: scenes from the life of an obsessive-compulsive.* New York: Atria Books.

Dooley, J.M., Brna, P.M., & Gordon, K.E. (1999). Parent perceptions of symptom severity in Tourette's syndrome. *Arch Dis Child, 81*, 440-441.

Dornbush, M.P. & Pruitt, S.K. (1995). *Teaching the tiger: a handbook for individuals involved in the education of students with attention deficit disorders, Tourette syndrome or obsessive-compulsive disorder.* Duarte, CA: Hope Press.

Drug Information FullText. (2002a). *Pimozide* [online]. Available: www.library.ucsf.edu/db/dif.html

Drug Information FullText. (2002b). *Fluoxetine* [online]. Available: www.library.ucsf.edu/db/dif.html

Edell, B.H. & Motta, R.W. (1988). The emotional adjustment of children with Tourette's syndrome. *J Psychol, 123*, 51-57.

Edell-Fisher, B.H. & Motta, R.W. (1990). Tourette syndrome: relation to children's and parents' self-concepts. *Psychol Rep, 66*, 539-545.

Findling, R.L., Schulz, S.C., Reed, M.D., & Blumer, J.L. (1998). The antipsychotics: a pediatric perspective. *Pediatr Clin North Am, 45*, 1205-1232.

Fireman, B., Koran, L.M., Leventhal, J.L., & Jacobson, A. (2001). The prevalence of clinically recognized obsessive-compulsive disorder in a large health maintenance organization. *Am J Psychiatry, 158*, 1904-1910.

Freeman, R.D., et al. (2000). An international perspective on Tourette syndrome: selected findings from 3500 individuals in 22 countries. *Dev Med Child Neurol, 42*, 436-447.

Freud, S. (1909/1973). *Three case histories* (P. Rieff, Trans.). New York: Macmillan.

Gadow, K.D., Sverd, J., Sprafkin, J., Nolan, E.E., & Grossman, S. (1999). Long-term methylphenidate therapy in children with comorbid attention-deficit hyperactivity disorder and chronic multiple tic disorder. *Arch Gen Psychiatry, 56*, 330-336.

Garvey, M.A., et al. (1999). A pilot study of penicillin prophylaxis for neuropsychiatric exacerbations triggered by streptococcal infections. *Biol Psychiatry, 45*, 1564-1571.

Geller, D. (1998). Juvenile obsessive-compulsive disorder. In M.A. Jenike, L. Baer, & W.E. Minichiello (Eds.), *Obsessive-compulsive disorders: practical management* (pp. 44-64). St Louis: Mosby.

Geller, D., et al. (1998). Is juvenile obsessive-compulsive disorder a developmental subtype of the disorder? A review of pediatric literature. *J Am Acad Child Adolesc Psychiatry, 37*, 420-427.

Geller, D.A., et al. (2002). Attention-deficit/hyperactivity disorder in children and adolescents with obsessive-compulsive disorder: Fact or artifact? *J Am Acad Child Adolesc Psychiatry, 41*, 52-58.

Goodman, W.K., et al. (1989). The Yale-Brown Obsessive Compulsive Scale I: development, use, reliability. *Arch Gen Psychiatry, 46*, 1006-1011.

Greene, R.W. (2001). *The explosive child: a new approach for understanding and parenting easily frustrated, chronically inflexible children* (2nd ed.). New York: HarperCollins.

Grimaldi, B.L. (2002). The central role of magnesium deficiency in Tourette's syndrome: causal relationships between magnesium deficiency, altered biochemical pathways and symptoms relating to Tourette's syndrome and several reported comorbid conditions. *Med Hypotheses, 58*, 47-60.

Handler, L. (1998). *Twitch and shout: a Touretter's tale.* New York: Dutton.

Hanna, G.L. (1995). Demographic and clinical features of obsessive-compulsive disorder in children and adolescents. *J Am Acad Child Adolesc Psychiatry, 34*, 19-27.

Hanna, G.L. (2000). Clinical and family-genetic studies of childhood obsessive-compulsive disorder. In W.K. Goodman, M.V. Rudorfer, & J.D. Maser (Eds.), *Obsessive-compulsive disorder: contemporary issues in treatment* (pp. 87-103). Mahwah, NJ: Lawrence Erlbaum Associates.

Hasstedt, S.J., Leppert, M., Filloux, F., van de Wetering, B.J., & McMahon, W.M. (1995). Intermediate inheritance of Tourette syndrome, assuming assortative mating. *Am J Hum Genet, 57*, 682-689.

Hollenbeck, P. (2000). TSA prompts National Institutes of Health roundtable meeting: experts focus on PANDAS phenomenon. *Tourette Syndrome Association Newsletter, 28*, 5.

Jankovic, J. (1997). Phenomenology and classification of tics. *Neurol Clin North Am, 15*, 267-276.

Jankovic, J. & Sekula, S. (1998). Dermatological manifestations of Tourette syndrome and obsessive-compulsive disorder. *Arch Dermatol, 134*, 113-114.

Jankovic, J. (2001). Differential diagnosis and etiology of tics. In D.J. Cohen, C.G. Goetz, & J. Jankovic (Eds.), *Tourette's syndrome* (pp. 15-27). Philadelphia: Lippincott Williams & Wilkins.

Jenike, M.A., Baer, L., & Minichiello, W.E. (1998). An overview of obsessive-compulsive disorder. In M.A. Jenike, L. Baer, & W.E. Minichiello (Eds.), *Obsessive-compulsive disorders: practical management* (3rd ed.). St Louis: Mosby.

Kadesjo, B. & Gillberg, C. (2000). Tourette's disorder: epidemiology and comorbidity in primary school children. *J Am Acad Child Adolesc Psychiatry, 39*, 548-555.

Keuthen, N.J., O'Sullivan, R.L., & Jefferys, D.E. (1998). Trichotillomania: clinical concepts and treatment approaches. In M.A. Jenike, L. Baer,

& W.E. Minichiello (Eds.), *Obsessive-compulsive disorders: practical management* (3rd ed., pp. 162-186). St Louis: Mosby.

Kiessling, L.S. (2001). Tourette's syndrome: it's more common than you think. *The Brown University Child and Adolescent Behavior Letter*, 6-7.

King, R.A., Leckman, J.F., Scahill, L., & Cohen, D.J. (1999). Obsessive-compulsive disorder, anxiety, and depression. In J.F. Leckman & D.J. Cohen (Eds.), *Tourette's syndrome—tics, obsessions, compulsions: developmental psychopathology and clinical care* (pp. 43-61). New York: John Wiley & Sons.

King, R.A., Leonard, H.I., March, J., & American Academy of Child and Adolescent Psychiatry Work Group on Quality Issues. (1998). Practice parameters for the assessment and treatment of children and adolescents with obsessive-compulsive disorder. *J Am Acad Child Adolesc Psychiatry, 37*, 27S-45S.

Kurlan, R. (2001). New treatments for tics? *Neurology, 56*, 580-581.

Lajonchere, C., Nortz, M., & Finger, S. (1996). Gilles de la Tourette and the discovery of Tourette syndrome. *Arch Neurol, 53*, 567-574.

Landau, E. (1998). *Tourette syndrome*. New York: Franklin Watts.

Latitudes. (2002). Letters from patients and families: Tourette syndrome. *Latitudes* [online]. Available: www.latitudes.org/articles/letters_patients_families.htm

Leckman, J.F. & Cohen, D.J. (1999). Evolving models of pathogenesis. In J.F. Leckman & D.J. Cohen (Eds.), *Tourette's syndrome—tics, obsessions, compulsions: developmental psychopathology and clinical care* (pp. 155-175). New York: Wiley & Sons.

Leckman, J.F., King, R.A., & Cohen, D.J. (1999). Tics and tic disorders. In J.F. Leckman & D.J. Cohen (Eds.), *Tourette's syndrome— tics, obsessions, compulsions: developmental psychopathology and clinical care* (pp. 23-42). New York: Wiley & Sons.

Leckman, J.F., et al. (1999). Yale approach to assessment and treatment. In J.F. Leckman & D.J. Cohen (Eds.), *Tourette's syndrome—tics, obsessions, compulsions: developmental psychopathology and clinical care* (pp. 285-308). New York: Wiley & Sons.

Leckman, J.F., Peterson, B.S., King, R.A., Scahill, L., & Cohen, D.J. (2001). Phenomenology of tics and natural history of tic disorders. In D.J. Cohen, C.G. Goetz, & J. Jankovic (Eds.), *Tourette's syndrome* (pp. 1-14). Philadelphia: Lippincott Williams & Wilkins.

Leckman, J.F., et al. (1989). The Yale Global Tic Severity Scale (YGTSS): initial testing of a clinical-rated scale of tic severity. *J Am Acad Child Adolesc Psychiatry, 28*, 566-573.

Leckman, J.F., et al. (1998). Course of tic severity in Tourette syndrome: the first two decades. *Pediatrics, 102*, 14-19.

Leonard, H.I., Goldberger, E.L., Rapoport, J.L., Cheslow, D.L., & Swedo, S.E. (1990). Childhood rituals: normal development or obsessive-compulsive symptoms? *J Am Acad Child Adolesc Psychiatry, 29*, 17-23.

March, J., Frances, A., Carpenter, D., & Kahn, D. (1997). The Expert Consensus Guideline Series: treatment of obsessive compulsive disorder. *J Clin Psychiatry, 58* (Suppl. 4), 1-72.

March, J.S. & Mulle, K. (1998). *OCD in children and adolescents: a cognitive-behavioral treatment manual*. New York: The Guilford Press.

Marras, C., Andrews, D., Sime, E., & Lang, A. E. (2001). Botulinum toxin for simple motor tics: a randomized, double-blind, controlled clinical trial. *Neurology, 56*, 605-610.

Martin, H. & Ammerman, S.D. (2002). Adolescents with eating disorders: primary care screening, identification, and early intervention. *Nurs Clin North Am, 37*, 537-551.

Miguel, E.C., et al. (2001). The tic-related obsessive-compulsive disorder phenotype and treatment implications. In D.J. Cohen, C.G. Goetz, & J. Jankovic (Eds.), *Tourette's syndrome* (pp. 43-55). Philadelphia: Lippincott Williams & Wilkins.

Milos, G., Spindler, A., Ruggiero, G., Klaghofer, R., & Schnyder, U. (2002). Comorbidity of obsessive-compulsive disorders and duration of eating disorders. *Int J Eat Disord, 31*, 284-289.

Muller, N., et al. (2001). Increased titers of antibodies against streptococcal M12 and M19 proteins in patients with Tourette's syndrome. *Psychiatry Res, 101*, 187-193.

Müller-Vahl, K.R., Schneider, U., Kolbe, H., & Emrich, H.M. (1999). Treatment of Tourette's syndrome with delta-9-tetrahydrocannabinol. *Am J Psychiatry, 156*, 495.

Murphy, M.I. & Pichichero, M.E. (2002). Prospective identification and treatment of children with pediatric, autoimmune neuropsychiatric disorder associated with group A streptococcal infection (PANDAS). *Arch Pediatr Adolesc Med, 156*, 356-361.

National Center for Complementary and Alternative Medicine [online]. Available: http://altmed.od.nih.gov/clinicaltrials

Nolte, J. (2002). *The human brain: an introduction to its functional anatomy* (5th ed.). St Louis: Mosby.

O'Connor, K.P., et al. (2001). Evaluation of a cognitive-behavioural program for the management of chronic tic and habit disorders. *Behav Res Ther, 39*, 667-681.

Oesterheld, J.R. & Shader, R.I. (1998). Cytochromes: a primer for child and adolescent psychiatrists. *J Am Acad Child Adolesc Psychiatry, 37*(4), 447-450.

Packer, L. (1997). Social and educational resources for patients with Tourette syndrome. *Neurol Clin North Am, 15*, 457-473.

Papadopoulos, R.B., Shady, G.A., Wand, R., & Furer, P. (1992). Your child's development. In T. Haerle (Ed.), *Children with Tourette syndrome: a parents' guide* (pp. 139-168). Rockville, MD: Woodbine House.

Perlmutter, S.J., et al. (1999). Therapeutic plasma exchange and intravenous immunoglobulin for obsessive-compulsive disorder and tic disorders in childhood. *Lancet, 354*, 1153-1158.

Peterson, B.S., Pine, D.S., Cohen, P., & Brook, J.S. (2001). Prospective, longitudinal study of tic, obsessive-compulsive and attention-deficit/hyperactivity disorders in an epidemiological sample. *J Am Acad Child Adolesc Psychiatry, 40*, 685-695.

Phillips, K.A. (2000). Connection between obsessive-compulsive disorder and body dysmorphic disorder. In W.K. Goodman, M.V. Rudorfer, & J.D. Maser (Eds.), *Obsessive-compulsive disorder: contemporary issues in treatment* (pp. 23-42). Mahwah, NJ: Lawrence Erlbaum.

Piacentini, J. & Chang, S. (2001). Behavioral treatments for Tourette syndrome and tic disorders: state of the art. In D.J. Cohen, C.G. Goetz, & J. Jankovic (Eds.), *Tourette syndrome* (vol. 85, pp. 319-331). Philadelphia: Lippincott Williams & Wilkins.

Pigott, T.A. & Seay, S. (2000). Pharmacotherapy of obsessive-compulsive disorder: Overview and treatment-refractory strategies. In W.K. Goodman, M.V. Rudorfer, & J.D. Maser (Eds.), *Obsessive-compulsive disorder: contemporary issues in treatment* (pp. 277-302). Mahwah, NJ: Lawrence Erlbaum.

Rapin, I. (2001). Autism spectrum disorders: relevance to Tourette syndrome. In D.J. Cohen, J. Jankovic, & C.G. Goetz (Eds.), *Tourette syndrome* (vol. 85, pp. 89-102). Philadelphia: Lippincott Williams & Wilkins.

Rapoport, J.L. (1989). *The boy who couldn't stop washing: the experience and treatment of obsessive-compulsive disorder*. New York: E.P. Dutton.

Rapoport, J.L., et al. (2000). Childhood obsessive-compulsive disorder in the NIMH MECA study: parent versus child identification of cases. *J Anxiety Disord, 14*, 535-548.

Rappaport, N. & Chubinsky, P. (2000). The meaning of psychotropic medications for children, adolescents, and their families. *J Am Acad Child Adolesc Psychiatry, 39*, 1198-1200.

Rauch, S.L. & Savage, C.R. (2000). Cortico-striatal pathology in OCD. In W.K. Goodman, M.V. Rudorfer, & J.D. Maser (Eds.), *Obsessive-compulsive disorder: contemporary issues in treatment*. Mahwah, NJ: Lawrence Erlbaum.

Rauch, S.L., Whalen, P.J., Dougherty, D.D., & Jenike, M.A. (1998). Neurobiological models of obsessive-compulsive disorders. In M.A. Jenike, L. Baer, & W.E. Minichiello (Eds.), *Obsessive-compulsive disorders: practical management* (pp. 222-253). St Louis: Mosby.

Riddle, M.A. & Carlson, J. (2001). Clinical psychopharmacology for Tourette syndrome and associated disorders. In D.J. Cohen, J. Jankovic, & C.G. Goetz (Eds.), *Tourette syndrome* (vol. 85, pp. 343-362). Philedelphia: Lippincott Williams & Wilkins.

Robertson, M.M. (1992). Self-injurious behavior and Tourette syndrome. *Adv Neurol, 58*, 105-114.

Rosenberg, D.R. & Hanna, G.L. (2000). Genetic and imaging strategies in obsessive-compulsive disorder: Potential implications for treatment development. *Biol Psychiatry, 48*, 1210-1222.

Samuels, J., et al. (2002). Hoarding in obsessive compulsive disorder: results from a case-control study. *Behav Res Ther, 40*, 517-528.

Scahill, L., King, R.A., Schultz, R.T., & Leckman, J.F. (1999). Selection and use of diagnostic and clinical rating instruments. In J.F. Leckman & D. J. Cohen (Eds.), *Tourette's syndrome—tics, obsessions, compulsions: developmental psychopathology and clinical care* (pp. 310-323). New York: John Wiley & Sons.

Scahill, L., et al. (1997). Children's Yale-Brown Obsessive Compulsive Scale: reliability and validity. *J Am Acad Child Adolesc Psychiatry, 36*, 844-852.

Schapiro, N.A. (2002). Dude, you don't have Tourette's: Tourette's syndrome, beyond the tics. *Pediatr Nurs, 22*, 243-253.

Schreier, H. (1999). Hallucinations in nonpsychotic children: more common than we think? *J Am Acad Child Adolesc Psychiatry, 38*, 623-625.

Sherman, E.M., Shepard, L., Joschko, M., & Freeman, R.D. (1998). Sustained attention and impulsivity in children with Tourette syndrome: comorbidity and confounds. *J Clin Experimental Neuropsychiatry, 20*, 644-657.

Shimberg, E.F. (1995). *Living with Tourette syndrome*. New York: Simon & Schuster.

Shoaf, T.L., Emslie, l.J., & Mayes, T.L. (2001). Childhood depression: diagnosis and treatment strategies in general pediatrics. *Pediatr Ann, 30*, 130-137.

Silver, A.A., Shytle, R.D., & Sanberg, P.R. (1999). Clinical experience with transdermal nicotine patch in Tourette's syndrome. *CNS Spectrum, 4*, 68-76.

Silver, A.A., et al. (2001). Multicenter, double-blind, placebo-controlled study of mecamylamine monotherapy for Tourette's disorder. *J Am Acad Child Adolesc Psychiatry, 40*, 1103-1110.

Singer, C. (1997). Coprolalia and other coprophenomena. *Neurol Clin North Am, 15*, 299-308.

Singer, H.S., Wendlandt, J., Krieger, M., & Giuliano, J. (2001). Baclofen treatment in Tourette syndrome: a double-blind, placebo-controlled, crossover trial. *Neurology, 56*, 599-604.

Snider, L.A., et al. (2002). Tics and problem behaviors in schoolchildren: prevalence, characterization, and associations. *Pediatrics, 110*, 331-336.

Spencer, T., et al. (1998). Disentangling the overlap between Tourette's disorder and ADHD. *J Child Psychol Psychiatry, 39*, 1037-1044.

Spencer, T.J., et al. (2001). Impact of tic disorders on ADHD outcome across the life cycle: findings from a large group of adults with and without ADHD. *Am J Psychiatry, 158*, 611-617.

Stephens, R.J. & Sandor, P. (1999). Aggressive behavior in children with Tourette syndrome and comorbid attention-deficit hyperactivity disorder and obsessive-compulsive disorder. *Can J Psychiatry, 44*, 1036-1042.

Thienemann, M., Martin, J., Cregger, B., Thompson, H.B., & Dyer-Friedman, J. (2001). Manual-driven cognitive behavioral therapy for adolescents with obsessive-compulsive disorder: A pilot study. *J Am Acad Child Adolesc Psychiatry, 40*, 1254-1260.

The Tourette's Syndrome Study Group. (2002). Treatment of ADHD in children with tics: a randomized controlled trial. *Neurology, 58*, 527-536.

Walkup, J.T. (2002). Tic disorders and Tourette's syndrome. In S. Kutcher (Ed.), *Practical child and adolescent psychopharmacology* (pp. 382-409). Cambridge, UK: Cambridge University Press.

Waltz, M. (2000). *Obsessive-compulsive disorder: help for children and adolescents*. Sebastopol, CA: O'Reilly & Associates.

Waltz, M. (2001). *Tourette's syndrome: finding answers and getting help*. Sebastopol, CA: O'Reilly & Associates.

Waters, T.L., Barrett, P.M., & March, J.S. (2001). Cognitive-behavioral family treatment of childhood obsessive-compulsive disorder. *Am J Psychother, 55*, 372-387.

Weintrob, N., Cohen, D., Klipper-Aurbach, Y., Zadik, Z., & Dickerman, Z. (2002). Decreased growth during therapy with selective serotonin reuptake inhibitors. *Arch Pediatr Adolesc Med, 156*, 696-701.

Wewetzer, C., et al. (2001). Long-term outcome and prognosis of obsessive-compulsive disorder with onset in childhood or adolescence. *Eur Child Adolesc Psychiatry, 10*, 37-46.

Wilensky, A.S. (1999). *Passing for normal: a memoir of compulsion*. New York: Broadway Books.

Wu, L., Li, H., & Kang, L. (1996). 156 cases of Gilles de la Tourette's syndrome treated by acupuncture. *J Tradit Chin Med, 16*, 211-213.

Zohar, A.H., et al. (1999). Epidemiological studies. In J.F. Leckman & D.J. Cohen (Eds.), *Tourette's syndrome—tics, obsessions, compulsions: developmental psychopathology and clinical care* (pp. 177-192). New York: Wiley & Sons.

Zohar, A.H., et al. (1997). Obsessive-compulsive disorder with and without tics in an epidemiological sample of adolescents. *Am J Psychiatry, 154*, 274-276.

INDEX

Ribavirin, 249

Rickets with bronchopulmonary dysplasia (BPD), 288

Right upper quadrant (RUQ) syndrome, 755

Riley Articulation and Language Test, Revised (RALT-R), 34t

Riley Preschool Development Screening Inventory (RPDSI), 35t

Rimantadine, 416

Risperidone (Risperdal), 223, 223t, 224, 614t

Ritalin. *See* Methylphenidate (Ritalin)

RITQ. *See* Revised Infant Temperament Questionnaire (RITQ)

Robert Wood Johnson Foundation Model for Effective Chronic Illness Care, 106

Rodents, control of, 183

Rofecoxib, 587t

Rolandic epilepsy, 475

Roof of mouth, anatomy of, 353f

ROP. *See* Retinopathy of prematurity (ROP)

Rowasa enema. *See* Mesalamine (Rowasa enema)

RPDSI. *See* Riley Preschool Development Screening Inventory (RPDSI)

S

SAARD. *See* Slow-acting antirheumatic drugs (SAARD)

Safe Haven, 539

Safety
  with allergies, 165-166
  with asthma, 187
  with attention deficit hyperactivity disorder (ADHD), 209
  with autism, 228-229
  with bleeding disorders, 251
  with bone marrow transplantation, 272-273
  with bronchopulmonary dysplasia (BPD), 290
  with cancer, 318
  with cerebral palsy, 337
  with chronic renal failure (CRF), 735
  with cleft lip and palate, 357-358
  with congenital adrenal hyperplasia (CAH), 373
  with cystic fibrosis, 415
  with diabetes mellitus, 436
  with Down syndrome, 460
  ensuring, 83-84
  with epilepsy, 485-486
  with fragile X syndrome, 505
  with head injury, 519-520
  with human immunodeficiency virus (HIV) infection, 533
  with hydrocephalus, 553
  with inflammatory bowel disease, 574-575
  with juvenile rheumatoid arthritis (JRA), 593
  with mood disorders, 620
  with myelodysplasia, 635-636
  with obsessive-compulsive disorder (OCD), 775-776
  with organ transplantation, 656-657
  with phenylketonuria, 675
  with prenatal cocaine exposure, 714
  with preterm infants, 696
  with sickle cell disease, 757
  with Tourette syndrome, 775-776

Salmeterol (Serevent)
  for asthma, 182
    dosage of, 180t
  for exercise-induced bronchospasms (EIB), 183

Salmonella, 749, 759
  with bone marrow transplantation, 275

Salt depletion with cystic fibrosis, 411-412

Sandifer syndrome, 488

Sandimmune. *See* Cyclosporine (Sandimmune)

Scalp infections with hydrocephalus, 556

SCHIP. *See* State Children's Health Insurance Program (SCHIP)

School(s), 71-86
  facilitating, 81-84
  fostering psychosocial health, 36-37
  legal issues in, 71-80
  resources for, 85-86

School(s) (*Continued*)
  responsibility for medical services
    in IDEA 97, 78-79
  role of, 71
  role of health professionals in determining, 80-81
  and terminally ill student, 84-85

School absenteeism, 82

School-age children
  developmental tasks, 25

School buses, 84

Schooling
  with allergies, 168-169
  with asthma, 192-193
  with attention deficit hyperactivity disorder (ADHD), 212-213
  with autism, 232
  with bleeding disorders, 253
  with bone marrow transplantation, 276-277
  with bronchopulmonary dysplasia (BPD), 293-294
  with cancer, 322
  with cerebral palsy, 341
  with chronic renal failure (CRF), 737-738
  with cleft lip and palate, 359
  with congenital adrenal hyperplasia (CAH), 376-377
  with congenital heart disease (CHD), 397
  with cystic fibrosis, 419
  with diabetes mellitus, 439
  with Down syndrome, 463
  with epilepsy, 491
  with fragile X syndrome, 507
  with head injury, 521-522
  with human immunodeficiency virus (HIV) infection, 537
  with hydrocephalus, 557
  with inflammatory bowel disease, 577-578
  with juvenile rheumatoid arthritis (JRA), 595-596, 595t
  with mood disorders, 624
  with myelodysplasia, 639
  with organ transplantation, 660
  with phenylketonuria, 677-678
  placement in, 109
  with premature birth, 699-700
  with prenatal cocaine exposure, 716
  with sickle cell disease, 761
  with Tourette syndrome and obsessive-compulsive disorder (OCD), 777-778

School nurses
  with asthma, 192-193
  role in determining special education services, 81

School programs, assessing family use of, 109

School reentry, 84

School to Work Opportunities Act (PL 103-239), 138t

SCID. *See* Severe combined immunodeficiencies (SCID)

Scissoring, 330f

Scoliosis with sickle cell disease, 758

Screening
  with allergies, 166
  with asthma, 188-190
  with attention deficit hyperactivity disorder (ADHD), 209
  with autism, 220-221, 229
  with bleeding disorders, 251-252
  with bone marrow transplantation, 273-275
  with bronchopulmonary dysplasia (BPD), 291
  with cancer, 319-320
  with CDH, 394
  with cerebral palsy, 338-339
  with chronic renal failure (CRF), 735-736
  with cleft lip and palate, 358
  with congenital adrenal hyperplasia (CAH), 374
  with cystic fibrosis, 415-416
  with diabetes mellitus, 436-437
  with Down syndrome, 461-462
  with epilepsy, 486-487